Clinical Nutrition

Clinical Nutrition

DAVID M. PAIGE, M.D., M.P.H.

Professor,
Department of Maternal and Child Health,
School of Hygiene and Public Health, and joint appointment in
Department of Pediatrics,
School of Medicine, Johns Hopkins University,
Baltimore, Maryland

Second Edition

With illustrations

The C. V. Mosby Company

St. Louis   Washington, D.C.   Toronto   1988

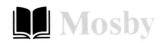

Editor: Terry Van Schaik
Assistant Editor: Patricia L. Gregory
Manuscript Editor: George B. Stericker, Jr.
Design: Rey Umali
Production: Ginny Douglas

Second Edition

The C. V. Mosby Company
11830 Westline Industrial Drive, St. Louis, Missouri 63146

Library of Congress Cataloging-in-Publication Data

Clinical nutrition.

Rev. ed. of: Manual of clinical nutrition c1983-
    Includes bibliographies and index.
    1. Diet therapy—Handbooks, manuals, etc.   2. Nu-
trition—Handbooks, manuals, etc. I. Paige, David M.
II. Manual of clinical nutrition. [DNLM: 1. Diet
Therapy—handbooks. 2. Nutrition—handbooks.
3. Nutrition Disorders—handbooks. QU 39 C641]
RM217.2.C56 1988   615.8′54   88-5219
ISBN 0-8016-3873-9

GW/GW/MV   9 8 7 6 5 4 3 2 1

Consulting Editors

Contributors

Lindsay H. Allen, Ph.D., R.D.
Professor, Department of Nutritional Sciences,
University of Connecticut, Storrs, Connecticut

David H. Alpers, M.D.
Professor and Chief, Gastroenterology Division,
Washington University School of Medicine, St. Louis,
Missouri

Marvin E. Ament, M.D.
Professor of Pediatrics, Department of Pediatrics,
University of California, Los Angeles Medical School,
Los Angeles, California

Arnold E. Andersen, M.D.
Associate Professor, Department of Psychiatry and
Behavioral Sciences, Johns Hopkins University;
Attending Physician, Department of Psychiatry, Johns
Hopkins Hospital, Baltimore, Maryland

William R. Beisel, M.D.
Adjunct Professor in Immunology and Infectious
Disease, Johns Hopkins University School of Hygiene
and Public Health, Baltimore, Maryland

Edwin L. Bierman, M.D.
Professor of Medicine and Head of the Division of
Metabolism, Endocrinology, and Nutrition, University
of Washington, School of Medicine, Seattle,
Washington

S. Allan Bock, M.D.
Department of Pediatrics, National Jewish Center for
Immunology and Respiratory Medicine, Denver,
Colorado

M. J. Bunk, Ph.D., M.P.H.
Department of Medicine, Memorial Sloan-Kettering
Cancer Center, New York Hospital–Cornell Medical
Center, New York, New York

Alan Chait, M.D.
Professor of Medicine, Department of Medicine,
Division of Metabolism, Endocrinology, and Nutrition,
University of Washington, School of Medicine,
Seattle, Washington

William Dietz, M.D., Ph.D.
Tufts University, School of Medicine, Boston,
Massachusetts

Johanna T. Dwyer, D.Sc.
Professor of Medicine and Community Health, Tufts
University School of Medicine; Director, Frances
Stern Nutrition Center, New England Medical Center
Hospital, Boston, Massachusetts

Phyllis L. Fleming, Ph.D.
President, Fleming & Associates, Minnetonka,
Minnesota

Alan J. Gelenberg, M.D.
Associate Professor, Department of Psychiatry,
Harvard Medical School; Chief, Special Studies,
Department of Psychiatry, Massachusetts General
Hospital, Boston; Psychiatrist-in-Chief, The Arbour
Hospital, Jamaica Plain, Massachusetts

Cleon W. Goodwin, M.D.
Associate Professor of Surgery, Department of
Surgery, Cornell University Medical College; Director,
Burn Center, New York Hospital, New York, New
York

Victor Herbert, M.D., J.D.
Professor of Medicine, Department of Medicine,
Mount Sinai School of Medicine, New York; Chief,
Hematology and Nutrition Research Laboratory, Bronx
Veterans Administration Medical Center, Bronx, New
York

David L. Horwitz, M.D., Ph.D.
Clinical Associate Professor, Department of Medicine;
Associate Professor, Department of Nutrition and
Dietetics, University of Illinois at Chicago; Attending
Physician, Department of Medicine, University of
Illinois Hospital, Chicago, Illinois

Howard N. Jacobson, M.D.
Director, Institute of Nutrition, University of North
Carolina, Chapel Hill, North Carolina

Robert B. Johnston, M.D.
Assistant Professor of Pediatrics and Neurology,
JohnsHopkins University School of Medicine; Staff
Pediatrician, Kennedy Institute, Baltimore, Maryland

Eileen T. Kennedy, D.Sc., M.S.
Visiting Associate Professor and Research Fellow,
Tufts University School of Nutrition and International
Food Policy Research Institute, Washington, D.C.

Mary Bess Kohrs, Ph.D., R.D.
Associate Professor, Department of Community Health
Sciences, University of Illinois, Chicago, Illinois

Natalie Kurinij
Collaborative Clinical Vision, Research Branch,
National Eye Institute, National Institutes of Health,
Bethesda, Maryland

Alan M. Lake, M.D.
Baltimore, Maryland

Fima Lifshitz, M.D.
Professor of Pediatrics, Department of Pediatrics,
Cornell University Medical College, New York; Chief,
Division of Pediatric Endocrinology, Metabolism, and
Nutrition; Associate Director of Pediatrics, Department
of Pediatrics, North Shore University Hospital,
Manhasset, New York

Esteban Mezey, M.D.
Professor of Medicine, Department of Medicine, Johns
Hopkins University School of Medicine; Active Staff,
Department of Medicine, Johns Hopkins Hospital,
Baltimore, Maryland

Grant A. Mitchell, M.D.
Research Fellow, Department of Pediatrics, Johns
Hopkins University School of Medicine, Baltimore,
Maryland

Kenneth H. Neldner, M.D.
Professor and Chairman, Department of Dermatology,
Texas Tech University Health Sciences Center,
Lubbock, Texas

David A. Newsome, M.D.
Professor, Department of Ophthalmology, LSU Eye
Center; Louisiana State University School of
Medicine, New Orleans, Louisiana

George M. Owen, M.D.
Medical Director, Bristol-Myers International Group;
Clinical Professor of Pediatrics, Cornell Medical
Center, New York, New York

Hugo da Costa Ribeiro, Jr., M.D.
Assistant Professor of Pediatrics, Facultade de
Medicina, Universidade Federal da Bahia, Salvador,
Bahia, Brazil

Richard S. Rivlin, M.D.
Professor of Medicine, Department of Medicine,
Cornell University Medical College; Chief, Nutrition
Service, Memorial Sloan-Kettering Cancer Center;
Chief, Nutrition Division, New York Hospital–Cornell
Medical Center, New York, New York

Robert M. Russell, B.A., M.D.
Associate Professor of Medicine and Nutrition,
Department of Medicine, Tufts University; Staff
Gastroenterologist, Department of Medicine, New
England Medical Center, Boston, Massachusetts

Nadine R. Sahyoun, M.S., R.D.
Research Dietition, Nutrition Services Department,
USDA–Human Nutrition Research Center on Aging,
Tufts University, Boston, Massachusetts

†Lloyd S. Schloen, Ph.D.
Formerly, Nova Pharmaceutical Corporation,
Baltimore, Maryland

Roger Sherwin, M.B., B.Chir.
Professor of Epidemiology and Preventive Medicine,
University of Maryland School of Medicine,
Baltimore, Maryland

Noel W. Solomons, M.D.
Senior Scientist and Coordinator, Center for Studies of
Sensory Impairment, Aging, and Metabolism
(CeSSIAM), Research Branch of the National
Committee for the Blind and Deaf of Guatemala,
Guatemala City, Guatemala

Edward A. Sweeney, D.M.D.
Professor of Pediatric Dentistry, Department of
Pediatric Dentistry School of Dentistry, University of
Texas Health Science Center at San Antonio; Chief,
Pediatric Dentistry, Department of Surgery, Santa
Rosa Children's Hospital, San Antonio, Texas

Benjamin Torún, M.D., Ph.D.
Department of Nutrition and Health, Institute of
Nutrition of Central America and Panama (INCAP),
Guatemala City, Guatemala

† Deceased.

Frederick L. Trowbridge
Director, Division of Nutrition, Center for Health
Promotion and Education, Centers for Disease
Control, Atlanta, Georgia

David Valle, M.D.
Professor of Pediatrics, Medicine, and Molecular
Biology and Genetics, Johns Hopkins University
School of Medicine, Baltimore, Maryland

José Villar, M.D., M.P.H., M.Sc.
Visiting Scientist, Prevention Research Program,
National Institute of Child Health and Human
Development (NICHD), National Institutes of Health,
Bethesda, Maryland

Fernando E. Viteri, M.D., D.Sc.
Department of Nutritional Sciences, University of
California, Berkeley, California

Mackenzie Walser, M.D.
Professor of Pharmacology and Molecular Sciences
and Professor of Medicine, Johns Hopkins University
School of Medicine; Physician, Johns Hopkins
Hospital, Baltimore, Maryland

Douglas W. Wilmore, M.D.
Professor of Surgery, Department of Surgery, Harvard
Medical School; Director, Nutrition Support Services,
Department of Surgery, Brigham and Women's
Hospital, Boston, Massachusetts

E. David Wright, M.D., D.Sc.
Intern, Department of Medicine, University of
Vermont College of Medicine, Burlington, Vermont

Vernon R. Young, Ph.D., D.Sc.
Professor of Nutritional Biochemistry, School Science,
Massachusetts Institute of Technology, Cambridge,
Massachusetts

Preface

Clinical Nutrition remains a widely consulted and up-to-date compendium of information in the field of nutritional management. It integrates basic elements of the field with the principles of patient assessment and care. This second edition reflects advances that have been made over the past decade and their application to clinical practice. Each of the chapters has been reviewed and, in some cases, extensively revised. Specific attention has been given to restating the basic principles and exploring relevant research, along with integrating information that is pertinent. New chapters have been added reflecting the increased attention to nutrition and exercise as well as home parenteral nutrition, and the interaction of nutrition and allergy. The book can be used as both a text and a ready reference for students and practitioners of clinical nutrition.

Each section of the book provides information in easily assimilated and useful form pertaining to an important facet of nutrition. The initial sections—"Principles of Nutrition," "Nutrition in the Normal Life Span," and "Evaluating Nutritional Status"—review the fundamentals of nutrient metabolism and the assessment of nutritional health during specific stages of life. Subsequent sections focus on the interactions of nutrition and disease: "Systemic Disorders" covers the nutritional events that parallel or follow a patient's disease. "Specific Disease States" focuses on the nutritional management and interventions necessary to improve the patient's outcome. In this section are discussions of various pathologic states (including cancer, infections, diarrhea, and the surgery of burn patients) from a nutritional management point of view. "Nutritional Deficiencies" addresses the consequences of abnormal intakes. The pathophysiology, diagnosis, and treatment of patients with vitamin-mineral deficiencies, anemias, protein-energy malnutrition, obesity, and other nutritional abnormalities are reviewed and discussed. Completing the text is the section entitled "Exercise, Diet, and Counseling." Following this section are the Appendices, which furnish detailed and practical standards, tables, diets, food analyses, and other pertinent clinical materials.

This book represents the vision and work of a dedicated group of individuals who recognized the need for a comprehensive and authoritative text. The judgment, wisdom, and diligence of the Consulting Editors in developing its content and format were indispensable. Their dedication, however, has been matched in every respect by the commitment to excellence of each of the contributors, whose thoughtful and critical papers distill the essence of the assigned topic while incorporating attention to detail and complying with the objectives of the book. The result is complete and comprehensive chapters fully integrated into the content and purpose of the book.

The critical endorsement of, and enthusiastic support for, the first edition of this book served to underscore the importance of the project and our continued responsibility for maintaining its character and excellence. We are indebted to all of our colleagues for assisting us in meeting this objective.

No work of such a scope can come to fruition without a dedicated staff of persons willing to give of themselves unselfishly, often without recognition. The Editor has been indeed fortunate to have had the opportunity to work with the professional staff of The C.V. Mosby Company, a publishing enterprise with a long tradition and outstanding reputation in the field. The quality of the Publisher is reflected in the excellence of its Editorial Staff. Ms. Terry Van Schaik, Acquisition Editor, guided this project with great skill, sensitivity, understanding, patience, and warmth. She is unique insofar as she was able to orchestrate the seemingly endless elements of the project into a final integrated, coherent, and unified book. Mr. George Stericker, Senior Manuscript Editor, combined skill, judgment, and background with an uncommonly encountered dedication to the book. Finally, as in the first edition, and as all who know her and have worked with her will attest, the conscientious and dedicated, indefatigable, Lenora Davis was invaluable. She handled innumerable contacts with authors, editors, publishers, and others, always infusing grace and warmth into the relationship.

Everyone associated with the project has expressed gratitude for the cooperation of contributors, publisher, and staff. The common objective was to produce a book of high scholarship and excellence. We hope we have met this expectation.

DAVID M. PAIGE
Baltimore, Maryland

To Nancy, Tara, and Danny, and to all people
who share a vision of food for all and peace on Earth

Contents

Clinical Nutrition

I

PRINCIPLES OF NUTRITION

CHAPTER 1
Human Metabolism

Noel W. Solomons

The human body needs a continuous and regulated supply of nutrients for normal growth, physiologic functioning, and health maintenance. Human metabolism embraces the processes by which nutrients are acquired from the environment (in food, water, and air) and are transported, utilized, and disposed of. Combined with the metabolism of nutrients per se are the synthesis, use, and degradation of endogenous compounds (whose elemental components are derived from the diet), the production of energy to warm and run the organism (the fuels, again, derived from dietary sources), and the integration and regulation of all physiologic processes. The control of these processes may be within the cell or between cells, the latter governed by hormonal signals.

Fig. 1-1 illustrates the principal components of human metabolism, specifically those relating to the acquisition, utilization, and elimination of dietary nutrients. To understand the biology of individual nutrients, it is necessary to understand the overall scheme of human metabolism. This chapter therefore is organized to summarize our understanding of human metabolism in general terms.

ALIMENTARY TRACT FUNCTIONING

The alimentary tract is a specialized mechanism for extracting nutrients from food. Its specific functions include motility, secretion, digestion, absorption/excretion, and nutrient production. Under normal conditions, appetite regulation is as important as appropriate food selection and the mechanical and physiologic status of the intestinal tract in supporting adequate nutrition. Appetite and the rate of eating are normally regulated by metabolic coordination, cultural factors, a person's psychologic status, and the degree of hunger and satiety experienced.[1,2] These regulatory influences can be bypassed by "mechanical" (enteral or parenteral) alimentation (Chapter 31) or by various appetite disorders, such as anorexia nervosa or hyperphagia (Chapters 3 and 26). Exactly *how* the human appetite and eating rate are regulated is not fully understood, but several biochemical and neurophysiologic mechanisms have been proposed.[1,2]

Motility

In general terms, foods, beverages, and secretions flow caudally along the alimentary tract (i.e., from the mouth to the lower gut).

Mouth. Nutrient utilization of ingested food or drink begins at the mouth, where teeth and tongue reduce solid elements to smaller particles (mastication) that are mixed with saliva. The food then is swallowed (deglutition) and propelled into the stomach both by gravity and by the coordinated peristaltic contractions of the esophagus. Dysfunctions of the oral cavity, including loss or disease of the teeth, impaired oral sensation or secretion, neuromuscular disease of the pharynx or larynx, and mechanical or neuromuscular disorders of the esophagus, compromise these two critical first steps in providing nutrients to satisfy physiologic needs (Chapter 20).

Stomach. The rate of gastric emptying is governed by the nature of the meal (solid or liquid) and the total volume ingested. The stomach acts as a reservoir for recently consumed food and beverage. Mechanical factors and hormonal feedback mechanisms regulate the flow of gastric contents into the small intestine. Compromise of the reservoir's capacity may lead to early satiety, vomiting, or regurgitation. Loss of gastric emptying regulation leads to the excessively rapid entry of osmotically active solutes into the small bowel, with a consequent "dumping syndrome" and/or development of diarrhea.

Small bowel. The flow of chyme through the small intestine also is assisted by peristalsis. The dietary elements flow through the gut as dis-

3

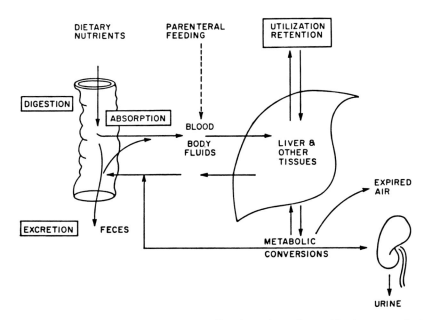

Figure 1-1 Various physiologic processes (e.g., digestion, absorption, utilization, excretion) comprise the major phases in the metabolism of nutrients.

persed liquids. Spastic or flaccid loss of coordinated propulsion is rare, but when it occurs the interruption of intestinal flow results in a pseudoobstruction that has all the characteristics (visceral pain, distension, vomiting) of a true mechanical obstruction.

Colon. The colon exhibits several types of motor responses. A gentle propulsive peristalsis, similar to that of the upper gut, carries the increasingly solid fecal material toward the sigmoid colon. Defecation involves a coordinated and powerful contraction of the sigmoid colon and rectum with the reflex relaxation of the anal sphincter. Constipation can result from psychologic or neuromuscular inhibition of the defecation response or from mechanical obstruction. As with impaired transit at any other stage, delayed colonic emptying will reduce spontaneous nutrient intake and eventually produce pain and distension of the upper gastrointestinal tract.

Diarrhea erroneously has been thought to result from intestinal hurry, secondary to propulsive disorders of the small and large bowels. In fact, it generally results from excessive net accumulation of fluid in the intestinal lumen as a consequence of an imbalance in fluid absorption and secretion rates.[3] Primary changes in transit time as a cause of diarrhea are rare (Chapter 29).

Secretion

Throughout the length of the alimentary tract, various secretions are produced either by specialized exocrine glands or by the surface mucosa. These secretions are necessary for lubrication, immune protection, and digestive functions of the gastrointestinal system as well as for the regulation of body stores of certain nutrients and to maintain the acid/base balance of the body.

The major components of gastrointestinal secretions are water, electrolytes, hydrochloric acid, a base (HCO_3^-), digestive enzymes, emulsifiers (bile salts), immunoglobulins (primarily IgA), and various specialized products, such as intrinsic factor. These are contained in the main secretory elements along the gastrointestinal tract—saliva, gastric juice, bile, pancreatic juice, and intestinal secretions.

Nervous reflexes and hormonal signals partially control the secretion rate and the composition of the fluids. At the level of the intestinal epithelia, various active cellular processes (pumps) absorb or extrude ionic substances to facilitate the transmucosal flow of water, electrolytes, minerals, and organic compounds, including essential nutrients. The total daily turnover of water among the secretions at the various levels of the alimentary tract may be 4 liters or more; however, water and electrolytes are efficiently reabsorbed by the colon and returned to the vascular compartments of the body.

Digestion

Foods and beverages in the diet are chemically complex, and most nutrients are bound up in forms that do not permit their direct entrance into the body. The process of digestion reduces dietary elements to substances that can cross the epithelial barrier and reach either the lymphatic or the venous portal circulation. Mechanical processes in the mouth and stomach and the emulsifying properties of bile acids assist in reducing foods to their simplest components. Although the pH and ionic conditions in the alimentary tract lead to spontaneous hydrolysis of some substances, digestive enzymes play the dominant role in preparing dietary nutrients for absorption and transport across the intestinal mucosa.

Enzymes. The digestive enzymes can act in the bulk phase of the chyme, on the brush-border surface, or within the cells of the alimentary mucosa. For example, saliva contains a soluble amylase that begins the digestion of dietary starch. In newborn infants a "lingual lipase" in saliva plays an important role in the digestion of the fat in breast milk at a time when the infant's gastric and biliary secretory responses are still immature. The stomach produces pepsin, a proteolytic enzyme. The pancreas secretes a family of enzymes tailored for the array of chemical substances ingested with meals: endo- and exopeptidases; lipases for triglycerides, phospholipids, and cholesterol esters; amylase; elastase; collagenase; and nucleases.

To protect the body from autodigestion, nature has provided two specialized devices to contain enzymes: (1) most soluble enzymes are formed in the exocrine glands as *proenzymes* and (2) *molecular modification* (usually partial digestion of the molecule) is required for them to exert their full catalytic activity. Thus, pepsin is secreted as pepsinogen and subsequently is hydrolyzed by acid in the gastric lumen to yield an activated enzyme that is most efficient in the low pH environment of the stomach; chymotrypsin is packaged in the pancreatic acinar cell as chymotrypsinogen, is activated by trypsin in the duodenal lumen, and is most active in the more

alkaline pH conditions of the small intestine. Secretion, therefore, plays a vital role in digestion by making the soluble bulk-phase exocrine enzymes efficient through regulation of the pH values in various levels of the gastrointestinal tract.

Bile salts. The effective digestion of dietary fats depends on the secretion of pancreatic lipases, the presence of an appropriate pH value in the duodenum, and the excretion of bile salts from the gallbladder and liver into the lumen. Bile salts first act as detergents to emulsify lipids and then help to form mixed micelles containing fatty acids, phospholipids, and/or sterols. (Since lipids are not miscible with water, they can achieve significant concentrations in an aqueous phase only in the form of *mixed micelles.*) Bile salts obtain their nonpolar hydrophilic properties through conjunction with either glycine or taurine and are conserved avidly through enterohepatic recycling. Once conjugated, they are excreted in the bile, reabsorbed in the ileum, and returned to the liver for reexcretion in bile. Any pathologic process that promotes the deconjugation of bile salts (e.g., bacterial overgrowth of the upper gut) or their malabsorption (ileal disease) will deplete the body of these essential participants in fat absorption and contribute to steatorrhea.

Membrane-bound enzymes. In addition to the hydrolyses catalyzed in the bulk phase by secretory enzymes, membrane-bound enzymes, attached to the brush border of the intestinal mucosal cells, play a significant role in digestion, primarily with respect to carbohydrates. Table sugar (sucrose) and milk sugar (lactose) are 12-carbon disaccharides and must be broken down into their component hexoses before absorption. They are hydrolyzed by the mucosal enzymes sucrase-isomaltase and lactase, respectively. Starch is digested by amylase to a two-glucose disaccharide (maltose) and to branched oligosaccharides; these products then are hydrolyzed to simple glucose at the membrane by maltase and isomaltase.

Additional components. Other dietary components, such as folic acid, usually are joined to a polyglutamic acid chain in foods. These glutamate residues are removed enzymatically during folate absorption. Similarly niacin, riboflavin, and thiamine are thought to be linked to phosphates in the diet; thus, specific or non-specific phosphatase enzymes in the intestine may participate in the uptake of these B-complex vitamins.[4]

Absorption

Once nutrients have been liberated in forms suitable for passage across the mucosal membrane, absorption can commence. This requires sufficient absorptive surface for contact, healthy mucosal cells for uptake, and an intact system of intracellular and postcellular transport for transferring nutrients into the body. Thus, loss of intestinal surface (e.g., from congenital atresia, surgical ablation, or pathologic atrophy) will compromise absorption.

Classically, three processes account for nutrient transport from the intestinal lumen into the enterocyte and beyond: (1) passive diffusion, (2) energy-dependent active transport, and (3) facilitated diffusion. Passive diffusion is governed by the permeability of the membrane or the perimembranous environment. Its nutrient uptake rate is related linearly to the concentrations of soluble substrate in the lumen and the blood. Certain nutrients, such as glucose and specific amino acids, are absorbed at high rates when present in low concentrations in the lumen but at lower rates (or at rates attributable to passive diffusion alone) at higher luminal concentrations (saturation kinetics). When such regulation can be modified by agents that block specific metabolic steps, it is assumed that the absorptive mechanism is energy-dependent (active transport). Facilitated diffusion occurs when saturation kinetics are evident but when the process is insensitive to metabolic inhibition, as in fructose absorption.

Permeability. The characteristics of the membrane, as well as the shape, size, and electrical charge of the nutrient molecule, can influence permeability. The cell membrane is largely a nonpolar lipid structure. Diffusion of the charged (salt) forms of organic acids is restricted to a greater degree than diffusion of the protonated (acid) forms. Although the bulk phase of the chyme has a pH value of 6 to 8, the microcalyx adherent to the brush border is considerably more acidic. This favors the uptake of nutrients such as folic acid or pantothenic acid. On the other hand, lipid-soluble nutrients (fatty acids, fat-soluble vitamins, cholesterol) pass easily through the membrane, which is itself nonpolar. Since the luminal contents are in liquid form, the movement of lipids is restricted prior to entry into the enterocyte. Mixed micelle formation allows the components of dietary fat to approach the intestinal wall, but an *unstirred layer* of water coats the mucosa. Lipid passage from its micelle to the intestinal cell membrane through the unstirred aqueous "cap" above the mucosa is the limiting step in the cellular uptake of dietary lipids.[5]

Cellular factors. A number of cellular factors also influence the absorption of various nutrients. In the absorption of dietary calcium two vitamin D–dependent mechanisms, a surface ATPase and a lateral border calcium-binding protein, assist in calcium mucosal uptake and in its transfer to the circulatory system. Iron is taken up into the cell by two distinct pathways, depending on its form as an inorganic ion (nonheme iron) or as a part of the hemoglobin or myoglobin heme ring. Inside the cell the release of both forms of iron into the body is governed by a regulatory mechanism that is sensitive to the levels of body iron stores. Fatty acids, phospholipids, and fat-soluble vitamins are deesterified in the process of luminal digestion but, once inside the enterocyte, are reesterified. Finally, in association with the rough endoplasmic reticulum and the Golgi apparatus, newly absorbed fats are packed with lipoproteins into the chylomicra and are released into the lymphatic lacteals of the intestine. There are other specialized intracellular mechanisms in nutrient absorption, but they are not described here.

Nutrients synthesized in the alimentary tract. In addition to the nutrients ingested with meals, several nutrients are synthesized by bacteria of the normal colonic flora. These include vitamin K, biotin, vitamin B_{12}, and folic acid. Colonic flora bacteria apparently produce vitamin K and biotin in amounts adequate to satisfy the body's physiologic needs, but folic acid and vitamin B_{12} are produced in inadequate amounts because the colon cannot absorb them. The vitamin B_{12} supply is augmented in two ways: (1) dental plaque in the mouth synthesizes some vitamin B_{12}; and (2) in a person with a colonic bacterial reflux (backwash) into the distal ileum, synthesis of vitamin B_{12} can occur in the region of its absorption, since gastric intrinsic factor, trypsin, and the conditions necessary for vitamin

B_{12} uptake are available in the lumen. It has been suggested that, in the vegetarian Hindu population of southern India, oral and ileal bacterial synthesis may be critical to vitamin B_{12} nutriture.

Colonic absorption. The colon has long been recognized as a site for water and electrolyte absorption. In recent years a number of additional absorptive capacities of the large bowel have been identified. As just mentioned, colonic bacteria synthesize both vitamin K and biotin. Indirect evidence from patients treated with enemas and/or oral antibiotics suggests that the biotin and vitamin K of colonic origin can serve as sources of these nutrients for the body. However, the precise mechanism by which the colonic mucosa absorbs the large molecules is not well understood.

When carbohydrates such as lactose (in lactase-deficient persons), raffinose, and stachyose (from legumes) and cellulose, hemicellulose, and pectin (components of dietary fiber) escape absorption in the small bowel and reach the colon, they encounter bacterial enzymes capable of hydrolyzing the substrates and fermenting their monosaccharide components. This fermentation produces short-chain volatile fatty acids. Observations in laboratory animals and in humans[6] suggest that the colon absorbs the products of carbohydrate fermentation in a highly efficient manner. Thus "malabsorption" of dietary carbohydrates by the small intestine does not imply a total loss of the available energy via the stools.

Excretion

The absorptive surface of the alimentary tract serves as a two-way system, transporting nutrients across the mucosa from the lumen into the body and, conversely, promoting passage of nutrients to the lumen in bulk form as components of intestinal, biliary, or pancreatic secretions. Substantial quantities of vitamin B_{12}, folic acid, and copper, for example, enter the duodenum via the bile. Although these two vitamins are reabsorbed efficiently by the intestine, biliary copper is absorbed poorly and essentially is excreted completely in the feces. Indeed, bile represents the principal route of copper excretion from the body.[7] Large quantities of zinc—equivalent to the amount ingested in meals—enter the intestinal lumen as part of meal-stimulated pancreatic secretions.[8] Some of this zinc is reab-

sorbed; but, again, the gastrointestinal tract also represents the major route of zinc excretion. Calcium also reenters the alimentary tract in various secretions; obligatory endogenous loss of calcium into the fecal stream amounts to between 70 and 150 mg/day. Finally, protein from exfoliated cells and pancreatic secretions may not be digested and reabsorbed completely. The feces normally contain 1 to 2 g of nitrogen, corresponding to 6 to 12 g of protein even when individuals ingest very low-protein or protein-free diets.[9]

PLACENTAL NUTRIENT TRANSPORT IN PREGNANCY

Novel metabolic processes are related to the events surrounding pregnancy and lactation. In both circumstances the transport of nutrients from the mother to the offspring is an essential consideration.

In human pregnancy the placenta is the organ that assures adequate nutriture of the fetus. Munro et al.[10] state that placental function involves "transmission of nutrients, gases, and water to the fetus, excretion of waste products of fetal metabolism into the maternal bloodstream, and adaptation of maternal metabolism to different stages of pregnancy by means of hormones." An obvious requirement of the placental system is to maintain gradients in nutrient concentrations between maternal and fetal circulations. For instance, plasma levels of glucose and amino acids are higher in the fetal plasma than in the maternal. Another requirement is an adaptive and graded response of delivery (maternal-to-fetal transfer) of nutrients depending on fetal demand. Calcium and trace metals, for instance, have their highest rates of transfer in late pregnancy.

The uterine and placental tissues that support the development of the human fetus have their own unique nutritional demands, also supplied from the maternal diet and nutrient stores. About two thirds of the glucose and half the oxygen delivered to the uterine circulation are consumed by placental and uterine tissues, with only a third of the glucose and half the oxygen entering fetal metabolism.[11] Moreover, Faber and Thornburg[12] find it useful to separate the nutrient costs of energy production and life maintenance in the fetus from those of incorporating nutrients into new tissue as part of fetal growth. They estimate

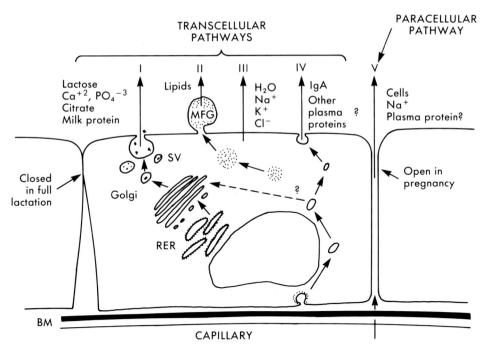

Figure 1-2 Milk secretion. *MFG*, Milk fat globules; *SV*, secretory vesicle; *RER*, rough endoplasmic reticulum; *BM*, basement membrane.

From Bauman DE, Neville MC: Fed Proc **43**:2430-2431, 1985.

that over a third of all combustible nutrients (carbohydrate, protein, fat) are, in fact, not used as fuel but are laid down as fetal tissue.

The production of placental hormones and the consumption of nutrients in the uterus have distinct effects on maternal nutrition. The adaptations are aimed at optimizing fetal nutrition. Clearly, *severe* maternal malnutrition, such as that seen in famine, can influence the nutrition of the fetus via the placenta. Milder degrees of protein-energy malnutrition and specific micronutrient deficiencies (e.g., of iron) have been postulated to influence adversely fetal nutriture, but the findings in human pregnancy are inconsistent. Since blood flow is a major determinant of nutrient availability, maternal nutritional factors that limit plasma volume expansion or that increase viscosity of maternal blood may act to diminish the nutriture of the fetus as well.

LACTATION

The other transport function to sustain life of the human offspring is the provision of water and nutrients to the milk. The mammary glands produce and secrete milk of a genetically determined composition, presumably tailored to the nutritional requirements of the infant.[13] Suckling by the infant stimulates two neural hormones: prolactin and oxytocin.[14] The former is responsible for the production of milk and its accumulation in the acini. The latter causes contraction of the myoepithelial cells, forcing milk into the ducts so it is available to the suckling action of the infant.

The supply/demand issues have a circular relationship in lactation and nursing. The stronger more vigorous infant provides a greater hormonal stimulus and more milk availability. More milk intake provides for greater infant growth and strength. A survey of 24-hour test weighings in 3-month-old infants[15] showed little geographic variance: Hungary, 714 ml; Sweden, 787 ml; Guatemala, 674 ml; Philippines, 689 ml; and urban Zaire, 666 ml. Only the rural Zaire infants had a substantially lower average intake (409 ml).

The cellular scheme for milk secretion is shown in Fig. 1-2. The cells are approximated by tight junctions in full lactation. The fat is packaged into fat droplets and has a variable content of fatty acids of differing chain lengths and degrees of saturation. Milk proteins are produced along the endoplasmic reticulum of the mammary cell and secreted into milk via the Golgi apparatus. Milk contains various plasma proteins and IgA in a secretory (bimolecular) form. Whether these proteins reach the milk by a transcellular or paracellular pathway, or both, is unclear. The concentration of sodium in mature human milk, 14 mM, is one tenth that in the plasma whereas the potassium concentration, 16 mM, is four times that in the blood.[16] Lactose is a disaccharide of glucose and galactose united by a 1-4 beta linkage, unique to mammalian milk. Its concentration is fairly constant at 170 mM (6.5 g/100 g of milk) in mature breast milk.

Milk produced by mothers who give birth to preterm infants differs from that of term milk[16]: it is richer in protein and lipids and poorer in lactose. These modifications may be the casual result of an immaturity of the mammary gland of the mother, providing more paracellular transport of nutrients from the bloodstream and less glandular synthesis, but the composition appears suited to the special needs of immature newborns.[16]

CELL GROWTH

After essential nutrients and energy-yielding substrates are absorbed from the intestinal tract, they are transported to the cells, which they often enter via specialized processes. In the cells nutrients and substrates either are modified further to carry out their biochemical functions or enter biochemical pathways, leading to cellular accumulation or elimination via degradation processes. An account of all metabolic events that occur during nutrient utilization is not feasible within the confines of this chapter, but a few important points will present a working basis for further discussion.

Regulatory Mechanisms

In amounts in excess of tissue needs, glucose and fatty acids (or their precursors or products) and amino acids are the quantitatively important energy-yielding substrates at the organ and cellular levels[17] (Table 1-1). The pattern of fuel sources changes markedly if food is withheld for

Table 1-1 Fuels of Individual Tissues

Source	Tissue
Glucose	Erythrocytes, leukocytes, renal medulla, brain, skeletal muscle (exercise), some malignant tumors, fetal tissues, intestinal mucosa
Free fatty acids*	Liver, kidney cortex, cardiac muscle, skeletal muscle (except in severe exercise)
Ketone bodies*	Cardiac muscle, renal cortex, skeletal muscle, brain

Other
  Amino acids (minor)
  Lactate (derived from glucose)
  Ethanol, glycerol, and pentoses (minor)	

From Young VR: Cancer Res **37**:2336-2347, 1977.
*These sources can be used in quantitatively significant amounts by the tissues shown.

a period that significantly exceeds the usual overnight fast. Therefore a fast extending for 2 or 3 days or longer decreases glucose oxidation in accordance with reduced rates of gluconeogenesis.[18] At the same time triglyceride mobilization from adipose tissue and utilization of fatty acids in peripheral tissues, particularly muscle, are increased and the brain utilizes ketone bodies as its major fuel source. This pattern of change in fuel utilization during short- and long-term fasts is achieved by alterations in substrate availability and hormonal balance. Furthermore, these responses emphasize that the body's nutritional state will determine, in part, the mixture of substrates used for meeting the energy needs of the cells and organs.

Similarly, the body's requirements for and intakes of other essential nutrients, such as the essential amino acids, will determine the degree of efficiency with which those nutrients are used. With high dietary protein intakes the amino acids consumed in excess of physiologic needs enter pathways of amino acid catabolism and are eliminated from the body in the forms of carbon dioxide, water, and urea. This elimination is achieved by amino acid–catabolizing enzymes and ensures that acutely high amino acid intakes do not result in sustained elevations of the levels

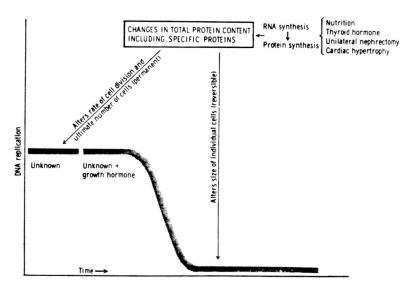

Figure 1-3 Mechanisms by which certain stimuli can affect cellular growth in adult and infant tissues.

From Winick M: Fed Proc **29:**1510-1515, 1970.

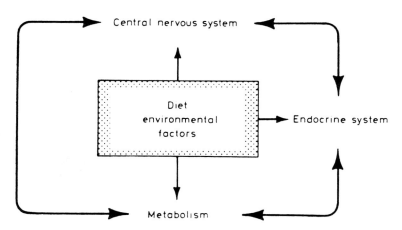

Figure 1-4 Interrelationships among the central nervous system, the endocrine system, and the nutritional and metabolic status of the intact organism.

From Young VR: In Buttery PJ, Lindsay D, editors: Protein deposition in farm animals, London, 1980, Butterworth & Co (Publishers) Ltd, pp 167-191.

of these amino acids in body fluids. Such sustained high levels can result in untoward effects on tissue metabolism and body function, as occurs, for example, in phenylketonuria or maple syrup urine disease,[19] both of which are inborn errors of amino acid metabolism.

The two examples given show that the nutrient intake level and the body's nutritional status determine the metabolic fate of any nutrient that enters the circulatory system. Thus the efficiency with which absorbed nutrients meet physiologic requirements also depends initially on those two factors.

The effects of nutritional factors can be ob-

Table 1-2 Major Organization of the Mammalian Immune Defense System

Component	Tissue or Cellular Elements	Mediators/Effectors	Function
Protective barrier	Skin and mucosa, gastric acid		Prevents entry of pathogens
Phagocytic	Polymorphonuclear leukocytes, monocytes, macrophages	Opsinins, complement	Engulfs and kills pathogens
Humoral	B-lymphocytes, plasma cells	Antibody, immunoglobulins	Recognizes pathogens as foreign
Cellular	T-lymphocytes	Lymphokines, interferon	Inflammatory response Kills intracellular pathogens
Acute phase response	Liver, other tissues	Endogenous pyrogen, interleukin-1, cachectin, other peptides	Unclear

served most readily in the rapidly growing body. A deficiency in dietary protein or energy, for example, inhibits normal growth and development and can lead to profound clinical deterioration, as evidenced by kwashiorkor and marasmus in infants and young children (Chapter 32). The effects of nutritional deficiency on the body's growth, development, and ability to recover from earlier malnutrition depend on many factors, including the time at which the deficiency was introduced, its severity, and its duration. Malnutrition early in growth and development inhibits cell mitosis and DNA replication, potentially leading to a smaller organism with fewer cells.[20] Later malnutrition, on the other hand, affects the size of cells or their content more profoundly than cell number (Fig. 1-3).

Thus the normal functioning and growth of cells and organs require an adequate supply of nutrients. Deficiencies or excesses can lead to altered function and, if severe or prolonged, permanent changes.

Hormonal Interrelationships

The body's hormonal balance is affected by diet and by nutritional status. Conversely, nutrient intake influences the activity and metabolic state of the neuroendocrine system[21] (Fig. 1-4). Thus, fasting and feeding produce changes in the sympathetic nervous system, in catecholamine release, and in the availability of insulin.[22] Hormones play a key role in regulating metabolism; changes in hormone balance and in the hormone responsiveness of tissues affect, in part, interactions between the body and its nutritional environment.

In addition, nutrient utilization may depend directly on the functioning of specific endocrine systems. The intimate relationships between (1) calcium absorption and utilization in bone metabolism and (2) parathormone and calcitonin functions are an obvious example.[23] Changes in parathyroid status may be responsible for changes in vitamin D metabolism, calcium absorption, and the calcium content of bones during progressive aging in humans, and for crippling osteoporosis in postmenopausal women.

IMMUNITY

People are in constant and intimate contact with potential pathogenic organisms and form antigens. Thus an elaborate system of immune protection has evolved (Table 1-2). Classically it has been divided into the *protective barrier system,* consisting of epithelial membranes and other systems (nasal cilia, gastric acid, intestinal proteases), to prevent the entry of pathogens; the *phagocytic system,* of fixed and mobile macrophages, to provide a mechanism for engulfing and then killing circulating viral, bacterial, and fungal organisms once they have been "recognized" as foreign and suitably coated with opsinins; and the *humoral system,* based on the B-lymphocyte, and *cellular system,* based on the T-lymphocyte (the former producing the various classes of immunoglobulin antibodies that recognize and attach to specific antigens, the latter being involved in the inflammatory response and killing of intracellular pathogens). Recent studies[24] have shown how complex the T-lymphocyte system is, with a mixture and interaction of effect cells, inhibitor cells, and cells that are themselves cytotoxic. The various subclasses of

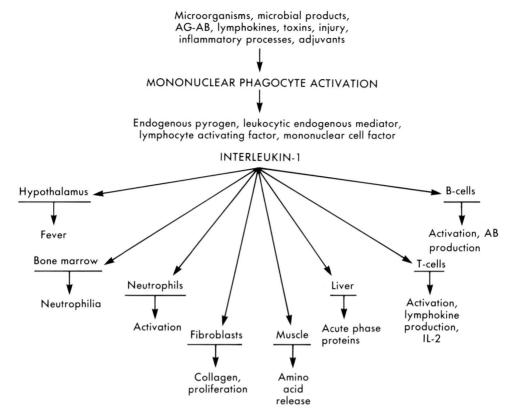

Figure 1-5 Initiation of the acute-phase response and the diverse effects of interleukin-1 on host nutrition and immune responses. *AG-AB* is antigen-antibody complexes.

From Dinarello CA: N Engl J Med **311**:1413-1418, 1984.

cells communicate via a network of soluble lymphocytes and interferons, and the phagocytic system communicates with the cellular immune system via a series of monokines. These soluble messengers have been termed the "interleukins,"[25,26] and an important member of this class, formerly known by other designations (Fig. 1-5), is interleukin-1.

The effects of the soluble mediators of the inflammatory response are both local and systemic. They give rise to the *acute-phase response*[27] (APR), which itself has many implications for nutrition and metabolism. There are, among other features, changes in glucose metabolism, attained synthetic priorities for proteins, and a redistribution of circulatory micronutrients. Most mediators of the APR are pyrogenic; that is, they give rise to the fever that accompanies infection and inflammatory processes.

A recently characterized soluble peptide of white cell origin, tumor necrosis factor or cachetin, is of importance at the interface of immunity and nutrition. It shares many of the effects of the other endogenous mediators of the acute phase response. Its special characteristic is that it disrupts fatty acid clearance (by inhibiting the production of lipoprotein-lipase) and impairs fatty acid synthesis within adipocytes. It both produces anorexia and enhances catabolic energy wasting. It has raised renewed interest concerning the teleologic significance of the anorexia accompanying infectious illness. If this is part of the cachetin-mediated response to infection, it might in some way be protective, raising doubts about the wisdom of parenteral feeding, tube feeding, forced feeding, or even early convalescent refeeding in the case of certain classes of microbial diseases.[29]

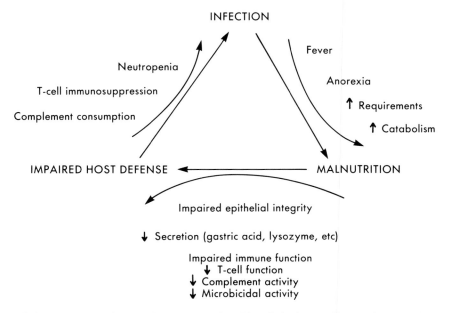

Figure 1-6 The triangle of interaction among malnutrition, infection, and host defense. Malnutrition may be initiated by primary or secondary deficiency (e.g., malabsorptive states) or by the metabolic effects of infection. The consequence of this is impairment of host defenses, which in turn leads to an increased burden of infection and further malnutrition.

From Keusch GT, Farthing MJ: Annu Rev Nutr **6**:131-154, 1986.

INTERACTION OF NUTRITION AND INFECTION

In their classic monograph, Scrimshaw, Taylor, and Gordon[32] illustrated the complex interaction of malnutrition and infection. Infection would predispose to a deterioration of nutritional status (synergistic relationship). Undernutrition would increase problems of infection (synergistic relationship) or, in certain instances, enhance resistance to infection (antagonistic relationship).

In the past two decades an immunologic perspective has been placed on the interaction of nutrition and infection.[30,31] The role of immune deficiencies in the mediation of the synergistic relationships is shown in Fig. 1-6. Chandra[30] has pointed out that overnutrition can also interfere with immune defenses, altering the host's resistance or response to infections.

Synergistic Relationships

Infections produce anorexia and catabolic stress. Thus it is not surprising that nutritional status suffers as a consequence. The occurrence of kwashiorkor, the edematous form of infantile protein-energy malnutrition, has often been noted to occur after outbreaks of measles.[32] In Bangladesh the diarrheal disease burden negatively influences the linear growth of preschool children.[33] Longitudinal data from northeast Brazil[34] quantify the impact of a bout of chickenpox on hepatic vitamin A reserves. Thus, it has been advanced[35] that controlling childhood infections will reduce the prevalence of malnutrition in developing countries.

Animals fed nutrient-restricted diets and exposed to specific pathogens in experimental infection models generally—although not always—exhibited greater morbidity and mortality than did well-nourished controls. Studies[36,37] have allowed the distinction to be made of specific lesions in one or another component of the immune system (Table 1-2) produced by mild to severe deficiencies of specific vitamin or mineral micronutrients. In malnourished human infants some clinical elements of the immune response (phagocytosis, T-cell function, secretory IgA production) become defunct while others (B-cell function, acute-phase response) remain relatively intact.[38] The translation of this roster of in vitro and in vivo reactions into a clinical response to naturally acquired infection at the level of the whole organism is not straightforward. Epidemiologic studies in malnourished populations,[39] however, have shown that generally the severity and duration—but not the incidence—of infections are greater in children with preexisting protein-energy malnutrition. That this is mediated through immune deficiency is suggested by the higher in-hospital mortality rates of these malnourished individuals with demonstrable impairment of cell-mediated immunity.[40]

Nutritional Antagonism of Pathogens

Nutritional impairment of specific components of the immune system tends to reduce resistance to infections or to their metabolic sequelae. However, Scrimshaw et al.[32] also found situations in which undernutrition actually appeared to have the opposite effect; that is, it reduced the effects of pathogens. This occurred most often with intracellular organisms. In some human infections nutritional depletion may favor the processes of host resistance.

Iron deficiency has been the most discussed of the antagonistic situations.[31] The mild ferropenic anemia of infants may protect them against septicemia, since unsaturated transferrin is possibly an effective retardant of bacterial proliferation in the bloodstream. Vigorous iron therapy to newborns exposes them to increased risk of gram-negative infections. Iron deficiency also may reduce the incidence of fulminant systemic amebiasis in populations with high rates of intestinal *Entamoeba histolytica* infections. Tissue depletion of iron has been reported to check the recrudescence of latent infections with intracellular organisms (e.g., brucellosis, tuberculosis, malaria).

Based on experiments in rats, it has been postulated that vitamin E deficiency, which increases red cell fragility, can block the proliferation of malaria by fostering the rapid elimination of parasitized red cells via the reticuloendothelial system. Protein-energy nutrition, finally, may reduce the inflammatory response to schistosomiasis, and hence reduce fibrosis, which mediates the vascular hypertension of that parasitic infection.

REFERENCES

1. Stricker EM: Biological bases of hunger and satiety: therapeutic implications, Nutr Rev **42**:333-340, 1984.
2. Grossman SP: The role of glucose, insulin, and glucogen in the regulation of food intake and body weight, Neurosci Biobehav Rev **10**:295-315, 1986.
3. Binder HJ: The pathophysiology of diarrhea, Hosp Pract **10**:107-113, 116-118, 1984.
4. Rose RC, et al: Transport and metabolism of water-soluble vitamins in intestine and kidney, Fed Proc **43**:2423-2429, 1984.
5. Wilson FA, et al: Unstirred water layers in intestine: rate determinant of fatty acid absorption from micellar, Science **174**:1031-1033, 1971.
6. Rerat AA: Contribution of the large intestine to digestion of carbohydrates. In Delmont J, editor: Milk intolerances and rejection, Basel, 1983, S Karger AG, pp 17-21.
7. Van Berge Henegouwen GP, et al: Biliary secretion of copper in healthy man: quantitation by an intestinal perfusion technique, Gastroenterology **72**:1228-1231, 1977.
8. Matseshe JW, et al: Recovery of dietary iron and zinc from the proximal intestine of healthy man: studies of different meals and supplements, Am J Clin Nutr **33**:1946-1953, 1980.
9. Young VR, Scrimshaw NS: Nutritional evaluation of proteins and protein requirements. In Milner M, et al, editors: Protein resources and technology: status and research needs, Westport Conn, 1978, AVI Publishing Co Inc, pp 136-173.
10. Munro HN, et al: The placenta in nutrition, Annu Rev Nutr **3**:97-124, 1983.
11. Battaglia FC: Placental transport and utilization of amino acids and carbohydrates, Fed Proc **45**:2508-2512, 1986.
12. Faber JJ, Thornburg KL: Fetal nutrition: supply, combustion, interconversion, and deposition, Fed Proc **45**:2502-2507, 1986.
13. Bauman DE, Neville MC: Nutritional and physiological factors affecting lactation, Fed Proc **43**:2430-2431, 1985.
14. Neville MC, et al: The mechanisms of milk secretion. In Neville MC, Neifert MR, editors: Lactation: physiology, nutrition, and breast feeding, New York, 1983, Plenum Press Inc, pp 49-103.
15. The quantity and quality of breast milk. Report of the WHO collaborative study on breast-feeding, Geneva, 1985, World Health Organization.
16. Anderson GH: The effect of prematurity on milk consumption and its physiological basis, Fed Proc **43**:2438-2442, 1985.
17. Young VR: Energy metabolism and requirements in the cancer patient, Cancer Res **37**:2336-2347, 1977.
18. Crabtree B, Newsholme EA: A quantitative approach to metabolic control, Curr Top Cell Regul **25**:21-76, 1985.
19. Scriver CR, Rosenberg LE: Amino acid metabolism and its disorders, Philadelphia, 1973, WB Saunders Co, p 491.
20. Winick M: Nutrition and nerve cell growth, Fed Proc **29**:1510-1515, 1970.
21. Young VR: Hormonal control of protein metabolism with particular reference to body protein gain. In Buttery PJ, Lindsay D, editors: Protein deposition in farm animals, London, 1980, Butterworth & Co (Publishers) Ltd, pp 167-191.
22. Landsberg L, Young JB: Fasting, feeding, and regulation of the sympathetic nervous system, N Engl J Med **298**:1295-1300, 1978.
23. DeLuca HF: The metabolism and functions of vitamin D, Adv Exp Med Biol **196**:361-375, 1986.
24. Schlossman SF: The human T-cell circuit—biologic and clinical implications, Harvey Lect **79**:31-49, 1983-84.

25. Dinarello CA: Interleukin-1 and the pathogenesis of the acute-phase response, N Engl J Med **311**:1413-1418, 1984.
26. Dinarello CA: Interleukin-1, Rev Infect Dis **6**:51-95, 1984.
27. Powanda M, Beisel WR: Hypothesis: leukocyte endogenous mediator/endogenous pyrogen/lymphocyte-activating factor modulates the development of nonspecific and specific immunity and affects nutritional status, Am J Clin Nutr **35**:762-768, 1982.
28. Beutter B, Cerami A: The endogenous mediator of endotoxic shock, Clin Res **35**:192-197, 1987.
29. Keusch GT: Interaction of nutrition and infection. Memorias: Inauguration of the "Leonardo Mata" Microbiological Laboratories, May 1986, Guatemala City, Institute of Nutrition of Central America and Panama. (In press.)
30. Chandra RK: Immunodeficiency in undernutrition and overnutrition, Nutr Rev **39**:225-231, 1981.
31. Keusch GT, Farthing MJ: Nutrition and infection, Annu Rev Nutr **6**:131-154, 1986.
32. Scrimshaw NS, et al: Interactions of nutrition and infection, Geneva, 1968, World Health Organization.
33. Black RE, et al: Effect of diarrhea associated with specific enteropathogens on the growth of children in rural Bangladesh, Pediatrics **73**:799-805, 1984.
34. Campos FACS, et al: Effect of an infection on vitamin A status of children as measured by the relative dose response (RDR), Am J Clin Nutr **46**:91-94, 1987.
35. Keusch GT, Scrimshaw NS: Selective primary health care: strategies for control of disease in the developing world. XXIII. Control of infection to reduce the prevalence of infantile and childhood malnutrition, Rev Infect Dis **8**:273-287, 1986.
36. Beisel WR: Single nutrients and immunity, Am J Clin Nutr **35**:417-478, 1982.
37. Corman LC: The relationship between nutrition, infection and immunity, Med Clin North Am **69**:519-531, 1985.
38. Suskind R: Malnutrition and the immune response, New York, 1975, Raven Press.
39. Brown RE, et al: Malnutrition is a determining factor in diarrheal duration, but not incidence, among young children in a longitudinal study in rural Bangladesh, Am J Clin Nutr **39**:87-94, 1984.
40. Brown KH, et al: Infections associated with severe protein-calorie malnutrition in hospitalized infants and children, Nutr Res **1**:33-46, 1981.

CHAPTER 2
The Major Nutrients

Noel W. Solomons
Vernon R. Young

The earliest forms of life were probably simple bacterium-like organisms capable of synthesizing all the compounds they needed from salts, nitrogen, water, and simple sources of carbon. When animal cells developed about one billion years ago, they needed certain additional carbon compounds supplied by their environment. These exogenous compounds were the essential dietary nutrients. Although the various animal species have developed many specific metabolic differences, the general quantitative and qualitative patterns of required nutrients are strikingly similar throughout the animal kingdom.

The first essential nutrient to be identified was gaseous oxygen, shown in the eighteenth century by Priestley to be essential for mammalian life. Oxygen, however, is atypical insofar as it is absorbed across the lungs (not the gut) and death ensues within minutes following severe oxygen deficiency. The remaining nutrients in mammalian metabolism are taken up from foods and beverages across the intestinal tract. The simplest of these are water and soluble ions; the most complex is vitamin B_{12}. The nutritional and health significance of vitamins was not appreciated until the earlier part of the twentieth century. Most of the dietary compounds and elements now recognized as essential for growth and health maintenance were discovered and identified only during the past 60 years.

Because the body depends on a consistent supply of dietary nutrients, it has developed regulatory biochemical mechanisms that enable it to adjust successfully to low or excessive nutrient intakes; thus the metabolism of essential nutrients is under constant control. When this control is upset by metabolic disorders, infectious diseases, trauma, medications, or other factors, dietary nutrient requirements are altered. Unless the dietary supply and balance of nutrients can compensate for these changes, health will deteriorate.

The six major classes of nutrients: proteins, fats (or lipids), carbohydrates, vitamins, minerals, and water will be discussed. A review of each of these classes, and of energy, will provide the framework for ensuing discussions of nutrition and dietary factors in relation to various physiologic and pathologic states.

ENERGY

All the biochemical and physiologic processes associated with utilizing nutrients for growth and for maintenance of normal cell composition and function, tissue repair, host defense, and body movement require energy.

The major dietary sources of energy-yielding substrates are carbohydrates, lipids, and proteins. An optional source of energy in regions is ethanol (alcohol). These substrates, through the course of their catabolism, liberate energy that is either trapped in the form of high-energy phosphate compounds, principally adenosine triphosphate (ATP), or lost directly as heat. Thus ATP is the central chemical intermediate involved in the many processes that require energy, and its rate and regulation of formation are fundamental aspects of the fuel homeostasis of the body. Since the amount of ATP present in body tissues and organs is limited, ATP must be generated continually to supply the required energy. As a result, the body's fuel stores are used continually and must be replenished via food ingestion.

The major endogenous source of substrate for ATP synthesis is body fat (Table 2-1), but carbohydrates in the form of glycogen and body proteins also serve a fuel sources. On a short-term basis, such as after an overnight fast or during a period of acute exercise, the carbohydrate reserve may account for a significant source of available energy. However, body fat plays the major role if the dietary energy supply continues to be inadequate for more than a day.

Extended dietary energy deprivation triggers biochemical mechanisms that mobilize fat from adipose tissue cells in the form of fatty acids and ketone bodies[1] to meet tissue energy needs. These mechanisms enable the body successfully to withstand relatively long periods of low dietary energy intake,[2] provided the fuel stores were replete initially.

Metabolically the process of energy transformation, either from tissue fuel reserves or from dietary sources, can be divided into three major stages (Fig. 2-1): (1) the hydrolysis of triglycerides, polysaccharides, and proteins to their primary components—fatty acids and glycerol, glucose, and amino acids, respectively; (2) the conversion of these components to two- or three-carbon fragments; and (3) the entrance of the fragments into the citric acid (Krebs) cycle, which, in this third stage, serves as the final common pathway for their metabolism. The major generation of ATP is achieved in the third stage, along with production of carbon dioxide and water. In the case of amino acids the liberated ammonia is converted to urea, providing for the elimination of the nitrogen moiety during oxidative catabolism.

The processes that integrate energy intake from the environment with the body's needs are poorly understood. Since obesity often accompanies affluence, it is clear that the regulatory controls on this process do not match precisely an individual's energy needs. In fact, fuel stores can expand to the point of impairing the body's health.

Overall energy requirements for most individuals vary with age, sex, body weight, and climate; they also can be influenced by various drugs and hormones and by disease. For young

adult women normal energy requirements range from 1600 to 2200 kcal/day (6700-9200 kJ); men normally need between 1800 to 3000 kcal/day (7500-12,500 kJ).[3] Starvation, however, reduces these figures.[2] Likewise, age causes a general lowering of the energy requirements. The needs of a rapidly growing child or adolescent are higher than those of an adult. At birth the approximate daily need is 118 kcal/kg, but this declines by 10% at the end of the first year. Over the next 10 years, until adolescence, it averages about 80 kcal/kg; and in young adulthood it approximates 50 kcal/kg in men and 40 in women. On an absolute basis, there is a gradual decline in energy requirements through the remainder of adult life.[4,5]

Carbohydrates

About 45% of total energy intake is derived from carbohydrates, which may be classified according to their chemical forms: (1) the monosaccharides, including glucose, fructose, galactose, and mannose; (2) the disaccharides, sucrose accounting for as much as one third of the total carbohydrate intake, maltose, and lactose; and (3) the polysaccharides, consisting of repeating units of monosaccharides. From a nutritional standpoint, starch is the most important carbohydrate. It is a plant polysaccharide consisting principally of two types of compounds: (1) amylose, long chains of glucose units joined via an alpha-1,4 linkage; and (2) amylopectin, a branched-chain polysaccharide in which chain branching occurs via an alpha-1,6 linkage between glucose units. Two other polysaccharides to be discussed are dextrins (hydrolytic products of amylopectin) and cellulose (cellobiose repeating units in which the glucose units are linked via a beta-1,4 bond). Since the human intestinal tract does not secrete an enzyme capable of hydrolyzing the beta-1,4 bond, cellulose is digested only by intestinal microflora (Chapter 3).

Metabolism

Digestion of the complex carbohydrates results in the liberation of di- and trisaccharides and, ultimately, via the action of enzymes located in or on the brush border of the epithelial cell of the intestinal mucosa, in the appearance of monosaccharides that cross the cells via specific transport processes. Intestinal tract disor-

Table 2-1 Fuel Reserves in the Average (70 kg) Human

		Reserve	
Fuel	Tissue	g	kcal
Triglyceride	Adipose tissue	15,000	1,000,000
Glycogen	Liver	70	200
	Muscle	120	400
Glucose	Body fluids	20	40
Protein	Muscle	6000	25,000

From Newsholme EA: Clin Endocrinol Metab **5**:543-578, 1976.

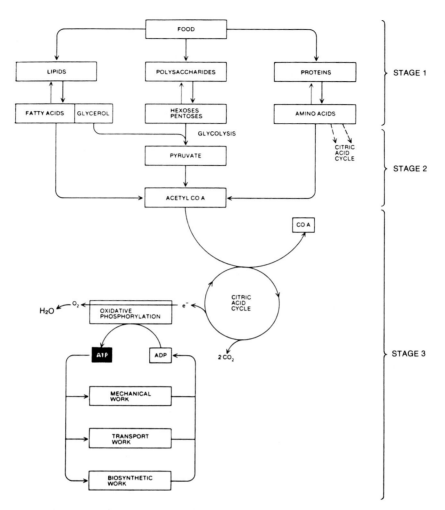

Figure 2-1 The metabolism of nutrients in the body can be divided into three stages: *STAGE 1,* Digestive enzymes in the alimentary tract degrade large nutrient molecules into their main building blocks. *STAGE 2,* These breakdown products are absorbed through the intestinal wall and transported by the blood to tissue cells, where they are either incorporated into cellular molecules by anabolic pathways or converted into a small number of intermediates by catabolic pathways. The inter-mediates—glucose, glycerol, fatty acids, and many amino acids—play a central role in metabolism. They are converted into the two-carbon acetyl group of the carrier molecule coenzyme A (CoA). *STAGE 3,* In this stage, localized to the mitochondria of cells, the CoA brings acetyl units into the citric acid cycle, where they are completely oxidized to carbon dioxide. Concurrently, four pairs of electrons are released. The energy-rich compound adenosine triphosphate (ATP) is generated in this stage as the electrons flow along a transport chain of oxygen atoms, the ultimate electron acceptor. Oxidation of a single glucose molecule can result in the formation of 36 molecules of ATP. Once generated, the ATP provides energy for the numerous physiologic and synthetic activities of the cells.

From Scrimshaw NS, Young VR: Sci Am **235**:50-64, 1976.

ders, either acquired or congenital, such as intestinal disaccharidase deficiency due to protein-energy malnutrition or to an inherited deficiency of sucrase-isomaltase activity, will affect the efficiency of carbohydrate utilization.

The importance of glucose in the energy metabolism of tissues is well established; indeed, some tissues, such as the erythrocyte and kidney medulla, have an obligatory need for glucose as a fuel source. Therefore it may be asked whether there is a specific dietary requirement for carbohydrate. This question is not easy to answer, particularly in relation to long-term health and the efficient utilization of essential nutrients (including amino acids). Available evidence indicates that neither carbohydrate nor glucose is essential for an adequate diet. For example, rapid growth in chicks can be achieved when they are fed carbohydrate-free diets. This is possible provided that an adequate source of glucose precursor such as glycerol or additional protein is available from which gluconeogenic amino acids can be used to satisfy tissue needs for glucose and other carbohydrates (i.e., ribose for nucleic acid synthesis, galactose for the formation of some glycoproteins). Similarly, Eskimos subsist on a carbohydrate-free protein-and-fat diet of marine mammals and fish during the Arctic winter.

Monosaccharides follow different metabolic pathways and therefore may not necessarily be equivalent in terms of nutrition or health. As an example, sucrose and starch, or glucose and fructose, have been shown[4] to exert different effects on plasma and tissue lipid levels and metabolism. High intakes of fructose relative to glucose lead to increased rates of triglyceride (triacylglycerol) synthesis in the livers of experimental animals and to elevated concentrations of cholesterol and triacylglycerols in the blood.[6] However, the different effects of various carbohydrates on lipid metabolism may be modified by the level or amount of carbohydrate in the diet and also by the amount and type of fat that is consumed. Thus it is difficult to judge the effect of sucrose as a dietary source of fructose by the level and type of blood lipids in free-living humans. Nevertheless, these experimental observations provide a partial basis for considering the role of dietary carbohydrate, and particularly the specific carbohydrate form, in the etiology of degenerative disease (especially coronary artery disease).

Lipids

Dietary fats (lipids) are a major source of human energy,[7] and there have been interesting trends in the consumption of fat during the present century (as revealed by data from the United States Department of Agriculture[18]): per capita intake of fat increased from 125 to 170 g over the years 1909-13 to 1984; the contribution of fat to total energy in the diet rose from 32% to 43% during those same years; and the percentage of fat in the diet from animal sources fell (from 83% to 58%) across those seven decades while the proportion from vegetable oil sources rose (from 17% to 42%).

Lipids exist mainly in the form of triacylglycerols, composed of fatty acids of varying chain length that may be saturated, monounsaturated, or polyunsaturated. The relative proportions and intake levels of these acids are of primary importance in determining their nutritional and health significance. Their obligatory nutrient function is to serve as a source of the essential fatty acids linoleic (18:2,n-6) and alpha-linolenic (18:3,n-3), which are required for normal growth and function of all tissues.* Since humans lack the enzymatic capacity to insert double bonds at the no. 6 and no. 3 carbon positions (n-6 and n-3) from the methyl end of the molecule, these fatty acids must be supplied by a dietary source. They are needed to form cell structures and to act as precursors for prostaglandins, prostacyclines, and thromboxanes (formed by the cyclooxygenase pathways) and leukotrienes (formed via the lipoxygenase pathways) (Fig. 2-2). These compounds can be regarded as "local hormones" insofar as they are not stored but are synthesized on demand after an appropriate stimulus and are immediately released and rapidly metabolized.

Prostaglandins have been implicated in numerous physiologic and pathophysiologic processes in every organ of the body. Leukotriene B_4 is the most potent chemotactic factor attracting leukocytes to the site of inflammation, and its release from white cells may represent a control mechanism for the accumulation of inflammatory cells at the point of injury.[19]

Animal experiments have shown that the young are more susceptible to essential fatty acid

---

*Arachidonic acid (gamma-linolenic) is manufactured in the body from linoleic acid.

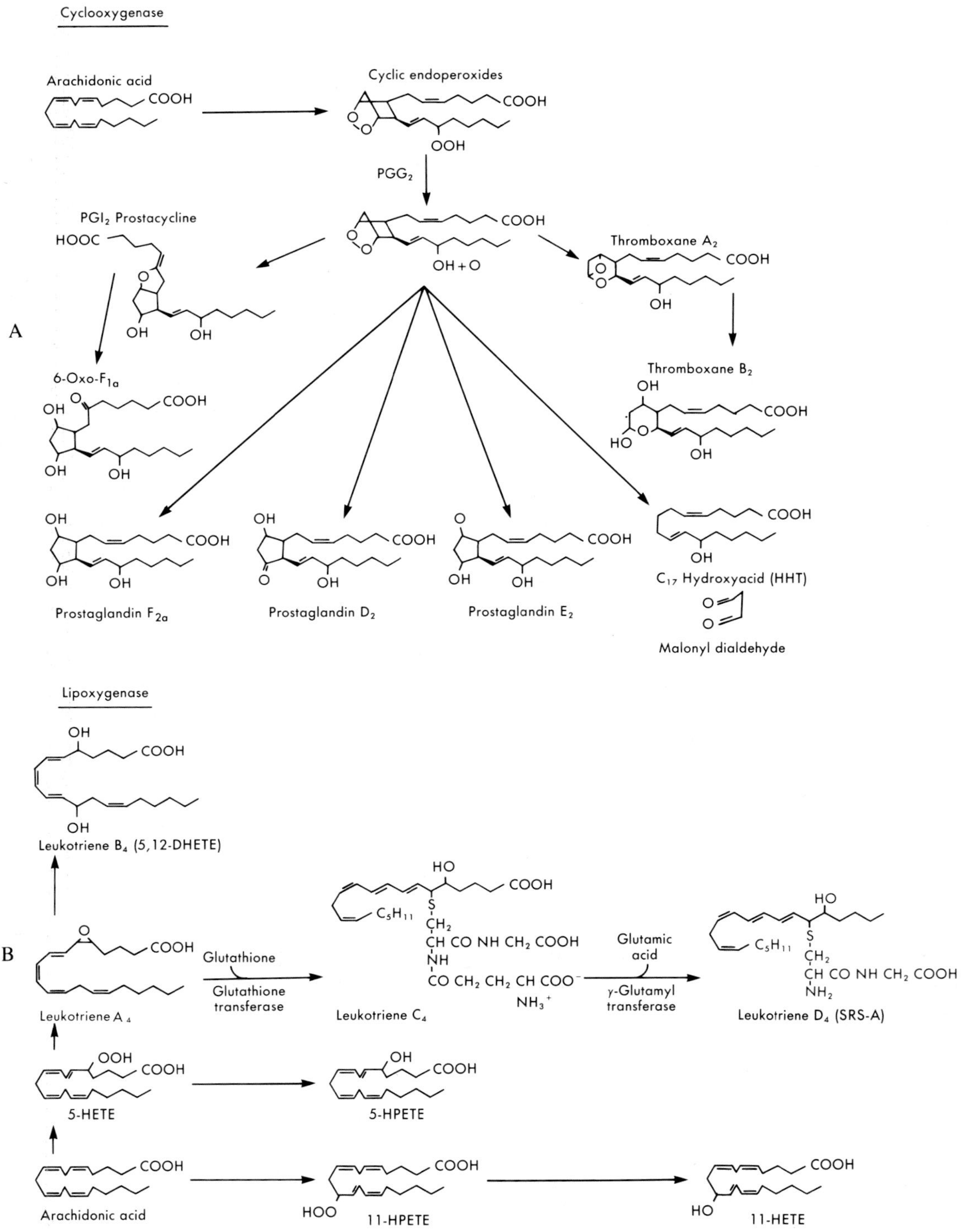

Figure 2-2 Metabolism of arachidonic acid by, **A,** cyclooxygenase and, **B,** lipoxygenase pathways. *6-Oxo-F*$_{1a}$, 6-Oxoprostaglandin F$_{1a}$; *HHT,* hydroxyheptadecatrienoic acid; *SRS-A,* slow-reacting substance of anaphylaxis; *HETE,* hydroxyeicosatetraenoic acid; *DHETE,* dihydroxyeicosatetraenoic acid; *HPETE,* hydroperoxyeicosatetraenoic acid. The 11-HPETE and 11-HETE, the 12- and 15-HPETE, and the 12- and 15-HETE may be formed by similar routes.

From Higgs GA: Proc Nutr Soc **44:**181-187, 1985.

(EFA) deficiency from lack of dietary fat than are adults. Similarly, body stores of EFAs are limited in low–birth-weight human infants, resulting in a deficiency state more rapidly evident in these infants than in adults. In young animals and human infants the EFA deficiency syndrome includes diminished growth, dermatitis, anatomic and degenerative histologic changes in the kidney, lung, fatty liver, impaired water balance, and defects in reproductive performance.

The intake of both *n*-3 and *n*-6 fatty acids has been implicated as a protective factor against coronary artery disease and myocardial infarction. Fish oils are a good source of the 20-carbon *n*-3 fatty acid eicosapentaenoic. Epidemiologic studies[10] have shown that consumption of large amounts of marine fish or fish oils is apparently protective against human coronary morbidity and mortality. Recent work in a swine model fed a high-cholesterol–high-fat diet[11] showed that cod-liver oil reduced luminal encroachment by the atherosclerotic occlusive process in the porcine coronary system; the platelet levels of eicosapentaenoic acid increased, and serum thromboxane decreased, both factors impeding the adherence of platelets to the wall and plaque formation. The natural sources of *n*-3 fatty acids, however, contain such high levels of vitamins A and D (six times the RDA in 30 ml of cod-liver oil) that toxicity may result from their long-term administration.

Fats in foods have a number of desirable qualities in addition to furnishing essential fatty acids: (1) they are concentrated sources of energy substrate; (2) their physical characteristics are responsible for improving the palatability of food for many people; and (3) they act as a source of fat-soluble vitamins. Dairy fats contain significant amounts of vitamins A and D, as do marine oils; vegetable oils are good sources of vitamin E; and a few oils (e.g., red palm) contain substantial amounts of carotenoids (beta-carotene or provitamin A).

Proteins and Amino Acids

For survival and health it is necessary to maintain adequate amounts of protein in the organs and tissues, including a wide variety of structural proteins and functional proteins such as enzymes, transport molecules, and polypeptide hormones. The substrates that form these compounds are the amino acids obtained through digestion of proteins present in foods.

Specifically, the nutritional protein requirement consists of two components: (1) the indispensable (essential) amino acids, which cannot be made by the mammalian organism at rates commensurate with needs, and (2) a source of utilizable nitrogen, usually in the form of the dispensable (nonessential) amino acids.[10] Understanding these nutrition issues begins with an explanation of dietary protein and amino acid metabolism.

Metabolism

Amino acids represent the currency of body protein metabolism (Fig. 2-3). Those that enter the tissue free amino acid pools are (1) incorporated into proteins; (2) catabolized via transamination and oxidative reactions, leading to their elimination from the body as carbon dioxide, water, and nitrogen (principally as urea and ammonia); or (3) converted to other physiologically important compounds, such as nucleic acids, porphyrins, glutathione, and creatine. The continued synthesis and subsequent breakdown

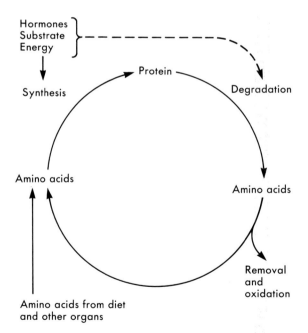

Figure 2-3 Amino acids serve as the currency of body protein metabolism. Tissue and organ proteins undergo constant synthesis and breakdown. Liberated amino acids are either recycled for protein synthesis or catabolized via oxidative metabolism. Diet (substrate and energy) and hormones affect the incorporation of amino acids into proteins and the rate at which proteins are degraded.

of protein within cells and organs enable the body to adapt to internal and/or external environmental alterations. This overall process is usually referred to as protein turnover. The balance between incorporation of amino acids into proteins and their later release via proteolysis will determine the size of the body and the organ protein mass. These rates, in turn, affect the total daily requirements for protein and amino acids.

Classification

Proteins usually consist of 18 amino acids. Approximately half of these can be synthesized by various tissues in the body from carbon and nitrogen precursors. The remainder cannot be synthesized because body tissues lack the necessary enzymatic capacity to promote their formation. These indispensable or essential amino acids must be supplied as part of an adequate diet (Table 2-2). Two amino acids, tyrosine and cystine, are termed semiessential because they can be supplied via the metabolism of phenylalanine and methionine, respectively, when the latter are consumed in adequate amounts. Conversely, when tyrosine and cystine are present in the diet, they can satisfy the requirement for phenylalanine and methionine. Protein nutrition, therefore, is based fundamentally on providing an adequate intake and balance of the essential amino acids and a sufficient source of nitrogen to form the nonessential ones.[3]

Dietary proteins contain essential amino acids in varying concentrations. A high concentration yields a protein value high enough to maintain adequate nutritional status; a relatively low concentration of one or more of the essential amino acids will give the protein a low nutritional quality; for example, wheat gluten contains a low content of lysine. Therefore, the nutritional values of food proteins differ and these values usually are related to the levels of the essential amino acids that the proteins contain. Animal food sources generally yield high-quality proteins whereas plant sources may yield lower-quality protein. However, combining plant proteins that contain low or limiting levels of specific essential amino acids with others that are not limiting in the same amino acids can produce a high-quality plant protein mixture. Thus, mixing corn and beans can yield high nutritional value because the lower lysine content of corn proteins is bal-

Table 2-2 The Common Amino Acids in Human Nutrition

Essential (indispensable)	Semiessential	Nonessential (dispensable)
Leucine		Glycine
Isoleucine		Arginine
Valine		Proline
Lysine		Glutamic acid
Threonine		Aspartic acid
Methionine	Cystine	Serine
Phenylalanine	Tyrosine	Alanine
Tryptophan		
Histidine		

Table 2-3 Estimates of Amino Acid Requirements at Different Ages (mg/kg/da)*

	Infants (3-4 mo)	Children (2 yr)	Schoolboys (10-12 yr)		Adults
Histidine	28	?	?	?	(8-12)
Isoleucine	70	31	30	28	10
Leucine	161	73	45	44	14
Lysine	103	64	60	44	12
Methionine + cystine	58	27	27	22	13
Phenylalanine + tyrosine	125	69	27	22	14
Threonine	87	37	35	28	7
Tryptophan	17	12.5	4	3.3	3.5
Valine	93	38	33	25	10
TOTAL	742	352	261	216	84

From FAO/WHO/UNU: WHO Tech Rep Ser 724, 1985.
*The pattern of essential amino acid requirements in infants differs somewhat from the pattern in human milk, which is richer in sulfur amino acids and tryptophan. The decision to base the scoring pattern for the protein quality of infants' diets on the pattern in human milk will, by comparison with this table, lead to a different estimate. It must be remembered, however, that measurements of the requirements for single amino acids are subject to uncertainty.

anced by the higher lysine concentration in beans. Similarly, the relatively low concentrations of methionine and crystine in beans are improved by the higher level of these sulfur amino acids in corn. From the standpoint of protein nutrition alone, it is not absolutely necessary to include animal protein foods in a diet.

Requirements

The requirements for specific essential amino acids and for total nitrogen (or protein) change with physiologic states and are affected by other factors, including infection, trauma, and disease. During early growth and development, requirements (expressed per unit body weight per day) are high, and they decline with approaching adulthood. Table 2-3 presents a recent assessment produced by an Expert Committee of United Nations organizations[3] of the protein and amino acid requirements of healthy infants, children and adults.

Vitamins

Vitamins are organic compounds required for growth and maintenance of normal cell and organ functions as defined in the box. Their primary function is to promote physiologic processes necessary for life.[12,13] Because they cannot be made by the body in sufficient quantities, they must be supplied by the diet. However, some vitamins, such as biotin and vitamin K, may be synthesized by the intestinal microflora in amounts that meet the body's physiologic requirements.

The basic reason that vitamins are essential constituents of an adequate diet is the lack of the enzymatic machinery necessary to achieve rates of synthesis in accordance with the body's needs.

VITAMINS

An organic compound required in small amounts for complete health and well-being

Not utilized primarily to supply energy or as a source of structural tissue components

Function to promote physiologic processes vital to continued existence

Cannot be synthesized by the organism and must be supplied *de novo*

Deficiency causes a well-defined disease that is prevented or cured by the appropriate vitamin

---

From Young VR, Newberne PM: Cancer **47**:1226-1240, 1981.

An example will emphasize the impact of a species-specific enzyme deficiency and the essential role of vitamins in the human diet. Humans now depend on *dietary* sources for ascorbic acid because the enzyme L-gulonolactone oxidase, which would have catalyzed the last step in the conversion of glucose to ascorbic acid,[13] has been lost through evolution. Therefore it is incorrect to consider that the development of scurvy with continued inadequate ascorbic acid intake is a consequence of a "hereditary metabolic disease" since *all* humans share this genetic lack of ascorbic acid synthesis.[14]

Fourteen vitamins have now been identified in human nutrition. Their common names, generic descriptors, and related compounds are listed in Table 2-4. They are the only compounds currently recognized as being vitamins for humans.

Functions

Vitamins participate in a variety of biochemical and physiologic processes; a brief summary of the major functions is given here (Table 2-5).

The B-complex vitamins serve as *precursors of coenzymes* in many enzyme systems. Each coenzyme is involved in the catalysis of a specific enzyme reaction associated with the metabolism of carbohydrates, lipids, proteins, and/or nucleic acids. For this reason the utilization of energy substrates, the formation of cellular constituents (e.g., proteins), the deposition of energy reserves (carbohydrate, triacylglycerols), and the integrity of the repair and defense mechanisms involve vitamin participation. In addition, a single metabolic pathway, such as that associated with the oxidation of an amino acid, simultaneously may require the active coenzyme forms of many vitamins.

A second function, met by some vitamins, is related to the *expression of genetic information.* Vitamins may affect (1) the synthesis of mRNA and/or its transport to the cytoplasm *(transcription),* (2) the formation of proteins at the *translation* stage of protein synthesis, including involvement of ribosomes, protein factors, and aminoacyl-tRNA, (3) the addition of a prosthetic group to a newly made protein *(post-translation modification),* or (4) a cell surface component that might regulate cell division, differentiation, or function. For example, vitamin D, by its conversion to 1,25-dihydroxycholecalciferol vitamin D_3, induces the transcription

Table 2-4 Generic and Common Names for Vitamins and Related Compounds in Human Nutrition

	Use
Fat-Soluble Vitamins and Related Compounds	
Vitamin A	Beta-ionone derivatives with retinol activity
Provitamin A carotenoids	Carotenoids with beta-carotene activity
Vitamin D	Steroids with cholecalciferol activity
Vitamin E	Tocol and tocotrienol derivatives with activity of alpha-tocopherol
Vitamin K	2-Methyl-1,4-naphthoquinone and derivatives with phylloquinone activity
Water-Soluble Vitamins and Related Compounds	
Folacin	Folic acid and compound with folic acid activity (e.g., THFA)
Niacin	Pyridine-3-carboxylic acid and derivatives with nicotinamide activity
Riboflavin (B_2)	
Thiamine (B_1)	
Vitamin B_6	2-Methylpyridine and derivatives with pyridoxine activity
Vitamin B_{12}	Corrinoids exhibiting cyanocobalamin activity
Vitamin C	Compounds with ascorbic acid activity
Pantothenic acid	
Biotin	

From CAB International: Nutr Abstr Rev **40**:395-400, 1970.

Table 2-5 Major Functions of Vitamins

	Vitamin
Precursor of coenzyme	Biotin
	Nicotinic acid
	Pantothenic acid
	Vitamin B_6
Transmission of genetic information (i.e., transcription, posttranslation)	Vitamin A
	Vitamin K
	Vitamin D
Antioxidant and electron transport	Vitamin E
	Vitamin C
"Specialized" properties	
Photosensitive reactions	Vitamin A
Neural transmission	Thiamine
Macromolecular structure	Vitamin B_6

of specific mRNAs that code for the synthesis of proteins responsible for calcium transport*; vitamin K participates in the posttranslation modification of prothrombin precursors, involving carboxylation of glutamate residues, with the

formation of active prothrombin*; and vitamin A induces the differentiation of epithelial cells.

Vitamins E and C carry out *antioxidant or electron transport* functions. Antioxidants are reducing substances that help maintain a low oxidation-reduction potential in tissues. Cellular lipids are protected from free-radical attack, and vitamin E interferes with the chain reactions by which these reactive molecular species multiply. In relation to normal physiology, vitamin C's main electron transfer role is the reduction of metals so the associated enzyme system can act in the transport of molecular oxygen (e.g., in the hydroxylation of proline during collagen synthesis and in formation of the catecholamine noradrenaline).

Finally, a number of vitamins perform *specialized* functions that cannot be grouped into one of the major categories in Table 2-5. For example, vitamin A is associated with the formation of rhodopsin, the light-sensitive pigment of the retina. A role for thiamine triphosphate in

---

*It has also been shown [16] that skeletal muscle is a target organ for vitamin D, whose effect may be mediated at the genome level (i.e., in transcription or translation) or at the membrane level.

*In fact, this carboxylation reaction is more universal than was previously thought, with other interactive proteins being formed through the action of vitamin K. The bone matrix protein, osteocalcin, is an example of a molecule modified by the action of this vitamin. [17]

nerve excitation has been proposed. It also is possible that pyridoxal phosphate modulates the binding of receptor-steroid complexes to cell nuclei.

Thus it is clear that vitamins play vital roles in cellular metabolism and in the maintenance of physiologic processes; and for these reasons, deficiencies or excesses can lead to changes in the status of the immune, detoxification, protective, repair, and differentiation systems of body cells and organs.

Vitamin-like Substances

The concept of "vitamin" for human nutrition is that of a substance *indispensable* for the function of the body, and *not synthesized* in the body. For our true vitamin needs we are therefore dependent on exogenous (dietary) sources. Three substances—taurine, carnitine, and choline—can be classified as "vitamin like." They differ from the 13 "true" vitamins insofar as the human body is genetically capable of their biosynthesis. They are similar to vitamins in that for each of them endogenous synthesis may not meet the full demand and a complementary, exogenous, dietary source may be needed for normal nutriture. Stated another way, diets severely restricted in any of these three items may load to a state of deficiency, despite maximal operation of the biosynthetic process.

Taurine. Taurine (beta-amino-ethanesulfonic acid) is an analogue of beta-alanine in which a sulfonic acid group replaces the carboxyl group. Its biochemical and nutritional features have recently been reviewed.[18-20] It plays a role (along with glycine) as a conjugator of bile acids, but it is also present in most cells.[18] Its biochemical action is not fully understood, although in the central nervous system and retina it is thought to stabilize neural membranes.

Cow's milk is low in taurine, but human colostrum and early mature milk are rich in this amino acid. It is absent in plant foods and abundant in flesh foods, especially shellfish.

In human metabolism the precursors of taurine are methionine and cysteine. The enzyme cysteinesulfinic acid–decarboxylase is the key regulatory step in its biosynthesis.

Reduced levels of circulating taurine and decreased renal excretion of the acid have been seen in babies fed taurine-free formulas[21] and in patients undergoing total parenteral nutrition (TPN).[22] In cats and primates retinal damage has been ascribed to dietary restriction.[19] In patients receiving taurine-free TPN, plasma levels decline and retinal function abnormalities are detectable.[22] Stress and disease may increase demand, and therefore these states require a greater external (dietary) supply; as such, taurine can be classified as a "conditionally essential" nutrient.[23]

Carnitine. Carnitine (beta-hydroxy-gamma-N-trimethylammonium butyrate) is an organic acid vital to human energy metabolism. Reviews of its metabolism and physiologic roles have recently been published.[24,25] Its principal role is in the transport of long-chain fatty acids from the cytoplasm across the mitochondrial membrane for their intramitochondrial oxidation. The carnitine content of a given cell type is related to the cell's optimum rate of long-chain fatty acid oxidation.[24]

Preformed carnitine is contained in foods of animal-flesh origin. In human metabolism the ultimate precursors are methionine and lysine. The endogenous synthesis of carnitine begins with the trimethylation of peptide-linked lysine in the liver and kidney. Since both methionine and lysine are essential amino acids, two that are often the *limiting* amino acids in cereal-based human diets, a derivative risk of reduced precursor availability is presented.

In states of metabolic stress a greater proportion of energy is derived from fat. For example, in liver cirrhosis, renal dialysis, and organic acidurias, carnitine becomes a conditionally essential nutrient.[26] In newborns the sudden release of fatty acids is not met by a release of ketones, suggesting that the neonatal liver is not fully mature in its fatty acid–oxidizing capacity. Hahn and Novak[27] argue that this is related to immaturity of carnitine metabolism; the problem is exaggerated in premature infants and infants fed a soybean-based formula.

Choline. Choline (trimethyl-beta-hydroxyethylammonium hydroxide) is a biologically important quaternary amine. Its primary role is in the synthesis of the cholinergic neurotransmitter, acetylcholine, in central and peripheral nervous tissue. It is also a component of membrane phospholipids (e.g., phosphatidylcholine) in pulmonary surfactant and of sphyngomyelin in neuronal axons.[30] Choline deficiency in animals is characterized by fatty liver.

Breast milk has a substantial amount of choline, as does cow's milk and infant formula.[30] Adult humans ingest between 300 and 1000 mg of choline per day,[31] largely in the form of phosphatidylcholine (lecithin). Liver, eggs, and legumes are rich in this compound.

New choline can be formed in the liver and other tissues of mammals. The synthetic reaction is catalyzed by the enzyme phosphatidylethanolamine-methyltransferase (PEMT).[32] In the absence of endogenous intake of choline, the synthetic process cannot meet the metabolic demand, especially if stores are depleted. Evidence from observations in malnourished patients receiving TPN suggests that choline, too, for humans is a conditionally essential nutrient.

Utilization

The supply of vitamins available to the body's cells and organs depends on, in addition to dietary content, the cooperative action of various physiologic processes, including digestion, absorption, inter- and intracellular transport, activation and/or conversion to active forms, and, finally, degradation and elimination via excretory pathways. These processes are regulated by complex mechanisms that involve both the nervous and the endocrine system. Furthermore, the major methods of vitamin utilization are integrated at the whole-body level to minimize any toxic accumulation when vitamin ingestion exceeds physiologic needs or to help conserve body stores when vitamin intake is deficient. Finally, the conversion of some of the vitamins to their active forms is specifically organ dependent. Vitamin D provides an example of this,[31] as shown in Fig. 2-4. Hence, an adequate vitamin D status depends on the coordinated activities of two organs, the liver and kidney, and is affected by several hormones[32] and by the concentration of phosphate ions in the kidney cells.

Many factors may affect nutrient utilization and requirements[32] (Table 2-6), and these change with the age and health status of the adult. Interaction between the coenzyme form of a vitamin and its apoenzyme, for example, depends on the surface and spatial configuration of the apoenzyme. Therefore it would be of interest to know whether age-dependent molecular changes in apoenzymes can lead to changes in the normal steric relationship between the coenzyme form of a vitamin and its apoenzyme. Although this topic has received only limited investigation, molecular changes in enzymes have been studied

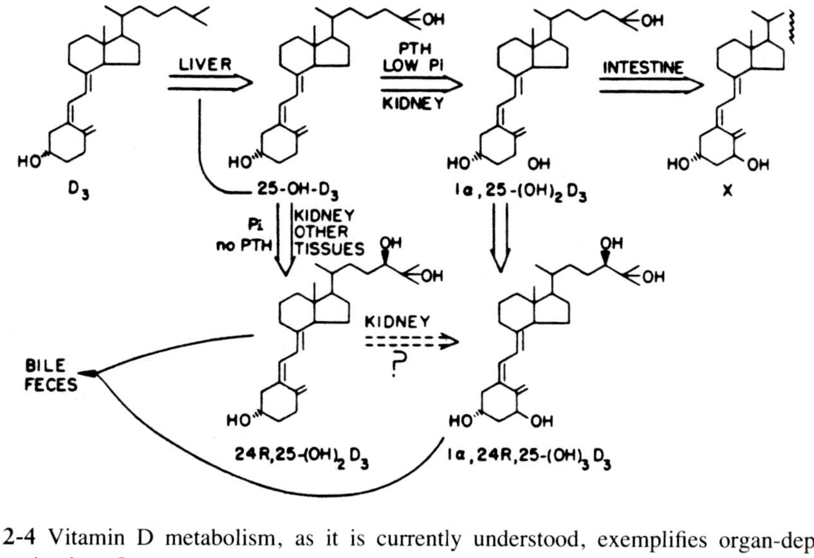

Figure 2-4 Vitamin D metabolism, as it is currently understood, exemplifies organ-dependent vitamin activation. Open arrows represent the major known reactions; dotted arrows show reactions that are probably not physiologically significant. Wording over the arrows represents the site and/or regulators of conversion. *PTH,* Parathyroid hormone.

From DeLuca H: In Alfin-Slater RB, Kritchevsky D, editors: Nutrition and the adult: micronutrients, New York, 1980, Plenum Press Inc, pp 205-244.

Table 2-6 Factors that May Affect
Nutrient Utilization and Requirements

	Affected Function
Chemical form in diet Components and composition of diet Absorption digestion Cellular and intracellular transport Conversion to metabolically active form	Delivery to cells and organs
Renal clearance Intestinal secretion and elimination Oxidation and metabolism Chemical or drug inactivation	Loss of nutrients
Size and activity of organs Binding to enzymes	Cellular activity

Modified from Brown RR: J Agric Food Chem **20**:498-505, 1972.

as a basis for a number of vitamin-dependent disease states.[33]

The absorption of many vitamins from the gastrointestinal tract occurs via active and regulated processes. The subsequent movement of vitamins through the circulatory system also may involve participation of specific transport proteins. The influence of physiologic and pathologic factors on vitamin absorption and metabolism, however, has not been studied extensively. For example, the absorption and fate of the various dietary forms of folacin during the aging process remain unexplored in spite of the conclusion that folate deficiency is widespread in some populations of elderly people.

Minerals

There are more than 25 minerals and trace minerals important to the body's nutrition and health. Nineteen of these are essential nutrients, ranging in amounts from calcium (at 1200 g in the 70 kg adult man) to selenium and chromium (less than 10 mg in an adult man). The human body also contains trace amounts of elements that are either neutral (rhodium) or potentially toxic (cadmium, mercury, arsenic) and their biologic effects.

In humans the elemental nutrients act in four ways: (1) as structural components, (2) as charged ions, (3) as components of metalloen-

zymes, and (4) as miscellaneous effectors in small molecules. Calcium and phosphorus combine to form the crystalline elements of skeletal and dental structures. Substantial proportions of the body's magnesium and zinc are incorporated into bones, but their physiologic roles in this context are not well understood.

Sodium, potassium, and chloride represent the major, charged, soluble elements (electrolytes) involved in electrochemical neutrality. Calcium and magnesium also play important roles as charged ions in the extracellular space, in muscular contraction, and in neuromuscular conduction. Magnesium and probably manganese are cofactors in a number of carboxylation reactions involving thiamine pyrophosphate (TPP) in intermediary energy metabolism.

Certain trace elements[35] (Table 2-7) are indispensable components of metalloproteins and metalloenzymes: hemoglobin (iron), alkaline phosphate (zinc), ceruloplasmin (copper), glutathione peroxidase (selenium), pyruvate carboxylase (manganese), and xanthine oxidase (molybdenum). Other trace elements are found in various small molecules: vitamin B_{12} (cobalt) and thyroxine/triiodothyronine (iodine). Others function as a soluble complex (chromium).

The minerals and trace elements are so ubiquitous in nature that the likelihood of their being deficient in humans was at one time considered remote. However, the total daily consumption of food has declined significantly in individual societies as the population assumed more sedentary activity patterns. Furthermore, the density of certain nutrients in some foods is so low that contemporary intakes of total calories may be insufficient to provide the recommended allowances.

The zinc content of a mixed diet in the United States, for example, is about 3 mg/1000 kcal.[36] An adult would have to consume 5000 kcal to ingest 15 mg of zinc as specified by the RDA.[37] Moreover, some dietary forms of nutrients are poorly absorbed and a nutrient's biologic availability varies according to its source. For example, calcium is highly absorbable from milk and most dairy products but may be poorly absorbed from spinach, where it forms a complex with oxalic acid. Muscle meats and blood are good sources of available iron, but iron from vegetable sources is less well absorbed. Similarly, phosphorus is absorbed more efficiently

Table 2-7 Classification of the Essential Trace Elements

Element	Function	Deficiency Signs		Occurrences of Imbalances
		Animals	Humans	
Fluorine	Structure of teeth, possibly of bones, possible growth effect	Caries, possibly growth depression	Increased incidence of caries, possible risk factor of osteoporosis	Deficiency and excess known
Silicon	Calcification, possible function in connective tissue	Growth depression, bone deformities	Not known	Not known
Vanadium	Not known	Growth depression, change of lipid metabolism, impairment of reproduction	Not known	Not known
Chromium	Potentiation of insulin	Relative insulin resistance	Relative insulin resistance, impaired glucose tolerance, elevated serum lipids.	Deficiency known in malnutrition, aging, total parenteral alimentation
Manganese	Mucopolysaccharide metabolism, superoxide dismutase	Growth depression, bone deformities, beta-cell degeneration	Not known	Deficiency not known, toxicity by inhalation
Iron	Oxygen, electron transport	Anemia, growth retardation	Anemia	Deficiencies widespread, excesses dangerous in hemochromatosis, acute poisoning
Cobalt	As part of vitamin B_{12}	Anemia, growth retardation in ruminant species	Only as vitamin B_{12} deficiency	Inability to absorb vitamin B_{12}, low B_{12} intake from vegetarian diets
Nickel	Interaction with iron absorption	Growth depression, anemia, ultrastructural changes in liver, impairment of reproduction	Not known	Not known
Copper	Oxidative enzymes, interaction with iron, cross-linking of elastin	Anemia, rupture of large vessels, disturbances of ossification	Anemia, changes of ossification; possibly elevated serum cholesterol	Deficiencies in malnutrition, total parenteral alimentation
Zinc	Numerous enzymes involved in energy metabolism and in transcription and translation	Failure to eat, severe growth depression, skin lesions, sexual immaturity	Growth depression, sexual immaturity skin lesions, depression of immunocompetence, change of taste acuity	Deficiencies in Iran, Egypt, and in total parenteral nutrition, genetic diseases, traumatic stress
Arsenic	Not known	Impairment of growth and reproduction, sudden heart death in third-generation lactating goats	Not known	Not known
Selenium	Glutathione peroxidase, interaction with heavy metals	Different depending on species: muscle degeneration (ruminants), pancreatic atrophy (chicken)	Endemic cardiomyopathy (Keshan disease)	Deficiency and excess in areas of China, cases resulting from total parenteral alimentation

From Mertz W: *Science* **213**:1332-1338, 1981.

Table 2-7 Classification of the Essential Trace Elements—cont'd

Element	Function	Deficiency Signs		Occurrences of Imbalances
		Animals	Humans	
Molybdenum	Xanthine, aldehyde oxidases	Difficult to produce, growth depression	Signs not known	Excessive exposure in parts of Soviet Union associated with goutlike syndrome
Iodine	Constituent of thyroid hormones	Goiter, depression of thyroid function	Goiter, depression of thyroid, cretinism	Deficiencies widespread, excessive intakes may lead to thyrotoxicoses

from meat and milk than it is when present as a component of phytic acid.

Elemental nutrients are important in fulfilling the body's requirements for growth and maintenance. However, the dietary levels of certain elements may influence health in other ways. Excessive sodium intake is associated with hypertension,[38] and various levels of fluorine in the diet and environment can influence the dental health of a community.[39] The content of calcium and magnesium in the water supply has been associated with increased incidence of cardiovascular disease,[40] as has the dietary intake of chromium.[41] Furthermore, it has been suggested[42] that the dietary ratio of zinc to copper may influence cholesterol concentrations and atherogenesis, with high zinc:copper ratios being detrimental. Seleniferous soils are associated with lower rates of certain malignancies in humans.[43] The evidence for all the aforementioned associations is of variable conclusiveness, but suggestive enough to warrant more detailed scientific evaluations.

WATER, ELECTROLYTES, AND ACID/BASE BALANCE

Called the "silent nutrient," water is taken for granted in most nutritional considerations. A deficient intake, however, can produce death more rapidly than that of any other nutrient. Normally water constitutes about 60% of the body weight, but the proportion may vary depending on body composition. Lean body tissues are approximately 75% water, yet adipose tissue is nearly anhydrous; thus the percentage of total body weight contributed by water is greater in lean than in obese individuals.

The body has three sources of water: beverages, food, and the metabolism of carbohydrates, lipids, and proteins. In adults the provision of water from these sources generally oscillates from 2 to 4 liters/day. During earliest historic times humans had basically four dietary sources of water: pure water, the juice of berries and fruits, the blood and body fluids of animals, and breast milk. The subsequent domestication of dairy animals, fermentation of fruits and grains, and improved processes of distribution and marketing have made liquids more freely available for consumption. Water, along with the other major classes of nutrients, is essential for growth, maintenance, and health.

To sustain an equilibrium of liquids, the losses of water (via urine, feces, sweat, menstrual bleeding, semen, and expired air) should equal the intake and endogenous formation of water (i.e., 2 to 4 liters/da). However, the body turns over from two to four times this amount. Plasma volume accounts for approximately 3.5 liters, saliva formation about 1.5 liters, and daily intestinal, biliary, and pancreatic secretions about 4 liters.

Water balance is controlled sensitively by the physiologic mechanisms of thirst that regulate a human's water intake when there is free access to liquid.[44] With normal posterior pituitary and renal function, however, the kidney can regulate the plasma volume by either conserving or excreting water as required. A starvation or carbohydrate-restriction regimen is associated with an acute loss of body water (1 to 1.5 liters), which represents the water normally held by glycogen storage in the tissues.

The concentration of hydrogen ions in extracellular fluid must be regulated within a narrow range (pH 7.35-7.45) to ensure normal health. Two mechanisms regulate the blood pH. (1) As dissolved CO_2 produces a weak acid (carbonic), which increases hydrogen ion concentration, respiratory excretion of the CO_2 reduces it. (2) A more potent regulator is the renal tubule, which excretes excess basic or acidic products formed in metabolism or absorbed by the body. In addition to these two mechanisms, the blood contains three buffering systems based on the plasma concentrations of bicarbonate, phosphate, and protein. Thus the maintenance of a constant volume of fluid in the extracellular space, of an appropriate blood pH, and of the normal hydration of cells is an essential component of nutritional health.

NUTRIENT INTERACTIONS

The metabolism of individual nutrients can be affected by the intake of other nutrients. For example, the efficiency with which dietary protein is utilized to meet protein needs is influenced by the level of energy intake.[45] The rate at which the body's vitamin B_6 stores are utilized is increased by high protein intakes.[46] The utilization of copper appears to be affected by the level of zinc intake.[47] It follows, then, that nutrient metabolism is a function of a complex set of interacting factors that determine the dietary intakes of the individual nutrients necessary to maintain adequate nutritional status.

Nutrients are important regulators of metabolism itself. Deficiencies or excesses can bring about profound changes in the biochemical activities of cells. For example, a zinc deficiency in a pregnant woman may lead to the development of teratogenic abnormalities,[48] possibly by influencing the processes involved in cell division and subsequent development. A vitamin B_6 deficiency may impair the normal functioning of the body's immune mechanisms, perhaps through an alteration in nucleic acid metabolism that affects enzyme reactions associated with amino acid interconversions and metabolism.[49] Metabolism is responsive not only to inadequate or excessive intakes of specific nutrients but also to the timing of nutrient intake. Indeed, many of the diurnal rhythms of metabolism are generated by the feeding and fasting cycles that characterize the nutritional behavior of both animals and humans.

PRINCIPLES FOR ESTIMATING DIETARY REQUIREMENTS
Dietary Method

The sequence of events incurred with the progressive development of a nutritional deficiency as a result of all factors (Fig. 2-5) forms the basis for determining human requirements for specific nutrients. One approach uses a diet survey to determine the nutrient intake of individual members in adequately nourished populations. This intake estimate then is compared to intake data obtained from individual members in populations with a nutrient deficiency. The method gives an estimate of the approximate range of nutrient intake that is associated with health maintenance; however, it is not an exact method for estimating minimum requirements for a nutrient and it is difficult to determine precisely the nutrient intake level by populations of free-living humans. Agent, host, and environmental factors must also be considered in estimating minimum nutrient requirements.

Metabolic Method

If, however, the amount of a nutrient in the diet is low or its availability interfered with, and if this diet continues, then biochemical and pathologic changes will develop eventually. These changes may include altered activities of blood enzymes or lower levels of excretion of the nutrient, or its metabolites, in the urine. Because some of these changes can be measured readily, they provide a basis for the design of metabolic studies conducted to determine minimum requirements for essential nutrients in humans. In these metabolic studies, volunteers receive experimental diets in which the level of a particular nutrient is altered during a specific diet period. In this way the researchers can determine the minimum intake level of that nutrient necessary to meet a given criterion, such as the maintenance of a normal blood level, rate of excretion in urine, or in some cases the amount sufficient to prevent symptoms of deficiency. For example, Table 2-8 presents results obtained in experiments using various criteria to estimate the thiamine requirements in adult subjects; there is general agreement in the requirement estimations obtained. However, the choice of different criteria may result in wide differences in a requirement value as noted in assessing vitamin A requirements in laboratory animals.[11]

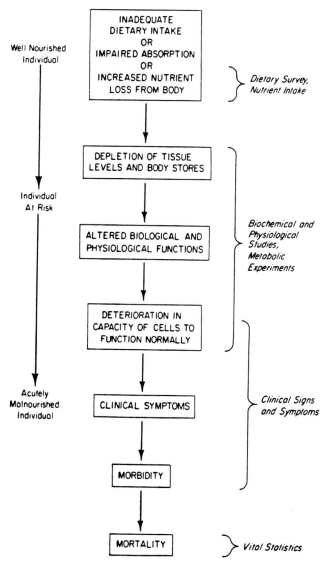

Figure 2-5 Major stages in the development of nutritional deficiency disease. First, a nutrient is not available or is available only in amounts that are inadequate for body cells and organs. Various factors can be the cause of the inadequacy, including both low dietary intake and relatively high rates of bodily loss. Then, biochemical deterioration occurs, with the appearance of clinical symptoms. Knowledge of these phases aids in designing different approaches that may be used to assess human nutrient requirements.

Table 2-8 Estimates of the Minimum Thiamine Requirement in an Adult Man

Criteria	Mean Requirement (mg/1000 kcal)
Clinical deficiency[16]	0.18
Urinary B₁ clearance[17]	0.35
Comprehensive[18]	0.23
Carbohydrate metabolism index, comprehensive[19]	0.18
Erythrocyte transketolase activity, urinary excretion[20]	0.3

Although the metabolic study approach is a more precise method than the dietary method, experiments with humans are often laborious, time-consuming, and expensive. Furthermore, they may involve monotonous experimental diets and may impose restrictions on volunteers, making it difficult for them to be followed for extended periods. For this reason such studies are frequently of short duration and usually involve small population groups. Therefore the data obtained may not be extrapolated easily for general application to large free-living populations. Nevertheless, this method has been used extensively to determine nutrient requirements in humans.

Experimental Extrapolation

For some nutrients it has not been possible to utilize human studies. In such cases it may be necessary to rely on the extrapolation of data obtained in animal experiments or in epidemiologic studies. The accuracy and precision of the various methods for estimating human requirements are usually not known. Rarely are repeat studies conducted within the same member or population to determine the reproducibility of a given nutrient's estimated requirement, and rarely are studies repeated over an extended time.

INTERNATIONAL STANDARDS OF INTAKE FOR PROTEIN AND ENERGY

A joint expert consultation panel met in 1981 in Rome to update the international standards of intake for protein and energy intake. This process had not been undertaken since the emission of a protein and energy intake recommendation in 1973. United Nation units, including the Food and Agriculture Organization (Rome), the World Health Organization (Geneva), and the United Nations University (Tokyo), participated in the drafting of the document.[3] They adopted aspects of the aforementioned principles for estimating requirements and applied new procedures to the determination of recommendations for individuals and populations.

Estimation of Energy Requirements

As is true of all nutrients, for which safe minimum levels on a group basis are established by age, sex, and physiologic status, the daily requirements of energy can be determined only on an individual basis. This is due to the fact that both a chronic excess and a chronic deficit of total dietary energy can produce progressive and undesirable changes in body composition. Thus, energy nutriture is a truly individual issue, and the FAO/WHO/UNU committee[3] has provided a method to estimate a given person's energy needs based on a factorial sum of basal energy requirements and physical activity. First, for adults, an estimation of basal metabolic rate (BMR) is made in relation to weight and height. (A nomogram exists to estimate BMR from these two anthropometric indices.) Then, a factor is added for the level of habitual activity. Totally sedentary activities during waking hours would result in an addition of about 40% above basal requirements. Thus one would apply a factor of 1.4 BMR for such a person according to the FAO/WHO/UNU scheme. For light activity the factor would be 1.6 BMR, for moderate activity 1.8 BMR, for heavy activity 2.0 BMR, and for very heavy activity 2.2 BMR. A detailed analysis of specific activities over the course of the waking day can lead to a more refined estimate for a given individual.

Estimation of Protein Requirements

Because there is a loss of tissue from the body (skin, hair, nails, intestinal cells), and there is excretion in the urine of nitrogen liberated as creatinine from muscle breakdown and as urea from the oxidation of amino acids, it is necessary to replace body protein daily with exogenous building blocks in the form of amino acids from the diet. In infancy and childhood, and during pregnancy, there is tissue growth that requires much more than a steady-state balance of nitrogen gained from and lost to the environment. Similarly, in lactation, nitrogen is lost in the secretion of breast milk. The deliberations of the FAO/WHO/UNU joint panel established average values per kilogram of body weight for populations up to 18 years of age. In the first 6 months the safe level of protein to be consumed is 1.86 g/kg. At age 17, girls require 0.80 g/kg and boys 0.86 g/kg. For adults of all ages and both sexes, the safe intake level is universal, 0.75 g/kg per day. Thus a 70 kg adult man would require 52.5 g of good-quality protein daily, and a 55 kg adult woman 41 g. If the protein is not of the highest quality, corrections for less complete utilization are included.[3]

DIETARY STANDARDS FOR THE UNITED STATES (the Recommended Dietary Allowances)

In the United States a distinct process has been undertaken to establish the levels of nutrients to be included in a nutritionally adequate diet. Determining the mean requirement for a nutrient in a population group provides a basis for developing a recommended dietary allowance (RDA). The steps are (1) to determine the mean requirement and degree of variability in the group, (2) to increase the average requirement by an amount sufficient to cover the needs of nearly all members of the group, (3) to increase the allowance for inefficient utilization of nutrients

consumed, and (4) to judiciously interpret and extrapolate the allowances when data are limited. It follows that, in addition to estimating the mean requirement for a nutrient in a given age and sex group, one must determine the extent to which requirements vary among apparently similar members within that population. Based on this estimate, the RDA will cover the needs of nearly all healthy subjects within the population but will actually exceed the requirements for most members so the few with extraordinary or demanding conditions are covered.

This task, embodying these operational principles, has been undertaken periodically by a committee of experts convened by the Food and Nutrition Board of the National Research Council. The most recent, ninth, edition of *Recommended Dietary Allowances* was published in 1980, based on deliberations concluded nearly a decade earlier. (A committee was formed to produce the tenth edition, to have been published in 1985, but scientific and policy differences led to the cancellation of its release.) The ninth edition committee felt that sufficient information was available to establish formal RDAs for 17 nutrients (Table 2-9). For an additional three vitamins and nine elemental nutrients, however, it

Table 2-9 Recommended Dietary Allowances

Nutrient	Young Adult (19-22 yr)		Mature Adult (51 + yr)	
	Male	Female	Male	Female
Energy (kcal/da)	2500-3300	1700-2500	2000-2800	1400-2200
Protein (g/da)	56	44	56	44
Vitamins				
A (μg RE)	1000	800	1000	800
D (μg)	7.5	7.5	5	5
E (mg α-TE)	10	8	10	8
C (mg)	60	60	60	60
Thiamine (mg)	1.5	1.1	1.2	1.0
Riboflavin (mg)	1.7	1.3	1.4	1.2
Niacin (mg)	19	14	16	13
B_6 (mg)	2.2	2.0	2.2	2.0
Folacin (μg)	400	400	400	400
B_{12} (μg)	3	3	3	3
Minerals				
Calcium (mg)	800	800	800	800
Phosphorous (mg)	800	800	800	800
Magnesium (mg)	350	300	350	300
Iron (mg)	10	18	10	10
Zinc (mg)	15	15	15	15
Iodine (μg)	150	150	150	150

From Committee on Dietary Allowances, Food and Nutrition Board, National Research Council: Recommended dietary allowances, ed 9, Washington DC, 1980, National Academy of Sciences.

Table 2-10 Estimated SADDIs (in mg)
of Selected Vitamins and Minerals

Vitamins	
Vitamin K	70-140*
Biotin	100-200*
Pantothenic acid	4-7
Trace elements	
Copper	2.0-3.0
Manganese	2.5-5.0
Fluoride	1.5-4.0
Chromium	0.05-0.2
Selenium	0.05-0.2
Molybdenum	0.15-0.5
Electrolytes	
Sodium	1100-3300
Potassium	1875-5625
Chloride	1700-5100

Abstracted from Committee on Dietary Allowances, Food and
Nutrition Board, National Research Council: Recommended
dietary allowances, ed 9, Washington DC, 1980, National Academy of Sciences.
*Measured in micrograms.

found insufficient data to establish precise intake
recommendations, so it established "safe and adequate daily dietary intakes" (SADDIs), expressed as a minimum-maximum range of values
(Table 2-10).

The RDAs represent allowances for healthy
people; they are not intended to be therapeutic
levels, although if followed they should prevent
the development of nutritional deficiency disease
and should maintain nutritional status in most
healthy individuals. A diet based on a wide selection of foods will likely ensure nutrient intakes that equal or exceed these allowances; but
supplements of vitamins, iron, and trace minerals that furnish levels approximately equivalent
to the RDAs may be considered as "insurance"
against the possible development of deficiencies
arising from a poorly selected diet. Nutrient intakes that are considerably in excess of these
allowances cannot be recommended as a broad
public health policy. The estimates in the ninth
edition of *Recommended Dietary Allowances* are
somewhat outdated, and new values are needed.
Moreover, the energy and protein recommendations have largely been superceded by those
of the FAO/WHO/UNU Joint Committee.[3]

REFERENCES

1. Newsholme EA: Carbohydrate metabolism in vivo: regulation of blood glucose level, Clin Endocrinol Metab **5**:543-
   578, 1976.
2. Cahill GF Jr: Starvation in man, Clin Endocrinol Metab
   5:397-415, 1976.
3. FAO/WHO/UNU. Energy and protein requirements: report of a Joint FAO/WHO/UNU Expert Consultation,
   WHO Tech Rep Ser 724, 1985.
4. Bray GA: Energy requirements of the aged. In Hawkins
   WW, editor: Nutrition of the aged. Quebec, 1978, Nutrition
   Society of Canada.
5. Shock NW: Energy metabolism, caloric intake, and physical activity in aging. In Carlson LA, editor: Nutrition in
   old age, Uppsala, 1972, Swedish Nutrition Foundation, pp
   12-21.
6. Cohen AM: Metabolic responses to dietary carbohydrates:
   interactions of dietary and hereditary factors, Prog Biochem
   Pharmacol **21**:74-103, 1986.
7. Food and Agricultural Organization: Dietary fats and oils
   in human nutrition. FAO Food and Nutrition Paper 3,
   Rome, 1977, FAO.
8. Raper NR, Marston RM: Levels and sources of fat in the
   U.S. food supply, Prog Clin Biol Res **222**:127-152, 1986.
9. Higgs GA: The effects of dietary intake of essential fatty
   acids on prostaglandin and leukotriene synthesis, Proc Nutr
   Soc **44**:181-187, 1985.
10. Kromhout D, et al: The inverse relation between fish con-
    sumption and 20-year mortality from coronary heart dis-
    ease, N Engl J Med **312**:1205-1209, 1985.
11. Weiner BH, et al: Inhibition of atherosclerosis by cod-liver
    oil in hyperlipidemic swine model, N Engl J Med **315**:841-
    846, 1986.
12. Young VR, Scrimshaw NS: Nutritional evaluation of pro-
    teins and protein requirements. In Milner M, et al, editors:
    Protein resources and technology: status and research
    needs, Westport Conn, 1978, AVI Publishing Co Inc, pp
    136-173.
13. Young VR, Newberne PM: Vitamins and cancer preven-
    tion: issues and dilemmas, Cancer **47**:1226-1240, 1981.
14. Reference deleted in proofs.
15. CAB International: Tentative rules for generic description
    and trivial names of vitamins and related compounds, Nutr
    Abstr Rev **40**:395-400, 1970.
16. Boland R: Role of vitamin D in skeletal muscle function,
    Endocr Rev **7**:434-448, 1986.
17. Hauschka PV: Osteocalcin: the vitamin K–dependent
    Ca^{+2}-binding protein of bone matrix, Haemostasis **16**:258-
    272, 1986.
18. Chesney R: Taurine: its biological role and clinical impli-
    cations, Adv Pediatr **32**:1-42, 1985.
19. Hayes KC: Taurine requirements in primates, Nutr Rev
    43:65-70, 1985.
20. Write CE: Taurine: biological update, Ann Rev Biochem
    55:427-453, 1986.
21. Okamoto E, et al: Role of taurine in feeding the low–birth-
    weight infant, J Pediatr **104**:936-940, 1984.
22. Vinton NE, et al: Visual function in patients undergoing
    home TPN, Am J Clin Nutr **45**:598, 1985.

23. Rudman D, Williams PJ: Nutritional deficiency during total parenteral nutrition, Nutr Rev **43**:1-13, 1985.

24. Bremer J: Carnitine-metabolism and function, Physiol Rev **63**:1420-1480, 1983.

25. Rebouche CJ, Paulson DJ: Carnitine metabolism and function in humans, Annu Rev Nutr **6**:41-66, 1986.

26. Borum P, Bennett SG: Carnitine as an essential nutrient, J Am Coll Nutr **5**:177-182, 1986.

27. Hahn P, Novak M: How important are carnitine and ketones for the newborn infant? Fed Proc **44**:2369-2373, 1985.

28. Sheard NF, Zeisel SH: Choline: an essential dietary nutrient? Nutrition. (In press.)

29. Wurtman J: Sources of choline and lecithin in the diet. In Wurtman RJ, Wurtman J, editors: Nutrition and the brain, vol 5, New York, 1979, Raven Press, p 73.

30. Schneider WJ, Vance DE: Conversion of phosphatidyl-ethanolamine to phosphatidylcholine in the rat liver, J Biol Chem **254**:3886-3891, 1979.

31. DeLuca H: Vitamin D. In Alfin-Slater RB, Kritchevsky D, editors: Nutrition and the adult: micronutrients, New York, 1980, Plenum Press Inc, pp 205-244.

32. Christakos S, Norman AW: Interaction of the vitamin D endocrine system with other hormones, Miner Electrolyte Metab **1**:231-239, 1978.

33. Elsas L, McCormick DB: Genetic defects in vitamin utilization. I. General aspects and fat soluble vitamins, Vitam Horm **43**:103-144, 1986.

34. Brown RR: Normal and pathological conditions which may alter the human requirement for vitamin B_6, J Agric Food Chem **20**:498-505, 1972.

35. Mertz W: The essential trace elements, Science **213**:1332-1338, 1981.

36. Solomons NW: Recent progress in zinc nutrition research. In Weininger J, Briggs GM, editors: Nutrition uptakes, New York, 1982, John Wiley & Sons Inc.

37. Committee on Dietary Allowances, Food and Nutrition Board, National Research Council: Recommended dietary allowances, ed 9, Washington DC, 1980, National Academy of Sciences.

38. Dahl LW: Salt and hypertension, Am J Clin Nutr **25**:231-244, 1972.

39. Ast DB, et al: Newburgh-Kingston caries fluorine study. XIV. Combined clinical and roentgenographic dental findings after ten years of fluoride experience, J Am Dent Assoc **52**:314-325, 1956.

40. Seeling MS, Heffveit HA: Magnesium interrelationships in ischemic heart disease: a review, Am J Clin Nutr **27**:59-79, 1974.

41. Mossop RT: The geography of diabetes and vascular occlusive disease in relation to chromium, Cent Afr J Med **32**:137-140, 1986.

42. Klevay LM: Interaction of copper and zinc in cardiovascular disease, Ann NY Acad Sci **355**:140-151, 1980.

43. Schrauzer GM: Trace elements, nutrition and cancer: perspectives of prevention. In Schrauzer GN, editor: Inorganic and nutritional aspects of cancer, New York, 1977, Plenum Press Inc, pp 323-344.

44. Anderson B: Regulation of water intake, Physiol Rev **58**:582-603, 1978.

45. Young VR, Bier DM: Protein metabolism and nutrition state in man, Proc Nutr Soc **40**:343-359, 1985.

46. Linkswiler HM: Vitamin B_6 requirements of man. In Sauberlich HE, Brown ML: editors: Human vitamin B_6 requirements, Washington DC, 1978, National Academy of Sciences, pp 279-290.

47. Patterson WP, et al: Zinc-induced copper deficiency: megamineral sideroblastic anemia, Ann Intern Med **103**:385-386, 1985.

48. Hurley LS: Teratogenic aspects of manganese, zinc, and copper nutrition, Physiol Rev **61**:249-295, 1981.

49. Sauberlich HE, Brown ML, editors: Human vitamin B_6 requirements, Washington DC, 1978, National Academy of Sciences.

50. Beaton GH, Patwardhan VH: Physiological and practical consideration of nutrient function and requirements. In Beaton GH, Bengoa JM, editors: Nutrition in preventive medicine, Geneva, 1976, World Health Organization, pp 445-481.

51. Elsom KO, et al: Studies of the B vitamins in the human subject. V. The normal requirements for thiamine; some factors influencing its utilization and excretion, Am J Med Sci **203**:569-577, 1942.

52. Melnick D: Vitamin B_1 (thiamine) requirement of man. J Nutr **24**:139-151, 1942.

53. Keys A, et al: The performance of normal young men on controlled thiamine intakes, J Nutr **26**:399-415, 1943.

54. Horwitt MK, Kreisler O: The determination of early thiamine-deficient states by estimation of blood lactic and pyruvic acids after glucose administration and exercise, J Nutr **37**:411-427, 1949.

55. Sauberlich HE, et al: Thiamine requirement of the adult human, Am J Clin Nutr **32**:2237-2248, 1979.

CHAPTER 3

Nonnutrient Factors in Metabolism

Noel W. Solomons

Many national and international bodies have found it convenient to estimate the dietary requirements of individuals and to provide advice to the public about what is a sound and satisfactory diet. The methods used to estimate dietary requirements, as just reviewed, do not consider the nonnutrient factors that influence metabolism. When final considerations of *diet* are made, however, a series of contributing factors related to the host, environment, or foods must be taken into account. The present chapter discusses nonnutrient factors that can alter the nutritional requirements of individuals and defines the basic elements of an adequate diet.

NONNUTRIENT FACTORS

Nutrient requirements and, in turn, a person's nutritional status are affected by various agent (dietary), host, and environmental factors (see box on p. 37) that must be considered in the design and evaluation of diets and nutritional therapies for patients.

Agent (Dietary) Factors

Chemical form. The chemical form of a nutrient influences its biologic availability. A classic example is iron: the organic (heme) form in foods is considerably more absorbable than the inorganic (nonheme) form.[1] A similar difference in bioavailability exists between organic and inorganic forms of dietary selenium[2] and chromium. The chemical form of a nutrient also influences its possible protective value as a cofactor modifying the effect of adverse environmental influences. Dietary vitamin A activity exists both as preformed (retinol) vitamin and as provitamin A (carotenoids). A specific antioxidant antimutagenic role for *carotene* in conferring protection against environmental carcinogens has been proposed.[3] Vitamin C in the form of reduced ascorbic acid (AA) but not as oxidized dehydroascorbic acid (DHAA) will neutralize carcinogenic nitrosamines in the stomach.[4] The partition of vitamin C in foods between reduced and oxidized forms varies considerably. Moreover, protection of the ocular lens from photooxidation damage by ultraviolet light is conferred by ascorbic acid (reduced).[5] The influence of the dietary proportions of AA and DHAA on ocular tissue partition is under investigation.

Total energy intake. Total energy intake is also a determinant of the utilization of specific nutrients, notably protein.[6] The amount of dietary protein necessary to maintain nitrogen balance is greater in more hypocaloric diets. Energy balance also plays a role in the expression of essential hypertension.[7]

Ethanol intake. Alcohol, a beverage in many human diets, is a source of metabolizable energy. In excess consumption, however, it can have many antinutritional consequences, which have been documented.[8] The most overt consequence is the toxic production of alcoholic hepatitis and chronic cirrhosis. Ryle[9] has shown that chronic alcoholism leads to (1) reduced or imbalanced dietary intake, (2) decreased uptake of ingested nutrients, (3) decreased utilization of absorbed nutrients, and (4) deranged metabolism. He also notes that, although spirits contain virtually no vitamins, niacin is required for the reduction of ethanol in the liver and pantothenic acid, biotin, and riboflavin are required for the synthetic metabolism of the derived acetate.

Food processing and preparation. Food processing and preparation may increase or decrease dietary demands for certain nutrients. Raw meat, for instance, reduces copper absorption. On the other hand, the treatment of corn meal with lime, as practiced in Mexico and Central America, increases the availability of niacin. Cast-iron cookware contributes iron to foods and decreases the amount that must be consumed to maintain acceptable iron nutriture. Iron contamination during food preparation can be carried to an extreme, however, as is the case with the native (kafir) beer consumed in large quantities by the Bantu of southern Africa; the brewing of this beer in iron receptables imparts such an excess of this metal to the beverage that many consumers develop an iron overload (nutritional siderosis), which in turn influences the utilization of other nutrients.

In commercial food production, and to a lesser extent in household preparation, food additives are used for enhancing flavor, preservation, or coloring. Moneret-Vautrin[10] provides rough estimates of the range of intakes of food additives daily in industrialized nations: saccharin (1-100 mg), gum arabic (1-50 g), metabisulfites (1-100 mg), azo dyes (100-400 mg), sodium nitrate (1-50 mg), sodium benzoate (1-400 mg), sodium glutamate (100-2000 mg), and both butylated hydroxytoluene (BHT) and butylated hydroxyanisole (BHA) (1 mg).

Processes of cooking and storage can destroy or alter nutrients in foods. Vitamin C and certain B-complex vitamins are subject to loss during cooking. Fat and fat-soluble vitamins will become rancid if sufficient natural or artificial antioxidant is not provided. Cooking foods also produces organic reactions that result in new dietary substances. An important example is the carcinogenic heterocyclic amines, formed when dried fish or ground meats are broiled or charred. These substances have induced tumors in rodents.[11] A similar process can result with fermentation or pickling of soybeans, Chinese cabbages, etc. The mutagenic reaction with *Salmonella typhimurium* (Ames test) and tumor responses with laboratory animals have been used to predict the carcinogenicity of dietary substances in human diets.[11,12] Table 3-1 lists a comprehensive series of substances found in or with foods that have produced tumors in animals. Of course, species differences and differences in the levels of exposure and the amount and frequency of consumption make extrapolation to humans an inexact undertaking. The epidemiologic evidence in human populations cited by Palmer and Mathews,[12] however, adds concern about the adverse potential of many constituents of and additives in the diet.

Dietary fiber. Since dietary fibers consist, in part, of polysaccharides, they are usually included in discussions of carbohydrates as nutrients. Dietary fibers include plant cell constituents that are not digested by the endogenous secretions of the human digestive tract. Therefore dietary fiber does not have a defined composition but varies with the type of foodstuff and makeup of the diet.

AGENT, HOST, AND ENVIRONMENTAL FACTORS INFLUENCING NUTRIENT REQUIREMENTS AND NUTRITIONAL STATUS

Agent (Dietary) Factors
Chemical form of nutrient
Total energy intake
Ethanol intake
Food processing and preparation
    Influence on nutritive value
    Destruction/transformation of nutrients
    Additives
    Carcinogens
Dietary fiber
Effect of other dietary components
    Intrinsic toxicants and inhibitors
    Megadose vitamins and minerals

Host Factors
Aging and senescence
Gender
Genetic makeup
Psychologic state
Physical activity
Allergy and food intolerance
Drugs and medicinal agents
Pathologic states
    Infection
    Physical trauma
    Chronic disease and cancer

Environmental Factors
Climatic conditions
    Ambient temperature
    Humidity
    Altitude
Physical environment
    Housing
    Crowding
Biozootic environment
    Microbial pathogens
    Parasites
    Protozoa
Socioeconomic conditions
    Poverty
    Poor dietary habits
    Poor food choices

Table 3-1 Carcinogenic Properties of Some Nonnutritive Dietary Components

| Substance | Source | Carcinogenicity | | Epidemiologic Evidence |
		Tumor Site	Species	
Acrylonitrile	Food packaging materials	Forestomach, central nervous system, Zymbol's gland	Rats	Limited; occupational exposure associated with high overall cancer risk
Aflatoxins	Moldy cereals, milk, peanuts, corn	Liver, kidney, stomach, lung, colon	Multiple (mice, rats, hamsters, others)	Correlated with high liver and esophageal cancer incidence in Africa and Far East
Arsenic	Contaminant or residue in seafoods, meats, vegetables, drinking water	Negative despite tests in multiple species		Occupational, medicinal, and drinking water exposure associated with high risk of skin or lung cancer
Aspartame	Nonnutritive sweeteners	Mostly negative	Mice, rats, dogs	No studies
Bracken fern toxin(s)	Bracken fern	Bladder, intestine, kidney	Multiple	Limited and inconclusive
Butylated hydroxyanisole	Preservative in fats and oils, baked goods, chewing gum, nonalcoholic beverages	Forestomach	Rats	No studies
Butylated hydroxytoluene	Preservative in fats and oils, baked goods, chewing gum, nonalcoholic beverages	Lung (promoter and possible initiator)	Mice	No studies
Cadmium	Contaminant in food and drinking water	Skin (nondietary route only)	Mice and rats	Occupational exposure and increased cancer risk and mortality in some studies
Cycasin	Cycad nuts	Liver, kidney, intestine	Rats	No conclusive evidence
Cyclamate	Nonnutritive sweeteners	Bladder (unlikely initiator, possible promoter or co-carcinogen)	Rats and mice	Nonnutritive sweeteners associated with higher risk of bladder cancer in some subgroups
FD & C Blue no. 2	Fruit, water ices, baked goods, chewing gum	Negative in recent definitive studies	Rats and mice	No relevant studies
FD & C Red no. 3	Condiments, chewing gum, gelatin, puddings, baked goods	Thyroid	Rats	No relevant studies
FD & C Yellow no. 5	Candy, beverages, frozen dairy desserts, baked goods	Negative	Multiple	No relevant studies
FD & C Yellow no. 6	Gelatins, puddings, snack foods, beverages, imitation dairy products	Negative in mice, incomplete in rats		No relevant studies
Hydrazines	Certain cultivated mushrooms	Lung, skin, blood vessels, liver	Primarily mice	No relevant studies
Lead	Canned foods; water, auto exhausts, some paints	Kidney	Mice and rats	Limited evidence of increased cancer risk by occupational exposure
Nitrosamines	Nitrate and nitrite in foods	Multiple sites	Multiple	Indirect evidence of high gastric and esophageal cancer risk

Modified from Palmer S, Mathews RA: Surg Clin North Am **66:**891-915, 1986.

Table 3-1 Carcinogenic Properties of Some Nonnutritive Dietary Components—cont'd

Substance	Source	Carcinogenicity		Epidemiologic Evidence
		Tumor Site	Species	
Polybrominated biphenyls	Accidental contamination of foods	Liver	Rats and mice	Inadequate
Polychlorinated biphenyls	Freshwater fish, meat, dairy foods	Liver (may be promoter)	Rats	Limited evidence of carcinogenicity
Polycyclic aromatic hydrocarbons	Charcoal-broiled and smoked foods, contaminated fish, air pollution	Multiple sites	Multiple	Occupational exposure and higher skin cancer risk; dietary exposure associated with stomach cancer risk
Pyrrolizidine alkaloids	Herbal medicines, teas	Liver	Rats	No direct evidence
Saccharin	Nonnutritive sweeteners	Bladder	Rats and mice	Nonnutritive sweeteners associated with higher risk of bladder cancer in some subgroups
Various organochlorine pesticides	Residues in food	Liver	Primarily mice	No definitive studies
Vinyl chloride	Food packaging materials	Multiple sites	Multiple	Occupational exposure associated with higher risk of brain, liver, and respiratory tract cancer

Table 3-2 presents a summary of the principal components of dietary fiber.[13] The structural features of the plant cell polysaccharides[14] are described in Table 3-3. In addition to the polysaccharides, lignin, a complex aromatic polymer whose precise chemical structure has not been established, contributes to the dietary fiber intake. The properties of dietary fiber are difficult to define because the chemical composition of fiber depends not only on the specific food or combination of foods in question but also on food preparation methods used. However, fiber serves a number of physiologic purposes within the intestinal tract,[15] and a summary of these actions is presented in Table 3-4. Although dietary fiber cannot be considered a nutrient by definition, it appears that optimum physiologic functioning of the intestinal tract requires a certain level and mixture of fibers.

The various chemical features and physiologic actions of fiber translate into consequences for human health, especially for persons on high-fiber (or, conversely, for those on low-fiber)

Table 3-2 Components of Dietary Fiber

Principal Source	Description	Classic Nomenclature
Structural materials of plant cell wall	Structural polysaccharides	Cellulose Hemicelluloses Pectic substances
Nonstructural materials, natural or used as food additives	Noncarbohydrate Polysaccharides from variety of sources	Lignin Storage polysaccharides Gums Mucilages Algal polysaccharides Fungal chitins Chemically modified polysaccharides

From Trowell H: Am J Clin Nutr **31**:S3-S11, 1978.

Table 3-3 Structural and Chemical Features of the Components of Dietary Fiber

Major Groupings	Principal Structural Types	Male Variations
Structural		
Noncellulosic	Galactguronans	Methoxy groups, side chains
Polysaccharides	Arabino- and glucuronoxylans	Branched and linear xylan chain, number and distribution of side chains
	Gluco- and galactomannans	Number and distribution of side chains
	Arabino galactans	Branching and side chains
Cellulose	β-D-glucan	Degree of polymerization
Lignins	Aromatic polymer	Type of polymer, functional groups
Unstructural		
Pectin	Galacturonans, polymers	Methoxy group, side chains
Gums, mucilages	Great variety, including arabi-noxylans and gluco- and galactomannans	Branching and side chains
Algal polysaccharides	Sulfated galactans and gulu-ronomannuronans	Variations in composition of backbone chain
Modified celluloses	Esters and ethers	Cross-linking

Modified from Southgate DAT: Am J Clin Nutr **31:**S107-S110, 1978.

Table 3-4 Physiologic Actions of Fiber As It Passes Along the Gastrointestinal Tract

	Type of Fiber	Modifying
Gel formation	Pectin	Gastric emptying
	Mucilages	Mouth-to-cecum transit
	Gums	Small intestinal absorption
Water-holding capacity	Polysaccharides	Mouth-to-rectum transit
	Lignins	Fecal weight
		Intraluminal pressure
		Fecal electrolytes
Bile-acid adsorption	Lignin	Fecal steroids
	Pectin	Cholesterol turnover
Cation exchange	Acidic polysaccharides	Fecal minerals
Antioxidant	Lignin	Free radical formation and action
Digestibility	Polysaccharides	Energy availability
		Chemical environment of colon
		Other physicochemical properties

Modified from Eastwood MA, Kay RM: Am J Clin Nutr **32:** 364-367, 1979.

diets. In the past decade both metabolic studies and epidemiologic investigations[16] have begun to reveal solid conclusions about the influence of dietary fiber in human health. Three points are essential to the formulation of questions and interpretation of data: (1) the systemic effects of fiber derive from the intraluminal effects on intestinal motility, secretion, and absorption; (2) the distinct fiber components, alone or in combination, have distinct functional consequences; and (3) the outcomes of acute administration of dietary fiber and of chronic consumption can be markedly different.

Fiber components with water-holding and gel-forming capacity tend to slow intestinal transit in the upper gut and to decrease residence time in the colon. There are secondary effects of high-fiber diets, specifically in the area of glucose and lipid metabolism. In acute as well as some long-term studies[16,17] various dietary fiber sources have been shown to improve glucose tolerance in both diabetic and nondiabetic subjects. Fiber also exerts a hypocholesterolemic effect, which can be seen early in the course of enriching a diet with fiber; the lipoprotein profile tends to regress to normal with sustained fiber administration.[16] Much of the carbohydrotic fiber that reaches the colon is digested by the action of colonic bacterial enzymes.[18] The fermentation of this substrate liberates short-chain fatty acids that can, in turn, be absorbed and used as energy by the organism.[19] Fermentation leads to an acidification of cecal pH, which has been speculated[20] to play a protective role for colonic tissue against carcinogenic and noxious dietary agents.

Effect of other dietary compounds. Largely harmful effects on human metabolism can result from other compounds occurring in the diet. Toxic substances occur in many foods. The high oxalate content of rhubarb and other leafy plants can lead to oxalate stone formation.[21] Hallucinogenic and poisonous substances occur in mushrooms. Microalgae in the periodic "red tides" of Pacific coastal fishing areas contain a potent nueromuscular toxin; consumption of shellfish feeding during red tides can result in fatal respiratory paralysis. Other substances are antinutrients. Natural enzymes in foods can destroy dietary thiamine or inactivate pancreatic amylase and proteases. Avidin in egg white binds dietary and endogenous biotin. Caffeine has a host of metabolic and endocrine consequences.[22]

A variety of other dietary compounds, nutrient and nonnutrient, can reduce or enhance the biologic availability of essential nutrients. Ascorbic acid and meat increase the absorption of inorganic iron[23]; red wine improves zinc absorption[24]; and lactose improves the uptake of dietary calcium.[25] The polyphenols (tannins) in tea and coffee, on the other hand, reduce the availability of iron.[26] Plant components (fiber, phytate, oxalate, etc.) variably reduce the absorption of certain mineral ions.[27]

Finally, the custom of taking specific vitamins and minerals in excess of usual requirements has led to the ingestion of "megadoses" of nutrients that are tenfold or more above the RDA.[28] Caution is advised with this practice since individual micronutrients in excess can produce toxicity. For example, excess vitamin A may cause hepatic fibrosis, ascitis, and increased intracranial pressure (pseudotumor cerebri); vitamin B overdose may induce a hypercalcemia; nicotinic acid is a potent vasodilator; vitamin C is laxative; iron overload can develop from excess oral iron; megadose zinc blocks the absorption of dietary copper.

Host Factors

Factors intrinsic to the host and to individual conduct and behavior can influence nutrient needs or aspects of human metabolism affecting nutrition.

Aging and senescence. The *Recommended Dietary Allowances*[29] and most other national or international dietary intake standards recognize that nutrient requirements change with advancing age in adulthood. The aging process involves physiologic changes that alter nutrient requirements.[30] Calcium is a notable example of a problem nutrient in elderly persons since the efficiency of intestinal calcium absorption decreases with age.[31] Iron stores, on the other hand, accumulate over a lifetime, and the intestine adapts to *down*-regulate the efficiency of dietary iron absorption. Often, however, the economic and constitutional circumstances associated with aging are accompanied by changes that alter nutrient requirements.

Gender. Sex differences, generally appearing after puberty, influence nutrient demands and metabolism. There is a clear divergence in energy requirements, with men needing more calories.[29] The body composition of the two sexes is different, however, with women having 40% more body fat.[32] Iron requirements are elevated for women during the fertile years.

Genetic makeup. Both specific gene abnormalities in particular individuals and multiple genetic variations influence human nutritional requirements. Nutritionists are now becoming aware, for instance, that variation in nutritional requirements across a healthy population may be the consequence of multiple genetic influences not yet completely understood.[33] Interest in thermogenesis and its role in obesity has led to the suggestion that a "thrifty" gene promotes the storage of energy more efficiently and hence leads to excess adiposity[34]; Pi-Sunyer,[35] however, reviewed the literature and tested the assump-

Table 3-5 Dose and Route of Vitamins Used to Treat Inherited Vitamin Dependency Disorders

Vitamin*	Units/day	Route†	Dosage Range
Retinol (A)	μg	p.o., i.m.	7500-25,000
Cholecalciferol (D₃)	μg	p.o., i.m.	1250-5000
2-Methylnaphthoquinones (K)	μg	p.o., i.m., iv	1000-6000
α-Tocopherol (E)	mg	p.o.	200-2000
Lipoic acid	mg	p.o.	200
Thiamine (B₁)	mg	p.o., i.v.	10-1000
Riboflavin (B₂)	mg	p.o.	20-300
Niacin	mg	p.o.	40-200
Pyridoxine (B₆)	mg	p.o.	10-1000
Pantoghenic acid	mg	p.o	10-1000
Pantothenic acid	mg	p.o.	100-1000
L-Carnitine (B_T)	mg	p.o., i.v.	1000-2000
Biotin (H)	μg	p.o.	10,000
Folacin	μg	p.o.	200-10,000
Cobalamin (B₁₂)	μg	p.o., i.m.	5-500
Ascorbate (C)	mg	p.o.	1000-10,000

From Elsas L, McCormick DB: Vitam Horm **43:**103-144, 1986.

*Actual forms administered depend on route (e.g., a retinyl ester is given i.m. or menadione is given i.v.).

†Route symbols: *p.o.*, per os; *i.m.*, intramuscular; *i.v.*, intravenous.

MECHANISMS PRODUCING INHERITED VITAMIN DEPENDENCY SYNDROMES

Intestinal malabsorption
  Reduced availability of lipid emulsants
  Defective intrinsic factors
  Impaired active transepithelial transport
  Impaired cleavage from natural protein
Impaired transport by blood protein or lymphatic chylomicrons
Defective plasma membrane uptake
Defective release from cytosolic transfer protein
Impaired production of active cofactors (coenzymes)
Impaired covalent bonding of vitamin to apoenzyme
Defective noncovalent binding of coenzyme to apoenzyme
Rapid degradation of holoenzyme
Slowed recycling of covalently bound vitamin
Rapid excretion

From Elsas L, McCormick DB: Vitam Horm **43:**103-144, 1986.

tions regarding thermogenesis and human metabolism. He found *no* evidence for a genetically determined "thriftiness" in fuel utilization.

Common genetically transmitted disorders (e.g., diabetes mellitus, cystic fibrosis, celiac disease) not only produce alterations in nutrient absorption but also require dietary restrictions. Various trace mineral deficiencies have been associated with sickle cell disease; recent data from Jamaica[36] suggest that glycine metabolism may be altered in this genetic disorder, common among blacks. A host of inherited metabolic disorders of vitamin metabolism have been described. Elsas and McCormick[37] outline the variety of metabolic defects that influence vitamin handling (box). The dosages of vitamins required to treat vitamin-dependency conditions are listed in Table 3-5.

Finally, the presence or persistence of activity in the genes for the expression of certain digestive enzymes can influence dietary intake, mediated by carbohydrate intolerance, leading to food avoidance. The most common example is lactase nonpersistence,[38] the condition of involuted intestinal lactase-digesting and reduced lactose-digesting capacity, which affects most of the world's population. An individual's intake of milk and dairy products is often reduced or eliminated entirely to avoid gastrointestinal discomfort. Hereditary sucrose deficiency is another example; descendants of Eskimos in Greenland have a substantial prevalence of this disaccharidase deficiency, limiting their consumption of table sugar, carbonated drinks, sweets, and pastries.[35]

Psychologic state. Psychologic factors play a role in determining nutritional status. Depression and social isolation can reduce spontaneous dietary intake. Anorexia nervosa and bulimia are the most widely discussed of the eating disorders, but situational stress and anxiety may also act to influence nutrient intake. Psychic factors are known to produce overeating (hyperphagia), leading to obesity.

Physical activity. A return to vigorous physical activity—not in industrial or agricultural work, but rather in jogging and long-distance racing—has emerged in Western nations. Nutritional consequences of such intense physical activity have been uncovered in the form of iron deficiency anemia and trace metal deficiencies as athletes, marathon runners, and swimmers consume prodigious amounts of metabolic fuel. Intake of the vitamins, thiamine, riboflavin, and niacin should *at least* be in proportion to the total calories consumed. Whether extra vitamin intakes are needed in sports participants has yet to be established.

Allergy and food intolerance. Food intolerance refers to any symptom or sign of discomfort related to the consumption of a specific food. *Allergy* refers to an immunologically mediated hypersensitivity to an antigen. In food allergies the antigens are contained in the diet. However, it is important to recognize that even in systemic allergies the uptake of foreign proteins by the gut is an inciting event.[40] The haptens (low–molecular weight compounds that attach to proteins to produce immunogenicity) as well as the antigenic proteins for the production of food allergy are found in the diet.[10] Allergies and food intolerance have obvious implications for selection of dietary items, and hence nutrient composition. These issues are discussed in detail in Chapter 26.

Drugs. Elderly persons consume a large number and variety of pharmaceutic agents.[41] This places them at risk of adverse consequences, including those involving their diet, nutrition, and gastrointestinal function. The interaction of drugs and medications with nutrients can profoundly affect the nutritional status of an individual and, possibly, the dietary requirement for a particular nutrient. Drugs interact with nutrients by (1) impairing nutrient absorption, (2)

increasing nutrient excretion in the urine, (3) directly competing with or antagonizing nutrients, (4) displacing nutrients from carrier proteins, (5) inducing microsomal enzymes, and/or (6) having hormonal effects on nutrients.[42]

Pharmacologic agents can reduce the intestinal absorption of nutrients (e.g., tetracyclines reducing iron absorption, phosphorus antacids reducing phosphorous absorption, megadoses of ascorbic acid reducing vitamin B_{12} absorption, salicylazosulfapyridine reducing folic acid absorption). Furthermore, various drugs can enhance the urinary excretion of nutrients (thiazide diuretics producing depletion of body potassium; aspirin, barbiturates, and other drugs increasing the excretion of ascorbic acid, human growth hormone reportedly causing hyperzincuria).

An important type of interaction is direct drug antagonism of nutrient metabolism. This is best illustrated by the folic acid antagonists, of which methotrexate is a classic example. Methotrexate inhibits the activity of the enzyme dihydrofolate reductase, which is essential for the normal intracellular metabolism of folates. In addition, several drugs can compete with nutrients for their carrier proteins.

The induction of hepatic microsomal enzymes by barbiturates can enhance the degradation of warfarin anticoagulants. This drug-drug interaction has consequences for vitamin K–dependent synthesis of clotting factors. Finally, hormones can alter the metabolism of nutrients; for instance, estrogen-containing oral contraceptive agents interfere with the metabolism of vitamin B_6, and, in the practice of clinical medicine, the prescription of drugs for patients inadvertently can be the cause of, or an aggravating factor in, various types of nutritional deficiencies. An extensive, but by no means exhaustive, listing of drug-nutrient interactions is presented in Table 3-6.

In addition to internal metabolic actions and malabsorptive problems, certain drugs and medicinal agents produce direct gastrointestinal injury that impedes successful alimentation.[43] Esophagitis is caused by various antibiotics, by potassium chloride, and by vasopressin and quinidine. Chemotherapy agents such as 5-fluorouracil injure the mucosa. Other drugs induce ischemia. Finally, a host of antibiotics can lead to pseudomembranous colitis.

Pathologic states. A most important factor

Table 3-6 Mechanisms of Drug-Nutrient Interaction

Drug	Nutrients Affected	Presumed Mechanism of Action	Possible Clinical Consequences
Antacids	Phosphate	Chelation	Hypophosphatemia (may be desirable in renal impairment, undesirable in other cases)
Colchicine	Vitamin B_{12}	Intestinal malabsorption, mucosal damage	Macrocytic anemia, neurologic dysfunction
PAS	Vitamin B_{12}	Intestinal malabsorption, mucosal damage	Macrocytic anemia, neurologic dysfunction
5-Fluorouracil	Protein	Intestinal malabsorption, mucosal dipeptidase activity	Altered mucosal structure and function, amino acid imbalance, oral hypoglycemia
Metformin Phenformin	Glucose Vitamin B_{12}, disaccharides	Intestinal malabsorption	Decreased blood glucose level Vitamin B_{12} deficiency
Cholestyramine	Triglyceride (also calcium soaps and fat-soluble vitamins)	Intestinal malabsorption (due to bile acid sequestration)	Steatorrhea, tetany, deficiency of fat-soluble vitamins
Neomycin	Triglyceride (also calcium soaps and fat-soluble vitamins)	Bile acid sequestration (also mucosal damage)	Steatorrhea, tetany, deficiency of fat-soluble vitamins
Thiazide	Sodium, potassium	Increased urinary excretion (also impaired gastrointestinal transport)	Hypokalemia, muscle weakness
Ethanol	Zinc	Increased zinc loss in urine	Altered sense of taste and smell
Aspirin, barbiturates, paraldehyde, hydantoins, aminopyrine, ether	Vitamin C	Increased urinary excretion (probably due to displacement from binding sites)	Clinical or subclinical vitamin C deficiency (scurvy)
Penicillamine	Vitamin B_4	Increased urinary excretion due to chelation of vitamin	Mood changes, peripheral neuritis, convulsions
Methotrexate, pyrimethamine, triaminopteridine, trimethoprum	Folate	Direct antagonism, competition for active site on enzyme due to similarities in chemical structure	Reduced serum folate level, macrocytic anemia, megaloblastic bone marrow
Isoniazed	Vitamin B_4, tryptophan, niacin	Direct antagonism, competition for active site on enzyme due to similarities in chemical structure	Peripheral neuritis, convulsions, pellagra-like syndrome
Chloramphenicol	Phenylalanine	Compete for attachment to tRNA	Abnormal protein synthesis
Alpha-Methyldopa	Vitamin B_4	Metabolic antagonism	May nullify beneficial effect of drug in Parkinson's disease
Coumadin	Vitamin K	Suppresses synthesis of vitamin K–dependent coagulation factors	Hypoprothrombinemia, hemorrhage if excessive
Oxyphen-butazone	Vitamin K	Enhances warfarin effect by displacing it from albumin-binding site	Less warfarin required
Barbiturates	Vitamin K	Lowers warfarin effect by induction of hepatic enzymes to inactivate	More warfarin required

From Butterworth CE: Pract Gastroenterol **2:**55-58, 1978.

Table 3-6 Mechanisms of Drug-Nutrient Interaction—cont'd

Drug	Nutrients Affected	Presumed Mechanism of Action	Possible Clinical Consequences
Ethanol	Vitamin B$_4$	Impaired conversion of pyridoxine to pyridoxal phosphate	Impaired iron utilization for heme-ringed sideroblasts in bone marrow
Ethanol	Folate	Uncertain	Increased requirement, megaloblastic anemia, fatty-acid–responsive impairment in iron utilization
Ethanol	Magnesium	Excessive magnesium loss in stool	Hypomagnesemic tetany
Oral contraceptive agent	Vitamin A	Impaired hepatic storage, increased plasma binding	Uncertain
	Copper	Increased plasma ceruloplasmin	?
	Iron	Increased transferrin	?
	Folate	Increased folate-binding protein	?
	Vitamin B$_4$	Altered vitamin B$_4$ and tryptophan metabolism	Mood changes, abnormal protein metabolism
	Vitamin B$_{12}$	Reduced serum concentration	Uncertain
	Folate	Reduced red cell concentration	Megaloblastic anemia, other effects uncertain
	Zinc	Reduced serum concentration	Uncertain
Diphenylhydantoin, primidone	Folate	Uncertain	Macrocytic anemia
Tetracyclines	Calcium	Drug binds to calcium in bones	Growth retardation in premature infants, pigmentation of teeth
Tricyclic antidepressants	Various	Stimulate appetite	Weight gain (in children)
Imipramine	Various	Stimulate appetite	Weight gain (in children)

is the host's state of physical health. Illness places a stress on nutritional reserves and is a barrier to normal alimentation. The qualitative effects of acute infection on nutrient utilization and requirements have been well described[44] for some infections (Chapter 23). Recently, more and more quantitative information on the interaction of nutrition and infection has been developed.[45] An important new concern is acquired immunodeficiency syndrome, which leads to a wasting diathesis even in the absence of overt opportunistic infections. Negative nitrogen balance develops in infectious stress. In infections and other major disease states the dietary protein requirement may be increased twofold.[46]

Hospitalization is associated with a risk of nutritional depletion. Surgical patients are at increased risk.[47] Barch et al.[48] have catalogued the various adverse nutritional effects that a variety of chronic diseases afflicting the elderly can exert. Finally, by virtue of its metabolic cost, its interference with normal alimentation, and the effects of both chemical and radiation therapy applied to combat it, human malignancy has a major negative effect on nutritional status.[49]

Environmental Factors

Environmental factors can influence the demand for nutrients and their utilization from the diet.

Climatic conditions. The ambient temperature may play a direct role in determining nutritional requirements. Excessive cold, uncompensated by adequate clothing and housing, will increase the need for dietary energy, for vitamin C, and possibly for certain B-complex vitamins associated with energy metabolism. Excessive heat, in the Tropics or at the workplace, leads to large sweat losses, producing additional demands for water and electrolytes. Minerals such as zinc and iron may also be affected by major tegmental losses of fluid. Living at high altitude definitely influences metabolism[50,68] and may also affect nutritional needs. Part of the influence is the associated cold temperature; another is the lower oxygen tension and the more intense ionizing radiation and ultraviolet exposure. The amount of iron in the erythron is increased at high altitudes. To the extent that ascorbic acid protects against photooxidation of the lens,[5] this nutrient may be needed in increased amounts. Finally, short stature seems to provide a selective advantage for high-altitude living.

Physical environment. The construction of homes adequate to compensate for any adversity of climate is needed, along with adequate sanitation. Local crowding within the community is another factor that might influence individual metabolism due to psychic stress and contamination. It is important to realize that the entire world's population, developed and developing countries alike, is rapidly urbanizing.[51]

Biozootic environment. Poor sanitation and inadequate hygiene often lead to fecal contamination of the home, school, or workplace. This causes an increased incidence of acute gastrointestinal infections, with losses of water and electrolytes, and general impairment of nutriture. The degree to which usual parasite loads stress the nutritional status of individuals has been discussed.[52]

Socioeconomic conditions. The prevalent socioeconomic conditions of a community or nation can act synergistically with many of the other factors discussed in this chapter to produce impaired nutrition. Poverty deprives individuals of the resources to obtain safe food, a varied diet, and a sanitary home. Poor education and illiteracy interfere with the development of sound dietary and hygienic practices. Many adverse consequences disappear as groups achieve more education, social integration, and material wealth.[53]

ELEMENTS OF AN ADEQUATE DIET

Identification of the essential nutrients and estimations of the quantitative requirements for them provide a basis for the implementation of national food and nutrition programs, the assessment of nutritional adequacy of food sources, and the formulation of diets. In addition, with this knowledge it is possible to consider what and how much should be eaten to maintain an adequate nutritional status.

Composition

The requirements for essential nutrients can be satisfied by the various foods consumed. The principal categories of foods are (1) cereals, (2) starchy roots, (3) sugars and syrups, (4) pulses, nuts, and seeds, (5) vegetables, (6) fruits, (7) meat, fish and eggs, (8) milk and milk products, (9) oils and fats, and (10) beverages. Some of these foods, such as wheat, may serve as dietary staples and thus potentially have an important effect on nutritional health. Other foods may be used in lesser amounts (e.g., for flavoring or other culinary purposes).

Although all foods provide some nutrients, no single food can satisfy all nutrient needs. An ideal diet, then, must use a wide variety of foods to guarantee that the requirements for energy and all essential nutrients are satisfied. For example, a dietition might suggest the following four steps in selecting an adequate diet: (1) choose and eat a wide variety of foods; (2) be moderate in your consumption of fat, saturated fat, cholesterol, sugar, and sodium; (3) try to maintain your ideal body weight; and (4) if you enjoy alcohol, consume it moderately. When many foods are readily available, nutritional deficiency disorders rarely arise. Many basic diet plans, using varying selections from the same food groups, can be individualized while maintaining nutritional balance by taking into account not only physiologic requirements but also psychologic, emotional, social, and economic factors. For example, some people like meat, but others do not. Similarly, some people show preferences for foods prepared in particular ways. (See Chapters 41 and 43.)

Because different foods provide different nutrients, an adequate diet would be planned by selecting foods from each group, although it is not essential that every food group be represented in the diet. For example, cereals serve as significant sources of calories, iron, thiamine, and niacin in most human diets. Sugars, sweets, and fats add appreciably to total energy intake but make little contribution to protein, mineral, and B-complex vitamin intakes. Milk and dairy products make important contributions toward meeting protein, calcium, and riboflavin requirements; however, they are generally poor sources of vitamins A and C. The meat group, beans, peas, nuts, poultry, and fish rank as good sources of protein and many vitamins and minerals. Therefore some diets may contain little or no meat but, when planned wisely, be nutritionally adequate. However, strict vegetarian diets (i.e., those based only on plant foods) for infants, young children, and pregnant women may be nutritionally deficient; great care must be taken in planning diets for the needs of these groups (for details, see Chapters 4, 5, and 45).

Amount

Exactly how much of each of these foods should be consumed is a difficult question to answer, because some people require more than others. Furthermore, it may be difficult to determine a person's ideal body weight, although a reasonable weight to maintain would be whatever that person weighed between the ages of 20 and 25 years. Additional nonnutrient factors, as just detailed, must also be considered.

It is likely that, when an excess calorie intake leads to increased body fat, the chances of developing diabetes, heart disease, and high blood pressure will be increased. Foods that are high in fat and cholesterol, when eaten to excess, also can increase risk of heart attack; therefore they should be eaten in moderation. Again, although this does not necessarily apply to all people, high intakes of fat, especially saturated fat and cholesterol, should be avoided. Lean cuts of meat, a moderate consumption of eggs and organ meats, and perhaps the use of skim milk in partial replacement of whole milk will ensure some of the nutritional qualities of these foods (e.g., adequate vitamins and minerals and good-quality protein) without any of the undesirable consequences of excessive fat intake. Similarly, carbohydrate foods should be chosen with care; and although there is no convincing evidence that sucrose causes heart and blood vessel diseases or diabetes, it does increase the risk of tooth decay (dental caries), especially if eaten between meals; therefore sugar intake also should be moderate.

Flexibility

All these composition and measurement factors make it unwise to be rigid about recommending specific foods. It is important to remember that considerable flexibility is possible in food choices. Again, a balanced intake of the various foods is the best guarantee of an adequate diet and, therefore, of meeting the body's nutrient requirements.

REFERENCES

1. Cook JD: Absorption of food iron, Fed Proc **36**:2028-2031, 1977.
2. Barbezat GO, et al: Selenium. In Solomons NW, Rosenberg IH, editors: Absorption and malabsorption of mineral nutrients, New York, 1984, Alan R Liss, pp 321-258.
3. Peto R, et al: Can dietary beta-carotene materially reduce human cancer rates? Nature **290**:201-208, 1981.
4. Kim YK, et al: Effects of ascorbic acid on the nitrosation of dialkyl amines. In Seib PA, Tolbert BM, editors: Ascorbic acid: chemistry, metabolism and uses, Washington DC, 1982, American Chemical Society, pp 571-585.
5. Chandra DB, et al: Vitamin C in the human aqueous humor and cataracts, Int J Vit Nutr Res **56**:165-168, 1986.
6. Garza C, et al: Human protein requirements: the effects of variations in energy intake within the maintenance range, Am J Clin Nutr **29**:280-287, 1976.
7. Mancini M: Energy balance and blood-pressure regulation: update and future perspectives, J Clin Hyperten **2**:148-153, 1986.
8. Halsted CH, editor: Alcoholism and malnutrition. Introduction to the symposium, Am J Clin Nutr **33**:2705-2708, 1980.
9. Ryle P: Nutrition and vitamins in alcoholism. In Rosalli SB, editor: Clinical biochemistry of alcoholism, New York, 1984, Churchill Livingstone Inc, pp 190-191.
10. Moneret-Vautrin DA: Food antigens and additives, J Allergy Clin Immunol **78**:1039-1046, 1986.
11. Sugimura T: Past, present, and future of mutagens in cooked foods, Environ Health Perspec **67**:5-10, 1986.
12. Palmer S, Mathews RA: The role of non-nutritive dietary constituents in carcinogenesis, Surg Clin North Am **66**:891-915, 1986.
13. Trowell H: The development of the concept of dietary fiber in human nutrition, Am J Clin Nutr **31**:S3-S11, 1978.
14. Southgate DAT: Dietary fiber: analysis and food sources, Am J Clin Nutr **31**:S107-S110, 1978.
15. Eastwood MA, Kay RM: An hypothesis for the action of dietary fiber along the gastrointestinal tract, Am J Clin Nutr **32**:364-367, 1979.
16. Bijlani RL: Dietary fiber: consensus and controversy, Prog Food Nutr Sci **9**:343-393, 1985.
17. Jenkins DJA, Jenkins AL: The clinical implications of dietary fiber, Adv Nutr Res **6**:169-202, 1984.
18. Rerat AA: Contribution of the large intestine to digestion of carbohydrates. In Belmont J, editor: Milk intolerance and rejection, Basel, 1983, S Karger AG, pp 17-21.
19. Ruppin H, et al: Absorption of short-chain fatty acids by the colon, Gastroenterology **78**:1500-1507, 1980.
20. Farthing MJG, et al: Tropical diseases of the colon. In Alexander Williams J, Binder HJ, editors: Gastroenterology 3. Butterworths International Medical Reviews, London, 1983, Butterworth & Co (Publishers) Ltd, pp 155-195.

21. Hagler L, Herman RH: Oxalate metabolism. II, Am J Clin Nutr **26:**882-889, 1973.

22. Workshop on caffeine, Nutr Rev **37:**124-126, 1979.

23. Monsen ER, et al: Estimation of available dietary iron, Am J Clin Nutr **31:**134-141, 1978.

24. McDonald JT, Margen S: Wine versus ethanol in human nutrition. IV. Zinc balance, Am J Clin Nutr **33:**1096-1102, 1980.

25. Allen LH: Calcium bioavailability and absorption: a review, Am J Clin Nutr **35:**783-808, 1982.

26. Disler PB, et al: The effect of tea on iron absorption, Gut **16:**193-200, 1975.

27. Rosenberg IH, Solomons NW: Physiological and pathophysiological mechanisms in mineral absorption. In Solomons NW, Rosenberg IH, editors: Absorption and malabsorption of mineral nutrients, New York, 1984, Alan R Liss, pp 1-14.

28. Council on Scientific Affairs, American Medical Association: Vitamin preparations as dietary supplements and as therapeutic agents, JAMA **257:**1929-1936, 1987.

29. Committee on Dietary Allowances, Food and Nutrition Board, National Research Council: Recommended dietary allowances, ed 9, Washington DC, 1980, National Academy of Sciences.

30. Munro HN: Nutrition and the elderly: a general overview, J Am Coll Nutr **3:**341-350, 1984.

31. Ireland P, Fortrand JS: Effect of dietary calcium and age on jejunal calcium absorption in humans studied by intestinal perfusion, J Clin Invest **52:**2672-2681, 1973.

32. Behnke AR: Anthropometric evaluation of body composition throughout life, Ann NY Acad Sci **110:**450-463, 1963.

33. Vasquez A, Bourges H, editors: Genetic factors in nutrition, New York, 1984, Academic Press Inc.

34. Daniels RJ, et al: Obesity in the Pima Indians, Am J Clin Nutr **35:**835, 1982.

35. Pi-Sunyer FX: Thermogenesis in human obesity, Curr Concepts Nutr **15:**51-66, 1986.

36. Jackson AA: The use of stable isotopes to study nitrogen metabolism in homozygous sickle cell disease. In Vasquez A, Bourges H, editors: Genetic factors in nutrition, New York, 1984, Academic Press Inc, pp 297-314.

37. Elsas L, McCormick DB: Genetic defects in vitamin utilization. I. General aspects and fat soluble vitamins, Vitam Horm **43:**103-144, 1986.

38. Solomons NW: An update on lactose intolerance, Nutr News **49:**1-3, 1986.

39. Gudmond-Hoyer E, et al: Sucrose deficiency in Greenland. Incidence and genetic aspects, Scand J Gastroenterol **22:**24-28, 1987.

40. Walker WA: Allergen absorption in the intestine: implications for food allergy in infants, J Allergy Clin Immunol **78:**1003-1009, 1986.

41. Lamy PP: The elderly and drug interactions, J Am Geriatr Soc **34:**586-592, 1986.

42. Butterworth CE: Drug-nutrient interactions, Pract Gastroenterol **2:**55-58, 1978.

43. Lewis JH: Gastrointestinal injury due to medicinal agents, Am J Gastroenterol **81:**819-834, 1986.

44. Scrimshaw NS, et al: Interactions of nutrition and infection, Am J Med Sci **237:**367-403, 1959.

45. Keusch GT, Farthing MJ: Nutrition and infection, Ann Rev Nutr **6:**131-154, 1986.

46. Munro HN, Young VR: Protein metabolism and requirements. In Exton-Smith AN, Caird FI, editors: Metabolic and nutritional disorders in the elderly, London, 1980, John Wright & Sons Ltd.

47. Meguid MM: Risk-benefit analysis of malnutrition and perioperative nutritional support: a review, Nutr Int **3:**25-34, 1987.

48. Barch DH, et al: Effects of chronic disease on nutrition, Nutr Int **3:**78-86, 1987.

49. Brennan MF: Malnutrition in patients with gastrointestinal malignancy. Significance and management, Dig Dis Sci **31**(suppl 9):775-905, 1986.

50. Arnaud J, et al: Haematology and erythrocyte metabolism in man at high altitude: an Aymara-Quecha comparison, Am J Phys Anthropol **67:**279-284, 1985.

51. Gross R, Solomons NW, editors: Tropical urban nutrition, Eschborn, Germany, 1987, Gesellschaft fur Technische Zusammenarbeit (GTZ).

52. Keusch GT, editor: The biology of parasitic infection. Workshop on interactions of nutrition and parasitic disease, Rev Infect Dis **4:**735-911, 1982.

53. Schensul S: Organizing research in the urban context. In Gross R, Solomons NW, editors: Tropical urban nutrition, Eschborn, Germany, 1987, Gesellschaft fur Technische Zusammenarbeit (GTZ), pp 79-106.

II

NUTRITION IN THE
NORMAL LIFE SPAN

CHAPTER 4

Pregnancy and Lactation

Howard N. Jacobson
José Villar

NUTRITION AND THE PHYSIOLOGY OF REPRODUCTION

Puberty

The attainment of sexual maturity in nearly all species is related to the attainment of adult body size and dimensions. Normal girls who have early menarche are generally well advanced in physical development from early childhood onward.[1] For the past 150 years there has been a trend toward an earlier onset of menarche in a number of Western European countries and in the United States. The advance in age has been about 4 to 6 months per decade, with the average age of menarche today being 12.7 years of age. Although improved nutrition and better control of infection in childhood certainly have played a large part in the accelerated development, there are a number of factors, such as environmental changes and improved health care, that also may be influential.

Fertility

Maternal nutrition, fertility, and population growth were linked together by a 1967 report on the world food supply[2] in which it was postulated that "the necessary preconditions for reducing fertility rates in developing countries are low infant and child mortality and a public awareness that mortality is low: We have the apparent paradox that a reduction in childhood mortality will reduce rather than raise the rate of population growth." Since this report was published, and despite intensive study of these factors, there continue to be uncertainty and doubt about the validity of the assumptions. The most critical area of doubt concerns the relationships between the nutrition of the mother and the survival of her offspring. It is now accepted that one of the most important factors in neonatal and infant mortality is the birth weight of the infant. There is also very little dispute over the importance of

an adequate supply of nutritious food for the mother during her entire lifetime, including pregnancy itself. There continues to be uncertainty, however, about the most effective approaches to improving nutritional status during pregnancy.[3]

Adolescence and Pregnancy

In adolescence the girl experiences a surge in physical, sexual, and physiologic development that is more pronounced than in any other single period in her life. An adolescent girl whose nutritional reserves have been depleted by poor diet and increased demands for growth and development will be ill-prepared for pregnancy. The potential consequences of this situation are illustrated by the finding that pregnant teenagers in the United States select diets similar to those of their nonpregnant peers.[4]

In general, the adolescent does not reach full stature until 4 years after the onset of menstruation.[5] Adolescents who become pregnant within 4 years after menarche are considered to be at biologic risk. During pregnancy such immature girls are more likely to develop complications such as toxemia, excessive or limited weight gain, and anemia. They also face a higher risk of perinatal mortality, with increased risks of prematurity and infants of low birth weight.[4] That these risks can be reduced has been demonstrated.[6]

Maternal Nutrition and Fetal Development

Animal evidence. Experiments in animals have demonstrated that alterations in maternal diet can have profound effects on size of the litter, survival rates, size at birth, growth patterns, and behavior of the progeny. The timing and duration of the dietary restriction also may influence the results.[7] The severity of dietary restriction used in most animal studies is greater than that commonly encountered in human populations, although from time to time individual women may consume comparably restricted diets. Moreover, the generational effect of malnutrition has been proved. For example, colonies of rats living under conditions of suboptimal protein intake for more than ten generations had a proportion of malnourished offspring ten times higher than that of the well-nourished control generations.[8] The need for caution in extrapolating the detailed results of animal studies to the human has been pointed out.[5] Nevertheless, important basic knowledge has come, and will continue to come, from animal experimentation.

Human evidence. Almost 40 years ago, an association was reported between protein intake during pregnancy and the infant's physical condition at birth. Catastrophic circumstances, like those experienced in Leningrad in 1942-43, and Holland in 1944-45, caused reductions of the average fetal weight. In the Leningrad experience these averaged 600 g. In Holland, when the birth weights were examined by percentile distribution in women starved during their last trimester, it was found that large and small infants showed approximately the same percentage reduction and that the weights of infants of medium size were reduced by about 240 g. The lengths of the children also were reduced but only by a small amount. This is reflected in the finding of another study in Holland during this same period[9] that the number of newborns under 3000 g at birth was 41% of the whole whereas in 1942 it had been only 24%.

Epidemiologic evidence is available also on the influences on birth weight of the maternal environment, social class, prepregnancy weight, and weight gained during pregnancy. Studies have indicated consistently that increases in average birth weight are independently related to maternal weight gain. Furthermore, field studies in India, Guatemala, and Canada[10,11] report that provision of supplemental foods during pregnancy both increases birth weight and reduces the incidence of low–birth-weight infants.

Brain Development

The relation of nutrition to brain development has been reviewed,[12] and it has been shown that the effects of malnutrition depend on the age when deprivation occurs as well as on its dura-

tion and severity. Pregnancy is considered one of the critical periods because it is during this time that maximum neuronal growth occurs. Nevertheless, a report on intelligence testing in 19-year-old men born during the Dutch famine of 1945[13] showed no measurable differences between men whose well-nourished mothers had been exposed to a relatively brief period of famine during pregnancy and those whose mothers had not. This observation bears out the conclusion that malnutrition is detrimental in both good and poor environments, "but not necessarily equivalently so."[12]

Maternal Nutrition and Educational Dysfunction

Evidence from many studies and reviews[14] indicates that the smaller a baby is at birth the greater is the likelihood that it will have neurologic or mental dysfunction. It is pointed out that, before planning suitable prevention or treatment measures to remedy neurologic or mental dysfunction, one must clarify the influence of maternal nutrition on birth weight.

In summary, studies consistently have shown that factors related to maternal nutrition, particularly the mother's weight gain and prepregnancy weight, have a strong influence on birth weight, on infant mortality and morbidity, and, through these factors, on physical and social development. Nonetheless, the precise relationship of maternal nutrition to these outcome factors remains unclear. Any attempt to clarify the situation should provide a more rational basis for nutrition practices in maternity care.

CALORIC (ENERGY) REQUIREMENTS
Pregnancy

Adequate caloric intake is important for the growth and development of the fetus and for the mother's ability to adapt to stresses such as infections. Needs for additional energy during pregnancy are related to the production of new fetal and maternal tissues, the additional metabolism that the new tissues require, and the increased energy demanded to move the additional body mass during physical activity. Since the body mass of a woman increases about 20% during pregnancy, work involving great movement will cost as much as 20% more in energy.[15] Given these considerations, the total caloric cost of pregnancy has been calculated to be about 80,000 kcal.[16] Table 4-1 indicates how this cost is partitioned.

Increases in caloric requirements related to fetal and maternal resting metabolism appear primarily during the second part of gestation. In contrast, maternal fat stores are produced early in the course of pregnancy and do not follow the overall pattern of weight gain. A further adjustment of energy requirement should be based on the woman's physical activities. Thus the expenditure of energy has been found to vary from 38 to 50 kcal/kg/day.[17]

Since energy expenditure varies so widely, the best index of adequate intake is a satisfactory weight gain.[18] Measurement of weight gain in conjunction with estimates of activity and intake, therefore, is one way in which the adequacy of the diet and the woman's ability to comply with dietary instructions can be assessed. A 24-pound (10.9 kg) weight gain may be produced by only 1800 kcal/day in a sedentary woman whereas in an active growing teenager 3000 kcal/day may be required to produce the same increase. Therefore the 80,000 kcal needed during an entire pregnancy represents an average increment of about 300 kcal/day. This increment might be distributed into 150 kcal/day during the first trimester and 350 kcal/day during the second and third trimesters.

Lactation

The additional energy requirements of lactation are determined by the quantity of milk produced, and this varies widely from one woman to another. The energy content of breast milk is reported to be approximately 67 to 77 kcal/100 ml. The efficiency of the conversion of maternal energy to milk energy has

Table 4-1 Caloric Needs During Pregnancy (kcal)

Fetus	5000-6000
Maternal rest	40,000
Maternal lean tissue growth (breast, blood protein, uterus, placenta, amniotic fluids)	2000
Maternal fat storage	9000-18,000
Physical activity	14,000
TOTAL	70,000-80,000

been reported to be 80%.[19] The production of 100 ml of milk requires approximately 90 kcal of energy.

Women achieving 11 to 12.5 kg of weight gain during pregnancy will have stored from 2 to 4 kg of body fat that may be drawn on to supply part of the additional energy needed for lactation. This fat deposit will provide from 200 to 300 kcal/day during a lactation period of about 100 days, or roughly one third the cost of an average milk production of approximately 850 ml/day. Thus energy allowances should be increased by nearly 500 kcal/day during the first 3 months of lactation. The allowance should be increased if lactation continues beyond this period or if maternal weight falls below the ideal for height. Allowances need to be much larger for women suckling more than one baby.

From all of these calculations some conclusions can be drawn: First, mothers with low fat deposits who plan to breast-feed should increase their caloric intake during early lactation by at least 750 kcal/day. Second, mothers who have accumulated large fat deposits but do not plan to breast-feed may have gained additional weight that could contribute to future obesity. Finally, severely malnourished women may produce less milk than well-nourished women.[20] Food supplementation of malnourished women has been beneficial.

PROTEIN REQUIREMENTS
Pregnancy

Complex new tissues are produced in pregnancy at a rate greater than at any other time during a woman's life. Protein is essential for this purpose, but during pregnancy protein metabolism cannot be separated from the needs for calories and other nutrients. Because energy needs take priority in metabolism during pregnancy, protein will be used for energy if carbohydrates and fat are not consumed in sufficient amounts. Conversely, increasing energy intake will improve utilization of protein. Adequate intake of both energy and protein is necessary for nitrogen retention. In favorable circumstances women tend to consume 70 to 90 g of protein/day and between 2300 and 2800 kcal/day.[21]

The usual estimate for deposition of protein during pregnancy is 925 g, and the efficiency of its utilization in pregnancy has been considered to remain unchanged (i.e., approximately 75% in the case of the average American diet[18]). Studies[22] have shown that the observed nitrogen retention greatly exceeds the amount predicted and that protein is utilized less efficiently than has been generally assumed. Thus it is recommended that an additional 30 g of protein/day and an increased energy intake above 36 kcal/kg of pregnant body weight be allowed for adequate utilization of protein during pregnancy.[18]

If a negative caloric balance is present, protein will be metabolized for energy, resulting in a shortage of protein for storage or growth. Recommended dietary allowances (RDAs) are designed for maintaining health, not for treatment or rehabilitation. Too often they are used for the latter purposes. Methods for quantitatively estimating protein deficiency must be improved before the precise amounts of protein needed by malnourished women can be specified with confidence. Another question that arises is whether protein is also stored during pregnancy or whether all the unaccounted-for weight gain can be considered fat. Although there is evidence that women can store more nitrogen than is found in the products of conception, this remains an area of intense research.

Lactation

The needs for additional protein during lactation depend on the amount of milk protein produced. Average daily milk yields for well-nourished mothers are estimated[18] to range from 850 ml to 1.2 liters, with a protein content of about 1.2%. Average protein yield therefore is some 10 g/day, with an upper limit of 15 g. The 20 g protein increase (to a total of 64 g/day) in the RDA for lactating women covers the requirement for milk production with an allowance for the approximate 70% efficiency of protein utilization as well as the biologic quality of dietary protein.

Protein/Energy Interrelations in Pregnancy

Protein recommendations generally are made on the assumption that energy needs will be satisfied by the diet. In field studies on nitrogen retention during pregnancy the influence of protein and energy cannot be separated, because as food intake increases energy and protein intakes increase as well. These studies have shown that increases in energy intake or protein intake alone can improve nitrogen balance within reason. An additional intake of 100 kcal or of 0.28 g nitrogen will have an equivalent effect on nitrogen retention. Thus, in studies on energy supplementation during pregnancy, increased caloric intake has allowed improved protein retention.

VITAMINS AND MINERALS

Blood levels for most vitamins are generally lower during pregnancy, and the application of standard norms for nonpregnant women results in higher percentages of abnormal findings. Indeed, laboratory methods suggest that such changes reflect only normal physiologic adjustments to pregnancy. One publication on laboratory indices of nutritional status in pregnancy, including vitamins,[23] offers a series of reported values that can be used as standards.

Fat-Soluble Vitamins

Vitamin A. Since fetal requirements for vitamin A increase maternal needs, a 25% increase over prepregnancy intake is advised.[18] To allow for fetal needs and storage, 1100 μg of retinol* during pregnancy and 1200 μg during lactation are recommended. However, there is some evidence[24] that either excessive amounts or a complete lack of vitamin A can produce teratogenic conditions. Therefore care should be exercised to ensure that dietary intake covers the daily needs for this nutrient. The typical North American diet can provide sufficient levels of vitamin A, and routine supplementation is not considered essential.

Vitamin D. Vitamin D facilitates calcium absorption and participates in bone metabolism. Studies[25] have shown that it plays a role in promoting positive calcium balance in pregnant women. One of its metabolites, 25-hydroxyvitamin D, freely crosses the placenta.[25] Reflecting these findings, the RDA for vitamin D has been increased by 200 IU (5 μg) for pregnant women. Whether maternal vitamin D deficiency is related to neonatal hypocalcemia remains to be determined.

Vitamin E. To maintain a level that will permit its deposit in fetal tissues, 15 IU of vitamin E/day is recommended. The association between vitamin E deficiency and miscarriage is

---

*1 IU of vitamin A = 0.3 μg of retinol.

not well established; therefore the use of vitamin E supplements for the prevention or treatment of spontaneous abortion has no foundation.[26]

Water-Soluble Vitamins

Two physiologic characteristics should be taken into account in any consideration of water-soluble vitamins: (1) blood levels generally decline during pregnancy and (2) fetal levels exceed those in the mother, reflecting active transport across the placenta.

Vitamin B₆. A clear reduction in the concentration of pyridoxal phosphate has been observed in pregnant women; observations also have shown that the excretion of xanthurenic acid increases when tryptophan is administered. The two factors related to the etiology of this deficiency[27] are (1) an increase in the levels of tryptophan oxygenase as attributed to estrogen increase during pregnancy and (2) a real state of deficiency near the end of the gestational period dut to fetal absorption of the nutrient. Since one study[28] has shown a significant correlation between serum levels at 20 weeks and the levels in cord serum and maternal milk, this may be a suitable time for assessment.

Nonetheless, vitamin B₆ needs tend to increase during pregnancy, particularly among women whose diets are rich in protein. The recommended daily increment of 0.5 mg is designed to be sufficient to satisfy basic needs.[18] This amount is not enough to "normalize" blood concentrations, however; for that purpose 6 to 10 mg/day is required.[29] More studies on the possible clinical implications of this process seem to be warranted.

Other B vitamins. Other B vitamins are required in greater amounts during pregnancy. Higher needs for thiamine, riboflavin, pantothenic acid, and vitamin B₁₂ have been determined. The RDAs for each are presented in Tables 2-9 and 2-10. Low levels of vitamin B₁₂ have been found in intrauterine growth-retarded infants.[30] Therefore, to avoid hematologic and growth alterations, vitamin B₁₂–supplemented formula is advised. Pregnant rats with pantothenic acid deficiency have been shown to develop litters with congenital malformations and brain defects.[31] Immunologic alterations in the presence of pantothenic acid deficiency have been reported in other laboratory animals as

well.[32] Thus, if these results are confirmed in humans, supplementation during pregnancy and for low–birth-weight infants may be considered.

Vitamin C. Insufficient information has accrued on vitamin C metabolism during pregnancy; however, there is general agreement that its intake should be increased during gestation and lactation.[18,26] To this end, a 20 mg/day increase above the 60 mg allowance for the nonpregnant woman is proposed.

Trace Elements

Zinc. There is a gradual reduction of plasma or serum zinc levels during pregnancy, reaching values about 25% of the prepregnancy levels by the third trimester. This could be as a consequence of the blood volume expansion, reduction of serum albumin, increased estrogen levels, and/or transfer of zinc from plasma to red blood cells. Some evidence of teratogenic association of low zinc plasma has been suggested.[33] During gestation an increase of 20 mg/day in zinc is recommended,[18] which represents 5 mg more than the RDA for nonpregnant women.

Calcium. The RDA for calcium is 1200 mg/day during gestation, compared to 800 mg for nonpregnant women. This increase (400 mg) takes into account the maternal absorption and provides the 30 g of calcium deposited in the fetus, particularly in the last trimester of gestation. However, studies[34] have determined that requirements can go as high as 2 g/day.

Human milk has 25 to 35 mg calcium/100 ml; for a lactating woman this represents an increment of 150 to 300 mg, depending on the amount of milk produced. The RDAs for lactating women are the same as those for women who are pregnant (1200 mg).[18] The best sources of calcium are milk and milk products. Cow's milk has 120 mg calcium/100 ml. It is very difficult to reach 1200 mg/day without milk products. Thus milk is considered a particularly valuable item of the diet during pregnancy. Women who do not like milk or who malabsorb it and do not need the RDAs from other milk products should receive calcium supplementation.

Sodium. The role of sodium in pregnancy long has been a controversial one. For a number of years the possibility of its having a primary role in inducing toxemia was the focus of attention, almost to the point of overlooking its normal physiologic role. Today it is recognized that sodium is required in the normal depots of fetal and maternal tissues. Nevertheless, pregnant women require only small additional quantities of salt to meet these added needs. An increase of 90 mg/day, or 25 g for the total pregnancy, will suffice. Typical diets in the United States contain 6 to 18 g of sodium per day.

Data derived from animal studies[35] show that low-sodium diets produce hyponatremia in organic fluids and reductions in the expansion of the physiologic intravascular volume. Furthermore, there is no evidence available to support the routine use of salt-restricted diets in the prevention of edemas and preeclampsia. Therefore neither salt-restricted diets nor diuretics have any place in the routines of healthy pregnant women.

Iron and Folic Acid

Hematologic changes. As shown in Fig. 4-1, the blood volume increases throughout pregnancy, starting as early as the sixth week, peaking at about 34 weeks, and expanding more slowly thereafter. In a singleton pregnancy the increase in plasma represents almost 50% of the average level found among nonpregnant women.[36] This figure represents an increase of approximately 1500 ml in multigravidas[16] and 2000 ml in multiple pregnancies.[37] Low plasma volume and low–birth-weight infants have been shown to be related; since diuretics can lead to reduced plasma volume, this is another reason to avoid their use during gestation.

Fig. 4-1 also shows a progressive increase in red cell volume during pregnancy but one that is usually less marked than the increment in plasma volume. This is a consequence of increased red cell production rather than of changes in the survival of existing cells.

After delivery the red cell volume declines because of blood loss and partial erythroid hypoplasia; it reaches normal nonpregnant levels

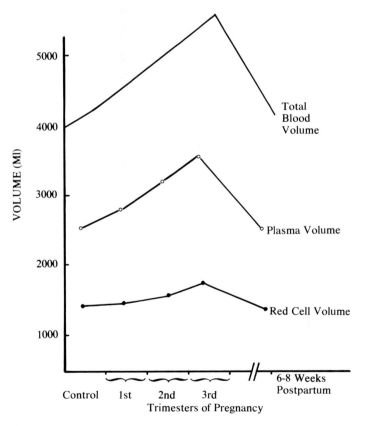

Figure 4-1 Changes in total blood volume, plasma volume, and red cell volume during pregnancy and postpartum.

Modified from Walters W, Lim YL: Clin Obstet Gynaecol **2:**301-320, 1975.

Table 4-2 Iron Requirements During Pregnancy (mg)

	First Half	Second Half	Total	Net Cost
Red cell mass expansion	—	500	500	—
Blood loss during delivery and puerperium	—	—	—	250
Fetal iron	—	290	290	290
Placental iron	—	25	25	25
Basal losses	110	110	220	—
TOTAL	110	925	1035	565

From FAO/WHO Expert Group: WHO Tech Rep Ser 452, 1970.

around the third week postpartum. The average increase in red cell volume is approximately 250 ml at term; with iron supplementation this figure rises to 400 ml.[5]

In the typical study[23] at 33 weeks the mean value for hemoglobin is 10.5 to 11 g/dl, for hematocrit 32% to 34%, and for erythrocyte count 3.7 million to 4.1 million/mm³. This phenomenon, called dilutional anemia, has the following characteristics:

It is due to an increase in plasma volume that is greater than the increase in red cell mass.
It begins early in pregnancy.
The red cells are normochronic and normocytic.
It is reversed postpartum.
It can be abolished or reduced by supplementation with iron and vitamins.

Iron requirements in pregnancy. During the course of a complete gestation a total of 1035 mg iron is required[38] (Table 4-2). However, the 470 to 500 mg corresponding to the expansion of the red cell mass is "saved." Thus the actual iron cost is 565 mg, or an average of 2 mg/day, nonuniformly distributed throughout the pregnancy: during the first trimester the increase is 0.8 mg/day; in the middle trimester it goes to 4.4 mg/day (the 0.8 mg base and an additional 3.6 mg for red cells); and in the third trimester it reaches 8.4 mg/day (0.8 base, plus 3.6 mg for red cells, plus 4.0 mg for fetus and placenta).[38]

Data from Canada, the United States, and Sweden[38] show that nearly 30% of women between the ages of 15 and 45 years do not have adequate iron deposits. Iron stores of nulligravid

women are about 300 mg, and almost 33% of them have no measurable stores at all. Women with low serum ferritin levels, consistent with very low iron stores, may require twice as much iron during pregnancy.

All these considerations lead to the conclusion that iron supplementation is essential to meet the requirements of almost all pregnancies. The individual woman's nutritional status will affect the amount of iron required; however, as a general rule, with very low iron reserves, 30 mg to 60 mg/day is required for the average patient.

Iron requirements in lactation. The production of breast milk requires about 0.5 to 1 mg of iron daily. Since menstruation generally is not present during lactation, the iron requirements during this state are similar to those of nonpregnant women.

Folic acid. A high prevalence of folic acid deficiencies has been reported. About 25% of normal pregnant women in the United States have marginal to low serum folate levels. In less developed countries 20% of hospital users have megaloblastic anemia and more than 50% have some kind of megaloblastic alterations.[38] Infertility and sterility as well as fetal and placental malformations have been associated with folic acid deficiency. Routine supplementation with 200 to 400 μg/day is suggested. Patients with a history of inadequate dietary intake, anemia in previous pregnancies, or multiple pregnancies and those receiving anticonvulsant drugs may require additional amounts.

Vitamin Supplementation

Multivitamin supplementation is widespread among pregnant women in the United States. Yet, for women who are economically capable of purchasing enough good-quality food, diet should meet most of their increased nutritional requirements, except for iron and folic acid. Thus, routine multivitamin supplementation during pregnancy has not been shown to be essential. Furthermore, the reported association between excessive doses of vitamins A, C, and D and some neonatal complications lends support to this conclusion. High doses of vitamins should not be prescribed during pregnancy. Moreover, low-income patients could be further handicapped if they use their restricted funds to cover the cost of vitamins instead of food.

WEIGHT GAIN DURING PREGNANCY
Desirable Gain

The objective of a program of guided weight increase during pregnancy is to help ensure the best outcome for the mother and her infant. The question of how to estimate a desirable increase in weight for a woman can, at present, be answered more confidently on the basis of three parameters: (1) the total weight gain measured during normal pregnancies, (2) the mother's weight gain relative to the birth weight of her infant, and (3) the weight of the components of a normal pregnancy.

With regard to the first, it has been found that normal patients without dietary restrictions gain about 24 pounds (10.8 kg). With regard to the second, it is known that elevated birth weights are directly related to increasing maternal weight gains during pregnancy (within the range of 24-32 lb). As regards the third, refinements in technique have made it possible to measure accurately the maternal and fetal components of weight gain during pregnancy. They show that the average weight at term of the fetus, placenta, amniotic fluid, and uterus, plus the increase in breast tissue, maternal blood volume, and interstitial fluid, comes to 20.5 pounds (9.2 kg). If 24 pounds (10.8 kg) is the average weight gained, then the 3.5-pound (1.6 kg) difference from 20.5 pounds must be accounted for. It is probably the measure of maternal storage of nutrients, particularly of fat, though maybe also of protein, and may be considered a "margin of safety" when planning a diet for the healthy pregnant woman.

Thus each of the preceding approaches suggests that the desirable gain for a pregnant woman should be about 24 pounds, or 10.8 kg, total.

Major Problems in the Management of Weight Gain

Now that minimal weight gain can be estimated with confidence, there are some reservations and conditions that must be considered. In the past, restricted weight gains generally were advised; and some now maintain that the recommendation for weight gains of as much as 24 to 30 pounds during pregnancy is tantamount to abandoning any sort of nutritional guidance whatsoever—in short, a license to overindulge. Furthermore, some experts have interpreted the recommendation of an average weight increase of 24 to 30 pounds as sufficient reason for doing away with weight control or with any recommendation for a desirable weight gain because there is such a wide range of normal gains. Finally, other experts encourage women to eat to appetite as a logical reply to the new data on the relation between mean maternal weight gain and average birth weight. Each of these replies deserves consideration.

A weight control program begins with an estimation of the patient's desirable weight and her nutritional status and it ends with an estimate of what would constitute an adequate gain for her. Thus, in the case of a seriously underweight woman, prenatal care might call for a carefully supervised large increase in weight to achieve a total gain during pregnancy of, say, 40 pounds (18 kg). Such women are known to present greater obstetric hazards and more difficult management problems.[39]

Although the wide range of normal weight gain often is used as justification for doing away with any recommendations for a desirable increase, there are limits at both ends of "desirable." At the low end a gain of less than 18 to 20 pounds in a woman producing an 8-pound fetus means that the mother must, to some degree, break down her own tissues to provide for the needs of pregnancy. The harmful consequences of low weight gains in underweight women are shown in Table 4-3. Furthermore, because precise information is not always available on a given patient's nutritional status or her nutritional stores, to provide a margin of safety there must be a lower limit to the positive control of weight gain. At the upper end there are also definable limits. One serious kind of excess weight gain is that due to the intake of too much carbohydrate. In this case the energy intake is more than sufficient and the protein intake is so low that the mother consumes her own lean body mass to support the growth of the fetus. The situation commonly is found among pregnant women who make unwise food selections or who have a limited budget. Another serious form of excessive weight gain is that due to edema. Women can accumulate 10 to 15 pounds of fluid and still have a small total weight gain, since there may be a matching loss of fat and body tissues. Weight gain by itself tells nothing about its components. The question to be answered

Table 4-3 Percentage of Low Birth Weight in Underweight Women by Level of Weight Gain at Term

Weight Gained (kg)	Percentile*	Low Birth Weight† (%)
<3.5	<3	60.0
3.5-4.5	3-5	33.3
4.5-6.5	5-10	30.3
6.5-8.0	10-16	15.6
8.0-11.0	16-25	12.7
11.0-12.5	25-50	12.6
12.5-14.0	50-75	12.6
>14.0	>75	6.8

Modified from Lechtig A, Klein RE: Bol Of Sanit Panam **89:**489, 1980.

*Based on 7061 caucasian mothers with prepregnancy weights between 50 and 60 kg.

†Based on 934 black mothers with prepregnancy weights less than 46 kg.

clinically is who is gaining the weight—the mother, the fetus, or both? Careful assessment is required, and the increasing use of physical anthropometry can be of assistance.[40]

Women whose knowledge of nutrition is scanty or whose income is low may, if they eat to appetite, come to depend on nutritionally inadequate food. In this connection there is increasing concern that pregnant women should learn to deal wisely with an increasingly sophisticated food supply, including more processed and formulated foods.

REFERENCES

1. Tanner JM: Growth at adolescence, ed 2, Oxford, 1962, Blackwell Scientific Publications.
2. President's Science Advisor Committee: Report. The world food problem, vol 1, Washington DC, 1957, Government Printing Office.
3. Rush D, et al: A randomized controlled trial of prenatal nutritional supplementation in New York City, Pediatrics **65:**683-697, 1980.
4. Zackler J, Brandstadt W, editors: The teenage pregnant girl, Springfield Ill, 1975, Charles C Thomas Publisher.
5. Committee on Maternal Nutrition, Food & Nutrition Board, National Research Council: Maternal nutrition and the course of pregnancy, Washington DC, 1970, National Academy of Sciences.
6. Hansen CM, et al: Effects on pregnant adolescents of attending a special school, J Am Diet Assoc **68:**538-541, 1976.
7. Simonson M, et al: Neuromotor development in progeny of underfed mother rats, J Nutr **98:**18-24, 1969.
8. Stewart RJC, et al: Twelve generations of marginal protein deficiency, Br J Nutr **33:**233-253, 1975.
9. Dean RFA: The size of the baby at birth and the yield of breast milk. In Department of Experimental Medicine, Cambridge: Studies of undernutrition, Wuppertal, 1946-9, Medical Research Council, Special Report Series 275, London, 1951, Her Majesty's Stationery Office.
10. Pitkin RM, Barness LA: Symposium on nutrition, Clin Perinatol **2:**205-206, 1975.
11. Lechtig A, et al: Effect of food supplementation during pregnancy on birth weight, Pediatrics **56:**508-520, 1975.
12. Committee on International Nutrition Programs, National Research Council: The relationship of nutrition to brain development and behavior, Washington DC, 1973, National Academy of Sciences.
13. Stein Z, et al: Nutrition and mental performance, Science **178:**708-713, 1972.
14. Richmond JB: Epidemiology of learning disorders. In Menkes JH, Schain RJ, editors: Learning disorders in children, Columbus Ohio, 1971, Ross Laboratories.
15. Blackburn ML, Calloway DH: Energy expenditure of pregnant adolescents, J Am Diet Assoc **65:**24-30, 1974.
16. Hytten FE, Leitch I: The physiology of human pregnancy, ed 2, Edinburgh, 1971, Blackwell Scientific Publications.
17. Committee on Maternal Nutrition, National Research Council: Nutritional supplementation and the outcome of pregnancy, Washington DC, 1973, National Academy of Sciences.
18. Committee on Dietary Allowances, Food and Nutrition Board, National Research Council: Recommended dietary allowances, ed 9, Washington DC, 1980, National Academy of Sciences.
19. Thompson AM, et al: The energy cost of human lactation, Br J Nutr **24:**565-572, 1970.
20. Hanafy MM, et al: Maternal nutrition and lactation performance, J Trop Pediatr **18:**187-191, 1972.
21. Calloway DH: Nitrogen balance during pregnancy. In Winick M, editor: Nutrition and fetal development, New York, 1974, John Wiley & Sons Inc, p 79.
22. King JC: Protein metabolism in pregnancy. In Pitkin R, editor: Symposium on nutrition, Clin Perinatol **2:**243-254, 1975.
23. Committee on Nutrition of the Mother and Preschool Child, National Research Council: Laboratory indices of nutritional status in pregnancy, Washington DC, 1978, National Academy of Sciences, p 109.
24. Bernhardt IR, Dorsey DJ: Hypervitaminosis A and congenital renal anomalies in a human infant, Obstet Gynecol **43:**750-755, 1974.
25. Pitkin RM, et al: Calcium metabolism in pregnancy: a longitudinal study, Am J Obstet Gynecol **133:**781-787, 1979.
26. Pitkin RM: Vitamins and minerals in pregnancy, Clin Perinatol **2:**221-232, 1975.
27. Rose DP, Braidman IP: Excretion of tryptophan metabolites as affected by pregnancy, contraceptive steroids, and steroid hormones, Am J Clin Nutr **24:**673-680, 1971.
28. Roepke JLB, Kirksey A: Vitamin B_6 supplementation during pregnancy: a prospective study, Am J Clin Nutr **32**(11):2249-2256, 1979.
29. Lumeng L, et al: Adequacy of vitamin B_6 supplementation during pregnancy: a prospective study, Am J Clin Nutr **29:**1376-1383, 1976.

30. Baker H, et al: Vitamin levels in low birth weight newborn infants and their mothers, Am J Obstet Gynecol **129:**521-524, 1977.
31. Rajalakshmi R, Nakhasi HL: Effects of neonatal pantothenic acid deficiency on brain lipid composition in rats, Am J Neurochem **24:**979-981, 1975.
32. Axelrod AE: Immune processes in vitamin deficiency states, Am J Clin Nutr **24:**265-271, 1971.
33. Tafari N, et al: Failure of bacterial growth inhibition by amniotic fluid, Am J Obstet Gynecol **128:**187-189, 1977.
34. Duggin GG, et al: Calcium balance in pregnancy, Lancet **2:**926-927, 1974.
35. Pike RL, et al: Juxtaglomerular degranulation and zona glomerulosa exhaustion in pregnant rats: induced by low sodium intakes and reversed by sodium load, Am J Obstet Gynecol **95:**604-614, 1966.
36. Walters WAW, Lim YL: Blood volumes and haemodynamics in pregnancy, Clin Obstet Gynaecol **2:**301-320, 1975.
37. Rovinsky JJ, Jaffin H: Cardiovascular hemodynamics in pregnancy. I. Blood and plasma volumes in multiple pregnancy, Am J Obstet Gynecol **93:**1-13, 1965.
38. World Health Organization: Requirements of ascorbic acid, vitamin D, vitamin B$_{12}$, folate, and iron: report of a joint FAO/WHO Expert Group, WHO Tech Rep Ser 452, 1970.
39. Naeye R: Weight gain and the outcome of pregnancy, Am J Obstet Gynecol **135:**3-9, 1979.
40. Maternal Nutrition Assessment Committee, National Research Council: Nutritional assessment in health programs, Am J Public Health **63**(suppl):57-63, 1973.

CHAPTER 5

Infants

David M. Paige
George M. Owen

At delivery the fetus is transported from a regulated environment in which nutritional and other support systems are available to one in which rapid adaptation is necessary for survival. This survival requires, in addition to a number of physiologic modifications, nutritional adequacy and immunologic defenses.

INFANT GROWTH

Average weight gain in the first year is 7.0 kg, about half of which occurs in the first 4 months of life. To achieve the 3.5 kg growth between birth and 4 months of age, approximately 61,000 kcal is required.[1]

Of the calories consumed, about 33% are utilized for growth during the first 4 months. The typical infant expends 7.5 kcal of energy to synthesize 1 g of protein and 11.6 kcal to synthesize 1 g of fat. This high proportion of energy required for growth drops to 7.4% of the required 180,000 calories consumed from 4 to 12 months of age.

The rapid growth of the healthy term infant during the first 4 months of life requires more energy, protein, and other essential nutrients per unit of body weight than are required at any other time in infancy or childhood. These needs can be met completely through the use of human milk or infant formula, since the gastroenteric and renal systems are still maturing and the types of foods and levels of nutrients that the infant safely can handle are limited.

At about 5 months of age the infant enters a transitional period characterized by a decreased rate of growth and an increased level of caloric expenditure for physical activity, developmental readiness, and increased physiologic capacity. While total calorie and nutrient requirements continue to increase as a result of growth, the decreasing need for energy and protein per unit of body weight reflects the progressive slowing of the rate of growth.

By age 8 or 9 months solid foods provide a significant source of energy and other nutrients necessary to supplement the basic intake from human milk or formula. The maturing gastroenteric and renal systems enable the infant to digest a variety of foods, to metabolize the components, and to excrete unneeded metabolites. As a result attention must be directed at the types and amounts of food being consumed by the older infant to ensure that nutritional needs are being met.

MINIMUM REQUIREMENTS, ADVISABLE INTAKES, AND DIETARY ALLOWANCES

Nutrient requirements for infants less than 6 months of age usually are based on the intakes of healthy thriving babies being breast-fed by healthy well-nourished mothers. In Table 5-1 these requirements are summarized. The minimum is the smallest amount of a nutrient needed to protect the individual from undernutrition attributable to deficiency.

The term advisable intake[2] applies to levels somewhat in excess of the estimated requirement. The margin between these two figures reflects the "degree of confidence in the estimated requirement and the likelihood of hazard from excess intake." The RDA for most nutrients represents a value well above the average estimated requirement and encompasses the range of variability observed in individual requirement estimates.

RDAs for infants up to 6 months of age are based primarily on the amounts provided by human milk but in some cases may exceed those levels to provide for infants receiving formula. RDAs for infants 6 months to 1 year of age are

Table 5-1 Minimum Requirements, Advisable Intakes, and Recommended Allowances of Selected Nutrients for Infants: 0-6 Months and 6-12 Months

	Minimum		Advisable		Recommended	
	(0-6)	(6-12)	(0-6)	(6-12)	(0-6)	(6-12)
Protein (g/100 kcal)	1.6	1.4	1.9	1.7	1.9	1.9
Protein (g/kg)	1.8	1.5	2.2	1.8	2.2	2.0
Vitamins						
A (µg RE)	75	75	150	150	420	400
D (µg cholecalciferol)	2.5	5	10	10	10	10
E (mg α-TE)	2	2	3	3	4	4
K (µg) ·	5	5	15	15	12	15
C (mg)	10	10	35	35	20	20
B_1 (mg)	0.1	0.2	0.2	0.2	0.3	0.5
B_2 (mg)	0.1	0.4	0.4	0.4	0.4	0.6
Niacin (mg NE)	2.0	4.5	5	5	6	8
B_6 (mg)	0.1	0.2	0.4	0.4	0.3	0.6
Folacin (µg)	50	50	50	50	30	45
Minerals						
Sodium (mEq)	2.5	2.1	8	6	10	21
Chloride (mEq)	2.3	2.1	7	6	8	13
Potassium (mEq)	2.4	2.0	7	6	16	21
Calcium (mg)	388	289	450	350	360	540
Phosphorus (mg)	132	110	160	130	240	360
Magnesium (mg)	16.5	13.5	25	20	50	70
Iron (mg)	7	7	7	7	10	15

Table 5-2 Ranges of Daily Intakes of Nutrients by 3-Month-Old Infants*

	Breast-Fed		Formula-Fed†	
	10th Percentile	90th Percentile	10th Percentile	90th Percentile
Protein (g/kg)	1.4	2.0	2.0	3.2
Vitamins				
A (µg RE)	380	600	455	715
D (µg)	0.4	0.6	7	11
E (mg α-TE)	1	1.5	7	11
K (µg)	10	16	22	34
C (mg)	30	45	35	65
B_1 (mg)	0.1	0.2	0.4	0.6
B_2 (mg)	0.3	0.4	0.6	0.9
Niacin (mg NE)	1	1.5	5.5	8.5
B_6 (mg)	0.05	0.08	0.3	0.4
Folacin (µg)	35	56	56	87
Minerals				
Sodium (mEq)	4.5	7.2	10.5	16.7
Chloride (mEq)	7.5	12	13.1	20.7
Potassium (mEq)	8.5	13.5	15.7	24.6
Calcium (mg)	225	360	415	650
Phosphorus (mg)	95	150	323	509
Magnesium (mg)	27	42	32	50
Iron (mg)	0.4	0.6	9	14

Based on data from Beals VA: In McCammon RW, editor: Human growth and development, Springfield Ill, 1970, Charles C Thomas Publisher.

*Estimates of intake levels of various nutrients are based on the average composition (amount of nutrients) of human milk and formulas relative to the 10th and 90th percentiles of energy intakes of infants involved in a longitudinal growth study.

† Iron-fortified Enfamil or Similac.

based on consumption of formula and increasing amounts of solid foods. In contrast to the allowances for specific nutrients, the allowance for energy is based on average needs of the population group under consideration and no adjustment is made for individual variability. For the infant 0 to 6 months old average energy needs are met by an intake of 115 kcal/kg/day, and for the 6-to-12-month-old infant by 105 kcal/kg/day. The range of intakes observed among healthy growing infants extends from 95-145 kcal/kg/day for infants 0 to 6 months old to 80-135 kcal/kg/day for infants 6 to 12 months old. The lower end of the range, approximately the 10th percentile, is slightly more than half the 90th percentile value. Thus there are substantial differences in infants' apparent energy needs. Physical activity is the dominant factor in varied energy needs during the latter part of infancy (and thereafter), since the maintenance energy requirement (basal metabolism) remains fairly stable (45% to 50% of calories) throughout the first year. Rate of growth, age, and environmental conditions such as temperature also influence energy needs.

SOURCES OF NUTRIENTS

Ranges of nutrient intakes for healthy infants who are exclusively breast-fed or formula-fed during the early months of life are shown in Table 5-2.[1,3] Breast-fed infants at the lower end of the energy intake distribution consume several nutrients in amounts very close to the estimated requirements. Nutrients in human milk tend to be more bioavailable than the same nutrients in formula, cow's milk, or solid foods.

Human Milk

Two nutrients that appear to be low in human milk are vitamin D and iron. It has been suggested[4] that a previously unidentified sulfate analogue of vitamin D in human milk is present in sufficient quantities to meet the young infant's needs, but this observation has not been confirmed.[5] Vitamin D_3, the naturally occurring form in animal tissues, is produced by the action of sunlight on 7-dehydrocholesterol in the skin. The amount produced depends on a number of variables, including length and intensity of exposure and color of the skin. For these reasons it is difficult to specify a dietary requirement for vitamin D. There is ample evidence[6] that infants who are breast-fed and have limited exposure to sunlight may develop nutritional rickets.

It is also difficult to specify a dietary requirement for iron during early infancy because of variations in levels of total body iron at birth, rates of growth, and bioavailability of iron in foods. The healthy term infant exclusively breast-fed by a well-nourished mother is not likely to be anemic by age 6 months, even though it may be in negative iron balance.[7] In the usual hematologic and biochemical measures of iron nutriture, it is difficult to distinguish this infant from one fed an iron-fortified formula for the same period.[8]

Levels of some nutrients secreted in human milk vary with maternal diet, stage of lactation, duration of lactation, and individual biochemical variability among women.[9] Caloric density and relative proportions of protein, fat, and carbohydrate in colostrum, transitional milk, and mature human milk vary considerably. The relative proportions of protein, fat, and carbohydrate in mature human milk are little influenced by maternal diet or nutritional status. The malnourished woman may be able to produce milk of acceptable quality though quantity may be limited. In the healthy and well-nourished mother the fatty acid composition of milk fat is determined primarily by diet.[10] Human milk fat represents a blend of fatty acids provided by maternal diet, maternal depot fat, and synthesis in the mammary gland. Lactating women with poor nutritional histories and evidence of undernutrition produce milk with a fatty acid composition that reflects predominantly depot (subcutaneous) fat.

There is a 30% decrease in protein content of human milk between the first and sixth months of lactation.[11] During the same time, lactose content increases slightly (10%); fat content does not change; and concentrations of calcium, phosphorus, zinc, iron, sodium, potassium, and chloride all decrease 10% to 20%. Studies of the mineral content of milk from women 1 to 31 months postpartum[12] showed that levels of some trace metals, particularly zinc, declined substantially over time. Most of the zinc in human milk is associated with protein fractions of low molecular weight whereas zinc in cow's milk is associated with fractions of high molecular weight.[13] This may explain the higher plasma zinc levels in breast-fed infants than in infants fed zinc-supplemented formulas.[14] Levels of copper and iron decrease only moderately after the first 6 months. There are no data to indicate that maternal diet or nutritional status significantly influences the levels of major minerals (calcium, phosphorus, magnesium), electrolytes (sodium, potassium, chloride), or trace metals (iron, copper, zinc, iodine, manganese, fluoride, selenium) in human milk.

Vitamin and mineral supplements are used widely during pregnancy and postpartum, especially during lactation. Thus variations in maternal diet appear to have a limited effect on levels of fat-soluble vitamins (A, D, E, K) in human milk. Variations in maternal intake of water-soluble vitamins (B vitamins and ascorbic acid) are reflected in levels of these vitamins in human milk.[14] Vitamin B_{12} deficiency has been reported in a 6-month-old infant breast-fed by his vegan mother.[15] Thiamine deficiency can occur in breast-fed infants of thiamine-deficient mothers but appears to be a problem only in some developing countries. Although it may be appropriate to recommend that infants being breast-fed by mothers who themselves are malnourished receive multivitamin supplements,[6] formula feeding in some instances represents an appropriate choice for these infants.

The changing composition of human milk during extended lactation, especially the decrease in protein content, argues for supplementation of human milk with other foods, especially those that are sources of protein, calcium, and iron, after the fifth or sixth month. Healthy infants who are exclusively breast-fed for 5 or 6 months appear to grow satisfactorily, at least during the first 5 to 7 months.[16] After this age exclusive breast-feeding appears to be associated with less adequate growth.

Immunologic Benefits of Breast-Feeding

In the past decade there has been considerable research on the nonnutritional aspects of human milk, especially its immunologic and other protective constituents. Secretory immunoglobulin A activity in mammary glands and human milk is largely derived from maternal gut-associated lymphoid tissue.[17] Secretory IgA resists the proteolytic action of the infant's gastroenteric secretions, diminishing antigen contact with the intestinal mucosa until the infant's own antibody responses develop. Human milk contains as many leukocytes as does maternal blood except

that 80% of them are macrophages. These phagocytic cells kill bacteria, viruses, and virus-infected mammalian cells. In addition, they secrete lysozymes, which mediate the inflammatory response and host defense.[18]

Available evidence indicates that lymphocytes comprise the majority of other cells in human milk. About half are B cells, which are identified by specific antibody molecules on their surface. These antibody molecules have specificity for potential antigens in the gastroenteric tract and respiratory passages. When the B cells meet antigens, they proliferate and differentiate to antibody-producing plasma cells. T cells comprise the other half of lymphocytes in human milk. They attach to the infant's intestinal mucosa and produce secretory IgA in response to bacterial, viral, and food (protein) antigens.

Lysozymes, lactoperoxidases, and lactoferrin are protein macromolecules in human milk that may be important host resistance factors for the infant. They act antimicrobially in a number of ways, including lysis of the bacterial cell membrane and chelation of the iron necessary for growth of certain microorganisms. Samples of human milk with the highest lipase activity have the highest antiviral effects.[19] The bacteriostatic effect of human milk, with unsaturated iron-binding capacities between 50% and 90%, can be abolished in vitro if the iron-binding proteins (primarily lactoferrin) are saturated with iron.[20]

The importance of these immunologic, cellular, and enzymatic components of human milk to the infant are indisputable whenever circumstances preclude the preparation, storage, and feeding of a nutritionally adequate and hygienically safe formula.

Other Nonnutrient Components of Human Milk

Drugs taken by the lactating woman may reach her infant via the milk she produces. The amount of drug secreted into human milk depends on the lipid solubility of the medication, mechanism of transport, degree of ionization, and changes in plasma pH. The higher the lipid solubility of the drug is, the greater will be its concentration in human milk. Drugs with a molecular weight of more than 600 (e.g., heparin) do not cross lipid barriers. Weakly alkaline drugs are secreted in higher concentrations in human milk than are weakly acidic ones. Nonionized drugs enter mammary alveolar cells more easily than do ionized ones, and their concentration in milk equals or exceeds their concentrations in plasma.[21] The possible consequences to the nursing infant of drugs excreted in human milk have been summarized by Hollingsworth and Kreutner.[22]

Although it may be possible to control the use of drugs by the lactating woman and to evaluate the acute or immediate potential hazard to the infant, environmental pollutants such as polybrominated (PBB) and polychlorinated (PCB) biphenyls, which are secreted in human milk, pose hazards to the nursing infant that are unknown over the long term. It has been suggested[23] that the woman whose milk contains PCBs in excess of 2.3 to 2.5 ppm (fat basis) should limit the duration of breast feeding to allow the infant the early advantages associated with breast-feeding but lessen the infant's body burden of the compound.

Immunoreactive prostaglandins have been detected in fresh human milk samples but not in cow's milk–based formulas.[24] It is known that prostaglandins are distributed throughout the gastroenteric tract and affect many physiologic functions, including gastric acid secretion, smooth muscle contraction, zinc absorption, and the release of brush border enzymes as well as water, glucose, and iron transport. Their relative importance in development and maturation of the infant's gut and early nutritional well-being requires additional study.

Limitations

Acquired knowledge about the nutritional, biochemical, microbial, and immunologic properties of human milk serves to underscore earlier assumptions of its benefit. There are, however, limitations of breast-feeding. Vitamin D deficiency has been reported in infants with limited exposure to sunlight. Deficiencies of pyridoxine, thiamine, and vitamin B_{12} have been reported in infants whose mothers consumed insufficient amounts during lactation.[25] Similarly, iron and fluoride supplements are required in fully breast-fed infants.

In addition, critical weight loss, feeding failures, and insufficient milk syndrome may occur in breast-feeding.[26,27] The need to remain alert to the possibility of inadequate lactation, especially among primigravidas, as a cause of infant weight loss has been emphasized.[28-30]. It is noted that breast-feeding failure in certain instances

can be an important cause of underweight. The infant who is fretful, irritable, frequently anxious, colicky, or vomiting may be taking frequent short feeds, resulting in a mother who is exhausted and who has an associated poor milk letdown reflex. On the other hand, critical weight loss may occur in the placid, passive, exclusively breast-fed infant who has a reduced suckling drive or defective appetite control.

Scrimshaw and Underwood,[31] in an overview of the timing of complementary feeding of breast-fed infants, observe that misunderstanding of the limitations of exclusive breast-feeding and the resultant failure to provide complementary foods at the appropriate time may lead to increased risk. They also note that there is no single time when exclusive breast-feeding is no longer adequate. They recommend that weight-for-age charts be used in making a decision, noting that there is considerable variability in the adequacy of breast-feeding alone and that dogmatic statements about the length of time it is appropriate should be avoided. Jelliffe and Jelliffe[32] observe that the growth of breast-fed infants is generally satisfactory for the first 5 months. A report by Ahn and MacLean[16] examines the growth of exclusively breast-fed infants in the United States, drawing on growth reports of 96 infants of upper-income mothers in La Leche League International. No significant differences were found during the first year in overall weight gained or length achieved between infants breast-fed exclusively for less than 6 months and those breast-fed longer. In male infants, however, after 4 months the weight and length fell below the original 75th percentile, females exhibited this shift at 6 months. Between 6 and 9 months the rate of weight gain was significantly lower in male infants exclusively breast-fed, with no significant difference in linear growth detectable at this time.

Suckle Feeding

The movements of the mother or caregiver at feeding time are important. The way she moves the infant's head, body, and limbs is significant, as are the sounds she makes and, to the extent that human infants are similar to lower mammals,[33] the odor she emits and the general smell of the maternal environment.

If the infant is in a feeding-ready state, touch stimulation in the perioral areas elicits rooting, which is a positional response of the lips and face and also of the head and neck. By this response the infant moves its mouth toward the nipple or similar object, whether the nipple touch has occurred on the cheek or on the upper or lower lip away from the mucosal margin. The rooting response is continuous with the motion of latching, by which the infant encloses the nipple and grasps it in the mouth between the lips and superior to the midline of the tongue.[34]

The infant's initial actions of suckle feeding are often irregular and ineffective, even in the feeding-ready state when the infant has participated fully in the preliminaries of rooting and latching. The posteriorward rippling protrusion of the tongue and the negative pressure about the nipple tip may be lacking. The barrier between the mouth and pharynx may not be stably closed, and thus milk may enter the pharynx before the pharynx is ready for swallowing. The infant may gasp or slightly choke before graduating into the rhythmic oral and pharyngeal actions of established suckle feeding. Suckling is a distinctive performance involving all the oral motor structures. Pressure recordings from the mouth, pharynx, and esophagus are useful in demonstrating the motor effectiveness of each stage and the timing of the stages. However, the most strategic evaluation of the internal feeding performance in feeding impairment is by cine- or videoradiography.[34]

Depending on the circumstances of suckle feeding, the infant may incidentally swallow a significant volume of air along with the milk. This enters the swallow bolus in the pharynx, and it may markedly distend the eosphagus and, in some infants, the stomach as well. Its release, by belch, is accomplished painlessly but may be associated with spill of the swallowed milk into the pharynx and mouth.[34]

The duration of a suckle feeding episode depends on the available flow of milk and the ingestion volume.[35] In breast-feeding, most of the intake from each offered breast is obtained in the first 4 mintues, but the mere performance of suckling is satisfying to the young infant, aside from the satisfaction derived from nutritional intake.

Prepared Formulas

In 1984, 45% of newborns in hospitals were fed prepared formula; and this percentage increased at 2, 3-4, and 5-6 months to 61%, 70%, and 72%, respectively. The majority of these infants received formulas derived from nonfat cow's milk or a mixture of nonfat milk and demineralized whey. Milk-based formulas marketed for full-term infants provide about 67 kcal/dl or 20 kcal per fluid ounce, with approximately 1.5 g of protein per deciliter, a level in the upper range of mature human milk. Protein provides about 9% of total calories in milk-based formula, lactose about 40%, and fat about 50% of the total calories. The lactose and fats are added along with vitamins and minerals to the basic ingredients to approximate human milk and assure good infant growth.

Soy-based formula has been given to large numbers of infants in the United States as a substitute for cow's milk–based formula. Deficiencies of certain vitamins (thiamine, vitamin K) and the occurrence of goiter were reported with earlier types of soy-based formulas.[36] When a water-soluble soy-protein isolate (acid-precipitated fraction of soy flour) became available in the 1960s, the major commercial formula manufacturers promptly used the soy isolate to reformulate existing products (e.g., Sobee to Prosobee) and to develop new soy-based formulas (Isomil, Nursoy). In addition to fortifying the products with appropriate levels of vitamins and minerals, DL- or L-methionine was added to achieve an appropriate amino acid composition.

These new soy isolate formulas promote satisfactory growth and nutritional status in healthy infants[37] as well as in infants recovering from malnutrition.[38] During the past decade an increasing proportion of healthy infants in the United States have been fed soy isolate formulas and apparently have thrived.[39] The reformulation of one product in 1978 resulted in deficient levels of chloride, and hypochloremic metabolic alkalosis developed in a number of infants.[40] Many who were fed the product, however, did not become chloride-deficient because they were receiving other foods that provided chloride. Nevertheless, the product was withdrawn from the market.

Cow's Milk

Despite substantial changes in the prevalence and duration of breast-feeding and the use of proprietary formulas in the past 10 years, approximately 9% of 6-month-old infants in the United States consume whole cow's milk or evaporated milk and the proportion increases steadily with age[41] (Table 5-3). The major dif-

Table 5-3 Infants Receiving Different Milks and Formulas at Selected Ages and Original Weights

Age and Feeding Preference	1971	1982	1983	1984	Percent Point Change 1971-82	Percent Point Change 1983-84
In hospital						
Breast*	24.7	61.9	61.4	62.5	+37.2	+0.6
WCM/EM†	0.9	0.1	0.1	0.1	−0.8	0
Prepared formula	77.4	44.9	45.6	45.1	−32.5	+0.2
TOTAL	103.0	106.9	107.1	107.7	+3.9	+0.8
At age 2 mo						
Breast*	13.9	47.2	46.5	47.5	+33.3	+0.3
WCM/EM†	14.8	1.5	1.2	0.9	−13.3	−0.6
Prepared formula	74.1	59.6	61.0	60.8	−14.5	+1.2
TOTAL	102.8	108.3	108.8	109.2	+5.5	+0.9
At age 3 and 4 mo						
Breast*	8.2	37.5	36.5	37.0	+29.3	−0.5
WCM/EM†	39.2	4.4	3.7	2.6	−34.8	−1.8
Prepared formula	54.4	66.9	68.7	69.8	+12.5	+2.9
TOTAL	101.8	108.9	108.9	109.4	+7.1	+0.5
At ages 5 and 6 mo						
Breast*	5.5	28.8	27.3	27.5	+23.3	−1.3
WCM/EM†	68.1	12.7	10.8	8.7	−55.4	−4.0
Prepared formula	28.0	66.4	69.8	72.3	+38.4	+5.9
TOTAL	101.6	107.9	107.9	108.4	+6.3	+0.5

From Martinez GA, Krieger FW: Pediatrics **76:**1004-1008, 1985.

*Includes supplemental bottle-feeding (i.e., formula in addition to breast-feeding).

†*WCM*, White cow's milk; *EM*, evaporated milk.

ferences between cow's milk and human milk are the greater concentrations of proteins and minerals and the lower concentration of lactose in cow's milk. The higher ratio of whey proteins (lactalbumin, lactoglobulin) to casein in human milk than in cow's milk has not been shown to be of nutritional significance. The butterfat in cow's milk is less well digested and absorbed than the fat in human milk. Cow's milk (or evaporated milk) meets the infant's needs for most of the B vitamins and for vitamins A and K. Most cow's milk is fortified with vitamin D, but it contains insufficient amounts of vitamins C and E, iron, and copper to serve as the only source of these nutrients for the infant. In addition, there are problems related to curd formation (relatively high casein content), digestibility of fat, and potential excess renal solute load because of the relatively high levels of protein (urea) and minerals (sodium, potassium, chloride, phosphorus) excreted in the urine.[42]

INFANT FEEDING PRACTICES
Breast-Feeding

Until the early 1940s, breast-feeding was the dominant mode of nutrient intake for infants in the United States; about 75% of all babies were breast-fed.[43] Ten years later, in the early 1950s, fewer than half of all babies were breast-fed. This figure dropped to fewer than one third by the early 1960s and to a low of about 22% to 25% in the early 1970s.[44]

During that period the declining incidence of breast-feeding in the population was accompanied by a decline in the duration of lactation in mothers of infants who were never breast-fed. In one study of firstborn infants[45] it was estimated that the average length of breast-feeding dropped by almost half in the period 1931 to 1951, from a mean of 4.2 months in 1931-35 to 2.2 months in 1951-59.

The first evidence of the reversal of this downward trend in breast-feeding appeared in 1972,[46]

Table 5-4 Percentages of Infants Breast-Feeding

	In Hospital			At 5-6 Months		
	1983*	1984*	1985†	1983*	1984*	1985† (at 5 mo)
Ethnicity						
White	64.4	65.0	64.3	28.9	28.6	29.0
Black	29.8	33.3	30.0	9.7	11.7	10.8
Maternal age (yr)						
Less than 20	39.3	36.8	37.3	8.7	10.2	9.0
20-24	55.5	58.0	55.2	19.1	19.7	20.1
25-29	65.3	66.6	64.9	31.1	30.6	30.3
	67.8	69.4	70.1	38.0	39.1	39.1
35 or older	60.7	64.7	62.8	34.9	38.5	38.8
Family income ($)						
Less than 7000	36.2	36.6	NA	12.3	12.4	NA
7000-14,999	54.0	54.5	NA	20.4	21.1	NA
15,000-24,999	63.8	64.8	NA	29.2	29.2	NA
25,000 and over	71.3	71.8	NA	33.9	33.4	NA
Maternal education						
Noncollege	49.1	50.7	NA	17.8	19.2	NA
College	76.7	77.5	76.4	39.8	38.8	39.5
Maternal employment						
Employed full time	55.5	56.2	56.2	12.2	12.3	12.9
Employed part time	65.9	67.6	63.8	28.6	28.9	28.4
TOTAL						
Employed	59.3	60.3	NA	17.5	18.2	NA
Not employed	58.0	58.6	57.9	29.0	29.2	29.9
United States census region						
New England	57.8	58.5	60.8	27.4	25.8	28.4
Middle Atlantic	48.9	50.9	49.6	23.1	23.4	23.1
East North Central	57.1	57.7	55.8	24.1	24.9	24.8
West North Central	62.3	66.0	65.6	26.9	28.2	27.7
South Atlantic	50.2	50.5	50.4	20.2	20.2	20.4
East South Central	42.7	45.9	44.5	16.1	17.3	17.6
West South Central	55.4	55.9	51.5	20.0	20.2	19.0
Mountain	75.8	77.6	76.8	36.4	37.6	37.4
Pacific	77.4	77.7	76.1	34.8	36.0	36.0
WIC						
Yes	NA	NA	40.9	NA	NA	14.3
No	NA	NA	66.1	NA	NA	30.7

*Martinez GA, Krieger FW: Pediatrics **76**:1004-1008, 1985.

†Martinez GA, Stahl D: Presented at the APHA Annual Meeting, Washington DC, November 20, 1985. (These data are preliminary through the third quarter of the year.)

NA, Data not available; *WIC*, women, infants, and children.

and the positive upturning has continued into the 1980s. In 1985, 64% of white women in the United States elected to breast-feed in hospital and 29% reported continuing until their infants were 5 months of age. Nevertheless, the proportion of women breast-feeding varies considerably by race, education, family income, maternal employment, and geographic region (Table 5-4).

Introduction to Solid Foods

In sharp distinction to contemporary practices, at the turn of the century the introduction of solid foods did not occur until the infant had reached the tenth month, and it often occurred even later. In 1895, Holt's recommendations (Cone[47]), like those of his contemporaries, were

Nothing but milk until the infant is 8 or 9 months old

At 10 months beef juice, beginning with 1 Tbsp and increasing to 4 to 6 Tbsp daily by 12 months age

Also at 10 months thin gruel made from the grains of oats, wheat, or barley, from farina, or from arrowroot; 1-3 Tbsp may be added to each feeding

A number of foods, such as bananas, liver, and bacon, were prohibited until 4 years of age. In 1909 Jacobi (Cone[47]) suggested that no vegetable of any kind be given to a child prior to 2 years of age.

Today, many infants receive solid foods by 6 weeks of age. Studies conducted by the New York City Department of Health revealed that 47% of randomly selected infants attending child health stations had received solid foods within their first month of life and by 4 months foods other than formula or milk constituted about 40% of their daily energy intake.[26]

In another study of 270 New York infants in 1980 from varying socioeconomic backgrounds, one third were given nonmilk foods by age 1 month. By age 3 months, all were receiving solid foods. Prior to 3 months, non–breast-fed infants were more likely to receive solid foods than were breast-fed infants.[48]

In a study of feeding practices in 403 Toronto and Montreal infants at intervals between 1 and 18 months of life,[49] foods were generally introduced in the following progression: cereal, sugar, fruits, vegetables, meats, dinners, and desserts. Solid foods were introduced early to bottle-fed infants. In a cross-sectional study of 250 infants in Sydney, Australia,[50] 46% of infants received solid food before 2 months and 98% received it prior to 4 months of age. Maryland studies also reflect early high intakes of solid foods and high nutrient intakes during the first year.[51] Dietary histories of 130 full-term infants on predominantly iron-fortified infant formula and utilizing health department well-baby services in six counties on the Eastern Shore of Maryland were obtained at approximately 2 and 7 months of age. The mean age of mothers was 22.2 years. In this population, new foods were generally introduced rapidly and multiple foods, rather than a single category of one or two foods, were fed. By age 1 week over 20% of infants had been introduced to one or a combination of any of 15 foods. By 2 weeks the number of foods had increased to 20 for 40% of the infants, and by 60 days it had

climbed to 40 foods, with over 90% of the infants having been introduced to many of these foods by this age. Early introduction of solid foods appeared to be responsible for the higher than necessary intake of nutrients among the 2.3-month-old infants in the Maryland study. An average intake of human milk or iron-fortified infant formula would have been adequate to meet the RDAs for all essential nutrients in these infants.

Nutrient intake greater than the age-specific RDA was noted again when the same subjects were reevaluated at mean age 7.3 months. Mothers were interviewed at their homes by a dietitian, using a 24-hour recall in combination with a frequency checklist. Mean reported daily energy intake exceeded the RDAs by 25% and mean protein intake was approximately 75% above the RDAs. Mean iron intake was twice the level recommended by the AAP Committee on Nutrition. Other selected nutrients were reported to be fed in excess of RDA levels.

In making a decision about the most appropriate time to introduce non-milk foods to the young infant, it seems advisable to monitor the growth of the infant as well as consider the infant's level of activity, environmental circumstances, and sex. Clearly, dogmatic recommendations about the introduction of nonmilk foods are inappropriate. Nevertheless, agreement seems to be emerging as to the need for additional foods between the fourth and sixth months of age.

If poor growth is observed, appropriate remedial steps should be taken regardless of age. During the subsequent months, as solid foods are introduced, human milk or formula accounts for a decreasing level of daily caloric intake. By age 9 months solid food accounts for one third of calories, but by 12 months it accounts for half the caloric intake. Furthermore, at age 9 months solid food may supply nearly half the total protein and iron intake, even though the infant continues to receive an average of 600 kcal of iron-fortified formula. If an isocaloric amount of human milk is substituted for the iron-fortified formula, the approximate total daily intakes of protein, iron, and calcium will be reduced by 20%, 50%, and 39%, respectively; solid foods will account for one half the calcium, two thirds of the protein, and essentially all the iron in the infant's diet. This example illustrates the importance of evaluating the older infant's diet to ensure food selection that complements the basic item in the diet (i.e., human milk or formula) and to provide for the shifting pattern of growth that occurs in infants during the second half of the first year.[25]

Feeding Development

The graduation from suckle feeding of milk to the ingestion of a physically varied postsuckling diet of other foods is accomplished by developmental changes in the central nervous system, with little anatomic change in the mouth, pharynx, and esophagus. These peripheral structures grow but are not much changed in form or proportion. The tongue continues to fill the central, or lingual oral, chamber; the pharyngeal palate is large within the upper pharynx; and the arytenoid apparatus is large within the larynx. The human-distinctive enlargement of the oral cavity about the pharyngeal palate and of the larynx about the arytenoid apparatus does not begin until the third or fourth year.[35]

The most notable change in the peripheral apparatus during transitional feeding is in the eruption of the incisors (usually at 6-16 months), molars (13-32 months), and cuspids (16-23 months). The role of the teeth as biting and chewing implements is difficult to assess and is probably overrated. The actions of biting and chewing, particularly in the age of feeding transition, can be accomplished effectively without teeth. The erupted teeth are probably of greater significance as sensory resources than they are for chewing. Their sensory inputs may be strategic in the development of central control of the feeding process.

The ability to ingest physically varied foods is acquired in parallel with the development of articulate speech and stability of the postural mechanisms of the head and neck. Suckle feeding continues to alternate with the current patterns of transitional feeding, being employed at the border of sleep or during distress or illness.[35] The continuation of breast- or bottle-feeding after mature feeding performance is acquired varies with local customs and with nutritional needs. Prolonged breast-feeding extends the attachment bonds of mother and infant and also provides nutritional support for the infant, which may be critical during periods of famine.[52]

If the nutrition of the mother is marginal, prolonged lactation delays the return of ovulation and thus diminishes the chance of pregnancy.[53] Prolonged breast-feeding has been indicted as a cause of dental caries[54]; however, this has been effectively challenged.[55] Prolonged bottle-feeding has been more clearly identified as a cause of dental caries, particularly if a sweetened formula is fed and if the feeding is intermittent during the sleeping period.[56] Candy pacifiers have a similar cariogenic effect and are not prohibited from being sold in the United States.

The entire suckle feeding sequence is retained throughout life, although its corollary reflexes of rooting and nipple latching are lost (to reappear only in circumstances of extensive suprabulbar brain damage). In fact, in some circumstances of feeding impairments resulting from surgery of the oral or pharyngeal area or from neurologic impairment of the oral and/or pharyngeal feeding actions, suckle feeding may be the only effective manner of voluntary oral intake.[57]

Recommendations: Birth to 6 Months

There is a general agreement that human milk is the most appropriate source of nutrients for the healthy infant during the first 5 to 6 months of life. The renewed emphasis on human milk as the ideal food has raised questions concerning supplementation with vitamins and/or minerals.

All newborns, and especially breast-fed infants, should receive vitamin K (0.5-1 mg intramuscularly or 1-2 mg orally) to protect them against hemorrhagic disease. If the infant is exclusively breast-fed by a healthy well-nourished mother and has adequate exposure to sunlight, no vitamin supplementation is necessary after the newborn period. If there is limited exposure to ultraviolet light (due to dark skin and/or limited time in sunlight), 10 mg (400 IU) of vitamin D daily is indicated. Adequate exposure to sunlight means an area of body surface equivalent to the infant's head should be in the sun for 15 minutes daily. The vitamin D supplement can be continued for the duration of breast-feeding. When formula or vitamin D–fortified cow's milk replaces human milk in the diet, vitamin D supplementation should be discontinued.[58] If the mother's nutritional status is in doubt, the infant should receive a multivitamin preparation that includes vitamins D and B_{12}.

If exclusive breast-feeding is continued past midinfancy, the infant should begin to receive iron supplements (5-10 mg daily) at 4 to 6 months of age. Iron-fortified precooked cereal is a good source of iron if food other than human milk is to be offered.

When a woman chooses not to breast-feed or to limit her lactation period, iron-fortified formula is recommended. This is a complete food for the healthy infant and requires no vitamin or mineral supplements. There are few indications for feeding commercially prepared formulas that are not fortified with iron. Some physicians oppose iron fortified formulas because they believe such feedings cause colic, spitting-up, diarrhea, or constipation. However, there is no evidence that iron-fortified formulas produce gastrointestinal side effects in infants.[59]

Unmodified cow's milk is not appropriate for infant feeding. It contains too much protein, phosphorus, and sodium for the infant's needs and is deficient in iron, vitamin C, and copper. Cow's milk not subjected to heat treatment equivalent to that employed in terminal sterilization can cause protein-losing enteropathy[60] and gastroenteric blood loss.[61] Skim milk poses the same nutritional problems for the infant as does whole cow's milk and may lead to deficiencies of essential fatty acids and total energy.[62] The 4-month-old infant fed skim milk and solid foods ad libitum may consume large quantities but achieve a caloric intake of only 80 kcal/kg/day. As a result weight gain will be slower than that of an infant fed formula or whole cow's milk and skinfold thickness will decrease rapidly, suggesting that body energy stores are being depleted.

Recommendations: 6 Months to 1 Year

For the thriving breast-fed infant, breast-feeding may be continued throughout the first year of life. Vitamin D supplements should be given as outlined, and the gradual introduction of other foods should be encouraged to provide sources of iron, protein, and other nutrients, account being taken of the changing composition of human milk as lactation continues. For most infants commercially prepared infant foods may be appropriate.

Infant cereals are prepared by precooking and partial enzyme (diastase) hydrolysis of cereal grain flour. The flour is milled to retain a maximum of naturally occurring vitamins, minerals, protein, and fiber. Such cereals are fortified with thiamine, riboflavin, and niacin. Electrolytic iron powder of small particle size and high bioavailability is used to fortify these products. Meats prepared in a sterile finely divided form are readily accepted by the infant and are good sources of protein, iron, zinc, riboflavin, niacin, and vitamins B_{12} and B_6. Vegetables and fruits supply vitamins A, C, E, folacin, and the other Bs. Strained and juice fruits are fortified with vitamin C.

If breast-feeding is discontinued in midinfancy, an iron-fortified formula is recommended and preferably continued throughout the first year, just as for the infant who is formula-fed from birth. When formula replaces human milk in the infant's diet, vitamin D and iron (medicinal) supplements may be unnecessary.[63] As with the breast-fed infant more than 6 or 7 months of age, attention must be given to the selection of solid foods. This may be less critical for the formula-fed infant, at least with respect to essential nutrients, but total calorie intake should be monitored; it may be appropriate to limit the quantity of formula to 900 ml daily.[58]

Fluoride supplementation is recommended during the first year for the breast-fed infant (0.25 mg daily starting in the first month of life), especially if breast-feeding is continued past midinfancy as the only source of nutrition.[64] If a ready-to-use formula is selected, fluoride supplementation should follow that recommended for the breast-fed infant since the ready-to-use products are manufactured with water low in fluoride content. If concentrated (or powdered) formula is used, fluoride supplements (0.25 mg) should be administered only when the water used to prepare the formula contains less than 0.3 ppm.

REFERENCES

1. Owen AL: Feeding guide: a nutritional guide for the maturing infant, Bloomfield NJ, 1979, Health Learning Systems.
2. Fomon SJ: Infant nutrition, ed 2, Philadelphia, 1974, WB Saunders Co, pp 109-117.
3. Beals VA: Nutritional intake. In McCammon RW, editor: Human growth and development, Springfield Ill, 1970, Charles C Thomas Publisher.
4. Lakdawola DR, Widdowson EM: Vitamin D in human milk, Lancet **1:**167, 1977.
5. Greer FR, et al: Bone mineral content and serum 25-hydroxyvitamin D concentration in breast-fed infants with and without supplemental vitamin D, J Pediatr **98:**696-701, 1981.

6. Committee on Nutrition, American Academy of Pediatrics: Vitamin and mineral supplement needs in normal children in the United States, Pediatrics **66:**1015-1021, 1980.

7. Garry PJ, et al: Iron absorption from human milk and formula with and without iron supplementation, Pediatr Res **15:**822-828, 1981.

8. Owen GM, et al: Iron nutriture of infants exclusively breast-fed the first five months, J Pediatr **99:**237-240, 1981.

9. Jelliffe DB, Jelliffe EFP: Early infant nutrition. In Winick N, editor: Nutrition, pre- and postnatal development, New York, 1979, Plenum Press, pp 259-299.

10. Guthrie HA, et al: Fatty acid patterns of human milk, J Pediatr **90:**39-41, 1977.

11. Lonnerdal B, et al: A longitudinal study of the protein, nitrogen, and lactose contents of human milk from Swedish well-nourished mothers, Am J Clin Nutr **29:**1127-1133, 1976.

12. Vaughn LA, et al: Longitudinal changes in the mineral content of human milk, Am J Clin Nutr **32:**2301-2306, 1979.

13. Hurley LS, Duncan JR: Intestinal absorption of zinc: a role for a zinc binding ligand in milk, Fed Proc **37:**253, 1978.

14. FAO/WHO: Requirements of ascorbic acid, vitamin D, vitamin B_{12}, folate, and iron: report of a joint FAO/WHO Expert Committee, WHO Tech Rep Ser 452, 1970.

15. Higgenbottom MC et al: A syndrome of methylmalonic aciduria, homocystinuria, megaloblastic anemia, and neurologic manifestations in a vitamin B_{12}–deficient breast-fed infant of a strict vegetarian, N Engl J Med **299:**317-323, 1978.

16. Ahn CH, MacLean WC: Growth of the exclusively breast-fed infant, Am J Clin Nutr **33:**183-192, 1980.

17. Ogra SS, Ogra PL: Immunologic aspects of human colostrum and milk, J Pediatr **92:**546-555, 1978.

18. Welsh JK, May JT: Anti-infective properties of breast milk, J Pediatr **94:**1-9, 1979.

19. Kabara JJ: Lipids as host-resistance factors of human milk, Nutr Rev **38:**65-73, 1980.

20. Bullen JJ, et al: Iron-binding proteins in milk and resistance to Escherichia coli infections in infants, Br Med J **1:**69-74, 1972.

21. Hervada AR, et al: Drugs in breast milk, Perinatal Care **2:**19-25, 1978.

22. Hollingsworth D, Kreutner AK: Drugs excreted in human milk. In Adolescent obstetrics and gynecology, Chicago, 1978, Year Book Medical Publishers Inc, pp 620-639.

23. Wickizer TM, et al: Polychlorinated biphenyl contaminators of nursing mothers' milk in Michigan, Am J Public Health **71:**132-137, 1981.

24. Reid B, et al: Prostaglandins in human milk, Pediatrics **66:**870-872, 1980.

25. Foman JT, Strauss RG: Nutrient deficiencies in breast-fed infants, N Engl J Med **299:**355-356, 1978.

26. Paige DM: Infant growth and nutrition, Clin Nutr **2**(5):14-18, 1983.

27. The Nutrition Foundation: Critical weight loss in breast-fed infants, Nutr Rev **41:**53-56, 1983.

28. Grey E: Underweight breast-fed babies, Lancet **1:**977, 1976.

29. Gilmore HE, Rowland TW: Clinical malnutrition in breast-fed infants, Am J Dis Child **132:**885-887, 1978.

30. Davies DP: Is inadequate breastfeeding an important cause of failure to thrive? Lancet **1:**541-542, 1979.

31. Scrimshaw NS, Underwood B: Timely and appropriate complementary feeding of the breast-fed infant. An overview, UN Univ Food Nutr Bul **2**(2):19-22, 1980.

32. Jelliffe DB, Jelliffe EFP: Adequacy of breast feeding, Lancet **2:**691-692, 1979.

33. Gryboski JD: The swallowing mechanism of the neonate. I. Esophageal and gastric motility, Pediatrics **35:**445-452, 1965.

34. Bosma JF: Development of feeling, Clin Nutr **5**(5):210-218, 1986.

35. Blass EM, Teicher MH: Suckling, Science **210:**15-20, 1980.

36. Committee on Nutrition, American Academy of Pediatrics: Appraisal of nutritional adequacy of infant formulas used as cow milk substitutes, Pediatrics **31:**329-338, 1963.

37. Fomon SJ, et al: Requirements for protein and essential amino acids in early infancy: studies with a soy-isolate formula, Acta Paediatr Scand **62:**33, 1973.

38. Graham GG, et al: Dietary protein quality in infants and children. IV. Isolated soy protein milk, Am J Dis Child **120:**419-423, 1970.

39. Fomon SJ: What are infants fed in the United States? Pediatrics **56:**350-354, 1975.

40. Roy S III, Arant BS Jr: Hypokalemic metabolic alkalosis in normotensive infants with elevated plasma renin activity and hyperaldosteronism: role of dietary chloride deficiency, Pediatrics **67:**423-429, 1981.

41. Martinez GA, Krieger FW: 1984 milk feeding patterns in the United States, Pediatrics **76:**1004-1008, 1985.

42. Ziegler EE, Fomon SJ: Fluid intake, renal solute load, and water balance in infancy, J Pediatr **78:**561, 1971.

43. Faden RR, Gielen A: Contemporary breast feeding patterns: focus on disadvantaged women, Clin Nutr **5**(5):200-209, 1986.

44. Hendershot GE: Trends in breastfeeding, Pediatrics **74**(suppl):591-602, 1984.

45. Hirschman C, Butler M: Trends and differentials in breastfeeding: an update, Demography **18:**39-54, 1981.

46. Martinez GA, Nalezienski JP: Recent trends in breast feeding: 1980 update, Pediatrics **67:**260, 1981.

47. Cone TE Jr: History of infant and child feeding. In Bond JT, et al, editors: Infant and child feeding, New York, 1981, Academic Press, Inc.

48. Andrew EM, et al: Infant feeding practices of families belonging to a prepaid group practice health care plan, Pediatrics **65:**978-988, 1980.

49. Yeung DL, et al: Infant feeding practices, Nutr Rep Int **23:**249-260, 1981.

50. Allen J, Haywood PF: Infant feeding practices in Syndey, Aust Pediatr J **15:**113-117, 1979.

51. Paige DM, Palmer NH: WIC food packs: analysis and recommendations. Child Nutrition Amendments of 1978, Washington DC, 1978, Government Printing Office, pp 371-402.

52. Jelliffe D, Jelliffe EFP: Human milk in the modern world, New York, 1978, Oxford University Press Inc.

53. Knodel J: Breast-feeding and population growth, Science **198:**1111-1115, 1977.

54. Kotlow LA: Breast feeding: a cause of dental caries in children, J Dent Child **44:**192-193, 1977.

55. Countryman BA, et al: Recommendation on breastfeeding [letter], J Dent Child **44:**498, 1978.

56. Gardner DE, et al: At-will breast feeding and dental caries: four case reports, J Dent Child **44:**186-191, 1977.

57. Ramsey WO: Suckle facilitation of feeding in selected adult dysphagic persons, J Dysphagia **1:**7-12, 1986.

58. Fomon SJ, et al: Recommendations for feeding normal infants, Pediatrics **63:**52-59, 1979.

59. Oski FA: Iron-fortified formulas and gastrointestinal symptoms in infants: controlled study, Pediatrics **66:**168-170, 1980.

60. Woodruff CW, Clark JL: The role of fresh cow milk in iron deficiency, Am J Dis Child **124:**18-30, 1972.

61. Walker-Smith J, et al: Cow's milk-sensitive enteropathy, Arch Dis Child **53:**375-380, 1978.

62. Fomon SJ, et al: Skim milk in infant feeding, Acta Paediatr Scand **66:**17-30, 1977.

63. Fomon SJ, et al: Cow milk feeding in infancy: gastrointestinal blood loss and iron nutritional status, J Pediatr **98:**540-545, 1981.

64. Committee on Nutrition, American Academy of Pediatrics: Fluoride supplementation: revised dosage schedule, Pediatrics **63:**150-152, 1979.

CHAPTER 6
Children and Adolescents

David M. Paige
George M. Owen

Nutrition is concerned directly with the provision of energy and nutrients needed for cellular structures in various metabolic systems and is critical to the growth, health, well-being, and intellectual development of children. It is operative at many levels. On the most primitive plane, it is essential for survival. On the most advanced level, it is critical to realizing the fullest intellectual performance. Between these two extremes, nutrition affects the child's perception of his home and environment, integration with his family, identification with his culture, and his social and cognitive development.[1]

CHILDHOOD

Changing nutritional requirements through childhood are closely related to growth. Nutrient intake must meet the requirements not only for growth, maintenance, and repair but also for increasing physical activity.

In addition to age- and sex-specific variability in human growth and nutritional requirements, there are individual variations in growth rate and in timing of maturational events. Repeated measurements of height and weight provide the simplest and best index of physical growth. By plotting a child's body measurements on a reference growth chart the clinician can determine how consistently the child is maintaining his percentile relationship to others of his chronologic age and sex. Hence, nutritional requirements in the individual child are determined by sex, physical size, rate of growth, amount of physical activity, and biologic maturation.

Children should be assessed not only for height and weight but also for rate of growth, relative proportions, and maturity in relation to chronologic age. Radiologic examination may be used to evaluate development. The appearance of centers of ossification and fusion of epiphyses will usually show whether an individual child's osseous development is delayed or advanced for his age. The dentition can be used to help confirm such observations.

The rate of growth at any age clearly is influenced by the interaction of genetic and environmental factors. A child's pattern of growth and potential adult structure are genetically determined, but environment significantly affects patterns of growth and the extent to which predetermined adult stature will be achieved. In an environment where nutrition is always adequate both quantitatively and qualitatively, where the parents are caring, and where social factors are stable, the genetic profile largely determines individual differences in growth and adult physique. In an environment that is suboptimal or unstable, differences in growth patterns and adult stature reflect individuals' health and social and economic status as much as their genetic endowment.

Growth and Nutritional Requirements

As a result of individual variations in growth, physiology, metabolism, and energy expenditure during childhood, there can be no single definition of an optimal diet. Nevertheless, population-based age-specific recommended allowances are a useful starting point, keeping in mind that recommended dietary allowances ensure sufficient intake for 97.5% of the healthy population.[2] Nutrient intakes below specified levels may be compatible with adequate nutrition. Recommended allowances also assume that the requirement for one nutrient is complemented by an adequate intake of energy and other nutrients. Individual differences in nutrient requirements, coupled with variability in levels of recommended nutrients and heterogeneity of diets, complicate the task of providing meaningful dietary counsel for the child.

The growth rate, already decelerating in late

infancy, continues its decline through the second year. It then remains relatively constant throughout the preschool years. During the second year the reference child will gain 2.5 kg of body weight, 12 cm in length, and less than 2.5 cm in head circumference. Average increments per year from ages 3 to 5 years are 2 kg of body weight and 7 cm in height. During early school years, average annual gain is 3 kg and 6 cm, but this relatively constant rate is interrupted at age 10 in girls and age 12 in boys in the adolescent growth spurt. Paralleling these shifts in growth patterns is a corresponding shift in energy and nutrient requirements. Clearly, growth velocity influences energy needs.[4] The precise body composition of the reference boy and girl from birth to age 10 years is presented in Table 6-1. Data on fat-free body mass at each age interval are also presented.

Energy. Energy requirements in a child must allow for (1) basal metabolism, (2) specific dynamic action of food, (3) losses in excreta, (4) muscular activity, and (5) growth. The average energy requirement for basal metabolism during the first 12 to 18 months of life is 55 kcal/kg of body weight. Thereafter, the requirement on a weight basis declines to an adult level of 25 to 30 kcal/kg. Specific dynamic action of food in the average U.S. diet is approximately 6 kcal/kg. High protein intakes may more than double this figure. For the average child, losses in urine and feces approximate 10% of daily intake. Energy required for physical activity obviously varies considerably from child to child. Energy allocated to activity on a weight-specific basis rises initially with age, from 20 to 28 kcal/kg between the first and fourth years. By 9 to 10 years it has dropped back to 20 kcal/kg. This contrasts with 6 kcal/kg in a moderately active adult.[5]

The energy requirements for growth decline with increasing age.[5] At age 3 months the infant requires 28 kcal/kg, at 9 to 12 months 6 kcal/kg, from 2 to 5 years 2 kcal/kg, and from 9 to 17 years 1 kcal/kg[6] (Table 6-2).

Protein. At birth nitrogen comprises approximately 2% of the body mass. When adult levels are reached at about 4 years of age, the body's nitrogen content is 3%. On an average diet, nitrogen retention decreases to a level of 11.0 mg/kg/day at age 4 years from a maximum of 204 mg/kg/day at age 1 month.

On a weight-specific basis, protein require-

ments decrease from the first month of life through childhood and adolescence. The decrease is most precipitous during the first six months of life. Safe levels of protein intake[7] approximate 2.2 g/kg/day (below age 6 mo), 2.0 g/kg/day (at 6-11 mo), and 1.76, 1.50, and 1.20 g/kg/day (at ages 1-3, 4-6, and 7-10 yr, respectively) (Fig. 6-1).

The quality of dietary protein also must be considered. Eight amino acids are essential for all human beings. Since the body cannot synthesize them, they must be obtained from the diet. In addition to isoleucine, leucine, lysine, methionine, phenylalanine, threonine, tryptophan, and valine, histidine is essential for growth in normal infants, during certain disease states, and possibly for tissue repair at other times.[5] Estimated requirements for essential amino acids as a proportion of total amino nitrogen decline progressively from infancy through childhood to adult life. The requirements for essential amino acids are greater for growth than for repair. Thus, the diet with protein composition appropriate for adults may not be suitable for young children.[6,8]

Lipids. Fat levels vary with the individual. Fat in the diet and that derived from excess carbohydrate and protein contributes to repair and building of many body tissues. It also plays a role in absorption of fat-soluble vitamins (A, D, E, K). Fat spares protein and is critical to the synthesis of steroid hormones. In addition, it is a source of concentrated energy.

According to some evidence, highly unsaturated fatty acids may be essential and cannot be synthesized by the body. Experimentally, diets deficient in linoleic and arachidonic acids may be responsible for poor growth and eczema. Low-fat diet experiments in children indicate that fat may be essential to normal growth.

During the early months of life, fat provides nearly one-half the calories in the infant's diet. This is especially true during the period of exclusive breast feeding.

Generally, after the nursing period, about one third of calories should be in the form of fat. Very low fat diets usually lead to high carbohydrate intake, as in the cases of celiac disease or cystic fibrosis. It is not clear whether diets low in saturated fats reduce the likelihood of adult atherosclerosis in children without a family history of hyperlipidemia. Despite the absence of direct evidence, it seems prudent to recom-

Table 6-1 Body Composition of Reference Children

						Components of FFBM (% of body wt)						
			Fat				Water			Minerals		
Age	Length (cm)	Wt (g)	(g)	(%)	FFBM* (g)	Protein	Total Body	Extra-cellular	Cellular	Osseous	Non-osseous	Carbo-hydrate
Boys												
Birth	51.6	3545	486	13.7	3059	12.9	69.6	42.5	27.0	2.6	0.6	0.5
1 mo	54.8	4452	671	15.1	3781	12.9	68.4	41.1	27.3	2.6	0.6	0.5
2 mo	58.2	5509	1095	19.9	4414	12.3	64.3	38.0	26.3	2.4	0.6	0.5
3 mo	61.5	6435	1495	23.2	4940	12.0	61.4	35.7	25.8	2.3	0.6	0.5
4 m0	63.9	7060	1743	24.7	5317	11.9	60.1	34.5	25.7	2.3	0.5	0.4
5 mo	65.9	7575	1913	25.3	5662	11.9	59.6	33.8	25.8	2.3	0.5	0.4
6 mo	67.6	8030	2037	25.4	5993	12.0	59.4	33.4	26.0	2.3	0.5	0.4
9 mo	72.3	9180	2199	24.0	6981	12.4	60.3	33.0	27.2	2.3	0.6	0.5
12 mo	76.1	10150	2287	22.5	7863	12.9	61.2	32.9	28.3	2.3	0.6	0.5
18 mo	82.4	11470	2382	20.8	9088	13.5	62.2	32.3	29.9	2.5	0.6	0.5
24 mo	87.2	12590	2456	19.5	10,134	14.0	62.9	31.9	31.0	2.6	0.6	0.5
3 yr	95.3	14675	2576	17.5	12,099	14.7	63.9	31.1	32.8	2.8	0.6	0.5
4 yr	102.9	16690	2656	15.9	14,034	15.3	64.8	30.5	34.2	2.9	0.6	0.5
5 yr	109.9	18670	2720	14.6	15,950	15.8	65.4	30.0	35.4	3.1	0.6	0.5
6 yr	116.1	20690	2795	13.5	17,895	16.2	66.0	29.6	36.4	3.2	0.6	0.5
7 yr	121.7	22850	2931	12.8	19,919	16.5	66.2	29.1	37.1	3.3	0.6	0.5
8 yr	127.0	25300	3293	13.0	22,007	16.6	65.8	28.3	37.5	3.4	0.6	0.5
9 yr	132.2	28130	3724	13.2	24,406	16.8	65.4	27.6	37.8	3.5	0.6	0.5
10 yr	137.5	31440	4318	13.7	27,122	16.8	64.8	26.7	38.0	3.5	0.6	0.5
Girls												
Birth	50.5	3325	495	14.9	2830	12.8	68.6	42.0	26.7	2.6	0.6	0.5
1 mo	53.4	4131	668	16.2	3463	12.7	67.5	40.5	26.9	2.5	0.6	0.5
2 mo	56.7	4989	1053	21.1	3936	12.2	63.2	37.1	26.1	2.4	0.6	0.5
3 mo	59.6	5743	1366	23.8	4377	12.0	60.9	35.1	25.8	2.3	0.6	0.5
4 mo	61.9	6300	1585	25.2	4715	11.9	59.6	33.8	25.8	2.3	0.5	0.4
5 mo	63.9	6800	1769	26.0	5031	11.9	58.8	33.0	25.9	2.2	0.5	0.4
6 mo	65.8	7250	1915	26.4	5335	12.0	58.4	32.4	26.0	2.2	0.5	0.4
9 mo	70.4	8270	2066	25.0	6204	12.5	59.3	32.0	27.3	2.3	0.5	0.4
12 mo	74.3	9180	2175	23.7	7005	12.9	60.1	31.8	28.3	2.3	0.5	0.5
18 mo	80.2	10780	2346	21.8	8434	13.5	61.3	31.5	29.8	2.4	0.6	0.5
24 mo	85.5	11910	2433	20.4	9477	13.9	62.2	31.5	30.8	2.4	0.6	0.5
3 yr	94.1	14100	2606	18.5	11,494	14.4	63.5	31.3	32.2	2.5	0.6	0.5
4 yr	101.6	15960	2757	17.3	13,203	14.8	64.3	31.2	33.1	2.5	0.6	0.5
5 yr	108.4	17660	2949	16.7	14,711	15.0	64.6	31.0	33.6	2.5	0.6	0.5
6 yr	114.6	19520	3208	16.4	16,312	15.2	64.7	30.8	34.0	2.6	0.6	0.5
7 yr	120.6	21840	3662	16.8	18,178	15.2	64.4	30.3	34.1	2.5	0.6	0.5
8 yr	126.4	24840	4319	17.4	20,521	15.2	63.8	29.6	34.2	2.5	0.6	0.5
9 yr	132.2	28460	5207	18.3	23,253	15.1	63.0	28.9	34.1	2.5	0.6	0.5
10 yr	138.3	32550	6318	19.4	26,232	15.0	62.0	28.1	33.9	2.5	0.6	0.5

From Fomon SJ, et al: Am J Clin Nutr **35:**1169-1175, 1982.
FFBM, Fat-free body mass.

Table 6-2 Estimated Energy Expenditure of Males per Kilogram of Body Weight

Age	Reference Weight (kg)	Maintenance		Growth		Activity	
		kcal	MJ*	kcal	(MJ)	kcal	MJ
<3 mo	4.6	79	0.33	28	(0.12)	12	0.04
9-12 mo	9.6	83	0.35	6	(0.03)	16	0.06
2-3 yr	13.6	75	0.31	2	(0.01)	23	0.10
4-5 yr	17.4	69	0.29	2	(0.01)	28	0.12
9-10 yr	31.3	56	0.23	1	(0.004)	21	0.09
16-17 yr	60.3	42	0.17	1	(0.004)	9	0.04
Adult (average activity)	65	40	0.17	—	—	6	0.03

Modified from World Health Organization: WHO Tech Rep Ser 522, 1973.

*MJ, Megajoules, equivalent to 737.5 ft-lb of energy.

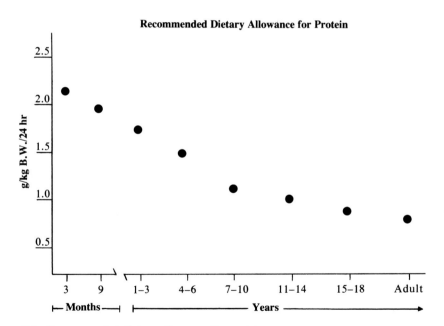

Figure 6-1. Recommended dietary allowance for protein.

From Committee on Dietary Allowances, Food and Nutrition Board, National Research Council: Recommended dietary allowances, ed 9, Washington DC, 1980, National Academy of Sciences.

mend limiting the ingestion of saturated fats.[5]

Minerals. During childhood there is a progressive increase in both absolute and relative mineral content of the body; thus in the adult 4.35% of body weight is mineral ash compared to 3% at birth.

The three major groups of minerals include (1) sodium, potassium, calcium, and magnesium; (2) chlorine, phosphorus, and sulfur; and (3) iron, iodine, and trace elements.

Mineral requirements are covered in Chapters 1 and 34 and are referred to only briefly here. Sodium and potassium requirements for growing children are met easily, since most foods contain an abundant supply. Calcium required during growth is estimated to be 50 to 70 mg/kg/day. A calcium intake of 1 g/day provides an ample margin of safety. Exact magnesium requirements are not known. About 16% of ingested magnesium is retained.[2] The usual diet is assumed to contain an adequate amount of magnesium.[5]

Phosphorus intake should be approximately 1.5 g daily in growing children, with an appropriate intake of vitamin D. Chlorine is abundantly supplied in food, and sulfur intake is sufficient with adequate protein intake.[6,8] Iron, trace elements, and vitamins are reviewed elsewhere in this manual.

The gains in length and weight and the components of weight gain are presented in Table 6-3. Information on the given fat-free body mass and the component gain in FFBM are also presented.

Feeding Patterns in Children

Food habits, patterns, practices, and preferences evolve during childhood. In reviewing the food habits of any child, it is important to keep in mind nutritional requirements, culture, socioeconomic status, and family dynamics as they influence the individual.

With the youngster's developing motor skills, less assistance is required in eating. By age 18 months to 2 years many toddlers are quite adept at feeding themselves. Individual dietary preferences appear and children should be allowed to choose the foods they like. Toddlers often prefer small frequent feedings of finger foods and will reject, or simply pick at, a prepared meal. This behavior should not alarm the parent, not should it be misperceived as a challenge to parental authority.

Parents distraught over eating patterns of 2- and 3-year-old children frequently can be reassured that personal problems such as psychogenic anorexia and atypical (by adult standards) eating behavior are normal during this period of experimentation.

Toddlers usually will ingest appropriate levels of nutrients if offered a balanced diet. Parents should be aware that the period of maximum growth has been completed by the end of the first year; between ages 1 and 5 years growth slows and is reflected by a proportional decline in nutrient intake on a weight-adjusted basis.

By age 5 years children can effectively use a knife and fork. Although they may need occasional assistance, they are fairly self-sufficient in obtaining and ingesting food. There are increased opportunities for socialization through school experiences, with exposure to new foods and new practices. Asking children to assist in preparing or serving a new food will permit them to overcome their reluctance to experiment with new foods.

School programs. Many children in the United States currently participate in Department of Agriculture–sponsored food programs. These include the special Supplemental Food Program for Women, Infants, and Children (WIC) and the School Nutrition Programs (School Lunch, School Breakfast, and Special Milk) as well as the Child Care Food Programs and the Summer Food Assistance Program. Over 90% of all schools in the United States participate and more than 23 million children are involved.

The National School Lunch Program utilizes a meal pattern intended to adjust both energy and nutrient intakes to the age of the child (Table 6-4). Minimum requirements are specified and periodically updated by the USDA. The pattern is designed to provide about one third of recommended dietary allowances. The school breakfast consists of milk, fruit or juice, and bread or cereal and furnishes approximately one sixth of the RDAs for a 10-to-12-year-old child.[9,10]

The impact of these programs on the nutritional well-being and behavioral activity of students within the classroom has been studied,[11] but results are inconclusive. Yet, nutritional supplementation of disadvantaged elementary school children does result in improved growth.[12] Additional information is needed to evaluate

Table 6-3 Length and Weight Gains in Reference Children

Age	Length (mm/da)	Weight (g/da)	Fat (g/da)	Fat (%)	FFBM* (g/da)	Protein (g/da)	Protein (%)	Water (g/da)	Minerals (g/da)	Carbohydrate (g/da)
Boys										
0-1 mo	1.03	29.3	6.0	20.4	23.3	3.7	12.5	18.6	0.9	0.1
1-2 mo	1.13	35.2	14.1	40.2	21.1	3.5	10.0	16.6	0.8	0.1
2-3 mo	1.06	29.9	12.9	43.2	17.0	3.0	10.0	13.3	0.6	0.1
3-4 mo	0.80	20.8	8.3	39.6	12.6	2.3	10.9	9.8	0.5	0.1
4-5 mo	0.65	16.6	5.5	32.9	11.1	2.0	12.1	8.6	0.4	0.1
5-6 mo	0.57	15.2	4.1	27.3	11.0	2.0	13.2	8.5	0.4	0.1
6-9 mo	0.52	12.6	1.8	14.2	10.8	2.0	15.8	8.4	0.4	0.1
9-12 mo	0.42	10.7	1.0	9.0	9.7	1.8	17.0	7.5	0.4	0.1
12-18 mo	0.34	7.2	0.5	7.2	6.7	1.3	18.4	5.0	0.3	<0.1
18-24 mo	0.26	6.1	0.4	6.6	5.8	1.1	18.7	4.3	0.3	<0.1
2-3 yr	0.22	5.7	0.3	5.8	5.4	1.1	19.1	4.0	0.2	<0.1
3-4 yr	0.21	5.5	0.2	4.0	5.3	1.1	19.7	3.9	0.3	<0.1
4-5 yr	0.19	5.4	0.2	3.2	5.3	1.1	19.9	3.9	0.3	<0.1
5-6 yr	0.17	5.5	0.2	3.7	5.3	1.1	19.8	3.9	0.3	<0.1
6-7 yr	0.15	5.9	0.4	6.3	5.5	1.1	19.5	4.1	0.3	<0.1
7-8 yr	0.14	6.7	1.0	14.8	5.7	1.2	17.9	4.2	0.3	<0.1
8-9 yr	0.14	7.8	1.2	15.2	6.6	1.4	17.9	4.8	0.4	<0.1
9-10 yr	0.15	9.1	1.6	18.0	7.4	1.6	17.5	5.4	0.4	<0.1
Girls										
0-1 mo	0.94	26.0	5.6	21.4	20.4	3.3	12.5	16.3	0.8	0.1
1-2 mo	1.10	28.6	12.8	44.9	15.8	2.8	9.8	12.3	0.6	0.1
2-3 mo	0.94	24.3	10.1	41.5	14.2	2.6	10.6	11.0	0.5	0.1
3-4 mo	0.77	18.6	7.3	39.3	11.3	2.1	11.3	8.7	0.4	0.1
4-5 mo	0.65	16.1	5.9	36.7	10.2	1.9	11.8	7.9	0.4	0.1
5-6 mo	0.63	15.0	4.9	32.4	10.1	1.9	12.6	7.8	0.4	0.1
6-9 mo	0.51	11.2	1.7	14.9	9.5	1.8	16.0	7.3	0.4	0.1
9-12 mo	0.43	10.0	1.2	11.9	8.8	1.7	16.7	6.8	0.3	<0.1
12-18 mo	0.32	8.7	0.9	10.7	7.8	1.5	17.0	6.0	0.3	<0.1
18-24 mo	0.29	6.2	0.5	7.8	5.7	1.1	17.5	4.4	0.2	<0.1
2-3 yr	0.24	6.0	0.5	7.9	5.5	1.0	17.6	4.2	0.2	<0.1
3-4 yr	0.20	5.1	0.4	8.1	4.7	0.9	17.5	3.6	0.2	<0.1
4-5 yr	0.19	4.7	0.5	11.3	4.1	0.8	17.0	3.2	0.2	<0.1
5-6 yr	0.17	5.1	0.7	13.9	4.4	0.8	16.6	3.3	0.2	<0.1
6-7 yr	0.16	6.4	1.2	19.6	5.1	1.0	15.6	3.9	0.2	<0.1
7-8 yr	0.16	8.2	1.8	21.9	6.4	1.2	15.2	4.9	0.2	<0.1
8-9 yr	0.16	9.9	2.4	24.5	7.5	1.5	14.8	5.7	0.3	<0.1
9-10 yr	0.17	11.2	3.0	27.2	8.2	1.6	14.3	6.2	0.3	<0.1

From Fomon SJ, et al: Am J Clin Nutr **35:**1169-1175, 1982.
FFBM, Fat-free body mass.

Table 6-4 Age-Specific School Lunch Pattern Requirements

Food Components	Preschool Children		Elementary School Children		Secondary School Children ⩾12 yr
	1-2 yr	3-5 yr	6-8 yr	9-11 yr	
Meat and Meat Alternatives					
Meat (1 serving of cooked lean meat, poultry, or fish, or meat alternative)	1 oz equivalent	1½ oz equivalent	1½ oz equivalent	2 oz equivalent	3 oz equivalent
Cheese	1 oz equivalent	1½ oz equivalent	1½ oz equivalent	2 oz equivalent	3 oz equivalent
Eggs* (1 large egg replaces 1 oz lean meat)	1	¾	¾	1	1½
Cooked dry beans/peas* (1 cup replaces 1 oz lean meat)	¼ c	⅜ c	⅜ c	½ c	¾ c
Peanut butter* (2T replaces 1 oz lean meat)	1 T	1½ T	1½ T	2 T	3 T
Vegetables and Fruits					
Two or more servings (full-strength vegetable or fruit juice can meet not more than ½ of total requirement)	½ c	½ c	½ c	¾ c	¾ c
Bread and Bread Alternates					
One serving (1 slice) of enriched or whole grain bread; or a serving of biscuits, rolls, muffins, etc. made with whole grain or enriched meal or flour; or a serving (1½ c) of cooked enriched or whole grain rice, macaroni, or noodle products	5 slices/wk	8 slices/wk	8 slices/wk	8 slices/wk	10 slices/wk
Milk or Fluid					
An option to fluid whole milk or flavored milk must be offered	½ c	¾ c	¾ c	½ pint	½ pint

Modified slightly from Frankle RT, Owen AY, editors: Nutrition in the community, St. Louis, 1978, The CV Mosby Co, p 115. Originally published in *Federal Register,* volume 42, number 7, September 9, 1977.

*May meet one half of the meat/meat alternate requirement.

fully the school feeding programs as a means of improving the nutritional status of children. However, the inability at present to demonstrate conclusively that such programs improved intellectual function of children does not obviate the potential short-term benefits to classroom performance or long-term improvement in nutrition.

ADOLESCENCE

Adolescence is the phase of growth that is sex hormone–induced. At a particular biologic age, which usually correlates with bone age, estrogen or androgen (produced in very small amounts during childhood) no longer suppresses the hypothalamic gonadotropin-releasing centers. There is consequently a slow but progressive in-

crease in sex hormones that integrates the individual's sexual development and the growth spurt.

Etymologically adolescence means no more than "becoming adult"; and, in fact, it begins when 80% to 85% of final stature, 53% of weight, and 52% of skeletal mass are achieved. Many adolescents almost double their weight while experiencing a 15% to 20% increase in height. In girls a relatively large component of this weight gain is increased body fat whereas in boys more of it is increased muscle mass. During peak adolescent growth the requirements for calories, proteins, and minerals exceed those of both earlier and later life.

Because of differences in biologic maturation among adolescents of similar chronologic age,

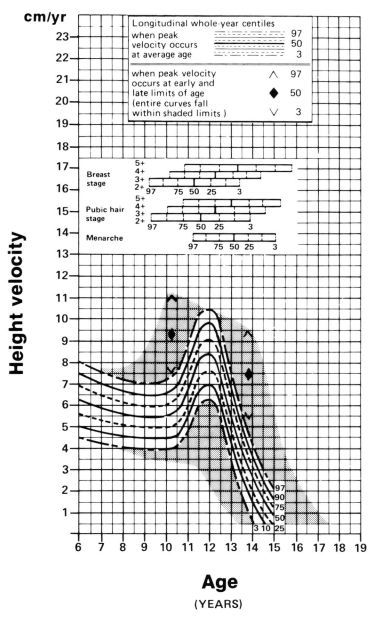

Figure 6-2. Height velocity and stage of puberty in girls.

Redrawn from Tanner JM, Whitehouse RH: Arch Dis Child **51**:170-179, 1976.

there are wide variations in caloric requirements. Growth may be as rapid as 1.2 g dry weight per day and 0.25 cm height increase per day. The 12-year-old girl growing rapidly and approaching menarche requires and consumes an appropriately higher level of calories than does a similarly matched peer who has not yet entered her maximum adolescent growth spurt. Age-specific nutrient requirements therefore must be tempered by the clinician's awareness of the biologic stage through which the adolescent is passing. As an average, in normal healthy girls, the growth spurt begins at 9.6 years of age; peak height velocity is seen at 11.8 years; stage 2 breast development occurs at 11.2 years; and menarche at 12.4 years. Normal variations around the mean are noted, as for any biologic phenomenon, but menarche before 9 years or after 16 years of age is considered outside the normal range[13] (Fig. 6-2).

Menarche

During the past 125 years mean age of menarche has decreased at a rate of 3 to 4 months per decade. Although mean age over this period has declined from 17 to below 13 years, mean weight at menarche in whites is reported to have remained constant at approximately 47 kg. This has led to a critical mass hypothesis[14] that initiation of the growth spurt, peak growth velocity, and menarche occur at certain invariant weights regardless of chronologic age. An important element in achieving this stage of reproductive maturity appears to be a progressive deposition of fat.

The sharp increase in body fat in the prepubescent girl appears to be a preliminary step for menarche. A minimal level of fat deposit in relation to height in girls is considered important not only for menarche but also to sustain normal menstruation.[14] Reports of amenorrhea in women athletes and ballet dancers with decreased body fat[15] suggest an association between the two events. Amenorrhea and infertility associated with periods of famine may partly result from a loss of body fat and associated metabolic changes. Clearly, other environmental and psychogenic factors also must influence such a complex hormonal and physiologic interrelationship. Garn[16] has disputed the hypothesis regarding body fat and menarche, noting the high fertility rates among some ethnic groups in which small body size precludes reaching the critical weight figure suggested. More recently, Scott and Johnston[17] have rejected the critical weight (fat) hypothesis.

Puberty in Boys

Boys begin their pubescent growth spurt approximately 2 years later than girls. In addition, their rate of growth is more variable than in girls. The onset of adolescence is initiated by gonadotropin-stimulated enlargement of the testes in the 9-to-12 year age range. In turn, testosterone is responsible for an increase in the size of the penis and growth of axillary, pubic, and facial hair. Skeletal growth continues at an accelerated rate, reaching a peak of approximately 10.3 cm/ year at age 14.1 years (Fig. 6-3). Associated changes in muscle mass, voice, and physical skills also are noted. Linear growth almost ceases at approximately 18 years, although some individuals continue to grow taller well into their twenties.

Hormones and Growth

The adolescent growth spurt and accompanying changes in nutritional needs are produced by joint and integrated actions of growth hormone, adrenal androgens, and testosterone. The precise role of each remains unclear, yet they do stimulate and influence morphologic events. Testosterone and growth hormone are essential for the male growth spurt. Each appears responsible for approximately half the spurt. In normal puberty growth hormone probably continues to be produced at a rate similar to that in childhood, accounting for a preadolescent growth velocity of 4 cm/year. Testosterone and adrenal androgens extend this yearly velocity during puberty by an additional 5 cm/year at peak growth. In girls the integrated effect of growth is less clear, but adrenal androgens may be responsible for the extra velocity.[18]

Increased muscle mass in boys may be due to testosterone, which is responsible for less fat, particularly in the limbs. Growth of the chest and shoulders in boys is a result of increased androgens, which stimulate cartilage in the coracoid and acromial processes of the scapula, in the sternal end of the clavical, and in the heads and tubercles of the ribs. In girls a new center of ossification, the os acetabuli, is seen between the ilium and pubis in the acetabular floor. Cells of the cartilage multiply in the pubescent girl, presumably due to estrogen, and lead to the increased width of hips and pelvic inlet.

Testicular or adrenal androgens stimulate the growth of facial, axillary, and pubic hair. This is a result of the differing thresholds for hormonal stimulation as well as the predilection of hair follicles at each site for differing hormonal stimulation. Sparse growth of pubic hair, chiefly along the labia or base of the penis, is seen on average at age 11 in girls and age 12 in boys. Axillary hair appears approximately 2 years after pubic hair. Facial hair begins to grow at about the time axillary hair appears. In boys facial hair

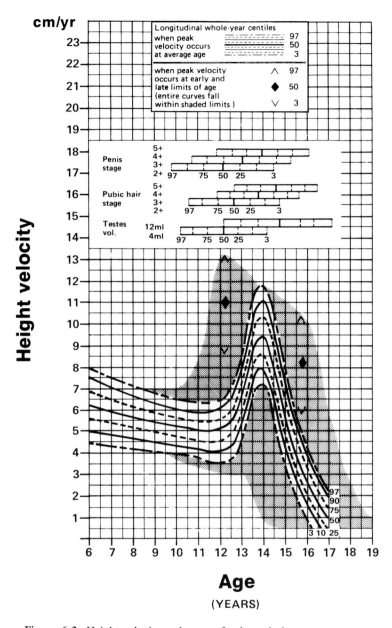

Figure 6-3. Height velocity and stage of puberty in boys.

Redrawn from Tanner JM, Whitehouse RH: Arch Dis Child **51**:170-179, 1976.

appears first at the corner of the upper lips, then on the full upper lip, upper part of the cheek, and the chin.

Hormonal control of skeletal maturation remains poorly understood, but the final stages of pubescent bone maturation, along with epiphy-sial closure, are hormone-dependent. In the absence of the onset of puberty, bone age in both boys and girls remains at approximately 13 years.

Hormonal influences on maturation and nutritional needs do not surface abruptly. Experiments in rats indicate that the immature male testes produce testosterone during the first few days after birth and this causes male differentiation. In humans the comparable maturational period would occur prenatally. Small amounts of sex hormone have been administered experimentally to inhibit the hypothalamus, which normally secretes gonadotropin releasers. This feedback mechanism operates at very low levels during infancy and childhood. At puberty, hypothalamic sensitivity to sex hormones is reduced, causing a resetting of this circuit at higher levels of sex hormone production. Evidence in humans[19] suggests that the prepubertal hypothalamic gonadostat may be about ten times as sensitive to estrogen feedback as the adult gonadostat.

Nutritional Requirements

Dietary recommendations for adolescents must take into account known and estimated individual differences. The adolescent may be particularly vulnerable to poor nutrition. It is difficult to estimate energy and nutrient needs, since both are closely related to the adolescent growth spurt and are greater than at almost any other time of life. Since these escalating needs are a function of sex, biologic age, and maturational stage rather than simply of chronologic age, recommendations that are age-specific may be inappropriate for the individual adolescent. Body mass almost doubles, making adolescents particularly vulnerable to aberrant eating patterns, unusual dietary practices, and food fads that may interfere with a steady availability of appropriate macro- and micronutrients. Accelerated anabolic needs are responsible for the adolescent's increased sensitivity to even modest levels of energy restriction, a fact not always fully appreciated by clinicians.

Energy. Peak caloric intake closely tracks peak growth spurts in both girls and boys. In girls, at 7 years of age, mean intake is 1670 calories, rising to 1970 at 8 years, 2152 at 9 years, and 2556 at 12 years before dropping to 2343 and 2260 at 14 and 17 years, respectively. Average intakes for a number of studies parallel the 1980 RDAs.

An average increase with age should be applied cautiously to the individual, however, because somatic growth and caloric intake are more clearly functions of biologic than of chronologic

age. In the 12.4-year-old girl, menarche is occurring, height velocity has peaked, weight velocity is peaking, and caloric intake is at a maximum. Another girl with chronologic age of 12.4 years who is retarded or advanced in biologic age will have caloric requirements correspondingly altered. A similar pattern of caloric intake is seen in adolescent boys. Peak intake is shifted to the right of that in girls, reflecting the 2-year delay in peak growth velocity in boys. At age 7 years the average intake in boys is 2070 calories, rising to 2431 at age 11 and to 3474 at age 16. Values of 3249 and 2966 calories are reported at ages 18 and 19, respectively.

Precise individual energy requirements are estimates at best. The most constant phenomenon is the great variability in food intake from one adolescent to another, regardless of adjustments for weight, height, surface area, age, and sex. Even when energy output is considered, differences remain. Calculations based on height may come closest to reflecting a growing child's true energy needs since they reflect the anabolic state of the growing child.[6]

Sex-specific energy requirements often are given for adolescents, since boys consume more calories per day than girls do. An increasing difference is seen through adolescence. The typical 10-year-old boy consumes 200 calories more than a girl of similar age. At 12, 14, 16, and 18 years energy intake for boys continues to exceed that for females—by 300, 400, 630, and 930 calories.

Protein. Protein requirements in childhood and adolescence parallel the individual's caloric needs. Muscle mass, blood volume, and blood constituents all increase and there is a positive nitrogen balance throughout adolescence. Adequate growth and nitrogen retention will occur if the diet provides enough essential amino acids and other required nutrients, along with adequate calories from nonprotein foods, to permit the protein to be used for tissue synthesis. Inadequate or poor-quality intake may interfere with growth and lead to increased metabolic risk, decreased physical activity, and susceptibility to infection.[7]

By age 4 years the adult body protein content (15% to 19% by weight) has been reached. Thereafter, maintenance requirements represent a gradually increasing proportion of the total protein requirement. Recommended allowances for

Table 6-5 Dietary Recommendations for Adolescents

Nutrient and Source	Males			Females				
	11-14	15-18	19-22	11-14	15-18	19-22	Pregnant	Lactating
Recommended Dietary Allowances (1980)								
Energy (kcal)*	2700	2800	2900	2200	2100	2100	+300	+300
Protein (gm)	45	56	56	46	46	44	+ 30	+ 20
Vitamin A (μg RE)	1000	1000	1000	800	800	800	+200	+400
Vitamin D (μg)	10	10	7.5	10	10	7.5	+ 5	+ 5
Vitamin E (mg α-TE)	8	10	10	8	8	8	+ 2	+ 3
Vitamin C (mg)	50	60	60	50	60	60	+ 20	+ 40
Thiamine (mg)	1.4	1.4	1.5	1.1	1.1	1.1	+ 0.4	+ 0.5
Riboflavin (mg)	1.6	1.7	1.7	1.3	1.3	1.3	+ 0.3	+ 0.5
Niacin (mg NE)	18	18	19	15	14	14	+ 2	+ 5
Vitamin B_6 (mg)	1.8	2.0	2.2	1.8	2.0	2.0	+ 0.6	+ 0.5
Folacin (μg)	400	400	400	400	400	400	+400	+100
Vitamin B_{12} (μg)	3.0	3.0	3.0	3.0	3.0	3.0	+ 1.0	+ 1.0
Calcium (mg)	1200	1200	800	1200	1200	800	+400	+400
Phosphorus (mg)	1200	1200	800	1200	1200	800	+400	+400
Magnesium (mg)	350	400	350	300	300	300	+150	+150
Iron (μg)	18	18	10	18	18	18	30-60 mg	30-60 mg
Zinc (mg)	15	15	15	15	15	15	+ 5	+ 10
Iodine (μg)	150	150	150	150	150	150	+ 25	+ 25

Estimated Safe and Adequate Daily Dietary Intakes (Food and Nutrition Board)	All Adolescents (11+ yr)
Vitamin K (μg)	50-100
Biotin (μg)	100-200
Pantothenic acid (mg)	4-7
Copper (mg)	2.0-3.0
Manganese (mg)	2.5-5.0
Fluoride (mg)	1.5-2.5
Chromium (mg)	0.05-0.2
Selenium (mg)	0.05-0.2
Molybdenum (mg)	0.15-0.5
Sodium (mg)	900-2700
Potassium (mg)	1525-4575
Chloride (mg)	1400-4200

Modified slightly from Dwyer J: Nutr Rev **39**:56-72, 1981.

*Mean values/light work.

children and adolescents are calculated from information on growth rates and body composition and decline from 2.0 g/kg during the last 6 months of the first year of life to 0.8 g/kg at 18 years of age. In general, protein should constitute 12% to 15% of total caloric intake.

Today protein consumption among girls and boys generally exceeds the recommended daily dietary levels. In girls at age 7 years the reported mean intake is 60 g/day, and it rises to 72 g/day at 10 years and to 80 g at 12. Then it declines to approximately 70 g/day through the remainder of the adolescent period. In boys the mean intake of protein rises from 80 g/day at 10 years to a peak of 104 g at 15 years and then it declines to 89 g at 19 years of age (Table 6-5).

Fat. In both sexes fat consumption tends to parallel caloric intake, with fat accounting for 40% to 43% of calories. Despite differences in absolute intake of fat between girls and boys, the percentage of energy derived from fat consumption is relatively constant. There is a reported rise from ages 8 to 12 years among girls, appearing to parallel the sharp increase in body

Table 6-6 Daily Increments in Body Content Due to Growth

Mineral		Average for Period 10- 20 yr (mg)	At Peak of Growth Spurt (mg)
Calcium	M	210	400
	F	110	240
Iron	M	0.57	1.1
	F	0.23	0.9
Nitrogen*	M	320	610 (3.6 g protein)
	F	160	360 (2.2 g protein)
Zinc	M	0.27	0.50
	F	0.18	0.31
Magnesium	M	4.4	8.4
	F	2.3	5.0

From Dwyer J: Nutr Rev **39**:56-72, 1981.
*Maintenance needs (2 mg/basal calorie) at age 18 years are 3500 mg and 2700 mg for males and females, respectively.

fat that takes place during this time. Approximately 17% of body fat deposit is considered necessary for the female adolescent growth spurt. Fat intake usually levels off after 12 years of age, ranging from 111 g at age 9 to 118 g at age 18. Among boys there appears to be a continuous rise in fat consumption from 9 through 18 years of age. Fat intakes range from 118 g daily at 9 years to 170 g daily at 18.

Calcium and phosphorus. Mineralization of the skeleton occurs progressively throughout childhood and early adult life (Table 6-6). The skeleton continues to become heavier long after linear growth ceases. At puberty it has achieved half its adult mass. Vertebral growth continues into the third decade of life.

The body of a 70 kg adult contains about 1200 g of calcium, approximately 99% of it in the skeleton. Despite the seeming permanence of bone and its deposits, it is constantly being formed and resorbed. This occurs more frequently during early childhood and at a declining rate during maturity and aging.

To ensure adequate calcium and phosphorus for normal skeletal development from ages 1 to 10 years, calcium allowance is set at 800 mg/day. On a unit/weight basis, growing children may require two to four times as much calcium as adults. Higher intakes, 1200 mg/day, have been recommended in the pubescent and adolescent period. Between 10% and 33% of dietary calcium is absorbed from the gut and trans-

ported, bound to albumin or in an ionized form, to bone.[2]

Phosphorus, along with calcium, contributes to supportive structure of the body. Phosphorus is present in nearly all foods, and dietary deficiency is extremely unlikely in humans.

Iron. The daily iron allowances in boys increase to 18 mg after age 10 years and continue at that level throughout adolescence. They then decrease to the prepubescent recommended level of 10 mg. In girls the daily recommended levels increase to 18 mg after age 10 but remain at this level throughout the reproductive years. The high iron requirements during adolescence reflect marked increases in blood volume and muscle mass in boys. In girls the increased iron demands for menstruation and some increases in lean body mass and blood volume are responsible for the sustained increase in daily iron levels throughout the adolescent years.[20]

The amount of stored iron in females is about half that found in males. Results of The Ten-State Nutrition Survey in the United States[21] suggested that boys 12 to 16 years of age from high-income families usually meet their iron needs. This contrasts with iron deficiency in 20% of poverty-level adolescent males. Regardless of income level, 20% of all families were reported to be deficient in iron.

Depending on the form in which iron is consumed and the iron status of the individual, approximately 10% to 15% of dietary iron is absorbed. Knowledge of the existence of iron in two categories (heme and nonheme) and of dietary elements that influence absorption makes it possible to develop more precise estimates of absorption. This permits the replacement of estimates with more precise quantitative values. Iron absorption can be enhanced by appropriate food selection. Iron from animal sources generally is absorbed more readily than that from vegetable sources.

The heme and nonheme iron in a particular meal can be calculated separately.[22] Of iron in meats, liver, poultry, and fish 40% is heme and the remaining 60% is considered nonheme. All iron in cereal grain and vegetable products is considered nonheme iron. Absorption of nonheme iron is enhanced by ascorbic acid and animal tissue. Meals can be classified as having low, medium, or high iron availability based on the levels of heme and nonheme iron and the presence of enhancers. Iron absorption can be decreased by calcium and phosphorus salts, ethylene diamine tetraacetate, phytates, tannic acid, and antacids.

Vitamins. Vitamin D is essential for the optimum metabolism of calcium and phosphorus. The long-term effects of its excessive intake, however, are unknown. Because of the recognized toxicity and apparent absence of benefits from excessive amounts of the vitamin, intakes should closely parallel the allowances recommended for children and adolescents. Levels of intake for water-soluble vitamins such as thiamine, riboflavin, and niacin parallel caloric intake during childhood and adolescence. These levels gradually increase during childhood, as does caloric need, and reach their maximum during adolescence. Unlike most other nutrients, ascorbic acid intake is not predicted by caloric intake. This, no doubt, reflects the distribution of ascorbic acid in citrus fruits and some vegetables, which are not major sources of calories. The vitamin A requirement parallels body size, reaching a peak during adolescence and remaining at that level.[20]

NUTRITIONAL REQUIREMENTS FOR SPORTS

All adolescents have need for increased total calories, protein, and other nutrients to support their rapid growth. Adolescents who compete in athletics have increased nutritional needs, which are dependent on the specific energy and lean body composition required for their sport.

Although dietary plans for athletes may often seem obscure, the basic needs, regardless of athletic participation, center on adequate proportions of carbohydrate, fat, and protein calories along with water, vitamins, and minerals.[23]

The percentage of body fat has been found to be an important variable in determining the ideal competing weight for an athlete. According to Snyder and Walker,[23] greater accuracy is achieved when changes in weight are made based on percent body fat. Athletes usually have a greater proportion of muscle mass, which is more dense than fat, and they may appear to be "overweight" by standard height-weight tables. Furthermore, when changes are based on the percent body fat, normal lean body growth in adolescents can continue during the weight change. The optimum body fat values for males and fe-

Table 6-7 Optimum Body Fat Values (%) for Males and Females by Sport*

	Males	Females
Baseball, softball	12-14	16-26
Basketball	7-10	16-27
Football	8-18	—
Gymnastics	4-6	9-15
Ice hockey	13-15	—
Skiing	7-14	18-20
Soccer	9-12	14-26
Swimming	5-10	14-26
Track and field		
Sprinting	6-9	8-20
Middle distance running	6-12	8-16
Distance running	4-8	6-12
Discus throwing	14-18	16-24
Shot putting	14-18	20-30
Jumping and hurdling	6-9	8-16
Tennis	14-16	18-22
Volleyball	8-14	16-26
Wrestling	4-12	—

Data from Smith NJ: Pediatrics **66:**139-142, 1980.
*Normal adolescents: males 14-16, females 20-22.

males by sport is listed in Table 6-7. The ideal weight for sports competition can be derived from the following formula[23-25]:

Ideal weight = Present weight ×
    (1 − [present % body fat] − [desired % body fat])

Percent body fat can be obtained by skinfold thicknesses at one of several sites: biceps, scapula, or abdomen. For example, a 15-year-old 50 kg boy competing in gymnastics was found at consultation with his physician and nutritionist to have 14% body fat; a goal of 6% body fat was chosen as his ideal for competition. His ideal body weight then would be 46 kg.

$$50 \text{ kg} \times (1 - [0.14 - 0.06]) = 46 \text{ kg}$$

A diet can then be selected to provide both the nutritional requirements necessary for adolescent growth and the energy requirements for gymnastics. Caloric needs will vary by sport as well as by the weight and competitive conditioning of the athlete. Estimates of caloric requirements for growth and athletic participation are noted in Table 6-8. The optimum distribution of caloric intake for an athlete's diet should approximate 12% protein, 30% fat, and 58% carbohydrate, levels similar to those in the average American diet. The frequency of meals should be no less than three times per day; for exhaust-

Table 6-8 Caloric Requirements

Age (yr)	Normal Growth*		Two Hours of Strenuous Exercise†	Total (based on mean caloric requirements)	
	Males (mean)	Females (mean)		Males	Females
11-14	2000-3700 (2700)	1500-3000 (2200)	800-1700	3500-4400	3000-3900
15-18	2100-3900 (2800)	1200-3000 (2100)	800-1700	3600-4500	2900-3800
19-22	2500-3300 (2900)	1700-2500 (2100)	800-1700	3700-4600	2900-3800

*From Committee on Dietary Allowances, Food and Nutrition Board, National Research Council: Recommended dietary allowances, ed 9, Washington DC, 1980, National Academy of Sciences.
†From Smith NJ: JAMA **236:**149, 1976.

ing sports activity of long duration, up to five or six lighter meals per day may be preferable. Frequent moderate-sized meals can improve efficiency from a psychologic standpoint; long intervals between meals can have unfavorable effects. A comprehensive review of specific nutritional requirements for the athlete and the basics of muscle metabolism is covered elsewhere.[23,26]

Psychologic and Environmental Influences

Many factors infringe on and modify the adolescent's diet. Most teenagers are preoccupied with physical appearance and peer acceptance. A strong desire to be lean and to have a particular body image can result in inappropriate weight reduction, dietary aberrations, and selective or widely distributed nutrient deficiencies. In adolescent girls such behavior may lead to anorexia nervosa, discussed in detail in Chapter 26.

Another problem associated with inappropriate weight loss in girls is amenorrhea, thought to be caused by the change in the ratio of lean body mass to body fat. At particular risk are women athletes, especially swimmers, and dancers who train intensively, with loss of body fat and concomitant gain in lean body mass.

On the other hand, adolescents who exercise infrequently run a high risk of becoming obese. Lack of exercise, coupled with boredom that results in increased food intake, puts the adolescent in double jeopardy for excessive accumulation of body fat. Poor self-image may lead to social withdrawal and isolation, which in turn may cause further dietary distortion and even greater peer censure.

Fast foods, fad diets, skipped meals, snacking, and high-carbohydrate foods are facts of life

in our society. Condemnation of such dietary practices does little to win the adolescent's confidence or to identify nutritional consequences of a particular practice. Many fast foods are perfectly adequate sources of energy and of selected nutrients. Pizza, hamburgers, ice cream, fishburgers, and chocolate covered peanuts all may be appropriate elements in meeting the adolescent's dietary needs. (The nutrient profile of such foods can be found in Appendix III.) However, continued intake of a single class of foods eliminates variety and balance, and skipping meals habitually can result in a low intake of selected nutrients or uncontrolled eating binges. Both practices are unhealthy. Vegetarian diets that are not restrictive may be quite appropriate nutritionally, as fully discussed in Chapter 42.

In general, the clinician may assume that the healthy, properly growing, prepubescent or adolescent youngster is receiving the recommended age-specific allowances of nutrients. When nutritional guidance is needed, it should be provided without preconceived or culturally induced bias about the importance or quality of a particular food. A rational approach is to determine the nutritional contribution of the particular food to the adolescent's overall daily needs. If deficiencies or excesses exist in the youngster's usually preferred diet, modifications can then be suggested.

DIETARY PRACTICES FOR DISEASE PREVENTION

Several areas of dietary intervention for disease prevention continue to be discussed. Atherosclerosis is of great interest. Early reinforcement of prudent dietary practices, along with the modification of adverse dietary patterns most often associated with this disease are recommended.[27]

The American Academy of Pediatrics Committee on Nutrition[28] recommends a moderate approach to feeding normal children in view of the diet-heart hypothesis. Specific recommendations include the following:

1. After 1 year of age, a varied diet from each of the major food groups is the best assurance of nutritional adequacy.
2. Detection of obesity by measuring height and weight and detection of hypertension by measuring blood pressure will permit the early recognition and treatment of these conditions.
3. Maintenance of ideal body weight, a regular exercise program, and (in teenagers) counseling concerning the dangers of smoking should be part of all health supervision visits.
4. The family history for every patient should include information about family members who have had premature heart attacks or strokes, hypertension, obesity, and hyperlipidemia.
5. Screening of children more than 2 years old who are at risk because of family history should consist of at least two serum cholesterol measurements. The high-density lipoprotein cholesterol should be measured in those who consistently have levels above the 95th percentile for age and sex. If high-density lipoprotein cholesterol is not the cause of the hypercholesterolemia, the patient should be treated with an appropriate diet and/or medication.
6. Current dietary trends in the United States toward a decreased consumption of saturated fats, cholesterol, and salt and an increased intake of polyunsaturated fats should be followed with moderation. Diets that avoid extremes are safe for children.

No changes in current feeding practices of infants are recommended. Afterward the diet should reflect moderate limitations of fat, a balanced selection of vegetables, the reduction of animal fats, and an increase in complex carbohydrates. Salt intake may be unnecessarily high and in excess of need. There is no evidence that benefit is derived from high levels of salt intake. Parents should actively seek to moderate the amount of salt in the diet. Nutrition as a factor in the epidemiology of malignancies must also be considered in health-promoting dietary practices of children.

REFERENCES

1. Paige DM: Nutritional deficiency and school performance. In Haslam R, editor: Medical problems in the classroom: the teacher's role in diagnosis and management, Baltimore, 1975, University Park Press, pp 253-279.
2. Committee on Dietary Allowances, Food and Nutrition Board, National Research Council: Recommended dietary allowances, ed 9, Washington DC, 1980, National Academy of Sciences.
3. Johnson TR: Developmental physiology and physical growth. In Moore WM, Jeffries FE, editors: Children are different, Columbus Ohio, 1975, Ross Laboratories, pp 2-5.
4. Fomon SJ, et al: Body composition of reference children from birth to age 10 years, Am J Clin Nutr 35:1169-1175, 1982.
5. Lowrey GH: Growth and development of children, ed 6, Chicago, 1973, Year Book Medical Publishers Inc, pp 330-339.
6. Burman D: Nutrition in early childhood. In McLaren DS, Burman D, editors: Textbook of pediatric nutrition, New York, 1976, Churchill Livingstone Inc, pp 46-75.
7. World Health Organization: Energy and protein requirements, WHO Tech Rep Ser 522, 1973.
8. Passmore R, et al: Handbook on human nutritional requirements, WHO Mongr Ser 61, 1974.
9. Paige DM, Egan M: Community nutrition. In Walter WA, Watkins JB, editors: Nutrition in pediatrics, Boston, 1985, Little Brown & Co, p 183.
10. Frankle RT, Owen AY, editors: Nutrition in the community, St Louis, 1978, The CV Mosby Co, pp 114-116.
11. Read MS: Malnutrition, hunger, and behavior. II. Hunger, school feeding programs, and behavior, J Am Diet Assoc 63:386-391, 1973.
12. Paige DM, et al: Nutritional supplementation of disadvantaged elementary-school children, Pediatrics 58:697-703, 1976.
13. Tanner JM: Growth and maturation in adolescence, Nutr Rev 39:43-55, 1981.
14. Frisch RE, McArthur TW: Menstrual cycles: fatness as a determinant of minimum for height necessary for their maintenance or onset, Science 185:149-151, 1974.
15. Frisch RE, et al: Delayed menarche and amenorrhea of ballet dancers, N Engl J Med 303:17-19, 1980.
16. Garn SM: Continuities and changes in maturational timing. In Brim CO Jr, Kagan J, editors: Constancy and change in human development, Cambridge Mass, 1980, Harvard University Press, pp 113-116.
17. Scott EC, Johnston FE: Critical fat, menarche, and the maintenance of menstrual cycles, J Adolesc Health Care 2:249-260, 1982.
18. Smith DW: Basics and nature of growth. In Growth and its disorders: major problems in pediatrics, Philadelphia, 1977, WB Saunders Co, pp 1-17.
19. Tanner JM: Growth and endocrinology of the adolescent. In Gardner L, editor: Endocrine and genetic diseases of childhood and adolescence, Philadelphia, 1975, WB Saunders Co, pp 14-59.

20. Dwyer J: Nutritional requirements of adolescents, Nutr Rev **39:**56-72, 1981.
21. Ten State Nutrition Survey, DHEW Publ 72-8130, Atlanta Ga, 1972, Health Services and Mental Health Administration, Center for Disease Control.
22. Monsen ER, et al: Estimation of available dietary iron, Am J Clin Nutr **31:**134-141, 1978.
23. Snyder JD, Walker WA: Nutritional problems in adolescence: anorexia nervosa and nutrition for young athletes. In Walker WA, Watkins JB, editors: Nutrition in pediatrics, Boston, 1985, Little Brown & Co, pp 747-750.
24. Smith NJ: Excessive weight loss and food aversion in athletes simulating anorexia nervosa, Pediatrics **66:**139-142, 1980.
25. Smith NJ: Sports medicine for children and youth. In Report of the Tenth Ross roundtable on critical approaches to common pediatric problems, Columbus Ohio, 1979, Ross Laboratories.
26. Bullin B, et al: Athletic and nutrition, Am J Surg **98:**343, 1959.
27. Woodruff CW: Diet in the prevention of disease in otherwise healthy children. In Walker WA, Watkins JB, editors: Nutrition in pediatrics, Boston, 1985, Little Brown & Co, pp 210-212.
28. Committee on Nutrition, American Academy of Pediatrics: Toward a prudent diet for children, Pediatrics **71:**88, 1983.
29. Tanner JM, Whitehouse RH: Clinical longitudinal standards for height, weight, height velocity, weight velocity, and stages of puberty, Arch Dis Child **51:**170-179, 1976.

CHAPTER 7
Adults

Roger Sherwin

For most of human history, limitations on the type and amount of food have been the dominant nutritional hazards to health. In fact, better nutrition may be the single most important factor in the improvement of health during the nineteenth and twentieth centuries.[1] It was not until the present century that a general concept of micronutrients was developed. This provided the stimulus to identify the 12 vitamins that are now recognized as essential for humans. It is now possible to construct a chemically defined diet (Table 7-1) that will allow adult volunteers to maintain good health for at least a period of weeks. In the "classical" era of nutritional science, interest was focused on the minimum amounts of macro- and micronutrients needed to maintain body weight and nitrogen balance while at the same time preventing the clinical manifestations of deficiency diseases. Currently a series of more complex problems is being addressed.

Today the concept of positive health implies more than the absence of clinical disease. It conveys the notion of optimum mental and physical performance and resistance to infection, combined with a minimum risk of the major chronic diseases—notably atherosclerosis and certain cancers—that appear to be related to an excess of certain macronutrients. These more recently recognized hazards of nutritional excess have introduced the concept of cost/benefit in the definition of an optimum diet. For example, a diet that maximizes growth rate, adult stature, vitality, intelligence, and fertility might also increase the risk of heart disease, diabetes, and cancer. Fortunately, the objectives of optimum present and future health are not necessarily mutually exclusive. Responsible scientists disagree about the relative hazards of nutritional excess and nutritional deficiency. Some nutritionists believe that new policies to combat nutritional excess in

Table 7-1 A Chemically Defined Diet for a Sedentary Adult Man

Substance	Grams	Substance	Milligrams	Substance	Milligrams
Water	1800	Ascorbic acid	100	Zinc sulfate	50
Glucose	600	Vitamin E	20	Ferrous sulfate	20
Ammonium acetate	21	Niacin	20	Manganese sulfate	10
Cellulose	20	Pantothenate	10	Sodium silicate	10
Trilinolein	5	Pyridoxine	3.5	Chromium sulfate	5
Calcium acid phosphate	5	Riboflavin	2.5	Nickel sulfate	5
Sodium chloride	3	Thiamine	1.5	Sodium selenate	5
Potassium chloride	3	Vitamin A	1.0	Copper sulfate	5
Magnesium carbonate	1	Vitamin K	0.1	Sodium fluoride	2
L-Leucine	1.1	Folate	0.1	Sodium molybdate	2
L-Methionine	1.1	Biotin	0.1	Stannic sulfate	1
L-Phenylalanine	1.1	Vitamin D	0.01	Potassium iodide	1
L-Lysine	0.8	Vitamin B$_{12}$	0.01	Sodium vanadate	0.1
L-Valine	0.8				
L-Isoleucine	0.7				
L-Threonine	0.5				
L-Tryptophan	0.3				

From Olson RE: Nutr Rev **36:**161-178, 1978.

one part of the population will inevitably lead to deficiency in another part. This belief is based on the assumption of a one-dimensional distribution of nutritional adequacy that moves as a whole (i.e., a decrease in nutritional excess necessarily being accompanied by an increase in nutritional deficiency). However, the one-dimensional concept of nutritional adequacy is an oversimplification that produces inappropriate policies. In most cases encountered in practice the dietary constituents that carry hazards of deficiency do not carry hazards of excess, and vice versa (although both kinds of constituents may be combined in certain foods).

NUTRITIONAL EXCESS

To understand the principles of healthful diets, it is necessary to understand the relationships between particular nutritional excesses and the chronic diseases associated with them.

Atherosclerosis

Of all the diseases related to nutritional excess, atherosclerosis is the most important in terms of severity and frequency. Atherosclerosis is responsible for approximately half of all deaths in the United States. The relationship of atherosclerosis to diet is considered in detail in Chapter 14 and will be only summarized here. In general, Americans consume relatively large amounts of saturated fat and dietary cholesterol. These increase the serum low-density–lipoprotein (LDL) cholesterol level, which enables other important atherogenic agents (including hypertension, smoking, lack of physical activity, and stress) to operate. Epidemic atherosclerotic disease occurs only in populations that consume large amounts of animal fat and that consequently have high average blood levels of LDL cholesterol. In the United States the problem is exacerbated by widespread obesity.

Hypertension

Excessive consumption of sodium and obesity are the major determinants of high blood pressure in genetically susceptible individuals. Alcohol abuse and diets deficient in potassium and/or calcium also tend to elevate the blood pressure. These dietary factors are therefore associated with the complications of hypertension, which include thrombotic and hemorrhagic cerebrovascular events as well as coronary and peripheral arterial disease.

Colorectal Cancer

The rates of cancer of the large bowel show at least a tenfold range among countries for which reliable statistics are available. The most plausible explanations for these differences are dietary ones. In general, high rates of colorectal cancer occur where intakes of fat (both saturated and unsaturated) and dietary cholesterol are high but intakes of dietary fiber are low.[2] Obesity is also associated with an increased risk of death from colorectal cancer.

The association that has repeatedly been reported between low serum cholesterol levels and the future risk of colorectal (and several other) cancers appears to be unrelated to diet. Most if not all of this association is explained by the presence of "preclinical" cancer when the cholesterol is measured. Cancer of several organs, including the colon, appears to lower serum cholesterol before other clinical evidence is present. The association is thus explained by the cancer's causing low cholesterol levels rather than the opposite.[3]

Breast Cancer

Excessive dietary fat, regardless of the degree of saturation, is the most important known environmental determinant of breast cancer.[2] A high-fat diet increases the rate of breast cancer in rats and mice exposed to several types of mammary gland carcinogens. The differences in tumor yields in rats are related to prolactin levels, which are increased by dietary fat. High fat intake has also been shown[2] to increase prolactin levels in women. All of these relationships are reviewed by Kakar and Henderson.[4]

The failure by Willet et al.[5] to find any positive correlation between the fat intake of U.S. women and their future risk of breast cancer does not refute the hypothesis that dietary fat is a major etiologic factor in breast cancer. There are a number of reasons for this statement: the measurement of individual dietary intakes is notoriously imprecise; the range of variation within a given population is quite limited; and almost all of the women in the U.S. breast cancer study[5] reported a dietary fat intake of more than 30% of calories whereas the international data show the protective effect of fat against breast cancer to be mainly at levels below 30%.[4]

Obesity

The most obvious manifestation of overnutrition is the gradual increase in adipose tissue with age. Reports of the lack of association between moderate adiposity[6] and ill health are based on seriously biased nonexperimental data[7] and should not overshadow the experimentally proved effects of increased adiposity on blood levels of LDL cholesterol, glucose, and uric acid. Weight gain is also the most common precipitating factor in maturity-onset diabetes and in essential hypertension. Both conditions can frequently be controlled if normal body weight is restored. Obesity not only exacerbates the effect of saturated fat and cholesterol in increasing LDL cholesterol but also depresses the level of HDL cholesterol, low levels of which are associated with an increased risk of coronary disease. Obesity is also associated with increased risk of death from most cancers, except those related to smoking (which is itself related to low adiposity).[8] The best available estimate[7] suggests that minimum mortality occurs at relative weights at least 10% below the U.S. average.

Tooth Decay

The relationship between dietary sugar and tooth decay is well accepted. Dental caries is an infectious disease in which *Streptococcus mutans* is the main cariogenic microorganism. Sugar, especially sucrose, promotes the growth of this organism. Sticky sweet foods taken between meals are much more cariogenic than are less sticky ones, which in turn are more cariogenic than sticky foods eaten with meals.

PROTEIN

Even after the end of the growth period, the adult body is in a continuously dynamic state. More protein is turned over daily than is ordinarily consumed in the diet, and there is a continuous loss of nitrogen through the urine and other routes. Most of the 22 amino acids, of which all tissue is constituted, can be synthesized by humans in the presence of a sufficient supply of amino nitrogen. A minority, the *essential* amino acids, must be provided by the diet, since they cannot be synthesized in the body. Because they cannot be stored, these amino acids must be available in the circulation at the time when they are required.

Essential Amino Acids

The human adult can synthesize all but eight of the amino acids. Histidine can be synthesized, to some extent, by the adult (though not by the infant), but dietary histidine may be necessary for some adults in certain circumstances. Because cystine can replace part of the requirement for methionine, and tyrosine part of that for phenylalanine, it is usual to consider these two additional amino acids in determining the adequacy of a given diet. The RDAs of essential amino acids (Table 7-2)[9] are higher than those commonly reported, since they have been adjusted upward by 30% to allow for individual variability. Despite this adjustment, the present RDA for total high-quality protein supplies at least twice (and for several amino acids more than three times) the RDA for individual essential amino acids. The average adult requires only

Table 7-2 Amino Acids and the Recommended Diet

	Requirement for 70 kg Man (g/da)	Grams in RDA (56 g high-quality protein)	Multiple of Requirement
Isoleucine	0.8	2.4	2.8
Leucine	1.1	3.9	3.5
Lysine	0.8	2.9	3.4
Methionine Cystine	0.7	1.5	2.1
Phenylalanine Tyrosine	1.1	4.1	3.4
Threonine	0.6	2.0	3.5
Tryptophan	0.2	0.6	2.9
Valine	1.0	2.7	2.8
TOTAL	6.3	20.1	

From Committee on Dietary Allowances, Food and Nutrition Board, National Research Council: Recommended dietary allowances, ed 9, Washington DC, 1980, National Academy of Sciences.

about 20% of the total nitrogen available from essential amino acids, if these are well-balanced.

Total Amino Nitrogen

In addition to essential amino acids, the body requires nonspecific amino nitrogen to compensate for losses in urine, feces, sweat, saliva, sputum, semen, milk, hair, nails, and skin, as well as in menstrual and other bleeding. On a protein-free diet, these losses average about 54 mg of nitrogen per kilogram (equivalent to 0.34 g of protein/kg) per day, with a coefficient of variation of about 15%. A 30% increase in this mean value leads to an estimate of 0.45 g/kg/day. However, proteins are used less efficiently as nitrogen sources when consumed in amounts approximating these requirements. This loss of efficiency is about 30% for egg protein, so the requirement for egg protein should be increased from 0.45 to 0.59 g/kg/day.

The nitrogen requirement is also influenced by the levels of energy intake and expenditure. An inadequate total energy intake will cause a larger proportion of the protein to be diverted for use as energy. A further adjustment is necessary because the average efficiency of utilization for the mixed proteins typical of the U.S. diet may be only 75% of that for the reference protein. Thus the present RDA for adults in the United States is 0.8 g of protein per kilogram of body weight per day.

FAT AND CHOLESTEROL

Dietary fat is a carrier for the fat-soluble vitamins and provides certain essential fatty acids. However, the need for these can be met by diets containing much less fat than contained in the diets typically eaten in the United States. There is no other specific requirement for fat as a nutrient in the diet. Additional fat is used as a source of energy interchangeably with carbohydrate and protein. Dietary fat in excess of energy requirements is stored as fat in adipose cells.

Fat is present in the diet in the form of triacylglycerols (triglycerides), which consist of one molecule of glycerol and three molecules of fatty acid. The fatty acids are classified according to the number of double bonds between the carbon atoms—the degree of saturation. Saturated fats have no double bonds and contain the maximum amount of hydrogen. Monounsaturated fats contain one double bond between car-

bon atoms; polyunsaturated fats contain more than one double bond.

The degree of saturation of unsaturated fat may be increased by artificial hydrogenation, but some remaining double bonds are converted to the *trans* rather than the natural *cis* stereochemical configuration. Saturated fats tend to be solid, and polyunsaturated fats liquid, at room temperature. Hydrogenation is used commercially to lengthen the shelf life and to harden fats of vegetable origin (especially in vegetable shortening, which contains up to 58% *trans* fatty acids, and "stick" margarine, which contains up to 47% *trans* fatty acids). *Trans* fatty acids are incorporated in cell membranes, whose function is thereby altered in several respects. The possible impact of *trans* fatty acids on human health is not known, although they have been shown to promote the development of bowel cancer in rats.[10]

Saturated Fatty Acids

There is no requirement for saturated fatty acids, as such, in the human diet. Myristic and palmitic acids are the two most commonly consumed. They occur mainly in foods of animal origin, including meat, milk products, and eggs. However, coconut oil consists almost entirely of saturated fat (86%) and palm oil is 56% saturated fat. These vegetable fats are used increasingly in the manufacture of simulated dairy products. In addition to their contribution to the total fat content of the diet, saturated fats are of particular importance as determinants of the serum cholesterol level. The proportion of the total dietary calories provided by saturated fat has a direct and approximately linear effect on the level of serum cholesterol. The most important dietary factor increasing the serum cholesterol of the average American is saturated fat, which provides approximately 14% of the calories.

Monounsaturated Fatty Acids

As with saturated fatty acids, there is no special requirement for monounsaturated fatty acids in the human diet. The average American consumes primarily monounsaturated fatty acids, which make up about 50% of the total fat content and provide some 20% of the calories of the diet. Oleic acid is the most commonly occurring monounsaturated fatty acid. Olive oil is the most concentrated source, but animal fats also contain substantial amounts of these fatty acids. Monounsaturated fatty acids neither elevate nor lower the level of serum cholesterol, so a "high-fat" diet is not necessarily associated with a high average level of serum cholesterol in the population. Inhabitants of the Mediterranean littoral consume large amounts of olive oil but tend to have low levels of serum cholesterol.

There has been some recent suggestion that monounsaturated fats actively lower serum cholesterol. This stems in part from confusion over the definition of the phrase "lowering serum cholesterol." It is true that if monounsaturated fats are substituted for saturated fats in the diet the serum cholesterol will fall, but this is attributable to the *removal* of saturated fat rather than to the introduction of monounsaturated fat. Extensive data[11,12] indicate that serum cholesterol is independent of the amount of monounsaturated fat in the diet over a wide range of variation.

Polyunsaturated Fatty Acids

Some knowledge of the nomenclature of fatty acids is necessary to understand the roles of the various classes of polyunsaturated fatty acids. Carbon atoms may be numbered either from the carboxyl group (the "alpha" end of the chain) or from the methyl group (the "omega" end); the omega nomenclature is now becoming more widely used. The main characteristics of a fatty acid are the number of carbon atoms, the number of double (unsaturated) bonds between carbon atoms, and the position of the double bond closest to the methyl group (i.e., the omega end of the chain). Other relevant information is the stereochemical configuration of each double bond. In almost all naturally synthesized unsaturated fatty acids the double bonds are in the *cis* configuration (as opposed to hydrogenated fats, which have some of their double bonds converted to the *trans* configuration). Only *cis* isomers can function as essential fatty acids. The specification of the most common polyunsaturated fat, linoleic acid, as $18:2,\omega\text{-}6$* implies that it contains 18 carbon atoms and two double bonds, of which the first is between the sixth and seventh carbon atoms counting from the methyl group.

Animals (including humans) are not able to desaturate carbon-carbon bonds of fatty acids when the bonds are closer to the methyl group

than the omega-9 position. Thus two broad classes of biologically active polyunsaturated fatty acids, the omega-6 and omega-3 groups, cannot be synthesized by humans. The omega-6 group includes the one definitely essential fatty acid, linoleic, which is the principal component of polyunsaturated fats in the diet. Because linoleic acid is converted in the body to other necessary longer-chain fatty acids (including arachidonic) via gamma-linolenic acid, linoleic acid in sufficient amounts is able to fulfill the requirements for all of the omega-6 group. However, the rate of conversion of linoleic to gamma-linolenic acid may not always be adequate, in which case gamma-linoleic acid becomes essential. The Food and Nutrition Board of the National Research Council recommends that at least 3% of total energy be provided as polyunsaturated fat (but also recognizes that larger amounts may be desirable to control blood lipid levels in certain individuals).*

Interest has recently been focused on the other main class of polyunsaturated fatty acids—omega-3—which, although not known to be essential, may enhance resistance to coronary artery disease and possibly other health problems. This interest stems from two general types of observation. First, it was pointed out[13] that Eskimos have very low rates of coronary heart disease despite diets with a high overall content of fat. Then, it was found in prospective studies[14,15] that individuals who habitually consume relatively large quantities of fish have a lower risk of developing coronary artery disease than do otherwise comparable individuals who consume only small quantities of fish. Omega-3 fatty acids are present in substantial amounts in a number of species of cold-water fish and form an important component of the Eskimo diet. Polyunsaturated fatty acids of marine origin are formed in uni- and polycellular marine plants such as phytoplankton and algae. They eventually move up the food chain and are incorporated into fish oils and the lipids of higher marine animals. The omega-3 polyunsaturated fatty acids in marine animal fats are almost exclusively 20- and 22-carbon fatty acids, probably because of the low temperature of the environment. Longer molecules can contain more double bonds, which re-

---

*n is used by some authors in place of ω (omega), but the two are exactly equivalent.

*The average American diet provides about 6% of total energy as linoleic acid—nearly twice the recommended minimum amount.

sult in lower melting points. The omega-3 structure also allows one more double bond to be introduced into the chain than the omega-6 structure.

Although the evidence for the efficacy of a diet containing large quantities of fish in preventing heart disease is incomplete and the mechanism of the effect, if present, is unclear, there are also no good reasons to advise against it. The substitution of fish for red meat and, to some extent, poultry will generally result in a lowering of serum cholesterol, mainly by reducing the intake of saturated fat. Any additional benefit conferred by the omega-3 fatty acids does not appear to be mediated by a further reduction in serum cholesterol. It is more likely to result from a prolongation of bleeding time. Although benefits appear to accrue from consuming fairly modest amounts of fish (including varieties that do not contain large amounts of omega-3 fatty acids), it should be borne in mind that the consumption of two 4 oz servings of cold-water fish per day would provide only about one quarter of the amount of omega-3 fatty acids consumed by the average Eskimo.

Greater caution should be exercised in recommending fish oils as dietary supplements. The potentially deleterious effects of excessive oxidation, relative deficiency of vitamin E, excesses of vitamins A and D, prolonged bleeding time, and increased intake of contaminants (e.g., PCBs, DDT) should be considered.

The general effects of polyunsaturated fats in lowering serum cholesterol are well established and have been found to be proportional to the amount of polyunsaturated fatty acids in the diet.* In principle, the amount of these acids can be raised without limit to provide an increasingly favorable effect on serum cholesterol levels. Diets containing up to 20% of their total energy as polyunsaturated fat depress serum cholesterol levels in humans by the expected amount of about 20 mg/dl when fed isocalorically under metabolic ward conditions. However, enthusiasm for such diets has been tempered by several important considerations:

1. Diets with high levels of any type of fat, including polyunsaturated fat, are calorically dense and tend to lead to higher energy consumption, the deposition of adipose tissue, and hence a competing adverse effect on serum cholesterol levels.

2. No known human population habitually consumes more than about 10% of its energy requirements in the form of polyunsaturated fatty acids; there is thus no available model to demonstrate the long-term safety of very high levels of polyunsaturated fat in man.

3. Some specific concerns about the safety of very high levels of polyunsaturated fats have arisen from work in both animals and humans. Polyunsaturated fat is an even more potent promoter of carcinoma of the colon and breast in rodents than are other types of fat. In one large-scale study[16] of the effects on humans of diets containing about 20% of their calories as polyunsaturated fatty acids, there was an increase of marginal significance in the death rate from cancer; however, this effect has not been observed in several comparable studies. Diets very high in polyunsaturated fat have also been shown to be immunosuppressive under certain conditions in animal experiments.

Total Fatty Acids

The saturated, monounsaturated, and polyunsaturated fatty acids together constitute the total dietary fatty acids. Under isocaloric conditions there is no additional effect of the total fat intake on serum cholesterol levels, after allowances for the separate and opposite effects of the saturated and polyunsaturated components. However, there is a strong association between diets high in fat, regardless of the degree of saturation, and the prevalence of obesity. Obesity, in turn, is associated with increased levels of total serum cholesterol (and more strongly so with increased levels of VLDL and LDL cholesterol and reduced levels of HDL cholesterol). Thus, North Americans, with a high dietary intake of animal fat, have high average levels of both adiposity and serum cholesterol; Italians, with a high intake of vegetable fat, have high average levels of adiposity and intermediate average levels of serum cholesterol; and Japanese, with a low intake of all types of fat, have low average levels of both obesity and serum cholesterol.

---

*Each increment of polyunsaturated fat equal to 1% of total calories lowers serum cholesterol by an average of 1 mg/dl.

The population risk of cancer of the colon and breast is related to total dietary fat consumption rather than to the level of specific components (although animal experiments suggest that polyunsaturated fat may be a somewhat more potent promoter of cancer than saturated fat).

Cholesterol

Although it is a necessary constituent of many body tissues, cholesterol is not an essential nutrient; adequate amounts can be synthesized by humans. No deficiency state has been described, even in vegans (whose diets are completely free of cholesterol); cholesterol is present only in foods derived from animal sources.

The effect of dietary cholesterol on serum cholesterol is complex and subject to considerable individual variation. On average, however, the first few hundred milligrams per day of dietary cholesterol have a substantial effect on the serum cholesterol level. The average intake of about 500 mg/day in the United States probably raises the average serum cholesterol level about 22 mg/dl, but cholesterol consumption above this average level has relatively little additional effect on the serum cholesterol level.

Patients are often confused about the distinction between "cholesterol-lowering" and "low-cholesterol" diets. The first term is best used for any diet that tends to lower the serum cholesterol level, and the second term for a diet low in cholesterol content. The most important characteristic of a cholesterol-lowering diet is a reduction in the amount of saturated fat eaten; it may or may not include a reduction in dietary cholesterol, whose effect would be small unless the reduction were drastic. There is reluctance among many nutritionists to recommend such drastic reductions on a broad scale, because dietary cholesterol is associated with many of the preferred sources of protein (eggs, meat, dairy products).

CARBOHYDRATES AND FIBER

Dietary carbohydrate can be divided into sugars (monosaccharides and disaccharides), starches (polysaccharides digestible by humans), and indigestible and carbohydrate-like substances (collectively referred to as fiber). Because humans can convert both protein and fat to glucose, there is no specific dietary requirement for digestible carbohydrate; but a carbohydrate-free diet leads to ketosis and excessive breakdown of tissue protein. These effects can be prevented by consuming 50 to 100 g of digestible carbohydrate per day. Although fiber has no specific metabolic requirement (it is by definition not absorbed), it may nonetheless have considerable significance as a dietary component.

Sugars

The consumption of mono- and disaccharides, especially in refined form, has increased markedly during the present century. These sugars provide no essential nutrients and are certainly involved in tooth decay. Their role in the etiology of hypertriglyceridemia and atherosclerosis has probably been overestimated, and it is unlikely that they are important factors in these conditions. High sugar consumption has not been convincingly implicated in the etiology of diabetes (other than as a contributor to excessive energy intake leading to obesity).

Starches

As the consumption of sugar (and fat) has increased during the present century, the consumption of starches has decreased. Although there is no known requirement for starches per se, they are, so far as is known, harmless at any level of intake within the energy requirement of the individual. Contrary to popular opinion, diets high in starch are not particularly conducive to obesity; populations that habitually consume large amounts (e.g., rice-based diets) have characteristically low levels of adiposity. Starch should therefore be considered the preferred primary source of energy in the diet. Whole grain cereals and potatoes are major sources of starch; they also provide a variety of vitamins and minerals.

Fiber

The general term fiber includes the carbohydrates cellulose, hemicellulose, gums, and pectines, together with lignin, the noncarbohydrate "woody" substance in plants. The substantially reduced consumption of fiber in developed countries during the present century has been invoked with considerable plausibility (but without proof) as an etiologic factor in a number of diseases including diverticulosis, hyperlipidemia, atherosclerosis, colon cancer, and diabetes.[17] Although it seems prudent to recommend some increase in the amount of fiber habitually eaten by Americans, there is also the potential risk that minerals will be less well absorbed in diets containing large amounts of fiber.

ALCOHOL

The average American adult now consumes 210 kcal/day in the form of alcohol, excluding the energy from other constituents of alcoholic beverages. Since there is a substantial amount of carbohydrate in beer and wine, the total caloric contribution from alcoholic beverages is approximately 300 kcal/day. The average is calculated for all adults. About one third of this group does not drink at all, so those who do drink consume an average of about 300 kcal/day as alcohol and a total of about 400 kcal from alcoholic beverages. The amounts of alcohol and energy in several typical alcoholic beverages are shown in Table 7-3. Note that a typical serving of beer has less alcohol but more calories than a typical serving of gin, whiskey, or vodka.

The dangers to health of large intakes of alcohol are well known; these include psychiatric, neurologic, and hepatic disease, hypertension, and increased death rates from accidents, homicide, suicide, heart disease, pneumonia, and tuberculosis. Only more recently has it been recognized that moderate intakes of alcohol (up to about 50 g/da) are associated with decreased rates of coronary artery disease compared to rates for individuals who consume no alcohol. The elevating effect of alcohol on high-density lipoproteins may be one of the mechanisms by which alcohol exerts this apparently protective effect. Although the social and medical hazards of alcohol (and especially the tendency for intakes to increase progressively) are great enough to preclude recommending alcohol to those who do not consume it, there is no sound medical reason to proscribe its use in moderation at appropriate times by healthy nonobese individuals. However, alcohol, like sugar, is a source of "empty" calories. When total calories are held constant, energy consumed from alcohol limits the amount consumed from other macronutrients and the micronutrients associated with them.

ENERGY

The energy requirement of an adult man or woman is the amount necessary to support the basic metabolism and habitual physical activity of that individual without deviation from the "desirable" body weight. For those above or below the desirable body weight, the energy requirement will be lower or higher, respectively, until the desirable weight is restored. Because levels of physical activity both at work and during leisure vary so greatly, it is of little value to recommend standard caloric intakes, even for specific categories of age, sex, and body size. In practice it is much more effective for individuals to adjust their caloric intakes and/or physical activity in such a way as to achieve and maintain desirable body weight. Most individuals attain their desirable weight during periods of peak physical fitness in early adult life. There is no evidence to suggest that it is physiologically desirable for body weight to increase with age, and there is evidence for the adverse effects of increased adiposity on serum lipoproteins, glucose tolerance, and blood pressure. A useful estimate of desirable body weight, in pounds, is given by the following formula:

$$\text{Desirable body weight} = \frac{\text{Height (in)} \times \text{Wrist circum (in)}}{3}$$

Table 7-3 Sources and Approximate Amounts of Energy in Alcoholic Beverages

	Serving (oz)	Alcohol			Energy From Other Constituents (kcal)	Total Energy (kcal)
		Percentage by Weight	Grams	Energy (kcal)		
Regular beer	12	3.6	13	90	60	150
Table wine	4	10	13	90	20	110
Fortified wine (dessert or aperitif)	3	14	13	90	30	120
Spirits						
80 proof	1½	33	14	100	—	100
90 proof	1½	38	16	110	—	110

This formula obviates the need for tables of desirable body weight based on sex, height, and frame size. Median levels of the triceps skinfold for young adult Americans are 10 mm for men and 17 mm for women. Median levels are less affected than mean levels by the small proportion of frankly obese individuals.

Although it is theoretically possible to estimate energy input and output from knowledge of the diet and physical activity throughout the day, the errors arising from inaccurate recording and daily variation, combined with substantial individual variation in the resting metabolic rate and the efficiency of energy conversion, render such estimates somewhat crude. Attempts to match the inputs and outputs calculated in this way are much less accurate than observation of the trend in body weight as a measure of energy balance.

MINERALS
Sodium

The minimum daily losses of sodium in the adult under temperate conditions and light physical activity are approximately 100 mg/day. The current average consumption in the United States is about 50 times this amount. It is important to distinguish between weights of sodium and salt; 5 g of salt contain approximately 2 g of sodium.

Intakes of sodium above about 1 g/day tend to aggravate a genetically determined susceptibility to hypertension, and intakes above 7 g may induce hypertension even in individuals without specific genetic susceptibility. There are no known benefits of high sodium consumption. A diet consisting of natural foods and an average intake of water provides about 1 g sodium daily (i.e., considerably more than the minimum daily losses). The additional sodium consumed by the typical American is provided by salt added during cooking and at table and by the increasing use of processed foods, many of which contain a large amount of sodium.

There is no specific current RDA for sodium, since the likelihood of deficiency under normal conditions is negligible (except for individuals with salt-losing renal disease or adrenal insufficiency). Although levels at or below 1 g/day are probably desirable, these are unpalatable to persons accustomed to average U.S. levels and are quite difficult to achieve, except by using specially purchased and prepared foods. If pro-

cessed foods particularly high in sodium content are avoided and salt is not added at table, an intake of about 2 g/day is achievable without undue effort and is acceptable to most individuals, at least after a short period of adaptation. Only under conditions of hard physical labor (or athletic activity) in high ambient temperatures, when the loss of sodium in sweat may reach as much as 8 g/day, should larger dietary allowances be necessary.

Potassium

The minimum obligatory loss of potassium daily in the healthy adult is probably about 100 mg (2.5 mEq/da). The usual adult intake is 2 to 6 g/day. The likelihood of depletion under normal circumstances is therefore remote. However, evidence exists that an increased intake of potassium (within the usual range) tends to lower blood pressure in hypertensives.[18] Very high intakes of potassium (above 18 g/da) can cause hyperkalemia and cardiac arrest. The optimum intake appears to be at the upper rather than the lower end of the range or usual intake—about 6 g/day. A large banana or 1 cup of citrus fruit juice provides about 0.5 g potassium. Tomato juice furnishes a similar amount but also provides at least as much sodium (unless a special low-sodium variety is used).

Calcium

The present adult RDA for calcium is 800 mg/day, but the FAO/WHO daily allowance is 400 to 500 mg. The RDA is relatively high because of the possible effects of elevated intakes of protein and phosphate, in promoting urinary calcium excretion and enhanced bone resorption, and the risk of reduced calcium absorption with advancing age. The relationship of dietary calcium to osteoporosis has been reviewed by Allen.[19] Intakes above 1.5 g/day do not appear to be associated with any particular hazards. In the United States 60% of calcium intake is derived from milk and dairy products.

Phosphorus

The average daily intake of phosphorus is about 1.5 g, and dietary deficiency is extremely unlikely to occur in humans. The amount of phosphorus in any given diet almost always exceeds that of calcium. The RDA for phosphorus is the same as for calcium (800 mg/da), but relatively wide dietary variations in the calcium:phosphorus ratio can be tolerated provided the amount of vitamin D is adequate.

Magnesium

The magnesium content of the average American diet is about 240 mg/day. Estimates of requirements, based on balance studies, range from 200 to 700 mg/day. The present RDA for magnesium is 350 mg/day for men and 250 for women. There is thus some potential for deficit in the average diet, although it has not been specifically identified except in malabsorption syndromes and during periods of prolonged parenteral nutrition. The deficiency may be manifested as neuromuscular hyperexcitability, with tremor and convulsions, and as behavioral disturbance. Spasm of isolated coronary arteries in dogs has been shown to result when magnesium is withdrawn from the incubation fluid.[20]

Evidence suggests that the low levels of magnesium in soft water may contribute to the increased death rates from coronary artery disease, especially sudden death, in areas where the water is characteristically soft. The magnesium content of water may range from less than 2 to more than 50 mg/liter in different water supplies. Although no consistent differences can be shown between the serum magnesium levels in residents of hard- and soft-water districts,[21] significant differences in myocardial levels have been shown between those dying of ischemic heart disease and those dying of other causes within each type of district. There are no data yet available to show whether an increase in magnesium intake will reduce the risk of death from ischemic heart disease either in individuals or in communities. Cereals, nuts, and legumes are among the richest dietary sources of magnesium.

Iron

As a component of hemoglobin, myoglobin, and several enzymes, iron is an essential nutrient in humans. Up to 30% of total body iron is stored in other forms. An adult man loses about 1 mg/day and a woman in the reproductive years about 1.5 mg. Because the average availability of iron in food is only about 10%, the present RDA for dietary iron is 10 mg for men and 18 mg for nonpregnant women of reproductive age. In fact, absorption of iron as heme is greater than 20%

whereas that of nonheme iron is less than 10%. The absorption of nonheme iron is enhanced by the presence of protein and ascorbic acid, provided these are consumed simultaneously. The iron content of the typical American diet is about 6 mg/1000 kcal. Since most men consume more than 2000 kcal daily, they easily meet their requirement; but the lower caloric consumption and increased requirement for women frequently lead to marginal or deficient intakes.

Zinc

Zinc-containing enzymes are involved in nucleic acid synthesis and degradation. Deficiency is manifested by impaired wound healing, appetite, and taste acuity. In healthy adults equilibrium or positive balance is achieved with an intake of about 12 mg/day. Zinc from animal sources is absorbed more readily than that from vegetable sources; dietary fiber and phytates tend to interfere with absorption. The present RDA for zinc is 15 mg/day, but the average U.S. diet supplies only 6 to 12 mg. Meat and seafood are good sources of available zinc. The total requirement is increased when food is obtained mainly or exclusively from vegetable sources, and there is some potential for deficiency among individuals following such diets.

Iodine

The synthesis of the thyroid hormones thyroxin and triiodothyronine requires iodine. Iodine deficiency leads to goiter, whose prevalence in the United States has been sharply reduced by the use of iodized table salt. The present RDA for iodine is 150 mg/day. Dietary intakes in the U.S. range from about 60 to 700 mg/day. Seafood is the most reliable natural source of dietary iodine. The iodine content of milk and eggs depends on the composition of the animal feed. The average use of 3.4 g of iodized salt adds approximately 260 mg to the daily intake, but only about half the salt used in the United States is iodized. Some risk of thyroid disorders resulting from excessive iodine supplementation has been suggested.

Fluorine

The well-documented protective effect of fluoride against dental caries occurs only at a total dietary intake of about 1.5 mg/day. Intakes above 2.5 mg/day in children cause some mottling of the teeth. Adults living in areas where the drinking water contains more than 4 mg/liter may enjoy some protection against osteoporosis. High fluoride content of the water has a substantial influence on the fluoride content of foods produced in such areas. Thus, total daily intake can vary from about 1 mg/day in areas with water low in fluoride to 5 mg/day in areas where the water has a high fluoride content; but drinking water accounts for only a minor portion of the total intake. Adjusting local water supplies to a concentration of 1 mg/liter will provide a dietary intake of 1 to 4 mg/day for adults without exceeding 2.5 mg/day for children. To obtain the additional protection against osteoporosis, adults may wish to take some supplementary fluoride (unless the water supply naturally contains more than 4 mg/liter).

OTHER TRACE ELEMENTS

The requirements for trace elements are less well established, and although estimated daily requirements are suggested by the Committee on Dietary Allowances,[9] these are not official RDAs.

Copper

Balance studies show that adults remain in equilibrium or positive balance with intakes of copper averaging 1 to 2 mg/day. The average dietary intake appears to be about 2 mg/day. The suggested daily intake is 2 to 3 mg. Oysters, nuts, corn oil, and legumes are good sources of copper. Substantial amounts may be supplied by the drinking water, especially with copper piping. Some potential for deficiency may exist in the United States, but it has been observed only among premature infants fed cow's milk exclusively for long periods.

Manganese

Although many species require manganese, deficiency has not been observed in free-living human populations. Balance studies suggest a daily requirement of 1 to 2 mg to maintain equilibrium. The adult daily intake in the United States varies from 2 to 9 mg, and the suggested intake of 2.5 to 5 mg is thus easily met. Manganese occurs mainly in food or vegetable origin, especially nuts and unrefined grains.

Chromium

Balance studies suggest that about 1 μg/day of absorbable chromium is necessary to maintain equilibrium. However, the absorbability is so low that a dietary intake as high as 200 μg/day may be necessary to provide the required amount. The average daily intake in the United States is 60 μg, which is at the lower end of the presently suggested range of intake (50 to 100 μg/da). Some chromium-responsive disturbances of glucose metabolism have been described in Americans, especially among elderly persons. Yeast, meat, dairy products, and whole grains are good sources of available chromium.

Selenium

The human requirement for selenium is uncertain, since clinical manifestations of deficiency have not been described. Selenium deficiency occurs in animals when the diet contains less than 5 μg/100 g of food consumed. A selenium concentration of 10 μg/100 g dietary intake is associated with optimum growth and reproduction in mammals. Vitamin E deficiency appears to increase the requirement for selenium. The present suggested intake (50 to 100 μg/da) is easily achieved in a well-balanced U.S. diet. Seafood and meat are consistently good sources of selenium, but cereals vary with the conditions under which they are grown.

Molybdenum

Deficiency of molybdenum has been produced in animals when the intake is less than 5 μg/100 g of food consumed, but this has not been described in humans. The present suggested intake is 150 to 500 μg/day, which is met by a well-balanced U.S. diet. Some risk of toxicity exists because of increased urinary excretion of copper when dietary levels of molybdenum depend heavily on the region where the foods are produced.

FAT-SOLUBLE VITAMINS
Vitamin A

The activity associated with vitamin A occurs in the diet in two forms: preformed vitamin A (retinol) and provitamin A (carotenoids). The main carotenoid in the human diet is beta-carotene. The first evidence of deficiency is impaired visual adaptation to the dark, which may lead in time to ocular damage and eventual blindness. Vitamin A activity is now stated in "retinol equivalents." A retinol equivalent is 1 mg of retinol, 6 mg of beta-carotene, or 12 mg of other carotenoids. The RDA for men is 1000 retinol equivalents, and for women 800 retinol equivalents, with a maximum of 7500 equivalents as retinol, since larger amounts over long periods are potentially toxic. Carotenes are not toxic, but excessive amounts cause reversible yellow coloration of the skin.

Retinol, as such, occurs only in foods from animal sources (e.g., dairy products, organ meats). Carotenes are present in plant foods in proportion to the green or yellow coloring. Although a usual balanced diet contains about 1200 retinol equivalents, both dietary deficiencies and low serum levels have been found in a significant proportion of the U.S. population. The recently demonstrated inverse correlation between blood retinol and dietary beta-carotene levels, on the one hand, and the present or future risk of cancer, on the other, is of great interest but does not yet constitute ground for specific nutritional advice with respect to vitamin A.[22]

Vitamin D

Deficiency of vitamin D impairs the mineralization of bone matrix, leading to rickets in children and osteomalacia in adults. Vitamin D occurs in two forms: vitamin D_2 (ergocalciferol) and vitamin D_3 (cholecalciferol). Ultraviolet radiation produces vitamin D_2 from ergosterol, a plant sterol. Vitamin D_3, the naturally occurring form in animal tissues, is produced from 7-dehydrocholesterol in the skin by sunlight. Total vitamin D activity is expressed as micrograms of vitamin D_3 (including actual D_3 and equivalent amounts of D_2). The dietary requirement depends on the amount synthesized by the individual, which in turn depends on skin pigmentation, exposure to sunlight, and atmospheric pollution. The adult requirement can usually be met by adequate exposure to sunlight. The current RDA takes into account adverse conditions and specifies 7.5 mg/day for persons aged 19 to 22 years and 5 mg/day thereafter. The widespread use of milk fortified with vitamin D has rendered deficiency uncommon. There is some evidence of toxicity when dietary intake substantially exceeds the RDA. The major dietary sources of vitamin D include fish, eggs, liver, and butter.

Most milk is now fortified with vitamin D to provide 10 mg of vitamin D_3 per quart.

Vitamin E

Deficiency of vitamin E has been shown in long-standing steatorrhea and is manifested by increased fragility of red cells, loss of muscle tissue, and pigmentation of the small intestine. Vitamin E activity of diets is expressed as milligrams of alpha-tocopherol equivalents, alpha-tocopherol being the most potent form of the vitamin. Average intakes in the United States are in the range of 8 to 11 mg/day. The requirement for vitamin E increases as the intake of polyunsaturated fats increases; but this relationship is rarely of clinical significance, since polyunsaturated fats are among the richest sources of vitamin E. Clinical trials of diets with high levels of polyunsaturated fat have not resulted in lower serum levels of vitamin E. The present RDA is 10 mg of alpha-tocopherol equivalents per day for men and 8 mg for women. These allowances are generally attained in balanced diets typically eaten in the United States.

Vitamin K

Vitamin K occurs in two natural forms: vitamin K_1 (phylloquinone), found in green plants; and vitamin K_2 (menaquinone), found in bacteria and animals. Vitamin K is necessary for the synthesis of prothrombin and other blood-clotting factors in the liver, and deficiency leads to impairment of blood coagulation. An average mixed U.S. diet provides 300 to 500 mg/day, of which 10% to 70% is absorbed. A similar quantity, synthesized by the flora in the gut, is usually sufficient to satisfy the metabolic requirement of adults, except during long-term antibiotic therapy or in cases of steatorrhea. However, it is prudent for adults to consume about 1 mg/kg of body weight as a safety precaution. Green vegetables are the richest dietary source, and a diet containing average amounts of such vegetables easily provides the recommended amount.

WATER-SOLUBLE VITAMINS
Vitamin B_1 (thiamine)

Deficiency of thiamine is the specific cause of beriberi, a condition that, in the United States, is limited almost entirely to alcoholics. The heavy consumption of alcohol leads to decreased ingestion and absorption of thiamine, together with an increased requirement. The utilization of thiamine is approximately proportional to the caloric intake, and the requirement is usually expressed in this form. The minimum requirement has been estimated at 0.34 mg/1000 kcal, but the RDA is 0.5 mg/1000 kcal to allow a margin of safety. The average U.S. diet contains about 1 mg/1000 kcal. Whole grain cereals are one of the most important sources of thiamine, and the use of refined unenriched flour (or polished rice) is a classic cause of deficiency. The standard practice of enriching flour with thiamine has reduced the incidence of deficiency to very low levels in the United States.

Vitamin B$_2$ (riboflavin)

Deficiency of riboflavin leads to glossitis, angular stomatitis, corneal keratosis, and other lesions of the lips and skin. Balance studies suggest that a dietary intake of 0.6 mg/1000 kcal is necessary to prevent depletion of tissue reserves, but the dependence on caloric intake holds only at relatively low levels of energy expenditure. No special allowance of riboflavin needs to be made for individuals engaged in heavy manual labor or athletic activity. The RDA (1.6 mg/da for men, 1.3 mg for women) is expressed independent of caloric intake. The average U.S. diet contains about 1.5 mg/1000 kcal. Milk is the single richest source of riboflavin in the U.S. diet, but meat, poultry, and fish also provide important amounts. There is some evidence that the use of oral contraceptives increases the requirement for riboflavin, but no special official recommendation has yet been made with respect to increased riboflavin intake during such usage.

Niacin

Two substances, nicotinic acid and nicotinamide, that have similar (though not identical) properties together are denoted by the term niacin. Deficiency results in pellagra, which is characterized by the classic triad of dermatitis, diarrhea, and dementia. The dietary requirement for niacin is related to the amount of the amino acid tryptophan consumed, since tryptophan can be converted to niacin by humans. A dietary intake of 60 mg of tryptophan is considered equivalent to 1 mg of niacin (1 niacin equivalent). An intake of about 12 niacin equivalents per day is adequate to prevent depletion in adults. Average U.S. diets provide 16 to 34 niacin equivalents.

The RDA for niacin in adults, expressed in relation to the caloric intake, is 6.6 niacin equivalents per 1000 kcal (but not less than 13 niacin equivalents, regardless of caloric intake). Ingestion of very large amounts (3 g/da) of nicotinic acid (but not nicotinamide) lowers both the serum cholesterol and the serum triglyceride levels, but at the cost of unpleasant flushing, skin rash, and a variety of potentially unfavorable biochemical disturbances.[23] Nicotinic acid should be used as a lipid-lowering agent only for specific indications under close medical supervision.

Vitamin B$_6$

Three naturally occurring and functionally related pyridines are known collectively as vitamin B$_6$, and they appear to be equally active. Deficiency causes various disturbances of the central nervous system, including confusion, depression, and convulsions. The dietary requirement for vitamin B$_6$ depends on the protein intake and has been estimated at 0.02 mg/g of dietary protein. This leads to the current RDAs of 2.2 and 2 mg of vitamin B$_6$ per day for men and women who daily consume 120 and 100 g of protein, respectively. The average U.S. intake is about 2.2 mg/day, derived principally from meat, poultry, and fish.

Folacin

A group of substances with structure and properties similar to those of folic acid (pteroylglutamic acid) is known collectively as folacin. Deficiency leads to macrocytic anemia. Typical U.S. diets provide an average intake of about 700 mg daily, but there is considerable variation. The present RDA for adults is 400 mg/day. Dark green vegetables, beef, eggs, and whole grain cereals are good sources of folacin.

Vitamin B$_{12}$

Cobalamins, which are biologically active members of the group of cobalt-containing corrinoids, are known collectively as vitamin B$_{12}$ and correspond to the "extrinsic factor" of Castle. The usual commercially produced form, cyanocobalamin, is not the major natural form of the vitamin. The typical U.S. diet supplies 5 to 15 mg/day, but the observed range is much wider, varying from 1 to 100 mg/day. A specific binding glycoprotein (Castle's "intrinsic factor"), secreted by the stomach, is the main vehicle for absorption of the vitamin, although this factor is secreted in limited amounts and the system becomes saturated by single doses of the vitamin exceeding 5 mg. About 2% of vitamin B_{12} consumed in ordinary diets is absorbed by simple diffusion; this explains the response of pernicious anemia to large oral doses of the vitamin (or liver). Substantial body stores and an effective enterohepatic circulation tend to protect against manifestations of deficiency for several years after the loss of the intrinsic factor (e.g., following total gastrectomy) or a marked reduction in the intake of the vitamin (as with vegan diets). The present RDA for adults is set at 30 mg/day, an amount that is easily provided by almost all diets of which any significant part is derived from animal sources, whether in the form of meat, dairy products, or eggs.

Biotin

Spontaneous deficiency of biotin has not been observed in human adults but can be induced by feeding large amounts of a biotin-binding glycoprotein, avidin, present in raw egg white. Symptoms include anorexia, nausea, vomiting, glossitis, dermatitis, and depression. The intestinal microflora synthesizes a significant proportion of the amount of biotin required. A typical U.S. diet containing 100 to 300 mg of biotin daily appears to meet the needs of practically all healthy adults, but there is no official RDA.

Pantothenic Acid

As with biotin, spontaneous deficiency of pantothenic acid has not been observed in humans. Deficiency has been induced artificially, either with a synthetic diet or by using a metabolic antagonist of pantothenic acid. The average U.S. diet contains about 7 mg of pantothenic acid/day, but daily intakes as low as 1 mg have been observed in teenage girls. The recommended intake for adults is in the range of 4 to 7 mg/day. Meat, cereals, and legumes are good sources of pantothenic acid.

Vitamin C (ascorbic acid)

Deficiency of vitamin C results in scurvy, a disease characterized by widespread capillary hemorrhaging. A daily intake of 10 mg of vitamin C will cure the clinical signs of scurvy. Scurvy is associated with plasma ascorbate levels of about 0.13 mg/dl and a body pool of less than 300 mg. A typical U.S. dietary intake of 75 mg/day is associated with a serum level of approximately 0.75 and a body pool of about 1500 mg in men. An intake of 200 mg/day raises the serum level to a maximum of about 1.4 mg/dl and the body pool to 2500 mg. The renal clearance rises sharply at higher serum levels. The present RDA for vitamin C is 60 mg/day, which is easily provided by diets that include citrus fruit or fruit juice; green vegetables and potatoes also provide substantial amounts of the vitamin. Some investigators believe that much larger amounts of vitamin C (1 g/da or more) will both reduce susceptibility to the common cold[24] and increase serum levels of immunoglobulins and complement.[25] The reproducibility and magnitude of these effects have not yet been fully established.

OTHER NUTRIENTS

The so-called essential nutrients have been discussed in some detail. The word essential implies that some obvious and potentially serious physical or mental disturbance results from prolonged deficiency or absence of the nutrient in question. The evidence may be obtained directly, from observing or inducing the deficiency in humans, or indirectly, from experimental evidence in other species, especially primates. However, the word essential has not yet been extended to include substances that may confer a greater sense of well-being or enhanced protection against certain diseases not primarily attributable to deficiency of a given substance.

The Recommended Dietary Allowances of the essential nutrients do not, in general, encompass certain putative effects on well-being or protection from disease that some believe to ensue from ingesting quantities larger (and often much larger) than those necessary to prevent manifestation of the specific deficiency state that defines a particular nutrient as essential. Of course, other "essential" nutrients may yet be discovered. Such undiscovered essential nutrients might include substances that are necessary only in such small amounts that deficiency virtually never occurs or substances necessary to prevent diseases that have not yet been recognized as primarily nutritional in etiology.

Choline

The amounts of choline synthesized in the body depend on the availability of methionine, vitamin B_{12}, and folacin. A dietary requirement for choline has been demonstrated under certain conditions in several species. No particular clinical manifestations attributable to choline deficiency have yet been identified in man (but few attempts have been made to induce such deficiency). If indeed choline is necessary, the average intake of 400 to 900 mg/day must exceed the dietary requirement by a substantial margin. Egg yolk is usually the richest dietary source, but major proportions of the total intake of choline are also provided by meat, dairy products, legumes, and whole grain cereals.

Trace Elements

In addition to the minerals already discussed, small amounts of cobalt, nickel, vanadium, silicon, tin, arsenic, and cadmium have been reported as necessary both for optimum reproduction and growth and to prevent pathologic change in one or more species of higher animals. Because very strict control of dietary and environmental contamination is necessary to demonstrate deficiency of these elements, it appears that any need for them is easily met by the amounts present in virtually all diets.

Nutrients of Potential Pharmacologic Value

Both essential and nonessential nutrients may be of pharmacologic value. Several vitamins are widely recommended in doses considerably larger than the amounts necessary to prevent clinical manifestations of the primary deficiency state that defines each as essential. Nicotinic acid in doses several hundred times the RDA is known to lower serum cholesterol levels, but such doses frequently cause unpleasant (though apparently not dangerous) side effects. Large doses of vitamin C appear to have some value in preventing viral infections and may also lower serum cholesterol levels without apparent toxic effects. Large doses of vitamins A and D are frequently recommended but have no well-documented benefits and are potentially toxic.

Although a wide variety of nonessential nutrients has been recommended for the prevention or treatment of human disease, only a minority of these have been subjected to scientific investigation. Some nonessential nutrients may be beneficial or even, by certain definitions, essential for certain individuals (e.g., lithium as used to control manic-depressive illness in persons genetically predisposed to the condition). Other substances, such as alcohol, may have both beneficial and harmful effects. There is now consistent evidence that moderate intakes of alcohol are associated with a lower death rate from coronary heart disease, but even such moderate intakes are also associated with higher death rates from other causes and can predispose the individual toward alcoholism and its related mental and physical sequelae.

Several investigators[26,27] have found evidence of a cholesterol-lowering factor in both whole and skim milk. This appears to compensate for the cholesterol-raising property of the fat in whole milk and to enhance the value of skim milk.

As stated previously, intakes of potassium substantially above those necessary to maintain potassium balance result in decreased blood pressure in hypertensives.

Other Nutrients of Biologic Value

Various substances identified as growth factors for bacteria, insects, and other invertebrates are normally synthesized by higher animals. Despite the lack of hard evidence of their essential or beneficial function in humans, they have been recommended as health-promoting nutrients. Included in this category are asparagine, bifidus factor, biopterin, carnitine chelating agents, cholesterol, coenzyme Q (ubiquinones), hematin, lecithin, lipoic acid (thiotic acid), nerve growth factors, nucleotides, nucleic acids, para-aminobenzoic acid, pimelic acid, and various peptides, proteins, polyamines, and pteridines.

Substances Without Known Essential Biologic Function

The vast majority of other organic chemicals, either synthetic or naturally occurring, are without proved essential nutrient function for the support of any species. Nonetheless, many such substances have been recommended as beneficial for health. Examples include amygdalin or laetrile ("vitamin B_{17}"), chlorophyll, orotic acid, pangamic acid ("vitamin B_{15}"), and "vitamin U."

CIRCUMSTANCES AFFECTING DIETARY ADEQUACY
Alcohol Intake

As stated earlier, approximately two thirds of the adult population of the United States drinks alcoholic beverages—about 300 kcal/day as alcohol and an additional 100 kcal from the other constituents (mainly carbohydrate) of alcoholic beverages. There is, of course, great variation around this average. Intakes of 1000 kcal/day from alcoholic beverages, particularly beer, are not uncommon. The greatest nutritional hazard faced by such a heavy drinker is the difficulty of obtaining sufficient amounts of protein and vitamins from the other components of the diet. When the expenditure of energy by physical activity, and hence the overall energy requirement, is small, the problem can become acute. It is not uncommon for alcoholic beverages to provide more than half the caloric intake, with negligible amounts of protein and vitamins. The problem is compounded by the fact that high intakes of alcohol actually increase the requirements for vitamins B_1, B_6, and folacin. Although a person who consumes such quantities of alcohol should be advised to reduce alcohol intake and increase physical activity, such advice is often ignored. It may then be necessary to modify the diet in such a way as to maximize the intake of protein and vitamins and, in certain cases, to prescribe supplementary vitamins.

Oral Contraceptives

The use of oral steroid contraceptives causes a variety of metabolic disturbances that, in turn, affect the utilization of certain micronutrients. Some 15% to 20% of women who use oral contraceptives have direct biochemical evidence of a vitamin deficiency.[28] There is also evidence of increased requirements for riboflavin, niacin, and vitamin B_6 in some users of oral contraceptives, although no official recommendations have yet been made.

Physical Activity

Several of the effects of physical activity on dietary behavior and requirements have already been considered. In general, high levels of physical activity demand high caloric intakes. If such caloric demands are satisfied by a well-balanced diet, the risk of essential nutrient deficiency will be diminished since the requirements for almost all essential nutrients (with the possible exception of thiamine and niacin) tend to be a function of lean body mass rather than of caloric expenditure. Conversely, reduced levels of physical activity (as occur with aging) are associated with decreased caloric requirements and an increased hazard of deficiency of essential nutrients. If the caloric intake is not adjusted to reduced physical activity, then increased adiposity and its undesirable consequences result. Thus the maintenance of high levels of physical activity throughout adulthood is an important step toward continuing nutritional adequacy.

Temperature

Energy requirements are at a minimum in temperate climates and increase, at given levels of physical activity, when the environment is cool (below 14° C) or very hot (above 37° C). Hard physical work at high temperatures may cause the loss of up to 8 g of sodium per day. Whenever more than 3 liters of water/day are required to replace sweat, extra sodium chloride should be provided. Increased intakes of vitamin C are required to maintain normal serum levels of the vitamin in high temperatures. South African mine workers require 200 to 250 mg of vitamin C/day to maintain serum ascorbate levels of 0.75 mg/dl.

Vegetarianism

Some individuals and groups avoid certain types of food derived from animal sources. They do so for a variety of religious, ethical, humanitarian, cultural, economic, medical, and other reasons. The range of dietary practices that fall under the heading of vegetarianism is so wide that no broad generalizations can be made about safety and desirability. There are several subdivisions that can be made among individuals who refer to themselves as vegetarians: *Vegans,* or total vegetarians, avoid any food derived from animal sources. They consume no meat, poultry, fish, seafood, eggs, or dairy products. *Lactovegetarians* consume dairy products but proscribe meat, poultry, fish, seafood, and eggs. *Lactoovovegetarians* consume dairy products and eggs but proscribe all kinds of flesh. *Semi-* or *partial vegetarians* exclude only certain kinds of flesh, most often red meat, from their diet.

In addition to the listed categories, certain vegetarians follow what they call a macrobiotic diet. These individuals, who may or may not be vegans, also exclude various vegetable products and emphasize cereals, "natural" foods (which are unrefined and free of preservatives and other artificial ingredients), and "organic" foods (which are raised without pesticides and "chemical" fertilizers). Many "macrobiotic" diets also include special foods (e.g., seaweed) that are believed to possess health-giving properties and to protect against deficiencies of micronutrients.

The practice of most forms of vegetarianism is, in principle, compatible with good and perhaps superior health, but certain precautions are necessary to avoid specific deficiencies, particularly with vegan diets. Attention should be directed toward the following nutrients:

1. Protein is generally less well-balanced, less digestible, and less concentrated in vegetable than in animal foods. Vegetarians who consume milk and/or eggs, both of which contain substantial amounts of well-balanced protein, rarely encounter problems with protein deficiency. Vegans should give special attention to the use of "complementary" proteins, which reciprocally compensate for deficient amino acids in each protein separately. Cereals and legumes provide such complementarity in many vegetarian diets. Complementary proteins are discussed in detail in *Diet for a Small Planet*.[29]

2. Vitamin B_{12} is generally absent in foods of vegetable origin, but milk and eggs are good sources. Vegans should be careful to include a dietary source of vitamin B_{12} such as fortified soy- or sesame seed–based milk.

3. Vitamin D is also absent from plant foods but can be synthesized by adequate exposure to sunlight or provided by a fortified milk substitute.

4. Riboflavin tends to be marginal in vegan diets unless these include relatively large quantities of dark green vegetables. Nutritional yeast is a rich source.

5. Calcium is also marginal in vegan diets but, as with riboflavin, can be obtained in sufficient amounts from dark green vegetables or from fortified soybean milk.

6. Iron is both of limited quantity and less absorbable in diets that do not provide the heme form of iron present in flesh. Phytic acid reduces the absorption of iron whereas ascorbic acid enhances it. Zinc is present in substantial quantities in many plant foods but, as with iron, its absorption is reduced by phytates and by fiber, which tend to be prevalent in many types of vegetarian diets.

In addition to the types followed for reasons other than specifically medical ones, certain vegetarian diets may be advised for the prevention or treatment of atherosclerotic disease (Chapter 14). The traditional lactoovovegetarian diets do not necessarily lower serum lipid levels, since they may contain as much saturated fat and cholesterol as (or more than) diets containing meat. However, the potential health benefits of a vegan diet can be enjoyed while obtaining high-quality protein, together with vitamins and minerals, from skim milk and egg white, both of which are virtually free of saturated fat and cholesterol.

PRUDENT EATING PATTERNS

The minimum adult requirements for various nutrients and the hazards of excess associated with certain of these nutrients have been reviewed in some detail. It now remains to translate this information into simple and practical recommendations for palatable eating patterns that minimize the known hazards of both deficiency and excess.

Recommendations for avoiding potential dietary excesses in the typical U.S. diet are shown in Table 7-4. These do not proscribe any major classes of food and they minimize interference with traditional eating patterns and cuisines. There is no significant reduction in the amount of animal protein. In fact, if the recommended eating pattern is followed isocalorically, there will be an increase in the amount of protein consumed because of the reduction in non–protein-containing sources of energy such as trimmed fat, milk fat, and sugar.

Unlike a number of other comparable sets of recommendations, (e.g., those of the American Heart Association), these basic recommendations do not mandate a reduction in dietary cholesterol. This exception arises from the nonlinear relationship of serum cholesterol to dietary cholesterol. Reductions in dietary cholesterol to levels at or about the typical intake produce only modest reductions in serum cholesterol levels. If a reduction in dietary cholesterol is recommended as an integral part of the eating pattern, many individuals may be deterred from following the eating pattern as a whole. Reductions in saturated fat that do not involve deliberate reductions in dietary cholesterol, nonetheless, do lower serum cholesterol levels. However, major reductions in dietary cholesterol intake (up to and including the cholesterol-free diet consumed

Table 7-4 Recommendations for Avoiding Potential Dietary Excesses

Excess	Recommendations
Saturated fat	Emphasize poultry, veal, and seafood rather than red meat
	Use lean cuts of any red meat eaten and trim all visible fat before cooking
	Remove skin from poultry
	Broil rather than fry
	Substitute skim milk (ideally) or ½% milk (acceptably) for whole milk
	Use butter only occasionally and substitute a polyunsaturated margarine for regular use (if needed)
	Use polyunsaturated cooking oil in place of vegetable shortening or animal cooking fat
	Use regular cheese only occasionally and substitute low-fat cheese for regular use (if needed)
	Eat ice cream only occasionally
	Avoid products containing coconut or palm oil
Sodium	Minimize added salt at table or in cooking
	Avoid heavily salted commercially prepared food and snacks
Sugar	Minimize consumption of candy, sweet desserts, and snacks and beverages containing sugar
Total energy	Achieve and maintain desirable body weight by balancing intake and expenditure of energy; reduce excess energy intake by reducing intake of total fat, sugar, and alcohol; engage in physical activity to use at least 1000 kcal/day more than resting metabolism
Alcohol	Avoid intoxication; gradually increase consumption over time
Cholesterol	Minor reductions (e.g., one instead of two eggs/da) are neither useful nor generally recommended; however, _eliminating_ egg _yolks_ and organ meats will achieve substantial reduction in serum cholesterol levels in persons who do so
Hydrogenated fat	Replace vegetable shortening and margarine containing hydrogenated fat with polyunsaturated cooking oil and margarine

Table 7-5 Recommendations for Avoiding Potential Dietary Deficiencies

Deficiency	Recommendations
Iron	Include sources of vitamin C (citrus fruits and juices) with most meals to enhance absorption of nonheme iron; especially important for women of reproductive age
Potassium	Consume citrus fruits and juices, tomatoes, and bananas
Magnesium	Consume legumes, nuts, and whole grain cereals
Zinc	Consume adequate amounts of fruit and green vegetables, especially in areas where soil is deficient in available zinc

by a vegan) have substantial and important effects on the serum cholesterol level, as discussed in detail in Chapter 14. No specific risks of dietary deficiency are introduced by these recommendations.

Additional recommendations for avoiding the risks of potential dietary deficiencies associated with the typical U.S. diet are shown in Table 7-5. Each of these potential deficiencies can be offset by ensuring adequate daily intakes of fruits, vegetables, and cereals (which are, in fact, consistent with and complementary to the reduction in fat, sodium, sugar, and alcohol

shown in Table 7-4). The eating pattern is designed to be applicable and acceptable to the entire adult population of the United States. If the recommended changes were to be made, the risks of both excess and deficiency of nutrients would be reduced simultaneously. Direct experimental proof of the value of such changes in preventing chronic diseases will probably never be obtained because of the enormous cost of such an experiment. However, much indirect evidence suggests that the risk of a wide variety of cardiovascular and other disorders can be reduced substantially.

REFERENCES

1. McKeown T: The role of medicine: dream, mirage, or nemesis? Princeton NJ, 1979, Princeton University Press.
2. Weisburger JH, et al: Nutrition and cancer—on the mechanisms bearing on causes of cancer of the colon, breast, prostate, and stomach, Bull NY Acad Med **56:**673-696, 1980.
3. Sherwin RW, et al: Serum cholesterol levels and cancer mortality in 361,662 men screened for the Multiple Risk Factor Intervention Trial, JAMA **257:**943-948, 1987.
4. Kakar F, Henderson M: Diet and breast cancer, Clin Nutr **4:**119-130, 1985.
5. Willett WC, et al: Dietary fat and the risk of breast cancer, N Engl J Med **316:**22-28, 1987.
6. Keys A: Seven countries: a multivariate analysis of death and coronary heart disease, Cambridge Mass, 1980, Harvard University Press.
7. Manson JE, et al: Body weight and longevity: a reassessment, JAMA **257:**353-358, 1987.
8. Lew EA, Garfinkel L: Variations in mortality by weight among 750,000 men and women, J Chron Dis **32:**563-576, 1979.
9. Committee on Dietary Allowances, Food and Nutrition Board, National Research Council: Recommended dietary allowances, ed 9, Washington DC, 1980, National Academy of Sciences.
10. Awad AB: Trans fatty acids in tumor development and the host survival, J Natl Cancer Inst **67:**189-192, 1981.
11. Keys A, et al: Serum cholesterol response to changes in the diet, Metabolism **14:**747-787, 1965.
12. Hegsted DM, et al: Quantitative effects of dietary fat on serum cholesterol in man, Am J Clin Nutr **17:**281-295, 1965.
13. Bang HO, Dyerberg J: Plasma lipids and lipoproteins in Greenlandic west coast Eskimos, Acta Med Scand **192:**85-94, 1972.
14. Kromhout D, et al: The inverse relation between fish consumption and 20-year mortality from coronary heart disease, N Engl J Med **312:**1205-1209, 1985.
15. Shekelle RB, et al: Fish consumption and mortality from coronary heart disease, N Engl J Med **313:**820, 1985.
16. Dayton S, et al: A controlled clinical trial of a diet high in unsaturated fat in preventing complications of atherosclerosis, Circulation **39-40**(suppl 2):1-63, 1969.
17. Burkitt DP, Trowell HC: Refined carbohydrate foods and disease: some implications of dietary fibre, New York, 1975, Academic Press Inc.
18. Whelton PK, Klag MJ: Potassium in the homeostasis and reduction of blood pressure, Clin Nutr **6:**76-82, 1987.
19. Allen LH: Calcium and age-related bone loss, Clin Nutr **5:**147-152, 1986.
20. Turlapaty PDMV, Altura BM: Magnesium deficiency produces spasms of coronary arteries: relationship to etiology of sudden death ischemic heart disease, Science **208:**198-200, 1980.
21. Elwood PC, et al: Magnesium and calcium in the myocardium: Cause of death and area differences, Lancet **2:**720-722, 1980.
22. Peto R, et al: Can dietary detacarotene materially reduce human cancer rates? Nature **290:**201-208, 1981.
23. Margolis S: Treatment of hyperlipidemia, JAMA **39:**2696-2698, 1978.
24. Anderson TW, et al: Winter illness and vitamin C: the effect of relatively low doses, Can Med Assoc J **112:**823-826, 1975.
25. Prinz W, et al: The effect of ascorbic acid supplementation on some parameters of the human immunological defense system, Int J Vitam Nutr Res **47:**248-257, 1977.
26. Kritchevsky D, et al: Influence of whole or skim milk on cholesterol metabolism in rats, Am J Clin Nutr **32:**597-600, 1979.
27. Howard AN, Marks J: Hypocholesterolemic effect of milk, Lancet **2:**225, 1977.
28. Rose DP: Oral contraceptives and vitamin B_6. In Human vitamin B_6 requirements, Washington DC, 1978, National Academy of Sciences, pp 193-201.
29. Lappe, FM: Diet for a small planet, New York, 1975, Ballantine Books Inc.
30. Olson RE: Clinical nutrition, an interface between human ecology and internal medicine, Nutr Rev **36:**161-178, 1978.

CHAPTER 8
The Elderly

Robert M. Russell
Nadine R. Sahyoun

Nutritional counseling of the elderly is a perplexing task because of the lack of established dietary, anthropometric, and biochemical standards for the aged. Most of the work on developing standards has been focused on the very young or on young to middle-aged adults. The problem of lack of standards for the elderly is important to address, however, since the number of old people is increasing in all populations: in the United States there are presently 25 million people over 65 years of age.[1]

With increasing age a person's diet requires greater attention than during the younger years. Although there is a diminution of total caloric need as a person ages, the need for specific nutrients (proteins, vitamins, minerals) may not similarly decline. Thus the quality of diet becomes the key issue. The achievement of desired dietary intakes is made more difficult in the elderly because physical, social, and emotional problems may interfere with appetite and limit the ability to prepare nourishing meals.

GENERAL CONSIDERATIONS

In general, four key points need to be kept in mind regarding the nutritional care of the heterogeneous group of elderly patients: First, each elderly patient is a person, with highly individualized abilities and capabilities, and widely varying levels of functioning. Therefore, personal assessment is essential. Second, elderly patients are more likely to be at nutritional risk and may be in a state of marginal nutritional deficiency upon entry into the health-care system. Third, a marginally nourished elderly patient can become frankly deficient under the stress of a new physical problem or emotional upset. Fourth, elderly patients require the clinician's careful attention to nutritional status at the onset, a well-worked-out care plan, and the monitoring of progress. The simplest, and often neglected, measurement is weight determination at regular intervals. A major change in a patient's weight should always be investigated, the cause determined, and appropriate action taken.[2] In summary, elderly patients require very careful nutritional assessment, including a dietary history, description of activity pattern, and biochemical and anthropometric measurements.

DIETARY STANDARDS AND SURVEYS

Dietary standards for specific nutrients are mostly lacking for people over 50 years of age. The recommended nutrient intakes that are used for the elderly generally have been extrapolated from established values for younger adults. However, the recommended energy intakes have taken into account the lower basal metabolic rate and the reduction of physical activity of the older person. It is known that as people advance in age caloric intakes lessen. For example, from one study,[3] men aged 20 to 37 years had an average daily caloric intake of 2700 kcal whereas those aged 75 to 90 years had an average of 2100 kcal. Most of this decrease can be accounted for by reduced physical activity, although a minor part is due to reduced basal energy expenditure. The recommended caloric intakes for men and women aged 51 to 75 years are 2400 ±400 and 1800 ±400 kcal, respectively. For those over 75 years of age, the recommended intakes are 2050 ±400 and 1600 ±400 kcal.[4] The Committee on Dietary Allowances, National Research Council,[4] recommends that elderly persons receive 12.7% or more of their energy intake as protein. Whether this increase should be accompanied by an increase in dietary calcium is an important question that needs further investigation. Recently demonstrated adverse effects of increased dietary protein on calcium metabolism[5] raise the urgency of addressing this problem. Osteoporosis is a widely prevalent condition among elderly women: 26% of women over age 60 have suffered a vertebral fracture. To prevent or retard this, the National Institutes of Health Consensus Development Conference on Osteoporosis[8] recommended that postmenopausal women and possibly elderly men ingest 1000 to 1500 mg of elemental calcium daily. In the HANES (Health and Nutrition Examination Survey)[9] more than 95% of the elderly women consumed less than 1500 mg of calcium.

A range from 40% to 100% of the recommended dietary allowance (RDA) for micronutrients has been used as a standard when comparing the dietary intakes of older people in different surveys. For HANES participants the dietary micronutrient intakes of people aged 65 to 74 years were found to be less than two thirds of the 1980 RDA in about 50% for calcium and vitamin A.[6] However, there was some evidence that the vitamin A RDA had been set inappropriately high for older persons. In the HANES among black people, a significantly greater proportion (25%-55%) were eating less than two thirds the RDA for riboflavin, niacin, and vitamin C, regardless of economic status.[6,10] More research is needed on the functional significance of such decreased dietary intakes. Many elderly persons are not exposed to sunlight. For housebound elderly, increased sun exposure combined with low-dose (400 IU/da) vitamin D supplementation is the best approach to improving vitamin D nutriture.

THE ELDERLY PATIENT'S DIET HISTORY

Research is needed on the most accurate way of obtaining dietary data from older persons. Short-term memory problems may make the 24-hour recall method totally inappropriate. The usefulness of food intake diaries should also be confirmed by investigations that incorporate into the research plan actual observation of actual food intakes. The diet history should include information about the person's food habits and beliefs, so the plan will be based on meeting the patient's likes and dislikes, thereby increasing its likelihood of success. Special attention should be given to the patient's ability to eat, including dental status and any other constraints on food choices. Finally, the intake of dietary supplements and alcohol must be made an integral part of the diet history of the older person, since in

many past studies these factors have not been included. For now (with the notable exception of calcium), the 1980 RDAs should be used to define dietary adequacy for the elderly, realizing that these standards may be found inappropriate in the future.

The key questions that can alert the health-care practitioner that an older person may be having a dietary problem are as follows:

1. Do you live alone?
2. How many meals do you eat out?
3. Who cooks?
4. Who shops for your food?
5. What handicaps do you have that prevent you from cooking or going to the grocery store?
6. Do you have a problem chewing?
7. How much alcohol do you drink?
8. What and how many medications do you take?
9. Is your income adequate for buying food?

CLINICAL EXAMINATION

The clinician should look for the same signs and symptoms of malnutrition among the elderly that one looks for among younger adults (Chapter 6). However, the interpretation of such signs and symptoms may be less certain among the elderly, since some of the changes normally associated with malnutrition may be related to the aging process itself. For example, hair growth becomes more sparse with aging and the skin texture changes in elderly persons may mimic the flaking dermatitis of protein deficiency or micronutrient malnutrition. Bleeding gums may be the result of ill-fitting dentures. In the HANES absent ankle jerks (a sign of thiamine deficiency) were seen in more than 10% of the black elderly.[10] However, many clinical signs reported in HANES showed poor correlation with dietary intakes, making clinical interpretation uncertain. Further research is needed.

ANTHROPOMETRICS

Several studies have demonstrated a change of body composition with aging. These consist of decreased lean body mass and relatively increased body fat. In addition, there is a redistribution of body fat. Whereas in young people fat is deposited subcutaneously, in elderly people it accumulates intraabdominally and intramuscularly.[11,12] One study[13] demonstrated a reduction in lean body mass of 40% for those over 70 years of age as compared to young adult levels. Most of this loss was attributed to muscle loss. Another study[14] demonstrated that a loss of 1 kg of lean body mass occurs between ages 70 and 75. The loss in lean body mass accelerates with age, particularly among men. This knowledge makes it imperative that anthropometric standards reflecting body fat and protein stores be established for older people.

In the HANES, weight was shown to reach a maximum between ages 35 and 55 years for men and between 55 and 65 for women.[15] It fell thereafter in both sexes, but more gradually in women. It is also known that height decreases with age for both men and women; the average lifetime loss in men is 2.9 cm and 4.9 cm for women.[16] These facts imply that weight for height reference standards available from life insurance companies (e.g., the Metropolitan Life Insurance tables) based on data derived from people between the ages of 20 and 59 years may be inappropriate for judging the nutritional status of the older person.[17] However, values derived from the HANES are normative values that are age-specific and include data from elderly groups up to the age of 74.9 years. These normative weights from the HANES are heavier than the reference values reported from life insurance company data but are appropriate for use as reference values until better guidelines are developed (e.g., from actuarial data derived from people over 60 years old). One measurement used to assess the nutritional status is the Quetelet

Body Mass Index (BMI). It assesses relative body weight by dividing the weight (in kilograms) by the height squared (in meters). The advantage of this index is that it minimizes the contribution of the individual's height in estimating overweight or underweight. The BMI may be determined without performing calculations by using the nomogram for body mass index[18] (see Fig. 10-4).

The Ten State Nutrition Survey data and the HANES data show triceps skinfold thickness to be relatively independent of age for men up to 80, but a drop-off occurs in women after 50. Recent studies[11,12] that compared skinfold thickness with other techniques in assessing body fatness have shown that although skinfold thickness is predictive of body fatness in young people it is a poor predictor in elderly people. This is probably due to the redistribution of body fat that occurs with age.

Similar problems arise when using the arm muscle area (AMA) for assessing lean body mass in an elderly individual. For example, in women there is no diminution in AMA with advancing age in the HANES I and II although lean body mass is known to decline with age when more sophisticated methodology is used (e.g., [40]K counting).

Interpretation of Anthropometric Measurements

Table 8-1 provides guidelines that may be used for interpreting anthropometric data in malnutrition and obesity of the elderly. For evalu-

Table 8-1 Risk of Malnutrition and Obesity in Elderly Patients

Anthropometric Measure	Reference Standard Men/Women	Malnutrition (% of Standard) Men	Malnutrition (% of Standard) Women	Obesity (% of Standard) Men	Obesity (% of Standard) Women
Weight for height†	*	<80	<80	>120	>120
Body mass index (kg/m²)‡					
55-64 yr	25.8/25.3	<80	<75	>115	>125
65-74 yr	25.4/25.9	<75	<75	>115	>125
Triceps skinfold (mm)‡	12/25	<40	<50	>150	>130
Arm muscle area (cm²)‡	52/35	<65	<60	NA	NA

*Table 8-2 is used as the reference standard.

†Corresponding to less than the 15th percentile (for malnutrition) and greater than the 85th (for obesity) in the combined HANES I and II.

‡Corresponding to less than the 5th percentile (malnutrition) and greater than the 85th (obesity) in the HANES II (for the body mass index) and combined HANES I and II (for the triceps skinfold and arm muscle area).

NA, Not applicable.

ating weights for heights in elderly individuals, even those older than 75 years, it is recommended that the normative values from the combined HANES I and II data sets (Table 8-2) be used. The recommended BMI reference standards are the Hanes II 50th percentiles for age groups 55-64 and 65-74.9 years.[20] Triceps skinfold and bone free upper arm muscle circumference are derived from the 50th percentile of HANES I and II data sets for age group 55-74.9. These two indices should be used for people up to the age of 75 years. For those over 75 years old, data for triceps skinfold thickness and arm muscle area are unreliable or uncertain in assessing nutritional status.

These guidelines may be used by the health care provider in comparing the direct measurements obtained to the reference standard as follows:

$$\frac{\text{Actual measurement}}{\text{Reference standard}} \times 100 = \text{Percent of standard}$$

If the percent of standard is below or above the guidelines given, the patient may be at severe risk of undernutrition or overnutrition.

Laboratory Assessment

The same laboratory standard values are generally being applied to the elderly as to younger adults, and although the justification for this practice is questionable there are few data at present to warrant the application of different reference values. It is difficult to establish normal laboratory reference values for elderly persons since studies that have included the elderly have varied greatly in their makeup in terms of race, sex, economic status, and life-styles. For most nutrients a higher prevalence of abnormal laboratory values has been found among the poor, among blacks, and among institutionalized people.

Hemoglobin. Low hemoglobin levels have been frequently reported in elderly groups, and several studies[21-23] show that the prevalence is in the range of 7% to 20%. In the HANES a low hemoglobin (defined as <14 g/dl for men and <12 g/dl for women) was found in 7% of whites aged 60 to 74 and 28% of blacks.[23] It is possible, however, that these prevalences are inflated since the reference standard used was based on young adult values. Until better guidelines are estab-

Table 8-2 Average Weight for Height (Ages 55-74) from Combined HANES I and II Data Sets

Height		Weight			
		Men		Women	
(in)	(cm)	(lb)	(kg)	(lb)	(kg)
58	147	—	—	125.4	57
59	150	—	—	136.4	62
60	152	—	—	143.0	65
61	155	—	—	140.8	64
62	157	149.6	68	140.8	64
63	160	154.0	70	143.0	65
64	163	156.2	71	145.2	66
65	165	158.4	72	147.4	67
66	168	162.8	74	145.2	66
67	170	171.6	78	158.4	72
68	173	171.6	78	154.0	70
69	175	169.4	77	158.4	72
70	178	176.0	80	160.6	73
71	180	184.8	84	—	
72	183	178.2	81		—
73	185	193.6	88		—
74	188	209.0	95		—

From Frisancho AB: Am J Clin Nutr **40**:808-819, 1984.

lished for the different age decades, the 5th percentile of the normative values obtained from the HANES II 65-to-74.9-year-old population are suggested for use. These hemoglobin figures are 12.6 and 11.7 g/dl for males and females. Iron deficiency has been implicated as a causative factor for anemia among some groups of elderly, and in one study of elderly people admitted to a hospital geriatric unit for anemia[24] 10% were found to be frankly iron deficient. Metabolic studies[25] have shown that iron absorption from the gastrointestinal tract may be intact but transfer to the red blood cell defective. Folate deficiency is also common among elderly persons and can be a major cause of anemia in poor and/or sick individuals.

Vitamins. Levels of vitamin C and vitamin B (particularly riboflavin, thiamine, and pyridoxine) have been found by various measurements to be low in certain groups of elderly patients, but the percent has ranged greatly from sample to sample (1%-55%).[26-30] Also, as has been mentioned, the significance of lower than normal measured levels of one or another vitamin in an older person is uncertain, since functional correlates have not been made. Vitamin A levels of less than 20 μg/dl were found in only 0.5% of old people in the HANES, although a much higher prevalence of low levels has been found among Spanish and institutionalized groups.[26] Similarly, low 25-hydroxyvitamin D levels have been found with high frequency among the institutionalized elderly. There are few data on trace mineral status of old people.

Protein. Assessment of protein nutriture is complex. One measure, the creatinine height index, is influenced by declining creatinine clearance with age. However, serum albumin is known to remain fairly constant, with a mean value of 4.0 g/dl in those under 40 years of age and 3.6 g/dl in those over 80.[31] This drop of 0.4 g/dl may have some significance in people taking drugs if the metabolism of the drugs is influenced by albumin binding. However, a low albumin in the absence of liver disease (i.e., <3.2 g/dl) in all likelihood accurately reflects protein deficiency no matter the person's age. Research is needed to investigate how proteins that turn over more quickly than albumin (e.g., transthyretin, retinol-binding protein, transferrin) are affected by age. In addition, the effect

of age on immune function must be carefully studied so the influence of nutrition on immunologic status of the old person can be delineated.

CIRCUMSTANCES AFFECTING DIETARY ADEQUACY

In terms of diet, the most important aspect of aging is the decline in energy requirements. Eating habits may not readily adjust to decreased energy expenditure, so an increase in adiposity frequently results. If, however, the intake of a previously adequate diet is curtailed to match a much-reduced level of energy expenditure, there is a risk of encountering deficiencies in those essential nutrients for which the requirement is absolute rather than relative to caloric intake. For both of these reasons adults should be encouraged to maintain reasonably high levels of physical activity as aging occurs. Individuals who are unable or unwilling to engage in appropriate physical activity should be advised to reduce their caloric intake accordingly.

Menu Planning

To ensure that the curtailed diet provides adequate protein, vitamins, and minerals, a menu plan for the elderly should emphasize foods of high nutrient density. Caloric reductions should therefore be made primarily in sugar, alcohol, and fat groups. Since desserts are often important, rich ones may be replaced by fresh fruits, or smaller portions can be served. Adequate sources of fiber should be included from grains, fruits, and vegetables. Water and juices should always be available.

Although the RDAs of both thiamine and riboflavin are expressed in relation to energy intake, the consumption of both should be maintained at the level suggested in a daily diet of 2000 kcal, even when the actual caloric intake falls below this level.

Government Programs

Most local communities have taken steps to support the needs of elderly persons in conjunction with churches, service clubs, senior citizens' groups, retirement groups, or unions. Since services available to the elderly change from time to time, it is essential that all health-care professionals be familiar with both the programs and the local community back-up services. Among the programs currently available for the elderly is the federal Food Stamp program. Food Stamps are issued according to income and number of persons in a household and can be redeemed at participating grocery stores. Title III of the Older Americans Act provides a number of feeding programs for the elderly. Meals are served Mondays through Fridays in many communities and home-delivered meals may also be available through public or private programs. Group meals should be encouraged if possible because socialization enhances appetite and food intake and provides an opportunity for people to make new friends and develop new interests. Experience has shown that elderly persons may participate more actively if they make some kind of a voluntary contribution. Many nutrition programs also provide other support services, such as shopping assistance, legal aid, and nutritional education.[4]

Other Community Resources

Home health services. Home services may be provided by public or private agencies. They are available for the home-bound patient but usually require referral by a physician. Frequently these services offer assistance with food shopping and preparation and may help elderly persons obtain Food Stamps when appropriate.

Social service agencies. Public and church-related agencies often provide social workers who can help elderly patients gain access to appropriate programs and services. Local and district health offices can be expected to maintain a list of services available to the elderly.

CONCLUSIONS

There is much to be learned about how to assess the nutritional status of the older person. It is impossible to say at present what the most prevalent or important nutritional deficiencies are among the aged. Better dietary, anthropometric, and biochemical standards must be established and, ideally, correlated with measure of function. Standards should be established using well-defined groups of non-debilitated elderly people. A long-term research commitment needs to be made to enable the interplay between aging and nutrition on disease processes and disorders of the elderly to be understood (see also Chapter

30). Costly longitudinal studies on aging already underway need to have a nutritional component added on, and the role of drugs in nutritional metabolism needs investigation. Only recently has medical attention turned to the problems of the elderly.

REFERENCES

1. Department of Commerce, Bureau of the Census: Statistical abstract of the United States, ed 103, Washington DC, 1983, Government Printing Office.
2. Eckstein D: Common complaints of the elderly, Hosp Pract, pp 67-74, April 1976.
3. McGandy RB, et al: Nutrient intakes and energy expenditure in men of different ages, J Gerontol 21:581-587, 1966.
4. Committee on Dietary Allowances, Food and Nutrition Board, National Research Council: Recommended dietary allowances, ed 9, Washington DC, 1980, National Academy of Sciences.
5. Anand CR, Linkswiler HM: Effect of protein intake on calcium balance of young men given 500 mg calcium daily, J Nutr 104:695-700, 1974.
6. Bowman BB, Rosenberg IH: Assessment of the nutritional status of the elderly, Am J Clin Nutr 35:1142-1151, 1982.
7. Urist MR: Osteoporosis in postmenopausal women, Med Folio 3:1, 1971.
8. National Institutes of Health Consensus Development Conference statement: Osteoporosis, Bethesda Md, 1984, NIH.
9. Carroll MD, et al: Dietary intake source data: United States, 1976-80, Vital Health Stat [11], 231, 1983.
10. National Center for Health Statistics: Dietary intake source data, United States, 1971-74, Hyattsville Md, 1974, National Center for Health Statistics, National Research Council.
11. Cohn SH, et al: Comparison of methods of estimating body fat in normal subjects and cancer patients, Am J Clin Nutr 34:2839-2847, 1981.
12. Borkan GA, et al: Age changes in body composition revealed by computed tomography, J Gerontol 38(6):673-677, 1983.
13. Korenchevsky V: Physiological and pathological aging (GH Bourne, editor), Basel, 1961, S Karger AG.
14. Steen GB, et al: Body composition at 70 and 75 years of age: a longitudinal population study, J Clin Exp Gerontol 1:185-200, 1979.
15. Abraham S, et al: Weight by height and age for adults 18-74 years, United States, 1971-74, Vital Health Stat [11], 208, 1979.
16. Metropolitan height and weight tables, New York, 1983, Metropolitan Life Insurance Co.
17. Russell RM, et al: Reference weights, practical considerations, Am J Med 76:767-769, 1984.
18. Burton BT, et al: Health implications of obesity: an NIH Consensus Development Conference, Int J Obes 9:155-169, 1985.
19. Frisancho AB: New standards of weight and body composition by frame size and height for assessment of nutritional status of adults and the elderly, Am J Clin Nutr 40:808-819, 1984.

20. National Center for Health Statistics (MF Najjar, M Rowland): Anthropometric reference data and prevalence of overweight, United States, 1976-80, Vital Health Stat [11], 238, 1987.

21. Kohrs MB, et al: Nutritional status of elderly residents in Missouri, Am J Clin Nutr **31:**2186-2197, 1978.

22. Bailey LB, et al: Folacin and iron status and hematological findings in predominately black elderly persons from urban low-income households, Am J Clin Nutr **32:**2346-2353, 1979.

23. Abraham S, et al: Preliminary findings of the first Health and Nutrition Examination Survey, United States, 1971-72: Dietary intake and biochemical findings, DHEW publication (HRA) 76-1219-1, Rockville, Md, 1976, National Center for Health Statistics.

24. Batata M, et al: Blood and bone marrow changes in elderly patients, with special reference to folic acid, vitamin B12, iron, and ascorbic acid, Br Med J, pp 667-669, June 1967.

25. Marx JJM: Normal iron absorption and decreased red cell iron uptake in the aged, Blood **53**(2):204-211, 1979.

26. Vir SC, Love AHG: Nutritional status of institutionalized and non-institutionalized aged in Belfast, Northern Ireland, Am J Clin Nutr **32:**1934-1947, 1979.

27. Harrill I, Cervone N: Vitamin status of older women, Am J Clin Nutr **30:**431-440, 1977.

28. Stiedemann M, et al: Nutritional status of elderly men and women, J Am Diet Assoc **73:**132-139, 1978.

29. Fisher S, et al: Nutritional assessment of rural Utahns by biochemical and physical measurements, Am J Clin Nutr **31:**667-672, 1978.

30. Pollitt NK, Salkeld RM: Vitamin B status of geriatric patients, Nutr Metab **21**(suppl 1):24-27, 1977.

31. Greenblatt DJ: Reduced serum albumin concentration in the elderly: a report from the Boston collaborative drug surveillance program, J Am Geriatr Soc **27:**20-22, 1979.

III

EVALUATING
NUTRITIONAL STATUS

CHAPTER 9
Infants and Children

Frederick L. Trowbridge

Nutritional assessment techniques include anthropometry, clinical evaluation, laboratory assessment, and dietary evaluation. Each of these has important strengths and limitations and no single technique will provide a thorough assessment of nutritional health.

Anthropometric assessment, the measurement of body size and proportions, provides a rapid and quantitative means of nutritional assessment. The quantitative nature of anthropometry permits accurate and reliable measurements that are useful in monitoring normal growth and nutritional health in well-nourished individuals as well as in detecting nutritional inadequacies or excesses. However, anthropometry is limited in that it can detect only those nutritional abnormalities that have resulted in measurable changes in body size or proportions. It may not detect more subtle, subclinical changes.

Clinical examination for nutritional abnormalities provides an overall impression of nutritional status and can reveal specific signs of malnutrition when these exist. Observation of the patient will indicate obvious obesity, wasting, pallor, robustness, or apathy, providing essential information regarding general nutritional status. The accompanying family and medical history can provide essential information regarding environmental and psychosocial factors bearing on nutritional health, and may indicate the need for further specific nutritional evaluation. However, many early nutritional deficiencies may not be clinically evident, and require additional evaluation.

Laboratory evaluation can identify specific nutrition-related abnormalities such as anemia, iron deficiency, or hypoproteinemia. Biochemical tests may provide the first indication of a nutritional abnormality, before clinical or anthropometric changes occur. However, biochemical tests are specific for the particular nutrient being investigated, and therefore one must have

a suspicion on clinical grounds that a particular deficiency exists so the appropriate biochemical assessment may be undertaken. Moreover, laboratory results in isolation can be misleading and must always be interpreted in the context of an overall clinical, anthropometric, and dietary evaluation.

Dietary assessment is an important adjunct to anthropometric, clinical, and biochemical assessment, since it provides a description of the dietary background, which may help to explain observed clinical or biochemical abnormalities and may suggest proper remedial steps. However, it is difficult to measure dietary intake quantitatively and to ensure that the dietary pattern estimated by assessment techniques is representative of the individual's long-term dietary habits. Dietary evaluation is not a measure of nutritional status, but rather a guide to dietary habits, patterns, and practices.

No single measurement can define nutritional status adequately. Given the diverse forms that an inappropriate nutritional state may take, it is obvious that malnutrition is an inexact term encompassing conditions that range from protein-energy and micronutrient deficiency states to obesity. Thus a careful selection of assessment techniques must be made to suit both the specific type of nutritional evaluation being considered and the circumstances and purposes of the evaluation. Simple anthropometric assessment of growth in children or of weight changes in adults, coupled with clinical examination, will monitor nutritional status in generally healthy individuals. Monitoring of hemoglobin levels also is indicated to identify anemia. If these routine evaluations suggest abnormalities or changes in status, specific laboratory assessment may be appropriate to define abnormalities that may not be clearly evident on clinical grounds. Also, at this stage of a suspected nutritional abnormality, dietary assessment will be useful in defining whether the individual's dietary habits are compatible with the suspected nutritional abnormality and whether recommendations for dietary change seem indicated. Once a nutritional abnormality is identified, the regular assessment of anthropometric, clinical, and biochemical status will provide a basis for judging the response to therapy.

Techniques for the office assessment of nutritional status aimed at routine evaluation and monitoring of nutritional health differ from the more intensive and comprehensive assessment techniques that may be applied in the hospital setting. Nonetheless, practical and reliable information can be obtained by the careful use of simple quantitative anthropometric measurements, coupled with a practical approach to clinical, laboratory, and dietary assessment.

This chapter outlines the elements used in evaluating the nutritional status of infants and children. Chapter 10 focuses specifically on nutritional evaluation of adults. Practical approaches to dietary assessment for both children and adults are outlined in Chapter 11.

FAMILY AND MEDICAL HISTORY

Nutritional evaluation of infants and children should begin with a review of family and medical history. Factors to be considered include (1) parental size and the growth pattern of siblings: differences in genetic growth potential exist and characteristics such as obesity are often familial; (2) dietary practices: family dietary practices such as vegetarianism, megavitamin therapy, or food exclusion, whether prescribed or self-imposed, can affect nutritional status; (3) acute or chronic illness: recent or recurrent acute infections (e.g., gastroenteritis) or chronic illnesses (malabsorption, congenital heart disease, renal disease) or conditions involving long-term steroid therapy (severe asthma) may interfere with growth; (4) social and psychologic environment: factors such as socioeconomic level, home environment, knowledge and skill regarding child care, and attitudes toward the child can markedly affect the quality and regularity of child care and feeding.

ANTHROPOMETRIC ASSESSMENT

Anthropometry, the measurement of body size and proportions, is the simplest and most quantitative measure of nutritional status. It is especially useful in children, in whom deviation from normal patterns of growth, with due consideration to expected genetic and individual variability, can serve as a sensitive index of nutritional adequacy. Still, anthropometry often is underutilized; frequently an otherwise complete medical evaluation lacks a carefully documented growth assessment. Information on body weight is found commonly, but careful length or height data often are lacking. This omission severely limits the interpretation of growth status. Even more underutilized are skinfold and arm circumference measurements, which directly assess the adequacy of fat stores and of muscular development.

Weight

Weight is the most common and fundamental measurement for assessing nutritional status in children. However, the existence of significant day-to-day and within-day variability in weight indicates that accurate evaluation must be based on multiple measurements.

Weight should be measured on a beam balance or electronic scale rather than the less reliable spring-type or "bathroom" scale. The zero adjustment of the scale should be checked regularly, and children should be weighed in minimal clothing or nude to obtain the most accurate results.

Length or Height

Although length or height measurement is of fundamental importance in anthropometric assessment, it is less consistently and carefully done than weight assessment. Length and height data are useful indicators of long-term nutritional adequacy and are less sensitive to short-term variations than are weight measurements.

Young children. Children under 2 years of age should be measured supine on an apparatus with a fixed headboard and a sliding footboard (Fig. 9-1). Measurements should be made with the help of an assistant to ensure that the head is in contact with the headboard and the legs are fully extended. Repeated measurements will ensure accuracy.

Older children. Children over 2 years of age may be measured standing by means of a tape securely fixed to a vertical wall and a sliding 90 degree angle block (Fig. 9-2). The height-measuring rod on the back of an office-type scale is generally less reliable. The child's posture should be erect, with the eyes looking straight forward and the head tilted neither forward nor backward.

Head Circumference

The measurement of head circumference is particularly important in assessing the growth of infants and young children. It is a standard procedure in pediatric practice and is the most commonly used means of detecting pathologic conditions associated with either a disproportionately large head size (as in hydrocephalus) or a disproportionately small one (as in microcephaly). It may not add significantly to the nutritional information gained from weight, height, skinfold thickness, and arm circumference measurements; but its relation to chest circumference is useful in assessing protein-energy malnutrition, since in well-nourished children the circumference of the chest generally exceeds that of the head after the first 6 months of life. However, it is not likely that this relationship will provide more useful information regarding nutritional status than the other indicators to be discussed on the ensuing pages.

The measurement is made with a flexible nonstretch tape passed firmly around the frontal bones just superior to the supraorbital ridges and laid over the maximum occipital prominence at the back. Measurements should be made to the nearest 0.1 cm and, if carefully executed, are highly reproducible.

Skinfold Thickness

Skinfold or "fatfold" thickness provides a more direct estimate of body fat than does weight or weight-for-height assessment. However, skinfold thickness measurements vary significantly between observers and even with a single observer at different times. Variations in fatness also occur at differing sites on the body; thus, accurate assessment of body fat requires measurement of multiple skinfold sites by an experienced person.

Special calipers are available for skinfold thickness measurements. The two most common are the Harpenden and the Lange. The Harpenden caliper provides a finer reading (0.2 versus 1 mm) and has a zero adjustment feature not found on the Lange caliper. A plastic caliper often distributed to health professionals may be

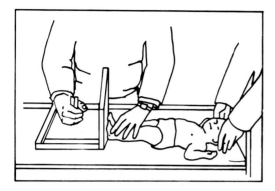

Figure 9-1 Length measurement of the infant.
From Jelliffe DB: WHO Monogr Ser 53, pp 63-78, 1966.

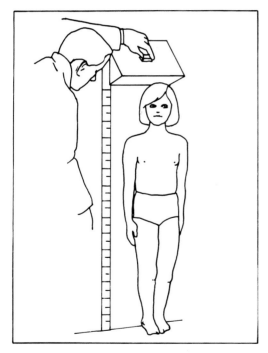

Figure 9-2 Height measurement of the child.
From Jelliffe DB: WHO Monogr Ser 53, pp 63-78, 1966.

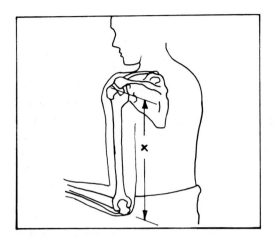

Figure 9-3 Assessing the midpoint of the upper arm. From Jelliffe DB: WHO Monogr Ser 53, pp 63-78, 1966.

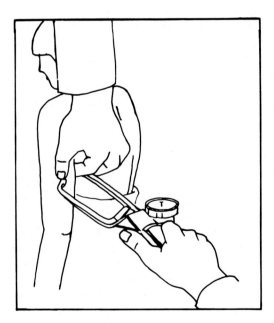

Figure 9-4 Triceps skinfold thickness measurement. From Jelliffe DB: WHO Monogr Ser 53, pp 63-78, 1966.

useful in office assessment since it is small, lightweight, and highly portable, but the Harpenden and Lange calipers give more accurate and reliable results.

The measurements are made at four sites: (1) triceps, the most common, along the posterior aspect at the midpoint of the upper arm (Fig. 9-3); (2) biceps, at the anterior aspect of the mid–upper arm over the body of the biceps muscle; (3) subscapular, immediately below the inferior angle of the scapula; and (4) suprailiac, 1 cm above and 2 cm medial to the anterior iliac spine (may be at or slightly anterior to the midaxillary line).

Skinfold measurements can be made on the right or left side, although the left side is more frequently illustrated. The exact site is located and marked with a felt-tip or ballpoint pen. A pinch of skin is grasped firmly between the thumb and forefinger of the left hand, with the hand coming down from above the site (Fig. 9-4). The pinch is retained with moderate firmness while the caliper is applied and released so the spring mechanism can exert a standard pressure. The reading is taken 2 to 3 seconds after caliper application, allowing time for the initial rapid decrease in skinfold thickness due to tissue compression. It is generally advisable to release the skinfold site and repeat the procedure two or three times to confirm results.

Arm Circumference

Arm circumference can serve as an index of nutritional status that is useful for screening large populations when speed, low cost, and portability of equipment are essential. It is useful when chronologic age is not specifically known. However, it is less useful than weight and height measurement for office or hospital assessment of individual children. In combination with triceps skinfold, the arm circumference can provide a useful estimate of arm muscle cross-sectional area as an indicator of the child's general muscular development.

The measurement is made with a metal or a fiberglass flexible tape. Recently an insertion-type tape has been developed that provides reliable readings.[1] The circumference is measured at the midpoint of the left upper arm (Fig. 9-3). The tape is pulled to contact the skin around the entire circumference, but care must be taken to avoid indenting the skin and fat (Fig. 9-5).

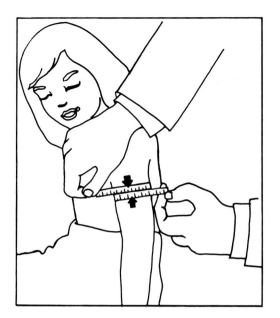

Figure 9-5 Arm circumference measurement.
From Jelliffe DB: Who Monogr Ser 53, pp 63-78, 1966.

Other Measures

Other techniques and measurements occasionally are useful in the assessment of nutritional status. Radiographic examination, usually of the hand and wrist, can be used in assessing the developmental stage of a child to judge biologic as opposed to chronologic age. Malnutrition may delay the developmental processes and retard the biologic age, which can be quantified by bone age status. Although bone age in relation to chronologic age is useful as an index of nutritional status, genetic and other nonnutritional factors also affect this relationship. Detailed guidelines for the evaluation of bone age are available.[2,3]

A variety of additional measurements are collected by anthropometrists to define particular aspects of growth. Chest circumference, abdominal circumference, biacromial and biiliac diameter, and sitting height or crown-rump length are among those used to define upper body growth. Thigh or calf circumference and tibial length are used to define growth of the lower limbs. Such measurements may be helpful in special studies but are of limited practical value in the general assessment of nutritional status. Beyond the technical difficulties and specialized equipment required for some of these measure-

ments, reference standards are not widely available for the definition of normal values. The more common measures of height, weight, head circumference, arm circumference, and skinfold thickness generally provide a practical and sufficiently complete assessment of growth as an index of nutritional status for use in clinical situations and population assessment.

Interpretation of Anthropometric Measurements

Interpretation of data generally involves comparing results from a test sample with those from a reference population or standard that is assumed to have normal nutritional status. In fact, "normal" may not be optimal, so the term reference population or reference data is preferred. Since genetic differences in growth patterns exist among children of diverse racial backgrounds, no absolute universal standard of growth can be established. For example, black children grow taller and have earlier skeletal maturation than white children when matched for socioeconomic status.[4] Body proportions also may be different among races: leg length relative to stature is greater in black, intermediate in white, and shorter in Mexican-American children.[5] Familial factors are highly significant in growth expectation, with parental size being an important predictor of child growth. Moreover, growth differences are observed in relation to birth weight: premature infants with normal weight for gestational age tend to achieve the weight and length of term infants by age 24 to 36 months,[6] although prematures who are small for gestational age tend to remain small and those large for gestational age to remain large later into childhood and perhaps to adulthood (as if following a predetermined channel of growth).[6,7]

The influence of racial, familial, and birth weight factors on growth expectation indicates the need to take these factors into consideration when using anthropometric measurements in nutritional assessment. However, from a practical standpoint, the use of a reference population specific to each racial, parental size, or birth weight group is a difficult and complicated process, even if reference data specific to the subgroup are available. Moreover, when different reference populations are used, comparisons among groups are complicated and the perplexing question is raised of which criteria to apply (e.g., in children with varying degrees of racial admixture, what is "normal" weight for age?). Thus the use of a single reference population is recommended, with due regard given to the possible racial, familial, and birth weight effects on growth outcome.

An additional factor in selecting a reference population is the secular change in growth attainment that has been observed over at least the last century. It is estimated, for example,[8] that height at the age of 5 to 7 years has increased by 1-2 cm per decade. Although the rate of change in growth may be slowing as maximum genetic growth potential is approached, the existence of these trends indicates how important it is to utilize reference data based on recent observations to assess the growth of children relative to that of their contemporaries.

Reference data for weight, height, and head circumference. The data that best represent the current weight, height, and head circumference status of a wide cross section of American children are those developed by the National Center for Health Statistics (NCHS) (Tables 9-1 to 9-6).[9] These reference data provide percentile distributions by age and sex, and they include weight-for-height percentiles not previously available. They come from two reference populations: In one, consisting of infants and young children 0 to 36 months of age (0-48 mo for the weight-for-height measurements) (Tables 9-1 to 9-3), recumbent length has been used. In

Table 9-1 Weight Percentiles (Birth to 36 mo)

Age (mo)	Boys (kg)							Girls (kg)						
	5th	10th	25th	50th	75th	90th	95th	5th	10th	25th	50th	75th	90th	95th
Birth	2.54	2.78	3.00	3.27	3.64	3.82	4.15	2.36	2.51	2.93	3.23	3.52	3.64	3.81
1	3.16	3.43	3.82	4.29	4.75	5.14	5.38	2.97	3.22	3.59	3.98	4.36	4.65	4.92
3	4.43	4.78	5.32	5.98	6.56	7.14	7.37	4.18	4.47	4.88	5.40	5.90	6.39	6.74
6	6.20	6.61	7.20	7.85	8.49	9.10	9.46	5.79	6.12	6.60	7.21	7.83	8.38	8.73
9	7.52	7.95	8.56	9.18	9.88	10.49	10.93	7.00	7.34	7.89	8.56	9.24	9.83	10.17
12	8.43	8.84	9.49	10.15	10.91	11.54	11.99	7.84	8.19	8.81	9.53	10.23	10.87	11.24
18	9.59	9.92	10.67	11.47	12.31	13.05	13.44	8.92	9.30	10.04	10.82	11.55	12.30	12.76
24	10.54	10.85	11.65	12.59	13.44	14.29	14.70	9.87	10.26	11.10	11.90	12.74	13.57	14.08
30	11.44	11.80	12.63	13.67	14.51	15.47	15.97	10.78	11.21	12.11	12.93	13.93	14.81	15.35
36	12.26	12.69	13.53	14.69	15.59	16.66	17.23	11.60	12.07	12.99	13.93	15.03	15.97	16.54

From Hamill PVV, et al: Am J Clin Nutr **32**:607-629, 1979.

Table 9-2 Length Percentiles (Birth to 36 mo)

Age (mo)	Boys (cm)							Girls (cm)						
	5th	10th	25th	50th	75th	90th	95th	5th	10th	25th	50th	75th	90th	95th
Birth	46.6	47.5	49.0	50.5	51.8	53.5	54.4	45.4	46.4	48.2	49.9	51.0	52.0	52.9
1	50.4	51.3	53.0	54.6	56.2	57.7	58.6	49.2	50.2	51.9	53.5	54.9	56.1	56.9
3	56.7	57.7	59.4	61.1	63.0	64.5	65.4	55.4	56.2	57.8	59.5	61.2	62.7	63.4
6	63.4	64.4	66.1	67.8	69.7	71.3	72.3	61.8	62.6	64.2	65.9	67.8	69.4	70.2
9	68.0	69.1	70.6	72.3	74.0	75.9	77.1	66.1	67.0	68.7	70.4	72.4	74.0	75.0
12	71.7	72.8	74.3	76.1	77.7	79.8	81.2	69.8	70.8	72.4	74.3	76.3	78.0	79.1
18	77.5	78.7	80.5	82.4	84.3	86.6	88.1	76.0	77.2	78.8	80.9	83.0	85.0	86.1
24	82.3	83.5	85.6	87.6	89.9	92.2	93.8	81.3	82.5	84.2	86.5	88.7	90.8	92.0
30	87.0	88.2	90.1	92.3	94.6	97.0	98.7	86.0	87.0	88.9	91.3	93.7	95.6	96.9
35	91.6	92.4	94.2	96.5	98.9	101.4	103.1	90.0	91.0	93.1	95.6	98.1	100.0	101.5

From Hamill PVV, et al: Am J Clin Nutr **32**:607-628, 1979.

Table 9-3 Weight-for-Length Percentiles (Birth to 48 mo)

Length (cm)	Weight (kg) Boys							Girls						
	5th	10th	25th	50th	75th	90th	95th	5th	10th	25th	50th	75th	90th	95th
48-50	—	—	2.86	3.15	3.50	—	—	—	—	3.02	3.29	3.59	—	—
50-52	—	—	3.16	3.48	3.86	—	—	—	—	3.25	3.55	3.89	—	—
52-54	—	—	3.52	3.88	4.23	—	—	—	—	3.56	3.89	4.26	—	—
54-56	3.49	3.65	3.95	4.34	4.76	5.13	5.33	3.54	3.64	3.93	4.29	4.70	5.02	5.21
56-58	3.90	4.09	4.43	4.89	5.23	5.69	5.88	3.93	4.05	4.37	4.76	5.20	5.55	5.77
58-60	4.37	4.58	4.94	5.38	5.84	6.28	6.47	4.38	4.50	4.85	5.27	5.73	6.12	6.36
60-62	4.88	5.10	5.49	5.94	6.42	6.88	7.08	4.85	4.99	5.37	5.82	6.30	6.70	6.95
62-64	5.43	5.65	6.05	6.52	7.02	7.50	7.72	5.35	5.50	5.91	6.39	6.89	7.30	7.55
64-66	5.99	6.20	6.62	7.11	7.63	8.13	8.36	5.87	6.03	6.47	6.97	7.48	7.90	8.15
66-68	6.55	6.76	7.19	7.70	8.23	8.75	8.99	6.38	6.56	7.02	7.55	8.07	8.50	8.75
68-70	7.10	7.31	7.75	8.27	8.82	9.35	9.62	6.89	7.08	7.56	8.11	8.64	9.08	9.33
70-72	7.63	7.84	8.28	8.82	9.39	9.93	10.21	7.37	7.58	8.08	8.64	9.18	9.63	9.88
72-74	8.13	8.33	8.78	9.33	9.92	10.48	10.77	7.82	8.05	8.56	9.14	9.68	10.15	10.41
74-76	8.58	8.73	9.24	9.81	10.43	10.99	11.29	8.24	8.49	9.00	9.59	10.14	10.63	10.91
76-78	9.00	9.21	9.68	10.27	10.91	11.48	11.78	8.62	8.90	9.42	10.02	10.57	11.08	11.39
78-80	9.40	9.62	10.09	10.70	11.36	11.94	12.25	8.99	9.29	9.81	10.41	10.97	11.51	11.85
80-82	9.77	10.01	10.49	11.12	11.80	12.39	12.69	9.34	9.67	10.19	10.80	11.37	11.93	12.29
82-84	10.14	10.39	10.88	11.53	12.23	12.83	13.13	9.68	10.04	10.57	11.18	11.75	12.35	12.72
84-86	10.49	10.76	11.27	11.93	12.65	13.26	13.56	10.03	10.41	10.94	11.56	12.15	12.76	13.15
86-88	10.85	11.14	11.67	12.34	13.07	13.69	14.00	10.39	10.78	11.33	11.95	12.55	13.19	13.57
88-90	11.22	11.53	12.08	12.76	13.50	14.13	14.44	10.76	11.17	11.74	12.36	12.98	13.63	14.01
90-92	11.60	11.94	12.52	13.20	13.94	14.58	14.90	11.16	11.58	12.17	12.80	13.45	14.10	14.45
92-94	12.00	12.37	12.97	13.63	14.40	15.05	15.39	11.59	12.02	12.63	13.27	13.95	14.61	14.92
94-96	12.42	12.81	13.45	14.14	14.88	15.54	15.90	12.05	12.48	13.12	13.77	14.48	15.14	15.42
96-98	12.88	13.28	13.96	14.66	15.39	16.06	16.43	12.55	12.98	13.64	14.31	15.04	15.71	15.99
98-100	13.37	13.78	14.50	15.21	15.94	16.62	17.00	13.10	13.51	14.19	14.87	15.63	16.32	16.64
100-102	13.90	14.30	15.06	15.81	16.54	17.22	17.60	13.68	14.08	14.77	15.46	16.25	16.96	17.39
102-104	14.48	14.85	15.65	16.45	17.18	17.87	18.24							

From Hamill PVV, et al: Am J Clin Nutr **32:**607-628, 1979.

Table 9-4 Weight Percentiles (1.5 to 18 yr)

Age (yr)	Boys (kg)							Girls (kg)						
	5th	10th	25th	50th	75th	90th	95th	5th	10th	25th	50th	75th	90th	95th
1.5	9.72	10.18	10.51	11.09	12.02	12.95	14.42	9.02	9.16	9.61	10.38	10.94	11.75	12.36
2.0	10.49	10.96	11.55	12.34	12.36	14.38	15.50	9.95	10.32	10.96	11.80	12.73	13.58	14.15
2.5	11.27	11.77	12.55	13.52	14.61	15.71	16.61	10.80	11.35	12.11	13.03	14.23	15.16	15.76
3.0	12.05	12.58	13.52	14.62	15.78	16.95	17.77	11.61	12.26	13.11	14.10	15.50	16.54	17.22
3.5	12.84	13.41	14.46	15.68	16.90	18.15	18.98	12.37	13.08	14.00	15.07	16.59	17.77	18.59
4.0	13.64	14.24	15.39	16.69	17.99	19.32	20.27	13.11	13.84	14.80	15.96	17.56	18.93	19.91
4.5	14.45	15.10	16.30	17.69	19.06	20.50	21.63	13.83	14.56	15.55	16.81	18.48	20.06	21.24
5.0	15.27	15.98	17.22	18.67	20.14	21.70	23.09	14.55	15.26	16.29	17.66	19.39	21.23	22.62
5.5	16.09	16.83	18.14	19.67	21.25	22.96	24.66	15.29	15.97	17.05	18.56	20.36	22.48	24.11
6.0	16.93	17.72	19.07	20.69	22.40	24.31	26.34	16.05	16.72	17.86	19.52	21.44	23.89	25.75
6.5	17.78	18.62	20.02	21.74	23.62	25.76	28.16	16.85	17.51	18.76	20.61	22.68	25.50	27.59
7.0	18.64	19.63	21.00	22.85	24.94	27.36	30.12	17.71	18.39	19.78	21.84	24.16	27.39	29.68
7.5	19.52	20.45	22.02	24.03	26.36	29.11	32.73	18.62	19.37	20.95	23.26	25.90	29.57	32.07
8.0	20.40	21.39	23.09	25.30	27.91	31.06	34.51	19.62	20.45	22.26	24.84	27.88	32.04	34.71
8.5	21.31	22.34	24.21	26.56	29.61	32.22	35.96	20.68	21.64	23.70	26.58	30.08	34.73	37.58
9.0	22.25	23.33	25.40	28.13	31.46	35.57	39.58	21.82	22.92	25.27	28.46	32.44	37.60	40.64
9.5	23.25	24.38	26.68	29.73	33.46	38.11	42.35	21.82	22.92	25.27	28.48	32.44	37.60	40.64
10.0	24.33	25.52	28.07	31.44	35.61	40.80	45.27	23.05	24.29	26.94	30.45	34.94	40.61	43.85
10.5	25.51	26.78	29.59	33.30	37.92	43.63	48.31	24.36	25.76	28.71	32.55	37.53	43.70	47.17
11.0	26.80	28.17	31.25	35.30	40.38	46.57	51.47	25.75	27.32	30.57	34.72	40.17	46.84	50.57
11.5	28.24	29.72	33.08	37.46	43.00	49.61	54.73	27.24	28.97	32.49	36.95	42.84	49.96	54.00
12.0	29.85	31.46	35.09	39.78	45.77	52.73	58.09	28.83	30.71	34.48	29.23	45.48	53.03	57.42
12.5	31.64	33.41	37.31	42.27	48.70	55.91	61.52	30.52	32.53	36.52	41.53	48.07	55.99	60.81
13.0	33.64	35.60	39.74	44.95	51.79	59.12	65.02	32.30	34.42	38.59	43.84	50.56	58.81	64.12
13.5	35.85	38.03	42.40	47.81	55.02	62.35	68.51	34.14	36.35	40.65	46.10	52.91	61.45	67.30
14.0	38.22	40.64	45.21	50.77	58.31	55.57	72.13	35.98	38.26	42.65	48.26	55.11	63.87	70.30
14.5	40.66	43.34	48.08	53.75	61.58	68.76	75.66	37.76	40.11	44.54	50.28	57.09	66.04	73.08
15.0	43.11	46.05	50.92	56.71	64.72	71.91	79.12	39.45	41.83	45.28	52.10	58.84	67.95	75.59
15.5	45.50	48.69	53.64	59.51	67.64	74.98	82.45	40.99	43.38	47.82	53.62	60.32	69.54	77.78
16.0	47.74	51.16	56.16	62.10	70.28	77.97	85.62	42.32	44.72	49.10	54.96	61.48	70.79	79.59
16.5	49.76	53.39	58.38	64.39	72.46	80.84	88.59	43.41	45.78	50.09	55.89	62.29	71.68	80.99
17.0	51.50	55.28	60.22	66.31	74.17	83.58	91.31	44.20	46.54	50.75	56.44	62.75	72.18	81.93
17.5	52.89	56.78	61.61	67.78	75.32	86.14	93.73	44.74	47.04	51.14	55.69	62.91	72.38	62.46
18.0	53.97	57.89	62.61	68.88	76.04	88.41	95.76	45.08	47.33	51.33	56.71	62.89	72.37	82.62

From Hamill PVV, et al: Am J Clin Nutr **32**:607-629, 1979.

Table 9-5 Height Percentiles (2 to 18 yr)

Age (yr)	Boys (cm)							Girls (cm)						
	5th	10th	25th	50th	75th	90th	95th	5th	10th	25th	50th	75th	90th	95th
2.0	82.5	83.5	85.3	86.8	89.2	92.0	94.4	81.6	82.1	84.0	86.8	89.3	92.0	93.6
2.5	86.4	86.5	88.5	90.4	92.9	95.6	97.8	84.6	85.3	87.3	90.0	92.5	95.0	96.6
3.0	89.0	90.3	92.6	94.9	97.5	100.1	102.0	88.3	89.3	91.4	94.1	96.6	99.0	100.6
3.5	92.5	93.9	96.4	99.1	101.7	104.3	106.1	91.7	93.0	95.2	97.9	100.5	102.8	104.5
4.0	95.8	97.3	100.0	102.9	105.7	108.2	109.9	95.0	96.4	98.8	101.6	104.3	106.6	108.3
4.5	98.9	100.6	103.4	106.6	109.4	111.9	113.5	98.1	99.7	102.2	105.0	107.9	110.2	112.0
5.0	102.0	103.7	106.5	109.9	112.8	115.4	117.0	101.1	102.7	105.4	108.4	111.4	113.8	115.6
5.5	104.9	108.7	109.5	113.1	116.1	118.7	120.3	103.9	105.6	108.4	111.6	114.8	117.4	119.2
6.0	107.7	109.6	112.5	115.1	119.2	121.9	123.5	106.6	108.4	111.3	114.6	118.1	120.8	122.7
6.5	110.4	112.3	115.3	119.0	122.2	124.9	125.6	109.2	111.0	114.1	117.6	121.3	124.2	126.1
7.0	113.0	115.0	118.0	121.7	125.0	127.9	129.7	111.8	113.6	115.8	120.6	124.4	127.6	129.5
7.5	115.6	117.6	120.6	124.4	127.8	130.8	132.7	114.4	116.2	119.5	123.5	127.6	130.9	132.9
8.0	118.1	120.2	123.2	127.0	130.5	133.6	135.7	116.9	118.7	122.2	126.4	130.6	134.2	136.2
8.5	120.5	122.7	125.7	129.6	133.2	136.5	138.8	119.5	121.3	124.9	129.3	133.6	137.4	139.6
9.0	122.9	125.2	128.2	132.2	135.0	139.4	141.8	122.1	123.9	127.7	132.2	136.7	140.7	142.9
9.5	125.3	127.6	130.8	134.8	138.8	142.4	144.9	124.8	126.6	130.6	135.2	139.8	143.9	145.2
10.0	127.7	130.1	133.4	137.5	141.6	145.5	148.1	127.5	129.5	133.6	138.3	142.9	147.2	149.5
10.5	130.1	132.6	136.0	140.3	144.6	148.7	151.5	130.4	132.5	136.7	141.5	146.1	150.4	152.8
11.0	132.8	135.1	138.7	143.3	147.6	152.1	154.9	133.5	135.6	140.0	144.8	149.3	153.7	156.2
11.5	135.0	137.7	141.5	146.4	151.1	155.6	158.5	136.8	139.0	143.5	148.2	152.6	156.9	159.5
12.0	137.6	140.3	144.4	149.7	154.6	159.4	162.3	139.8	142.3	147.0	151.5	155.9	160.0	162.7
12.5	140.2	143.0	147.4	153.0	158.2	163.2	166.1	142.7	145.4	150.1	154.6	158.8	162.9	166.6
13.0	142.9	145.8	150.5	156.5	161.8	167.0	169.8	145.2	148.0	152.8	157.1	161.3	165.3	168.1
13.5	145.7	148.7	153.6	159.9	165.3	170.5	173.4	147.2	150.0	154.7	159.0	163.2	167.3	170.0
14.0	148.8	151.8	156.9	163.1	168.5	173.8	176.7	148.7	151.5	155.9	160.4	154.6	168.7	171.3
14.5	152.0	155.0	160.1	166.2	171.5	176.6	179.6	149.7	152.5	156.8	161.2	165.6	169.8	172.2
15.0	155.2	158.2	163.3	159.0	174.1	178.9	181.9	150.5	153.2	157.2	161.8	166.3	170.5	172.8
15.5	158.3	161.2	166.2	171.5	176.3	180.3	183.9	151.1	153.6	157.5	162.1	166.7	170.9	173.1
16.0	161.1	163.9	168.7	173.5	178.1	182.4	185.4	151.6	154.1	157.8	162.4	166.9	171.1	173.3
16.5	163.4	166.1	170.6	175.2	179.5	183.6	186.6	152.2	154.6	158.2	162.7	167.1	171.2	173.4
17.0	164.9	167.7	171.9	176.2	180.5	184.4	187.3	152.7	155.1	158.7	163.1	167.3	171.2	173.5
17.5	165.6	168.5	172.4	176.7	181.0	185.0	187.6	153.2	155.6	159.1	163.4	167.5	171.1	173.5
18.0	165.7	168.7	172.3	176.8	181.2	185.3	187.6	153.6	156.0	159.6	163.7	167.6	171.0	173.6

From Hamill PVV, et al: Am J Clin Nutr **32**:607-629, 1979.

Table 9-6 Weight-for-Height Percentiles (Prepubescent Children)

Height (cm)	Weight (kg)													
	Boys							Girls						
	5th	10th	25th	50th	75th	90th	95th	5th	10th	25th	50th	75th	90th	95th
90-92	11.70	11.97	12.59	13.41	14.35	15.25	15.72	11.45	11.67	12.28	13.14	14.11	14.98	15.74
92-94	12.07	12.36	13.03	13.89	14.84	15.87	16.41	11.86	12.10	12.74	13.63	14.63	15.57	16.42
94-96	12.46	12.77	13.49	14.38	15.34	16.45	17.06	12.26	12.53	13.21	14.12	15.14	16.13	17.05
96-98	12.87	13.21	13.98	14.89	15.87	17.01	17.69	12.66	12.97	13.70	14.62	15.66	16.69	17.65
98-100	13.31	13.67	14.48	15.43	16.41	17.56	18.29	13.05	13.42	14.19	15.13	16.19	17.24	18.23
100-102	13.77	14.15	15.00	15.98	16.98	18.11	18.89	13.48	13.88	14.69	15.65	16.73	17.80	18.80
102-104	14.25	14.65	15.54	16.55	17.57	18.67	19.50	13.91	14.36	15.21	16.20	17.28	18.38	19.38
104-106	14.76	15.18	16.10	17.13	18.18	19.25	20.12	14.36	14.85	15.75	16.75	17.86	18.98	19.98
106-108	15.30	15.73	16.68	17.74	18.82	19.86	20.76	14.84	15.37	16.30	17.33	18.46	19.62	20.61
108-110	15.85	16.31	17.28	18.37	19.49	20.51	21.45	15.35	15.91	16.87	17.94	19.09	20.30	21.29
110-112	16.43	16.91	17.90	19.02	20.18	21.22	22.18	15.90	16.48	17.47	18.56	19.76	21.03	22.03
112-114	17.04	17.53	18.54	19.70	20.91	21.98	22.98	16.48	17.09	18.08	19.22	20.47	21.81	22.84
114-116	17.66	18.18	19.20	20.39	21.66	22.82	23.85	17.11	17.72	18.72	19.91	21.23	22.67	23.73
116-118	18.32	18.85	19.89	21.11	22.45	23.73	24.80	17.77	18.40	19.40	20.64	22.04	23.60	24.71
118-120	18.99	19.55	20.60	21.85	23.28	24.73	25.83	18.48	19.11	20.11	21.42	22.92	24.62	25.81
120-122	19.70	20.28	21.34	22.63	24.15	25.80	26.96	19.22	19.85	20.87	22.25	23.88	25.73	27.03
122-124	20.43	21.03	22.11	23.45	25.07	26.96	28.18	19.99	20.64	21.68	23.13	24.91	26.95	28.37
124-126	21.20	21.82	22.92	24.32	26.05	28.18	29.50	20.80	21.47	22.54	24.09	26.05	28.27	29.87
126-128	21.99	22.64	23.77	25.24	27.10	29.48	30.92	21.65	22.34	23.47	25.11	27.28	29.71	31.51
128-130	22.82	23.50	24.67	26.22	28.21	30.86	32.44	22.53	23.25	24.46	26.22	28.63	31.28	33.33
130-132	23.69	24.39	25.62	27.26	29.41	32.31	34.07	23.44	24.22	25.52	27.40	30.09	32.99	35.33
132-134	24.59	25.32	26.62	28.38	30.68	33.82	35.81	24.38	25.22	26.66	28.68	31.68	34.84	37.53
134-136	25.53	26.30	27.68	29.58	32.05	35.40	37.67	25.35	26.28	27.88	30.06	33.41	36.84	39.93
136-138	26.51	27.32	28.80	30.85	33.51	37.05	39.65	26.34	27.39	29.19	31.54	35.29	39.01	42.54
138-140	27.53	28.38	29.99	32.23	35.08	38.77	41.74	—	—	—	—	—	—	—
140-142	28.59	29.48	31.25	33.70	36.75	40.55	43.97	—	—	—	—	—	—	—
142-144	29.70	30.64	32.58	35.27	38.54	42.39	46.32	—	—	—	—	—	—	—
144-146	30.86	31.85	34.00	36.95	40.45	44.29	48.80	—	—	—	—	—	—	—

From Hamill PVV, et al: Am J Clin Nutr **32**:607-629, 1979.

the other, comprising children 2 years of age and older (Tables 9-4 to 9-6), standing height measurements are given. For children in the overlapping ages 24 to 36 months, either reference population can be used.

Reference data for growth velocity by age and sex[10] are also available. The adequacy of an individual child's growth velocity can be estimated by comparing the congruency between the curve for that child and the NCHS or another "distance" curve.[9] Interpreting growth velocity in adolescents is complicated by the wide range of variation in age of onset of puberty. Growth curves represent the average, and they can be misleading when children whose adolescent growth spurt begins earlier or later than average are evaluated.

The adequacy of growth attainment and velocity in individuals needs to be judged in relation to their stage of maturation or biologic age as indicated radiographically by their bone age or by the developmental stage of their secondary sexual characteristics.

Reference data for skinfold thickness and arm circumference. Data from the first Health and Nutrition Examination Survey (HANES I) provide a useful reference for evaluating triceps skinfold thickness and arm circumference (Table 9-7).[11] The measurements may be combined to give an estimate of the arm muscle area, a reasonably good indicator of muscular development (Table 9-8).

Formation of Indicators

Indicators of nutritional status commonly are formed by determining the percentile ranking of the individual child or by calculating the percentage of the median (50th percentile) value for the child's specific age/sex group. Percentile ranking can be determined using growth charts or tables to indicate the child's approximate place in the distribution of "normal" children in the reference population. However, percentile ranking only places a child within a broad range (e.g., 10th to 25th percentile or >95th percentile) and does not provide an exact quantitative index of nutritional status.

Unlike percentiles, percentage-of-median indicators do not show the child's standing among "normal" children but they do provide a quantitative index of growth useful in measuring nutritional status and in evaluating changes over time. For example, nutritional improvement could be quantified for a child whose weight was 75% of median but improved with nutritional therapy to 80% of median. The same child might have remained below the 5th percentile of weight-for-age both before and after therapy; and thus following the percentile ranking of the child would not have given as clear or quantitative an indication of improvement. The use of standard deviation units (Z-score) instead of percentages to express the distance of a child's growth from the median has been proposed.[12] Z-scores offer the advantage of relating deviation from the median to the expected distribution of values in the reference population. For example, a child with a weight that was 2 Z-scores below the median would be expected to be at about the 3rd percentile.

Weight-for-age. The most common nutritional index used in children, weight-for-age, provides a good general expression of growth status. It is the most widely used indicator of protein-energy malnutrition. However, weight-for-age will not distinguish between a fat child who is short, and a tall child who is slim if the two have the same weight at the same age, despite their obvious differences in nutritional status. For this reason it is wise to assess height-for-age and weight-for-height in addition to weight-for-age.

Height-for-age. Since height cannot decrease and does not increase rapidly, height-for-age provides an excellent index of long-term nutritional health. Height-for-age is not influenced by short-term changes in nutritional status.

Weight-for-height. Weight-for-height provides an index that reflects current nutritional status and is relatively independent of the child's long-term nutritional health. For example, a child with stunted linear growth because of chronic malnutrition but who recently has been rehabilitated nutritionally will have low height-for-age, reflecting previous chronic undernutrition, and may have low weight-for-age because of short stature. However, weight-for-height may be normal or even increased, reflecting the child's current nutritional well-being.

Additional growth indices. A number of other indices have been proposed for the assessment of nutritional status using anthropometric measurements. Several, including the ratio of weight to the square of height[13] and the ratio of

Table 9-7 Percentiles for Triceps Skinfold and Arm Circumference (mm)

Age Group (yr)	Triceps Skinfold							Age Group (yr)	Arm Circumference						
	5th	10th	25th	50th	75th	90th	95th		5th	10th	25th	50th	75th	90th	95th
								Males							
1-1.9	6	7	8	10	12	14	16	1-1.9	142	146	150	159	170	176	183
2-2.9	6	7	8	10	12	14	15	2-2.9	141	145	153	162	170	178	185
3-3.9	6	7	8	10	11	14	15	3-3.9	150	153	160	167	175	184	190
4-4.9	6	6	8	9	11	12	14	4-4.9	149	154	162	171	180	186	192
5-5.9	6	6	8	9	11	14	15	5-5.9	153	160	167	175	185	195	204
6-6.9	5	6	7	8	10	13	16	6-6.9	155	159	167	179	188	209	228
7-7.9	5	6	7	9	12	15	17	7-7.9	162	167	177	187	201	223	230
8-8.9	5	6	7	8	10	13	16	8-8.9	162	170	177	190	202	220	245
9-9.9	6	6	7	10	13	17	18	9-9.9	175	178	187	200	217	249	257
10-10.9	6	6	8	10	14	18	21	10-10.9	181	184	196	210	231	262	274
11-11.9	6	6	8	11	16	20	24	11-11.9	186	190	202	223	244	261	280
12-12.9	6	6	8	11	14	22	28	12-12.9	193	200	214	232	254	282	303
13-13.9	5	5	7	10	14	22	26	13-13.9	194	211	228	247	263	286	301
14-14.9	4	5	7	9	14	21	24	14-14.9	220	226	237	253	283	303	322
15-15.9	4	5	6	8	11	18	24	15-15.9	222	229	244	264	284	311	320
16-16.9	4	5	6	8	12	16	22	16-16.9	244	248	262	278	303	324	343
17-17.9	5	5	6	8	12	16	19	17-17.9	246	253	267	285	308	336	347
18-18.9	4	5	6	9	13	20	24	18-18.9	245	260	276	297	321	353	379
19-24.9	4	5	7	10	15	20	22	19-24.9	262	272	288	308	331	355	372
25-34.9	5	6	8	12	16	20	24	25-34.9	271	282	300	319	342	362	375
35-44.9	5	6	8	12	16	20	23	35-44.9	278	287	305	326	345	363	374
45-54.9	6	6	8	12	15	20	25	45-54.9	267	281	301	322	342	362	376
55-64.9	5	6	8	11	14	19	22	55-64.9	258	273	296	317	336	355	369
65-74.9	4	6	8	11	15	19	22	65-74.9	248	263	285	307	325	344	355
								Females							
1-1.9	6	7	8	10	12	14	16	1-1.9	138	142	148	156	164	172	177
2-2.9	6	8	9	10	12	15	16	2-2.9	142	145	152	160	167	176	184
3-3.9	7	8	9	11	12	14	15	3-3.9	143	150	158	167	175	183	189
4-4.9	7	8	8	10	12	14	16	4-4.9	149	154	160	169	177	184	191
5-5.9	6	7	8	10	12	15	18	5-5.9	153	157	165	175	185	203	211
6-6.9	6	6	8	10	12	14	16	6-6.9	156	162	170	176	187	204	211
7-7.9	6	7	9	11	13	16	18	7-7.9	164	167	174	183	199	216	231
8-8.9	6	8	9	12	15	18	24	8-8.9	168	172	183	195	214	247	261
9-9.9	8	8	10	13	16	20	22	9-9.9	178	182	194	211	224	251	260
10-10.9	7	8	10	12	17	23	27	10-10.9	174	182	193	210	228	251	265
11-11.9	7	8	10	13	18	24	28	11-11.9	185	194	208	224	248	276	303
12-12.9	8	9	11	14	18	23	27	12-12.9	194	203	216	237	256	282	294
13-13.9	8	8	12	15	21	26	30	13-13.9	202	211	223	243	271	301	338
14-14.9	9	10	13	16	21	26	28	14-14.9	214	223	237	252	272	304	322
15-15.9	8	10	12	17	21	25	32	15-15.9	208	221	239	254	279	300	322
16-16.9	10	12	15	18	22	26	31	16-16.9	218	224	241	258	283	318	334
17-17.9	10	12	13	19	24	30	37	17-17.9	220	227	241	264	295	324	350
18-18.9	10	12	15	18	22	26	30	18-18.9	222	227	241	258	281	312	325
19-24.9	10	11	14	18	24	30	34	19-24.9	221	230	247	265	290	319	345
25-34.9	10	12	16	21	27	34	37	25-34.9	233	240	256	277	304	342	368
35-44.9	12	14	18	23	29	35	38	35-44.9	341	251	267	290	317	356	378
45-54.9	12	16	20	25	30	36	40	45-54.9	242	256	274	299	328	362	384
55-64.9	12	16	20	25	31	36	38	55-64.9	243	257	280	303	335	367	385
65-74.9	12	14	18	24	29	34	36	65-74.9	240	252	274	299	326	356	373

From Frisancho AR: Am J Clin Nutr **34**:3540-3545, 1981.

Table 9-8 Percentiles for Arm Muscle Area (mm²)

	Males								Females						
Age Group	5th	10th	25th	50th	75th	90th	95th	Age Group	5th	10th	25th	50th	75th	90th	95th
1-1.9	956	1014	1133	1278	1447	1644	1720	1-1.9	885	973	1084	1221	1378	1535	1621
2-2.9	973	1040	1190	1345	1557	1690	1787	2-2.9	973	1029	1119	1269	1405	1595	1727
3-3.9	1095	1201	1357	1484	1618	1750	1853	3-3.9	1014	1133	1227	1396	1563	1690	1846
4-4.9	1207	1264	1408	1579	1747	1926	2008	4-4.9	1058	1171	1313	1475	1644	1832	1958
5-5.9	1298	1411	1550	1720	1884	2089	2285	5-5.9	1238	1301	1423	1598	1825	2012	2159
6-6.9	1360	1447	1605	1815	2056	2297	2493	6-6.9	1354	1414	1513	1683	1877	2182	2323
7-7.9	1497	1548	1808	2027	2246	2494	2886	7-7.9	1330	1441	1602	1815	2045	2332	2469
8-8.9	1550	1664	1895	2089	2296	2628	2788	8-8.9	1513	1566	1808	2034	2327	2657	2996
9-9.9	1811	1884	2067	2288	2657	3053	3257	9-9.9	1723	1788	1976	2227	2571	2987	3112
10-10.9	1930	2027	2182	2575	2903	3486	3882	10-10.9	1740	1784	2019	2296	2583	2873	3093
11-11.9	2016	2156	2382	2670	3022	3359	4226	11-11.9	1784	1987	2316	2612	3071	3739	3953
12-12.9	2216	2339	2649	3022	3496	3968	4640	12-12.9	2092	2182	2579	2904	3225	3655	3847
13-13.9	2363	2546	3044	3553	4081	4502	4734	13-13.9	2269	2426	2657	3130	3529	4081	4568
14-14.9	2830	3147	3586	3963	4575	5368	5530	14-14.9	2418	2562	2874	3220	3704	4294	4850
15-15.9	3138	3317	3788	4481	5134	5631	5900	15-15.9	2426	2518	2847	3248	3689	4123	4756
16-16.9	3625	4044	4352	4951	5753	6576	6980	16-16.9	2308	2567	2865	3248	3718	4353	4946
17-17.9	3998	4252	4777	5286	5950	6886	7726	17-17.9	2442	2674	2996	3336	3883	4552	5251
18-18.9	4070	4481	5066	5552	6374	7067	8355	18-18.9	2398	2538	2917	3243	3694	4461	4767
19-24.9	4508	4777	5274	5913	6660	7606	8200	19-24.9	2538	2728	3026	3406	3877	4439	4940
25-34.9	4694	4963	5541	6214	7067	7847	8436	25-34.9	2661	2826	3148	3573	4138	4806	5541
35-44.9	4844	5181	5740	6490	7265	8034	8488	35-44.9	2750	2948	3359	3783	4428	5240	5877
45-54.9	4546	4946	5589	6297	7142	7918	8458	45-54.9	2784	2956	3378	3858	4520	5375	5964
55-64.9	4422	4783	5381	6144	6919	7670	8149	55-64.9	2784	3063	3477	4045	4750	5632	6247
65-74.9	3973	4411	5031	5716	6432	7074	7453	65-74.9	2737	3018	3444	4019	4739	5566	6214

From Frisancho AR: Am J Clin Nutr **34**:3540-3545, 1981.

weight to height raised to the 1.6 power,[14] are intended to reflect weight-for-height status. Arm circumference in relation to height (the Quaker upper-arm circumference [QUAC] stick) also has been suggested as an indicator of nutritional status[15]; but it generally provides little information that is not included in the more common weight-for-height indicator. Although potentially useful in field situations when a rapid survey must be made using limited equipment, arm circumference–for–height does not appear to be more sensitive or more specific in identifying malnourished children than simple upper-arm circumference alone.[16]

A significant limitation of all these indicators is their lack of a well-defined reference population for judging normal values, particularly when compared to the availability of the NCHS standards for weight and height.[9] It is likely, therefore, that they will be less useful for practical application in clinical situations than height and weight indicators.

Indicators of obesity. Skinfold thickness, usually over the triceps muscle, has been the most widely used anthropometric technique for estimating body fatness. It is possible, using reference data from the HANES I, to determine the percentile ranking of a child's triceps skinfold thickness. Values exceeding the 90th percentile suggest obesity. Excess weight for age also has been used as an indicator of obesity, but it lacks specificity, since increased weight may reflect greater stature and/or lean mass as well as fat. Weight-for-height provides a potentially better index of obesity, since it corrects for height. However, increases in weight for height may reflect increased muscular development as well as excess fat so this indicator lacks specificity. A weight-for-height value exceeding 120% of median has been used as a criterion for obesity. Weight for height greater than the 90th percentile of the NCHS standards also may be used as a criterion for obesity. The 90th percentile corresponds to approximately 115% to 130% of median at different ages.

Muscular development. As reflected in up-

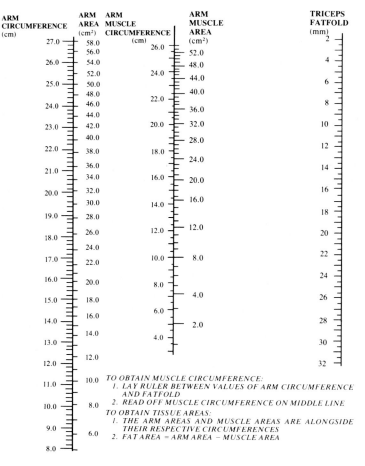

Figure 9-6 Arm anthropometry nomogram for children.

From Gurney JM, Jelliffe DB: Am J Clin Nutr **26:**912-915, 1973.

per-arm muscle size, muscular development may be estimated from arm circumference and skinfold thickness by calculating arm muscle diameter, circumference, or area according to the following formulas[17]:

Arm muscle diameter (mm) =
$$\frac{\text{Arm circumference (mm)}}{\pi} - \text{Triceps skinfold (mm)}$$

Arm muscle circumference (mm) =
$$\text{Arm circumference (mm)} - \pi \text{ (Triceps skinfold)}$$

$$\text{Arm muscle area (mm}^2) = \frac{\pi}{4} \text{ (Arm muscle diameter}^2)$$

Of these indicators, arm muscle area shows the most change during childhood and may be the most sensitive index. Arm muscle area and arm

muscle circumference can be calculated easily with a nomogram[18] (Fig. 9-6). Reference values for interpreting arm muscle area based on data from the HANES I are given in Table 9-8.

CLINICAL EXAMINATION

Clinical examination provides a valuable overall impression of nutritional health (e.g., is the child obese, thin, pale, robust, apathetic?); in addition, the child's general appearance may suggest the adequacy of care provided at home, which can directly influence nutritional well-being. Examination also may reveal specific signs suggesting malnutrition, although the classic deficiency syndromes such as scurvy or rickets rarely are seen. However, many physical findings relating to malnutrition, beyond obvious obesity or wasting, are nonspecific and stem from primarily nonnutritional causes: environmental exposure, drug use, or underlying infectious or metabolic disease. Another limitation of clinical examination is the subjective nature of many physical signs. Because of the potential variability and nonspecificity of clinical signs, diagnosis may not always be made on this basis alone. Rather, positive signs suggesting nutritional illness indicate the need for further specific anthropometric, biochemical, and/or radiologic investigation.

Clinical evaluation for determining nutritional status should include examination of the skin, hair, eyes, lips, tongue, teeth and gums, neck (thyroid gland), subcutaneous tissue, and musculoskeletal system. Specific signs that may be observed include the following, although the list is not intended to be exhaustive:

Skin. General dryness or, more specifically, roughness caused by follicular hyperkeratosis may suggest vitamin A or essential fatty acid deficiency. Petechiae or ecchymoses may be associated with vitamin C or vitamin K deficiency. Hyperpigmented areas bilaterally on sun-exposed areas may suggest pellagrous dermatosis.

Hair. Thin, dyspigmented, easily pluckable hair without normal luster may reflect protein or protein-energy deficiency.

Eyes. Pale conjunctivae suggest anemia. Dullness and dryness of the conjunctivae or corneas (xerosis) and Bitot's spots (dry grayish yellow or white foamy circumscribed areas) suggest vitamin A deficiency.

Lips. Cracks, redness (stomatitis), white or pink scars at the angles, or vertical fissures (often in the lower lip) may be associated with riboflavin and/or niacin deficiency.

Tongue. Glossitis (red painful tongue) or a smooth pale tongue with atrophic papillae may be associated with B vitamin deficiencies.

Teeth and gums. Caries and gingivitis may suggest high ingestion of sweets and poor supervision of the child's oral hygiene. Lack of fluorides also may contribute.

Thyroid. Enlargement may indicate iodine deficiency, but this is unlikely in American children today. Consider other causes of thyroid enlargement.[19]

Subcutaneous tissue. Edema of the extremities or face may suggest severe protein deficiency, but nutritional edema is an unlikely finding in children from a generally well-nourished population.

Musculoskeletal system. Muscle wasting suggests protein-energy deficiency. Skeletal deformities, including knock-knees, bowed legs, frontal and parietal bossing, and epiphyseal enlargement (e.g., of the wrists) suggest rickets.

LABORATORY EVALUATION

Some biochemical measures reflecting nutritional status are used frequently in routine screening examinations (e.g., hemoglobin, serum protein). Others have become more widely available because of automated microsample analysis (serum cholesterol, alkaline phosphatase). However, laboratory assessment remains principally a resource for the investigation and documentation of specific nutritional abnormalities suspected on anthropometric and/or clinical grounds and is not a substitute for careful clinical, anthropometric, and dietary evaluation. Biochemical tests may detect abnormalities before they become clinically evident, although results can be influenced by many factors and always must be interpreted in the light of supportive clinical information. When unusual or inconsistent results occur it is highly advisable to repeat the biochemical test to avoid drawing erroneous conclusions from faulty laboratory results.

A detailed review of the great variety of biochemical tests relating to nutritional status is beyond the scope of this manual. More complete reviews are available. The more relevant and useful of these tests are reviewed below, and normal values are summarized in Table 9-9.

Hemoglobin

Hemoglobin is a measure of iron deficiency or other nutritional anemias. It is decreased in protein-energy malnutrition because of the reduced production of globin frequently combined with iron deficiency. It also may be decreased in nonnutritional anemias.

Serum Albumin

Serum albumin is a useful general index of protein status and is considered to be more reliable than serum total protein, but the two tests are highly correlated. Nevertheless, albumin may remain in the low to normal range even in the presence of significant reduction of body protein reserves; therefore other estimates of pro-

Table 9-9 Guidelines for Interpreting Laboratory Values

Determination		Normal Range	
Hemoglobin (g/100 ml)			
Infant (1-23 mo)		10-15	
Child (2 yr–puberty)		11-16	
Thereafter: Male		14-18	
Female		12-16	
Serum albumin and total protein (g/dl)	Albumin		Total protein
Infant (1-23 mo)	4.4-5.3		6.1-6.7
Thereafter	4.0-5.8		6.2-8.1
Serum transferrin and iron	Transferrin (g/dl)		Iron (µg/dl)
Newborn	0.2-0.3		100-200
Infant/Child (4 mo–2 yr)	0.2-0.3		100-400
Thereafter	0.2-0.3		85-150
Transferrin saturation (%)			
Infant (6-23 mo)		>15	
Child (2-12 yr)		>20	
Child (>12 yr): Male		>20	
Female		>15	

From Mabry CC: In Vaughan VC III, McKay RJ, editors: Nelson Textbook of pediatrics, ed 10, Philadelphia, 1975, WB Saunders Co, pp 1783-1798.

tein status (creatinine/height index, arm muscle area) also should be used if protein deficiency is suspected.

Serum Transferrin

Serum transferrin may be a more sensitive index of protein deficiency than serum albumin because of shorter half-life and more rapid turnover. In combination with serum iron, serum transferrin provides a good index of iron status (percentage transferrin saturation).

Serum Iron

In iron deficiency anemia as well as in infections and nephrosis, serum iron is reduced.

Creatinine/Height Index

Urinary creatinine excretion reflects body muscle, but it may also reflect dietary creatine from meat consumption and show significant day-to-day variation. A 3-day collection of urine has been advocated to ensure reliable estimates,[21] but this is difficult outside a well-controlled hospital setting. Creatinine/height index (CHI)

based on a minimum 24-hour collection has been proposed as an indication of body protein status.[22] The index is calculated as follows:

$$CHI = \frac{\text{Excretion by subject per 24 hr}}{\text{Excretion by normal child of same height per 24 hr}}$$

The creatinine excretion expected of normal children may be estimated from tables[22] or can be approximated from the formula

Expected creatinine (mg/24 hr) =
$$252 - 8.01 \text{ (height)} + 0.0817 \text{ (height}^2)$$

The CHI should be close to 1.0 in normal children and in recovered malnourished ones.

Patient Assessment

The clinician has the responsibility of synthesizing the anthropometric values, laboratory data, and clinical assessment to determine whether the young patient is normal. The question of whether a child is growing appropriately is raised most often by parents of children who appear to deviate from the commonly observed patterns within the community.

Measurement	Result	Reference Standard	Approximate Percentile Rank	Percentage of Median
Weight	13.2 kg	Table 9-4	5th	82.7
Height	95.2 cm	Table 9-5	5th	93.7
Weight for height		Table 9-6	25th	93.4
Arm circumference	151 mm	Table 9-7	10th	91.1
Triceps skinfold	7 mm	Table 9-7	5th	70.0
Arm muscle area	1324 mm^2	Table 9-8	25th	94.1

To illustrate this, in one case a 4-year-old girl is brought to the office because her mother is concerned about the child's small size. Birth and developmental history are normal, and the child has had no major illnesses but has grown along the 5th percentile of height and weight since birth. The parents are in good health, with a maternal height of 152 cm (5'0") and a paternal height of 170 cm (5'7"). Dietary evaluation (see Chapter 6) suggests a well-balanced intake with adequate nutrients. The child is given daily multivitamin with iron supplements.

The physical examination shows a bright, active, neatly dressed girl in apparently good health. No clinical signs of malnutrition are found except for her short stature for age. The hemoglobin is 11.8 g/dl (normal), and the serum albumin 4.5 g/dl (normal).

Anthropometric measurements and calculated percentile ranking and percentage of median index are as shown in the box above, based on the indicated reference population.

The proportional weight and height, with weight-for-height in the normal range and normal skinfold, arm muscle, and laboratory values, suggest a normal 5th percentile child. The clinical examination and family and medical history indicate that the girl is well cared for and that her short stature may simply reflect the short stature of her parents.

In another illustration a 10-year-old boy is brought to the office because he is "chubby." He is otherwise well and has had no major illnesses. Growth has been between the 50th and 75th percentiles since birth. Dietary evaluation (see Chapter 6) suggests more than adequate nutrient intake, with a habit of frequent snacks between meals consisting of candy, soft drinks, and potato chips.

The physical examination suggests obesity in a prepubertal boy but no other positive findings. The hemoglobin is 12.8 g/dl (normal), and the serum albumin 4.5 g/dl (normal).

Anthropometric measurements and calculated percentile ranking and percentage of median index are shown in the box below, based on the reference population.

The findings in this case indicate increased fat deposition with muscle development apparently appropriate for age. Boys frequently put on fat in the prepubertal period, and it is likely that some of this will be lost after puberty. Reduced energy intake by curtailing snacks would be beneficial, as would regular exercise. The boy meets the criteria for obesity at present. Monitoring of anthropometric measurements would permit quantitative evaluation of therapeutic progress.

Measurement	Result	Reference Standard	Approximate Percentile Rank	Percentage of Median
Weight	41 kg	Table 9-4	90th	130
Height	141.4 cm	Table 9-5	75th	103
Weight for height		Table 9-6	90th	122
Arm circumference	223 mm	Table 9-7	75th	106
Triceps skinfold	21 mm	Table 9-7	95th	210
Arm muscle area	2220 mm^2	Table 9-8	25th	86

REFERENCES

1. Zerfas AJ: The insertion of tape: a new circumference tape for use in nutritional assessment, Am J Clin Nutr **28:**782-787, 1975.
2. Greulich WW, Pyle SI: Radiographic atlas of skeletal development of the hand and wrist, ed 2, Stanford Calif, 1959, Stanford University Press.
3. Roche AF: Bone growth and maturation. In Falkner F, Tanner JM, editors: Human growth, New York, 1978, Plenum Press, pp 317-351.
4. Garn SM, et al: Tendency toward greater stature in American black children, Am J Dis Child **126:**164-166, 1973.
5. Garn SM: The anthropometric assessment of nutritional status. In Smith MAH, editor: Proceedings of the Third National Nutrition Workshop for Nutritionists in University Affiliated Facilities, Memphis, 1976, Child Development Center, University of Tennessee Center for the Health Sciences, pp 3-16.
6. Brandt I: Growth dynamics of low–birth-weight infants, with emphasis on the perinatal period. In Falkner F, Tanner JM, editors: Human growth, New York, 1978, Plenum Press, pp 557-617.
7. Garn SM, Shaw HA: Birth size and growth appraisal, J Pediatr **90:**1045-1051, 1977.
8. Van Wieringen JC: Secular growth changes. I. The concept of secular changes in growth and maturation. In Falkner F, Tanner JM, editors: Human growth, New York, 1978, Plenum Press Inc, pp 445-473.
9. Hamill PVV, et al: Physical growth: National Center for Health Statistics percentiles, Am J Clin Nutr **32:**607-629, 1979.
10. Tanner JM, Whitehouse RH: Clinical longitudinal standards for height, weight, height velocity, weight velocity, and stages of puberty, Arch Dis Child **51:**170-179, 1976.
11. Frisancho AR: New norms for upper limb fat and muscle areas for assessment of nutritional status, Am J Clin Nutr **34:**3540-3545, 1981.
12. Waterlow JCR, et al: The presentation and use of height and weight data for comparing the nutritional status of groups of children under the age of 10 years, Bull WHO **55:**489-493, 1977.
13. Rao KV, Singh D: An evaluation of the relationship between nutritional status and anthropometric measurements. Am J Clin Nutr **23:**83-93, 1970.
14. Dugdale AE: An age-independent anthropometric index of nutritional status, Am J Clin Nutr **24:**174-176, 1971.
15. Arnhold R: The QUAC stick: a field measure used by the Quaker service team, Nigeria, J Trop Pediatr **15:**241-247, 1969.
16. Trowbridge FL, Staehling N: Sensitivity and specificity of arm cirumference indicators in identifying malnourished children, Am J Clin Nutr **33:**687-690, 1980.
17. Frisancho AR: Triceps skinfold and upper arm muscle size norms for assessment of nutritional status, Am J Clin Nutr **27:**1052-1058, 1974.
18. Gurney JM, Jelliffe DB: Arm anthropometry in nutritional assessment: nomogram for rapid calculation of muscle circumference and cross-sectional muscle and fat areas, Am J Clin Nutr **26:**912-915, 1973.
19. Trowbridge FL, et al: Iodine and goiter in children, Pediatrics **56:**82-90, 1975.
20. Sauberlich H, et al: Laboratory tests for the assessment of nutritional status, Cleveland, 1974, Chemical Rubber Co Press.
21. Forbes GB, Bruining GB: Urinary creatinine excretion and lean body mass, Am J Clin Nutr **29:**1359-1366, 1976.
22. Viteri FE, Alvarado J: The creatinine height index: its use in the estimation of the degree of protein depletion and its repletion in protein-calorie malnourished children, Pediatrics **46:**696-706, 1971.
23. Mabry CC: Tables of normal laboratory values. In Vaughan VC III, McKay RJ, editors: Nelson Textbook of pediatrics, ed 10, Philadelphia, 1975, WB Saunders Co, pp 1783-1798.
24. Jelliffe DB: The assessment of the nutritional status of the community, WHO Monogr Ser 53, pp 63-78, 1966.

CHAPTER 10
Adults

Robert M. Russell
Nadine R. Sahyoun

Nutritional evaluation is an important facet of the adult patient's clinical assessment. As discussed in the previous chapter, anthropometric, laboratory, and clinical evaluation of the growth and nutritional well-being of children has long been an important feature of pediatric practice. Recently professionals responsible for the health of the adult population have been increasingly concerned with nutritional assessment. This concern has its origins in a variety of factors—the increased association of diet with a number of chronic illnesses, the use of special foods and diets for patients with chronic diseases, the early clinical identification of nutritional disorders.

Malnutrition among adult patients has become an increasingly recognized and reported problem. The prevalence of protein-energy malnutrition has been reported as 48% among hospitalized medical adult patients[1] and 50% among hospitalized surgical adult patients.[2]

DIETARY HISTORY

The first step in the complete nutritional assessment of an adult patient is not unlike that required for a child. It necessitates taking a detailed family and medical history. From this the physician can detect reasons for an existing nutritional problem or assess the likelihood of a nutritional problem some time in the future. For example, a strong family history of heart disease will alert the physician to check serum lipid levels and to encourage the patient to decrease excess weight. Alternatively, recent appetite or weight changes, digestive problems, or difficulty in chewing or swallowing are symptoms of medical problems that can cause a patient's nutritional status to deteriorate.

A socioeconomic history may explain why the patient has a poor food intake or is noncompliant with a particular dietary regimen. A patient living alone may be unable to eat an adequate diet because of financial problems, lack of food preparation skills and facilities, disabling handicaps, depression and loneliness, poor dentition, or lack of nutritional knowledge. Such a patient may eat many meals in lunchrooms or from vending machines, or may skip meals altogether. Advice to improve dietary habits can be futile if such problems are not solved. Self-imposed dietary restrictions from allergies, ethnic or religious beliefs, or prolonged use of fad diets can be detrimental to nutritional status. The physician should be aware that these restrictions may cause symptoms such as lightheadedness, malaise, and weakness.

Key Questions to Ask Adults as Part of a Nutritional Assessment

1. Are there recent changes in appetite?
2. Are there difficulties in chewing or swallowing or symptoms suggesting a gastrointestinal disease or disorder?
3. Are there recent changes in weight?
4. Does the patient live alone? Does he/she know how to cook?
5. Are one or more meals eaten away from home?
6. Who prepares the meals?
7. Are there adequate food preparation and food storage facilities at the patient's residence?
8. Is the patient financially able to obtain food?
9. Are there any disabling handicaps that prevent the patient from obtaining an adequate diet?
10. Is the patient's dentition adequate—does he/she have poorly fitting dentures?
11. Is the patient under any dietary restrictions? Are they self-prescribed?
12. Are there any food allergies, intolerances, or ethnic or religious beliefs that prevent adequate food intake?
13. What is the patient's alcohol intake?
14. Does the patient take any diet supplements (e.g., vitamins)?
15. Does the patient add salt to his/her food during and after cooking?

With this background information the physician then may proceed to the anthropometric, clinical, and laboratory components of nutritional assessment with knowledge of possible problem areas to investigate.

ANTHROPOMETRIC ASSESSMENT

Anthropometric measurements can indicate the patient's protein and fat reserves and alert the physician to nutritional problems. The materials and methods are similar to those outlined for children. Virtually every clinician can perform these measurements in a few minutes and at little cost. The only equipment needed is a beam or lever balance scale with a tape measure fixed to the wall, and a constant-tension skinfold caliper. Plastic calipers, which may be less accurate, can be obtained at no cost from one or more pharmaceutical laboratories.

The components of anthropometric measurements include height in centimeters, weight in kilograms, triceps skinfold in millimeters, and mid-arm circumference in centimeters. From these measurements calculations can be performed to obtain actual weight as a percentage of reference standard, weight as a percentage of usual weight (within the last year), triceps skinfold thickness, and bone-free upper-arm muscle area as percentages of reference standards.

Weight and Height

Two bodies of data that are of interest in a discussion of weights for heights are the Metropolitan Insurance (MET) reference weights (Table 10-1)[3,4] and the Health and Nutrition Examination Survey (HANES) normative values. The MET table is derived from actuarial data on people 25 to 59 years old and, therefore, represents the recommended or desirable weights for heights for a young to middle-aged population. It is suggested that this table be used for the anthropometric assessment of such persons. The normative values obtained by the HANES I and II[5] are higher than the MET reference weights, indicating that the general population may be heavier than recommended according to the MET table. The HANES, however, may be used to indicate where a person's weight for height fits in comparison to the weights for heights of the general population in the United States. The HANES height and weight tables

Table 10-1 Metropolitan Insurance Reference Weights (Nude Without Shoes)

Height		Midpoint (medium frame)	
(in)	(cm)	(lb)	(kg)
Men			
62	157	133	60.4
63	160	135	61.4
64	163	137.5	62.3
65	165	140	63.6
66	168	143	65.0
67	170	146	66.4
68	173	149	67.7
69	175	152	69.1
70	178	155	70.4
71	180	158.5	72.0
72	183	162	73.6
73	185	166	75.4
74	188	174	79.1
Women			
58	147	114	51.8
59	150	116.5	53.0
60	152	119	54.1
61	155	122	55.4
62	157	125	56.8
63	160	128	58.2
64	163	131	59.5
65	165	134	60.9
66	168	137	62.3
67	170	140	63.6
68	173	143	65.0
69	175	146	66.4
70	178	149	67.7
71	180	165	75.0

From Metropolitan height and weight tables, New York, 1983, Metropolitan Life Insurance Co., and Russell RM, et al: Am J Med **76:**767-769, 1984.

may also be used for persons over age 55 (see Chapter 8).

Weight for height may provide important information on the nutrition assessment of a patient. For example, an adult patient who has lost over 10% of his/her body weight during the past 4-6 months or weighs less than 80% of desirable body weight (MET reference weight) may need extra nutritional support.[6-8] The rate of weight loss may affect the patient's functioning more than the total amount of weight lost. A recent rapid weight loss (within 6 mo) up to 10 pounds or 6% of body weight, even if the usual weight is above desirable body weight, may indicate a loss of muscle protein to meet caloric needs and the need for an immediate nutritional workup of the patient.[6] However, a patient who weighs more than 130% of the MET midpoint weight for height is considered obese.

The patient's height should be measured without shoes, using a vertical tape or rod; if using a rod, the lower border of the orbit should be in the same horizontal plane as the external auditory meatus. With arms relaxed at the patient's side and the patient facing away from the scale, the headpiece is lowered until it makes contact with the scalp. The patient's desirable body weight then is obtained from the MET reference table (Table 10-1) and the following calculations can be made:

$$\text{Percentage of desirable body weight} = \frac{\text{Actual weight}}{\text{Reference body weight (from Table 10-1)}} \times 100$$

$$\text{Percentage usual weight} = \frac{\text{Actual weight}}{\text{Usual weight}} \times 100$$

$$\text{Percentage weight change} = \frac{\text{Usual weight} - \text{Actual weight}}{\text{Usual weight}} \times 100$$

Although it is recommended that the MET reference weight table be used, the following formulas can also be employed for a quick approximate desirable body weight:

Male desirable body weight = 127 lb for first 5 ft + 3 lb for every inch over 5 ft

Female desirable body weight = 119 lb for first 5 ft + 3 lb for every inch over 5 ft

Height and weight measurements have their limitations. Alone they cannot serve as a complete nutritional evaluation, although they may be used as a screening tool. Edema and ascites can mask tissue weight loss and malnutrition. Obesity, which may look like overnutrition, actually may conceal depressed circulating protein (e.g., albumin) levels.

Skinfold Thickness

Triceps skinfold (TSF) is an objective indicator of a patient's fat reserves. Skinfold thickness can be measured at several sites: deltoid triceps, subscapular, lower thoracic, iliac, abdominal. The deltoid triceps usually is employed in assessing fat stores of adults, both for practical reasons (accessibility) and since edema is not usually present here (although gross obesity will

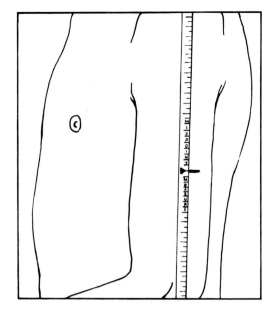

Figure 10-1 Determining the midpoint of the upper arm, halfway between the acromion and the olecranon.

increase the measurement error at this site). Triceps skinfold is measured by a caliper on the right arm, unless arm edema or paralysis is present. The patient should be standing erect with the arm and shoulder bare. A patient who cannot stand should sit on the edge of a chair or bed. The arm must not be resting on any surface.

Since fat overlying the triceps muscle is not uniform in thickness, the measurement is taken at a carefully measured reference site. Before measurement the midpoint between the acromion (of the scapula) and the olecranon (of the ulna) is determined with a tape measure. To measure the midpoint of the arm, the patient must bend the arm 90 degrees at the elbow and the measured midpoint must be marked on the patient's arm (Fig. 10-1). With the patient standing erect and the arm hanging free of tension, the marked midpoint is grasped posteriorly between the thumb and forefinger of the evaluator's hand. With fingers far enough apart to grasp a full fold firmly, the evaluator raises the fold, allowing the muscle to fall back to the bone. The remaining skinfold and subcutaneous fat then is held lightly during the entire measurement. Calipers are placed on the fold below the fingers and a reading is taken to the nearest 0.5 mm on the caliper (Fig. 10-2). The skinfold then is released. It is most ac-

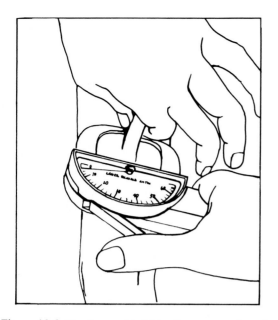

Figure 10-2 The Lange skinfold calipers measuring triceps skinfold thickness. Throughout the measurement the evaluator maintains light pinching pressure on the skinfold.

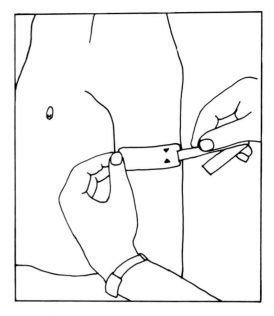

Figure 10-3 Measuring the midarm circumference with a Ross Laboratories insertion tape measure. The evaluator must be careful not to constrict the patient's arm.

curate to repeat the procedure three times and use the average of the three readings as the final measurement.

Arm Muscle Area

Bone-free upper arm muscle area (AMA) gives an indication of the patient's lean body tissue. The circumference of the arm is measured with a tape measure at the marked midpoint. The patient's right arm should be hanging free of tension, not resting on any surface, and the tape measure should be applied firmly but without constricting the arm (Fig. 10-3). Bone-free upper-arm muscle area then is derived by the following formulas:

$$\text{Male upper AMA (cm}^2) = \frac{[\text{Arm circumference (cm)} - 3.14 \times \text{TSF (cm)}]^2}{4\pi} - 10$$

$$\text{Female upper AMA (cm}^2) = \frac{[\text{Arm circumference (cm)} - 3.14 \times \text{TSF (cm)}]^2}{4\pi} - 6.5$$

Interpretation of Anthropometric Measurements

Reference standards for weight and height. The MET reference nude weight-for-height val-

ues, which are the recommended standards, have been derived from studies of factors affecting longevity and then adjusted for people of average frame.[12] Another measurement of interest, the Quetelet body mass index (BMI), which is weight (in kilograms) divided by height squared (in meters), may be used to assess relative body weight. It is determined by using the body mass nomogram (Fig. 10-4).[9] As a guideline in detecting obesity, the National Center for Health Statistics has set criteria for defining overweight. These have been adopted by the Consensus Conference on Obesity[10] and are the BMI values of ≥27.8 kg/m² and ≥27.3 kg/m² (for males and females), which correspond to the 85th percentile from the HANES II for ages 20-29 years.[11] The rationale for using this age group is that young adults are relatively lean and any later increase in body weight may be due to undesirable fat accumulation. These BMI values also correspond to 30% above the midpoint of the 1983 Metropolitan Life Insurance Company weight-for-height tables. In assessing underweight it is suggested that a figure 20% below the midpoint of the MET value be used as a guideline. This corresponds to less than the 5th

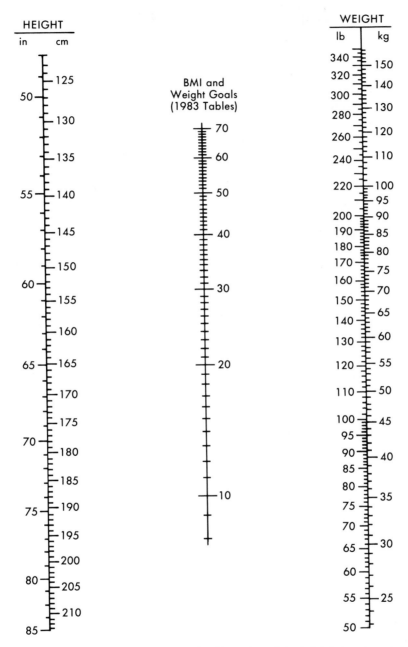

Figure 10-4 Nomogram for body mass (kg/m^2). The ratio weight/height^2 (metric units) is used from the central scale after a straightedge is placed between height and body weight.

From Burton BT, et al: Int J Obes **9:**155-169, 1985.

percentile in the combined HANES I and II data sets for age group 25-54 years. Also the BMI 5th percentile from the HANES II for ages 20-29 years may be used.

Reference standards for skinfold thickness and arm muscle area. The most frequently cited reference values for skinfold thickness and arm circumference are based in part on surveys done in Turkey, Greece, and Italy.[12] Since body composition may vary with environment and diet, these standards are not appropriate in determining the nutritional status of Americans. Local race-specific reference standards are needed, but few exist because recognition of the importance of nutritional assessment is relatively new and these standards are difficult to develop. In addition, separate standards are needed for different age groups, since fat distribution and muscle mass vary with age. Such standards are available for children, but not for elderly people, who are at high risk for malnutrition.[13] Age- and sex-specific American standards for skinfold measurements and bone-free arm muscle area have been compiled based on the combined HANES I and II data sets (1971-74 and 1976-80)[5] and are presently the most representative values for noninstitutionalized American adults. All races are included in the sample of 21,752, and the data are presented for two age categories, 25-54 and 55-74 years.

To simplify the interpretation of anthropometric measurements, certain criteria recommended for assessing the risk of malnutrition and obesity in adults are summarized in Table 10-2. These criteria pertain to adults up to age 54 years. Beyond that age the reference standards presented in Chapter 8 are more appropriate. The MET weight-for-height table is recommended as a standard for assessing adults up to age 54. The BMI reference standard is the HANES II 50th percentile for age group 20-29.[11] Triceps skinfold and bone-free upper AMA reference standards are derived from the 50th percentile of HANES I and II data sets for ages 25-54 years. Direct measurements can be compared to the reference standards by using the formula

$$\frac{\text{Actual measurement}}{\text{Reference standard}} \times 100$$

The percentages given in the table may help in assessing an individual's risk of malnutrition.

Any patient with two or more anthropometric and laboratory values in the severe category is classified as at high risk for malnutrition and deserves immediate attention.

Clinical Examination

Before deciding whether to begin specialized nutritional therapy or to administer extra nutritional support, the practitioner first must be able to recognize the malnourished individual. Unfortunately, many of the clinical signs and symptoms of malnutrition are not obvious or are relatively nonspecific. Moreover, clinical signs and symptoms of malnutrition often appear late in the process of undernutrition. Laboratory or functional (e.g., dark adaptation) evaluation of the patient may reveal a subclinical nutritional deficiency that would be missed by the history or physical examination. However, all three components of nutritional value assessments (anthropometric, clinical, laboratory) should become a routine part of the patient's workup to ensure an early diagnosis of malnutrition. Stud-

Table 10-2 Risk of Malnutrition and Obesity in Adults

Anthropometric Measure	Reference Standard Men/Women	Malnutrition (% of Standard)		Obesity (% of Standard)	
		Men	Women	Men	Women
Weight-for-height†	*	<80	<80	>130	>130
Body mass index (kg/m²)‡	23.7/22.0	<80	<80	>120	>120
Triceps skinfold (mm)‡	12/23	<40	<50	>170	>145
Arm muscle area (cm²)‡	55/31	<70	<70	NA	NA

*Table 10-1 is used as the reference standard.

†Corresponding to less than the 15th percentile (for malnutrition) and greater than the 85th (for obesity) in the combined HANES I and II.

‡Corresponding to less than the 5th percentile (malnutrition) and greater than the 85th (obesity) in the HANES II (for the body mass index) and combined HANES I and II (for the triceps skinfold and arm muscle area).

NA, Not applicable.

ies in Baltimore[14] indicate that only one quarter of moderately or severely malnourished hospitalized patients are given physician-prescribed nutritional supplements, implying a present failure to recognize nutritional depletion.

Recent experience suggests that physicians can be trained to review the nutritional status of the patient as well as consider the disease status. The physical examination for determining nutritional status is the same as the usual clinical exam except that the physician looks at the patient's physical signs and symptoms from a "nutritional point of view." Simple anthropometric and laboratory techniques can confirm or disprove a clinical impression of malnutrition. The more common clinical symptoms and signs of malnutrition in adults are listed in Table 10-3. Many of them have more than one cause, and it should be recognized that there are very few "key" signs that signify a deficiency of a single specific nutrient. For example, angular stomatitis may be caused by a lack of riboflavin, vitamin B_6, or folate; tetany by deficiencies of either magnesium or calcium. More specific signs of singular nutrient deficiencies include cheilosis, which is usually caused by a deficiency of riboflavin; spooning of the nails due to lack of iron; and Bitot's spots due to vitamin A deficiency.

LABORATORY EVALUATION

There are many laboratory tests that may be used to assess the nutritional status of patients. However, the most useful are those already being done in many hospitals and clinics as part of a

Table 10-3 Nutritional Deficiency in Adults*

	Sign or Symptom	Deficiency
General	Wasted, skinny	Calorie
	Loss of appetite	Protein, calorie
Head	Temporal muscle wasting	Protein, calorie
Eyes	History of night blindness (especially impaired visual recovery after glare)	Vitamin A
	Dryness, Bitot's spots	
Mouth	Glossitis	Riboflavin, niacin
	Bleeding gums	Vitamin C
	Cheilosis	Riboflavin
	Angular stomatitis	Riboflavin, vitamin B_6, folate
	Hypogeusia	Zinc
Skin	Pallor	Folate, iron, vitamin B_{12}
	Follicular hyperkeratosis	Vitamin A
	Perifollicular petechiae	Vitamin C
	Flaking dermatitis	Protein, calorie, niacin, zinc, riboflavin, vitamin B_6, essential fatty acids
Hair	Sparse and thin	Protein
	Easy to pull out	Protein
Nails	Spooning	Iron
	Transverse lines	Protein
Neck	Goiter	Iodine
	Parotid enlargement	Protein
Abdomen	Distention	Protein, calorie
	Hepatomegaly	Protein, calorie
Extremities	Edema	Protein
	Bone tenderness	Vitamin D
	Muscle wasting and weakness	Protein, calorie, vitamin D
	Calf muscle tenderness	Thiamine
Neurologic	Tetany	Calcium, magnesium
	Loss of reflexes	Thiamine
	Loss of vibratory and position sense	Vitamin B_{12}
	Dementia	Niacin

*Most signs and symptoms are not specific (i.e., not related to a deficiency of only one nutrient). Nevertheless, they are useful in recognizing the malnourished patient.

Table 10-4 Assessing the Severity of Malnutrition in Adults

Laboratory Test	Moderately Substandard	Severely Substandard
Albumin	2.8-3.5 g/dl*	<2.8 g/dl†
Transferrin	160-200 mg/dl*	<160 mg/dl†
Transthyretin	11-14 mg/dl*	<11 mg/dl†
Creatinine/height index	80%-90% of standard	<80% of standard
Skin antigen reactivity	No reaction to three antigens‡	No reaction to three antigens‡
Total lymphocyte count	<1500/mm³	<1200/mm³

*Or up to a 20% reduction from the lower limit of normal.
†Or greater than a 20% reduction from the lower limit of normal.
‡For example, mumps, PPD, *Candida,* or streptokinase-streptodornase.

basic laboratory data base or profile for all patients, and it is simply a matter of interpreting those laboratory results with the nutritional status of the patient in mind. For example, serum albumin may be used as a liver function test and, in patients without liver disease, as a parameter of protein nutriture.

Esoteric vitamin and mineral laboratory measurements are of limited use in the nutritional evaluation of patients except when the clinical presentation is highly suggestive of a specific micronutrient deficiency (e.g., zinc in a patient with hypogeusia). For sick patients, assessment of protein and calorie status is by far the most important issue.

Assessment of Protein Status

For purposes of nutritional assessment, body protein can be considered as divided about equally between muscle (somatic) and nonmuscle (so-called "visceral") compartments. In patients with protein malnutrition without calorie deprivation, the measures of nonmuscle or visceral protein (e.g., serum albumin) may be severely substandard while the anthropometric measure of somatic protein (arm muscle area) may be normal. The reverse is true in patients with calorie deprivation; that is, all anthropometric measurements may be severely substandard while the visceral protein measurements are normal. Thus, in assessing and classifying patients according to the type of malnutrition (e.g., marasmus [or calorically deprived] versus kwashiorkor [or protein-deprived]), it is useful to have measurements of both the somatic and the visceral protein compartments available.

Serum albumin. In almost all hospitals and clinics serum albumin values are readily obtained and serve as good indicators of visceral protein

nutriture. A patient whose serum albumin level is more than 20% below the lower limit of the normal range (e.g., <2.8 g/dl in a laboratory whose lower limit of normal is 3.5 g/dl) is regarded as severely depleted of visceral protein (Table 10-4). However, since the half-life of albumin is approximately 16 days, its measurement does not reflect acute protein deprivation and it cannot be used to reflect protein nutritional status in patients with chronic liver disease.

Serum transferrin. Serum transferrin has a shorter half-life (approximately 9 da) than does albumin[16] and currently is being used as a more rapid indicator of protein malnutrition. It may be measured directly by radioimmunodiffusion or derived indirectly from a measurement of the serum total iron binding capacity. The formula used to obtain a derived transferrin value[8] is

$$\text{Serum transferrin} = (0.8 \times \text{Total iron binding capacity}) - 43$$

There are conflicting data on how accurately the derived value reflects the directly measured value of transferrin by radioimmunodiffusion. Nevertheless, a derived or measured value that is more than 20% below the lower limit of the normal range is generally regarded as severely substandard.

Transthyretin. Transthyretin (prealbumin) has been used as an early indicator of protein nutritional status because, like albumin and transferrin, it has a short half-life.[17] However, although available commercially, it is not yet widely used in clinic or hospital laboratories.*

---

*Albumin, transferrin, and transthyretin all are synthesized in the liver and hence cannot be used to reflect protein nutriture in patients with hepatic disease.

Table 10-5 Standard Creatinine Values

Males		Females	
Height (cm)	Ideal (mg)	Height (cm)	Ideal (mg)
157.5	1288	147.3	830
160.0	1325	149.9	851
162.6	1359	152.4	875
165.1	1386	154.9	900
167.6	1426	157.5	925
170.2	1467	160.0	949
172.7	1513	162.6	977
175.3	1555	165.1	1006
177.8	1596	167.6	1044
180.3	1642	170.2	1076
182.9	1691	172.7	1109
185.4	1739	175.3	1141
188.0	1785	177.8	1174
190.5	1831	180.3	1206
192.0	1891	182.9	1240

From Blackburn G, et al: J Parenter Enter Nutr **1**(1):11-22, 1977.

Retinol-binding protein. Retinol-binding protein, with an even shorter half-life than transthyretin, also has been used as a nutritional assessment parameter, despite the fact that it likewise is influenced by liver status. In addition, it is subject to the vitamin A status of the patient.

Creatinine/height index. A convenient biochemical measurement that reflects the somatic or muscle protein compartment is the creatinine/height index. Creatinine is a metabolic product of muscle metabolism, and the amount appearing in the urine over 24 hours is proportional to lean body mass. Thus, in the protein-malnourished individual, urinary creatinine will decrease in proportion to the decrease in muscle mass. Tables have been derived giving standard values of 24-hour urine creatinine according to the height and sex of normal individuals.[7] To measure somatic protein status, one obtains a 24-hour urine sample for creatinine and then compares the result with the standards (Table 10-5). This measurement may be used to complement the anthropometric measurement of midarm circumference. The creatinine/height index is not useful in patients with renal disease; and because a 24-hour urine collection is required, the test usually is done only with hospitalized patients.

Immunologic Status

Delayed hypersensitivity is impaired in protein-energy malnutrition and may be assessed by placing skin tests (e.g., mumps, PPD, and *Candida*) on the patient's forearm.[18] Failure to react to these antigens is seen in patients with deprivation of both proteins and calories. The total lymphocyte count is low (i.e., $<1500/mm^3$), especially in patients with protein malnutrition. Levels of less than $1200/mm^3$ are regarded as severely substandard and correlate with the inability to react to skin antigens (Table 10-5). The total lymphocyte count can be derived from the following formula:

Total lymphocytes =
% in differential count × Total white count

Prognostic Nutritional Index

Using some of the foregoing nutritional indices, Buzby et al.[19] developed a model to predict operative morbidity and mortality and to identify the patient prospectively at increased risk of nutritionally based complications. This model, known as the prognostic nutritional index (PNI), can be obtained by the following formula:

$$PNI(\%) = 158 - 16.6 \,(Alb) - 0.78(TSF) - 0.20(TFN) - 5.8 \,(DH)$$

Where *PNI* is the risk of a complication or death in an individual patient, *Alb* the serum albumin level (g/100 ml), *TSF* the triceps skinfold (mm), *TFN* the serum transferrin level (mg/100 ml), and *DH* the cutaneous delayed hypersensitivity reactivity to any of three recall antigens (mumps, streptokinase-streptodornase, *Candida*) graded as 0 (nonreactive), 1(<5 mm induration), or 2 (≥5 mm induration).

Patients are classified as high risk (PNI $\geq$ 50%), intermediate risk (PNI = 40% to 49%), or low risk (PNI $<$ 40%). Although a greater number of surgical complications and greater mortality were seen in the patients with a high PNI, it was unclear whether the PNI could similarly be applied to medical patients.

Nitrogen Balance

In treating hospitalized patients who are protein malnourished, the physician must determine when the patient is getting enough protein. The anthropometric and biochemical measurements of the patient's protein nutritional status often are slow to improve, and the information usually is needed quickly for more effective patient management. An approximate measurement of nitrogen balance may be used to document the effectiveness or ineffectiveness of protein nutritional support being given. The only measurement required is that of urinary urea nitrogen in a 24-hour urine collection[20]:

$$\text{Nitrogen balance} = \frac{\text{Dietary protein intake (g/24 hr)}}{6.25} - \text{Urinary area nitrogen (g/24 hr)} + 4$$

In a patient receiving protein nutritional support, a positive balance of at least 4 g/24 hr is desirable. The formula is not useful in patients with protein-losing enteropathy (e.g., inflammatory diarrhea) or in patients with inflammatory skin disease or burns, since the unmeasured protein losses are great in these conditions. The measurement cannot be used in patients with renal disease, and since a 24-hour collection of urine is required, the test usually is carried out only in hospitalized patients.

Additional Laboratory Tests

Hematocrit, blood smear for red and white cell morphology, serum carotene, and serum folate values are all readily available laboratory tests for which the results are frequently abnormal in malnourished adults. Anemia is a sensitive indicator of malnutrition but is relatively nonspecific in that blood loss and chronic disease (without malnutrition) are often causative factors.

A blood smear is of great value in assessing the cause of an anemia, since the other red cell indices may be reported as normal when both folate and iron are deficient (a common finding among alcoholics). Whereas these other indices will not pick up a dimorphic anemia, the blood smear will. In some cases of folate and severe iron deficiency the red cells will appear hypochromic-microcytic. Then consideration of white cell morphology may lead to a diagnosis of folate deficiency as well, because iron deficiency cannot mask the multilobed nuclear changes of the polymorphonuclear leukocytes (i.e., >5 nuclear lobes in five out of 100 neutrophils counted).[21]

The serum carotene level classically has been used as a screening test for fat malabsorption. It also may be an indirect indicator of vitamin A

status, although it is highly dependent on the dietary intake of carotene; that is, the serum carotene level may be low (<60 μg/dl) in individuals who eat few leafy green or yellow vegetables while the serum vitamin A value is normal. Thus the serum carotene can be interpreted only if one has specific knowledge of the patient's dietary habits.

Serum folate is a useful indicator of malnutrition, for it has a rapid turnover and a small body store (approximately 10 mg). It takes about 20 days to develop a subnormal serum folate level on a folate-free diet.[22,23] Since folate is absorbed in the proximal small intestine, it is very useful to screen for malabsorption caused by proximal small intestinal disease (e.g., celiac sprue).

Functional or end organ tests also may be important in assessing the nutritional status of a patient. Bone density and dark adaptation are two examples of such tests, which may accurately diagnose subclinical vitamin D and vitamin A malnutrition, respectively.[24,25] Additional functional tests need to be developed as part of nutritional assessment. It is possible that stress or exercise testing may become more appropriate than anthropometric measurements in predicting the patient's ability to recover uneventfully from an operation.

At present, anthropometric, clinical, and biochemical measurements can give an adequate appraisal of the patient's nutritional status as well as inform the physician of the patient's response to nutritional intervention. Basic laboratory tests (albumin, transferrin, urinary creatinine and urea nitrogen, total lymphocyte count, hematocrit) should be repeated weekly, and anthropometric measurements every 3 weeks.

REFERENCES

1. Wiensier RL, et al: Hospital malnutrition: a prospective evaluation of general medical patients during the course of hospitalization, Am J Clin Nutr **32**:418-426, 1979.
2. Bistrian BR, et al: Protein status of general surgical patients, JAMA **230**:858-860, 1974.
3. Metropolitan height and weight tables, New York, 1983, Metropolitan Life Insurance Co.
4. Russell RM, et al: Reference weights. Practical considerations, Am J Med **76**:767-769, 1984.
5. Frisancho AR: New standards of weight and body composition by frame size and height for assessment of nutritional status of adults and the elderly, Am J Clin Nutr **40**:808-819, 1984.

6. Wilmore DW: The metabolic management of the critically ill, New York, 1977, Plenum Medical Book Co, p 44.

7. Blackburn GL, et al: Nutritional and metabolic assessment of the hospitalized patient, J Parenter Enter Nutr 1(1):11-22, 1977.

8. Butterworth CE, Blackburn GL: Hospital malnutrition, Nutr Today 19(2):8-18, 1975.

9. Burton BT, et al: Health implications of obesity: an NIH Consensus Development Conference, Int J Obes 9:155-169, 1985.

10. Van Itallie TB: Health implications of overweight and obesity in the United States, Ann Intern Med 103:983-988, 1985.

11. National Center for Health Statistics, Division of Health Examination Statistics: Data from the second National Health and Nutrition Examination Survey, 1976-80. (Unpublished.)

12. Jelliffe DB: The assessment of the nutritional status of the community, WHO Monogr Ser 53, pp 63-78, 1966.

13. Alfin-Slater RB: Nutrition and aging, Fed Proc 28(6):1993-2000, 1979.

14. Bushman L, et al: Malnutrition among patients in an acute care veterans facility, J Am Diet Assoc 77(4):462-465, 1980.

15. Eckart J, et al: The turnover of ^{125}I-labeled serum albumin after surgery and injury. In Wilkinson AW, editor: Parenteral nutrition, New York, 1972, Churchill Livingstone Inc, pp 288-298.

16. Awai M, Brown EB: Studies of the metabolism of ^{131}I-labeled human transferrin, J Lab Clin Med 61:363-396, 1963.

17. Ogunshina SO, Hussain MA: Plasma thyroxine binding prealbumin as an index of mild protein-energy malnutrition in Nigerian children, Am J Clin Nutr 33:794-800, 1980.

18. Menkins JL, et al: Delayed hypersensitivity: indicator for acquired failure of host defenses in sepsis and trauma, Ann Surg 186:241-249, 1977.

19. Buzby GP, et al: Prognostic nutritional index in gastrointestinal surgery, Am J Surg 139:160-167, 1980.

20. MacKenzie T, et al: Clinical assessment of nutritional status using nitrogen balance, Fed Proc 33:683, 1974.

21. Herbert V: Megaloblastic anemias. In Beeson P, et al, editors: Textbook of medicine, ed 15, Philadelphia, 1979, WB Saunders Co, pp 1719-1729.

22. Herbert V: Experimental nutritional folate deficiency in man, Trans Assoc Am Physicians 75:307-320, 1962.

23. Herbert V: Minimal daily adult folate requirement, Arch Intern Med 110:649-652, 1962.

24. Sorenson JA, Cameron JR: A reliable in vitro measurement of bone mineral content, J Bone Joint Surg (Am) 49:481-497, 1967.

25. Russell RM, et al: The use of dark adaptation as a reversible indicator of subclinical vitamin A deficiency in patients with chronic small intestinal disease, Lancet 2:1161-1162, 1973.

CHAPTER 11
Dietary Assessment

Eileen T. Kennedy

A comprehensive dietary history is an essential complement to the anthropometric, laboratory, and clinical assessment of the patient. Although many health professionals have minimum training in this area and a general skepticism of the reliability of the methods employed in obtaining a dietary history, the information retrieved is important in establishing dietary patterns and practices essential to making a proper nutritional diagnosis.

Understanding an individual's dietary practices and food consumption patterns allows the medical professional to identify nutrient deficiencies, imbalances, and excesses. This chapter illustrates methods that can be used in dietary assessment as part of a comprehensive nutritional status evaluation.

DIETARY STATUS VERSUS NUTRITIONAL STATUS

Dietary status is a measure of an individual's present and prior food and nutrient consumption; as such, it is one component of nutritional status. An inadequate dietary intake eventually will produce biochemical changes in the body that ultimately may lead to overt clinical manifestations of nutritional deficiency. For example, scurvy was the leading cause of death for many years among British sailors on long sea voyages.[1] This pathologic condition eventually was traced to insufficient intake of ascorbic acid. Later other diet/disease relationships were elucidated—thiamine/beriberi, niacin/pellagra, vitamin A/night blindness, iron/anemia, iodine/goiter. It is partially because of the established links between diet and certain diseases that clinicians began to use an assessment of dietary intake as an indirect measure of nutritional status.

Dietary status and nutritional status are not synonymous. An adequate dietary status is a necessary, but not a sufficient, criterion for optimum nutritional status, since the latter is influenced not only by what a person eats but also by how the food is digested, transported, metabolized, stored in the body, and excreted. An individual's nutritional status will not be better than the dietary status, but it may be significantly worse. For example, a person who consumes more than adequate quantities of iron can still be anemic because of an illness such as ulcerative colitis, yet assessment of dietary intake alone will not necessarily reveal the anemia.

Dietary data can be used in a clinical setting to identify individuals likely to be at risk of inadequate or improper nutrient intake. The information also can be used to interpret or clarify biochemical or clinical results. For research purposes dietary information can be used to compare nutrient intakes of treatment and nontreatment groups or individuals to assess changes in dietary status over time.

METHODS OF DIETARY ASSESSMENT

Some of the earliest studies on dietary assessment[2] were conducted using balance study techniques. Food intake was quantified exactly, and urinary and fecal outputs then were measured; however, these studies were expensive and could be done only on small samples of individuals. To make dietary assessment feasible in a clinical setting, dietary instruments were developed for measuring food intake. Two general classes of instruments have been used: the first involves weighing or estimating food intake; the second relies on a recall of food consumption.

Weighed Food Record

The weighed food record is one of the most accurate methods for determining nutrient consumption.[3] Food is weighed prior to eating and any leftover is recorded after the meal. The record can be kept for varying lengths of time, although commonly it is used for 4 to 10 days. In carefully controlled settings a duplicate meal may be prepared and sent to a laboratory for analysis of its nutrient content.

The weighed food record has been used extensively for nutrition surveys in developing countries. It is most practical when there is limited variety in the diet and when most of the meals are eaten at home. The major burden is on the individual required to keep the record. Although the weighed food record may give an accurate measure of food consumption, because of this burden it also may bias normal eating patterns. Individuals tend to eat less because of the difficulty in weighing each food item. In a 1-year study of dietary intake,[4] researchers found that caloric intake of men and women consistently decreased when subjects were asked to prepare a duplicate meal; the authors pointed out that intakes of respondents during food collection periods did not represent their habitual level of consumption reported throughout the year.

Other studies have reported similar findings. A consistently lower reported caloric intake was observed with a weighed food record than with dietary recall data[5]; the snacking patterns of women in the study changed when they were required to weigh each item. In another study[6] the caloric intake tended to decrease after the first week of keeping a weighed food record. Other investigators[7] found that the weighed food record gave a precise estimate of food intake but not necessarily a true picture of normal consumption. However, the dietary data collected from the weighed food record have generally correlated positively and significantly with certain biochemical measures.[8]

Estimated Food Record

With the estimated food record an individual is asked to keep a record of all food consumed for 1 to 14 days. Records can be kept for longer periods, but compliance is then low.[9] The quantities of food eaten are estimated by using common household utensils (e.g., cups and measuring spoons). For items like eggs or slices of bread, a simple count is used[3]; for candy bars and similar items the package weight is entered on the food record.

The accuracy of the estimated food record is a function of both the individual's ability to es-

timate portion sizes and his or her cooperation in recording foods as they are consumed. Studies indicate that individuals tend to record consumption information immediately before the record must be submitted. Thus the estimated food record is often simply a recall of the most recent food intake and not a continual record of foods consumed.

Some of the difficulties encountered in using the weighed food record also create problems for individuals using the estimated food record. Reported caloric intake tends to decrease after the first week, primarily because of the record-keeping burden on the individual.[3] Accuracy in estimating portion sizes is the main source of error in the estimated food record.[10] Foods that can be measured easily (milk) or itemized (slices of bread) show the least measurement errors.

The individual's ability to cooperate in keeping an estimated food record is inversely related to the length of time for which the record is to be kept. Subjects will be more willing to cooperate for a 2-to-3-day period than for a week or longer. If the estimated food record is kept accurately, however, data will correlate with some biochemical measures.[10]

Because of the burden placed on the individual and the problem of noncompliance in keeping either weighed or estimated food records, dietary recalls are often used in a clinical setting.

24-Hour Recall

The 24-hour recall is one of the most common methods of dietary assessment. As the name implies, the individual is asked to recall all foods and beverages consumed over the preceding 24 hours. If the recall were given at 2:00 PM, the information would cover the period from 2:00 PM on the previous day and would span a 2-day period. Alternatively, the recall could cover the previous full day using a midnight-to-midnight time period. The individual is asked to recall everything he or she has eaten or drunk on the previous day, beginning with the time of arising in the morning. The advantage in using the first approach is that the patient may be better able to recall the meal or snack immediately preceding the interview than the food intake from the previous day. This is especially true for individuals not exposed to recall methods prior to the interview. A sample 24-hour recall format is shown in Fig. 11-1.

Name: _____ Weight: _____

Date: _____ Height: _____

Age: _____ Sex: _____

Special condition of disease: _____

Day of week: _____

	Food	Amount	How Prepared
Meal:			
Time eaten:			
Location:			
Snack:			
Meal:			
Time eaten:			
Location:			
Snack:			
Meal:			
Time eaten:			
Location:			

Is this a typical day's intake? _____

Figure 11-1 Suggested 24-hour recall format.

The following protocol can be used to elicit information for the 24-hour recall:

Step 1. Ask the individual to recall the last meal or snack eaten prior to the interview. If the patient seems to have trouble recalling, prompt him or her with questions: "Did you eat or drink anything while you were waiting to see me?" "Did you eat or drink anything on the way to this examination?"

Step 2. Proceed backward from the last meal or snack:
- Lunch on the interview day
- Any snack between breakfast and lunch
- Breakfast on the interview day
- Any snack between supper and bedtime on the previous day
- Supper on the previous day
- Any snack between the midday meal and supper on the previous day

Step 3. For each item, record the food, amount eaten, how prepared (broiled, baked, fried), time eaten, and where eaten. Food models or measuring devices should be on hand to allow the patient to estimate portion sizes. It is best to allow the patient to recall all food and beverages for the previous 24 hours before any probing begins.

Step 4. After the individual has recalled all items, there may be some omissions or areas that need clarification. For example, the lunch menu may have been reported as

```
Meal:   Lunch
Time eaten:   12:30
Location:   Hospital cafeteria
Food:   Tuna sandwich (1 oz)
          whole wheat bread (2 slices)
          Vanilla ice cream (1 scoop)
How prepared:
```

Clarification is needed as to how the sandwich was prepared. Ask, "Was there anything on the tuna sandwich?" (butter, mayonnaise).

There also appear to be possible omissions in the menu. Ask, "Did you have anything to drink with your lunch?" The common omissions in recall tend to be
- Spreads used on sandwiches or breads
- Gravy and other condiments used on entrees and vegetables
- Beverages and items such as milk and sugar used in drinks
- Form of preparation
- Desserts

Probing for omissions always should be nondirective; never suggest the "correct" answer. For example, avoid asking, "Did you have milk with lunch?" Ask, "Did you have anything to drink with lunch?"

Step 5. Ask the individual if the 24-hour recall reflects a usual day's intake; if the present recall is not typical, record the reason why it is not.

The advantage of the 24-hour recall is that it can be completed in 20 to 30 minutes and requires little effort on the part of the respondent. However, the data provide information on only the past day's food intake; even if the intake is reported to be typical, it does not show day-to-day and season-to-season variations. The accuracy of one day's intake in reflecting usual consumption is low, particularly for nutrients like vitamin A, which can be ingested in widely varying amounts from day to day.

To reflect the intraindividual variation in caloric and nutrient intake accurately, a large number of recalls need to be collected for one person.[12] To determine an individual's usual diet pattern, the 24-hour recall is often used in conjunction with other methods, like food frequency or diet history, that reflect intake for a longer period.

The precision of the recall is directly affected by the person's ability to recollect accurately. Studies comparing the 24-hour recall to the weighed food record[13] or direct observation[14] show that the 24-hour method consistently tends to underestimate food consumption in certain categories (desserts) and to overestimate it in others (vegetables). The 24-hour recall method gives a representative picture of calorie and nutrient intake for large groups of subjects; however, it is not a sensitive measure of usual intake of an individual. It may be used in conjunction with a food frequency or diet history to obtain usual food consumption patterns. Alternatively, a series of 24-hour recalls may be administered over a 2- to 3-month period to measure the variability of intake and to enhance the validity of results.

Diet History

The diet history is used to collect data on food habits and practices for an extended time, typically 2 to 3 months. Unlike the 24-hour recall, it is designed to provide information on *usual* or average food patterns.

As shown in Fig. 11-2, the diet history contains three distinct components:

Part I.   Health history
Part II.   Usual food intake pattern
Part III. Frequency of consumption in selected food groups

Part I provides details on eating habits, food likes and dislikes, economic factors that affect food choices, and health factors that influence food patterns. This information is helpful in interpreting dietary consumption data and in tailoring counseling to the specific needs of the individual.

Part II provides information on the usual meal patterns of the patient. For each meal the clinician asks, "What do you usually eat?" If an individual has one type of breakfast during the work week but a different pattern on weekends, both are recorded. A complete record of every meal and snack, with the amount of each food, should be recorded.

Part III measures the frequency of consumption in selected food groups. This serves two purposes: it provides additional information on a broader range of food items, and it allows for a cross-check of items reported in Part II.

Although the diet history gives a comprehensive picture of an individual's eating habits, two main disadvantages often preclude its use in a clinical setting: (1) it may be valuable as a *qualitative* measure of dietary intake, but it has only limited usefulness as a *quantitative* measure[3]; it tends to overestimate food intake when compared to the 24-hour recall or the estimated food record[15]; (2) it requires, furthermore, a good deal of expertise if it is to yield accurate data and, more important, it takes approximately 1 hour to complete. If it is only one component of a longer examination, the time needed to complete the questionnaire may be prohibitive. An alternative is to have the patient complete the diet history at home; the completed questionnaire can be brought to the physician or other health professional at time of check-up. Again, however, this requires a well-motivated subject. A more realistic approach might be to use a rapid diet-appraisal method such as the food frequency.

Name: _____ Age: _____

Part I: Health History

Good _____

Number meals eaten per day: _____   Appetite: Fair _____

Poor _____

Has your appetite changed over the past several months? _____

If yes, specify how _____

Food likes and dislikes _____

Are you taking any vitamin or mineral supplements? _____ If yes, list _____

_____

Has your weight changed more than 5 pounds in the last year? _____

If yes, state reason _____

Sleep, hours per night _____ sound _____ or disturbed? _____ (check one)

Work, kind _____ hours per day _____

Leisure activities _____

Do you smoke? _____ If yes, number of cigarettes or cigars per day _____

Do you have dentures? _____ If yes, do they fit securely? _____

Are you on any type of special diet? _____

If yes, when was it prescribed and by whom? _____

_____

Number of persons living at home? _____

Income $ _____ Are you on Food Stamps? _____

Who is responsible for food purchasing? _____ Food preparation? _____

Do you own a stove? _____ Refrigerator? _____

Continued.

Figure 11-2 The diet history.
From Burke BS: J Am Diet Assoc **23:**1041-1046, 1947.

Part II: Usual Food Intake Pattern

Day of Week _____

	Food	Amount	How Prepared
Meal:			

Time eaten:

Location:

Snack:

Meal:

Time eaten:

Location:

Snack:

Meal:

Time eaten:

Location:

Snack:

Figure 11-2, cont'd. The diet history.

Part III. Frequency of Consumption in Selected Food Groups

Food Group	Average Intake	Never	Daily	Weekly	Monthly	Less than Once a Month
Milk: whole						
skim						
low fat						
Cheese						
Meat, fish, or poultry						
Luncheon meats						
Eggs						
Fruit: citrus						
dried						
others						
Vegetables: deep green or leafy						
dark yellow						
potato						
legumes						
other						
Cereals						
Bread: whole grain						
other						
Rice, pasta						
Butter, oil, or margarine						
Cake, cookies, or pastry						
Candy						
Nuts and peanut butter						
Ice cream						
Jam or jelly						
Salt (included in cooking and added at the table)						
Soups						
Alcohol						
Coffee or tea						
Soft drinks						

Heading: Frequency of Consumption (check one box)

Figure 11-2, cont'd. The diet history.

Food Frequency

The food frequency was devised as a modification of the diet history.[16] It measures the number of times certain foods are consumed over a 1-day, 1-week, 1-month, or longer period. The number of food groups and the length of observation can vary. The food frequency questionnaire used in the Health and Nutrition Examination Survey included 18 food groups[17] (Fig. 11-3). Participants were asked to recall their frequency of consumption in each group for the 3-month interval prior to the interview.

The food frequency can be simplified by condensing the number of food groups used. Questionnaires using as few as four groups (meat, milk, fruits and vegetables, bread and cereals) have been reported to yield valuable information.

The food frequency is simple to use and even can be self-administered with proper direction. It has been used extensively in epidemiologic studies to provide qualitative information on food intake. Since the data it provides are descriptive, it is not the appropriate instrument to use if precise nutrient intakes are required. However, it can aid in assessing the usual food consumption of the individual.

Name: _____

FOOD GROUP	Number of Times				
	Never	Daily	Weekly	Less than Once a Week	Unknown
(1) Milk, as beverage and on cereals					
(2) Meat					
(3) Poultry					
(4) Fish or shellfish					
(5) Eggs					
(6) Cheese and cheese dishes					
(7) Dry beans and peas (legumes, seeds, and nuts)					
(8) Fruits and vegetables (all kinds)					
(9) Fruits and vegetables rich in vitamin A (dark green and deep yellow)					
(10) Fruits and vegetables rich in vitamin C (grapefruit, orange, cantaloupe)					
(11) Bread					
(12) Breakfast cereals					
(13) Butter, margarine, and other fats and oils					
(14) Desserts such as cake, pie, cookies, puddings, and ice cream					
(15) Candy					
(16) Beverages (cold drinks, such as soda, lemonade, Kool-aid)					
(17) Artificially sweetened drinks					
(18) Coffee or tea					
(19) Salty snack foods (potato chips, corn chips)					

Figure 11-3 Food frequency questionnaire.

Adapted from Department of Health, Education, and Welfare: Food consumption profiles of white and black persons aged 1-74 years, United States, 1971-74, Washington DC, 1979, Government Printing Office.

ANALYSIS OF AN INDIVIDUAL'S DIETARY DATA

Dietary data collected from the weighed or estimated food record, the 24-hour recall, or the food intake portion of the diet history can be analyzed quantitatively and qualitatively.

Quantitative Analyses

Nutrient analysis of the dietary data is a two-stage process: *First,* the nutrient content of the foods identified from the dietary assessment must be calculated. The most complete sources of information on the nutrient content of foods are Handbooks no. 8[18] and no. 456,[19] developed by the U.S. Department of Agriculture. Nutrient analyses, including food-energy protein, fat, carbohydrate, calcium, phosphorous, iron, sodium, potassium, vitamins A and C, thiamine, riboflavin, and niacin, are provided for approximately 2500 foods. *Second,* after the nutrient content of each food item has been calculated, these val-

ues are combined to produce an estimate of the person's total nutrient intake. This then can be compared to an accepted standard. The Food and Nutrition Board of the National Academy of Sciences[20] publishes recommended dietary allowances (RDAs) that can be used to evaluate dietary data. The RDAs are the average daily amounts of calories and 17 nutrients that should be consumed by healthy individuals. Table 11-1 illustrates the most recent RDAs for specified groups by sex and age.

Some caution must be used in comparing a patient's nutrient consumption to the RDAs. Except for calories, the RDAs for nutrients are set at levels high enough to cover the needs of most individuals in the population. Therefore an intake below a particular RDA does not necessarily signify a deficiency. For example, most women do not achieve the RDA for iron yet are not anemic.[21] It is reasonable to assume that the farther below a specified RDA an individual's nu-

Table 11-1 Recommended Dietary Allowances

	Age (yr)	Weight (kg)	Weight (lb)	Height (cm)	Height (in)	Protein (g)	Vita-min C (mg)	Thia-mine (mg)	Ribo-flavin (mg)	Niacin (mg NE)	Vita-min B$_6$ (mg)	Fola-cin (µg)	Vita-min B$_{12}$ (µg)
Infants	0.0-0.5	6	13	60	24	kg × 2.2	33	0.3	0.4	6	0.3	30	0.5
	0.5-1.0	9	20	71	28	kg × 2.0	35	0.5	0.6	8	0.6	45	1.5
Children	1-3	13	29	90	35	23	45	0.7	0.8	9	0.9	100	2.0
	4-6	20	44	112	44		45	0.9	1.0	11	1.3	200	2.5
	7-10	28	62	132	52	34	45	1.2	1.4	16	1.6	300	3.0
Males	11-14	45	99	157	62	45	50	1.4	1.6	18	1.8	400	3.0
	15-18	66	145	176	69	56	60	1.4	1.7	18	2.0	400	3.0
	19-22	70	154	177	70	56	60	1.5	1.7	19	2.2	400	3.0
	23-50	70	154	178	70	56	60	1.4	1.6	18	2.2	400	3.0
	51 +	70	154	178	70	56	60	1.2	1.4	16	2.2	400	3.0
Females	11-14	46	101	157	62	46	60	1.1	1.3	15	1.8	400	3.0
	15-18	55	120	163	64	46	60	1.1	1.3	14	2.0	400	3.0
	19-22	55	120	163	64	44	60	1.1	1.3	14	2.0	400	3.0
	23-50	55	120	163	64	44	60	1.0	1.2	13	2.0	400	3.0
	51 +	55	120	163	64	44	60	1.0	1.2	13	2.0	400	3.0
	76 +	55	120	163	64								
Pregnant						+ 30	+ 20	+ 0.4	+ 0.3	+ 2	+ 0.6	+ 400	+ 1.0
Lactating						+ 20	+ 40	+ 0.5	+ 0.5	+ 5	+ 0.5	+ 100	+ 1.0

From Committee on Dietary Allowances, Food and Nutrition Board, National Research Council: Recommended dietary allowances,

trient intake falls, the higher is the probability of a deficiency. An intake falling below two thirds of a particular RDA is often taken to indicate a deficiency in consumption. However, any potential deficiency revealed by the dietary assessment should be corroborated with additional biochemical and clinical data, as pointed out in the preceding chapters on nutritional evaluation.

Historically the RDAs have been the standards for evaluating dietary adequacy. Initially they were used to project food needs of the population and to identify possible nutrient deficiencies in some population segments. Many of the deficiency diseases that occurred in the early part of the twentieth century have been eliminated in the United States; however, other diet-related problems still exist. Numerous Americans are overweight or obese, and a significant proportion are affected by hyperlipidemia. Although for many chronic degenerative diseases diet is but one of the causal factors, nevertheless, excesses in the American diet can contribute to poor health. As a result the National Research Council has developed dietary guidelines, particularly for those at high risk of coronary artery disease and obesity[20]: reduce total fat intake to 35% of calories; decrease intake of refined sugars and increase complex carbohydrate intake; reduce alcohol intake.

Manual computation of the nutrient content of food is time consuming, tedious, and as a result rarely done. Numerous computerized nutrient data bases have been developed to aid in the analysis of dietary data. Many of these systems are "user friendly." For example, Witschi et al.[22] have developed a simplified computer-based table of nutrient values and an interactive retrieval system for direct use by clinicians; this type of computerized analysis saves time and gives immediate results.

The type of system that is most appropriate

Fat-Soluble Vitamins			Minerals						Energy Needs (with range)	
Vita-min A (μg RE)	Vita-min D (μg)	Vita-min E (mg α-TE)	Calcium (mg)	Phos-phorus (mg)	Mag-nesium (mg)	Iron (mg)	Zinc (mg)	Iodine (μg)	(kcal)	(MJ)
420	10	3	360	240	50	10	3	40	kg × 115 (95-145)	kg × 0.48
400	10	4	540	360	70	15	5	50	kg × 105 (80-135)	kg × 0.44
400	10	5	800	800	150	15	10	70	1300 (900-1800)	5.5
500	10	6	800	800	200	10	10	90	1700 (1300-2300)	7.1
700	10	7	800	800	250	10	10	120	2400 (1650-3300)	10.1
1000	10	8	1200	1200	350	18	15	150	2700 (2000-3700)	11.3
1000	10	10	1200	1200	400	18	15	150	2800 (2100-3900)	11.8
1000	7.5	10	800	800	350	10	15	150	2900 (2500-3300)	12.2
1000	5	10	800	800	350	10	15	150	2700 (2300-3100)	11.3
1000	5	10	800	800	350	10	15	150	2400 (2000-2800)	10.1
									2050 (1650-2450)	8.6
800	10	8	1200	1200	300	18	15	150	2200 (1500-3000)	9.2
800	10	8	1200	1200	300	18	15	150	2100 (1200-3000)	9.2
800	7.5	8	800	800	300	18	15	150	2100 (1700-3000)	8.8
800	5	8	800	800	300	18	15	150	2000 (1600-2500)	8.8
800	5	8	800	800	300	10	15	150	1800 (1400-2400)	8.4
									1600 (1200-2000)	6.7
+200	+5	+2	+400	+400	+150		+5	+25	+300	
+400	+5	+3	+400	+400	+150		+10	+50	+500	

ed 9, Washington DC, 1980, National Academy of Sciences.

Table 11-2 Qualitative Dietary Evaluation Using the Four Food Groups

	Adults			Pregnant Women		Children		Preteens		Adolescents		
	Women	Men	Servings	Pregnant Women	Servings	1-6 yr	Servings	1-12 yr	Servings	Girls	Boys	Servings
Meat, fish, poultry Legumes, peanut butter, eggs	4 oz	6 oz	2	4 oz	2	1-3 oz	2	3-4 oz	2	4 oz	2 6 oz	2
Milk, cheese	16 oz	16 oz		32 oz		24 oz		24-32 oz		32 oz	32 oz	
Fruits, vegetables Vitamin C foods (1 medium-size fruit or fruit juice)	½ c	½ c	1		1		½-1		1			1-1½
Dark green or yellow vegetable	½ c	½ c	1		1	2-4 Tbsp		¼-½ c				1
Other vegetables and fruits			2 to 3		2		2 (small)	¼-½ c	2			2-3
Bread (slice)	1	1	4-6	1	3-4	1	4	1	4	1	1	4-5 (girls) 6-9 (boys)
Cereal (whole grain enriched)	or ½ c	or ½ c		or ½ c		or ½ c		or ½ c		or ½ c	or ½ c	

in a given setting varies depending on the needs of the individual clinician. One good resource is the National Nutrient Data Bank Directory,[23] which has an extensive list of available computerized nutrient data bases including their strengths and limitations.

Qualitative and Semiquantitative Analyses

Computing the nutrient content of the total diet can be time-consuming, even with a computer-assisted system. Several rapid diet-appraisal methods can be used to supplement the most in-depth nutrient analyses. For example, a qualitative evaluation of food frequency can be done using the four food–group standard. Table 11-2 illustrates the recommended quantities in each of the major groups. Selection of a variety of foods in the proper amounts from each of the categories will minimize the possibility of an inadequate nutrient intake. (However, appropriate intake of nutrients may also be achieved from other dietary combinations.)

In addition, there are several semiquantitative scoring systems that have been developed to evaluate dietary adequacy. A food frequency scoring system based on the Basic Four Food Guide[24] is shown in Table 11-3. Points are assigned according to the number of servings in each food group. This simple scoring method has compared well with more detailed calculations of nutritional adequacy. A maximum score of 16 met the RDAs for 7 of the 12 nutrients

Table 11-3 Dietary Score Based on the Basic Four Food Groups

	Points per Serving	Possible Food Group Score
Milk and milk products (up to maximum of 2)	2	4
Meat and meat alternatives* (up to maximum of 2)	2	4
Fruit and vegetables (up to maximum of 4)	1	4
Bread and cereals† (up to maximum of 4)	1	4
TOTAL		16

From Guthrie HA, Scheer JC: J Am Diet Assoc **78**:240-245, 1981.
*Includes animal protein foods, legumes, and nuts.
†Includes enriched and whole grains.

examined and exceeded 80% of the RDAs for the remaining five nutrients. The scoring system was not sensitive in identifying low intakes of iron, however.[24]

Other rapid dietary screening methods taking 2 to 10 minutes to administer have also been used successfully.[25]

DIETARY ASSESSMENT OF INFANTS

The dietary assessment methods just presented assume that respondents will report their own food intake patterns. For infants and preschoolers, information on dietary intake is collected from the primary caretaker and different techniques are appropriate.

A questionnaire (Fig. 11-4) used for assessing food intake and dietary practices in infants should cover caloric intake, iron sources, introduction of solid foods, infant caries, food preparation facilities, and inappropriate dietary practices.

Caloric Intake

The adequacy of caloric intake for a breast-fed infant cannot be assessed directly. It is evaluated indirectly by monitoring the changes in weight and length of the infant. A breast-fed infant who is receiving adequate calories will grow normally.

For a bottle-fed infant, up to 32 ounces of formula is sufficient to promote normal growth and development. Intakes of more than 32 ounces per day usually are excessive. A cross-check with anthropometric data will reveal whether the infant is outside weight-for-length norms. Intakes of less than 16 ounces daily are, by and large, inadequate. One cause may be improper formula dilution. A cross-check of formula consumption with weight and length data will disclose the problem. (Further information on formula dilution can be obtained from question *3* in Fig. 11-4.) Use of skim or low-fat milk also may contribute to caloric inadequacy.

Introduction of Solid Foods

Questions *5* and *8* (Fig. 11-4) will allow an assessment to be made of whether solid foods have been introduced at the most appropriate time for the infant. Introduction of solid foods at 4 to 6 months appears desirable in many cases. Prior to 4 months of age the infant is not developmentally ready to handle solid foods: neuro-

(1) Is the baby breast-fed or bottle-fed? _____

    If breast-fed, does the baby also receive formula? _____

    If bottle-fed, does the baby receive (check all that apply):

		Times per day
Ready-to-feed formula	_____	_____
Concentrated liquid	_____	_____
Other _____		_____
2% milk _____		_____
Skim milk _____		_____
Whole milk _____		_____
Evaporated milk _____		_____

(2) If the baby drinks milk or formula, what is the usual amount per day?

    Less than 16 ounces _____

    17 to 32 ounces _____

    More than 32 ounces _____

(3) How is the formula prepared, especially details on dilution? _____

_____

(4) Is the formula iron-fortified: _____

(5) Does the baby eat or drink any of the following (check all that apply):

Food	Usual Amount Eaten	How Often	Age When First Began Eating This Food
Eggs			
Dried beans or peas			
Meat, fish, poultry			
Bread, cereal, rice, pasta			
Fruits or fruit juices			
Vegetables			

(6) Do you have a working stove? _____ Refrigerator? _____ Indoor water? _____

(7) Does the baby take vitamin or mineral drops (specify)? _____

    How often? _____

(8) Is the baby on a special diet? _____ Why? _____

    Who prescribed the diet? _____

(9) Does the baby eat paint chips, dirt, or any other nonfood item? _____

    If yes, what and how often? _____

(10) Does the baby have any particular feeding problems? _____

(11) Does the baby fall asleep with a bottle? _____ If yes, what is in it? _____

Figure 11-4 Infant dietary assessment questionnaire.

From Fomon SJ: Nutritional disorders of children: prevention, screening, and follow-up, Washington DC, 1976, US Department of Health, Education, and Welfare, Public Health Service.

(1) Does the child drink any of the following: _____   How often?

    Whole milk _____   _____

    Skim milk _____   _____

    Low-fat milk _____   _____

    Other, specify _____   _____

(2) How much milk is consumed daily?

    Less than 8 ounces _____

    Eight to 32 ounces _____

    More than 32 ounces _____

(3) Does the child take a bottle to bed? _____ If yes, what is in it? _____

_____

(4) How many times a day does the child usually eat? _____

(5) Does the child eat the following:

	How Often	Amount
Cheese, yogurt		
Eggs		
Legumes or peanut butter		
Bread or cereal		
Rice or pasta		
Fruit or fruit juice		
Vegetables		

(6) Do you have a working stove? _____ Refrigerator? _____

    Indoor water? _____

(7) Is the child on a special diet? _____ Why? _____

    Who recommended it? _____

(8) Does the child eat paint chips, dirt, or any other nonfood item? _____

    If yes, what and how often? _____

(9) Is the child's appetite good _____ fair _____ poor _____ ?

(10) Does the child have any health-related problems (specify) _____

_____

Figure 11-5 Preschooler dietary assessment questionnaire.

From Fomon SJ: Nutritional disorders of children: prevention, screening, and follow-up, Washington DC, 1976, US Department of Health, Education, and Welfare, Public Health Service.

muscular control is poorly developed and salivary, gastric, and intestinal secretions are not yet produced in sufficient quantity to metabolize these foods effectively. Delaying the introduction of solid foods beyond 6 months of age may lead to insufficient intake of calories and other nutrients. By 4 to 6 months of age the infant usually requires an additional iron source—iron-fortified formula, iron-fortified cereal, or iron drops.

Other questions will permit assessment of food preparation facilities, feeding practices, and the use of vitamin and mineral preparations. If the initial dietary assessment indicates a potential problem, the clinician should follow up with a more thorough investigation of dietary consumption patterns and practices.

DIETARY ASSESSMENT OF PRESCHOOLERS

Many of the questions included in the infant dietary assessment questionnaire are appropriate for a young preschooler. However, a different questionnaire (Fig. 11-5) is used for the dietary assessment of an older preschool child. It is designed to identify any dietary intake deficiencies as well as any practices that may be inappropriate for normal growth and development.

SUMMARY

There are several methods that can be used for dietary assessment in a clinical setting. No one method is perfect under all circumstances. The choice of technique will be contingent on the assessment objectives, the time allotted, and the precision of information needed.

REFERENCES

1. Lind J: Treatise on the scurvy, Edinburgh, 1753, Sands, Murray, & Cochran, p 456.
2. Burke BS: The dietary history as a tool in research, J Am Diet Assoc 23:1041-1046, 1947.
3. Burke MC, Pao EM: Methodology for large-scale surveys of household and individual diets, Washington DC, 1976, US Department of Agriculture.
4. Kim WW, et al: Effect of making duplicate food collection on nutrient intakes calculated from diet records, Am J Clin Nutr 40:1361-1367, 1984.
5. Ohlson MA, et al: Nutrition and dietary habits of aging women, Am J Public Health 40:1101-1108, 1950.
6. Yudkin J: Dietary surveys: variation in the weekly intake of nutrients, Br J Nutr 5:177-194, 1951.
7. Marr JW: Individual dietary surveys: purposes and methods, World Rev Nutr Diet 13:105-164, 1971.
8. Dieckmann WJ, et al: Observations on protein intake and the health of the mother and baby. II. Food intake, J Am Diet Assoc 27:1053-1058, 1951.
9. Sprauve ME, Dodds ML: Dietary survey of adolescents in the Virgin Islands, J Am Diet Assoc 47:287-291, 1965.
10. Young CM, Trulson MF: Methodology for dietary studies in epidemiological surveys. II. Strengths and weaknesses of existing methods, Am J Publ Health 50:803-814, 1960.
11. Beaton GH, et al: Source of variance in 24-hour dietary recall data: implications for nutrition study design and interpretation, Am J Clin Nutr 32:2546-2559, 1979.
12. Balogh M, et al: Random repeat 24-hour dietary recalls, Am J Clin Nutr 24:304-310, 1971.
13. Linusson E, et al: Validating the 24-hour recall method as a dietary survey tool, Arch Latinoam Nutr 24:277-293, 1974.
14. Madden J, et al: Validity of the 24-hour recall: analysis of data obtained from elderly subjects, J Am Diet Assoc 68:143-147, 1976.
15. Young CM, et al: A comparison of dietary study methods. I. Dietary history versus seven-day record, J Am Diet Assoc 28:124-128, 1952.
16. Trulson MF: Assessment of dietary study methods. I. Comparison of methods for obtaining data for clinical work, J Am Diet Assoc 30:991-995, 1954.
17. Department of Health, Education, and Welfare: Food consumption profiles of white and black persons aged 1-74 years, United States, 1971-74, Washington DC, 1979, Government Printing Office.
18. Agricultural Research Service: Composition of foods. Agriculture handbook 8, Washington DC, 1975, US Department of Agriculture.
19. Agricultural Research Service: Nutritive value of American foods in common units, Washington DC, 1975, US Department of Agriculture.
20. Committee on Dietary Allowances, Food and Nutrition Board, National Research Council: Recommended dietary allowances, ed 9, Washington DC, 1980, National Academy of Sciences.
21. Monsen ER, et al: Estimation of available dietary iron, Am J Clin Nutr 31:134-141, 1978.
22. Witschi J, et al: Analysis of dietary data: an interactive computer method for storage and retrieval, J Am Diet Assoc 78:609-613, 1981.
23. Hoover LW: Nutrient data bank directory, ed 4, Columbia, 1984, University of Missouri Printing Services.
24. Guthrie HA, Scheer JC: Validity of a dietary score for assessing nutrient adequacy, J Am Diet Assoc 78:240-245, 1981.
25. Strohmeyer SL, et al: A rapid dietary screening device for clinics, J Am Diet Assoc 84:428-432, 1984.
26. Fomon SJ: Nutritional disorders of children: prevention, screening, and follow-up, Washington DC, 1976, US Department of Health, Education, and Welfare, Public Health Service.

IV

SYSTEMIC DISORDERS
AND NUTRITION

CHAPTER 12

Gastrointestinal Disorders

David H. Alpers

NUTRITIONAL ASSESSMENT TECHNIQUES

Gastrointestinal disorders often are accompanied by nutritional deficiencies of two general types: calorie or protein, and vitamin or mineral. Since the proper treatment of these deficiencies depends on their cause, the physician's first responsibility should be to determine the reason for the deficiency.

Calorie or Protein Deficiency

The possible cause of calorie or protein deficiency in gastrointestinal disease may be assessed by several standard methods, depending on the etiology of the disorder. When food intake has decreased, a diet history or a calorie count is suggested. The diet history usually is based on 24-hour recall and often is inaccurate. Somewhat more accurate is a two- or three-day food record, which can be compiled by the patient. Best of all available methods is the calorie count performed in the hospital.

When increased utilization of caloric intake is suspected, the amount of energy used can be gauged by estimating the caloric and protein requirements in disease. These can be projected by percentage additions to the basal metabolic requirements for calories and protein, shown in Table 12-1. (See Chapter 2 for BMR computations.) Although these estimates are reasonable if applied to surgical disorders (e.g., fractures, severe burns), they may overestimate the needs in severe medical disease. Patients receiving total parenteral nutrition for gastrointestinal disease uncommonly have a measured energy requirement in excess of their estimated basal requirement.[2] The reason for this seeming paradox is unclear but may be related in part to malnutrition with a lowered body muscle mass and to decreased basal muscle activity.

Tests for fat or calorie malabsorption often

are underutilized because of the difficulty in obtaining stool samples. The 72-hour collection of fecal fat remains the standard test for evaluating fat (and calorie) malabsorption. However, if the stool is solid or semisolid, assessment of fecal weight alone provides useful information. Normal stool weight is up to 200 g/day. In the absence of watery diarrhea, any increase in this daily weight strongly suggests malabsorption. If stool fat is to be measured, it is important that the intake of fat be measured during the stool collection. Thus a true absorption coefficient can be calculated as follows:

$$\frac{\text{Intake} - \text{Excretion}}{\text{Intake}} \times 100$$

Vitamin or Mineral Deficiency

Vitamin or mineral deficiency in intestinal disease may be assessed on the basis of intake or absorption, on the one hand, and in terms of the state of body stores, on the other. Frequently these two aspects of nutrient metabolism are measured by different techniques. Tests that may be useful in gastrointestinal disease are outlined in Table 12-2, together with the normal values for adults.

When the Schilling test for vitamin B_{12} absorption is performed in the presence of intestinal

Table 12-1 Caloric and Protein Requirements in Disease

Severity	Percentage of Basal Requirement	
	Caloric	Protein*
Mild	110	130
Moderate	125	160
Severe	150-300†	200

*Range 0.6-0.8 g/kg/day.
†Rarely exceeds twice the basal requirement.

Table 12-2 Tests for Vitamin and Mineral Deficiency

Nutrient	Tests Reflecting Intake or Absorption	Normal Adult Values	Tests Reflecting Body Stores	Normal Adult Values
Folic acid	Serum (*Lactobacillus casei*)	>6 ng/ml	Red cell	>140 ng/ml
Vitamin B$_{12}$	24-hour urinary excretion of ^{57}Co B$_{12}$ (Schilling test)	>7%	Serum	220-900 pg/ml
Vitamin A	Plasma vitamin A	>20 µg/dl >80 µg/dl	Plasma vitamin A	>20 µg/dl
Vitamin D	—		Alkaline phosphatase Serum 25-hydroxy-vitamin D	<85 IU/dl >10 ng/dl
Vitamin K	—		Prothrombin time	<2 sec prolonged
Iron	Serum iron	>50 µg/dl	Hemoglobin	Men, 14-17 ng/dl Women, 12-15 g/dl
			Iron binding capacity	15-60%
			Serum ferritin	Men, 10-275 ng/ml Women, 5-100 ng/ml
			Narrow staining	Abundant
Calcium	24-hour urinary calcium	100-300 mg/day (2-4 mg/kg)	Bone densitometry	
	Total serum calcium	9-11 mg/dl		
	Ionized serum calcium	4-4.5 mg/dl		
Magnesium	Serum magnesium	1.5-2 mEq/l	—	
Zinc	—		Serum zinc	>100 µg/dl

From Alpers DH, et al: Manual of nutritional therapeutics, ed 2, Boston, 1987, Little Brown & Co.

disease, intrinsic factor can be added orally to assess ileal function.* As is the case for most vitamin or mineral deficiencies caused by malabsorption, the absorptive defect can be detected before the body stores are depleted. Accordingly, deficiencies in which body stores already are depleted are more severe and deserve more rapid replacement. Both vitamin A and carotene are ingested in food, but only vitamin A is stored in the body. Therefore carotene levels reflect little more than the most recent intake of carotene whereas vitamin A levels reflect both intake and body stores. There are conditions that cause hypercarotinemia (e.g., diabetes mellitus) in which serum carotene levels are not related to intake.[4]

Tests for mineral deficiency, in contrast to those for vitamin deficiency, do not divide so neatly into measures of intake and body stores. This is due to the fact that many factors other than availability within the body determine the circulating plasma levels. For example, red cell production is altered by chronic illness or by protein or serum iron depletion; the amounts of calcium and magnesium are affected by such factors as parathormone levels, renal function, and pH. In general, serum levels are low when malabsorption is severe, but the tests are insensitive to moderate degrees of malabsorption. In the steady state, urinary calcium equals net intestinal absorption; however, for accurate test results calcium intake must be kept at a constant level for at least a few days prior to the 24-hour collection. Except for iron, assessment of body stores for other minerals is either insensitive (e.g., bone x-rays for calcium) or nonexistent (magnesium).

Treatment of nutritional deficiencies in most gastrointestinal disorders depends on the underlying mechanism of the disease. Although some diseases are characterized by increased caloric utilization (e.g., inflammatory bowel disease), most disorders are characterized by either decreased nutrient intake or decreased nutrient absorption. The problems presented by fat, car-

*However, the one-stage Schilling test can provide, unaccountably, inaccurate results.[3] Therefore the use of cobalamin (vitamin B$_{12}$) alone is still the standard for the Schilling test.

bohydrate, or protein malabsorption are somewhat different and will be discussed separately.

DISORDERS CHARACTERIZED BY DECREASED NUTRIENT INTAKE

Decreased nutrient intake can occur with (1) loss of appetite, (2) vomiting, (3) a swallowing disorder, (4) an obstructing lesion of the esophagus, stomach, or proximal small intestine, or (5) severe diarrheal illness. Because food intake is such an emotionally important event, the therapy chosen must be socially and psychologically acceptable to the patient.* Obviously, any diet that is marginal in calories and protein will require careful replacement of vitamins and minerals. Specific suggestions for replacement will be discussed separately.

Nausea and/or Vomiting

Nausea or vomiting is managed most effectively by understanding its etiology and, when possible, removing the causative agent (Table 12-3). Drugs are a common cause, and virtually all medications can induce these symptoms. A careful review of the patient's medications (including over-the-counter drugs) and the elimination of unnecessary ones are important steps in controlling nausea. The next most common causes, in the absence of an obstructing lesion, are chronic diseases (e.g., malignancy, hepatic inflammation). Although antiemetic medications can be used in these conditions, they produce sedation and are more effective in prophylaxis than in treatment of chronic nausea or vomiting. In the patient with a malignancy, the use of pain medication, radiation, or chemotherapy may be responsible for nausea or vomiting. Depression, too, in such patients may be a common cause of decreased appetite, a symptom that is often interpreted as nausea. Associated symptoms of fatigue, altered sleep patterns, or emotional lability can assist the physician in distinguishing depression as the cause of nausea.

In treating nausea or vomiting, every attempt should be made to provide food that is acceptable to the patient, and oral intake should be recorded carefully. If intake is not adequate, parenteral

*For example, a feeding tube or forced enteral feedings may not be acceptable to many patients, necessitating placement of a gastrostomy tube either endoscopically or surgically.

Table 12-3 Factors that Increase Nausea and Vomiting

	Suggested Countermeasure
Medication	Decrease dose or eliminate if possible
Chemotherapy	Antiemetics to prevent nausea
Radiotherapy	Antiemetics to prevent nausea
Hepatitis	Bed rest
Fever	Antipyretics
Acidosis from diarrhea	Oral or parenteral bicarbonate
Depression	Antidepressants, psychotherapy

nutrition can be provided (see Chapter 31). If intake is limited and high caloric density is desired, a complete food supplement can be offered. Since many of these are hypertonic, however, they tend to delay gastric emptying and may exacerbate nausea and vomiting. Chronic vomiting itself can lead to deficiencies not only of potassium and chloride but also of sodium. When vomiting complicates nausea, the oral route is not always possible and replacement must be parenteral.

Dysphagia

Dysphagia interferes with food intake. Either the stricture should be dilated or its cause removed, depending on the etiology. If obstruction is incomplete or if the dysphagia is due to neurologic (stroke, achalasia) or myopathic (muscular dystrophy) disorders, mechanically soft or low-residue foods may be used. (See "Alteration in Fiber Intake," p. 183.) Certain characteristics of soft and low-residue diets must be kept in mind for their successful long-term use:

Foods need not be bland.

Milk-based foods form an important part of the diet.

Flavoring is helpful for some liquids, but vanilla is tolerated best for long periods.

Medication should be given in liquid form if possible.

Caloric intake must be maintained at or close to the estimated requirement levels.

Mechanical assistance for food delivery may

be needed when an esophageal stricture is too narrow to allow the passage of even blended foods or liquids. Available methods include bougienage with or without the placement of an indwelling plastic tube, laser or radiation therapy for exophytic tumors, and gastrostomy.

Bougienage is the simplest technique and can be used even during radiotherapy for esophageal tumor. When the stricture does not permit passage of the soft-tipped Maloney dilators, rigid olive dilators may be passed over a metal guide and will be especially helpful for high strictures.

A laser can be used to enlarge the lumen compromised by exophytic tumor to provide temporary relief, but it requires considerable experience on the part of the physician and should be reserved for an advanced stricture that is unresponsive to other therapy or for "palliative" measures in inoperable cases.[5] Problems with its use include perforation and bleeding. The primary indication should be to allow removal of oral secretions, not the maintenance of long-term nutrition. When the stricture presents early in the course of a malignancy and is not exophytic, other therapies (radiation, bougienage) are preferable.

Gastrostomy certainly is useful for long-term delivery of calories when the esophagus is obstructed. The availability of percutaneous endoscopic gastrostomy has made this form of therapy more acceptable[6]; but the esophageal lumen must be sufficiently patent to allow this technique, which is more commonly used for nonobstructing causes of dysphagia (neurologic or muscular disorders). When obstruction is severe, a gastrostomy can be placed surgically.

Altered Gastric Emptying

Delayed emptying. The major causes of delayed emptying are *mechanical* (peptic disease, neoplasm) and *neurologic* (diabetes mellitus, vagotomy).

Mechanical obstructions tend to be treated surgically. However, some benign strictures can be improved enough by endoscopic balloon dilation to allow satisfactory resolution of the obstruction. Even when gastric tumor is metastatic, reestablishing an available intestinal tract is important as palliative therapy. If the obstruction is incomplete, premixed low-residue enteral feedings can be utilized in preparation for surgery. (See Chapter 31.) If feeding produces

symptoms by stimulating motility, oral ingestion may need to be discontinued and parenteral delivery used perioperatively.

Neurologic causes of delayed emptying include *diabetes* of long duration, especially when peripheral neuropathy also is present. Diarrhea is often an associated symptom further complicating nutritional management. Since specific therapy is not always successful, diabetic complications are difficult to treat. The use of small frequent feedings is the most satisfactory approach. Gastric emptying improves with 10 mg of parenteral metoclopramide. Metoclopramide is not always successful orally when the delayed emptying becomes severe, however. In this case absorption of medications as well as calories is delayed by the physiologic abnormality. Diabetic diarrhea can be managed in some patients with the alpha-adrenergic agonist clonidine (0.1-0.3 mg/da).[8] The delayed emptying that follows *vagotomy* takes two forms: postoperative ileus and gastric retention of solid foods. After gastric surgery, ileus occasionally is prolonged for 1 to 2 weeks. Parenteral delivery of calories is the procedure of choice in this situation. Rarely does the ileus last for many weeks, especially if dense adhesions from prior surgery are present. After vagotomy, particularly that performed in conjunction with gastric resection, solid foods may empty slowly. The coordinated peristaltic motion of the antrum is impaired after vagotomy; liquids empty but solid food resides longer in the stomach. In some cases a residual ball (bezoar) is formed.[9] Usually no routine preventive treatment is required, because bezoar formation is uncommon. However, patients should be cautioned not to eat excessive amounts of citrus fruits, which often form the core of a gastric bezoar.

Rapid emptying. The rapid emptying of liquids after vagotomy produces a series of symptoms known as the dumping syndrome. In the first half hour after eating, the symptoms are related to distention of the small bowel, with release of vasoactive peptides, including bradykinin, and to hypovolemia resulting from the delivery of hypertonic fluid to the proximal bowel, with subsequent secretion of fluid to restore isotonicity in the intestinal lumen. Delayed symptoms are related to reactive hypoglycemia. They can be controlled by dietary measures and by medication.

The low–available carbohydrate diet is employed in an attempt to decrease the osmolarity of ingested food. Since most meals are hypertonic and since the intestinal fluid reaches iso-osmolarity within a few centimeters of the pylorus, ingestion of hypertonic food leads to increased intraluminal volume and distention of the bowel. This distention causes the release of active peptides. Although the low–available carbohydrate diet is helpful, ingestion of any food, especially carbohydrate or protein, includes large–molecular weight substrates that can be hydrolyzed to small osmotically active substances, with subsequent effects. Therefore most foods have the potential to cause dumping, and the diet per se is only part of the therapeutic program, which includes besides the low-carbohydrate diet* the following measures:

Small frequent feedings, to control symptoms
Liquids ingested at different times from solids, to limit the total fluid load
Anticholinergics, to delay gastric emptying

Since the purpose of such a program is to limit symptoms, the degree to which these measures are followed will depend on the severity of symptoms.

Gastric bypass. Gastric bypass is sometimes performed in the treatment of excessive obesity. It involves creating a small fundic gastric pouch anastomosed to the small bowel. The postoperative diet consists of liquids and small amounts of solids. Vitamin and mineral supplementation may be necessary, depending on the contents of the diet. Since many of the patients are female, special attention should be given to calcium and iron replacement.[10]

DISORDERS CHARACTERIZED BY DECREASED NUTRIENT ABSORPTION
Fat Malabsorption

The treatment of fat malabsorption may be divided into two types of therapy: symptomatic and specific.

Symptomatic Therapy

Low-fat diet. Steatorrhea from any cause will diminish when triglyceride (triacylglycerol) intake is decreased. Diarrhea also will improve, since part of the pathogenesis of diarrhea with steatorrhea is the formation of hydroxy fatty acids in the colon. If fewer fatty acids reach the colon, less diarrhea will result. Therefore absorption of other nonfat caloric sources will improve, provided the intestine is intact and capable of carbohydrate and protein absorption. The low-fat diet is richer in these other caloric sources (especially carbohydrate).

Low-fat diets are used to control symptoms, not to reverse abnormal physiology. Therefore, no single amount of restriction can be prescribed for every patient. The best approach is first to determine the patient's usual fat intake. If this exceeds 100 g/day, a fat intake that is 50% of normal ingestion is recommended. For example, if intake is less than 100 but more than 75 g, then 40 to 50 g is the suggested limit. Restriction to less than 40 g/day is severe and difficult to maintain. A low-fat diet is not easy to achieve in the United States. Most protein sources also are rich in fat, and fat is responsible for the taste that many people associate with meat and fish. Thus there may be difficulty in reducing fat intake.

Triglycerides are the type of fat that causes most symptoms. Therefore the cholesterol content of foods will not be considered in this discussion. Triglycerides are found in large amounts in a number of common foods—cooking oil (27 g/oz), butter or margarine (24 g/oz), American cheese (8.4 g/oz), sausage (14.5 g/oz raw, 5.8 cooked), lunch meats (6.4-10.2 g/oz).[11]

Dietary fats (cooking oils, butter, margarine) contain large amounts of triglycerides. Thus the preparation of food becomes very important on a low-fat diet, since the addition of fat markedly alters the fat content of foods. To calculate the amount of fat in cooking oils, the following equation can be used:

$$\text{Grams} = \text{Milliliters of oil} \times \text{Specific gravity (0.91)}$$

For example, 2 tablespoons of olive oil contains 30 ml × 0.91 or 27 g of fat. It is thus apparent that on a low-fat diet all foods must be broiled, boiled, or baked. Moreover, since long-chain triglycerides provide 9 kcal/g, a low-fat diet can be low in calories. In fact, making the low-fat diet adequate in calories is often as large a challenge as avoiding fatty foods.

Eggs and many meats, especially luncheon

---

*See the discussion "Lactose Intolerance" (p. 175) for details. This diet is low in lactose as well as in dextrose and sucrose, so it limits milk products, sweets, and liquids with sugar.

RESTRICTED-FAT DIET	
Fat Intake (g/da)	**Foods Allowed**
40	Vegetables, most fruits, bread, cereals with skim milk, two 3-ounce servings of lean meat, one egg, one teaspoon of margarine
60	The above plus 2 cups of 2% milk *or* 1 additional ounce of meat per serving *or* 1 egg *or* 4 teaspoons of margarine or oil
75	The above plus 2 cups of whole milk instead of 2% milk *or* 2 slices of bacon *or* 4 ounces of ice cream *or* 2 servings of lean meat (6 oz each)

meats, have high fat contents and should be discouraged. Chicken and turkey contain less fat, especially if the skin is removed, and should form the meat staples of the low-fat diet. Fish that can be eaten as steaks contain the most fat. The flat fish (sole, flounder) contain less fat, and need to be served with a sauce to enhance their flavor. Dairy products made with whole or 2% milk contain triacylglycerols in large amounts, as do desserts (cakes, cookies, pies, pastry, candy), cream sauces, and gravies. A general table of foods allowed on a restricted-fat diet is presented above.

Medium-chain triglycerides (MCTs). Theoretically MCTs are useful in treating steatorrhea because they are hydrolyzed more rapidly by pancreatic enzymes, they do not require bile acid micelles for absorption of their hydrolysis products, and the products are taken into the portal blood (not the lymph). Therefore the defects present in many of the causes of steatorrhea can be bypassed by feeding MCTs. However, there are a number of problems with using MCTs. *First,* they provide only 8.3 kcal/g of energy (not 9 as the long-chain triglycerides do).[12] *Second,* they undergo omega oxidation in the body; that is, a second carboxyl group is formed on the first carbon. The resulting dicarboxylic acids cannot be utilized and are excreted. (It is not known how much of ingested MCTs are metab-

olized this way, but the effective caloric content of 1 tablespoon of MCT is probably less than expected from the theoretical value.) *Finally,* MCTs in large amounts cause diarrhea because of their osmotic effects, although when used appropriately they can deliver a small but perhaps important caloric addition to a marginal diet. (Moreover, since MCTs have a detergent action, they help solubilize and enhance the absorption of fat-soluble vitamins.)

Medium-chain fatty acids are delivered best as the oil (Mead Johnson) in a dose of up to 15 ml by mouth three times per day. This provides over 300 effective kilocalories per day. The oil is ingested most easily undiluted as a medication, although it may be mixed with a strong-flavored fruit juice (tomato or grape).

Low-fat caloric supplement. When table foods must be restricted severely to control calories, low-fat dietary supplements may be needed to deliver adequate calories. A representative sampling of such supplements is presented in Table 12-4. All these preparations can be used as complete nutritional supplements since they contain adequate protein, vitamins, and minerals. Since they do not taste especially good when used alone, they are better ingested as supplements, especially chilled. Vivonex contains largely digested nutrients and is especially appropriate for use in pancreatic insufficiency, *if* diet and enzyme replacement are not adequate.

Fat-soluble vitamins. When steatorrhea is present, fat-soluble vitamins need to be replaced. These often are offered in water-miscible forms (i.e., with detergent added). However, when the vitamins enter the intestinal tract, they still require bile acid micelle formation for absorption. Therefore, if the cause of steatorrhea involves bile acid depletion (e.g., short bowel) large doses of vitamins will be needed to achieve some absorption. The exception is vitamin K, which is available in a water-soluble form, menadione. Contents of some fat-soluble vitamin preparations are listed in Table 12-5. When bile acid absorption is intact, fat-soluble vitamin requirements can be managed by the use of preparations that offer fat-soluble vitamins alone or that are combined with other vitamins and minerals. Only the preparations limited to fat-soluble vitamins are listed in Table 12-5.

Note that the large doses of fat-soluble vitamins needed to treat fat malabsorption are avail-

Table 12-4 Selected Low-Fat Supplements

Product	Formulation for Serving (final volume)	kcal/100 cc	Osmolality (mOsm/1)	Calories (%)		
				Carbohydrate	Fat	Protein
Citrotein	1.18 oz packet + 6 oz water (200 ml)	63	496	73.5	2.3	24.2
Precision LR	3 oz packet + 8 oz water (285 ml)	111	525	89.9	0.6	9.5
Precision HN	2.93 oz packet + 8 oz water (285 ml)	105	557	83.0	0.4	16.6
Vivonex flavored	80 g packet + 8.5 oz water (300 ml)	100	617-678	90.5	1.3	8.2
Vivonex HN	80 g packet + 8.5 oz water (300 ml)	100	850-920	83.1	0.8	16.1

Table 12-5 Vitamins Provided by Selected Fat-Soluble Vitamin Preparations

Trade Name	A (IU)	D (IU)	E (IU)	C (mg)	K_3 (mg)
Aquasol A	25,000				
	50,000				
Calciferol		50,000			
Aquasol E			30		
			100		
			400		
Synkayvite					5
ADC Drops	5000	400		50	
Cod Liver Oil Concentrate (caps)	10,000	400			
Super D Cod Liver Oil	4000	200			
Super D Perles	10,000	400			
Tri-Vi-Sol	2500	400		60	
ViPenta Drops	5000	400	2	50	
ViSynerel Drops	5000	400	5	60	
ViZac	5000		50	500	

Table 12-6 Enzyme Activities in Selected Pancreatic Enzyme Preparations (units per capsule or tablet)

	Lipase	Protease	Amylase
Pancrease	4000	25,000*	20,000*
Ilozyme	3600	6600	330,000
Ku-Zyme HP	2300	6100	594,000
Festal	2100	1800	219,000
Cotazyme	2000	5800	499,000
Viokase	1600	4400	277,000

Modified from Graham D: N Engl J Med **296:**1314-1317, 1977.
*Manufacturer's estimates; all other determinations made independently.

able only as the individual vitamin, not as part of a multivitamin preparation. Moreover, vitamin K is not present in any multivitamin preparation. Since vitamin E deficiency is uncommon in most adult diseases, except with severe cholestasis (e.g., biliary cirrhosis) or severe fat malabsorption (e.g., abetalipoproteinemia),[13] and since the vitamin is available in virtually all dietary fats, this supplement usually does not need to be provided.

Specific Therapy

Pancreatic enzymes. Pancreatic enzymes are used in pancreatic insufficiency to relieve symptoms (diarrhea). This also will lead to increased efficiency of absorption because of prolonged transit time. It is difficult to return fat absorption to normal by this means, however, because the delivery of enzymes is not coordinated with gastric emptying, as it is physiologically. Nevertheless, fat malabsorption usually is decreased some 50% (e.g., from 60% to 80% absorption of fat) by enzyme replacement. On a 100 g fat diet, about 5 pancreatic enzyme tablets need to be used with each meal, and 1 or 2 with snacks. Table 12-6 compares the enzyme activities of the most potent commercial preparations.

All of these preparations are available as tablets or capsules. Festal and Cotazyme are enteric-coated, and Pancrease is a microencapsulated, preparation. Both of these modifications are intended to decrease the availability of the enzymes to gastric acid, which irreversibly destroys enzyme activity. No single preparation has been demonstrated superior to the others, despite the theoretical advantage of reducing exposure to gastric acid. This may be the result of decreased acid production in many patients with alcoholic pancreatitis, the usual cause of pancreatic insufficiency. If fecal fat and diarrhea are not decreased adequately by enzyme replacement, either the dose can be increased (up to 7 or 8 tablets/meal) or histamine₂ receptor antagonists can be added with each meal in an attempt to deliver more enzyme to the small intestine.[14] The maximum benefit to be achieved in any individual still will be short of complete correction and will vary. Thus, if no further improvement in symptoms is noted, one should return to the original dosage.

Pancreatic enzyme replacement is not useful as a nonspecific treatment and should be reserved for documented cases of pancreatic insufficiency. Some preparations contain bile acids and should not be used. If bile acid malabsorption is present, orally administered bile acids will not correct the defect, because the amounts contained in the tablets are insufficient to increase bile acid concentration above the critical micellar concentration needed to assist in fat absorption.

Gluten-free diet. The gluten-free diet is used to treat specific conditions (e.g., nontropical sprue[15]). It is less effective when used as nonspecific therapy. In addition, since adherence to it outside the hospital is more difficult and response to it may take a few weeks, it is best started immediately after a small bowel biopsy demonstrating villous atrophy has been obtained. It is a rather restrictive diet, and the physician needs to understand its principles to be better able, in this era of increasing reliance on prepackaged foods, to assess patient compliance with it.

Foods containing gluten from wheat, rye, barley, and probably oats should be eliminated from the diet. Wheat gluten is the component that gives form to dough and allows the ingredients to maintain shape during baking. The flours allowed on a gluten-free diet (corn, rice) do not contain these sticky proteins, so breads and other baked products are flat or crumbly. Any product that rises during baking (e.g., bread) must contain some proscribed gluten and thus is not permitted on the diet.

Cereal beverages (Postum, Ovaltine, beer, ale) are not allowed, although distilled alcohol may be ingested. Some commercial ice creams contain gluten stabilizers. Since there is much local variation in manufacturing, one should check with area suppliers about individual brands. Ice cream cones and commercial cakes, cookies, doughnuts, and pastries prepared with the offending glutens cannot be used.

Many commercial salad dressings contain gluten stabilizers. Canned meat products often contain gluten, as do cold cuts, sausages, and frankfurters. Although some brands of these products are free of stabilizers, their gluten content must be determined on an individual basis.

Commercial soups often contain cereal additives. Many instant coffees, catsups, mustards, and candy bars contain wheat flour. Processed frozen foods with sauces frequently are made with gluten stabilizers.

Labels must be read with great care. Any product containing wheat, rye, barley, or oats should be avoided. Other words to check for are flour, starch, emulsifiers, stabilizers, and hydrolyzed vegetable protein. Products with these words in the label may contain wheat or related glutens.

Useful recipes and detailed instructions for preparing gluten-free meals are available from a number of publications.[16,17]

Antibiotics. There is specific therapy for some illnesses associated with steatorrhea, but it may or may not be curative. Thus, often a low-fat diet is used in conjunction with a more specific therapy such as antibiotics. The underlying diseases for which antibiotics are used (Whipple's, or stagnant loop syndrome) are controlled rather than cured by the antibiotics. Steatorrhea in the stagnant loop syndrome is related to the growth of microorganisms that deconjugate bile acids and have a direct toxic effect on the mucosa. Theoretically the constant use of antibiotics could lead to overgrowth of other bacteria that also might produce symptoms. For this reason antibiotics often are used in cyclic fashion, either on a 2-week pattern (12 da on treatment, 2 da off) or on a longer cycle (4 to 6 wk on treatment,

1 wk off). Giardiasis can present with steator-rhea, but in this case treatment with antibiotics should be curative, and nonspecific therapy is used only during the acute phases of the illness.

Carbohydrate Malabsorption
Lactose Intolerance

Lactose intolerance defines the syndrome of diarrhea, bloating, and gas following ingestion of lactose.[18] It can be due to lactase deficiency or to decreased time of exposure to mucosa with a normal or low enzyme level. The latter situation is seen with short bowel syndrome, acute gastroenteritis, or dumping syndrome. Often lactose intolerance and irritable bowel syndrome are present in the same patient. Thus a low-lactose diet must be used in conjunction with other treatment for irritable bowel.

Low-lactose diet. Treatment for lactose intolerance is usually a low-lactose diet. Individual susceptibility varies greatly but the average patient develops symptoms after ingesting 12 g of lactose (the contents of an 8-ounce glass of milk). A few patients, however, will have symptoms after ingesting 3 g and their diets must be more restricted. When lactose intolerance is due to the dumping or short bowel syndrome, diarrhea and bloating may have other causes, and lactose restriction usually does not resolve all symptoms.

A low-lactose diet will contain very few dairy products. It may therefore be low in calcium. Supplements of calcium are usually necessary, especially in postmenopausal women. Patients on this diet should become label readers and should avoid all packaged foods that have any of the following words on the label: milk products, milk solids, whey, lactose, milk sugar.

Milk in all its forms is restricted in a low-lactose diet. Lactose actually is added to some skim milks to increase their caloric content. Buttermilk, even when naturally fermented, contains large amounts of lactose. Milk or cream is added to commercial yogurt after fermentation to avoid the sour taste produced by the fermenting lactose; thus the lactose content per ounce is similar to that of milk (about 1.5 g). However, the active culture in yogurt leads to partial hydrolysis of the lactose, allowing yogurt to be ingested without symptoms, even by many lactose-intolerant individuals.[19] Ice cream also is very rich in lactose because the milk solids are concentrated.

Sherbets contain about half as much lactose. Ice milks are even higher than ice cream, since lactose is the major caloric source. In cheese, lactose separates into the whey. Harder pressed cheeses contain less whey and consequently less lactose; soft cheeses, especially spreads to which milk or cream is added, contain more lactose than harder cheeses. The lactose content of most cheeses is only about 0.5 to 1 g/ounce. Since the average patient can tolerate 3 g of lactose, it is likely that at least a few ounces of cheese will not cause problems. Many desserts are made with milk and milk chocolate, and sauces or stuffings often contain milk, cream, or cheese. Table 12-7 lists the lactose content of selected foods.

Lactose-hydrolyzing enzymes. The lactose in milk can be hydrolyzed by yeast enzyme preparations (Lact-Aid, Lactrase). Mixture of a packet of Lact-Aid (containing lactase from the yeast *Kluyveromyces lactis*) with milk at 4°C results in 70% hydrolysis of the lactose in 1 day and 90% hydrolysis in 2 or 3 days. Patients with

Table 12-7 Lactose Content of Selected Milk Products

	Unit	Lactose Content (g/unit)
Milks		
Whole	c	11
2%	c	9-13
Skim	c	11-14
Chocolate	c	10-12
Sweetened condensed	c	35
Reconstituted dry	c	48
Buttermilk	c	9-11
Cream		
Light	Tbsp	0.6
Half-and-half	Tbsp	0.6
Whipped	Tbsp	0.4
Solid confections		
Ice cream	c	9
Sherbet	c	4
Ice milk	c	10
Yogurt (low fat)	c	11-15
Cheeses		
Hard (e.g., Parmesan)	oz	0.6-0.8
Semihard (e.g., cheddar)	oz	0.4-0.6
Soft (e.g., Brie)	oz	0.1-0.2
Spreads	oz	0.8-1.7
Cottage	oz	5-6
Cottage, low fat	oz	7-8
Butter	Tbsp	0.15

Adapted from Welsh JD: Am J Clin Nutr **31**:592-596, 1978.

limited tolerance of lactose can use this milk, which is sweeter than regular milk but is well accepted, in cooking or on cereal. Dairy products other than milk cannot be treated in this way at home. However, preparations are available as tablets that can be ingested along wtih lactose-containing foods.

Substitute milk products. Commercial non-dairy products are available that do not contain lactose. They include nondairy creamers and liquid milk substitutes. The latter utilize corn solids and syrup as their carbohydrate sources and thus are high in carbohydrate content. They are useful for lactose-intolerant patients, in whom generalized carbohydrate intolerance (e.g., dumping syndrome) is not a problem.

Sucrase/Isomaltase Deficiency

Sucrase/isomaltase deficiency rarely is encountered in the United States, but it occurs in about 10% of Eskimos. The principles of dietary management are similar to those for lactose intolerance, except that the foods involved differ. Sucrose is contained in many naturally occurring fruits and, most important, in sugar cane. Thus table sugar and foods cooked with it are not allowed. A detailed list of foods and their sucrose content is available.[20] Isomaltose residues are found in dextrans after amylase digestion of starch. These dextrans will not be digested in sucrase deficiency, but form a small part of the total sucrose/isomaltose intake of a normal diet. Thus starch restriction is not usually necessary.

Starch Intolerance

It is uncertain how many gastrointestinal symptoms are related to malabsorption of starch. The processing of starch may play a role in the digestion of dietary starches.[21] Some persons develop symptoms of flatus and cramping, along with increased breath hydrogen production, indicative of carbohydrate malabsorption. This syndrome is incompletely understood at present, and starch restriction remains a diet only for limited purposes. Some individuals with troublesome flatus notice a marked change in symptoms following dietary restriction of carbohydrates. However, in most persons flatus is a symptom of altered motility in addition to, rather than because of, increased gas production. In pancreatic insufficiency, salivary amylase remains and ac-

counts for partial hydrolysis of starch. Since a low-fat diet often is required to control symptoms, starch restriction would prevent adequate caloric intake, and thus is prescribed rarely.

Protein Loss and/or Malabsorption

Virtually every intestinal disease can be associated with increased protein loss, since approximately 10 g of protein normally is secreted or lost into the intestine each day. Thus disorders characterized by increased loss of cells or secretions or by decreased efficiency of digestion or absorption will have increased protein losses. These losses range from 4 to 40 g/day.

Treatment for protein loss or malabsorption differs greatly from that for fat or carbohydrate malabsorption, since fats and carbohydrates are not essential nutrients (except for the small need for essential fatty acids). Moreover, malabsorption of fat or carbohydrate causes symptoms. Protein must be ingested in large quantities each day (0.5-1 g/kg) to provide enough essential amino acids for growth and maintenance of tissues. No protein is stored in the body, since each protein has a function. Unlike fat and carbohydrate, then, because there is no storage pool in the body to call on when dietary intake is inadequate, protein must be ingested in excess, to allow for the decreased efficiency of reabsorption.

Dietary Treatment Using Table Foods

Although sound in principle, dietary treatment using table foods is difficult in practice, because foods that are rich in protein usually contain large amounts of triglycerides.[11] Most of the diseases that produce protein malabsorption or loss also present with steatorrhea. Even in a disorder characterized primarily by protein loss (e.g., severe congestive heart failure, intestinal lymphangiectasia), increased dietary fat enhances lymph flow, causing increased secretion of protein into the intestine. This occurs because the lymphatic flow from the intestine into the body is blocked in these disorders. Thus, available protein sources often are limited to those that contain little triglyceride—skim milk, shellfish, skinless chicken or turkey, water-packed tuna, and legumes. It should be noted that legumes contain large amounts of nonabsorbable carbohydrates, such as raffinose, which can cause bloating and gas.

Table 12-8 Supplemental Protein Sources in Common Foods

	Serving Size	Approximate Protein Content (g)	Comment
Whole milk	c	8.5	All milk products contain lactose
			Commercially available lactase (Lact-Aid) treated milk to hydrolyze over 90% of disaccharide
Skim milk	c	9	Skim milk and nonfat dry milk contain <1 g of fat per cup; other milk products contain 4-5 g of fat or more per serving
Nonfat dry milk	c	43	
Ice cream	c	6	
Ice milk	c	6	
Cottage cheese	c	30	
Yogurt (low-fat)	c	8	
Cheese (slice)	oz	6-8	Harder cheeses have less lactose; all cheeses are high in fat content
Egg	1 large	7	
Eggnog	c	12	
Peanut butter	Tbsp	4	50% of weight is fat (8 g/Tbsp)
Lean beef	oz	7	
Fresh fish	oz	7	Flat fish have lowest fat content
Tuna	oz	8	
Chicken/turkey (without skin)		8	

When fat absorption is not a problem, regular dietary sources of protein may be used (milk, meat, cheese, eggs, peanut butter, ice cream).

Protein Supplements

To supply adequate protein in the diet, it is frequently necessary to use supplements. Total protein ingested often must exceed 1 g/kg/day to produce positive protein balance. Although it is not usually possible to determine when positive balance is achieved, the protein requirement and status of visceral protein can be assessed as described at the beginning of this chapter and in Chapter 2.

Any of the low-fat supplements listed in Table 12-4 may be used as sources of protein and carbohydrate. It is important to remember that, when protein is ingested, enough additional calories must be provided so the protein is used as a source of amino acids and not converted into a source of energy. Usually this protective effect requires a nonprotein calorie/gram of protein ratio of about 25 to 35:1. Selected dietary protein supplements are analyzed in Table 12-8.

It is sometimes better to provide protein as a nonfood supplement, along with nonprotein calories in the form of carbohydrate. Such supplements include Casec and PVM powders (pro-

viding 4 g of protein/Tbsp and 8.5 g of protein/scoop, respectively). These are mixed with water and/or flavored with added table sugar or corn solids (e.g., Polycose) to make a palatable drink. Often it is best to use both food and nonfood supplements to avoid taste fatigue.

DISORDERS CHARACTERIZED BY MALABSORPTION OF VITAMINS AND MINERALS

Although malabsorption caused by diffuse mucosal disease or loss of mucosal surface area can produce deficiency of any vitamin or mineral, certain deficiencies associated with intestinal disorders are seen more commonly than others. This common association may be due to many factors: (1) an organ uniquely involved in absorption may be diseased or bypassed (ileum for cobalamin, duodenum for iron); (2) body stores may be low and requirements great so a clinical deficiency frequently occurs (e.g., folic acid); (3) an essential mechanism for absorption may be lost (e.g., bile salt absorption for fat-soluble vitamins); (4) the body may be unable to compensate for intestinal losses (e.g., iron or zinc in the stool); (5) absorption may be inefficient under normal conditions (e.g., calcium, magnesium, iron); and (6) more than one mech-

Table 12-9 Replacement Therapy With Vitamins in Gastrointestinal Disease

Vitamin	Condition Commonly Producing Deficiency	Preparation Used	Dose
Folic acid	Gluten-sensitive enteropathy, tropical sprue, stagnant loop syndrome, alcoholism	Pteroylglutamic acid	1 mg/da p.o.
Cobalamin	Ileal disease or resection, subtotal gastrectomy	Cyanocobalamin	1000 μg/mo i.m.
Other water soluble	Decreased food intake, alcoholism	Multivitamin	1/da
A	Short bowel syndrome, ileal disease	Retinol	5000-10,000 IU/da
D	Short bowel syndrome, ileal disease	Vitamin D	50,000 IU 2-3 times/wk
E	Biliary obstruction, short bowel syndrome, abetalipoproteinemia	D-α-Tocopherol	100-200 IU/kg/da
K	Ileal disease or resection, chronic antibiotic therapy	Vitamin K_3	5-10 mg/da p.o.

Table 12-10 Replacement Therapy With Minerals in Gastrointestinal Disease

Mineral	Conditions Commonly Producing Deficiency	Preparation Used	Dose
Iron	Blood loss, Billroth II gastrojejunostomy	Inorganic iron (e.g., sulfate)	325 mg 3 times/da with meals
Calcium	Short bowel syndrome, ileal disease, steatorrhea of any cause	Calcium carbonate	500 mg 1-3 times/da p.o.
Magnesium	Short bowel syndrome, alcoholism	Magnesium oxide	250-600 mg 1-3 times/da p.o.
Zinc	Severe diarrhea (e.g., Crohn's), cirrhosis	Zinc sulfate	50 mg 1-3 times/da p.o.

anism for absorption may be lost (e.g., vitamin D and calcium malabsorption producing calcium deficiency). Tables 12-9 and 12-10 outline the major disorders leading to deficiency of vitamins and minerals commonly seen with intestinal diseases and offer representative treatment schedules. They do not cover all possible deficiency states or all replacement requirements, however. The reader is referred to other sources[20] for a more extensive discussion of vitamin and mineral deficiencies. Because the functions of the proximal and distal intestine differ, deficiency states that characterize disorders involving these two anatomic regions also differ. Thus it is helpful to consider the problems unique to disorders of the proximal and distal small bowel.

Bypass of the Proximal Small Intestine

Iron absorption. The major nutrient absorbed primarily by the duodenum is iron. However, iron absorption is not efficient (only about 10% in normal persons). Gastric surgery for peptic ulcer or obesity may result in duodenal bypass and unabsorbed iron. A Billroth I anastomosis or a gastroplasty procedure still leaves the duodeum in its normal anatomic relationship with the stomach, and thus bypass does not occur. However, when a Billroth II procedure or gastric bypass is constructed, the flow of food is from the stomach into the jejunum and the duodenum is bypassed, resulting in iron loss. In addition, excessive iron may be lost from the peptic disease for which the operation was performed, resulting in iron deficiency. Iron deficiency may also occur in gastrointestinal bleeding of any cause and in malabsorption where the proximal bowel is involved (e.g., nontropical sprue). Nongastrointestinal causes, such as menstrual loss or deficient iron intake, are other common reasons for an iron deficiency.

Treatment of iron deficiency usually involves the use of an oral iron preparation. Iron is included in many multivitamin and mineral preparations. The amount of inorganic iron in such products varies greatly, from 10 to 143 mg/tablet. Nearly all the preparations are available in forms that contain from 25 to 50 mg vitamin C. This reducing agent is needed in the case of hypo- or achlorhydria, when sufficient hydrogen ions are not present to ensure the existence of ferrous ions. For gastric bypass that excludes the acid-producing portion of the stomach vitamin C should be included with iron.

Normal daily iron requirements are about 1.2 mg for men and 2.5 mg for women. If 10% is absorbed normally, then 12 to 25 mg of oral inorganic iron daily should be sufficient. The RDA for iron, 10 and 18 mg for men and women, is intended to allow for differences in absorption and for the fact that food iron, especially in vegetables, is less available than heme or inorganic iron. Iron used for oral therapy is usually inorganic, but the elemental iron content varies according to the compound. The approximate content of iron is 20% for the sulfate, 30% for the fumarate, and 10% for the gluconate salt. To avoid the epigastric symptoms caused by direct chemical action on the gastric mucosa, oral iron preparations should be ingested with meals.

Calcium and vitamin absorption. Bypass of the proximal intestine does not commonly produce deficiencies other than of iron. The active transport region for calcium absorption is duodenal, but in humans the bulk of calcium is absorbed in the jejunum and ileum.[29] Folic acid and most other water-soluble vitamins are absorbed largely in the proximal bowel, but only because they are efficiently absorbed by the first segment of bowel to which they are exposed. Deficiencies of folic acid and vitamin B_{12} occur after ulcer surgery (26% and 20% of the time, respectively) although less frequently than does iron deficiency (48% of the time).[22] When there is mucosal disease, however, such that absorption is impaired throughout much or all of the intestine, deficiency of folic acid and other water-soluble vitamins can be seen more regularly. Support for this comes from results in patients who have undergone gastric bypass operations for obesity.

Gastric-Bypass for Obesity

Despite earlier expectations, gastric exclusion surgery for obesity results in anemia and iron, folate, and vitamin B_{12} deficiencies rather commonly. Anemia has occurred in from 18% to 36% of patients.[23] It develops rapidly, with a mean time of 20 months after bypass surgery; in contrast, postgastrectomy deficiencies usually take years to develop.[22] The reasons for the rapid development of anemia are not clear, but they suggest that factors other than malabsorption, maldigestion, and altered intake must be operative. Normal Schilling test results have been found in most patients with low serum vitamin B_{12} levels.[23] Perhaps the proteolysis of bound cobalamin is impaired after gastric bypass, although this has not been demonstrated in these patients, as it has in postgastrectomy patients. The other micronutrient deficiencies reported in gastric exclusion operations are probably of little clinical importance. A number of cases of Wernicke-Korsakoff syndrome have been reported following recurrent and profuse vomiting. Although thiamine deficiency has been suspected, only one report[24] shows a response to thiamine replacement.

Bypass or Resection of the Distal Small Intestine

The clinical disorders occurring with bypass or resection of the distal small intestine include Crohn's disease, recurrent adhesions (with resection), bowel infarction (with resection), and ileal bypass for hypercholesterolemia.[25] Treatment consists of a low-fat diet and fat-soluble vitamins, since bile acids are absorbed in the most distal portion of the small intestine. The extent of the ileum involved can make a marked difference in the degree of fat restriction needed.

Pure bile acid diarrhea is uncommon, but a few patients have presented with an abnormality that approximates this syndrome.[26] Some bile acid is lost, but not so much that the bile acid concentration in the small bowel falls below the critical micellar concentration. With normal bile acid micelles, fat absorption is normal. However, the small amount of bile acid that escapes into the colon causes net secretion of water and electrolytes, with resulting diarrhea. These patients usually have normal Schilling tests for vitamin B_{12} absorption, although test results can be mildly abnormal. They often respond to a low-fat diet, because bile acid production from the liver is decreased on such a diet. Therefore the absolute amount of bile acid malabsorbed will be less and diarrhea will abate. When the diarrhea persists, cholestyramine may be successful.

Fatty acid diarrhea is the more common syndrome, although occasionally a component of the diarrhea is due to bile acid–stimulated secretion. In this syndrome the diarrhea and steatorrhea are more severe because bile acid pools are lower than in bile acid diarrhea. Vitamin B_{12} absorption usually is abnormal because the area of the ileum that contains receptors for the intrinsic factor–B_{12} complex is large, encompassing the entire ileum. Thus only large areas of resected or diseased bowel eliminate most of the active uptake of vitamin B_{12}. Since much of the diarrhea is due to hydroxy fatty acids formed in the colon, decreasing the fatty acid load alleviates symptoms. Binding more bile acids with cholestyramine usually makes the steatorrhea worse.

Features of the low-fat diet and fat-soluble vitamin replacement are discussed in previous sections.

Cholestyramine. The resin cholestyramine binds bile acids as well as other structurally related compounds such as sterols (vitamin D) and drugs (digitalis). By further depleting bile acid stores, it can worsen steatorrhea and cause more malabsorption of fat-soluble vitamins. Thus its use should be restricted to cases in which the criteria for bile acid diarrhea seem to be met (i.e., mild steatorrhea, a normal Schilling test, a moderate response to fat restriction). The resin comes in 4 g packets, which can be mixed in tomato juice to decrease the somewhat disagreeable flavor of the particles. If the gallbladder is present, the bile acid pool is stored there during the night. Consequently 4 g of cholestyramine given at breakfast, in the middle of the morning, and with lunch will bind more of the pool than will evenly spaced doses. If the gallbladder is not present, doses can be given with meals. Sometimes a fourth dose is needed to control symptoms. If chronic cholestyramine therapy is needed, the replacement dose of fat-soluble vitamins should be doubled in an attempt to ensure absorption of adequate amounts. Serum vitamin A levels can be used to follow the efficacy of this replacement.

Vitamin B_{12} (cobalamin). When vitamin B_{12} therapy is required for ileal disease or resection, the Schilling test will become abnormal long before the serum level falls. The body contains sufficient stores of vitamin B_{12} to last at least 1 to 2 years, even in the face of malabsorption. Deficiency develops more slowly in pernicious anemia. The vitamin B_{12}, both administered and dietary (along with folic acid and vitamin A), undergoes enterohepatic circulation and is malabsorbed. Thus, deficiency occurs more rapidly with malabsorption. However, treatment should be started when malabsorption is detected, not when deficiency is detected. Since the enterohepatic circulation accounts for about 10 μg/day, total malabsorption would require 300 μg/month for replacement. Such complete malabsorption is uncommon. Nevertheless, it is recommended that 250 to 500 μg/month be used intramuscularly as replacement. Because the defect is a lack of ileal receptors, oral vitamin B_{12} is not effective in the low doses available in hematinics.

Low-oxalate diet. The degree of oxaluria and the risk of forming oxalate stones are inversely correlated with the degree of fat absorption.[28] The excess of free fatty acids in the lumen in steatorrhea binds calcium, which is thus unavailable to form a salt with oxalic acid. Consequently, sodium oxalate is formed, which is much more soluble than the calcium salt. In the presence of bile acid malabsorption, bile acids alter colonic permeability and the sodium oxalate is absorbed by the colon. A low-oxalate diet is used to limit oxaluria and decrease the risk of oxalate stones. The major drawback of the diet is that it is only partially effective in lowering urinary oxalate excretion since only about 10% of the body's oxalate pool derives from the diet. Therefore urinary oxalate should be measured again after initiation of the diet to assess its effectiveness. Foods that should be avoided because they are very high in oxalate include spinach, rhubarb, cocoa, chocolate, tea, and Ovaltine. Parsley, green beans, collards, kale, turnip greens, beets, brussels sprouts, bread, potatoes, raw nuts, strawberries, figs, oranges, some instant coffees, and cola beverages all are moderately high in oxalate and should also be avoided.

Addition of calcium supplements, which often are required in ileal disease or resection, helps to reestablish the calcium oxalate and to decrease hyperoxaluria. Such therapy may be useful along with the low-oxalate diet. A low-oxalate diet combined with a low-fat diet often is too restrictive. Therefore calcium supplements can sometimes be tried first for hyperoxaluria. Doses used are from 600 to 1000 mg of elemental calcium.

Calcium. Calcium is absorbed with the greatest efficiency by duodenal enterocytes. However, the bulk of calcium in humans is absorbed in the ileum. This is because the duodenum is so short, and calcium absorption even at best is only about 35% to 40% efficient. Many other factors play roles in calcium absorption, and some are affected by small bowel loss.[29]

Calcium ions are ingested complexed either with protein (e.g., caseinate from milk) or with organic anions (e.g., phytates from green leafy vegetables). Inorganic salts (carbonate, gluconate, lactate) are used for therapy. Indirect evidence suggests that in the stomach the calcium salt of any origin is partially converted to the chloride salt. As the calcium complex passes through the small intestine into fluid of increasingly alkaline pH, it becomes less soluble and more calcium forms complexes with PO_4 and other binding anions. In the short bowel syndrome phosphate is malabsorbed and the concentration of luminal PO_4 increases, thereby decreasing calcium solubility. However, increasing phosphorus intake up to 2000 mg/day, nearly double the average intake, does not adversely affect calcium absorption.[30] Nonphosphate anions, such as fatty acids, also are malabsorbed and decrease the availability of calcium for absorption. Transit time is shortened because of the loss of intestinal length and the regulatory function of the ileocecal valve. Finally, vitamin D is malabsorbed in short bowel syndrome because of the loss of bile acids. Vitamin D plays a permissive role in absorption of calcium throughout the small intestine. If the colon is in place, calcium balance is improved, but whether from slower transit or from colonic absorption is not clear.

Urinary calcium excretion is dependent on protein intake, although the precise relationship is not clear. An adequate protein intake (0.6-0.8 g/kg/da) is necessary to absorb and retain one third of the calcium intake when the calcium intake is in the usual range (800-1400 mg/da). Since urinary calcium is a measure of calcium absorption in the steady state, one must be mindful of the protein intake when this assessment is carried out. A low-fat diet, which can be a low-protein diet, often is used in the short bowel syndrome. Thus care must be given to maintaining an adequate protein intake along with calcium supplementation. Furthermore, these intakes should be constant for 5 to 7 days before assessing urinary calcium.

Since the form or salt of calcium is not usually an important variable in the absorption of calcium, any salt may be used for therapy. Table 12-10 analyzes some of the available preparations and the percentage of the salt that is elemental calcium. Because calcium carbonate contains more calcium per unit weight than other salts of calcium do, however, a $CaCO_3$ pill can be smaller than a pill containing the same amount of calcium bound in another salt. Thus calcium supplements in the carbonate form are generally preferred. Although absorption of calcium does not seem to require gastric acid,[31] the carbonate salt will sometimes not be effectively absorbed in elderly patients and a more water-soluble form must be used.

Low-lactose diets often are used in treating the short bowel syndrome. This removes the most available source of calcium from the diet. In short bowel syndrome therefore calcium supplements should be considered routine treatment. At intakes of less than 300 to 400 mg/day, however, negative calcium balance also occurs because of losses from the intestinal tract; thus calcium supplements are needed not only to produce positive calcium balance but also to prevent endogenous calcium losses. If calcium absorption is 33% efficient and calcium requirement 300 to 400 mg/day, then the daily requirement for a normal intake is about 1000 mg. If malabsorption decreases calcium retention by 50%, intake may increase to 2000 mg/day. This is probably the maximum required by any individual.

Magnesium. Unlike calcium, magnesium is not secreted to a great extent into the intestinal tract, and thus low intake normally is not associated with net negative balance. However, absorption is not efficient (25% to 30%) and is affected adversely by many of the factors that decrease calcium absorption in the short bowel syndrome.[29] In addition, serum magnesium is not necessarily a good measure of body stores. When absorption is severely impaired, serum magnesium levels are low. In severe magnesium deficiency a sequence of events occurs that is very important to recognize when caring for a patient with calcium deficiency. In magnesium deficiency, secretion of parathormone is markedly impaired. This then leads to decreased absorption of calcium, because of the permissive action of parathyroid hormone, and it further decreases serum calcium because of the loss of parathyroid hormone's action on bone. The importance of these observations for therapy is obvious. When magnesium deficiency is severe, hypocalcemia often cannot be corrected until magnesium is replaced. This is done by administering parenteral magnesium, 8 mEq of elemental magnesium every 4-6 hours depending on clinical status and serum levels.

When magnesium deficiency is not severe but the short bowel syndrome is present and intestinal losses are thought to be excessive, oral magnesium supplementation often is needed. Magnesium oxide or sulfate is the salt used most often, but it is very insoluble and in any considerable dose it produces diarrhea. Oral replacement doses of the oxide range from 130 to 360 mg of elemental magnesium (250-600 mg of MgO) depending on need and bowel pattern.

Zinc. The factors that control zinc balance in humans are not well understood. However, the major losses occur through the intestinal tract. Urinary excretion varies little no matter what the state of overall zinc balance. Therefore zinc absorption and balance are regulated by zinc intake. About 1 to 2 mg per day is absorbed from an average intake of 15 mg. In addition to the normal replacement of 15 mg/day, some 17 mg of zinc should be added for every kilogram of stool or 12 mg for every kilogram of gastric or duodenal fluid lost per day.[33] Zinc can be replaced orally as the sulfate in doses of 15 or 50 mg of elemental zinc per tablet.

Massive Resection or Bypass

The chronic changes and therapy described for distal small bowel resection all apply to massive proximal resection or bypass. The use of low–available carbohydrate or low-lactose diets also may be necessary. Then the diet can become extremely restrictive in terms of the table foods that are low in fat as well as in carbohydrate. However, when most of the small bowel is resected or bypassed, there are acute changes that differ from the problems encountered chronically. The acute problems develop within the first few weeks or months after surgery and are the same for both resection and bypass. In addition, special problems associated with the bypassed intestine presumably are related to the retained blind loop of small intestine.

Postoperative problems. There are three major problem areas that require care after resection or bypass of most of the small bowel: fluid, electrolytes, and protein loss.[25]

The small bowel absorbs not only the 2 liters of dietary fluid but also the approximately 7 liters of internal secretions. The volume of these secretions declines when no food is eaten but is still sufficient to create a negative fluid balance when that fluid is malabsorbed. The colon has a capacity to absorb 1.5 to 2 liters under normal circumstances. When required, this can increase to about 4 liters/day. This adaptation is important in short bowel syndrome.

The most common electrolyte problems postoperatively are sodium and potassium deficiency. Losses of both ions increase linearly with stool volume. In the early postoperative period diarrhea is uniformly present and persists until colonic compensation develops. In this period sodium and potassium must be replaced, first intravenously, and then by mouth. The major sodium and potassium losses are associated with losses not only of chloride, but also of bicarbonate. Thus the anion used will depend on serum Cl^- and HCO_3^- determinations.

Under normal circumstances endogenous protein enters the intestinal lumen from gastric, pancreatic, and intestinal secretions. About 10% of the catabolism of plasma proteins also is accounted for by secretion into the intestine. The secreted proteins then are digested and reabsorbed in the small intestine. After resection or bypass, this recovery of luminal protein is lost; in addition, protein catabolism increases as expected postoperatively. Serum albumin levels fall rapidly from the usual half-life of 16-17 days, and albumin replacement often is required. With the use of parenteral nutrition, amino acids can be provided for endogenous synthesis of albumin and other proteins. Thus parenteral delivery of amino acids is preferable to the use of albumin alone in this setting, unless edema secondary to hypoalbuminemia is a clinical problem.

Jejunoileal bypass for obesity. In addition to the problems discussed for other types of bypass or resection, anemia and liver disease develop in jejunoileal bypass surgery patients.[34]

The anemia is multifactorial but usually is caused by iron or folic acid deficiency. The liver disease develops in the first 24 months after the operation and is not seen in small bowel resection alone. It is thought that bacterial overgrowth in the long blind loop left in situ produces toxins that affect the liver. Liver damage can vary from the nearly universal finding of fatty accumulation to mild periportal inflammation to cirrhosis and even death. The latter two complications are uncommon, occurring in only a small percentage of patients with clinical liver disease. The severity of the liver disease cannot be appreciated by standard liver function tests but must be assessed by periodic liver biopsy in the first 2 years. Therapy for progressive inflammation and fibrosis is limited to reversal of the bypass. Since jejunoileal bypass operations no longer should be performed (because of the high rate of metabolic complications), the early progression of liver disease is likely to become uncommon. It is not clear what the long-term course of liver disease will be in patients who already have undergone such a procedure. Most patients seem to maintain stable hepatic function many years after their bypass surgery.

Colonic Resection with Ileostomy

The major function of the colon is to absorb water and sodium. Therefore ileostomy patients need to maintain adequate intake of these nutrients. The small bowel is able to compensate to some extent, but the average ileostomate has an output of 0.5 to 1 liter/day. When added to insensible water loss, intake of fluid should be about 2 liters/day. During the summer or when perspiring rapidly, fluid intake should be even higher. Salt intake can be increased in the diet or added as tablets (0.5-1 g NaCl each). Sufficient supplements should be given to maintain normal serum sodium. Maintenance of normal circulating intravascular volume will help prevent the formation of renal stones. Obligatory sodium loss from ileostomies is about 30 to 40 mEq/day, or 700 to 900 mg, in 0.5 liter. If volume loss exceeds 0.5 liter/day, sodium loss will increase proportionately.

ALTERATION IN FIBER INTAKE
Dietary Fiber

Dietary fiber includes all complex polysaccharides and other polymers that escape digestion in the small intestine. These substances may be divided into three classes: cellulose, noncellulosic polysaccharides, and lignins. Noncellulosic polysaccharides are further divided into gums, mucilages, pectins, and hemicelluloses. Dietary fiber contains many food groups or classes, and within each group there can be much variation. Measurement of fiber content involves complicated methods, most of which have not yet been made widely available.[35] One of the more commonly used, crude fiber content, is not particularly accurate. With time, other methods will be applied more frequently. At present, crude fiber gives only an approximation of fiber content. Certain foods with relatively low crude fiber values (carrots, peaches, white bread), in fact, contain moderate amounts of dietary fiber. (See Table 12-11.)

Further complicating the use of fiber content of foods is the fact that such content is based on unprocessed foods. Freezing and drying, freezing alone, grinding, and washing can alter content. Thus different preparations of the same food contain differing amounts of fiber. These considerations (measurement and preparation) lead to the widely divergent statements about the foods allowed or not allowed in high- or low-fiber diets.

The two best-documented functions of fiber are to increase the stool weight and shorten the

Table 12-11 Fiber Content of Commonly Used Foods

Approximate Content (g/serving)	Representative Foods*
5	Bran-containing cereals, stewed prunes, grapes, baked beans, raspberries
4	Peas, broccoli, pears, apples, potato skins, canned fruit, fruit pies
2	Citrus fruits, root vegetables, peanut butter, strawberries, cherries, wheat and corn cereals
1	Melons, white bread, salad vegetables, rice cereals
<0.2	Milk, egg, meat, sugar, fats, strained juices

Based on information contained in Southgate DA, et al: J Hum Nutr 30:303-313, 1976, and McCance RA, Widdowson EM: McCance and Widdowson's The composition of foods, revised ed 4, New York, 1978, Elsevier/North Holland Inc.
*NOTE: This categorization is based on the fiber content per *usual serving* not on the fiber contained within 100 g of the food.

bowel transit time.[36] In addition, fiber may decrease intraluminal sigmoid pressure and its absorbent properties may play a role in human nutrition; but these latter two functions are incompletely understood.[37]

High-Fiber Diet

The high-fiber diet is used in treating diverticular disease or irritable bowel syndrome, when alternating diarrhea and constipation are the predominant symptoms. Although it is not clear whether total dietary fiber intake is low in patients with these disorders, supplemental fiber is helpful. This can be supplied either in the diet or as psyllium seed or bran in a dose of 1 teaspoon two or three times per day. Psyllium seed is rich in hemicellulose; bran is largely cellulose and hemicellulose.

A high-fiber diet emphasizes whole grain breads and cereals, fresh fruits, and fresh vegetables. The result using either approach should be production of a regular pattern of defecation with formed stools. Too much dietary fiber can cause too frequent bowel movements or distention (if colonic spasm leads to incomplete evacuation of the fiber). A high-fiber diet should not be used for the symptoms of constipation alone or for obstructing lesions. In such cases it will only lead to distention and more obstipation. However, when constipation is associated with abdominal pain and is considered a symptom of irritable bowel syndrome, a high-fiber diet is occasionally helpful.

Low-Fiber Diet

The major indications for a low-fiber diet are acute diarrheal states, preparation for air contrast enema or colonoscopy, and preparation for intestinal surgery. The diet reduces intake of grains, fruits, and vegetables. Fat intake is diminished because fats are absorbed with only 95% efficiency. When fat intake is large, dietary fat enters the colon in considerable amounts and helps to maintain a large colonic bacterial population and thus stool bulk. However, the commonly applied restriction for all fats is unnecessary. The major problem with the low-fiber diet is that it is often calorically inadequate. This is a disadvantage when nutrition is marginal. In these circumstances, the diet can be supplemented by one of a variety of preparations designed for enteral feedings (see Chapter 31). Al-

though it was previously thought that a low-fiber diet was helpful in treating irritable bowel syndrome or diverticular disease, more recent experience confirms that such an approach is not helpful. A high-fiber diet is indicated in managing the symptoms of those disorders.

Bland Diet

The ulcer or bland diet has been favored in the past for the treatment of peptic disease. Despite much controversy, however, there is little evidence to favor its use. Moreover, during any illness, maintaining adequate calorie intake is critical. All aspects of food intake, from chemical composition (fat, protein, carbohydrate) to food preparation (spices, cooking method), are important in making food palatable. No rigid rules regarding food preparation should be used, since the perception of what makes a diet attractive will vary widely among patients. If an individual patient finds fried or spicy foods distasteful, he should be allowed to avoid them. A well-balanced and palatable diet is the objective.

REFERENCES

1. Kinney JM, Elwyn DH: Protein metabolism and injury, Ann Rev Nutr **3**:433, 1983.
2. Baker JP, et al: Randomized trial of total parenteral nutrition of critically ill patients: metabolic effect of varying glucose-lipid ratios as the energy source, Gastroenterology **87**:56, 1984.
3. Fairbanks VF, et al: Tests for anemia: the Schilling test, Mayo Clin Proc **58**:541, 1983.
4. Alpers DH, Clouse RE, Stenson WF: Manual of nutritional therapeutics, ed 2, Boston, 1988, Little Brown & Co.
5. Fleischer D, Sivak MV Jr.: Endoscopic Nd:YAG laser therapy as palliation for esophagogastric cancer. Parameters affecting initial outcome, Gastroenterology **89**:827, 1985.
6. Ponsky JL, et al: Percutaneous approaches to enteral alimentation, Am J Surg **149**:102, 1985.
7. Pinker RM, et al: Metoclopramide: a review of its pharmacological properties and clinical use, Drugs **23**:81, 1976.
8. Fedorak RN, et al: Treatment of diabetic diarrhea with clonidine, Ann Intern Med **102**:187, 1985.
9. Malagelada JR: Physiological basis and clinical significance of gastric emptying disorders, Dig Dis Sci **24**:657, 1979.
10. Halverson JD: Micronutrient deficiencies after gastric bypass for morbid obesity, Am Surgeon **82**:594, 1986.
11. United States Department of Agriculture: Nutritive value of American foods in common units, USDA Publication 456, Washington DC, 1975, Government Printing Office.
12. Kauenitz N: Clinical uses of medium chain triglycerides, Drug Therapy **8**:91, 1978.
13. Sokol R, et al: Vitamin E deficiency with normal serum vitamin E concentrations in children with chronic cholestasis, N Engl J Med **30**:1209, 1984.
14. Regan PT, et al: Comparative effects of antacid, cimetidine,

and enteric coating on the therapeutic response to oral enzymes in severe pancreatic insufficiency, N Engl J Med **297**:856, 1977.

15. Cole SG, Kagnoff MG: Celiac disease, Ann Rev Nutr **5**:241, 1985.

16. Allergy recipes. American Dietetic Association, 630 N. Michigan Ave., Chicago, Ill, 60611.

17. Hjortland M: Low gluten diet with tested recipes, ed 6, Ann Arbor, 1973, University of Michigan Medical School.

18. Paige DM, Bayless TM, editors: Lactose digestion: clinical and nutritional implications, Baltimore, 1981, John Hopkins University Press.

19. Kolers JC, et al: Yogurt—an autodigesting source of lactase, N Engl J Med **310**:1, 1984.

20. Hardinge MR, et al: Carbohydrates in foods, J Am Diet Assoc **46**:197, 1965.

21. Anderson IH, et al: Incomplete absorption of the carbohydrate in all-purpose wheat flour, N Engl J Med **304**:891, 1981.

22. Hines JD, et al: The hematologic complications following partial gastrectomy: a study of 292 patients, Am J Med **43**:455, 1967.

23. Amaral DF, et al: Prospective hematologic evaluation of gastric exclusion surgery for morbid obesity, Ann Surg **201**:186, 1985.

24. Fiet H, et al: Peripheral neuropathy and starvation after gastric partitioning for morbid obesity, Ann Intern Med **96**:453, 1982.

25. Weser E: The management of patients after small bowel resection, Gastroenterology **71**:146, 1976.

26. Hofmann AF: The syndrome of ileal disease and the broken entrohepatic circulation: cholerrheic enteropathy, Gastroenterology **52**:752, 1967.

27. Hofmann AF, Poley JR: Cholestyramine treatment of diarrhea associated with ileal resection, N Engl J Med **281**:397, 1969.

28. Earnest DL: Enteric hyperoxaluria, Adv Intern Med **24**:407, 1979.

29. Nordin BEC, editor: Calcium, phosphate, and magnesium metabolism, New York, 1976, Churchill Livingstone, Inc.

30. Bo-Linn GW, et al: An evaluation of the importance of gastric acid secretion in the absorption of dietary calcium, J Clin Invest **73**:640, 1984.

31. Spencer H, Kramer L: The calcium requirement and factors causing calcium loss, Fed Proc **45**:2758, 1986.

32. Rude RK, Singer SF: Magnesium deficiency and excess, Ann Rev Med **32**:245, 1981.

33. Wolman SL, et al: Zinc in total parenteral nutrition: requirements and metabolic effects, Gastroenterology **76**:458, 1979.

34. Hocking MP, et al: Jejunoileal bypass for marked obesity: late follow-up on 100 cases, N Engl J Med **308**:995, 1983.

35. Southgate DA, et al: A guide to calculating intake of dietary fiber, J Hum Nutr **30**:303-313, 1976.

36. Kelsey JL: A review of research on effects of fiber intake in man, Am J Clin Nutr **31**:142, 1978.

37. Trowell H, et al, editors: Dietary fibre, fibre-depleted foods, and disease, New York, 1985, Academic Press Inc.

CHAPTER 13
Liver and Biliary System

Esteban Mezey

The liver plays a central role in the handling of nutrients, and diseases of the liver and biliary tract often are associated with malnutrition. Although the principal cause of nutritional deficiency is decreased intake, frequently also there are decreases in absorption and abnormalities in metabolism. Thus alcoholism, a common cause of decreased absorption and abnormal metabolism, may be implicated in both malnutrition and liver disease.

ALCOHOLISM
Dietary Intake and Nutritional Status

Poor dietary intake is a principal cause of malnutrition in alcoholism. Decreased dietary intake is due to the high caloric value of alcohol, epigastric discomfort resulting from gastritis, limited finances, and a disrupted meal schedule in association with a disorganized family and social life. Alcohol has 7 calories per gram; however, chronic alcohol intake does not result in the same weight gain as isocaloric amounts of carbohydrate. This apparent lower energy value of alcohol stems from (1) its adverse effects on the absorption and metabolism of nutrients and (2) the fact that when present in high concentrations a greater proportion of it is metabolized by the non–energy-producing microsomal system that metabolizes drugs.

A history of grossly substandard diets, consisting of less than one meal a day, occurs in two thirds of patients who have been drinking for at least 10 days prior to arrival at the hospital in search of help for their alcoholism.[1] The dietary intake of the alcoholic patient consists mostly of carbohydrate with inadequate amounts of protein and vitamins. During drinking sprees food intake is negligible. A history of weight loss is found in most patients, and almost invariably there is a weight gain following abstinence and the reinstatement of a normal diet.

In one study[2] the circulating levels of two or more water-soluble vitamins were reduced in half the alcoholic patients admitted to the hospital. Folic acid is the vitamin most commonly deficient, followed by thiamine, riboflavin, nicotinic acid, and pyridoxine. Fat-soluble vitamins usually are not deficient unless the patient has advanced liver disease. Clinical stigmas of vitamin B deficiency regularly are associated with low serum vitamin levels. Macrocytosis, megaloblastic changes, or macrocytic anemia is found frequently in association with low serum folate levels.

Peripheral neuropathy in most patients is associated with thiamine deficiency and in a few patients with low pyridoxine, nicotinic acid, or pantothenic acid levels. Beriberi heart disease, now very rare in the United States, is associated with severe thiamine deficiency. The Wernicke-Korsakoff syndrome (presbyophrenia) is a manifestation of thiamine deficiency only when the individual also has an abnormality of the enzyme transketolase, consisting of a decreased affinity of the enzyme for thiamine pyrophosphate.[3] In those patients thiamine deficiency results in a much lower transketolase activity than in individuals who have no abnormality of this enzyme.

Glossitis, chelitis, or atrophy of the lingual papillae is associated with low nicotinic acid or riboflavin levels. Pellagra is found in a few patients with low nicotinic levels. Decreases in serum phosphorus and in cations such as potassium, magnesium and zinc (located prinically in the intracellular compartment) are frequent. Phosphorus deficiency can contribute to mental confusion and muscle weakness. Potassium deficiency results in muscle weakness and cardiac arrythmias. Magnesium deficiency may be responsible for irritability and seizures. Zinc deficiency results in delayed wound healing but is unassociated with other clinical symptoms.

Digestion and Absorption

Alcoholics frequently have pancreatic dysfunction and abnormalities in intestinal absorption after heavy alcohol ingestion. The substances that have been found to be malabsorbed are D-xylose, thiamine, folic acid, and vitamin B_{12}.[4] A decreased intestinal transport of sodium and water may contribute to diarrhea. Mild steatorrhea, which is common, is caused by reduced pancreatic function (and lowered lipase output) rather than by reduced intestinal absorption of fat. The abnormalities of intestinal absorption and digestion are readily reversible after abstinence and the institution of a normal diet. Both ethanol and dietary deficiencies (e.g., of folic acid) are causes of intestinal malabsorption.[4] Ethanol has been demonstrated to inhibit active transport of low concentrations of folic acid and thiamine by intestinal loops[6]; however, this inhibition can be overcome by administering large concentrations of these vitamins, which then are absorbed by passive movement.

Metabolism

Abnormalities in the metabolism of proteins, carbohydrates, lipids, vitamins, and minerals occur in alcoholism. Acute alcohol intake inhibits albumin synthesis,[7] whereas chronic intake increases urinary losses of urea nitrogen.[8] Hypoglycemia occurs in patients who have been drinking heavily and not eating. The mechanism for alcohol-induced hypoglycemia is a combination of depletion of liver-glycogen stores, which occurs after 2 or 3 days of fasting, and an inhibition of hepatic gluconeogenesis.[9] Liver and plasma triglycerides rise after the ingestion of moderate amounts of alcohol. The principal cause of the hypertriglyceridemia is increased synthesis as well as decreased degradation of fatty acids by the liver, leading to increased triglyceride synthesis.[10] The hepatic accumulation of plasma triglycerides is greater when ethanol is ingested with a diet of high fat content. In patients with Type IV hyperlipidemia, elevations of plasma triglycerides are particularly high after moderate intake of alcohol and remain high for up to 36 hours following cessation.[11] However, moderate alcohol consumption is associated with elevations of high-density lipoprotein (HDL) cholesterol and depressions of low-density lipoprotein (LDL) cholesterol in fasting blood.[12] The increases in plasma HDL cholesterol following moderate ethanol ingestion may be related to an induction of microsomal enzymes, or to an inhibition of cholesterol degradation to bile acids, by the ethanol. Epidemiologic studies[12] show lower levels of HDL cholesterol in patients with a history of myocardial infarction than in matched control subjects. The increased HDL cholesterol in association with ethanol consumption may explain the lower risk of nonfatal myocardial infarction and death from coronary artery disease reported to occur with moderate drinking.

The ingestion of ethanol also has been shown to interfere with the metabolism of folic acid and pyridoxine. In the case of folic acid the alcohol causes a fall in serum 5-methyltetrahydrofolate (the circulating form of the acid) by decreasing the enterohepatic circulation of the ester and thereby increasing the hepatic uptake and storage of folate (in polyglutamate form), which decreases biliary folate secretion[13] and inhibits intestinal folate absorption. In the case of pyridoxine metabolism, acetaldehyde accelerates the degradation of pyridoxal-5-phosphate (the active form of pyridoxine) by displacing pyridoxal-5-phosphate from albumin and making it susceptible to degradation by membrane-bound alkaline phosphatase.[14]

Alcoholic patients with fatty infiltration of the liver have decreased hepatic concentrations of vitamins and hence are more susceptible to vitamin deficiencies when ingesting marginal diets. Best documented is a study[15] showing that folate deficiency is induced more readily in alcoholics than in nonalcoholics when a folate-deficient diet is administered. Increased losses of urinary urea nitrogen and intracellular cations (as occur in chronic alcoholics) probably represent an alcohol-induced increase in cellular catabolism.

Dietary Management

Acute alcoholism. Mild to moderate degrees of intoxication require no treatment. In the case of alcoholic stupor or unconsciousness, the administration of glucose is recommended even prior to obtaining the results of blood studies, since this will prevent brain damage in the event of hypoglycemic coma. In most cases hypoglycemia responds to the intravenous administration of 50 ml of 50% glucose, although sometimes more than one injection is necessary. Thereafter, a 10% glucose infusion should be continued until the alcohol is completely eliminated from the blood. The administration of glucagon is ineffective in treating hypoglycemia because of the depletion of hepatic glycogen stores in these patients. Thiamine, 100 mg intramuscularly, and other vitamins (e.g., Solu-B sterile) should be added to the glucose infusion to prevent precipitous severe avitaminosis.

Because acute alcoholics generally are overhydrated and unless there has been vomiting, diarrhea, and excessive diaphoresis, limited fluids should be given. Electrolyte deficiencies, particularly of potassium and magnesium, can be corrected by adding 80 mEq of potassium chloride per 1000 ml of intravenous fluid and by administering 2 ml of 50% magnesium sulfate intramuscularly. Hypophosphatemia, if severe and symptomatic, can be corrected by administering 15 to 25 mEq of monobasic potassium phosphate per 1000 calories of nutrient. Many drugs have been tried, with varied success, in attempts to accelerate the rate of disappearance of alcohol from the blood. Administering insulin with glucose for this purpose has proved ineffective. Fructose (levulose) may be effective when given in large doses (1-2 g/kg of body weight).

Alcoholic withdrawal. Acute alcohol withdrawal often is associated with anorexia, epigastric distress, and nausea. These symptoms are usually the result of gastritis and subside within 2 to 3 days. Patients with them generally do not tolerate a regular hospital diet but are able to ingest a full liquid diet (e.g., 1700 calories containing 72 g of protein, 24 g of fat, and 293 g of carbohydrate for the first 1-2 da following admission to the detoxification unit).

In treating delirium tremens, the most severe form of alcohol withdrawal, it has been customary to give large quantities of fluids and electrolytes under the assumption that such patients were dehydrated. However, some of these patients may be overhydrated rather than dehydrated. The present recommendation is to administer fluids and electrolytes based on the estimated daily requirement, taking into account the losses that occur as a result of diaphoresis, agitation, fever, vomiting, and diarrhea. The fluid should provide a minimum of 1000 ml normal saline, 1300 ml of 10% dextrose and water, and 4 g of potassium chloride. Excessive loss from fever and perspiration can be replaced

readily with hypotonic normal saline. In addition, patients should be given thiamine, a B complex vitamin preparation, and magnesium sulfate as described for the treatment of severe acute alcohol intoxication.

Following recovery from acute intoxication and withdrawal, placing the patient on a diet having a minimum of 2600 calories and 100 g of protein will result in a positive nitrogen balance and adequate weight gain. Vitamin deficiencies are corrected by daily oral supplements of 1 mg folic acid and one multivitamin tablet.

Specific vitamin deficiency syndromes. Megaloblastic anemia resulting from folic acid deficiency is treated with a single intramuscular injection of 5 mg folic acid followed by 1 mg of folic acid per day for 4 to 5 weeks. Alcoholic polyneuropathy is treated with oral thiamine 10-15 mg/day; the prognosis for full recovery is good only if treatment is initiated early. Wernicke-Korsakoff syndrome requires therapy with thiamine (100 mg intramuscularly followed by 10-15 mg/da orally); the response is complete recovery if the treatment is started early in the course of the disease. Beriberi heart disease is treated with thiamine (100 mg intramuscularly once a day for 1 week followed by 10-15 mg/da orally); a rapid dramatic improvement in cardiac function results. Pellagra is treated with nicotinic acid (nicotinamide) in doses of 50 to 100 mg/day and replacement of fluid and electrolytes; the response to therapy is dramatic, and the symptoms tend to disappear in 2 to 3 days.

Chronic alcoholism. The ideal overall therapy, nutritional or otherwise, for the alcoholic is abstinence. Since this goal rarely is accomplished, persons who continue to ingest excessive amounts of alcoholic beverages should be encouraged to maintain adequate nutrient intake. Such a combination will result in maintenance of body weight, but there is no evidence that adequate nutrient intake will prevent many of the major complications of alcoholism such as cirrhosis and pancreatitis. Daily supplementation of nutrient intake with therapeutic amounts of B complex vitamins and folic acid will prevent the symptoms of vitamin deficiencies found in alcoholism. As just mentioned, it appears that alcohol-produced decreases in absorption of vitamins such as folic acid and thiamine can be overcome by increasing the amounts of these vitamins, which then are absorbed by passive movement. A daily capsule that contains adequate therapeutic amounts of B complex vitamins as well as 1 mg of folic acid is suggested for alcoholic patients.

ACUTE HEPATITIS

Acute hepatitis is a self-limited inflammatory condition of the liver that can be caused by viruses, alcohol, drugs, and toxins. Nutritional deficits in patients with acute hepatitis, regardless of etiology, are principally the result of decreased oral intake because of anorexia, nausea, and epigastric discomfort. In addition, vomiting and diarrhea often contribute to fluid and electrolyte abnormalities. In most cases the nutritional deficits in acute hepatitis are not serious because of the self-limited duration of symptoms. Fasting hypoglycemia is an occasional finding in patients with acute hepatitis.[16] The hypoglycemia results from decreased hepatic glucose production owing to decreased hepatic glycogen stores, a failure of glycogen repletion after high carbohydrate intake, and diminished gluconeogenesis. In patients with fulminant hepatitis, hypoglycemia is common and often persistent, requiring large quantities of parenteral glucose for maintenance of blood glucose.

Dietary Management

The patient with acute hepatitis usually is able to continue dietary intake despite symptoms. Since anorexia and nausea usually are minimal in the morning, the patient should be encouraged to eat a large breakfast. Intake of a normal-calorie high-protein diet is recommended. Fat should not be restricted unless the patient is intolerant of its intake. Persistent nausea can be controlled with Benadryl (25 mg t.i.d.) without danger of central nervous system depression. Intravenous fluids and dextrose, and even enteric and intravenous hyperalimentation in the most extreme cases, may be necessary if the patient has persistent nausea and vomiting. A preparation of B complex vitamins should be added to the intravenous fluids in such cases. Vitamin K (15 mg i.m.) is indicated if the prothrombin time is prolonged; repeat administration of vitamin K is contraindicated, for, paradoxically, it may prolong the prothrombin time.[17]

CHRONIC LIVER DISEASE
Nutritional Status and Dietary Intake

Decreased dietary intake is a principal cause of malnutrition in both alcoholic and nonalcoholic patients with cirrhosis. In patients with alcoholic cirrhosis surveyed in the United States and Great Britain,[18] the total daily calorie intake was normal but alcohol contributed 52% to 63% of the calories while protein intake (50-56 g) contributed to 6% to 10% of the calories. Decreased caloric intake was found in 44% of nonalcoholic patients with cirrhosis in another survey in Great Britain.[19] Anthropometric measurements often show decreased arm muscle circumference and triceps skin fold thickness.* Anergy, demonstrated by failure to respond to skin test antigens, was found in 42% of cirrhotics.[20] Deficiencies of water-soluble vitamins, particularly of thiamine, folic acid, and pyridoxine, occur in 30% to 60% of patients with alcoholic cirrhosis. Also common are decreases in the circulating levels of fat-soluble vitamins: vitamin A and vitamin E were decreased, respectively, in 43% and 17% of patients with alcoholic liver disease, and 25-hydroxyvitamin D was decreased in 44% of patients with alcoholic cirrhosis.[21] In contrast to alcoholic patients, nonalcoholic patients rarely manifest deficiencies of most water-soluble vitamins. However, in one study,[17] leukocyte ascorbic acid levels and serum folate were decreased in 35% and 17% of nonalcoholic patients, respectively. The principal deficiency in patients with nonalcoholic liver disease is of fat-soluble vitamins. Plasma levels of vitamins A and E were low in 42% and 38%, respectively, of these patients.[17]

Digestion and Absorption

Steatorrhea is the only common manifestation of malabsorption in patients with cirrhosis. It occurs in about 40% of patients and is usually mild, not exceeding 10 g/day; however, in 10% of cases it exceeds 30 g/day.[22]

Causes of steatorrhea in liver disease include decreased concentrations of intraluminal bile acids, pancreatic insufficiency, alterations of small intestinal absorption, and treatment with drugs. A decreased concentration of intraluminal bile acids leading to decreased formation of micelles is the principal cause of steatorrhea in cirrhosis. The reduced synthesis, diminished bile acid pool, and decreased biliary excretion of bile

---

*Arm muscle circumference =

Mid-arm circumference − Triceps skinfold × Pi (π)

acids are responsible for the lower bile acid concentrations.[23]

In patients with chronic enterohepatic obstructive jaundice (primary biliary cirrhosis) there is a marked reduction in the biliary excretion of bile acids and, as a consequence, marked steatorrhea with associated decrease in the absorption of fat-soluble vitamins.[24] Clinical symptoms associated with the deficiency of the following fat-soluble vitamins are likely: night blindness caused by vitamin A deficiency; osteoporosis and osteomalacia in association with vitamin D deficiency; and ecchymoses, hematomas, or hemorrhage caused by vitamin K deficiency. Vitamin E deficiency also is common but has not been associated clearly with any clinical symptoms. Pancreatic exocrine insufficiency has been demonstrated by secretin/pancreozymin stimulation in a number of patients with cirrhosis; however, there has been a poor correlation between this finding and steatorrhea.[25]

A diminished intestinal absorption of long-chain fatty acids from a perfused micellar solution was demonstrated in one study.[26] This abnormality as well as an increased gastrointestinal loss of albumin found in some patients with cirrhosis is probably the result of increased lymphatic congestion in association with postsinusoidal obstruction to portal blood flow.

Drugs that can cause steatorrhea are neomycin and cholestyramine. The following changes produced by neomycin may be responsible for steatorrhea; direct toxicity to the mucosal cell of the intestine, inhibition of intraluminal hydrolysis of long-chain triglycerides, and precipitation of bile acids and fatty acids.[27] Steatorrhea caused by cholestyramine is the result of its action in binding bile acids in the lumen of the intestine, which may lead to deficiency of bile acids necessary for micelle formation.

Metabolism

Abnormalities in the metabolism of proteins, carbohydrates, lipids, vitamins, and minerals occur in liver disease and often have significant effects on the nutritional status of the patient and on his or her ability to recover from liver injury.

The basal metabolic requirement is normal in cirrhosis. However, the source of fuel is altered and there is a rapid development of the catabolic state after an overnight fast. The changes observed are a decrease in the percentage of cal-

ories derived from carbohydrate and an increase in the calories derived from fat (to values obtained in normal subjects only after a 36-72 hr fast). The percentage of calories derived from protein is not altered but remains high despite the marked depletion of muscle mass observed in many patients.[28] The most likely mechanism for these changes is a decrease in the availability of glucose, because of diminished glycogen stores, leading to an increased gluconeogenesis with increased lipolysis and fatty acid oxidation as a source of energy.

For most patients with liver disease, the protein required to maintain nitrogen balance is no different from that for normal individuals. Patients with cirrhosis are in nitrogen equilibrium or positive nitrogen balance on a protein intake of 35 to 50 g/day,[29] which is in the range of the minimum protein requirement for normal adults. A high protein intake therefore is not necessary to maintain a positive nitrogen balance in cirrhotic patients. Although estimates of total body nitrogen do not seem to be altered significantly in cirrhosis, there are profound alterations in the distribution of nitrogen between the liver and other organs and in intermediary nitrogen metabolism. An increased demand for nitrogen after liver injury drains nitrogen from other organs and leads to deficiencies in those other organs.

Increases in plasma glucagon and a decrease in the plasma insulin:glucagon ratio cause increased gluconeogenesis with the release of amino acids from muscle.[30] This altered distribution of amino acids may contribute to the muscle wasting commonly observed in patients with cirrhosis. The normal breakdown of tissue proteins leads to a release of amino acids into the bloodstream. The catabolism of many amino acids occurs in the liver whereas essential branched-chain amino acids (e.g., valine, leucine, isoleucine) and many of the nonessential ones are taken up preferentially by extrahepatic tissues. In chronic liver disease there is a tendency for an increase in plasma concentrations of the amino acids normally removed by the liver and a fall in those principally taken up by extrahepatic tissues. Therefore the most common amino acid pattern observed in chronic liver disease consists of rises in the aromatic amino acids tyrosine and phenylalanine and in glutamic acid, methionine, and sometimes cystine and a fall in the branched-chain amino acids (valine, leucine, isoleucine).[31,32] The elevated plasma amino acids appear in the urine in increasing quantities; however, these urinary losses are not great enough to alter nutritional requirements.

Excess nitrogen is released from amino acids by the liver as ammonia and enters the urea cycle, eventually to become incorporated into urea. In patients with liver disease there is a decreased synthesis of urea, with the resultant accumulation of ammonia.[33]

The amount of protein synthesized by the liver frequently is reduced in patients with liver disease, as manifested clinically by the decreases in circulating proteins (e.g., albumin) and clotting factors.

Glucose intolerance is found in 50% to 80% of patients with cirrhosis.[34] The principal cause appears to be insulin resistance. This is suggested by findings of inappropriately high plasma insulin levels in response to glucose administered either orally or intravenously, increased insulin response even when glucose tolerance is normal, and a diminished glucose response to injected insulin.[35] Elevated levels of free fatty acids, fasting growth hormone, and glucagon, as well as hepatic damage, may be causes for the insulin resistance. Hypokalemia, a frequent finding in cirrhosis, is a contributory cause for glucose intolerance in some cases.[36] The mechanism for the glucose intolerance associated with hypokalemia is not well understood.

The liver is the principal source of cholesterol, very low-density lipoproteins (VLDL), and high-density lipoproteins (HDL). Low-density lipoproteins (LDL) are not synthesized by the liver but are derived from VLDL, and this conversion requires lipoprotein lipase. Patients with cirrhosis commonly have increased levels of free fatty acids and triglycerides. These elevations occur in association with decreased post-heparin lipolytic activity and decreased removal of fatty acids.[37] In addition, the percentage of serum cholesterol that is esterified often is depressed, owing to low activity of the enzyme lecithin/cholesterol acyltransferase, which is synthesized in the liver and catalyzes cholesterol esterification.[38]

Abnormalities in the metabolism of thiamine, pyridoxine, vitamin A, and vitamin D occur in chronic liver disease. Patients with cirrhosis appear to have a defect in the phosphorylation of thiamine to its active form, thiamine pyrophos-

phate. Administering thiamine to thiamine-deficient alcoholics with cirrhosis increases blood thiamine levels but produces no significant change in red blood cell transketolase activity, which is dependent on thiamine pyrophosphate.[39] Improvement in red cell transketolase activity and in peripheral neuropathy after therapy coincides with an improvement in liver function.

Acceleration in the degradation of pyridoxal-5-phosphate, the active form of pyridoxine, has been observed in cirrhotic patients independent of alcoholism,[40] but the mechanism for this remains unknown.

Decreased plasma vitamin A and impaired dark adaptation in cirrhosis are in part attributable to decreased release of vitamin A from the liver resulting from the decreased synthesis of retinol-binding protein and prealbumin necessary for its transport.[41] Administering vitamin A raises the levels of the transport proteins and plasma vitamin A and increases dark adaptation in most patients. A few patients, however, who are unresponsive to vitamin A and are zinc deficient will respond to the administration of zinc sulfate with improved laboratory parameters and dark adaptation. Decreased plasma retinol-binding protein[42] or decreased retinal alcohol dehydrogenase activity,[43] both of which have been demonstrated in zinc-deficient animals, may account for the association between zinc deficiency and impaired dark adaptation.

Patients with cirrhosis have a slower conversion of vitamin D to 25-hydroxyvitamin D in the liver, since large doses of vitamin D are needed for prolonged periods to restore abnormal plasma 25-hydroxyvitamin D levels.[44] Also, despite correction of serum levels of 25-hydroxyvitamin D to normal, these patients continue to have osteoporosis, suggesting that factors other than the slow conversion of vitamin D to 25-hydroxyvitamin D play a role in the development of bone disease. A defect in the formation of 1,25-dihydroxyvitamin D in the kidney or a decreased responsiveness to the action of this vitamin may account for the progression of bone disease in cirrhosis.

Liver disease also is associated with changes in the body concentrations, and in some cases the hepatic concentrations, of many minerals. The most extensively studied well-known changes are in sodium and potassium. Deficiencies in calcium, phosphorus, magnesium, and trace minerals also are common. Total body sodium usually is increased in patients with cirrhosis and ascites principally because of increased tubular absorption of sodium by the kidney. In patients with cirrhosis and ascites most of the sodium filtered by the glomeruli is absorbed by the tubules, so urinary sodium concentration is less than 10 mEq/liter. The mechanisms responsible for this retention of sodium are the absence of a not-yet-characterized natriuretic factor, which normally blocks sodium absorption in the proximal tubule during salt overload, and the presence of secondary hyperaldosteronism.[45] The increased aldosterone levels appear to be due to stimulation of the adrenal cortex by angiotensin, which is formed from angiotensinogen by the action of renin. In the cirrhotic patient large amounts of renin are released by the juxtaglomerular apparatus of the kidney in response to renal redistribution of blood flow and decreased perfusion of the renal cortex.[46]

Water retention occurs in association with sodium retention, although there is also impairment of free water clearance secondary to an increase in circulating antidiuretic hormone. The serum sodium usually is decreased, despite the increases in total body sodium stemming from the increased water retention with expansion of the extracellular volume. Only rarely is low serum sodium indicative of total body sodium depletion. This may occur without fluid retention in cirrhotic patients who recently have lost sodium either by vomiting or by increased urinary excretion following diuretics.

Hypokalemia is a common manifestation in chronic liver disease. The causes include decreased dietary intake, increased gastrointestinal losses because of diarrhea or vomiting, and increased urinary losses from hyperaldosteronism or diuretics. Hypokalemia often is associated with alkalosis. Hypokalemic alkalosis frequently precipitates hepatic encephalopathy because it favors the conversion of ammonium ion (NH_4^+) to ammonia, thus facilitating its diffusion across the blood-brain barrier.

Calcium deficiency is secondary to vitamin D deficiency and/or deficient binding of calcium in the intestine because of excess fatty acids in steatorrhea following biliary obstruction. Phosphorus deficiency is found in alcoholism and cirrhosis as well as in children with the syndrome of encephalopathy and fatty degeneration of the viscera.[47] Poor dietary intake, malabsorption, and increased urinary excretion of phosphorus have been suggested as causes of the hypophosphatemia. Magnesium deficiency also is common in patients with alcoholism and cirrhosis.[48] The possible causes include poor diet, diuretic therapy, and hyperaldosteronism, since aldosterone has been demonstrated to increase urinary excretion of magnesium.[49] The liver is the principal organ of storage for trace minerals. Many trace minerals are constituents of enzyme systems or important for optimum activity of various enzymes. However, in most cases their physiologic function remains unknown.

Zinc deficiency is common in cirrhosis.[50] A close relationship between total serum zinc and albumin, but not globulin-bound zinc, has been found in cirrhotic patients, suggesting that a fall in serum zinc may follow a reduction in albumin concentration.[51] Zinc deficiency in cirrhosis has been attributed to increased urinary excretion. The decrease in albumin concentration and the loss of other available binding sites for zinc and proteins would render zinc more available for urinary excretion. Although parameters of zinc metabolism do not correlate with measures of hepatic dysfunction, improved liver function usually is accompanied by a return of serum zinc concentrations to normal.

Nutritional Management

Patients with chronic liver disease not complicated by fluid retention or encephalopathy are encouraged to ingest a balanced diet high in carbohydrate (at least 300 g/da), high in protein (75 g/da), but low in salt. If fluid retention (edema, ascites, or both) complicates the picture, salt intake is restricted to 1 g (500 mg Na^+/da). Fluid intake is limited (to 1000 ml/da) only if there is dilutional hyponatremia (Na^+ less than 130 mEq/liter), indicating retention of fluid in excess of sodium. Patients with hepatolenticular degeneration (Wilson's disease), primary biliary cirrhosis, or chronic active hepatitis with increased liver copper (which contributes to the pathogenesis of liver disease) are started on a low-copper diet. Foods rich in copper that should be avoided include shellfish, organ meats (liver, kidney, brain), nuts, dried peas and beans, mushrooms, prunes, raisins, and cocoa. In addition, patients with hemochromatosis are told to avoid ingesting iron capsules or medicines that contain iron.

The diets of patients with chronic liver disease are supplemented by a capsule of B complex vitamins and folic acid (1 mg once a day) if the patient's intake does not appear to be adequate or if there is evidence of vitamin deficiencies. Vitamin K (15 mg parenterally) may improve abnormal prolongation of the prothrombin time. In addition, patients with chronic cholestatic liver disease, such as primary biliary cirrhosis, require supplementation of vitamins A, D, and K. This can be accomplished by monthly intramuscular injections of 100,000 IU each of vitamins A and D and 15 mg of vitamin K.

Potassium deficiency is difficult to assess because serum potassium concentration is a poor reflection of total body potassium; but when the serum potassium level falls below 3.5 mEq/liter, the body potassium deficit is approximately 300 to 500 mEq. This can be replaced over a period of a few days with oral solutions of 10% potassium chloride, which provides 40 mEq of potassium per ounce. Hypomagnesemia, which occasionally is the cause of weakness and cramps in patients with cirrhosis, can be corrected readily by the intramuscular injection of 2 ml of 50% magnesium sulfate. In patients who are severely ill and cannot be fed orally, fluid, electrolytes, glucose, and B complex vitamins are administered intravenously. Parenteral administration of amino acids (7% Aminosyn or 8.5% Travasol) for 4 weeks to patients with alcoholic hepatitis has been reported[52] to decrease morbidity and mortality.

HEPATIC ENCEPHALOPATHY

Hepatic encephalopathy consists of nonspecific changes in consciousness, behavior, and neurologic status in patients with liver disease. It can be the result of decompensated chronic liver disease, acute fulminating hepatic failure in patients without prior evidence of liver disease, or a portal-caval shunt. Its exact etiology is unknown, but the most widely accepted mechanism is that nitrogenous breakdown products and ammonia produced by bacteria in the colon reach the systemic circulation and brain because of the damaged liver and portal-systemic shunt.

Elevations of ammonia are common in patients with encephalopathy, and decreases in levels after treatment often correlate with improvement of the encephalopathy. Furthermore, administration of ammonia or substances that give rise to it often precipitates encepalopathy, although the correlation is far from perfect. In fact, about 10% of patients with encephalopathy have normal arterial levels of ammonia. Of course, it is likely that blood ammonia does not reflect intracellular brain ammonia concentration.

It has been suggested[53] that plasma, and hence brain amino acids, may influence the pathogenesis of hepatic encephalopathy by producing changes in central neurotransmitters. Fisher et al.[54] found a correlation between the degree of hepatic encephalopathy and the molar ratios of branched-chain amino acids (valine, leucine, isoleucine) to the aromatic amino acids phenylalanine and tyrosine in dogs and humans. These amino acids compete for entry across the blood-brain barrier; hence a decrease in the plasma concentrations of branched-chain amino acids would cause increased entry and elevated brain concentrations of the aromatic amino acids, which are the precursors of central neurotransmitters. Decreased brain concentrations of the normal neurotransmitter norepinephrine and increased concentration of the false neurotransmitters (β-hydroxylated phenylethylamines, octopamine) have been demonstrated in experimental hepatic encephalopathy.[55] In patients, elevations of serum octopamine were found to be correlated with the degree of hepatic encephalopathy.[56]

Medical Management

The main aims in the treatment of hepatic encephalopathy are to decrease the concentrations of nitrogenous substances and bacteria in the large intestine. All dietary protein is discontinued, a laxative (e.g., magnesium sulfate) and an enema are given, and intravenous glucose is administered to prevent excessive endogenous protein breakdown.

Lactulose has replaced neomycin as the principal therapy for hepatic encephalopathy. It is a nonabsorbable synthetic disaccharide that, when administered in doses of 20 to 30 g three or four times a day, reduces blood ammonia and improves encephalopathy in over 80% of patients. Improvement can be expected in 24 to 48 hours after therapy starts. The mechanism of its action is not well defined, but its effectiveness is related to its ability to trap nitrogen in the stool and to decrease ammonia production.[57] Neomycin (3-4 g/da orally in divided doses) is the antibiotic of choice to decrease bacterial flora in the colon and is an alternative therapy for hepatic encephalopathy. The combination of lactulose and neomycin may be synergistic.

Potassium deficiency is corrected by administering oral solutions of 10% potassium chloride, which provides 40 mEq of potassium per ounce, or, if the patient is comatose, by adding 80 mEq of potassium chloride to 1000 ml of intravenous solution as long as urinary output is adequate. A good way to follow the conscious patient and evaluate the response to therapy is by daily determinations of the presence or absence of asterixis and the patient's ability to write his or her name clearly or to draw a figure such as a five-pointed star.

Recently, efforts have been made to treat hepatic encephalopathy while maintaining an adequate nitrogen balance. This has been attempted by administering special mixtures of amino acids to normalize plasma amino acids or by administering keto analogues of amino acids to offset both hyperammonemia and protein deficiency. Parenteral administration of mixtures of amino acids, high in branched-chain but low in aromatic amino acids, has resulted in normalization of plasma amino acids and improvement in hepatic encephalopathy in some patients.[58] This therapy is effective only when the amino acids are infused with dextrose as an energy source, however. Administration of keto analogues of the essential amino acids valine, leucine, isoleucine, methionine, and phenylalanine, caused an increase in the plasma concentrations of these amino acids, corresponding to the infused analogues, and an increase to normal levels in the ratio of essential to nonessential plasma amino acids. There was a delayed, but only slight, decrease in blood ammonia. Clinical improvement, as assessed by mental and psychologic studies, was obtained in 8 of the 11 patients studied.[59]

More recently, it has been demonstrated[60] that ornithine salts of branched-chain keto acids are more effective than calcium salts of branched-chain keto acids or branched-chain amino acids in improving hepatic encephalopathy. Ornithine administered in the beta-ketoglutarate form had a deleterious effect. L-Dopa has been used in the therapy of hepatic encephalopathy with the idea that it might replenish the normal neurotransmitters dopamine and norepinephrine and displace the false neurotransmitters that accumulate. Although a few patients awakened from hepatic coma after the administration of L-dopa, no efficacy has been demonstrated in another recent study.[61]

For the more chronic types of hepatic encephalopathy frequently seen after portalsystemic anastomosis, in which mental deterioration manifested by loss of memory, apathy, periods of confusion, and personality changes are the principal symptoms, continuous medical therapy with lactulose is indicated. Orally administered branched-chain amino acids are of potential benefit in patients with chronic encephalopathy, but more information is needed regarding indications for their use and their effectiveness. A change from an animal-protein to a vegetable-protein diet has been found to decrease hepatic encephalopathy in association with decreased arterial ammonia levels in some of these patients. The exact mechanism whereby vegetable protein is tolerated better than animal protein is unknown. However, vegetable protein contains smaller amounts of ammonia, methionine, and aromatic amino acids and also results in alterations of small intestinal and colonic bacterial flora.[62] The beneficial effects of a vegetable protein and lactulose on hepatic encephalopathy are additive.

BILIARY DISEASES
Diseases of the Gallbladder

The formation of stones in the gallbladder is the principal cause of diseases of this organ. However, the majority of patients with gallstones have no symptoms. It is estimated that about 10% of the population has gallstones. The incidence increases with age, and the prevalence is higher in women. The majority of gallstones are cholesterol stones. Cholesterol is completely insoluble in water and maintained in solution in the bile by its incorporation into a micelle formed by bile acids and phospholipids. Cholesterol precipitates as gallstones whenever it is in excess relative to the bile acids and phospholipids. This usually occurs because of an increase in the hepatic secretion of cholesterol, a decreased bile concentration of bile acids, or a combination of both factors.

Acute cholecystitis is usually the result of gallstone obstruction of the cystic duct. The patient presents with symptoms of abdominal pain, nausea, vomiting, and fever. Chronic cholecystitis probably is caused by transient obstruction of the cystic duct by stones and is not necessarily associated with an inflammatory reaction in the gallbladder. Its symptoms are intermittent short-lived attacks of abdominal pain often radiating to the back and associated with vomiting. Many of these patients with chronic cholecystitis complain of flatulence and intolerance to fats and other foods.

Dietary Management

The therapy for acute and chronic cholecystitis with cholelithiasis is surgical removal of the gallbladder. In patients with acute cholecystitis, all oral feeding is discontinued and the stomach is maintained empty by continuous nasogastric suction. Intravenous fluids and electrolytes are administered to correct deficiencies caused by lack of oral intake and vomiting. This therapy is continued until the symptoms subside or the patient undergoes surgery. In chronic cholecystitis there is no evidence that dietary changes, such as the institution of a low-fat diet, alter the clinical course. Trials have demonstrated, however, that oral administration of chenodeoxycholic[63] or ursodeoxycholic[64] acid over a prolonged period can dissolve cholesterol gallstones. The mechanism of action of these bile acids is an increase in the bile acid pool coupled with a decrease in the cholesterol content of bile because of the inhibition of hydroxymethylglutaryl-CoA reductase (a rate-limiting enzyme in the hepatic synthesis of cholesterol). The bile acids are administered in daily doses of 12-15 mg/kg of chenodeoxycholic or 8-10 mg/kg of ursodeoxycholic acid. In one study[63] chenodeoxycholic acid therapy for 2 years produced complete or partial dissolution of stones in 41% of patients. Dissolution occcured more frequently in women, thin patients, and patients with floating gallstones. Medical therapy for gallstones should be reserved for patients who are without symptoms or have only mild symptoms and are poor operative risks because of their age or physical condition.

BILIARY OBSTRUCTION

The most common causes of biliary obstruction are gallstones, strictures, and neoplasms originating in the biliary tree or pancreas. Regardless of its cause, the principal nutritional consequence of biliary obstruction is related to the decrease in bile acids reaching the intestinal lumen. This leads to decreased formation of micelles and hence to malabsorption of fat and fat-soluble vitamins. Diarrhea often results from the action of excess unabsorbed fatty acids in stimulating water secretion upon reaching the colon. In addition, the excess fatty acids bind calcium and form insoluble salts, preventing calcium absorption and contributing to calcium deficiency caused by a lack of vitamin D.

Dietary Management

Little dietary management is necessary for biliary obstruction of short duration that can be remedied by surgery, other than replacement of fluid and electrolytes. Prolonged prothrombin time due to vitamin K deficiency is frequent and can be corrected readily by administering 15 mg of vitamin K intramuscularly prior to surgery. For patients with chronic biliary obstruction that cannot be remedied by surgery (i.e., with extensive strictures of the biliary tree) a diet low in fat should be prescribed, because this reduces troublesome steatorrhea and diarrhea if present. To maintain adequate caloric intake, the diet can be supplemented with medium-chain triglycerides. These contain fatty acids of chain length from 6 to 12 carbon atoms. Unlike triglycerides of longer chain length, which are present in a regular diet, medium-chain triglycerides are hydrolyzed rapidly and absorbed in the absence of bile acids via the portal vein.[65] The medium-chain triglycerides can be administered as Portagen (Mead Johnson), which provides 30 calories (protein, 1.4 g; fat, 1 g; carbohydrate, 3.4 g) per fluid ounce when the powder is reconstituted in water. A total of 16 ounces per day, given in four equal doses of 4 ounces with meals, provides an extra 480 calories/day. Medium-chain triglycerides also can be ingested in the form of oil (15 ml provides 115 calories), which can be added to salads or incorporated in sauces used for cooking fish or meats. These patients also require parenteral supplementation of vitamins A, D, and K. This can be accomplished by monthly intramuscular injections of 100,000 IU each of vitamins A and D and 15 mg of vitamin K. Deficiencies of calcium, which is malabsorbed because of its binding by fatty acids in the intestine, and vitamin D are supplemented by oral calcium gluconate (1 g t.i.d.).

REFERENCES

1. Mezey E, Faillace LA: Metabolic impairment and recovery time in acute ethanol intoxication, J Nerv Ment Dis **153**:445-452, 1971.
2. Leevy CM, et al: B-complex vitamins in liver disease of the alcoholic, Am J Clin Nutr **16**:339-346, 1965.
3. Blass JP, Gibson GE: Abnormality of a thiamine-requiring enzyme in patients with Wernicke-Korsakoff syndrome, N Engl J Med **297**:1367-1370, 1977.
4. Mezey E: Intestinal function in chronic alcoholism, Ann NY Acad Sci **252**:215-247, 1975.
5. Halsted CH, et al: Intestinal absorption in folate-deficient alcoholics, Gastroenterology **64**:526-532, 1973.
6. Hoyumpa AM Jr, et al: Thiamine transport across the rat intestine: effect of ethanol, J Lab Clin Med **86**:803-816, 1975.
7. Rothschild MA, et al: Alcohol, amino acids, and albumin synthesis, Gastroenterology **67**:1200-1213, 1974.
8. McDonald JT, Margen S: Wine versus ethanol in human nutrition. I. Nitrogen and calorie balance, Am J Clin Nutr **29**:1093-1103, 1976.
9. Freinkel N, et al: Alcohol hypoglycemia. I. Carbohydrate metabolism of patients with clinical alcohol hypoglycemia and the experimental reproduction of the syndrome with pure ethanol, J Clin Invest **42**:1112-1133, 1963.
10. Lieber CS, Spritz N: Effects of prolonged ethanol intake in man: role of dietary, adipose, and endogenously synthesized fatty acids in the pathogenesis of alcoholic fatty liver, J Clin Invest **45**:1400-1411, 1966.
11. Ginsberg H, et al: Moderate ethanol ingestion and plasma triglyceride levels: a study of normal and hypertriglyceridemic persons, Ann Intern Med **80**:143-149, 1974.
12. Moore RD, Pearson TA: Moderate alcohol consumption and coronary heart disease: a review, Medicine **65**:242-267, 1986.
13. Hillman RS, et al: Alcohol interference with the folate enterohepatic cycle, Trans Assoc Am Physicians **90**:145-156, 1977.
14. Lumeng L, Li TK: Vitamin B₆ metabolism in chronic alcohol abuse: pyridoxal phosphate levels in plasma and the effects of acetaldehyde on pyridoxal phosphate synthesis and degradation in human erythrocytes, J Clin Invest **53**:693-704, 1974.
15. Eichner ER, et al: Folate balance in dietary induced megaloblastic anemia, N Engl J Med **284**:933-938, 1971.
16. Felig P, et al: Glucose homeostasis in viral hepatitis, N Engl J Med **283**:1436-1440, 1970.
17. Weiner M, Farhangi M: The response of hypoprothrombinemia in cirrhosis to vitamin K₁ and K₃, Am J Med Sci **242**:207-210, 1961.
18. Mezey E: Nutritional state in liver disease. Assessment, incidence, and mechanisms of malnutrition. In Holm E, Kasper H, editors: Metabolism and nutrition in liver disease, Lancaster, England, 1984, MTP Press Ltd, pp 5-15.
19. Morgan AG, et al: Nutrition in cryptogenic cirrhosis and chronic aggressive hepatitis, Gut **17**:113-118, 1976.
20. Mills PR, et al: Assessment of nutritional states and *in vivo* immune responses in alcoholic liver disease, Am J Clin Nutr **38**:849-859, 1983.
21. Posner DB, et al: Effective 25-hydroxylation of vitamin D₂ in alcoholic cirrhosis, Gastroenterology **74**:866-870, 1978.
22. Linscheer WG: Malabsorption in cirrhosis, Am J Clin Nutr **23**:488-492, 1970.
23. Badley BWD, et al: Diminished micellar phase lipid in patients with chronic nonalcoholic liver disease and steatorrhea, Gastroenterology **58**:781-789, 1970.
24. Atkinson M, et al: Malabsorption and bone disease in prolonged obstructive jaundice, Q J Med **25**:299-312, 1956.
25. Baraona E, et al: Absorptive function of the small intestine in liver cirrhosis, Am J Dig Dis **7**:318-330, 1962.
26. Malgelada JR, et al: Impaired absorption of micellar long chain fatty acid in patients with alcoholic cirrhosis, Am J Dig Dis **19**:1016-1020, 1974.
27. Thompson GR, et al: Actions of neomycin on the intraluminal phase of lipid absorption, J Clin Invest **50**:319-323, 1971.
28. Owen OA, et al: Nature and quantity of fuels consumed in patients with alcoholic cirrhosis, J Clin Invest **72**:1821-1832, 1983.
29. Gabuzda GJ, Shear L: Metabolism of dietary protein in hepatic cirrhosis, Am J Clin Nutr **23**:479-487, 1970.
30. Soeters PB, Fischer JE: Insulin, glucagon, amino acid imbalance, and hepatic encephalopathy, Lancet **2**:880-882, 1976.
31. Zinneman HH, et al: Plasma and urinary amino acids in Laennec's cirrhosis, Am J Dig Dis **14**:118-126, 1969.
32. Rosen HM, et al: Plasma amino acid patterns in hepatic encephalopathy of differing etiology, Gastroenterology **72**:483-487, 1977.
33. Rudman D, et al: Maximal rates of excretion and synthesis of urea in normal and cirrhotic subjects, J Clin Invest **52**:2241-2249, 1973.
34. Megyesi C, et al: Glucose intolerance and diabetes in chronic liver disease, Lancet **2**:1051-1055, 1967.
35. Collins JR, et al: Glucose intolerance and insulin resistance in patients with liver disease. II. A study of etiologic factors and evaluation of insulin actions, Arch Intern Med **126**:608-614, 1970.
36. Conn HO: Cirrhosis and diabetes. IV. Effect of potassium chloride administration on glucose and insulin metabolism, Am J Med Sci **259**:394-404, 1970.
37. Swartz MC, et al: Fat transport in cirrhosis, Am J Med Sci **252**:701-708, 1966.
38. Simon JB, et al: Serum cholesterol esterification in human liver disease: role of lecithin-cholesterol acyltransferase and cholesterol ester hydrolase, Gastroenterology **66**:539-547, 1974.
39. Fennelly J, et al: Red blood cell–transketolase activity in

malnourished alcoholics with cirrhosis, Am J Clin Nutr **20**:946-949, 1967.

40. Mitchell D, et al: Abnormal regulation of plasma pyridoxal 5-phosphate in patients with liver disease, Gastroenterology **71**:1043-1049, 1976.

41. Russell RM, et al: Vitamin A reversal of abnormal dark adaptation in cirrhosis, Ann Intern Med **88**:622-626, 1978.

42. Smith JE, et al: The effect of zinc deficiency on the metabolism of retinol binding protein in the rat, J Lab Clin Med **84**:692-697, 1974.

43. Huber AM, Gershoff SN: Effects of zinc deficiency on the oxidation of retinol and ethanol in rats, J Nutr **105**:1486-1490, 1975.

44. Skinner RK, et al: 25-hydroxylation of vitamin D in primary biliary cirrhosis, Lancet **1**:720-721, 1977.

45. Epstein M: The sodium retention in cirrhosis. A reappraisal, Hepatology **6**:312-315, 1986.

46. Schroeder ET, et al: Plasma renin level in hepatic cirrhosis, Am J Med **49**:186-191, 1970.

47. Keating JP, et al: Hypophosphatemia in Reye's syndrome, Lancet **2**:39-40, 1975.

48. Lim P, Jacobs E: Magnesium deficiency in liver cirrhosis, Q J Med **41**:291-300, 1972.

49. Mader IJ, Iseri LT: Spontaneous hypopotassemia, hypomagnesemia, alkalosis, and tetany due to hypersecretion of cortisone-like mineralo-corticoids, Am J Med **19**:976-988, 1955.

50. Boyett JD, Sullivan JF: Zinc and collagen content of cirrhotic liver, Am J Dig Dis **15**:797-802, 1970.

51. Boyett JD, Sullivan JF: Distribution of protein-bound zinc in normal and cirrhotic serum, Metabolism **19**:148-157, 1970.

52. Nasrallah SM, Galambos JT: Amino acid therapy in alcoholic hepatitis, Lancet **2**:1276-1277, 1980.

53. Fischer JE, et al: The role of plasma amino acids in hepatic encephalopathy, Surgery **78**:276-290, 1975.

54. Fischer JE, et al: The effect of normalization of plasma amino acids on hepatic encephalopathy in man, Surgery **80**:77-91, 1976.

55. Fischer JE, Baldessarini RJ: False neurotransmitters and hepatic failure, Lancet **2**:75-79, 1971.

56. Manghani KK, et al: Urinary and serum octopamine in patients with portal-systemic encephalopathy, Lancet **2**:943-946, 1975.

57. Weber FL Jr: The effect of lactulose on urea metabolism and nitrogen excretion in cirrhotic patients, Gastroenterology **77**:518-523, 1979.

58. Fischer JE: Branched-chain amino acids in hepatic encephalopathy: results of parenteral trials. In Holm E, Kasper H, editors: Metabolism and nutrition in liver disease, Lancaster, England, 1984, MTP Press Ltd, pp 259-273.

59. Maddrey WC, et al: Effects of keto analogues of essential amino acids on portal systemic encephalopathy, Gastroenterology **71**:190-195, 1976.

60. Herlong HF, et al: The use of ornithine salts of branched-chain ketoacids in portal-systemic encephalopathy, Ann Intern Med **93**:545-550, 1980.

61. Michel H, et al: Treatment of cirrhotic hepatic encephalopathy with L-dopa: a controlled trial, Gastroenterology **79**:207-211, 1980.

62. DeBruijn KM, et al: Effect of dietary protein manipulations in subclinical portal-systemic encephalopathy, Gut **24**:53-60, 1983.

63. Schoenfield LS, Lachin JL: The steering committee and the National Gallstone Study Group: Chenodiol (chenodeoxycholic acid) for dissolution of gallstones: a controlled trial of efficacy and safety, Ann Intern Med **95**:257-282, 983.

64. Maton PN, et al: Ursodeoxycholic acid treatment of gallstones, Lancet **2**:1297-1301, 1977.

65. Holt PR: Medium chain triglycerides. A useful adjunct in nutritional therapy, Gastroenterology **53**:961-966, 1967.

CHAPTER 14
Cardiovascular System

Roger Sherwin

Cardiovascular diseases account for almost half of all deaths in the United States, as shown in Table 14-1. Atherosclerosis and hypertension, either separately or in combination, are involved in most of these deaths and probably also in many of the deaths attributed to diabetes mellitus, which is not classified as a cardiovascular disease.

Diet influences the development of atherosclerosis through three separate pathways:[4] the blood lipids and their associated lipoproteins,[2] hypertension,[3] and obesity. Lipid disturbances and hypertension will be discussed in this chapter. The main discussion of obesity appears in Chapter 39.

The general relationships among diet, hypertension, lipid disturbances, obesity, and atherosclerosis with its complications are shown schematically in Fig. 14-1. To facilitate the development of a rational approach to overall nutritional management, the natural history of

Table 14-1 Estimated Major Causes of Death in the United States, 1985-86*

	Percent of Total	
Cardiovascular disease, diabetes, renal disease		50
Heart disease		37
Ischemic (coronary) heart disease	26	
Other heart disease	11	
Stroke		7
Other cardiovascular diseases		3
Diabetes and renal disease		3
Cancer		22
Other diseases		21
Accidents, suicide, homicide		7

Based on data from Monthly Vital Statistics Report, vol 35, DHHS Publ (PHS) 87-1120, Hyattsville Md, Dec 24, 1986, Public Health Service.
*Based on a 10% sample.

diet-related cardiovascular disease will be considered as a series of stages, beginning with lipid disturbances and/or hypertension and ending with death from one or more clinical endpoints. Atherosclerosis, particularly in the coronary arteries (coronary artery disease), is distinguished from its complications, particularly coronary heart disease, a term that will be used in this chapter to denote some detectable impairment of myocardial function.

The diet-related aspects of cardiovascular disease (Fig. 14-1) account for an increasing proportion of the observed morbidity and mortality. The incidence and mortality of rheumatic heart disease have fallen dramatically in the twentieth century, and more recently the pharmacologic treatment of high blood pressure has greatly reduced the burden of hypertensive heart disease. Improved survival of the hazards of early life has produced a significant change in the age structure of the population, with a larger proportion of middle-aged and elderly individuals at risk of hypertension and atherosclerotic disease. Superimposed on these changes has been the increased risk of coronary heart disease — the "epidemic" of heart attacks that has affected most Western developed countries, especially the United States, in this century.

The strongest evidence that the increase in coronary disease is real rather than artificial is the change in the ratio of male to female deaths from all types of heart disease since 1900 (Fig. 14-2). Although only slightly more deaths were attributed to heart disease in men than in women until 1920, a gradual and steady rise began in men thereafter. This increase in the ratio was accompanied by an absolute increase in the male death rate from all types of heart disease between 1920 and 1950. Whether there was an absolute increase in the death rate from coronary disease in women before 1950 is more difficult to establish because of altered classifications, diag-

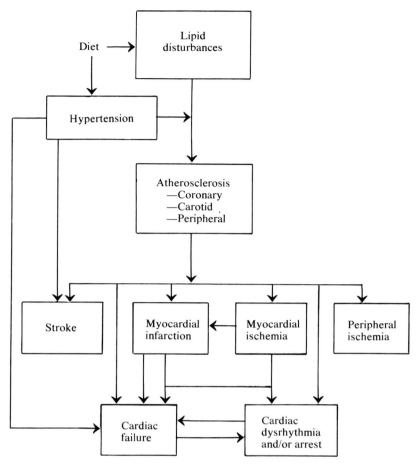

Figure 14-1 Causal relationships among diet, hypertension, lipid disturbances, atherosclerosis, and atherosclerotic complications.

nosis, and habits of certification. Data for coronary heart disease since 1950 suggest that the death rate increased in both men and women after 1950, reached a peak between 1963 and 1968, and then declined. The decline continues in the most recent provisional statistics for 1987.

Controversy about the etiology of atherosclerotic disorders and the "diet-heart hypothesis" is complicated by confusion over the exact question under discussion. The following lines of inquiry will be addressed in terms of the nutritional management and prevention of cardiovascular disease:

1. Why did an epidemic of coronary disease begin to affect American men in about 1920?

2. Why is the current rate of coronary heart disease higher in the United States than in many other countries?

3. Why has the U.S. death rate from coronary heart disease declined recently in American men and women?

4. What are the most promising approaches to preventing first heart attacks in the population at large, in hyperlipidemic individuals, and in individuals with other risk factors?

5. What is the most promising approach to preventing recurrent heart attacks?

It would be simple and intellectually satisfying to be able to answer each question in terms of a single etiologic factor, but the evidence does

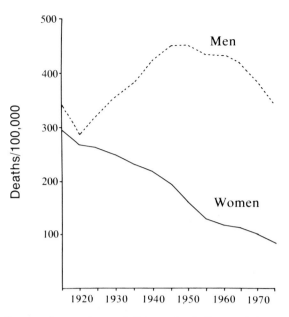

Figure 14-2 Deaths from cardiovascular-renal diseases (excluding stroke) among men and women aged 45-54 years.

HYPERTENSION

Elevation of the systolic and diastolic blood pressure is a major health problem in the United States and in many other countries. The prevalence of hypertension depends on its definition, and the division of individuals into normotensive and hypertensive groups involves an arbitrary decision. Furthermore, an individual's blood pressure varies substantially over time.

There are several possible approaches to defining elevated blood pressure. Prospective epidemiologic studies indicate an increasing risk of coronary disease and other complications from the lowest to the highest level of both diastolic and systolic blood pressure. There is thus no natural cutoff point in defining abnormal blood pressure, although risk begins to rise more steeply at a systolic of about 140 and a diastolic of about 90 mm Hg. Despite traditionally greater clinical interest in the diastolic blood pressure, the systolic is at least as good an indicator of prognosis, and in some instances a better one.

not support such an approach. The answer to each question may involve a different factor or combination of factors.

The clinical approach to defining hypertension has been to establish, by randomized clinical trials, the level of blood pressure above which drug therapy provides a net benefit in reducing the incidence of complications. The classic placebo-controlled study by the Veterans Administration[1,2] demonstrated a dramatic reduction in major complications within 1 year by treatment of "basal" diastolic pressure at levels above 114 mm Hg and substantial benefit within 3 years from treatment at levels above 104 mm Hg. The much larger Hypertension Detection and Follow-Up Program (HDFP) of the National Heart, Lung, and Blood Institute[3] showed a reduction in major complications over 5 years by the aggressive treatment ("Stepped Care") of diastolic pressures above 89 mm Hg, compared to the less consistent and less aggressive treatment prevailing in the community. The most recent and largest study of all, the Medical Research Council's trial in Britain,[4] generally confirmed the findings of the HDFP except that the benefit of treatment was confined to a reduction in cerebrovascular disease (as in most of the other trials). Existing data suggest that sustained diastolic pressures even lower than 90 mm Hg, especially in the young, should be considered abnormal and an indication for advice to control the dietary intake of sodium, energy, and alcohol and to prevent potassium and calcium deficiency in an effort to prevent or delay further elevation of the pressure and the need for drugs.

Nutritional and Other Etiologies

A number of definite causes of "secondary" hypertension have been isolated. These include renal arterial disease, renal parenchymal disease, aortic coarctation, adrenogenital syndrome, adrenal enzyme defects, primary aldosteronism, hyperdynamic circulation, and pheochromocytoma. Each of these conditions is rare; and even when taken together, they represent only a small fraction of the causes of hypertension.[5] Cases of secondary hypertension account for less than 6% of the total, and only a minority of these are curable by surgery. The remaining cases are considered "primary" or "essential" (with the exception of a small number whose etiology is related to oral contraceptives). Whereas essential hypertension is formally of unknown etiology, indirect evidence[6] suggests that several aspects of nutrition, especially the ingestion of excessive amounts of sodium, may be involved.

Sodium intake. Before the development of effective pharmacologic agents to lower blood pressure, it had been demonstrated[7] that drastic reductions in sodium intake lower the blood pressure in patients with essential hypertension. Populations eating less than 30 mEq (0.7 g) of sodium per day and about 200 mEq of potassium have virtually no hypertension and no rise in blood pressure with age. However, when members of such populations migrate and become acculturated within populations consuming more than 100 mEq (2 g) of sodium per day and prone to hypertension, they develop hypertension at a similar rate and their blood pressure increases with age. Experimental diets containing up to 1500 mEq of sodium per day produce a rise in blood pressure, and populations that consume more than 360 mEq daily have an unusually high incidence of both hypertension and stroke.

The sodium intake typical of most Western industrialized societies ranges from about 90 to 200 mEq/day (2-5 g). Within this range it has not been possible to demonstrate a correlation between salt intake and blood pressure levels,

which suggests that such intakes are sufficient to permit the development of hypertension in genetically susceptible individuals but not sufficient to induce it in genetically resistant individuals. Both chickens and rats can be made hypertensive by the addition of 1% to 2% sodium chloride to their drinking water. The hypertension induced in rats by deoxycorticosterone is enhanced by high-sodium diets and prevented by very low-sodium diets.

The physiologic requirement for sodium is small, and the usual intake appears to bear no relationship to need. Minimum daily losses are about 2 to 8 mEq. These are increased by sweating, and daily losses as high as 350 mEq of sodium have been observed during hard physical work in high ambient temperatures. Many nonindustrialized societies in regions as diverse as the Tropics and the Arctic subsist on less than 43 mEq of sodium per day without evidence of deprivation. Infants require no more than 9 mEq/day. The average daily sodium intake in the United States is clearly several times greater than the requirement.

Obesity. A second important nutritionally related etiologic factor in hypertension is obesity. The association between relative body weight and blood pressure also extends to the complications of hypertension. This implies that the rise in blood pressure associated with obesity is not a "benign" variety of hypertension to be distinguished from essential hypertension in the lean and treated less aggressively. The possible effect of an inappropriate cuff size for measuring blood pressure in obese patients has been excluded as a major cause of the observed association. It is estimated that up to half the cases of hypertension in the United States are attributable to excess adiposity. Recent studies demonstrate that weight loss results in a fall of blood pressure often great enough to return blood pressure levels to normal.

Alcohol consumption. A third nutritionally related factor in the etiology of hypertension is alcohol. The importance of this factor has been recognized only recently.[8] Individuals who habitually consume more than 60 g of absolute alcohol per day (equivalent to four mixed drinks, five 12 oz bottles of beer, or five glasses of wine) are approximately twice as likely to be hypertensive as those who consume less than 30 g/

day. The effect of alcohol persists after adjustment for other known risk factors. However, there is no evidence that moderate intakes of alcohol (up to about 30 g/da) have any adverse effects on blood pressure.

Potassium intake. A fourth possible nutritional factor in the etiology of hypertension is a low intake of potassium. Population comparisons are complicated by the fact that low average sodium intakes are usually associated with relatively high potassium intakes. However, potassium salts have been shown to ameliorate the pressor effects of salt loading, and the ratio of sodium to potassium may have important implications for the development of hypertension. The role of potassium in the homeostasis of blood pressure has recently been reviewed by Whelton and Klag.[9] Several studies have found a low intake of potassium in blacks, a factor that may contribute to their high incidence of hypertension.

Calcium intake. A fifth possible nutritional factor that has received recent attention in the etiology of hypertension is a low intake of calcium. This controversial issue was recently reviewed in detail by Villar et al.,[10] who concluded that there is some association between increased blood pressure and low intake of calcium and that blood pressure could be reduced by increasing the amount of dietary calcium. However, further work is necessary before the clinical implications of this relationship are clear.

Correlation. In summary, although the overall pathogenesis of essential hypertension is not completely understood, certain useful generalizations now can be made: some 10% to 20% of individuals, depending on race, appear to be genetically susceptible to hypertension when their sodium intake is in the range typical of the United States; this level of susceptibility is increased by obesity, a high intake of alcohol, and possibly a low intake of potassium and/or calcium.

Screening and Diagnosis

Blood pressure should be measured by a standardized technique, such as that recommended by the American Heart Association,[11] at routine "well care" pediatric visits both to exclude secondary hypertension and to determine the percentile level compared to a population of normal children. A "tracking" phenomenon of blood pressure is well established: persons at the upper end of the distribution in childhood are likely to remain so in their adult years and to be at increased risk for the development of hypertension throughout life. The routine measurement between ages 20 and 30 years is necessary only for those above the 90th percentile in childhood, but in the absence of such information at least one reading should be taken in the third decade. After age 30 years an annual reading is of value to reestablish the percentile level and provide an overview of the long-term trend. A continuous record of such readings is more useful than sporadic readings that are recorded and acted on only when they rise above some predetermined level.

In general, hypertension should not be diagnosed at a single visit; usually it involves determinations on several separate occasions. Such determinations should be made at intervals of several weeks because of day-to-day correlation of blood pressure levels in a given individual. The closer the average level of blood pressure is to the boundary for defining hypertension, the more determinations will be necessary to decide whether an individual's "true" level is above or below some predetermined boundary point. Investigation for underlying causes is no longer considered necessary for hypertension that appears first in middle life. A thorough physical examination—including hematocrit, urinalysis, serum urea nitrogen or creatinine, serum potassium, serum cholesterol, and an electrocardiogram—will provide the minimum information needed for diagnostic purposes (although other serum electrolyte levels may be required before prescribing certain drugs, especially diuretics). The onset of hypertension earlier than age 30 years and of newly developed diastolic hypertension later than 60 years may warrant more extensive investigation. The diagnostic workup for hypertension is discussed in more detail in the 1984 report of the Joint National Committee on Detection Evaluation and Treatment of High Blood Pressure.[12]

Dietary Management

The value of lowering diastolic blood pressure in the range of 90-104 mm Hg to reduce the risk of stroke has been demonstrated by both the Hypertension Detection and Follow-up Program[3] and the Medical Research Council trial in Britain.[4] Although full-scale investigations of "hygienic" (nonpharmacologic) care have not been completed, a comparable reduction in blood pressure achieved by removing etiologic factors rather than by instituting pharmacologic regimens should prevent complications to at least the same degree without the hazards and expense of the drugs. The etiologic roles of diet in hypertension and dietary management of the condition have been comprehensively reviewed by Cohen.[13]

Whereas drug treatment is necessary for persons with sustained levels of diastolic pressure at or above 105 mm Hg, the vast majority of individuals with newly identified hypertension will have diastolic pressures in the range of 90 to 104 mm Hg. Most will be overweight, and a high intake of alcohol will be common. Liver enlargement and/or an elevated serum gammaglutamyltranferase provide strong presumptive evidence of a high alcohol intake in an otherwise healthy person. It is not often possible to identify an unusually high intake of sodium, by either dietary history or urinary excretion. A program of "hygienic" measures should be instituted for all hypertensives, and the effects of these measures should be evaluated for at least 2 months before the initiation of drugs when the pretreatment diastolic blood pressure is below 105 mm Hg. The program consists of (1) restricting dietary sodium to no more than 70 mEq/day, (2) reducing excess body fat to achieve desirable body weight, (3) reducing excess alcohol intake, and (4) increasing dietary potassium to at least 100 mEq/day.

Sodium restriction. A sodium intake of 70 mEq/day corresponds to 1.6 g of sodium or 4.1 g of sodium chloride. It is important in a sodium-restricted diet to make clear whether the amount of sodium or the amount of sodium chloride is being specified. The use of milliequivalents for the specification avoids this potential for confusion. A diet containing 70 mEq of sodium per day proscribes all salt added at the table and certain high-salt foods. A small quantity of salt can be used in cooking, and such a diet made reasonably palatable for most individuals. Restriction of sodium to less than 50 mEq/day is incompatible with the use of salt in cooking and entails major restrictions in the choice of foods, with consequent inconvenience and lack of palatability for individuals accustomed to the higher

intakes characteristic of Western societies. Although diets extremely low in sodium will control even malignant hypertension, the present effectiveness of diuretics has made the use of such diets generally unnecessary in managing hypertension.

The natural sodium content of most foods of animal origin is relatively high but fairly constant. In a sodium-restricted diet, red meat (including organ meats), poultry, fish, eggs, milk, and cheese are used in measured amounts. Shellfish are particularly high in sodium. Fruits, most vegetables, cereals, sugars, oils, shortenings, and unsalted butter and margarine have negligible amounts. Salt is used in the preparation of many processed foods, as are other sodium compounds. The physician must be aware of the sodium content of certain drugs — antibiotics, sedatives, laxatives, cough medicines, and alkalizers. Guides to mild,[14] moderate (1.0 g),[15] and severe (0.5 g)[16] sodium-restricted diets are published by the American Heart Association. A compact but comprehensive list of the sodium content of foods and nonprescription drugs is published by the U.S. Department of Agriculture.[17] The sodium content of common foods is included in Appendix III of this manual.

Weight reduction. The determination of desirable body weight and the nutritional approach to weight loss are discussed in detail in Chapter 39. The possibility of avoiding lifelong medication is often a powerful incentive for success in weight reduction. Caloric limitation should be combined with a program of increased physical activity that can be safely and regularly incorporated into the individual's daily routine. Evidence suggests that increased physical activity leads to some lowering of blood pressure independent of its effect on body weight.

Alcohol restriction. The levels of alcohol intake likely to cause a significant elevation of blood pressure are those associated with "problem" drinking and tend to involve some degree of addiction. Although limiting alcohol intake to less than 45 g/day (three 1.5 oz mixed drinks) may be satisfactory in terms of blood pressure, it is often impractical for a problem drinker to achieve such a sustained major reduction short of total abstinence. For behavioral reasons it may be necessary to recommend abstinence, but it is not critical for the control of the hypertension per se.

Potassium increase. Increases in the usual dietary intake of potassium by hypertensives under controlled experimental conditions have generally resulted in only small reductions of systolic and diastolic blood pressure. The effect has been most notable among hypertensives consuming large amounts of sodium, among blacks, and among elderly persons.[9] Potassium intakes of about 60 mEq/day (2.3 g) should be increased to more than 100 mEq/day (3.9 g) as a hygienic measure, even in the absence of diuretic therapy. Nuts, vegetables, whole-grain cereals, fruits, and fruit juices are rich sources of potassium, and intakes of 100 mEq/day can be achieved readily without the use of potassium salts (as substitutes for table salt or baking powders or as medicinal preparations). Specific potassium supplements are often necessary when thiazide, thiazide derivative, and loop diuretics are used, but they are contraindicated with the potassium "sparing" diuretics spironolactone, triamterene, or amiloride.[18]

Blood pressure reduction below a level at which treatment is believed to be desirable (e.g., 90 mm Hg) will in itself provide considerable reinforcement for continuing these measures. If recommendations to reduce consumption of sodium, alcohol, and excess calories and to add potassium do not normalize the blood pressure, a drug regimen is necessary. The physician should, nevertheless, emphasize the value of these nonpharmacologic measures both in minimizing the dosage of drugs and in making later weaning from therapy a possibility.

Prevention

It is probably not practical, at least in the foreseeable future, to reduce the sodium content in the diet of most people to a level that would achieve a significant reduction in the incidence of hypertension. To do so would mean reducing the average intake of sodium to below 100 mEq/day, which would entail major changes of lifestyle and processing techniques. It seems more realistic to identify a subgroup at particular risk for the development of hypertension and to provide appropriate nutritional advice.

A promising approach is to obtain periodic measurements of blood pressure in childhood and early adult life. Most middle-aged hypertensives generally have had pressures above the 80th percentile since their youth. These individuals can be advised of the risk of hypertension and the measures likely to reduce that risk. Many such persons should be able to decrease their sodium intake to approximately 70 mEq/day, increase their potassium intake above 100 mEq/day, and avoid the caloric excess and diminished physical activity that lead to obesity. The additional hazards of acquiring a habit of high alcohol intake should also be emphasized.

LIPID DISTURBANCES

Although disturbances of the blood lipids and of the lipoproteins that transport them are not disturbances of the cardiovascular system per se, they nevertheless accelerate the atherosclerotic process and hence the clinical complications of that process. The term "disturbances" has been chosen instead of "disorders" or something else that would imply a limited number of discrete types of abnormality, because most atherosclerotic complications are associated with quantitative rather than qualitative abnormalities of lipid metabolism. The terms hyperlipidemia and hyperlipoproteinemia are also too limited, since they embrace only elevations of these substances; an unusually low level of high-density lipoprotein is considered to have clinical significance.

General Approach

Not only are qualitative definitions of most lipid disturbances difficult or impossible, the quantitative definitions of hypercholesterolemia and hypertriglyceridemia present serious problems. The traditional approach to defining normal ranges for the blood levels of various substances has been to determine the distribution of values in apparently healthy individuals and to designate those that fall within a certain range (e.g., the central 90% or 95%) as "normal" and those outside this range as "abnormal." However, about half (rather than 5%-10%) of American men are destined to die of atherosclerotic disease. Thus a major emphasis in this discussion will be on the actual lipid values rather than on assigning the values within a particular range to a "normal" or "abnormal" category. Obviously the clinician, at some point, must decide whether therapeutic advice or treatment is needed, but such a decision should not be made on the basis of only one dimension (e.g., serum cholesterol) or even on the overall lipid profile. Rather, several dimensions of the risk of atherosclerotic complications should be considered before therapeutic decisions are made.

Blood Lipids and Lipoproteins

The two main lipids in the blood are cholesterol and triglyceride. As lipids they are not soluble in aqueous solutions, such as blood, and must therefore be transported by other macromolecular complexes known as lipoproteins. Lipoproteins are composed of an outer surface of specific peptides (apoproteins) and polar lipids (unesterfied cholesterol and phospholipid) and an inner core of nonpolar lipids (cholesterol ester and triglyceride). The five major classes of lipoproteins are shown in Table 14-2.[19] The nomenclature from ultracentrifugation is now most commonly used (although ultracentrifugation is rarely necessary for clinical purposes). The density and the cholesterol:triglyceride ratio increase as the size of the particles and the overall percentage of fat decrease. Chylomicrons carry triglyceride almost exclusively, and high-density lipoprotein (HDL) carries cholesterol almost exclusively. In fasting serum very low-density lipoprotein (VLDL) is the principal vehicle for triglyceride, but it also carries smaller quantities of cholesterol. Low-density lipoprotein (LDL) is the principal vehicle for cholesterol, but it also carries small amounts of triglyceride. The order by which lipoproteins migrate on paper or agarose gel electrophoresis (origin, β, pre-β) differs from their order of density and size (chylomicrons, VLDL, LDL, HDL): the VLDL (pre-β) and LDL (β) are reversed. Only three of the lipoprotein classes (VLDL, LDL, and HDL) are normally present in fasting serum. Usually the levels of these fractions are denoted by the amount of cholesterol carried in each fraction. The sum of the cholesterol carried by VLDL, LDL, and HDL is the total cholesterol.

Measurement of lipids and lipoproteins. The most commonly measured, simplest, and best-documented lipid index of the risk of atherosclerosis is the total blood cholesterol. It can be determined from the serum or plasma without fasting, since cholesterol is influenced primarily by the cumulative effect of the diet over several weeks and very little by that over the few hours preceding measurement. The next most commonly measured (though not the next most important) lipid index is the triglyceride. Because triglyceride levels depend heavily on food intake in the preceding few hours, this measurement is useful only after fasting (preferably for 12 hr).

Recently the measurement of cholesterol carried by HDL has become both routine and inexpensive in many laboratories. The method involves precipitating all the other lipoproteins by heparin and manganese and then remeasuring the cholesterol. A fasting specimen is not essential if HDL alone (and not triglycerides) is to be measured.

The presence of chylomicrons can be detected simply by allowing plasma to stand for 18-24 hours at 0° to 4° C (without freezing). Chylomicrons rise to the top of the tube as a creamy layer. They are always abnormal in fasting serum

Table 14-2 Major Classes of Plasma Lipoproteins

Lipoprotein	Density	Diameter (mm)	Approximate Percentage of Total Mass		Approximate Cholesterol:Triglyceride Ratio	Electrophoretic Mobility on Paper or Agarose Gel
			Cholesterol Ester	Triglyceride		
Chylomicrons	<0.95	120-1100	5	85	1:17	Origin
Very low density (VLDL)	0.95-1.006	30-90	15	45	1:3	Pre-β
Intermediate density (IDL)	1.006-1.019	25-30	30	30	1:1	"Broad" β
Low density (LDL)	1.019-1.063	21-25	40	10	4:1	β
High density (HDL)	1.063-1.21	7-10	20	5	4:1	α

Adapted from Miller NE: J Clin Pathol **32:**639-650, 1979.

Table 14-3 World Health Organization Classification of Lipoprotein Abnormalities

	WHO Type					
	I	IIa	IIb	III	IV	V
Chylomicrons present	+					+
"Elevated" VLDL (pre β)			+		+	+
IDL ("floating" or "broad" β) present				+		
"Elevated" LDL (β)		+	+			

and indicate either Type I or Type V hyperlipoproteinemia. Elevated VLDL levels produce diffuse turbidity throughout the tube.

A combination of these procedures gives as much information as is required for general clinical purposes. Because the VLDL cholesterol can be estimated as 20% of the triglyceride (for levels of triglycerides <300 mg/dl), it is possible to estimate LDL cholesterol from the expression

Total cholesterol = HDL chol + VLDL chol + LDL chol

where *LDL chol* is the only unknown. This procedure has almost eliminated the need for the more expensive ultracentrifugation and/or electrophoresis in clinical practice.

Classification of hyperlipoproteinemias. The World Health Organization classification has provided a useful framework for the management and investigation of lipid abnormalities.[20,21] However, it has been misinterpreted as the definition of a set of discrete, predominantly genetic, abnormalities of lipid metabolism. As shown in Table 14-3, the system is both qualitative, in that it depends on the presence or absence of chylomicrons and intermediate-density lipoproteins (IDL), and quantitative with respect to LDL and VLDL.

When the system is applied, only a relatively small proportion of a population (e.g., that of the United States) is identified as abnormal. Types I, III, and V hyperlipoproteinemias, which depend on qualitative abnormalities, are each rare and the "abnormal" levels of LDL and VLDL may be defined as being above the 90th or 95th percentile. Hence less than 20% of the population is identified, even though some degree of hyperlipidemia (in relation to optimum levels) is probably involved in the atherosclerotic disease that eventually affects at least half of all Americans. A number of other weaknesses of

the system have been described[19]: the patterns are not unique to particular inborn errors of metabolism, different genetic defects producing the same lipoprotein pattern but through different mechanisms; conversely, the phenotypic pattern of a given genotype depends heavily on other factors such as body weight and dietary composition; the system also fails to embrace reductions in the concentration of lipoproteins or to take into account the concentration of HDL.

For these reasons and because the clinical manifestations (including the risk of atherosclerosis) depend largely on the particular lipoprotein affected rather than on the WHO type or the etiologic mechanism, the present discussion classifies hyperlipidemias in terms of elevations or reductions within each of the major lipoprotein classes.

Clinical consequences of dyslipoproteinemias. There are three important clinical reasons for concern about disturbances of the blood lipids.[22] First, elevated levels of certain lipids and lipoproteins are causally implicated in atherosclerotic disease of blood vessels supplying the heart, brain, viscera, and legs. Second, hyperlipidemia may be a cause of a variety of clinical problems other than atherosclerosis. Third, hyperlipidemia may indicate the presence of an underlying disease. These clinical consequences are summarized in Table 14-4. As the table demonstrates, clinical manifestations are characteristic of the individual lipoproteins involved rather than of either the WHO type or the causal mechanism.

The presence of chylomicrons is always abnormal in fasting serum and may be due to genetic factors or to other disease states. Abdominal pain is a frequent presenting symptom both in children (usually Type I) and in adults (usually Type V). Often accompanied by enlargement of

Table 14-4 Clinical Consequences of Dyslipoproteinemias

Lipoprotein	Level in Fasting Plasma	WHO Type	Early Clinical Manifestations	Effect on Risk of Atherosclerosis
Chylomicrons	Present	I or IV	Eruptive xanthomas Lipemia retinalis Hepatosplenomegaly Abdominal pain Acute pancreatitis	None
LDL (β)	High	IIa or IIb	Tendinous xanthomas Xanthelasma Arcus senilis	Positive
LDL (β)	Low or absent	—	Malabsorption Retinitis pigmentosa Acanthocytic red cells	Negative
IDL (broad β)	Present	III	Tuberous and planar xanthomas	Positive
VLDL (pre-β)	High	IV or IIb	—	None or weakly positive
HDL (α)	High	—	—	Negative
HDL (α)	Low	—	—	Positive
HDL (α)	Very low or absent	—	Discolored tonsils Splenomegaly Neuropathy	Uncertain

the liver and spleen, it leads in many cases to acute hemorrhagic pancreatitis. Chylomicronemia does not appear to be associated with any increased risk of atherosclerosis.

Increased LDL levels are the most important abnormality of lipoproteinemia in terms of cardiovascular disease. This is consistent with the well-documented relationship between total serum cholesterol (of which LDL cholesterol is the principal component) and atherosclerosis. Whereas average levels of LDL cholesterol in the U.S. population are associated with increased risk of atherosclerosis, only the much higher levels, usually resulting from a specific genetic abnormality, lead to the other obvious clinical manifestations such as tendinous xanthomas. The reduced level or complete absence of LDL found in certain rare genetic disorders may be associated with a variety of clinical findings, but the risk of atherosclerosis is lower than average. This observation is consistent with the view that LDL is the principal atherogenic lipoprotein.

Whereas IDL (broad-β) is also atherogenic, its accumulation in the blood (Type III hyperlipoproteinemia) is rare; it probably is the most homogeneous of the WHO types. Its characteristic clinical manifestation is tuberous xanthomas. The disorder leads to premature atherosclerosis, and patients may present first with angina rather than skin lesions.

Isolated elevations of VLDL (or triglyceride) are the least critical of the lipid disturbances. Most authorities do not attribute either direct clinical manifestations or accelerated atherosclerosis to elevations of triglycerides in the absence of chylomicronemia. Although high VLDL levels are undoubtedly associated with an increased risk of atherosclerosis and its complications, this now appears explainable by the inverse association between VLDL and HDL.[23]

HDL displacements have been studied in detail only recently and do not enter into the WHO classification. Levels of HDL above the average do not produce untoward clinical manifestations and are associated with below-average risk of atherosclerosis. Low levels of HDL are associated with a sharply increased risk of atherosclerosis but do not appear to produce other clinical manifestations. A rare condition characterized by extremely low levels of an abnormal form of HDL (or a complete absence of HDL) has been given the name Tangier disease. It generally presents with hyperplastic tonsils and adenoid tissue of a characteristic orange-red color. Two thirds of the patients have an enlarged spleen, and almost 50% have neuropathy. Corneal infiltration occurs in patients over 40 years of age. The number of known cases is not sufficient to determine whether the risk of atherosclerosis is increased.

Etiology of Lipid Disturbances

The principal determinants of blood lipid and lipoprotein levels are genetic endowment, composition of the diet, and the degree of adiposity. Other factors, including certain disease states, hormone and drug therapy, physical activity, and stress may be involved in some individuals.

Genetic factors. There do not appear to be many important systematic genetic differences in average lipid and lipoprotein levels among the major ethnic and racial groups. Within such groups, however (whose members tend to eat similar diets), most of the individual differences in lipids are genetically determined. This substantial variation is not explained by the presence or absence of known genes of major effect. Although several such genes have been identified (Table 14-5), the least rare of these (causing heterozygous familial hypercholesterolemia) affects only about one in 500 individuals. Some other genes of major effect are believed to exist, but rigorous genetic analysis is impossible when the only means of definition is an arbitrary cutoff point on a quantitative measurement (e.g., levels of cholesterol or triglyceride above the 95th percentile). In the vast majority of individuals the genetic influence on lipid levels accrues from the cumulative effect of genes at a number of loci, each exerting a relatively small effect. For this reason the distributions of lipid and lipoprotein levels among individuals within populations appear as smoothly unimodal curves (and not as the bimodal or multimodal curves that would result if the lipid levels were dependent on the presence or absence of a small number of genes of major effect).

Dietary composition. The second most important determinant of the serum lipid and lipoprotein levels is the kind of food eaten. Dietary factors account for most of the variation in lipid and lipoprotein levels among populations. This effect (illustrated in Fig. 14-3) can be seen in the distributions of serum cholesterol for individuals of Japanese ancestry living in Japan, Hawaii, and San Francisco.

Of the major dietary components that affect

Table 14-5 Genetic Dyslipoproteinemias with Defined Metabolic Defect

Dyslipoproteinemia	Lipoprotein Disturbance	Occurrence
Familial hypercholesterolemia (heterozygous)	High levels of LDL	Rare (about 1/500)
Familial hypercholesterolemia (homozygous)	Very high levels of LDL	Very rare
Familial lipoprotein lipase deficiency	Chylomicronemia	Very rare
Apoprotein CII deficiency	Chylomicronemia	Very rare
Abetalipoproteinemia	Absence of chylomicrons, LDL, IDL, VLDL	Very rare
Tangier disease	Low levels of abnormal HDL	Very rare
Familial lecithin/cholesterol acyltransferase (LCAT) deficiency	Discoidal HDL	
	Abnormal chylomicron and VLDL remnants	Very rare
	Lipoprotein X	

Table 14-6 Major Chronic Effects of Nutritional Factors on Lipoproteins in Fasting Serum

Lipoprotein or Lipid	Nutritional Factor			
	Saturated Fat	Polyunsaturated Fat	Dietary Cholesterol	Caloric Excess (Obesity)
VLDL cholesterol				+
LDL cholesterol	+	−	+	+
HDL cholesterol				−
Total cholesterol	+	−	+	+
Triglycerides				+

the lipids and lipoproteins (Table 14-6), the most important is saturated fat, which increases serum cholesterol. Monosaturated fat has little effect on serum cholesterol (although the substitution of monounsaturated fat for saturated fat will lower cholesterol). Polyunsaturated fat decreases serum cholesterol. Dietary cholesterol increases serum cholesterol levels in most individuals, but the effect is not linear. The first few hundred milligrams per day of dietary cholesterol causes a substantial increase in the serum cholesterol level although increments above the average U.S. intake (about 500 mg/da) cause little further increase. The overall average net effect of the dietary composition on the serum cholesterol (in mg/dl), assuming constant body weight, can be approximated as

$$2\,S - P + \sqrt{C}$$

where S is the percentage of calories from saturated fat, P the percentage of calories from polyunsaturated fat, and C the milligrams of dietary cholesterol per day. The square root function of dietary cholesterol approximates the nonlinear relationship. The average diet in the United States contains about 15% of calories from saturated fat, 6% of calories from polyunsaturated fat, and some 400 mg/day of cholesterol.[24] When these figures are substituted in the formula, the calculated increase in blood cholesterol comes to 44 mg/dl. This increase occurs almost entirely in LDL cholesterol (the primary atherogenic fraction). Thus the average American has an additional burden of about 44 mg/dl of LDL (and total) cholesterol superimposed on his or her genetically determined level by the composition of the U.S. diet. The response of individuals to any given dietary composition is not uniform, and sensitivity to dietary factors, especially dietary cholesterol, appears to vary considerably, probably as a result of genetic differences.

High habitual or episodic intakes of alcohol are known to increase triglyceride (and hence VLDL cholesterol) levels in certain persons. Although alcohol also tends to increase HDL levels, it is not yet clear whether such elevations reduce the risk of coronary disease. Those who drink moderately are at somewhat lower risk of coronary disease than are those who do not drink at all, but heavy drinkers are at greater risk than either of the other groups. The effects of alcohol intake on blood lipids and mortality from coronary heart disease have been reviewed in detail.[25]

Fiber (indigestible carbohydrate) influences serum lipids in humans, depending on its type. The most widely used source of total fiber, bran, has little or no effect on the serum cholesterol;

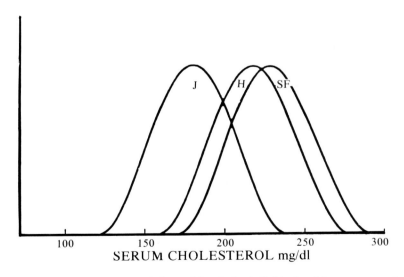

Figure 14-3 Distributions of serum cholesterol levels for individuals of Japanese ancestry living in *(J)* Japan, *(H)* Hawaii, and *(SF)* San Francisco.

Modified from Marmot NG, et al: Am J Epidemiol **102:**514-525, 1975.

but pectin, which is present in nuts and the peels of apples and pears, has been shown to lower serum cholesterol (though only at daily doses of 12 to 36 g, equivalent to 2.5 to 7.5 pounds of apples). Such intakes can be achieved by using the commercially available pectin powder with water or orange juice and swallowing rapidly before it has time to gel. Guar gum, which is obtained from the seeds of the cluster bean *(Cyanopsis psoralioides),* is also effective in lowering serum cholesterol; but again the required amounts (about 36 g/da) are not likely to be consumed naturally. Guar gum is available commercially as a powder and can be taken with water or orange juice. The specific effects on serum lipids of certain classes of fiber should be distinguished from the general association between diets high in fiber and low serum lipids; this association results primarily from the fact that diets high in fiber tend to be characterized by small amounts of saturated fat and cholesterol.

The influence of carbohydrates, both simple and complex, on serum lipid levels has been the subject of controversy. It now appears unlikely that either sugars or starches have any important long-term effect. Increased dietary carbohydrate does result in temporary elevation of triglyceride and VLDL cholesterol, but these measures return to baseline levels after several weeks despite continued high levels of dietary carbohydrate. Populations that consume up to 80% of calories as carbohydrates (and hence eat little fat) have characteristically low levels of lipids, obesity, and low rates of atherosclerosis.

No substantial effects in humans of adding different dietary proteins, minerals, vitamins, or lecithin to a normally balanced diet have been demonstrated convincingly. The one exception is niacin, which lowers serum cholesterol when given in doses 50 to 100 times greater than the nutritional requirement, but the side effects are often unacceptable.

Adiposity. In addition to the effect of dietary composition under conditions of caloric balance, the degree of adiposity has a major influence on the levels of individual lipoproteins and total triglycerides. However, because these influences are not all in the same direction, the net effect on the total serum cholesterol is less than that on some of the individual lipoproteins. Excess body fat characteristically increases triglyceride and VLDL cholesterol, but it also increases LDL cholesterol. The latter effect is more important because of the etiologic role of LDL cholesterol in atherosclerosis. Furthermore, adiposity decreases HDL cholesterol. Thus each of the effects of obesity on the individual lipoproteins is in a direction generally considered undesirable from the point of view of atherosclerotic risk. The effects of lipoproteins during periods of rapid weight gain or loss may be exaggerated and should be distinguished from the effect of a given degree of adiposity during periods of caloric balance.

Other factors affecting lipids and lipoproteins. The possible effects of certain diseases, hormones, and drugs on lipids and lipoproteins are summarized in Table 14-7. The effects on lipids of drugs used to treat hypertension are generally unfavorable and effects have been reviewed in detail.[26] Although the average effects on the individual are relatively small and hard to detect against the background of normal variation, they are of sufficient magnitude to cause concern when up to 40% of a population sample may meet the criteria for drug treatment of hypertension at some time in their lives.

Table 14-7 Disease States, Hormones, and Drugs Affecting Plasma Lipoproteins

Lipoprotein or Lipid	Diabetes Mellitus	Nephrotic Syndrome	Uremia	Hypothyroidism	Steroids	Thiazide Diuretics	Beta-blockers
Chylomicrons	+	+	+		+		
VLDL cholesterol	+	+	+	+	+	+	+
IDL cholesterol	+			+			
LDL cholesterol		+		+	+	+	
HDL cholesterol							−
Total cholesterol	+	+	+	+	+	+	
Triglycerides	+	+	+	+	+	+	

The recent widespread use of oral contraceptives and estrogen replacement therapy has shifted the lipoprotein patterns of women in the United States[23] (Fig. 14-4). Oral contraceptives increase the LDL cholesterol and decrease the HDL cholesterol—both unfavorable effects with respect to congenital heart disease (CHD). When estrogens are taken alone without the opposing effects of progesterone, the effects are reversed: estrogens decrease LDL cholesterol and increase HDL cholesterol—both favorable effects with respect to the risk of CHD. However, it must also be borne in mind that estrogens, whether taken in the form of oral contraceptives or alone, unfavorably affect the clotting system. Thus thromboembolic events are substantially more frequent in women taking oral contraceptives. The absence of consistent results in studies of the effect of unopposed estrogens on the risk of coronary heart disease probably reflects the varying dominance of these opposite effects.[27,28] In women who do not already have advanced coronary atherosclerosis, estrogens may help retard or prevent its development; but in women who do have advanced coronary atherosclerosis, estrogens may precipitate a thrombosis and consequent infarction, despite a long-term favorable effect on serum lipids and atherogenesis.

The influence of physical activity on serum lipids is hard to assess in view of the changes in body weight and body fat that are usually associated with any marked change in the level of habitual physical activity. However, high levels of aerobic exercise appear to increase the HDL cholesterol independently of changes in body fat.

Stress of various kinds has been associated

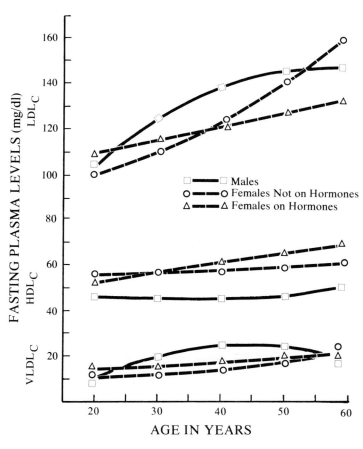

Figure 14-4 Mean plasma lipoprotein-cholesterol levels for American men and women.

Based on data from Heiss et al: Circulation **61**:302-315, 1980. (Reprinted by permission of the American Heart Association.)

with increased lipid values, but the lack of experimental data and adequate means to measure stress makes it difficult to draw firm conclusions, especially with respect to the levels of individual lipoproteins.

Screening and Diagnosis

Although there is general agreement that high levels of serum cholesterol and, in particular, LDL cholesterol are undesirable, there is lack of agreement as to how such levels should be defined, identified, and managed. At one extreme are scientists who believe that almost every American suffers from some degree of hyperlipidemia, that screening is neither necessary nor cost-effective, and that dietary change at a population level is the solution to the problem (the "public health" view). At the other extreme (the "clinical" view) are those who believe that only a minority of the population has any clinically significant lipid abnormality, that it is unnecessary (and possibly unsafe) to recommend dietary changes for all, and that persons specifically in need of dietary change should be identified by screening and treated accordingly. Various combinations of these views are expressed by many others.

The recommendation made here combines elements of both positions. Some decrease in the intake of saturated fat by the whole United States population appears to be desirable, not only because of the effect this would have on blood lipids but also because of favorable effects on obesity and possibly on the risk of certain cancers, notably of the colon and breast. However, the degree of dietary change that is likely for the whole population probably will not be sufficient to normalize the risk of individuals whose levels of total or LDL cholesterol are substantially above the average of the population. In view of the considerable potential for lowering the cholesterol level and the risk of atherosclerotic disease in these individuals by dietary and other means, effort should be made to identify those with high levels of serum cholesterol. The earlier in life that this can be achieved, the greater the potential for retarding, arresting, reversing, or, ideally, preventing the atherogenic effect of high levels of LDL cholesterol will be.

Total blood cholesterol should be determined on all children at least once before age 17 years. Initially, only a nonfasting cholesterol determination is necessary, in the absence of symptoms,

or a family history of hyperlipidemia with or without premature atherosclerotic disease. Further investigation should be undertaken only if the screening level of cholesterol exceeds 200 mg/dl, between the 90th and 95th percentile values for both boys and girls in the United States.[29] Because of the doubtful atherogenicity of triglycerides (as well as the usual lack of expression of familial hypertriglyceridemia in childhood), determination of triglycerides should not be undertaken routinely. The usefulness of the cholesterol determination is greatly increased by recording the value, together with the blood pressure and any other pertinent clinical information, on a card to be retained by the patient or the parents. This will avoid the need for future screening and will provide a valuable baseline against which to assess the clinical implications of future determinations.

If the childhood determination of serum cholesterol exceeds 200 mg/dl, it is useful to determine both the HDL cholesterol and the triglycerides (in the fasting state), and to examine for chylomicronemia. Estimates of the LDL and VLDL cholesterol then can be derived as described. Levels of LDL cholesterol above 150 mg/dl in this age group indicate seriously increased risk of future atherosclerosis and require further evaluation of the family for premature atherosclerotic disease and lipid abnormalities. The dietary management for such children is discussed in the next section.

Serum cholesterol should be remeasured at least once in males before the age of 30 years as part of a general assessment of atherosclerotic risk. At this time it is useful also to measure HDL cholesterol, but again routine measurement of triglycerides is not recommended. Both the total and the HDL cholesterol can be determined on a nonfasting specimen. Values of total cholesterol over 240 mg/dl (the approximate 90th percentile) are an indication for repeat determinations, including triglycerides in the fasting state, with examination of a standing specimen for chylomicronemia. Estimates of the LDL and VLDL cholesterol levels are derived as before. The frequency and content of future lipid determinations in males depend on the overall risk of atherosclerosis, the specific dietary measures introduced, or the diagnosis of hypertension.

Total nonfasting cholesterol should be determined in females before oral contraceptives are prescribed, and high levels should constitute a relative contraindication. Total cholesterol should be remeasured after about 1 year's use of oral contraceptives. It should also be measured when there are other risk factors for atherosclerosis (e.g., family history, hypertension, diabetes, heavy cigarette smoking) or before the planned introduction of long-term estrogen therapy. Hyperlipidemia, especially in combination with other major risk factors, may indicate existing coronary artery disease. Although unopposed estrogens have a favorable effect on the lipid profile, they may be hazardous in the presence of existing coronary artery disease because of the increased risk of thromboembolic events. Such risk was observed in a trial of estrogen therapy in men who had suffered a previous myocardial infarction.[30]

Dietary Management
General Approach

The reduction of elevated lipids by diet has been simplified in recent years. Most authorities no longer support the notion that different diets are necessary for each of the common types of hyperlipidemia. Apart from the rare cases of chylomicronemia (for which minimum levels of fat are indicated), the general dietary approach to hyperlipidemia is the same for the various types. However, the aggressiveness with which the approach is applied depends on both the degree of elevation and the lipoprotein(s) involved. Except in chylomicronemia, the primary objective of dietary management is to reduce elevated levels of LDL cholesterol. Elevated levels of triglyceride and VLDL cholesterol are no longer believed to contribute significantly to increased risk of atherosclerosis.

The principles of the dietary management of hyperlipidemia are inherent in the dietary etiology already discussed. The LDL cholesterol is increased by dietary saturated fat and cholesterol and reduced by polyunsaturated fat. Excess body fat tends to increase both the triglycerides and the VLDL and LDL cholesterol. The typical American diet promotes hypercholesterolemia directly, because of large amounts of saturated fat and cholesterol, and indirectly because of the high level of total fat, which promotes obesity. The first objective in managing hyperlipidemia should be to restore and/or maintain the desirable body weight.

Tables of desirable body weight in both men and women are given in Chapter 38. The weights in the tables can be closely approximated by the formula:

$$\text{Desirable body weight (lb)} = \frac{\text{Height (in)} \times \text{Wrist circum (in)}}{3}$$

The desirable weight generally corresponds closely to the weight at peak fitness, which is likely to have been achieved if the patient served in the armed forces or participated in competitive sports. The caloric restriction necessary for weight loss combines readily with the compositional changes necessary to reduce the serum cholesterol, since the cornerstone of these changes is the reduction of saturated fat (which is calorically dense). The compositional changes can be approached by the series of cumulative steps shown in Table 14-8. The number of steps that should be recommended depends both on the severity of hyperlipidemia and on the patient's willingness to make changes.

Step I. Moderate reduction of saturated fats. The first step represents a relatively minor modification of the typical United States diet that should be achievable without undue effort or social isolation. It is, in fact, recommended elsewhere in this manual as a desirable eating pattern for all adults and should not be regarded as a strictly therapeutic diet. Dietary cholesterol is not limited in Step 1 because moderate limita-

Table 14-8 Stepwise Approach to Reducing Serum Cholesterol by Dietary Change

	Recommended Change from Typical American Diet	Cumulative Approximate Reduction (mg/dl)
Step I	Reduce saturated fat to 10% of calories with partial substitution of polyunsaturated fat as needed	15
Step II	Reduce dietary cholesterol to 200 mg/da	24
Step III	Reduce saturated fat to 5% of calories and dietary cholesterol to 100 mg/da	35
Step IV	Vegan diet with addition of skimmed milk and egg white	50
Step V	Increase polyunsaturated fat to 15% of calories (maintaining caloric balance)	65

tion, although irksome to the patient, provides only a small improvement in the serum cholesterol response. It is important to avoid the common confusion between "low cholesterol" and "cholesterol-lowering" diets. The latter is the more general and preferred term. The following precepts should be adequate to limit saturated fat to 10% of calories:

1. Substitute poultry, fish, and veal for red meat as much as possible.
2. Use lean cuts of any red meat eaten; trim any remaining visible fat.
3. Remove skin from poultry.
4. Broil, roast, or stew rather than fry.
5. Substitute skimmed milk (ideally) or ½% milk (acceptably) for whole milk.
6. Use butter only occasionally and substitute a soft (tub) margarine, if needed, regularly.
7. Use oils for cooking, either monounsaturated (e.g., olive oil) or polyunsaturated (corn oil).
8. Use regular cheese only occasionally and substitute low-fat cheese, if needed, for more frequent use.
9. Eat ice cream only occasionally.
10. Avoid products containing coconut or palm oil (which are highly saturated).
11. Include whole grain breads and cereals, fruits, vegetables, beans, peas, and nuts daily.

These general precepts avoid the need for measuring the amounts of food and do not proscribe any common foods totally. The individual need not have the feeling of being "on a diet," but rather that the emphasis is shifted from some foods to others. The precepts are simple to apply at home but do require some care in the selection of food when eating out.

It should be recognized that many health-conscious persons have already made many of the recommended changes in response to widespread publicity in the mass media with regard to cholesterol-lowering diets. Reduction in serum cholesterol can of course be expected only to the extent that the application of these precepts represents a change from previous eating habits.

Step II. Reduction of dietary cholesterol. Step II can be added for individuals to whom eggs do not represent an important part of the diet. The precepts for Step II are

1. Eliminate egg yolks.
2. Eliminate organ meats (brain, pancreas, liver, kidney, heart).

Egg whites, obtained either by direct separation of the yolks or as a constituent of several commercial egg substitutes, are quite acceptable and an excellent source of protein. (A number of authorities, including the American Heart Association and the U.S. Departments of Agriculture and of Health and Human Services, recommend limiting dietary cholesterol as part of their "prudent" diets for all individuals regardless of risk of disease status.)

Step III. Major reduction of saturates. The Step III diet is, for the average American, a much more radical departure from the typical diet and, as such, should be regarded as a specifically therapeutic rather than a general recommendation. However, diets that approximate these specifications are eaten by choice in many parts of the world and are the basis of sophisticated cuisines.

The main precepts of Step III (over and above Steps I and II) are

1. Limit red meat, poultry, veal, fish, and low-fat cheese to a total of 3 ounces/day.
2. Minimize shellfish, sardines, and red meat (lean cuts only).
3. Use no butter.
4. Use only skimmed milk (and skimmed milk products).
5. Eat no ice cream.

Step IV. Vegan diets. A vegan diet represents an even more radical departure from the typical United States diet and is acceptable as a therapeutic diet only to a minority of patients. In its pure form, such a diet proscribes all foods of animal origin (i.e., meat, fish, eggs, all dairy products). Since cholesterol is present only in foods of animal origin, the diet is completely free of cholesterol. The level of saturated fat is very low and the net effect on the genotypic level of serum cholesterol is negative (depending on the proportion of polyunsaturated fat). Whereas vegan diets historically have been eaten for religious or ethical reasons, their application for therapeutic purposes allows certain modifications that otherwise would not be acceptable. Skimmed milk, skimmed milk products, and egg whites (including commercial egg substitutes) can be added to provide additional balanced protein with negligible amounts of saturated fat and cholesterol. Skimmed milk is also a useful source of vitamin B$_{12}$, which is liable to be deficient in strict vegan diets. A pint of skimmed milk daily provides sufficient vitamin B$_{12}$ for almost all individuals. Although evidence of vitamin B$_{12}$ deficiency does not appear for at least several years after the adoption of a strict vegan diet, it is prudent to take a supplement if the diet is to be adhered to rigorously.

When skimmed milk products and egg whites are not used regularly, special attention should be paid to including complementary vegetable proteins at each meal. Empirical ways of achieving this have been developed by the traditional cuisines of the Mediterranean, Middle Eastern, and Asian cultures. A useful guide to complementary proteins is provided in the widely available *Diet for a Small Planet*[31]; however, many recipes for meatless meals included in this book specify eggs and high-fat cheeses, which should not be used at all in Step III and IV diets.

Step V. Additional polyunsaturated fat. The further increase of polyunsaturated fat above that used to substitute partially for saturated fat is not now widely recommended. Polyunsaturated fat has a caloric density as high as saturated fat and is not therefore conducive to weight control. Furthermore, there are doubts about the safety of large amounts of polyunsaturated fat in the diet, since there is no well-established cultural model for such diets, as there is for all the other types of diet discussed so far. Concern about the safety of polyunsaturated fat per se is to be distinguished from concern about the safety of hydrogenated fat, in which *trans* bonds are formed in place of the naturally occurring *cis* forms; hydrogenation is a process used to increase the degree of saturation of commercial shortenings, margarines, and some salad and cooking oils.

Application of the Stepwise Approach

The general goal for managing hyperlipidemias other than chylomicronemia is to reduce serum cholesterol, in particular the LDL fraction. There is insufficient evidence of either the atherogenicity of triglycerides or any benefit from their reduction to warrant major dietary changes (other than the control of body weight and alcohol intake in susceptible individuals) because of isolated elevation of triglycerides in the absence of chylomicronemia.[22] Knowledge of the individual lipoprotein levels is useful (but by no means essential) for initiating dietary change. The serum cholesterol alone is adequate for monitoring the response to dietary management. The management of hypercholesterolemia depends on the following main criteria:

1. Level of total cholesterol and/or LDL cholesterol
2. Age of the individual
3. Presence of other risk factors
4. Presence of clinical manifestations of atherosclerosis
5. Presence of xanthomas
6. Willingness and ability of the patient to make dietary changes.

Some arbitrary estimates of acceptable, desirable, and possibly optimum lipid levels depending on age and the presence or absence of other risk factors are shown in Table 14-9. Two alternative lipid measures are indicated. The total cholesterol is the simplest and most generally used. Since the apparent source of risk and the

Table 14-9 Guidelines for Managing Hypercholesterolemia

	Before Age 20 Years		After Age 30 Years	
	Total Cholesterol (mg/dl)	LDL Cholesterol (mg/dl)	Total Cholesterol (mg/dl)	LDL Cholesterol (mg/dl)
Acceptable upper limit without other risk factors	200	140	220	160
Prudent upper limit, especially with other risk factors for atherosclerosis	180	120	200	140
Approximate average levels in populations at minimal risk of atherosclerosis	140	90	160	110

main target of dietary intervention are both LDL cholesterol, the decision to intervene ideally (but by no means necessarily) is based on this determination, as just described.

The objective of dietary management should be to use the number of steps necessary to control the total or LDL cholesterol below the chosen upper limit for the appropriate age and status with respect to risk factors. Certain individuals may wish to pursue goals close to those suggested by the lipid levels of populations at minimum risk of atherosclerosis. Others may be unwilling or unable to make the changes necessary to reduce cholesterol below even the acceptable upper limit. When the level achievable by dietary changes exceeds the upper acceptable limit substantially, it may be necessary to consider other measures (e.g., drugs) discussed later in this section. The feasibility and benefit of achieving substantial dietary change after age 60 years is questionable, and each case should be given individual consideration.

The five steps need not be interpreted as distinct increments in managing hypercholesterolemia. Many other types of dietary modifications could be devised, some of them perhaps more suitable for certain individuals. Table 14-10 shows the calculated effect of specific examples of dietary change. The patient can be shown directly the relative expected value of several alternative changes and is then in a position to make informed choices based on personal preferences. Active involvement of the patient in developing dietary specifications will maximize the motivation to comply with the final negotiated prescription.

Relationship of Diet to Other Therapy for Hyperlipidemia

Although it is beyond the scope of this manual to present a detailed account of therapy other than diet for hyperlipidemia, it is necessary to consider the possibilities presented by such therapy and their relationships to dietary therapy. Several classes of drugs are effective in lowering either serum cholesterol or triglycerides or both, together with their associated lipoproteins, and partial ileal bypass is being used experimentally in certain centers. In general, these other modes of therapy are considered only when diet has failed to bring the total or LDL cholesterol to an acceptable level. This failure occurs for three principal reasons (listed in order of frequency):

1. Failure to make sufficient dietary change
2. A serum cholesterol level that remains high even after reduction by diet
3. Metabolic resistance to the reduction of serum cholesterol by dietary change

Table 14-10 Impact of Dietary Precepts for Reducing Serum Cholesterol

	High-Fat Food	Fat-Controlled Substitute	Expected Reduction (mg/dl)
Eliminate organ meats	3 oz liver	3 oz tuna	23
Trim all visible fat	6 oz untrimmed porterhouse steak	6 oz trimmed porterhouse steak	22
Substitute egg whites for whole eggs	1 whole egg	1 egg white	19
Substitute polyunsaturated oils for solid cooking fats	1 oz lard	1 oz safflower oil	18
Substitute polyunsaturated margarine for butter	1 oz butter	1 oz corn oil margarine	16
Substitute poultry or fish for red meat	4 oz lamb chop	4 oz skinned chicken	13
Choose lean meats	4 oz hamburger (35% fat)	4 oz hamburger (10% fat)	13
Substitute low-fat for regular cheese	2 oz cheddar cheese	2 oz part skim mozzarella	10
Substitute low-fat desserts for ice cream	4 oz ice cream	4 oz skim yogurt	8
Substitute skim for whole milk	½ pint whole milk	½ pint skim milk	5

Adapted from Hulley SB, et al: West J Med **135**:25-33, 1981.

Major dietary change is difficult to achieve, especially in the patient who has no symptoms. Often it is only after a serious clinical manifestation of atherosclerosis has occurred that a patient is willing to act on dietary recommendations (i.e., at a stage of the a natural history when it may be too late to expect dramatic benefit from the reduction of serum lipids). In certain individuals cholesterol levels remain high after the most extensive dietary measures, because of a very high initial level or the lack of response to diet, or both. Heterozygotes for familial hypercholesterolemia (about 1 in 500 individuals) usually cannot be controlled at acceptable levels by diet alone, and homozygotes (about 1 in 1,000,000) never can. Type III hyperlipidemia ("broad" or "floating" β disease) and certain polygenic forms of hypercholesterolemia are also not fully controllable by diet. However, dietary change, to the fullest extent that the patient will accept it, should be recommended before resorting to more radical (and less physiologic) modes of therapy.

No ideal drug has been developed for the management of hyperlipidemia.

The drug that was previously widely used, clofibrate (Atromid-S), affects mainly the triglycerides and VLDL cholesterol, with a lesser effect on LDL cholesterol. Evidence from a large-scale clinical trial of clofibrate for the primary prevention of coronary heart disease[32] not only failed to show any benefit with respect to death from coronary heart disease but also demonstrated a highly significant increase in deaths from all causes during and after the trial. Clofibrate also failed to provide any benefit in a large-scale trial of the secondary prevention of coronary heart disease.[33] Clofibrate is still recommended by some authorities for the rare Type III hyperlipidemia, but its long-term benefit in this condition has not been established.

Niacin (nicotinic acid) given in pharmacologic rather than nutritional doses reduces total cholesterol and triglycerides, with corresponding reductions in both LDL and VLDL cholesterol. Such doses often result in flushing of the skin and other side effects that limit its usefulness. A large clinical trial of niacin in the secondary prevention of coronary heart disease[33] resulted in a significant decrease in recurrent nonfatal coronary events, and a 15-year follow-up of this study[34] has demonstrated a substantial and significant reduction in mortality.

The most potent cholesterol-reducing agents are the bile acid–sequestering resins cholestyramine and colestipol. Their effects occur on the LDL fraction, which is reduced by about 40%, with a consequent reduction of some 30% in total cholesterol, in persons who comply with the recommended dosage of about 24 g daily. The efficacy of cholestyramine in reducing coronary events as well as in lowering both total and LDL cholesterol has been demonstrated in the large randomized double blind Coronary Primary Prevention Trial of the Lipid Research Clinics.[35]

In another study, of 116 patients with elevated LDL cholesterol and angiographic evidence of coronary artery disease,[36] the 58 patients randomly assigned to receive cholestyramine demonstrated less progression of the disease by angiography (5 yr later) than those assigned a placebo.

The combination of niacin and colestipol has been shown to be synergistically effective in the management of heterozygous familial hypercholesterolemia.[37]

The most radical and probably most effective approach to managing hypercholesterolemia that persists after diet and drug therapy is partial ileal bypass. This major surgical procedure reduces the total cholesterol level by 40% to 50%.[38] A randomized clinical trial of the effectiveness of the procedure in the secondary prevention of coronary heart disease is in progress.

Management of Chylomicronemia

The rare condition chylomicronemia is the only lipid disturbance that requires a dietary approach different from the one just described. The cornerstone of dietary therapy for chylomicronemia is to reduce dietary fat regardless of the degree of saturation. The maximum level of dietary fat that can be tolerated varies from one patient to another and can be ascertained only by trial of different levels. A diet containing 20% of calories as fat should be tried first, but it may be necessary to reduce this to 10% or even 5% to control chylomicronemia. It is important also to ensure that such diets contain at least 1% of total calories as linoleic acid to meet essential fatty acid requirements. Medium-chain triglycerides can be added to increase palatability. It may be necessary to use a fat-free formula diet (in fruit juice) for short periods to prevent the risk of acute pancreatitis. Body weight should be maintained at, or restored to, desirable levels by calorie control, especially in the case of acquired (Type V) chylomicronemia. Alcohol should be avoided. In contrast to the diets for hypercholesterolemia, it is not necessary to control the intake of dietary cholesterol. Shellfish are therefore a useful substitute for meat in diets limiting the intake of total fat.

Prevention

The prevention of lipid disturbances is one of the principal considerations in the choice of diets most suitable to maintain health and is considered in Chapter 7 of this manual. Because of the major genetic component in most serious lipid disturbances, it is important to screen the relatives of patients so diagnosed. However, it is clear from the international epidemiologic data mentioned in the discussion of lipid disturbances that the most common and most serious lipid disturbance—elevated serum total cholesterol combined with Type II hyperlipoproteinemia—rarely occurs (at least by United States standards) in populations with a low intake of saturated fat and cholesterol and with a low prevalence of obesity. In this context it is important to reemphasize that the main burden of lipid disturbances in Western industrialized countries falls not on a few genetically unusual individuals but on approximately half the population whose cholesterol level falls above the average, an average that corresponds roughly to the 95th percentile of the Japanese population. The combination of low saturated and total fat in the diet and high levels of habitual activity are conducive to low adiposity as well as low LDL and high HDL levels, all of which appear to be favorable attributes in terms of the risk for the majority of cardiovascular diseases.

Summary of Lipid Disturbances

The single lipid disturbance of most importance in terms of both frequency and severity of consequences is elevated serum cholesterol. Increased levels of LDL cholesterol, the main atherogenic lipid, are reflected in increased levels of total cholesterol. Total cholesterol should be measured routinely at least once in childhood and again at about age 30 years in males and at menopause in females. Routine testing for triglycerides, chylomicronemia, and HDL cholesterol is not necessary (but each should be undertaken for certain indications). All lipid disturbances can be managed with two general types of dietary therapy:

1. Hypercholesterolemia is approached by losing excess weight, reducing saturated fat, reducing dietary cholesterol, and increasing polyunsaturated fat, in that order of importance.
2. The much rarer chylomicronemia is approached by sharply limiting amounts of normal dietary fat (regardless of saturation) and by using medium-chain triglycerides if necessary.

In addition, limiting saturated fat to not more than 10% of calories, and total fat to 30% of calories, is recommended as a prudent diet for all individuals in the absence of major lipid disturbances.

ATHEROSCLEROTIC DISEASE

Most cases of myocardial, cerebral, and peripheral ischemia result from the single underlying disease process atherosclerosis, which is a subcategory of the more general condition of arteriosclerosis. The term "arteriosclerosis" describes a group of arterial diseases characterized by degeneration, thickening, and induration of one or more layers of the vascular wall. Atherosclerosis is predominantly a disease of the arterial intima affecting large and medium-sized arteries.

There are three types of atherosclerotic lesion: the *fatty streak,* the *fibrous plaque,* and the *complicated lesion.*

Fatty streaks are flat or slightly raised accumulations of intimal smooth muscle cells that both contain and are surrounded by deposits of lipid. The streaks appear gradually in various parts of the arterial tree but are almost always present in the aorta by age 10 years, regardless of sex, race, or environment. The involvement of the aortic surface increases from about 10% at age 10 years to about 30% at age 30.

The fibrous plaque, which is characteristic of the disease, does not occur universally. It is an elevated lesion that consists mainly of lipid-laden smooth muscle cells, also surrounded by lipid, collagen, and elastic fibers. These components form a fibrous cap that covers a deposit of cell debris mixed with free extracellular lipid. It is widely believed that fatty streaks are the precursors of fibrous plaques, since both tend to occur at the same sites in the coronary and carotid arteries. In the aorta, however, fatty streaks and fibrous plaques may occur at different sites. So-called transitional fatty streaks, in which necrosis of some cells has led to the release of lipid, are present in the coronary arteries of adolescents from populations with high rates of symptomatic atherosclerotic disease.

Such symptomatic disease is usually a result of one or more types of complication of the fibrous plaque. These complications can cause partial or complete obstruction of the arterial lumen, with consequent ischemia or infarction of the affected area. The following are the most common complications:

1. Mural thrombosis that may evolve into a complete obstruction
2. Ulceration, with the release of debris into the bloodstream
3. Hemorrhage into the lesion
4. Calcification

The pathogenesis of the plaques and their complications is incompletely understood and controversial. Some of the more modern hypotheses have been reviewed by Ross and Glomset.[39] Although more complete understanding of the mechanism by which atherogenesis develops may be important in the future management and prevention of the disease, the present state of knowledge in this area is less relevant to the clinical management than is the large body of knowledge concerning the etiology.

Etiology

The relatively small amount of disagreement concerning the etiology of atherosclerosis receives much more publicity than the broad areas of general agreement that exist among workers in the field. Virtually all such scientists attribute the high U.S. rates of coronary heart disease to features of the American way of life: diet, smoking, physical inactivity, stress. Most scientists believe that all these factors are involved in the epidemic (although not in each individual case). The disagreement largely concerns the relative importance of the factors and is often compounded by failure to identify the precise question to be addressed. The present state of etiologic knowledge results from a merging of findings by pathologists, clinicians, animal experimentalists, and epidemiologists. These studies can be divided into four major categories: (1) studies of individuals within populations, (2) comparisons among populations, (3) studies of racial or ethnic groups that have emigrated from one environment to another, and (4) clinical trials of risk factor modification.

Several of the largest prospective studies in the United States (of which that conducted in Framingham, Massachusetts,[40] is the prototype) have been reanalyzed in a standardized fashion.[41] These studies provide consistent evidence that blood cholesterol level, cigarette smoking, and blood pressure are major predictors of clinical atherosclerotic disease, each accounting for roughly the same amount of variation in risk.

The most comprehensive and best standardized study among populations confirms the predictive value of the same three major risk factors in individuals.[42] It also allows a more fundamental generalization to be made: high rates of atherosclerotic disease are found only in countries with high average levels of blood cholesterol, which, in turn, are found only in countries with high levels of saturated fat and cholesterol in the diet. High average levels of cigarette smoking or blood pressure, either alone or in combination, do not result in high rates of atherosclerotic disease when average blood cholesterol blood levels are low, as in Japan and Italy.

The conclusions from the first two types of study are confirmed by studies of emigrants, which show that racial or ethnic groups acquire rates of atherosclerotic disease characteristic of their new environment (and in particular of its diet). These observations suggest that there are no major systematic genetic differences in susceptibility to atherosclerosis among the major racial or ethnic groups (although there are important genetic differences in susceptibility among individuals within such groups).

The general findings of the epidemiologic studies are consistent with those from the direct study of human atherosclerotic lesions, the experimental induction of atheroma-like lesions in laboratory animals, and the natural history of the more serious genetic disorders of lipid metabolism in humans. Although it would be desirable in principle to confirm these findings by experiments in humans, the long natural history of the disease and the lack of a safe and simple measure of preclinical atherosclerosis make such experiments impractical. However, the many sources of indirect evidence allow reasonably secure etiologic models to be built. Such a model for the natural history of coronary disease (Fig. 14-5) follows the general scheme of Fig. 14-1 and stresses the role of dietary elevation of LDL cholesterol as a prerequisite for epidemic atherosclerotic disease. The left side of the figure also emphasizes the many other indirect effects of diet on coronary disease mediated through obesity, physical inactivity, hypertension, diabetes, and depressed levels of HDL cholesterol. Other factors not closely associated with diet—stress (i.e., factors operating through the central nervous system) and smoking—are implicated at several stages in the natural history of coronary disease.

Fig. 14-5 presents the essential features of the diet-heart hypothesis. Despite frequent statements to the contrary, this hypothesis does not attribute the twentieth century epidemic of coronary disease in the United States to major changes in diet at the beginning of the century.

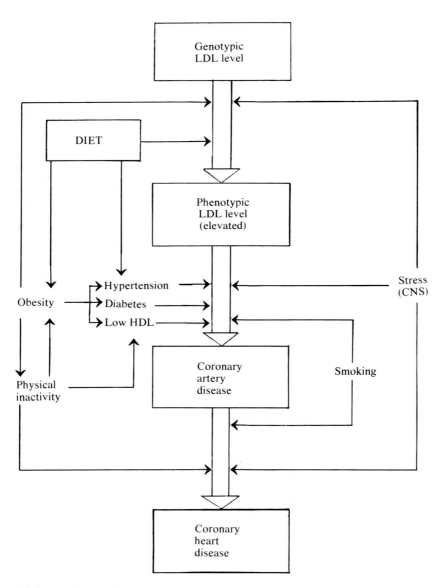

Figure 14-5 Causal model for the roles of diet and other factors in the natural history of coronary heart disease.

There is, in fact, no evidence for such change, especially with respect to the probable average consumption of saturated fats and cholesterol that had been high for many years preceding the epidemic. It is much more likely (though unproved) that the major changes that produced the epidemic were (1) the large scale adoption of cigarette smoking by American men in the early years of this century and (2) the declining levels of physical activity, both at work and in leisure, as portable sources of power and automobiles proliferated. The diet high in animal fat that was already characteristic of the United States merely furnished the prerequisite with which smoking and physical inactivity interacted. Smoking and declining physical activity have not resulted in epidemics of atherosclerotic disease in countries such as Japan and Italy, where the diets have remained low in animal fats, with correspondingly low average levels of serum cholesterol.

A comprehensive model for the etiology of atherosclerotic disease also must account for the substantial decline in mortality from coronary disease since about 1968, in both sexes and at all ages. No single factor adequately explains the rise and fall of coronary disease between 1920 and 1988. Furthermore, it seems that the factors operating in women have been somewhat different from those operating in men. Both sexes have altered their dietary habits in the past 25 years by reducing consumption of saturated fat and cholesterol and increasing consumption of polyunsaturated fat. These changes have reduced average serum cholesterol levels by about 20 mg/dl in women and 15 mg/dl in men. Although such changes would have little clinical significance in the individual because of normal variation, their impact on the population could account for a substantial part of the decline in coronary deaths. The reduction in cigarette smoking (especially among men), the major improvements in controlling hypertension (especially among women), and the increased amount of leisure time activity are each likely to have contributed further to the overall decline in mortality from coronary disease. There has also been a decline in fatalities because of improved medical care, which has contributed to the falling death rate independent of any reduction in incidence.

Although changes in diet and blood pressure have probably contributed to the decline in the epidemic of coronary disease, it is unlikely that converse changes in either of these factors have led to its rise. The absence of systematic changes in diet at the beginning of this century has been advanced as evidence against the "diet-heart hypothesis." Such an argument is based on a misunderstanding of the hypothesis, which holds only that a diet rich in animal fat is a necessary but not sufficient condition for epidemic coronary disease. The fact that dietary changes do not account for the rise of coronary mortality diminishes in no way the potential value of dietary change as an approach to preventing such mortality.

Screening and Diagnosis

One major shortcoming in the current diagnostic armamentarium is the lack of a safe, noninvasive, inexpensive, and accurate means of measuring the extent of atherosclerosis in the coronary, cerebral, or peripheral circulation. For the several decades during which the disease develops silently, there is no generally applicable method of demonstrating its presence directly. Not until clinical manifestations of ischemia appear is it feasible to detect the presence, location, and extent of atherosclerosis with any degree of assurance. In general, therefore, the best that can be achieved is to identify individuals at high risk of developing complications and clinically manifest disease. The importance of identifying such individuals depends, of course, on the extent to which the natural history can be changed by intervention at this stage of the disease. No fully controlled trial of dietary intervention before clinical manifestations of atherosclerosis has been conducted, and it is unlikely that one of sufficient size to produce definitive results will be carried out in the foreseeable future. It is, therefore, necessary to make decisions on the basis of incomplete and indirect evidence.

The major studies in the primary prevention of coronary heart disease in particular and cardiovascular disease in general have been recently reviewed.[43] Although the results of the Multiple Risk Factor Intervention Trial,[44] which involved combined interventions in hyperlipidemia, hypertension, and smoking, were indecisive, the Coronary Primary Prevention Trial[35] showed significantly reduced fatal and nonfatal coronary events following cholesterol reduction by cholestyramine in men with Type II hyperlipidemia. The applicability of these results to dietary intervention in men and women with lower levels of cholesterol has been questioned,[45] but most authorities agree that the case for dietary intervention in the general population has been strengthened.[46]

In the present state of knowledge, it is prudent to identify the major risk factors for atherosclerosis before any clinical manifestations of the disease occur. The profile should include total cholesterol, HDL cholesterol, fasting blood glucose, and information concerning smoking, physical activity, and family history. All Americans should limit their intake of saturated fat, but more specific dietary advice is necessary for those with the highest levels of cholesterol, particularly LDL cholesterol. Recommended thresholds of lipid levels about which specific cholesterol-lowering dietary advice should be given have been discussed in connection with hyperlipidemia (pp. 213 to 216) and are shown in Table 14-9. The maintenance of desirable weight should be encouraged for all individuals and stressed for those with lipoprotein disturbances (including HDL levels <40 mg/dl), hyperglycemia (fasting glucose >120 or repeatedly >110 mg/dl), and hypertension (SBP >140 or DBP >90). In children and young adults blood pressure above the 80th percentile should be regarded as a potential risk factor for future hypertension and hence of coronary heart disease; maintenance of desirable body weight and limited sodium intake should be stressed for these individuals.

Clinical Manifestations

Atherosclerosis is a silent disease throughout most of its natural history. In their unobstructed state the large arteries characteristically affected by the disease can accommodate rates of flow substantially greater than those required under even the most extreme conditions of oxygen demand by the tissues. Thus the symptoms of ischemia occur only after several decades of gradual progression of the disease (except in cases of major metabolic disturbance such as homozygous familial hypercholesterolemia). For this reason dietary management of hyperlipidemia aimed at the underlying atherosclerotic disease is unlikely to be curative at this late stage in the natural history of the disease.

Coronary heart disease. The principal clinical manifestations of atherosclerotic disease of the coronary arteries are angina pectoris, myocardial infarction, sudden death, and cardiac failure resulting from chronic ischemia. In the absence of symptoms evidence of myocardial ischemia on exertion may be obtained by electrocardiography and other noninvasive procedures. Symptomatic or latent atherosclerotic coronary disease generally implies at least 70% obstruction of the cross-sectional area of at least one major coronary artery. Myocardial infarction and/or sudden death may result from complete obstruction of a coronary vessel by thrombosis, hemorrhage, or ulceration of an atherosclerotic plaque, as well as by spasm of an artery already partially obstructed by atherosclerosis. Thrombosis is no longer considered to be a prerequisite for the occurrence of infarction (as implied by the previously interchangeable use of the terms coronary thrombosis and myocardial infarction). There is increasing evidence that much of the thrombosis observed at autopsy is a result rather than a cause of the coronary event. Spasm, on the other hand, is now believed to be a relatively common factor in the onset of angina, infarction, and death; but these events rarely occur in the absence of advanced underlying atherosclerosis.

Chronic coronary disease commonly leads to congestive heart failure (through loss of sufficient functioning myocardium), to mitral regurgitation resulting from dysfunction of the papillary muscle, and to various dysrhythmias. Failure is usually preceded by angina or clinically evident myocardial infarction, but it can also be the first clinical presentation of coronary heart disease.

Cerebral ischemia. Several types of vascular accident can compromise the blood supply to the brain, which involves the carotid, subclavian, and vertebral arteries as well as the intracranial vessels. Although there are some analogies with myocardial ischemia, they are not by any means complete. Gradual obstruction of the extracranial and larger intracranial vessels by atherosclerosis may reach a point at which there is episodic cerebral ischemia—transient ischemic attacks— characterized by temporary interference with motor function, monocular blindness, or loss of consciousness. Such attacks frequently precede a completed stroke, which may be defined as sudden neurologic deficit lasting more than 24 hours and due to ischemia. The possible pathogenic mechanisms for stroke include thrombosis, embolism, and hemorrhage (either intracerebral or subarachnoid).

Whereas atherosclerosis of the extracranial vessels appears to resemble that of the coronary arteries in morphology and etiology, disease of the intracranial arteries is different in both respects.[40] In the vessels of the circle of Willis and the larger vessels over the base of the brain, proliferative fibrosis of the intima rather than lipid infiltration appears to be the predominant lesion. In the larger intracerebral vessels the principal pathologic change is limited to the adventitia, which undergoes proliferative fibrosis and ultimately replaces the vessel wall. In the arterioles the chief degenerative change is limited to the media and consists of progressive medial fibrosis. Disease of the intracranial vessels has a much weaker association with lipid levels, both within and among populations, than does disease of the extracranial vessels and the coronary arteries. Hypertension appears to be the principal risk factor for disease of the intracranial arteries. Such disease may predispose to thrombosis or hemorrhage.

The contrast between the etiology and morphology of most cerebrovascular diseases, on the one hand, and atherosclerotic disease of the coronary, visceral, and peripheral arteries, on the other, is emphasized by the sex-specific incidence rates. Rates of cerebrovascular disease are similar in men and women after age 50 years, reflecting the similar incidence of hypertension in the two sexes.[40] However, the rates of cerebrovascular disease before age 50 and ischemia of all the other vascular territories are substantially higher in males than in females, reflecting the greater susceptibility of males to atherosclerosis of the large arteries.[40]

Visceral and peripheral ischemia. Atherosclerosis of the renal, splanchnic, and iliac arteries and of the aorta is strongly associated with disease of the coronary arteries and is much more frequent in men than in women (by a ratio of up to 10:1). Atherosclerosis of the renal artery is a surgically correctable cause of hypertension and should be considered in hypertensive patients whose disease remains progressive despite drug therapy or who have evidence of advanced atherosclerosis elsewhere in the vascular tree.

Acute mesenteric arterial occlusion is a severe disease that is fatal if not properly treated. About half the patients with preexisting atherosclerotic disease of the splanchnic vessels have warning symptoms of pain, called "abdominal angina." The pain occurs typically after meals, is located in the epigastrium, and radiates to the back; it may be associated with anorexia, nausea, vomiting, and weight loss. The disease should be corrected surgically before thrombosis of a mesenteric artery with consequent bowel infarction supervenes.

Atherosclerosis of the aorta and iliac arteries leads to the Leriche syndrome. If occlusion of both iliac arteries occurs, superimposed thrombosis causes complete occlusion of the distal aorta and may extend proximally toward the renal arteries. The severity of the ischemic symptoms depends on the speed with which the obstruction develops. Gradual occlusion tends to promote collateral circulation, which mitigates the symptoms.

More peripheral disease of the femoral, popliteal, and tibial arteries, though strongly associated with atherosclerosis in other parts of the vascular tree, is also associated with smoking and diabetes. The classic symptom is intermittent claudication ("angina of the legs"). In advanced stages gangrene often supervenes.

Dietary Management

The model for the etiology of atherosclerotic disease and its complications (Figs. 14-1 and 14-5) suggests that dietary intervention is much more likely to be effective if applied early in the natural history, since diet as a causal factor is mediated through the hyperlipidemia that commonly initiates and promotes the atherosclerotic process. Symptomatic disease implies advanced atherosclerosis that has usually occurred over a period of several decades.

Although animal experiments have demonstrated regression of lesions following withdrawal of an atherogenic diet fed over a period of months, these experiments do not provide substantial assurance that longstanding complicated atherosclerosis in humans is likely to regress with any but the most profound dietary or pharmacologic modifications of serum lipids. Thus the expectations for the results of dietary modification begun after symptomatic atherosclerotic disease should be modest. The primary goal of long-term therapy after an acute complication of atherosclerotic disease is to prevent a recurrence of the conditions that precipitated the acute event (usually the complete obstruction of a vessel already affected by longstanding atherosclerotic disease). The reduction of serum lipids by dietary intervention is a secondary goal that depends for its effectiveness on the survival of the patient over a period sufficient to allow some impact of altered serum lipid levels on the underlying artherosclerotic process.

Another aspect of dietary interventions may also be especially relevant to the management of artherosclerotic disease. A particular class of polyunsaturated fatty acids is typically present at relatively high concentrations in cold-water fish. These omega-3 fatty acids reduce platelet aggregability and prolong bleeding time. They are thus comparable in their effects to the "antiplatelet" drugs (e.g., aspirin, dipyridamole) that are now used in both the treatment and the prevention of atherosclerotic disease. The sources and possible hazards of omega-3 fatty acids are discussed in more detail in Chapter 7 beginning on p. 95.

Coronary heart disease. Randomized clinical trials of cholesterol-lowering diets in the prevention of recurrent myocardial infarction after at least one such event have not produced evidence of dramatic benefit (especially with respect to the most reliable endpoint, death). Nor have the largest trials of lipid-lowering drugs in similar patients been more encouraging. This is not surprising, since symptomatic coronary disease implies at least 70% obstruction of at least one major coronary vessel. An individual who has suffered one coronary event thus remains at risk of another, even if the progression of the underlying atherosclerotic disease is retarded or arrested.

Recent advances in the pharmacologic and surgical management of acute and chronic disease, and consequently prolonged survival, make it highly desirable to minimize further progression of the underlying disease, even if regression of atherosclerosis is unlikely. It should be standard clinical practice to adopt measures to reduce the total serum cholesterol levels (and cholesterol in particular) as much as the circumstances of each individual patient allow. In general, a myocardial infarction provides motivation to make dietary modifications that would not have been made before the event. Although the major lipid reductions achievable with a vegan diet, combination drug therapy, or a partial ileal bypass seem most likely to influence

the natural history of the disease, it is debatable whether such regimens should be recommended, given the current lack of direct evidence about their benefits. However, the compromise position of recommending milder dietary modification (Step I, II, or III in Table 14-8) is less likely to alter the natural history. The principal determinants in selecting a particular dietary approach to lipid reduction should be the level of LDL cholesterol and the patient's age. There is a natural and appropriate reluctance to urge major changes of life-style on an elderly patient with limited life expectancy unless there is substantial confidence in its benefit. The current randomized clinical trial of partial ileal bypass in patients who have already suffered a myocardial infarction will yield valuable information concerning not only the usefulness of the procedure but also the potential value of vigorous reduction of LDL cholesterol by diet or drugs. Only when the physician has full confidence in the efficacy of lipid reduction at this stage of the atherosclerotic process will it be possible to transmit that confidence to the patient and achieve the necessary degree of compliance with radical dietary change or with drugs that are unpleasant either to take or in their side effects.

Congestive heart failure. Although heart failure is a frequent complication of coronary heart disease, it may also result from heart disease of any other etiology. The objectives in the nutritional management of heart failure are similar, regardless of etiology, although other objectives (e.g., the reduction of hyperlipidemia) may be superimposed on the basic ones. The diet in heart failure should aim at minimizing both cardiac work and edema. The two main considerations in achieving these objectives are to eliminate excess body fat by caloric reduction and to control sodium in the diet. In contrast to the control of obesity in other situations, it is not usually possible to promote increased physical activity in patients with cardiac failure, so a negative energy balance must be achieved solely by reduced caloric intake. Sodium restriction to control edema in heart failure needs to be rigorous (i.e., 20 mEq of Na per da). This level of restriction proscribes added salt during cooking and calls for the careful selection of foods in measured amounts. The American Heart Association publishes a guide for patients following a diet limited to 500 mg of sodium (22 mEq) per day at 1200, 1800, or unrestricted caloric levels. However, these diets allow foods such as heavy cream and butter that should be proscribed, especially if cholesterol reduction is also indicated.

Cerebral ischemia. The dietary indications for either transient ischemia or a completed stroke due to thrombosis or embolism depend mainly on the site of the underlying arterial disease. Although this is best determined by arteriography, considerable circumstantial evidence is provided by the presence of other risk factors and of atherosclerotic disease elsewhere in the arterial tree. Hyperlipidemia, especially that associated with evidence of coronary or peripheral atherosclerosis, increases the likelihood that the cerebral ischemia is the result of extra- rather than intracranial arterial disease.[46] The control of serum lipids by diet is more strongly indicated for such extracranial disease. When hypertension is the predominant risk factor, the odds shift in favor of relatively distal intracranial disease, whose natural history is less likely to be influenced by lipid reduction. The stepwise approach to the reduction of serum cholesterol by dietary change (Table 14-9) and the suggested goals for such change (Table 14-8) are applicable when there is actual or presumptive evidence of an atherosclerotic basis for cerebral ischemia. Excess body weight is also a major risk factor for cerebral ischemia, and every effort should be made to normalize it.

Visceral and peripheral ischemia. Cigarette smoking is the most consistent risk factor for atherosclerosis of the abdominal and leg vessels, and complete smoking cessation should be the first objective of treatment. As in cerebral ischemia, the most proximal disease is more clearly associated with hyperlipidemia and more likely to be retarded by reducing blood lipid levels. When lipid levels exceed those shown in Table 14-9, reduction should be pursued by normalizing body weight and using the stepwise approach shown in Table 14-8.

Prevention

As has been stressed throughout this chapter, the role of diet in atherosclerosis begins at the earliest stages of the disease, in childhood. Many of the dietary habits that lead to hyperlipidemia, hypertension, obesity, and atherosclerosis are established in American children well before adolescence. The true primary prevention of atherosclerosis should begin in childhood when food preferences first develop, largely as a matter of habit. Although there can be no serious doubt about the role of diet and hyperlipidemia in the development of atherosclerosis, there also is no assurance that change after the onset of the clinical complications will effectively alter the natural history of the disease. The same is true of the advanced but still asymptomatic atherosclerosis characteristic of middle-aged American men.

For these reasons it is highly desirable to institute a diet appropriate for the prevention of atherosclerosis as early in life as possible. The approach to identifying hyperlipidemia in children and young adults described in the section "Screening and Diagnosis" for hyperlipidemia (p. 212) applies equally to the prevention of atherosclerosis. A shift toward reduced amounts of saturated fat and cholesterol in the diet of the whole population, together with the prevention of obesity and cigarette smoking, constitutes the most rational approach to preventing atherosclerosis and its complications.

REFERENCES

1. Veterans Administration Cooperative Studies Group on Antihypertensive Agents: Effects of treatment on morbidity. Results in patients with diastolic blood pressure averaging 115 through 129 mm Hg, JAMA **202:**1028-1034, 1967.
2. Veterans Administration Cooperative Studies Group on Antihypertensive Agents: Effects of treatment on morbidity in hypertension. II. Results in patients with diastolic blood pressure averaging 90 through 114 mm Hg, JAMA **213:**1143-1152, 1970.
3. Hypertension Detection and Follow-Up Program Cooperative Group: Five-year findings of the Hypertension and Detection and Follow-up Program, JAMA **242:**2562-2577, 1979.
4. Medical Research Council Working Party: MRC trial of treatment of hypertension: principal results, Br Med J **291:**97-104, 1985.
5. Bergland G, et al.: Prevalence of primary and secondary hypertension. Studies in a random population sample, Br Med J **2:**554-556, 1976.
6. Tobian L: The relationship of salt to hypertension, Am J Clin Nutr **32:**2739-2748, 1979.
7. Kempner W: Treatment of kidney disease and hypertensive vascular disease with rice diet, NC Med J **5:**125-133, 1944.
8. Klatsky AL, et al: Alcohol consumption and blood pressure: Kaiser-Permanente/multiphasic health examination data, N Engl J Med **296:**1194-1200, 1977.
9. Whelton PK, Klag MJ: Potassium in the homeostasis and reduction of blood pressure, Clin Nutr **6:**76-82, 1987.
10. Villar J, et al: Calcium and blood pressure, Clin Nutr **5:**161-166, 1986.

11. Kirkendall WN, et al: American Heart Association recommendations for human blood pressure determination by sphygmomanometer, Circulation 62(2):1146A-1155A, 1980.

12. United States Department of Health and Human Services: Report of the Joint National Committee on Detection, Evaluation, and Treatment of High Blood Pressure, NIH Publ 84-1088, September 1984.

13. Cohen JD: Role of nutrition in the management of hypertension, Clin Nutr 3:135-138, 1984.

14. American Heart Association: Your mild sodium restricted diet, Dallas, 1969, The Association.

15. American Heart Association: Your 1000 milligram sodium diet, Dallas, 1969, The Association.

16. American Heart Association: Your 500 milligram sodium diet, Dallas, 1969, The Association.

17. Marsh AC, et al: The sodium content of your food, Home and Garden Bulletin 233, Washington DC, 1980, United States Department of Agriculture.

18. Russell RP: Potassium supplementation, potassium-retaining diuretics, and the hazards of hyperkalemia, Clin Nutr 6:70-75, 1987.

19. Miller NE: Plasma lipoproteins, lipid transport, and atherosclerosis: recent developments, J Clin Pathol 32:639-650, 1979.

20. Beaumont JL, et al: Classification of hyperlipidemias and hyperlipoproteinemias, Bull WHO 43:891-908, 1970.

21. Frederickson DS, et al: Fat transport in lipoprotein—an integrated approach to mechanisms and disorders, N Engl J Med 276:34-44, 93-103, 148-156, 215-226, 273-281, 1967.

22. Connor WE, Connor SL: Nutrition management of hyperlipidemias, Curr Concepts Nutr 8:179-216, 1979.

23. Hulley SB, et al: Epidemiology as a guide to clinical decision. The association between triglyceride and coronary heart disease, N Engl J Med 302:1383-1389, 1980.

24. Schaefer EJ: Nutrition, lipoproteins, and atherosclerosis, Clin Nutr 5:99-111, 1986.

25. Hulley SB, Dzvonik ML: Alcohol intake, blood lipids, and coronary heart disease, Clin Nutr 3:139-142, 1984.

26. Sherwin RW, Cutler JA: The effect of antihypertensive agents on lipids, lipoproteins, and coronary heart disease, Clin Nutr 3:131-134, 1984.

27. Wilson PWF, et al: Postmenopausal estrogen use, cigarette smoking, and cardiovascular morbidity in women over 50, N Engl J Med 313:1038-1043, 1985.

28. Stampfer JJ, et al: A prospective study of postmenopausal estrogen therapy and coronary heart disease, N Engl J Med 313:1044-1049, 1985.

29. Heiss et al: Lipoprotein-cholesterol distributions in selected North American populations: Lipid Research Clinics program prevalence study, Circulation 61:302-315, 1980.

30. Coronary Drug Project Research Group: The Coronary Drug Project. Initial findings leading to modifications of its research protocol, JAMA 214:1303-1313, 1970.

31. Lappe FM: Diet for a small planet, New York, 1975, Ballantine Books, Inc.

32. Oliver MF, et al: W.H.O. cooperative trial on primary prevention of ischemic heart disease using clofibrate to lower serum cholesterol: mortality follow-up, Lancet 2:379-383, 1980.

33. Coronary Drug Project Research Group: Clofibrate and niacin in coronary heart disease, JAMA 231:360-381, 1975.

34. Canner PL, et al: Fifteen year mortality in Coronary Drug Project patients: long-term benefit with niacin, J Am Coll Cardiol 8:1245-1255, 1986.

35. Lipid Research Clinics Program: The Lipid Research Clinics Coronary Primary Prevention Trial results. I. Reduction in incidence of coronary heart disease, JAMA 251:351-364, 1984.

36. Brensika JF, et al: Effects of therapy with cholestyramine on progression of coronary arteriosclerosis: results of the NHLBI Type II Coronary Intervention Study, Circulation 69:313-324, 1984.

37. Kane JP, et al: Normalization of low-density lipoprotein levels in heterozygous familial hypercholesterolemia with a combined drug regimen, N Engl J Med 304:251-258, 1980.

38. Moore, RB, et al: Plasma lipoproteins and coronary arteriography in subjects in the program on the surgical control of the hyperlipidemias: preliminary report, Atherosclerosis 32:101-119, 1979.

39. Ross R, Glomset JA: The pathogenesis of atherosclerosis. I and II, N Engl J Med 295(7):369-377, 295(8):420-425, 1976.

40. Dawber TT: The Framingham Study, Cambridge Mass, 1980, Harvard University Press.

41. Pooling Project Research Group: Relationship of blood pressure, serum cholesterol, smoking habit, relative weight, and ECG abnormalities to the incidence of major coronary events. Final report of the Pooling Project, Dallas, 1978, American Heart Association.

42. Keys A: Seven countries, Cambridge Mass, 1980, Harvard University Press.

43. Sherwin RW: Recent clinical trials of the preventability of coronary heart disease, Clin Nutr 3:128-130, 1984.

44. Multiple Risk Factor Intervention Trial Group: Multiple Risk Factor Intervention Trial. Risk factor changes and mortality results, JAMA 248:1465-1477, 1982.

45. Consensus Conference, National Institutes of Health: Lowering blood pressure to prevent heart disease, JAMA 253:2080-2086, 1985.

46. Kuller L, Reisler DM: An explanation for variations in distribution of stroke and arteriosclerotic heart disease among populations and racial groups, Am J Epidemiol 93:1-9, 1971.

CHAPTER 15
Renal System

Mackenzie Walser

The spectrum of clinical disturbances that characterize renal failure results primarily from an imbalance between excretory capacity and the intake of nutrients. For many ingested substances intake becomes excessive in the patient with renal failure, leading to accumulation with resulting clinical disturbances and also to compensatory responses that often have their own deleterious side effects. For other ingested substances intake may become inadequate because of renal wastage, increased requirements, or overzealous dietary restriction.

Thus the goal of nutritional management in renal failure is to adjust the intake of nutrients to meet the profoundly altered needs and capacities of the patient. If this goal can be achieved, many of the clinical disturbances seen in renal failure can be relieved.

Nonexcretory functions of the kidney are also impaired in renal failure. Among these are the hormonal functions of the kidney, such as its role in hormonal excretion and degradation, blood pressure regulation, erythropoiesis, and vitamin D activation. Impaired substrate-fuel functions of the kidney also contribute to the uremic state, such as alterations in amino acid metabolism and gluconeogenesis. Correction of these abnormalities is more difficult and often not possible by nutritional management. Nevertheless, these abnormalities significantly modify the strategy of nutritional therapy in such patients.

In the patient on chronic dialysis, a different spectrum of problems may emerge. Many but by no means all of them are nutritional. They are not generally the result of imbalance between intake and excretory capacity, since they may persist even when excretory capacity is increased by more frequent dialysis. They may arise from the failure of nonexcretory functions of the kidney, from the accumulation of trace substances derived from the dialysis water or equipment, or from the removal by dialysis of important constituents of body fluids. For discussions of the relationship between nutritional management and the particular techniques and schedule of dialysis the reader is referred elsewhere.[1-6]

Conservative nutritional management in the predialysis stage may in some cases slow progression of renal insufficiency (as measured by the rate of decline of glomerular filtration rate). The aspects of management that are most important in this respect and the results that can be achieved in different types of renal disease are as yet ill-defined. However, the obvious merit of slowing or halting the progression of renal failure, especially when compared with the difficulties and expense of dialysis and/or transplantation, makes this an area of high priority for investigation.

NITROGEN RETENTION

Accumulation of the nitrogenous products of metabolism is the hallmark of renal failure, since excretion of such products is a function performed almost exclusively by the kidney. The formation of these substances generally is regarded as obligatory, for their production continues even when protein intake is inadequate or in severe protein deficiency. Thus complete correction of the azotemic features of renal failure by nutritional means appears to be an unattainable goal.

Yet, this traditional view may have been overstated. In renal failure the rates of formation for all of the urinary components of waste nitrogen excretion are often far below the usually accepted "obligatory" minima. Furthermore, in starvation[7,8] or during prolonged oral or parenteral feeding of elemental diets[9] fecal nitrogen becomes much lower than so-called "endogenous" fecal nitrogen.[10]

The absence of any obligatory ureagenesis is demonstrated most strikingly in infants with complete defects of one of the first four enzymes of the urea cycle. Although these children make some urea, it is evidently derived entirely from dietary arginine via arginase and therefore does not represent the excretion of waste nitrogen.[11] Despite complete inability to excrete waste nitrogen as urea, these infants may grow normally for months or years on a diet severely restricted in protein, supplemented with essential amino acids and their nitrogen-free analogues.[12] In a study of patients with chronic renal failure receiving a defined formula diet by continuous nasogastric alimentation,[13] it was shown that all components of waste N excretion fall below usually accepted "obligatory" minima.

Urea Retention and Metabolism

As the major nitrogenous waste product under almost all conditions, urea is retained in every case of renal failure. The degree of urea retention is a useful index of the severity of the disorder, for it correlates more closely with symptomatology than does any other single measure. This is probably not a reflection of the toxicity of urea, but rather of the fact that urea accumulation reflects the accumulation of all products of protein catabolism. The serum urea nitrogen (SUN) level is a function of two independent processes: the net rate of urea formation and the renal clearance of urea. Hence the severity of uremic symptoms is determined both by the rate of protein catabolism and by the degree of impairment in renal function.

Urea production exceeds urea excretion in normal as well as uremic subjects.[14-24] The difference is attributable to urea degradation by bacterial urease in the gastrointestinal tract, producing carbamate, which rapidly decomposes to ammonia and carbon dioxide. The rate of this process can be expressed in three ways: (1) as grams per day of urea nitrogen converted to ammonia nitrogen, (2) as the extrarenal clearance of urea (the preceding quantity divided by the SUN), or (3) as the fraction of urea produced that is metabolized (the first quantity divided by the rate of production of urea nitrogen).

In normal subjects urea nitrogen degradation averages about 3 g/day, and extrarenal clearance of urea about 25 liters/day. In chronic uremic patients urea degradation is also about 3 g/day. It is unclear why this value is not higher given the elevated SUN levels. The extrarenal clearance of urea is much reduced in renal failure. When the third method of expressing urea degradation is used, the percentage rises from about 20% in normal subjects to 50% or even higher in renal failure. This is because the renal clearance of urea in uremic subjects is reduced even more than the extrarenal clearance. Hence the ratio of extrarenal clearance to total clearance (which is equal to the ratio of urea degradation to urea production) rises, even though degradation is normal and extrarenal clearance is subnormal.

Urea Nitrogen Appearance

The difference between the production and degradation of urea nitrogen has been termed urea nitrogen appearance,[25] usually expressed in grams of nitrogen per day. This is the quantity of protein nitrogen irreversibly converted to urea nitrogen and is therefore one component of the nitrogen balance calculation. Since the other components of waste nitrogen excretion are much less subject to variation than urea nitrogen appearance, the latter is closely correlated with total nitrogen output. In fact, this correlation is sufficiently close[26] that one can estimate total nitrogen output (and hence nitrogen balance, if intake is known) by measuring urea nitrogen appearance, a procedure far less cumbersome than measuring total nitrogen output in urine and feces.

When SUN is not changing, urea nitrogen excretion is equal to urea nitrogen appearance. This is usually (though not always) the case in normal subjects, in whom day-to-day fluctuations in the body urea pool are generally small compared to the rate of urea excretion. This can be readily seen by comparing the usual body urea nitrogen pool (about 15 mg/dl × 500 dl = 7.5 g) with the usual rate of urea nitrogen excretion (13 g/da). Thus the pool turns over about twice a day. In the uremic patient, however, day-to-day fluctuations in the urea nitrogen pool are significant compared to the rate of urea nitrogen excretion. For example, in a uremic subject ingesting a 40 g protein diet with a SUN of 100 mg/dl, the urea nitrogen pool is about 100 mg/dl × 500 dl (50 g) and the rate of urea nitrogen excretion is about 4 g/day. Hence the pool turns over about once a fortnight. Thus urea nitrogen appearance seldom equals urea nitrogen excretion in severe or moderately severe renal failure.

To measure changes in the urea nitrogen pool with greatest accuracy, the volume of distribution of urea must be determined. This can be done by injecting labeled urea[22] or by comparing the fall in blood urea induced by dialysis with the amount of urea removed in the dialysis fluid.[27] However, a simpler method can be used, which is probably adequate for clinical purposes. The volume of distribution of urea is nearly equal to total body water. In uremic subjects total body water as a fraction of body weight averages 60% ± 16% (SD)[14]—somewhat less than in young healthy normal subjects but probably not different from a comparably aged group of normal individuals. This value and daily SUN determination may be used to calculate the urea nitrogen pool on consecutive days. Changes in the volume of distribution of urea should also be accounted for by obtaining daily weights. Weight change nearly equals change in body water, since body solids (weight minus total body water) remain constant, in the short term.

To gauge nitrogen balance from urea nitrogen appearance and nitrogen intake ($0.16 \times$ protein intake), it is necessary to estimate the rate of nitrogen excretion in forms other than urea. In patients with chronic renal failure receiving dietary therapy, this quantity is 37 mg/kg/day.[28] Urea nitrogen appearance also can be used to estimate the level at which SUN will stabilize when it is changing, since steady-state SUN equals urea nitrogen appearance divided by renal clearance of urea.

In summary, urea nitrogen appearance, a quantity useful in evaluating nutrition in renal failure, is obtained most simply by measuring SUN, body weight, and 24-hour urea nitrogen excretion on several successive days. Using an assumed value for body water on the first day, and estimating body water on each successive day as this value plus change in weight (if any), one can readily obtain values for urea space and hence urea nitrogen pool. The rate of change of this pool in grams of nitrogen per day then can be determined by drawing a line or curve through these points. The rate of change of the urea nitrogen pool plus the urea nitrogen excretion equals urea nitrogen appearance.

Urea Nitrogen Reutilization

For many years it was believed that urea nitrogen was reutilized (after degradation to ammonia nitrogen) in patients with renal failure, especially in those receiving protein-restricted diets and/or nitrogen-free analogues of essential amino acids. The evidence for this premise is now seen to have been faulty. Most of the data used to support it consisted of measurements of (1) circulating amino acids labeled with ^{15}N or (2) protein after the administration of ^{15}N-labeled urea or ammonia.[29] It was not appreciated that, even when the net flux of the glutamate dehydrogenase reaction (which must precede the utilization of ammonia for amino acid synthesis) was from glutamate to ammonia rather than the reverse, adding labeled ammonia would label the glutamate nitrogen. When degradation has been suppressed in uremic patients given such regimens, nitrogen balance improved rather than worsened.[30] Thus urea degradation serves no useful purpose in renal failure, and urea nitrogen is not reutilized in such subjects.

Urea Toxicity

The toxicity of urea has been a subject of debate for many years. Most workers now agree that urea is completely nontoxic at steady-state SUN levels below 100 mg/dl. Induction of such levels in normal subjects by urea loading causes a transient headache owing to osmotic disequilibrium across the blood-brain barrier. However, such levels maintained chronically exert no effects other than mild osmotic diuresis. On the other hand, SUN levels above 150 mg/dl usually are associated with symptoms. That these symptoms may be ascribed to urea itself was shown by adding urea to the dialysis bath in uremic patients undergoing regular dialysis[31]; a variety of symptoms, including nausea, vomiting, lethargy, and tremors, appeared as SUN levels increased above 150 mg/dl.

Creatine and Creatinine

Creatine and creatine phosphate, located chiefly in muscle, are continuously converted to creatinine nonenzymatically at a rate of about 1.7% per day.[32] The resulting creatinine is excreted nearly quantitatively in normal subjects and is thus a measure of muscle mass, provided dietary sources of creatine and creatinine are minor. In renal failure, however, a significant fraction of creatinine production (as is the case with urea) is not excreted in the urine.[33-35] Presumably it is metabolized by intestinal bacteria, though this never has been proved conclusively. Whether the metabolic products of creatinine are toxic is also uncertain, although there are reasons to believe that they are. The importance of this finding is that urinary creatinine output ceases to be a measure of lean body mass in renal failure (except in the early stages). In addition, serum creatinine underestimates the degree of reduction of glomerular filtration rate as renal failure approaches the end stage. In patients with severe renal failure, correction of the serum creatinine level for creatinine metabolism proportional to serum creatinine yields an estimate for creatinine clearance that closely correlates with the measured value[35] (Fig. 15-1). Nevertheless, the disparity between predicted and observed clearances in individual patients becomes substantial when clearances are very low.

It has been suggested that the ratio of SUN to serum creatinine can be used as an indicator of urea nitrogen appearance and thus of protein intake in chronic uremic subjects, since urea appearance reflects protein intake while creatinine excretion is only slightly affected.[36] However, this technique can give quite misleading results because creatinine appearance diminishes in severe renal failure and consequently the ratio tends to rise as renal failure progresses, even though urea appearance and the ratio of urea clearance to creatinine clearance remain constant.

A clinical dictum holds that creatinine production increases in acute renal failure when associated with rhabdomyolysis. This would be surprising, since the conversion of creatine to creatinine occurs by a nonenzymatic process that should proceed at the same rate whether creatine is intracellular or has leaked into the extracellular space. Furthermore, a recent study in dogs with experimental renal failure[37] has failed to support this dictum. Cell membrane damage should not release creatinine into the extracellular space[38] because creatinine is quite uniformly distributed throughout body water.[34] Noncreatinine chromogens may be responsible for part of the apparent increase in creatinine production.

Other Nitrogenous Waste Products

In addition to urea and creatinine, other components of nitrogen excretion are reduced in chronic renal failure. These include uric acid,

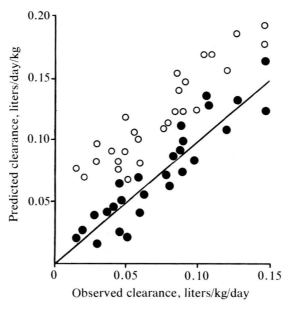

Figure 15-1 Creatinine clearance predicted from serum creatinine, age, and sex in relation to measured 24-hour clearances in 27 patients with chronic renal failure *(open symbols)*. The creatinine clearance is consistently overestimated, especially when it is severely reduced (normal 2.7 liters/kg/da). With a constant extrarenal clearance of 0.0475 liter/kg/day *(solid symbols)*, the prediction is improved.

From Mitch WE, et al: Clin Sci **58:**327-335, 1980.

which is metabolized in the gut at an increased rate in renal failure,[39] and ammonia, which is excreted at a high rate per unit of glomerular filtrate but a low rate in absolute terms.[40]

An important point to consider in designing nutritional therapy is proteinuria. The loss of 5 g/day of urinary protein, for example, must increase dietary protein requirements by at least 5 g/day (probably more, since protein synthesis is not 100% efficient).

Fecal nitrogen excretion in renal failure is usually normal or slightly higher than normal. An important source of abnormally high protein requirements is occult gastrointestinal bleeding. Not only are peptic ulcers more common in renal failure than they are in the general population, but slow oozing, usually from unidentified sources, also becomes very common in severely azotemic patients.[41] Fecal nitrogen may or may not be increased by bleeding; even if it is not, protein requirements are likely to increase because the digested and reabsorbed hemoglobin and plasma proteins cannot be resynthesized with complete efficiency. Tests for occult blood obviously become important in following such patients.

Protein Restriction

Since the average protein intake in developed countries exceeds the daily requirements, restriction of dietary protein is an obvious and time-honored technique for reducing the azotemic symptoms of renal failure. An intake of 40 g/day/70 kg of body weight will usually maintain nitrogen balance, provided requirements are not unusually large for one of the reasons just noted. Such a diet is readily tolerated by most patients. The resulting fall in SUN is proportionally greater than the reduction in protein intake, because the nonurea components of nitrogen excretion will be little affected and will remain at approximately 2.5 g/day (the amount of nitrogen found in about 15 g of protein). For example, reduction of protein intake from 80 to 40 g/day will reduce urea nitrogen appearance from $(80 \times 0.16) - 2.5$ or 10.3 g/day to $(40 \times 0.16) - 2.5$ or 3.9 g/day.

In designing low protein diets, a skilled dietitian should be consulted not only for the original diet prescription but also for periodic conferences to assess compliance and make modifications when needed.

Modification of Protein Quality

The limiting factor that determines protein requirements is the available essential amino acid content of the ingested protein. As is well known from nutritional studies in normal animals and humans, the quantity of protein (or the dose of a mixture of amino acids) needed to sustain nitrogen balance or to promote growth is determined by its content of one or more limiting essential amino acids. Using essential amino acids combined in proportions optimized for young healthy adults, it has been shown that as little as 7 g/day of this mixture, if supplemented by about 2.5 g of nitrogen from nonessential amino acids, will maintain nitrogen balance.[42] Larger amounts are required in growing children.

In patients with chronic renal failure nitrogen balance can be maintained on as little as 20 to 25 g of protein per day, if it is supplied almost entirely as protein rich in essential amino acids and balanced with respect to human needs, at least according to some workers.[43,44] However, these results have been disputed in other studies.

In practice the use of such high-quality protein diets has not proved popular, even when the diets have been modified for different cultural preferences, including vegetarianism. Their monotony has been the main obstacle to patient acceptance.

Essential Amino Acid Supplements

An alternative means of reducing azotemia involves providing essential amino acids as such, along with a nearly protein-free diet.[44] This also has proved unacceptable to most patients. However, a modification of the regimen has been much better tolerated and achieved nearly the same results. Essential amino acids are provided as a supplement to a diet containing 15 to 25 g of protein unrestricted as to quality.[45] The advantage of this regimen is that wide variety can be achieved in the diet, with the supplement providing most of the essential amino acid requirements. Indeed, patients may prefer this regimen to a diet containing 40 g of predominantly high-quality protein.[46]

In diets containing less than 40 g of protein, it may be helpful to provide a significant portion of caloric needs in the form of an electrolyte-free, nitrogen-free, oligosaccharide preparation. Many such products are available in liquid or powder form. They vary in their sweetness (some are nearly tasteless) and also in sodium content; some contain significant amounts of sodium.

Amino acid supplements containing all nine essential amino acids are available in tablet form (Aminess). A preparation is also on the market containing eight essential amino acids plus oligosaccharides, taken as a chilled slurry (Amin-Aid). To receive 3 g of essential amino acid nitrogen in this form, it is necessary to ingest 2700 calories. A higher proportion of amino acids would be more practical. In addition, many patients find the taste offensive.

Clinical results obtained in patients treated with a diet containing 15 to 25 g of protein unselected as to quality and supplemented with 10 to 20 g/day of essential amino acids have been impressive. Uremic symptoms abated rapidly, and patients noticed an increase in strength and vigor. Acidosis, which was occasionally troublesome when the basic amino acids in these supplements were given as chloride salts, ceased being a problem when histidine base and lysine acetate were used. Hyperkalemia was reported

in one series but has not been observed by other workers. Nutrition has been maintained on long-term therapy.[47] Children also have been maintained this way and exhibited improved growth,[48,49] although compliance was a problem with outpatients.

All of these essential amino acid supplements have contained either eight or nine amino acids in the proportions required by normal subjects. Despite the successful clinical results with this regimen, there are reasons to believe that these proportions are not optimal for the patient with renal failure. This evidence derives from three sources: (1) the plasma or intracellular concentrations of free amino acids in uremic patients, (2) the rate of disposal of loads of individual amino acids given as tracer injections or as unlabeled amino acids, and (3) the effect on plasma amino acid patterns of dietary restriction of one or more amino acids. Fig. 15-2 illustrates the plasma pattern in chronic renal failure calculated as percentages of normal values and displayed on a semilogarithmic scale so decreases are emphasized as much as increases. The results

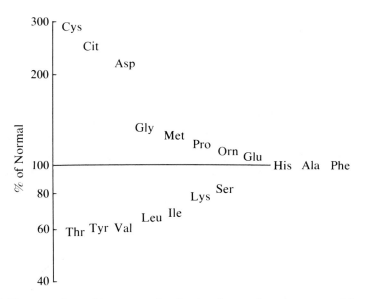

Figure 15-2 Plasma amino acid concentration in chronic uremic patients treated by protein restriction alone calculated as a percentage of normal and averaged over six published studies. To emphasize decreases as much as increases, a logarithmic scale has been used. The most abnormal values are shown on the left. In view of the variety of sources of the data, statistical significance cannot be evaluated.

From Mitch WE, Walser M: In Brenner BM, Rector FC, editors: The kidney, Philadelphia, 1986, WB Saunders Co, pp 1757-1790.

shown are means of several studies reported in the literature, using the normal values in each series for comparison. Included are patients on protein restriction alone and patients receiving supplements of essential amino acids and/or their nitrogen-free analogues, differences between results on these regimens being minor. The figure shows that, of the essential amino acids, the levels of branched-chain compounds (valine, leucine, isoleucine), lysine, and threonine are the lowest in plasma. Methionine is elevated, and cystine is increased substantially. Furthermore, other sulfur amino acids (including cystathionine, cysteic acid, homocysteic acid, taurine, N-monoacetylcystine, homocysteine, and cysteine-homocysteine disulfide) are markedly increased.[50-52] The two last-named compounds may contribute to vascular injury. Phenylalanine is normal but its metabolic product, tyrosine, is quite subnormal. Tryptophan, unlike other amino acids, is substantially protein-bound, and thus total tryptophan concentration may have little meaning. The protein-binding of tryptophan is decreased in renal failure, but studies of free tryptophan concentration[53-55] are contradictory. Histidine and arginine usually are found to be low normal or slightly subnormal.

One comparable study of intracellular amino acids in muscle[56] has been reported in adult patients, with somewhat different results. In particular, the apparent extracellular deficiency of valine was also found in muscle but the deficiency of leucine and isoleucine was not; histidine and ornithine were reported to be subnormal intracellularly. Erythrocyte patterns of free amino acid levels in uremic patients are not substantially different from the plasma pattern,[57] except for increased histidine and alanine. In leukocytes, branched-chain amino acids, methionine, and ornithine are subnormal.[58] Cerebrospinal fluid levels also tend to be altered in the same direction as the plasma levels.[59]

If intracellular patterns in these tissues reflect the disturbances intracellularly in more vital organs, such as liver, heart, or brain, it would be reasonable to design therapy based on these measurements. Analysis of liver and brain of uremic rats has been performed[60,61] but is obviously impractical in humans.

Tentative inferences may be drawn from these studies: uremic patients receiving a 20-25 g protein diet of unselected quality should receive a supplement relatively high in valine, lysine, and threonine, with some isoleucine and leucine, and containing tyrosine, histidine, and possibly arginine (or better yet its guanidine-free precursor, ornithine) but little or no methionine, phenylalanine, or tryptophan.

Addition of tyrosine to a complete essential amino acid supplement has led to improved protein nutrition in a study of patients with chronic renal failure.[62]

In another study[63] uremic subjects receiving a virtually protein-free diet supplemented by eight amino acids exhibited a rapid fall in plasma histidine and eventually negative nitrogen balance associated with malaise and an erythematous scaling rash, all corrected by the addition of histidine to the supplement.

A supplement modified to contain more valine, and with tyrosine added, has resulted in a more nearly normal muscle amino acid pattern[64] and positive nitrogen balance.[65] These data support the view that valine deficiency is more pronounced in chronic renal failure than are deficiencies of other essential amino acids.

Studies of experimental chronic renal failure in animals have attempted to define the ideal amino acid formulation. Although these are of substantial interest, their applicability to renal failure in humans is uncertain.

Supplements Containing Nitrogen-Free Analogues of Essential Amino Acids

The suggestion[29,66] to use alpha-keto analogues of essential amino acids instead of essential amino acids themselves was based on (1) animal studies showing that the analogues of all of the essential amino acids except lysine and threonine could support growth (though usually with reduced efficiency) in rats on diets devoid of the corresponding essential amino acids; and (2) the concept of urea nitrogen reutilization in uremia, now known to be incorrect. In these studies of animals as well as in early studies of the utilization of single ketoacids in humans an isonitrogenous source of nitrogen was added to the diet when the ketoacid replaced its corresponding essential amino acid. Thus a reduction in SUN would not have been expected and was not seen.

In chronic uremic patients treated with a supplement containing five to seven keto analogues of essential amino acids plus the remaining essential amino acids, urea nitrogen appearance fell and nitrogen balance improved, provided the initial SUN was not too high.[67]

Later it was found that the D,L-hydroxy analogue of methionine, long used as a supplement in animal feeds, could be substituted for the keto analogue, which is much harder to synthesize.[68]

Experience with supplements containing keto analogues of valine, leucine, isoleucine, the keto or hydroxy analogue of phenylalanine, the hydroxy analogue of methionine, and the four remaining essential amino acids has been summarized.[69] Some of these studies have included comparisons of the efficacy of this regimen with one in which all the essential amino acids were supplied as such. In general, the results have shown that neither supplement is particularly effective unless protein intake is restricted to about 25 g/day or less. When it is, the analogue-based supplement produces somewhat more favorable results in terms of SUN, nitrogen balance, and measures of protein nutrition, including selected serum proteins, hemoglobin, and nerve conduction velocity.

Gastrointestinal intolerance has been fairly common in these studies, perhaps because of the high calcium content of the supplement (the analogues were added as calcium salts). Dosage has varied from 9 to 16 g/day. The only other side effect noted has been hypercalcemia, occurring at one time or another in about 57 patients on long-term therapy with the higher dose in one study.[70] In only one of these 57 patients was hypercalcemia pronounced (12 mg/dl) or clinically significant.

Analogue-based supplements are not currently available commercially in the United States, although they are in Europe. Improved formulations in which the calcium salts of keto acids have been replaced with ornithine, lysine, and histidine salts of keto acids, tyrosine has been added, and phenylalanine and tryptophan have been omitted are currently under study.[71-73] The mixed salts formed between basic amino acids and branched-chain keto acids have the advantage of greater solubility and improved palatability. Since the keto analogue of leucine, in particular, spares nitrogen under circumstances in which leucine does not,[74] probably because it inhibits protein breakdown,[75] these analogue-based supplements may have some advantage over amino acids given as such.

Energy Requirements for Nitrogen Sparing

The recommended daily allowances of energy intake for adult men and women aged 23 to 50 years doing light work are 38 and 36 kcal/kg, respectively; for older men and women these figures are 34 and 33 kcal/kg respectively.[76] In children energy requirements are substantially higher because the energy cost of weight gain is about 5 kcal/g.[77]

The same energy requirements may apply to patients with chronic renal failure; however, in normal individuals higher energy intakes are needed to maintain nitrogen balance on protein-restricted diets. There is some evidence[78] that nitrogen balance continues to improve in uremic patients on low-protein diets up to and including 55 kcal/kg, although others[62] have failed to confirm these findings in studies of adults with chronic renal failure. There is no doubt that at least 35 kcal/kg is required for optimal nitrogen balance in uremic adults[79] and that caloric intake is a critical factor in the growth of uremic children.[80] As a practical matter, however, it is difficult to persuade patients to consume more calories than their appetite dictates; more progress can be made by improving the composition of the dietary regimen than by forcing calories.

Parenteral Nutrition with Essential Amino Acids

In predialysis uremic patients unable to consume adequate amounts of food, it is often advantageous to administer essential amino acids intravenously. This can be done via a peripheral vein without excessive fluid load and should be considered in any patient whose intake of essential amino acids by mouth is inadequate. The use of such solutions in acute renal failure often attenuates the rise in SUN,[81] but early reports that recovery of renal function or mortality rate is favorably affected have not been confirmed.

Tube Feeding with Essential Amino Acids and/or Keto Acids

Continuous nasogastric alimentation via a small-bore tube offers promise as an alternative approach in certain circumstances.[13] Connecting the tube to a portable infusion pump makes it possible for the patient to be ambulatory and to receive not only the needed amino acids but also optimum caloric intake throughout the 24 hours, thus suppressing nocturnal gluconeogenesis. Provision of about two thirds of caloric and nitrogen intake in this way along with three small meals can lead to substantial improvement in azotemia and nitrogen balance.[82] This approach is applicable only in hospitalized patients who are in a transition phase, such as those awaiting the maturation of an arteriovenous fistula. It should be noted, however, that either enteral or parenteral nutrition can induce a rapid reduction of hyperphosphatemia in renal failure[83] and this alteration itself may limit damage to the kidney by deposition of calcium phosphate.

Long-Term Effects of Dietary Therapy on Protein Nutrition

One objection to the nutritional therapy of uremia is that prolonged protein restriction may sap the patient's vitality and make him a poor candidate for dialysis and/or transplantation. There is, in fact, little evidence for this view. Patients treated with a 20 g protein diet plus essential amino acids for 1 year showed no change in lean body mass, as measured by total body potassium and total body water, except when illness prevented adequate caloric intake.[47] Other investigators[84] also have found normal total body potassium in conservatively managed patients.

Phosphate Retention and its Consequences

Hyperphosphatemia, hypocalcemia, secondary hyperparathyroidism, and vitamin D deficiency are all characteristic of severe uremia and major contributors to the clinical disturbances seen. Much debate has taken place as to which of these problems is primary and which are secondary.

The most widely accepted theory[85] holds that impairment in the renal activation of vitamin D occurs early in the course of renal failure and results in vitamin D deficiency with consequent hypocalcemia, hyperphosphatemia, and demineralization of bone. Hyperparathyroidism, according to this view, begins as a response to vitamin D deficiency and only later is perpetuated by phosphate retention. There is evidence to support this theory,[86] most workers agreeing that deficiency of 1,25-dihydroxycholecalciferol (the most active metabolite of vitamin D) can be detected early in renal failure in adults[87,88] as well as children.[89] According to the opposing view,[90] retention of phosphate, especially postprandi-

ally, is the initiating event causing secondary hyperparathyroidism, and vitamin D deficiency only appears later.

These differing theories have important implications for the therapeutic modalities chosen to correct the divalent ion abnormalities of chronic renal failure. These include dietary phosphate restriction and the oral administration of phosphate-binding antacids, calcium supplements, and the use of one of the available forms of vitamin D. Each of these measures tends to counteract secondary hyperparathyroidism and renal osteodystrophy. Each also can be hazardous when overdone.

Phosphate restriction alone rarely leads to significant phosphate depletion, but overzealous use of aluminum-containing antacids, particularly in early renal failure, can cause significant phosphate depletion. In general, serum phosphate levels of 2 mg/dl or higher are rarely if ever associated with symptomatic phosphate depletion, although there is the theoretical possibility of aggravating renal osteodystrophy by prolonged hypophosphatemia of this degree. Careful monitoring of serum phosphate generally will prevent any ill effects from phosphate depletion.

Hyperphosphatemia is much more common in the later stages of chronic renal failure. It is important to correct this abnormality, not only because it may contribute to secondary hyperparathyroidism but also because it may accelerate the progression of renal insufficiency. The use of basic aluminum salts without dietary phosphorus restriction is to be deplored. Significant aluminum absorption occurs and tissue levels of aluminum increase; osteomalacia, resistant to vitamin D, may develop on prolonged use.[91,92] A microcytic anemia may also occur.[93] Mild dietary phosphate restriction is accomplished readily by eliminating milk and milk products from the diet. Severe phosphate restriction is difficult but is facilitated by low-protein regimens.

Calcium supplementation can be provided as calcium carbonate. In children, an aqueous suspension of $CaCO_3$ can be used in place of tablets. Early in renal failure, this measure may help to prevent hyperparathyroidism and renal osteodystrophy and may reduce phosphate retention by inhibiting the intestinal absorption of phosphate as effectively as does $Al(OH)_3$.[94] However, when hyperphosphatemia is present there is a danger of aggravating renal insufficiency by oral calcium administration. This evidently occurs whenever the serum Ca × P product is elevated by such therapy and presumably reflects deposition of these minerals in the renal parenchyma.[95]

Vitamin D can be given as its most active metabolite, 1,25-dihydroxycholecalciferol, or one of the less potent but nevertheless efficacious derivatives now available. These are particularly useful in dialysis patients, but their administration in the predialysis phase is the subject of debate. Since serum phosphate rises as calcium rises during vitamin D administration, the progression of renal insufficiency can be accelerated by the use of these agents.[96-100] There are suggestions that this may occur even if hypercalcemia is avoided by frequent monitoring of serum calcium, which danger is greatest in the later stages of renal failure and in patients who are hyperphosphatemic. In such patients vitamin D should not be given unless hypocalcemia of significant degree persists despite control of serum phosphate. However, in early renal failure active forms of vitamin D appear to offer promise of preventing hyperparathyroidism with little risk of renal damage.

Magnesium deficiency, if present, should be corrected even if the patient is without symptoms. The use of antacids containing magnesium in patients with renal failure is risky because of the danger of hypermagnesemia, owing to limitation in the renal excretory capacity for magnesium.

MANAGEMENT OF ACID-BASE BALANCE

The degree of renal bicarbonate wastage varies widely among patients with chronic renal failure. It must be compensated by administering sufficient sodium bicarbonate to prevent symptomatic acidosis. This usually means keeping the serum bicarbonate level above 16 mM. In some patients no bicarbonate is required; in those with renal tubular acidosis as a component of their nephropathy, large amounts may be required. In children with renal tubular acidosis, giving sufficient bicarbonate to compensate for their renal losses leads to substantially improved growth as well as reduced symptoms.[101] The NaHCO₃ requirement in renal failure must take precedence over other electrolyte problems, because it in turn conditions the optimum intake of salt and of potassium. If acidosis cannot be counteracted without giving so much NaHCO₃ that clinically significant expansion of extracellular fluid volume occurs, dialysis must be initiated.

Calcium salts also have been used (especially in Europe) to combat acidosis. This approach is based on a very tenuous rationale: unless the NaHCO₃ content of the extracellular fluid volume is increased, acidosis will not improve. The only ways in which calcium salts can increase the NaHCO₃ content of the extracellular fluid are by calcium-sodium exchange at the bone surface and by suppression of secondary hyperparathyroidism, which contributes to bicarbonate wastage. If the administered calcium remained in the extracellular fluid, dangerous hypercalcemia would supervene. The temporary efficacy of calcium salts in combating uremic acidosis is attributable to one or the other of these mechanisms, but calcium-sodium exchange at the bone surface can continue only for a short time. Furthermore, the ability of calcium supplementation to suppress secondary hyperparathyroidism is limited. And finally, as noted earlier, calcium salts can damage the kidney unless the serum Ca × P product is prevented from rising to abnormal levels. Thus the use of calcium salts to treat uremic acidosis on a long-term basis is inadvisable and ineffective.

Management of Salt Balance

Although sodium retention often is viewed as characteristic of renal failure, renal excretion of an abnormally high fraction of the filtered sodium load is the rule. This does not mean salt wastage; on the contrary, total 24-hour salt output is commonly less than average. Rather, it reflects the fact that the glomerular filtration rate (GFR) is reduced more than the sodium clearance (C_{Na}). Consequently, the ratio C_{Na}:GFR, which equals the fraction of filtered sodium excreted, is almost invariably high. The mechanism that causes this adaptation has been postulated to involve an unidentified natriuretic hormone. It also has been shown[102] that very slow and cautious reduction of sodium intake eventually can correct this abnormality in some patients—at the cost of ingesting an extremely unpalatable diet. However, attempts to reduce salt intake or to promote diuresis, especially if vigorously pursued, lead to dehydration, with an attendant fall in GFR from which the patient may not recover. Dehydration occurs because the natriuresis per nephron often continues even as extracellular volume falls below optimal, especially when the reduction in volume is rapid. Thus the use of vigorous diuretic measures to reduce extracellular fluid volume in chronic renal failure can hasten the need for dialysis.

On the other hand, many or most patients appear to benefit from the addition of furosemide in doses of 80 to 240 mg/day. The drug maintains diuretic efficacy in renal failure (though larger doses are required). Its use permits the patient to ingest more salt, and adjustments in diuretic dosage are easier to accomplish than adjustments in salt intake. Thiazides also may be used for this purpose; their GFR-lowering effect is evidently only transient. The usual side effects occur with both classes of drugs, and deafness with furosemide can be a particularly troublesome problem. Contrary to some texts, this deafness is not always reversible on withdrawing the drug.[103]

Thus the dietary therapy of chronic renal failure usually entails some degree of salt restriction, determined by the patient's $NaHCO_3$ requirement and characteristic rate of sodium excretion and by the response to chronic diuretic therapy.

Overdiuresis can be detected early by a postural change in blood pressure; soon serum creatinine will increase. Overhydration should be judged not on the presence or absence of dependent edema but rather on the presence or absence of pulmonary rales or signs of increased systemic venous pressure such as pulsating neck veins at 60° or more.

Management of Water Balance

Most patients with chronic renal failure have an intact thirst mechanism, despite impairment of urinary concentrating and diluting ability. Consequently they usually maintain a normal or modestly low serum sodium concentration and effective plasma osmolality. In a minority of patients dilutional hyponatremia becomes a problem. In these individuals water intake must be restricted, sometimes severely (i.e., 800 to 1000 ml/da). Hypertonic saline never should be used to treat hyponatremia, since it may precipitate pulmonary edema.

Potassium

Total body potassium stores are reported to be normal in most adult patients with chronic renal failure,[84] although they are often reduced in uremic children despite a normal serum potassium level.[104] Extracellular hyperkalemia may be dangerous even if the intracellular potassium stores are subnormal. Hyperaldosteronism in renal failure[105] may aggravate potassium deficiency, and occasionally the opposite may occur. Therapy of hyperkalemia is generally not dietary, because these patients already are on a restricted diet, but consists instead of giving potassium-binding resins by mouth (or if necessary rectally) when serum potassium is high (over 5.5 mM). Oral potassium supplements may be used in rare cases when hypokalemia is a problem. Supplemental oral potassium is available in forms that release the ion slowly into the gut and entail no risk of inducing small bowel ulceration.

Vitamins

The vitamin needs of the patient with chronic renal failure are different from those of normal subjects. Vitamin A levels are usually above normal, and supplementation is not only unnecessary but probably harmful.

The use of supplementary vitamin D in the commonly available form (vitamin D_3) is generally ineffective, because activation of vitamin D occurs in the kidney. As mentioned previously, the active derivatives of vitamin D, such as 1,25-dihydroxycholecalciferol, 24,25-dihydroxycholecalciferol, 1-hydroxycholecalciferol, or dihydrotachysterol, all of which are effective in chronic renal failure patients, are potentially useful in early renal failure (before hyperphosphatemia occurs) but hazardous in severe renal failure in the predialysis phase because such patients are usually hyperphosphatemic and renal damage is readily induced. Even in the earlier stages careful monitoring of serum calcium, phosphate, and creatinine is important in the use of these agents.

Supplements of vitamin C and of the B vitamins are usually provided in restricted diets in which a major portion of the intake of carbohydrate and amino acids is given as "elemental" or defined products, which are free of vitamins. Pyridoxine and folic acid may be required in greater than usual amounts. Again, this is particularly true of patients receiving more or less defined diets.

Effect of Nutritional and Drug Therapy on Progression

Chronic renal failure usually is characterized by inexorable progression. The rate of progression varies widely among patients, but it tends to be slower in some conditions (e.g., polycystic disease), and faster in others (hypertension with arteriolar nephrosclerosis). Although this progression traditionally has been viewed as irreversible and attributable to the underlying disease process, there is also longstanding evidence in both animals and humans that high protein intakes can accelerate progression. More recently it has become clear that progression can be slowed or even arrested by a number of dietary and pharmacologic maneuvers.

Of the several mechanisms that may play a role in progression, one is phosphate retention. As noted nearly 50 years ago,[106] the kidneys of animals with chronic renal failure develop substantial deposits of calcium and phosphate in the renal parenchyma and this process can be ameliorated by parathyroidectomy. Evidently both a high serum Ca × P product and secondary hyperparathyroidism independently can promote the renal deposition of calcium and phosphate. Thus any therapeutic approach that reduces the Ca × P product or attenuates secondary hyperparathyroidism might offer some chance of slowing progression. Although this does occur in animals,[107] in patients with end-stage or near end-stage renal failure, controlling serum phosphate at a low normal level becomes difficult and slows or halts progression only in a minority of cases.[108] However, when serum calcium and phosphate are maintained at normal levels in early renal failure by the use of phosphate binders, calcium supplements, and in one study[109] an analogue of vitamin D, progression may be arrested for years in unselected groups of patients, including all the common types of chronic renal failure.[110]

Protein restriction may slow progression by reducing the stimulus to hyperfiltration and glomerular hypertension in residual nephrons.[111] At least in rats (though not in dogs), this compensatory response to loss of nephrons appears to induce progressive glomerulosclerosis.

Control of hypertension can have dramatic effects on the progression of renal failure in patients whose primary disorder is malignant hypertension. Even in the nonmalignant type of hypertension commonly seen as a secondary event in renal failure, control of blood pressure by drugs often slows progression.[112] Angiotensin-converting enzyme inhibitors appear to be particularly effective in slowing progression.[113]

Ketoacid supplements are more effective than amino acid supplements in slowing progression when added to a low-protein low-phosphorus diet.[114] The mechanism is unknown, but it could be related to one or more of the effects of these substances on the intermediary metabolism of the uremic state, which include suppression of secondary hyperparathyroidism,[115] reduction of protein degradation,[74,75] reduction of hypertriglyceridemia,[116] and decrease in glucose intolerance and insulin resistance.[117]

In diabetic nephropathy, antihypertensive therapy, notably with angiotensin-converting enzyme inhibitors, may slow progression toward the end stage,[118,119] but improved glycemic control does not seem to help.[120]

A variety of other mechanisms of progression have been suggested from experimental work and are now under clinical study, including thromboxane production, oxalate accumulation, and altered proportions of dietary fats.

REFERENCES

1. Kopple JD: Dietary requirements. In Massry SG, Sellers AL, editors: Clinical aspects of uremia and dialysis, Springfield Ill, 1976, Charles C Thomas Publisher, pp 453-489.
2. Guarnieri G, et al: Simple methods for nutritional assessment in hemodialyzed patients, Am J Clin Nutr 33:1598-1607, 1980.
3. Kluthe R, et al: Protein requirements in maintenance hemodialysis, Am J Clin Nutr 31:1812-1820, 1978.
4. Wolfson M, Kopple JD: Nutritional status in apparently healthy hemodialyzed patients, Kidney Int 19:160-161, 1981.
5. Farrell PC, Hone PW: Dialysis-induced catabolism, Am J Clin Nutr 33:1417-1422, 1980.
6. Mitch WE, Sapir DG: Evaluation of reduced dialysis frequency using nutritional therapy, Kidney Int 20:122-126, 1981.
7. Adibi SA, et al: Alteration in the urinary excretion rate of amino acids and nitrogen by dietary means in obese and normal human subjects, J Lab Clin Med 77:278-289, 1971.
8. Owen OE, et al: Liver and kidney metabolism during prolonged starvation, J Clin Invest 48:574-583, 1969.
9. Bury KD, et al: Chemically defined diets, Can J Surg 17:124-134, 1974.
10. Munro HN: An introduction to nutritional aspects of pro-

tein metabolism. In Munro HN, Allison JB, editors: Mammalian protein metabolism, vol 2, New York, 1964, Academic Press Inc, pp 3-39.

11. Walser M, et al: Nitrogen metabolism in neonatal citrullinaemia, Clin Sci Mol Med **53:**173-181, 1977.

12. Walser M: Urea cycle disorders and other hereditary hyperammonemic syndromes. In Stanbury JB, et al, editors: The metabolic basis of inherited disease, ed 5, New York, 1982, McGraw-Hill International Book Co, pp 402-438.

13. Abras E, Walser M: Nitrogen utilization in uremic patients fed by continuous nasogastric infusion, Kidney Int **22:**392-397, 1982.

14. Walser M, Bodenlos LJ: Urea metabolism in man, J Clin Invest **38:**1617-1626, 1959.

15. Jones EA: Enterohepatic circulation of urea nitrogen, Clin Sci **37:**825-836, 1969.

16. Murdaugh HV Jr: Urea metabolism and low protein intake: studies in man and dog. In Schmidt-Neilsen B, Kerr DNS, editors: Urea and the kidney, Amsterdam, 1970, Excerpta Medica Foundation, pp 471-477.

17. Walser M, Dlabl P: Urea metabolism. In Proceedings: Conference on Adequacy of Dialysis, sponsored by the Artificial Kidney–Chronic Uremia Program, National Institute of Arthritis, Metabolism, and Digestive Diseases, Monterey, Calif, March 20-22, 1974.

18. Varcoe R, et al: Efficiency of utilisation of urea nitrogen for albumin synthesis by chronically uraemic and normal man, Clin Sci Mol Med **48:**379-390, 1975.

19. Gibson JA, et al: The role of the colon in urea metabolism in man, Clin Sci Mol Med **50:**51-59, 1976.

20. Long CL, et al: Metabolism and recycling of urea in man, Am J Clin Nutr **31:**1367-1382, 1978.

21. Robson AM: Urea metabolism in chronic renal failure. Thesis submitted for the degree of Doctor of Medicine, University of Newcastle Upon Tyne, England, 1964.

22. Walser M: Urea metabolism in chronic renal failure, J Clin Invest **53:**1385-1392, 1974.

23. Walser M: Use of isotopic urea to study the distribution and degradation of urea in man. In Schmidt-Neilsen B, Kerr DNS, editors: Urea and the kidney, Amsterdam, 1970, Excerpta Medica Foundation, pp 421-429.

24. Mitch WE, et al: Effects of oral neomycin and kanamycin in chronic uremic patients. I. Urea metabolism, Kidney Int **11:**116-122, 1977.

25. Walser M, et al: The effect of keto-analogues of essential amino acids in severe chronic uremia, J Clin Invest **52:**678-690, 1973.

26. Grodstein GP, et al: Nutritional and metabolic response to catabolic stress in uremia, Am J Clin Nutr **33:**1411-1416, 1980.

27. Sargent J, et al: Urea kinetics: a guide to nutritional management of renal failure, Am J Clin Nutr **31:**1696-1704, 1978.

28. Maroni BJ, et al: A method for estimating nitrogen intake of patients with chronic failure, Kidney Int **27:**58-65, 1985.

29. Richards P, et al: Utilization of ammonia nitrogen for protein synthesis in man and the effect of protein restriction and uremia, Lancet **2:**845-848, 1967.

30. Mitch WE, Walser M: Effect of oral neomycin and kanamycin in chronic uremic patients. II. Nitrogen balance, Kidney Int **11:**123-128, 1977.

31. Johnson WJ, et al: Effects of urea loading in patients with far-advanced renal failure, Mayo Clin Proc **47:**21-29, 1972.

32. Heymsfield SB, et al: Measurement of muscle mass in humans: validity of the 24-hour urinary creatinine method, Am J Clin Nutr **37:**478-494, 1983.

33. Jones JD, Burnett PD: Creatinine metabolism in humans with decreased renal function, Clin Chem **30:**1204-1212, 1974.

34. Mitch WE, et al: Creatinine metabolism in chronic renal failure, Clin Sci **58:**327-335, 1980.

35. Mitch WE, Walser M: A proposed mechanism for the reduced creatinine excretion in severe chronic renal failure, Nephron **21:**248-254, 1978.

36. Kopple JD, Coburn JW: Evaluation of chronic uremia: importance of serum urea nitrogen, serum creatinine, and their ratio, JAMA **227:**41-44, 1974.

37. Swenson RS, et al: Evidence that creatinine generation is not increased in experimental rhabdomyolysis–acute renal failure [abstract], Kidney Int **16:**777, 1979.

38. Grossman RA, et al: Nontraumatic rhabdomyolysis and acute renal failure, N Engl J Med **291:**807-811, 1974.

39. Sorensen LB, Levinson DJ: Origin and extrarenal elimination of uric acid in man, Nephron **14:**7-20, 1975.

40. Welbourne T, et al: The effect of glutamine administration on urinary ammonium excretion in normal subjects and patients with renal disease, J Clin Invest **51:**1852-1860, 1972.

41. Bailey GL: Uremia as a total-body disease. In Bailey GL, editor: Hemodialysis: principles and practice, New York, 1972, Academic Press Inc, pp 1-58.

42. Rose WC, Wixom RL: The amino acid requirements of man. XVI. The role of the nitrogen intake, J Biol Chem **217:**997-1004, 1955.

43. Giovannetti S, Maggiore Q: A low-nitrogen diet with proteins of high biological value for severe chronic uraemia, Lancet **1:**1000-1003, 1964.

44. Giordano C: Use of exogenous and endogenous urea for protein synthesis in normal and uremic subjects, J Lab Clin Med **62:**231-246, 1963.

45. Bergström J, et al: Treatment of chronic uremic patients with protein-poor diet and oral supply of essential amino acids. I. Nitrogen balance studies, Clin Nephrol **3:**187-194, 1975.

46. Kampf O, et al: Efficacy of an unselected protein diet (25g) with minor oral supply of essential amino acids and keto analogues compared with a selective protein diet (40g) in chronic renal failure, Am J Clin Nutr **33:**1673-1677, 1980.

47. Attman P-O, et al: Body composition during long-term treatment of uremia with amino acid supplemented low protein diet, Am J Clin Nutr **33:**801-810, 1980.

48. Jones RWA, et al: Oral essential amino acid supplements in children with advanced chronic renal failure, Am J Clin Nutr **3:**1696-1702, 1980.

49. Sigstrom L, et al: Growth during treatment with low-protein diet in children with renal failure, Clin Nephrol **21:**152-158, 1984.

50. Wilcken DEL, et al: Accumulation of sulphur-containing amino acids including cysteine-homocysteine in patients on maintenance hemodialysis, Clin Sci **58:**427-430, 1980.

51. Wilcken DEL, Gupta VJ: Sulphur containing amino acids

in chronic renal failure with particular reference to homocystine and cysteine-homocysteine mixed disulphide, Eur J Clin Invest 9:301-307, 1979.

52. Gejyo F, et al: Identification of N-monoacetylcystine in uraemic plasma, Clin Sci 60:331-334, 1981.

53. Cernacek P, et al: Plasma tryptophan level in chronic renal failure, Clin Nephrol 14:246-249, 1980.

54. Saito A, et al: Tryptophan and indolic tryptophan metabolites in chronic renal failure, Am J Clin Nutr 33:1402-1406, 1980.

55. Gulyassy PF, De Torrente A: Tryptophan metabolism in uremia, Kidney Int 7:S311-S313, 1975.

56. Bergström J, et al: Intracellular free amino acids in uremic patients as influenced by amino acid supply, Kidney Int 7:S345-S348, 1975.

57. Jontofsohn R, et al: Amino acid content of erythrocytes in uremia, Am J Clin Nutr 31:1956-1960, 1978.

58. Metcoff J, et al: Effects of amino acid infusions on abnormal cell metabolism in uremics, Clin Res 29:754A, 1981.

59. Pye IF, et al: Studies of cerebrospinal fluid and plasma amino acids in patients with steady-state chronic renal failure, Clin Chim Acta 92:65-72, 1979.

60. Schmid G, et al: Intracellular histidine content of various tissues (brain, striated muscle and liver) in chronic renal failure, Klin Wochenschr 55:583-585, 1977.

61. Shear L: Selective alerations of tissue protein and amino acid metabolism in uremia. In Dialysis and renal transplantation, Proceedings of the Fourth International Congress of Nephrology (Stockholm, 1969), Basel, 1970, S Karger AG, pp 233-241.

62. Young GA, et al: The effects of calorie and essential amino acid supplementation on plasma proteins in patients with chronic renal failure, Am J Clin Nutr 31:1802-1807, 1978.

63. Kopple JD, Swendseid M: Evidence that histidine is an essential amino acid in normal and chronically uremic man, J Clin Invest 55:881-891, 1975.

64. Alvestrand A, et al: The effect of nutritional regimens on branched chain amino acid antagonism in uremia. In Walser M, Williamson JR, editors: Metabolism and clinical implications of branched chain amino and ketoacids, New York, 1981, Elsevier North-Holland Inc, pp 605-613.

65. Alvestrand A, et al: Clinical results of long-term treatment with a low protein diet and a new amino acid preparation in patients with chronic uremia, Clin Nephrol 19:67-73, 1983.

66. Schloerb PR: Essential amino acid administration in uremia, Am J Med Sci 252:650-659, 1966.

67. Walser M, et al: The effects of keto-analogues of essential amino acids in severe chronic uremia, J Clin Invest 52:678-690, 1973.

68. Walser M: Ketoacids in the treatment of uremia, Clin Nephrol 3:180-187, 1975.

69. Mitch WE, et al: Treatment of chronic renal failure with branched chain ketoacids plus the other essential amino acids or their nitrogen-free analogues. In Walser M, Williamson JR, editors: Metabolism and clinical implications of branched chain amino and ketoacids, New York, 1981, Elsevier North-Holland Inc, pp 587-592.

70. Mitch WE, et al: Hypercalcemia and hypophosphatemia in uremic patients receiving essential amino acids or N-free analogues, Kidney Int 12:530, 1977.

71. Abras E, et al: Mixed salts of basic amino acids with branched chain ketoacids as the basis for new supplements designed to improve nutrition in chronic renal failure. In Walser M, Williamson JR, editors: Metabolism and clinical implications of branched chain amino and ketoacids, New York, 1981, Elsevier North-Holland Inc, pp 593-598.

72. Mitch WE, et al: Long-term effects of a new ketoacid—amino acid supplement in patients with chronic renal failure, Kidney Int 22:48-53, 1982.

73. Mitch WE, et al: The impact on the progression of chronic renal failure of a ketoacid/amino acid supplement to a restricted diet, N Engl J Med 311:623-629, 1984.

74. Mitch WE, et al: Nitrogen-sparing induced by leucine compared with that induced by its keto-analogue, alpha-ketoisocaproate, in fasting obese man, J Clin Invest 67:553-562, 1981.

75. Tischler ME, et al: Does leucine, leucyl-tRNA, or some metabolite of leucine regulate protein synthesis and degradation in skeletal and cardiac muscle? J Biol Chem 257:1613-1621, 1982.

76. Committee on Dietary Allowances, Food and Nutrition Board, National Research Council: Recommended dietary allowances, ed 9, Washington DC, 1980, National Academy of Sciences.

77. Ashworth A: Energy balance and growth: experience in treating children with malnutrition, Kidney Int 14:301-305, 1978.

78. Hyne BB, et al: The effect of caloric intake on nitrogen balance in chronic renal failure, Clin Sci 43:679-688, 1972.

79. Kopple JD, et al: Effect of energy intake on nitrogen metabolism in nondialyzed patients with chronic renal failure, Kidney Int 29:734-742, 1986.

80. Abitbol CL, Holliday MA: The effect of energy and nitrogen intake upon urea production in children with uremia and undernutrition, Clin Nephrol 10:9-15, 1978.

81. Abel RM, et al: Improved survival from acute renal failure after treatment with intravenous L-essential amino acids and glucose, N Engl J Med 288:695-699, 1978.

82. Meng HC: Beneficial effects of tube feedings with essential amino acids and adequate calories in uremic patients, Z Ernahrungswiss S19:34-35, 1977.

83. Kleinberger G, et al: Hypophosphatämie bei der parenteralen Ernährung niereninsuffizienter Patienten, Wien Klin Wochenschr 90:169-172, 1978.

84. Letteri JM, et al: Serial measurement of total body potassium in chronic renal disease, Am J Clin Nutr 31:1937-1944, 1978.

85. Massry SG, Ritz E: The pathogenesis of secondary hyperparathyroidism of renal failure, Arch Intern Med 138:853-856, 1978.

86. Maschio G, et al: Long-term effects of dietary phosphate restriction in chronic renal failure. Third Capri Conference on Uremia, August 31, 1980.

87. Slatopolsky E, et al: Low serum levels of $1,25(OH)_2D_3$ are not responsible for the development of secondary hyperparathyroidism in early renal failure [abstract], Kidney Int 14:733, 1978.

88. Kimura Y, et al: Interrelations between 1,25-dihydroxyvitamin D_3 [$1,25(OH)_2D_3$], phosphorus (Pi), calcium (Ca), and creatinine clearance (Ccr) in chronic renal failure, Miner Electrolyte Metab 2:238, 1979.

89. Portale AA, et al: Effect of dietary phosphorus on plasma 1,25-(OH)₂D in children with moderate renal insufficiency (MRI). Abstr 12A, Fourteenth Annual Meeting, American Society of Nephrology, 1981.

90. Slatopolsky E, et al: How important is phosphate in the pathogenesis of renal osteodystrophy? Arch Intern Med **138:**848-852, 1978.

91. Ott SM, et al: The prevalence of bone aluminum deposition in renal osteodystrophy and its relation to the response to calcitriol therapy, N Engl J Med **307:**709-713, 1982.

92. Ihle BU, et al: Clinical and biochemical features of aluminum-related bone disease, Kidney Int **29:**S80-S86, 1986.

93. Touam M, et al: Aluminum-induced, reversible microcytic anemia in chronic renal failure: clinical and experimental studies, Clin Nephrol **19:**295-298, 1983.

94. Fournier A, et al: Calcium carbonate, an aluminum-free agent for control of hyperphosphatemia, hypocalcemia, and hyperparathyroidism in uremia, Kidney Int **29:**S114-S119, 1986.

95. Walser M: Calcium carbonate–induced effects on serum Ca × P product and serum creatinine in renal failure: a retrospective study. In Massry SG, et al, editors: Phosphate and minerals in health and disease, New York, 1980, Plenum Press Inc, pp 281-287.

96. Nielsen HE, et al: 1-Alpha-hydroxy-vitamin D₃ treatment of non-dialyzed patients with chronic renal failure. Effects on bone, mineral metabolism, and kidney function, Clin Nephrol **13:**103-108, 1980.

97. Christiansen C, et al: Decreased renal function in association with administration of 1,25-dihydroxyvitamin D₃ in uremia, Contrib Nephrol **18:**139-146, 1980.

98. Postlethwaite RJ, Houston IB: Impairment of renal function in patients on 1-alpha-hydroxycholecalciferol, Lancet **2:**427-428, 1978.

99. Christiansen C, et al: Is 1,25-dihydroxycholecalciferol harmful to renal function in patients with chronic renal failure? Clin Endocrinol **15:**229-236, 1981.

100. Naik RB, et al: Effects of vitamin D metabolites and analogues on renal function, Nephron **28:**17-25, 1981.

101. McSherry E, Morris RC: Attainment of normal stature with alkali therapy in infants and children with classic renal tubular acidosis, J Clin Invest **61:**509-527, 1978.

102. Danovitch GM, et al: Reversibility of the "salt-losing" tendency of chronic renal failure, N Engl J Med **296:**14-19, 1977.

103. Gallagher KL, Jones JK: Furosemide-induced ototoxicity, Ann Intern Med **91:**744-745, 1979.

104. Weber H-P, et al: Total body potassium in children with chronic renal failure, Int J Pediatr Nephrol 1:42-47, 1980.

105. Berl T, et al: Role of aldosterone in the control of sodium excretion in patients with advanced chronic renal failure, Kidney Int **14:**228-235, 1978.

106. Donohue W, et al: The calcium content of the kidney as related to parathyroid function, J Exp Med **66:**697-704, 1937.

107. Ibels LS, et al: Preservation of function in experimental renal disease by dietary restriction of phosphate, N Engl J Med **298:**122-126, 1978.

108. Walser M, et al: Essential amino acids and their nitrogen-free analogues in the treatment of chronic renal failure. In Schreiner G, editor: Controversies in nephrology, Washington DC, 1979, Georgetown University Press, pp 404-413.

109. Maschio G, et al: Early dietary phosphorus restriction and calcium supplementation in the prevention of renal osteodystrophy, Am J Clin Nutr **33:**1546-1554, 1980.

110. Johnson WJ, et al: The influence of maintaining normal serum phosphate and calcium on renal osteodystrophy. In Norman AW, et al: editors: Vitamin D and problems related to uremic bone disease, New York, 1975, Walter de Gruyter Inc, pp 513-524.

111. Brenner BM, et al: Dietary protein intake and the progressive nature of kidney disease: the role of hemodynamically mediated glomerular injury in the pathogenesis of progressive glomerular sclerosis in aging, renal ablation, and intrinsic renal disease, N Engl J Med **307:**652-659, 1982.

112. Alvestrand A, et al: The effect of blood pressure reduction on the progression rate of chronic renal failure [abstract], Kidney Int **31:**189, 1987.

113. Ruilope LM, et al: Control of hypertension (HPN) with a converting enzyme inhibitor (CEI) slows progression of renal insufficiency in human chronic renal failure (CRF) [abstract], Kidney Int **31:**215, 1987.

114. Walser M, et al: Progression of chronic renal failure in patients given ketoacids following amino acids, Kidney Int **32:**123-128, 1987.

115. Schaefer K, von Herrath D: The striking effect of ketoacids on the serum phosphate and parathyroid hormone in patients with chronic uremia [abstract], Kidney Int **31:**357, 1987.

116. Ciardella F, et al: Effects of a low-phosphorus low-nitrogen diet supplemented with essential amino acids and ketoanalogues on serum triglycerides of chronic uremic patients, Nephron **42:**196-199, 1986.

117. Mak RHK, et al: The effect of a low-protein diet with amino acid/keto acid supplements on glucose metabolism in children with uremia, J Clin Endocrinol Metab **63:**985-989, 1986.

118. Hasslacher C, et al: Blood pressure and metabolic control as risk factors for nephropathy in Type 1 (insulin-dependent) diabetes, Diabetalogia **28:**6-11, 1985.

119. Bjorck S, et al: Beneficial effects of angiotensin converting enzyme inhibition on renal function in patients with diabetic nephropathy, Br Med J **293:**471-474, 1986.

120. Bending JJ, et al: Intermittent clinical proteinuria and renal function in diabetes: evolution and the effect of glycaemic control, Br Med J **292:**83-87, 1986.

CHAPTER 16
Neurologic System

Robert B. Johnston

Nutrition plays an important role in establishing and maintaining normal neurologic structure and function; and the brain, through its functions of intelligence, cognition, and emotion, influences the nutritional experiences of the individual. These interactions serve as the fundamental basis for the organization of this chapter, which addresses the following:

1. The differential vulnerability of the nervous system to nutritional insults, depending on the degree and location of the insult and on the person's age
2. The effect of the nutritional insult on the neurologic system, whether a deficiency (malnutrition or vitamin inadequacy) or an excess (amino acid overloads in certain inborn errors of metabolism or the alleged toxic effects of food additives)
3. The types of interventions directed toward resolution of the insult through dietary enrichment or restriction
4. The fact that nutritional insults may affect nervous system structure and/or neuropsychiatric function (e.g., cognition, motivation, attention, and other behaviors)
5. Neurologic conditions not related to nutrition (e.g., the ketogenic diet used to control seizures) that may require nutritional management

The psychologic influences that strongly affect nutritional status, as seen in classic anorexia nervosa, are discussed in Chapter 26.

DEVELOPMENTAL CENTRAL NERVOUS SYSTEM VULNERABILITY

It is clear from both human and animal studies that the central nervous system is most vulnerable during the time of intensive metabolic activity. In humans this corresponds to the prenatal period and extends into the second year of life. Insults in early life can affect the cell number, cell size, and brain composition, depending on the timing and duration of their occurrence.

Some human brain maturation processes are not completed until the second decade of life. Cell division and proliferation are 75% complete by birth, but increases in cell size and changes in metabolism (especially carbohydrate metabolism, enzymatic interactions, synapse proliferation, and increases in myelin content) occur primarily in the postnatal period.[1,2] Brain growth is only one component of the overall changes that occur during maturation. The effects of insults depend on their timing (i.e., when they occur in the maturational spectrum). This subject has been studied extensively by Winick and Noble.[1,3]

An insult that occurs early in the period of rapid cell division will result in a decreased number of cells. If it is removed during this critical period, which is thought to extend into the second year in humans, there may be some recovery; otherwise, the number of cells (DNA content) remains irreversibly decreased. However, if the insult occurs during a period of hypertrophy, a decrease in cell size results, as evidenced by a decreased ratio of protein to DNA. The latter phenomenon is less sensitive to critical periods and may be reversed when the insult is removed. The specific cell type involved, its location in the brain, its subsequent effect on function, and thus the degree of vulnerability depend on which area of the brain is metabolically most active at the time of insult.

In addition to affecting cell size and number, insults during a vulnerable period may influence the chemical composition of the brain. Myelination, active during the brain growth spurt, is subject to insults that may result in a reduced rate of myelination and ultimately reduce the amount of myelin in the brain. The potential effects on function are addressed below.

NEUROLOGIC REACTIONS TO NUTRITIONAL DEFICIENCIES
Severe Protein-Energy Malnutrition

Severe protein-energy malnutrition is estimated to be present in 0.5% to 20% of the world's population. Its major manifestations, marasmus and kwashiorkor, represent two extremes on a continuum: marasmus involves mainly a decrease in protein intake, kwashiorkor a deficiency of both calories and proteins. (See also Chapter 33.)

Marasmus is a chronic condition that typically begins in the early months of life, following early and abrupt weaning. It is associated with poor hygiene that results in contaminated intake and acute gastroenteritis. Treatment of gastroenteritis usually involves restricting dietary intake, which compounds the emaciation and growth retardation seen in the irritable, hungry, crying child. Reduced brain weight, cortical atrophy, hypotonia, irritability, and diminished volitional activity are the neurologic sequelae in marasmus.

Kwashiorkor is an acute condition that usually is found after the first 6 to 8 months of life. It may be secondary to late gradual weaning and subsequent dependence on a high-carbohydrate low-protein diet. Increased susceptibility to acute infections leads to the additional physiologic stress of illness, which, in association with the low-protein diet, produces the classic features of kwashiokor. The child is edematous, anorectic, and apathetic and often has a monotonous whine or cry. In severe cases the child lies immobile, essentially unresponsive to any environmental stimuli. Neurologic sequelae have been documented in physiologic, anatomic, and functional spheres. They include electroencephalographic abnormalities, cortical and subcortical brain atrophy, hypotonia, and delayed psychomotor skill development.

The neurologic findings of the two conditions are not mutually exclusive and may occur in any form of severe protein-energy malnutrition. In fact, individuals may have characteristic features of both kwashiorkor and marasmus concurrently.

The reduced activity and inattention to their surroundings characteristic of malnourished infants can affect intellectual and behavioral development. In a very real sense these children experience a severe form of sensory deprivation. Their apathy limits their response to a given environmental stimulus and results in deficient or absent learning experiences. In addition to limiting cognitive development, this apathy and short attention span jeopardize maternal/child bonding, so important in normal psychosocial development. When the mother is not reinforced for giving attention to the infant, she subsequently may diminish her efforts to stimulate or interact with the child. Thus intellectual and social development, which depend heavily on interaction with the environment, are at considerable risk in the severely malnourished child.

Pollitt and Thompson[4] conclude that severe protein-energy deficiency occurring throughout the first year of life in a population where malnutrition is endemic results in a severe deficit of intellectual functioning as compared to standards for that population. Severe acute protein-energy deficiency occurring in the second year may but generally does not result in intellectual retardation compared to standards for that same population.

Mild to Moderate Protein-Energy Malnutrition

There is no definite set of neurologic signs or symptoms that characterize mild to moderate malnutrition. Although retarded physical growth is an expected finding, aberrant brain growth (microcephaly) and function (mental deficiency) have not been well documented and are not proved sequelae. Since malnutrition often is associated with such factors as limited genetic endowment, poverty, large families, deprivation, chronic illness, and prolonged hospitalization, it is difficult to isolate the influence of nutrition on neuropsychologic development.

Studies of humans born under famine conditions provide useful insights into the effects of mild to moderate malnutrition. Although the Dutch famine of 1944-45 caused malnutrition in the entire western part of the country, there was no evidence 20 years later of any difference in the incidence of mental retardation among those born of malnourished mothers.[5] It appears that postnatally the dietary intake of these individuals was sufficient.

A study of a group of Korean orphans, some of whom suffered severe malnutrition during the first year of life, provides insight into the multifactorial nature of intellectual development.[2] The orphans had been placed in American homes at 2 years of age and were studied at 7 to 16 years of age. The previously well-nourished children scored significantly better in IQ and achievement tests than the previously malnourished children. However, the latter attained levels of IQ and school achievement that were average for American children of their age and grade.

A review of the literature in this area[4] indicates that cognitive development in populations where malnutrition is endemic appears to be more related to stature and socioeconomic status. Mild protein-energy malnutrition may retard the rate of developmental change, but it does not appear to impair the ultimate level of psychosocial development. There is little evidence to support the contention that older children and adolescents have significant aberrations in intellectual development when subjected to mild or moderate degrees of malnutrition.

The subsequent poor performance of previously malnourished children on cognitive testing may be more a reflection of their intellectually and educationally deprived environments than of basic neurologic deficits.[6] Poverty and malnutrition coexist frequently. It is impossible to ferret out individual contributions. Both conditions serve to isolate the child from appropriate stimulation.

Vitamin Deficiency

In animals deficiencies of vitamins A, B_1, B_2, B_{12}, E, and folic acid have been implicated as teratogenic to the nervous system and have resulted in such abnormalities as microphthalmia, anophthalmia, hydrocephaly, anencephaly, and microcephaly. Limited experimental evidence in humans has failed to implicate an isolated vitamin deficiency as a cause of such malformations.

A number of neurologic and psychiatric conditions or symptoms have been associated with specific vitamin deficiencies in humans.[7,8] (Table 16-1). However, neurologic involvement associated with specific vitamin deficiency is difficult to isolate. Other elements of malnutrition, such as calorie and/or protein deficiency and the subsequent predisposition of the nervous system to damage from other insults, may accompany vitamin deficiency. Neurologic sequelae range from isolated nerve lesions to extensive demyelination of spinal cord tracts and focal cortical lesions.

Vitamin A. The earliest clinical manifestation of vitamin A deficiency may be night blindness. Rhodopsin, a substance in the rods of the retina that is involved with vision in dim light, contains a derivative of vitamin A, retinene. Other man-

Table 16-1 Neurologic and Psychiatric Conditions Associated with Vitamin Deficiency

Vitamin	Neurologic	Psychiatric
A	Xerophthalmia	
B_1 (thiamine)	Peripheral neuropathy	Depression
	Wernicke's encephalopathy	Apathy
	Polyneuritis	Anxiety
	Cerebellar ataxia	Korsakoff's psychosis
B_2 (riboflavin)	Hydrocephalus	
	EEG changes	
B_3 (niacin)	Neurologic degeneration	Dementia (pellagra)
	Bulbar palsy	Depression
	Tremor	Anxiety
	Spasticity	
B_6 (pyridoxine)	Infantile seizures	
	Ataxia	
	Mental retardation	
	Carpal tunnel syndrome	
	Peripheral neuropathy	
B_{12} (cyanocobalamin)	Posterolateral sclerosis	
	Peripheral neuropathy	
Biotin	Myalgia	Somnolence
	Hyperesthesia	
Folic acid	Brain malformation	Apathy
		Forgetfulness
		Insomnia

ifestations of vitamin A deficiency include metaplasia of epithelial structures, resulting in keratinization of the cornea, conjunctiva, and lacrimal ducts. Additional neurologic sequelae can result from overgrowth of bone within the skull foramina, causing nerve compression symptoms. In infants vitamin A deficiency can lead to mental and physical retardation, facial palsy, or hydrocephalus, but the mechanisms are unclear. (See Chapter 21.)

B Vitamins. As a group, the B vitamins are instrumental in cellular catabolic reactions that incorporate carbohydrate as a source of energy for nervous system function. Therefore such vitamin deficiencies affect both the peripheral and the central nervous system. Although striking changes in neurologic function are found in a wide variety of vitamin B deficiencies, there is seldom a direct relationship to a single vitamin, (e.g., ophthalmoplegia and ataxia in Wernicke's disease [thiamine]). More often, the pathology can be attributed to a combination of factors, as in the polyneuropathy due to B_1, B_6, and/or B_{12}. Deficiencies of four of the B vitamins (thiamine, niacin, pyridoxine, and cyanocobalamin) significantly influence neurologic dysfunction.

Thiamine deficiency (beriberi), usually associated with high alcoholic intake for at least 3 months, has been implicated in a number of neurologic conditions. It manifests itself in three identifiable forms: the wet form, with serous effusions and edema; the cardiac form, with cardiovascular abnormalities; and the dry form, classically associated with polyneuropathy, which is usually symmetric and involves paresthesias and weakness in the extremities. Thiamine has been implicated in Wernicke's encephalopathy, characterized by disturbed mental functions, paralysis of eye movements, and ataxic gait. The oculomotor paralysis responds rapidly to thiamine, whereas the other two symptoms respond less rapidly. Korsakoff's psychosis, characterized by memory deficit and confabulation, is one extreme of the disturbed mental function. In addition, thiamine deficiency has been associated with retrobulbar neuropathy, diminished visual acuity, nerve deafness, laryngeal paralysis, trigeminal anesthesia, anosmia, and cerebellar degeneration.

Niacin (B_3) deficiency results in the classic symptoms of pellagra—dermatitis, diarrhea, and dementia. The mental symptoms often are vague and suggestive of a neurosis. They may include fatigue, weakness, irritability, headache, and emotional lability in the early stages. Advanced stages are characterized by toxic confusional states, catatonia, and/or mania. Lesions of the nervous system are nonspecific and may be neuritic, myelitic, or encephalitic.

Pyridoxine (B_6) deficiency, though rare, can occur in association with antitubercular drugs (isoniazid and cycloserine). The sensory polyneuropathy is characterized by paresthesias. In addition, there may be symptoms of somnolence, headache, tremor, dysarthria, or seizures.

Cyanocobalamin (B_{12}) deficiency is present in pernicious anemia, which is characterized by macrocytic anemia, megaloblastic hyperplasia, gastric achlorhydria, and subacute combined degeneration of the spinal cord tracts. This symptom complex rarely is a result of a dietary deficiency of B_{12}; it usually is caused by a defect in absorption. Neurologic involvement depends on the degree of pathology in specific areas. Degeneration of the dorsal and/or lateral columns of the spinal cord results in decreased vibration sense and gait disturbances. A sensory neuropathy causes parethesias and shooting pains. Involvement of the brain may cause mild to moderate mental disturbance with irritability, confusion, amnesia, and/or depression.

Vitamin-Dependent Metabolic Abnormalities

Over the past years a number of specific vitamin-dependent inborn errors of metabolism have been identified. Although rare, these conditions are clinically important because they are treated easily with pharmacologic doses of the relevant vitamin. The inherited disorders usually entail a single biochemical reaction and are corrected by administering a single vitamin. Rosenberg[9] noted neurologic sequelae with at least 14 such vitamin-responsive disorders involving six different water-soluble vitamins— B_1, B_2, B_{12}, folic acid, biotin, and nicotinamide.

In certain rare instances classic psychotic symptoms have been relieved by appropriate vitamin therapy. For example, psychosis has been manifested in pyridoxine-responsive homocystinuria and folate-responsive homocystinuria with hypomethioninemia. In patients with increased amounts of urinary homocystine and a defect in folate coenzyme synthesis, delusions, hallucinations, withdrawal, and catatonic posturing can be improved by administering large amounts of folic acid.[10] (See Chapter 27.)

Pyridoxine-responsive seizures in the neonatal period highlight the importance of early identification and subsequent prevention of symptoms associated with vitamin-dependent conditions. In 1954 there was a report of twins who had neonatal seizures; although the first child died of uncontrolled seizures on day three, the second, with seizures starting on day five, responded to a multivitamin preparation given for possible neonatal sepsis; it was determined that pyridoxine played a specific protective role since the seizures were controlled on a pharmacologic dosage of 1 to 3 mg/day (normal physiologic range, 0.3 mg/da); the seizures were well controlled, but the child subsequently demonstrated mental retardation. In more recent cases infants have been spared mental deficiency when replacement therapy was started early in the clinical course.

Some rare vitamin-responsive disorders may account for an occasional case of seizures, mental retardation, cerebellar ataxia, and/or coma, but there is no scientific evidence to suggest the widespread use of vitamin therapy in these conditions. It does not follow that all, or even many, of the symptoms are related to a vitamin deficiency or dependency. A similar statement can be made for the treatment of psychiatric symptoms.

Orthomolecular Psychiatry

The terms megavitamin therapy and orthomolecular psychiatry are used synonymously by workers who believe that schizophrenia is caused by a vitamin deficiency. Proponents of this theory contend that schizophrenic symptoms respond to high doses of niacin (nicotinic acid), which acts as a methyl acceptor and inhibits the methylation of norepinephrine to the alleged hallucinogen adrenochrome. This initial formulation has now been expanded, and therapeutic regimens currently include ascorbic acid, pyridoxine, thyroid, B_{12}, lecithin, and some phenothiazines. In addition, claims of megavitamin efficiency have been made for other conditions—autism, dyslexia, hyperactivity, mental retardation, Down's syndrome, alcoholism, heroin addiction. However, these claims have not been substantiated by other investigators.

Nevertheless, despite numerous formal reports (including one by the National Advisory Committee on Hyperkinesis and Food Additives, 1980) that criticize this approach as lacking in scientific merit, megavitamin therapy remains popular with the public.

It is difficult to assess such an approach accurately. Practitioners of orthomolecular psychiatry resist submitting this policy to analysis, claiming that to do so would be unethical since some patients would be denied necessary and beneficial therapy. Evaluation is hampered further since proponents do not use standard criteria for diagnosis or for assessment of results. In addition, therapeutic regimens are quite varied. Lipton et al.[8] conclude that properly controlled studies indicate no significant benefits from megavitamin therapies in the treatment of schizophrenia, alcoholism, or drug abuse.

It should be recognized that some vitamins can have toxic effects when given in large doses. For example, nicotinic acid in excess has caused flushing, pruritis, decreased blood pressure, somnolence, activation of ulcers, and liver or cardiac damage. Long-term consumption of pharmacologic doses of vitamins, as in megavitamin therapy, has a significant potential for toxicity, has not proved useful in the large majority of patients, and is not considered a sound approach to treating a complex set of symptoms.

The American Academy of Pediatrics[11] has stated unequivocally that there is no evidence suggesting that vitamins in large doses have any beneficial effect on children except in cases of vitamin-dependent disease. Few studies have been published on the topic.

FOOD COMPONENTS AS A SOURCE OF ILL EFFECTS

Under certain circumstances the components of foods can cause undesired structural or functional abnormalities. This negative influence may occur in a variety of ways. Dietary substances that are normally innocuous, or are even essential, may achieve *toxic status* when the body fails to metabolize them properly and there is a resultant buildup of metabolites that act as cellular poisons (e.g., inborn errors of amino acid metabolism). A second instance occurs when *certain substances* interact idiosyncratically with an otherwise normal body system. A number of food additives, preservatives, and artificial colors have been implicated as potential poisons to the nervous system of certain individuals. A third possible mechanism involves an *allergic reaction* between food and host that mediates an insult to the nervous system. Treatment in all three instances is based on decreasing or removing the offending substance(s) through dietary manipulation.

Inborn Errors of Amino Acid Metabolism

An increasing number of inborn errors of amino acid metabolism that affect the nervous system have been identified (Table 16-2). Dietary treatment, started early enough, may reverse biochemical changes and allow normal physical and mental development. The restriction of essential amino acids (e.g., leucine, isoleucine, valine, phenylalanine) requires close monitoring to support normal growth.[12]

A discussion of phenylketonuria illustrates the overall approach to clinical management of amino acid deficiencies with neurologic involvement. Phenylketonuria is an inherited autosomal recessive metabolic disorder caused by a deficiency of the enzyme phenylalanine hydroxylase, which leads to a failure to change phenylalanine to tyrosine. As a result there is a buildup of metabolic substances that act as toxins to the developing nervous system. Children with phenylketonuria characteristically are blond and blue-eyed because of the tyrosine deficiency. In untreated cases a high percentage have microcephaly, severe or profound mental retardation, and associated hyperkinesis and seizures.

Intervention involves identification and prevention of sequelae through dietary means. Since the nervous system has developed normally in utero, the major vulnerability occurs in the neonatal period when phenylalanine is introduced into the diet. Early identification and treatment are the keys to preserving normal neurologic function. In the United States, newborn screening programs have been developed in each state toward this end. Diagnosis is confirmed by the quantitative measurement of phenylalanine blood levels and a 24-hour urinalysis for metabolites.

Dietary restriction of the amount of phenylalanine should be started as soon as the diagnosis is confirmed. Because phenylalanine is an essential amino acid, it cannot be eliminated totally. A blood level of 3 to 10 mg/100 ml must be maintained to support normal cellular functions. Levels below 3 mg/100 ml are associated with defective growth and other sequelae (e.g., hepatomegaly, hypoglycemia).

The basic component of the diet is a high-protein low-phenylalanine food such as Lofenalac, a synthetic casein-based powdered formula from which most of the phenylalanine has been removed. It is fortified with fat, carbohydrate, vitamins, and minerals. The addition of milk and subsequent other natural foods to the diet requires careful regulation based on protein and calorie needs.

Dietary control usually requires close collaboration of parents and the pediatrician, nutritionist, psychologist, and other members of the team. Serum phenylalanine levels are monitored

Table 16-2 Inborn Errors of Amino Acid Metabolism

	Amino Acid	Neurologic Manifestations
Phenylketonuria	Phenylalanine	Mental retardation Convulsions
Maple sugar urine disease	Leucine Isoleucine Valine	Mental retardation
Hyperprolinemia	Proline	Seizures Deafness Mental retardation
Homocystinuria	Methionine Homocystine	Mental retardation
Hyperammonemia	Ammonia	Coma, death
Propionicacidemia	Propionic acid	Mental retardation

weekly during the first year and biweekly or monthly thereafter. No age has been established at which the diet can be discontinued. It is clear that the mature nervous system is not sensitive to the buildup of metabolites in phenylketonuria, but the exact timing of this invulnerability is not well understood. Some centers discontinue the diet at 4 years; in general, the current practice is to maintain the diet until 8 years of age, at which time the brain has essentially reached adult size and myelination has been completed. Careful monitoring of psychologic and intellectual performance should continue following cessation of the diet to assure that discontinuation was not premature.

Offspring of phenylketonuric mothers not under treatment during their pregnancy are affected by high levels of phenylalanine and may have serious deficits. Intrauterine growth retardation, microcephaly, and mental retardation can occur. Attention to maternal levels of phenylalanine is mandatory during pregnancy, and maintenance of normal levels can result in normal offspring. (See Chapter 36.)

Food Additives

An association has been suggested between the increasing frequency of learning and behavior problems in our society over the past decades and the increased use of food additives. Specifically, artificial colorings and flavors, preservatives, and extenders have been alleged to be toxic to the nervous system and responsible for learning and attention problems.

In 1965 Dr. Benjamin Feingold treated a woman suffering from hives with a diet that omitted artificial flavors and colors. She experienced clearing of her skin as well as dramatic improvement in a number of chronic behavioral problems, including hostility and aggression. This initial observation was extended to a group of learning-disabled and behavior-disordered children who were treated with a similar elimination diet, known as the Kaiser-Permanente (K-P) or Feingold diet.[13] The original diet eliminated naturally occurring salicylates (Group 1) and artificial food flavors and colorings (Group 2). Examples of the wide range of foods that were eliminated are shown in Table 16-3.

Table 16-3 The K-P or Feingold Elimination Diet

Group 1 (foods containing natural salicylates)	
Almonds	Mint flavoring
Apples (cider and cider vinegars)	Nectarines
Apricots	Oil of wintergreen
Blackberries	Oranges
Cherries	Peaches
Cloves	Prunes, plums
Cucumbers and pickles	Raspberries
Currants	Strawberries
Gooseberries	Tea, all varieties
Grapes and raisins (wine and wine vinegars)	Tomatoes

Group 2 (foods containing artificial flavors and colors)	
Bacon and sausage	Candies
Commercial ice cream	Diet drinks
Margarine	Toothpastes and powders
Vitamins	Colored butter
Chocolate syrup	Dessert mixes
Prepared mustard	Instant breakfast preparations
Luncheon meats	Frozen fish
Cereals	Cough drops
Soft drinks	Snacks
Cake mixes	Chips
Catsup	Prepared chocolate drink
Bakery goods	Instant gelatin
Powdered puddings	

Unfortunately, this type of unidimensional approach to such multifaceted problems has met with little well-substantiated success. Children with learning and/or attentional problems represent a very heterogeneous population. Some may be harboring neurologically based deficiencies whereas others may have a specific learning disorder; still others may have school performance difficulties based on emotional problems. Poor teaching techniques have also been implicated. It is generally accepted now that such disorders represent one or a combination of these neurologic, psycholosocial, and environmental factors and that resolution involves selecting a multifaceted approach if success is to be achieved. Isolated and unilateral therapy, such as the use of diet or medication alone, rather than enlisting other resources at home and in the school is shortsighted.[14]

The K-P diet mandates that all prohibited foods (including most pills and vitamin preparations, which contain artificial colors and/or flavors) be kept out of the home. To help ensure success, the entire family must actively participate in the dietary restrictions.

According to Feingold[14] response to the diet may be demonstrated within days or weeks. Younger children apparently react more quickly than do older children. Slight infractions can lead to reversal of progress lasting for days. If improvement is noted initially, the diet may be gradually liberalized by reintroduction of Group 1 foods (containing salicylates). However, foods with artificial colors and flavorings remain excluded. In addition, it is recommended that preservatives, particularly BHT (butylated hydroxytoluene) and BHA (butylated hydroxyanisole), commonly found in butter or margarine, bread, and potato chips, be eliminated from the diet.

Feingold submits that children who react to these synthetic additives have a genetic sensitivity predisposing them to hyperkinetic reactions, and he claims dramatic improvement in 50% of the children prescribed the diet, with at least some positive response in 75% (who can then be removed from drug management).[14] Improvement is cited in a number of areas—including decreased hyperactivity and clumsiness, better responses to the environment, and marked improvement in scholastic abilities. It also has been claimed that the diet produces effective resolution of enuresis, antisocial behavior, epilepsy, mental retardation, juvenile delinquency, headaches, and eye problems; however, there has been no published substantiation of these claims.

Acceptance by parents and the lay press has been more vigorous than by the scientific community. The support by these parents indicates that some improvement is being experienced, but the question remains whether it is a response to the specific diet or a placebo response. With incorporation of the diet into the family dynamics, a number of changes take place over and above the diet itself: the entire family is doing something about the problem and has mobilized its total resources; parental and child anxieties are likely to be allayed when something definite finally is being done; attitudinal and emotional changes can be positive in influencing the child's behavior beyond the effect (if any) of the diet; the child is now the object of increased attention; parental guilt and blame, which may have been present throughout a previously difficult time, can be transferred to a food toxin.

There has been little if any direct scientific research on the potential behavioral toxicity of specific food additives either in animals or in humans. Feingold and his followers have not conducted rigorous controlled clinical trials, since they feel that parents and children cannot be expected to await scientific proof for a treatment that is working. Studies that have been generated have fallen into three categories[15]: (1) uncontrolled open clinical trials with the additive-free diet, (2) blind clinical trials of the diet, and (3) double-blind challenges. Open clinical trials, conducted with no controls, and with parental, teacher, and child awareness of who is on the diet, generally have been supportive of the Feingold hypothesis; but controlled clinical trials and blind challenge studies have not supported Feingold's claim that 50% to 75% of hyperactive children dramatically improve when placed on the diet.

In a review of research literature on the Feingold diet, Mattes[16] concludes that no single controlled study has demonstrated a consistent dietary effect on such characteristics as hyperactivity, distractability, and/or impulsiveness. When positive effects were noted, they were often sporadic, unreproducible, inconsistent between studies, and thought to be due to chance.

Scientific studies by Weiss et al.[17] and Mattes and Gittelman-Klein[18] also have shown no dietary effects even when parents were strong supporters of the diet. Furthermore, reports from national study groups[19,20] have not found any evidence of a clinical effect of artificial additives on "hyperkinetic" behaviors in the vast majority of children.

On the other hand, one NIH-sponsored group[21] has concluded that there is evidence that a small percentage of affected children do indeed respond to artificial coloring agents. The fact that certain hyperkinetic children of preschool age are affected by the diet more than a comparable group of school-age children suggests the possibility that a very small subgroup of children may benefit from the additive-free diet and react adversely to the challenge substances. Specific characteristics of the population have not been delineated clearly.

In either case there remain serious questions regarding the Feingold diet and its effectiveness. Continued careful analysis, research, and study may be warranted, but at present the evidence does not seem to favor its overenthusiastic utilization. It is very difficult to maintain for the general group of children with learning and behavior disorders and, when used, should not be taken as a substitute for necessary and appropriate educational, medical, and/or psychologic support for the child and family.[13]

Sugar

Perhaps the widest gap between public knowledge and the existing facts rests with the effects of sugar on children's behavior.[22] Sugar has been indicted as the culprit in behaviors ranging from anxiety through learning disabilities to juvenile delinquency. Although some studies suggest an association between sucrose ingestion and poor school performance[23] and/or hyperactivity,[24] there is no proof of a relationship. At this time difficulties in measuring behavioral change and inconsistent or conflicting results among studies leave the question of sugar effect unanswered.

ALLERGY

The role of food allergy has been suggested in pediatric migraine[25] and hyperkinesis[26] (ADDH, attention deficit disorder with hyperactivity). In both instances an oligoantigenic diet consisting of two specific meats, two starches, two fruits, and one vegetable plus water, calcium, and

multivitamin tablets was associated with improvement in migraine or hyperkinetic status. Subsequent challenges with potential offending foods, however, were noted to cause symptoms in more than a fourth of the subjects—for example, milk, soy, chocolate, grapes, wheat, oranges, eggs, corn, fish, and oats. It would thus appear that these preliminary findings are tentative and require replication, and this approach needs to be addressed with caution. The unsupervised diet is dangerous, expensive, disruptive of social and family life, and difficult to maintain. In fact, it almost makes the "rigorous" Feingold diet seem like a "carefree picnic."[27]

KETOGENIC DIET AND EPILEPSY

The relationship between nutrition and neurologic function has a particular application in the treatment of epilepsy. The nutritional-neurologic interface has been identified for centuries in the treatment of epilepsy. Biblical references recommended prayer and fasting. Other dietary "cures" have had short-lived popularity over the last two centuries, involving recommendations for either an excess or a strict limitation of specific animal, vegetable, or mineral nutritive sources. The beneficial effects of fasting and dehydration in the control of seizures led to the development over 50 years ago of the ketogenic diet, which attempted to maintain the body in a chronic state of ketosis.

Such a regimen initially requires a period of starvation to induce ketosis. The state is maintained through a stringent diet that contains three to four times as much fat by weight as the total carbohydrate and protein diet. It is most effective in children between the ages of 2 and 5 years. Although its indications are not absolute, more beneficial results have been noted in myoclonic and major motor forms of epilepsy. It usually is attempted when other, more traditional, medication regimens have failed to control the seizures. It has received varying degrees of acceptance within the neurologic community.

The mechanism of action of the ketogenic diet is not entirely clear. There is evidence that the physiologic effects of ketosis, acidosis, and dehydration play key roles in seizure control. It has also been proposed that ketone bodies, particularly acetoacetic acid, have mildly anesthetic anticonvulsant properties. It has been suggested, in fact, that mild acidosis and decreased water content influence seizure control physiologically and that the elevation of plasma lipids has a specific anticonvulsant effect.

The diet regimen is based on maintaining a 4:1 ketogenic/antiketogenic ratio, which requires careful calculation to ensure sufficient calories to maintain growth.[28] Consultation with a nutritionist or dietitian and ample medical support are needed since the regimen is individualized to ensure growth.

The 4:1 ratio is maintained over a three-meal daily schedule, and the diet relies heavily on fat in the forms of whipped cream, butter, mayonnaise, and margarine. Carbohydrates and protein are limited. The diet has low bulk and often is low in water-soluble vitamins B and C as well as in calcium. The ketogenic diet is not particularly palatable and is rejected frequently on this basis. Children often break from the restrictions of the diet, and such indiscretions severely limit its effectiveness.

The discovery that medium-chain triglycerides (MCTs) are more ketotic than ordinary dietary fats has led to the MCT diet, which appears to be more palatable and less hypercholesterolemic than the regular ketogenic diet. Depending on the individual case, 50% to 70% of calories are provided by the use of MCT oil, which is blended with skim milk, fruit juices, cocoa, and other foods. Appropriate vitamin and mineral supplements are necessary.

Children receiving the ketogenic diet must avoid medications with a high sugar content, such as the broad group of cough medicines, cough drops, and laxatives. Even toothpaste can diminish the effectiveness of this diet. Protein needs must be monitored, particularly during periods of rapid growth, in light of the low amounts of protein usually recommended.

Complications, although usually rare, include growth retardation, persistent vomiting, and renal calculi. When the diet is effective in controlling seizures, motivation remains high despite the negative aspects. Follow-up includes daily urinalysis and monthly monitoring of the nutritional status.

REFERENCES

1. Winick M: Malnutrition and brain development, New York, 1976, Oxford University Press Inc.
2. Hurley LS: Developmental nutrition, Englewood Cliffs NJ, 1980, Prentice-Hall Inc.
3. Winick M, Noble A: Qualitative changes in DNA, RNA, and protein during prenatal and postnatal growth in the rat, Dev Biol **12:**451-466, 1965.
4. Pollitt E, Thompson C: Protein-calorie malnutrition and behavior: a view from psychology. In Wurtman RJ, Wurtman JJ, editors: Nutrition and the brain, vol 2, New York, 1977, Raven Press, pp 261-306.
5. Stein Z, et al: Famine and human development, New York, 1975, Oxford University Press Inc.
6. Levitsky DA, Strupp BJ: Malnutrition and tests of brain function. In Miller SA, editor: Nutrition and behavior, Philadelphia, 1981, Franklin Institute Press.
7. Dodge PR, et al: Nutrition and the developing nervous system, St Louis, 1975, The CV Mosby Co.
8. Lipton MA, et al: Vitamins, megavitamin therapy, and the nervous system. In Wurtman RJ, Wurtman JJ, editors: Nutrition and the brain, vol 3, New York, 1977, Raven Press, pp 183-264.
9. Rosenberg L: Vitamin-responsive inherited diseases affecting the nervous system. In Plum F, editor: Dysfunction in metabolic disorders, New York, 1974, Raven Press, pp 263-272.
10. Freeman J, et al: Homocystinuria presenting as reversible "schizophrenia," Pediatr Res **6:**163-168, 1972.
11. American Academy of Pediatrics: Megavitamins and mental retardation. Policy statement, 1981.
12. Stansbury JB, et al: The metabolic basis of inherited disease, ed 4, New York, 1978, McGraw-Hill Book Co.
13. Feingold BF: Why is your child hyperactive? New York, 1975, Random House Inc.
14. Johnston RB: Learning disabilities: medicine and myths, Boston, 1987, Little Brown & Co.
15. Lipton MA, et al: Hyperkinesis and food additives. In Wurtman RJ, Wurtman JJ, editors: Nutrition and the brain, vol 4, New York, 1979, Raven Press, pp 1-28.
16. Mattes JA: The Feingold diet: a current reappraisal, Learning Disabil **16:**319-323, 1983.
17. Weiss B, et al: Behavioral response to artificial food colors, Science **207:**1487-1489, 1980.
18. Mattes JA, Gittelman-Klein R: Effects of artificial food coloring in children with hyperactive symptomatology, Arch Gen Psychiatry **38:**714-718, 1981.
19. National Advisory Committee on Hyperkinesis and Food Additives: Final report to the Nutrition Foundation, New York, 1980, The Nutrition Foundation.
20. Stare FJ, et al: Diet and hyperactivity: is there a relationship? Pediatrics **66:**521-525, 1980.
21. Office for Medical Application of Research, National Institutes of Health: Defined diets and childhood hyperactivity, JAMA **245:**290-292, 1982.
22. Levitsky DA, Strupp BJ: Nutrition and the behavior of children. In Walker WA, Watkins JB, editors: Nutrition in pediatrics, Boston, 1985, Little Brown & Co.
23. Lester ML, et al: Refined carbohydrate intake, hair cadmium levels, and cognitive functioning in children, Nutr Behav **1:**3, 1982.
24. Prinz RJ, et al: Dietary correlates of hyperactive behavior in children, J Consult Clin Psychol **48:**760-768, 1980.
25. Egger J, et al: Is migraine food allergy? Lancet **2:**865-869, 1983.
26. Egger J, et al: Controlled trial of oligoantigenic treatment in the hyperkinetic syndrome, Lancet **1:**540-545, 1985.
27. Podell RN: Food, mind, and mood: hyperactivity revisited, Postgrad Medicine **78:**119-123, 1985.
28. Livingston S: Comprehensive management of epilepsy in infancy, childhood and adolescence, Springfield Ill, 1972, Charles C Thomas Publisher.

CHAPTER 17
Endocrine System

David L. Horwitz
Mary Bess Kohrs

By itself or in conjunction with other regulatory mechanisms, the endocrine system regulates many aspects of growth, intermediary metabolism, stress responses, and calorie and mineral balance. Therefore disruptions of endocrine function may have adverse nutritional consequences. Conversely, altered nutritional states affect a number of endocrine responses. This chapter will consider endocrinopathies in which nutritional intervention can play a therapeutic role, endocrine disorders with signs or symptoms that suggest nutritional diagnoses, and the effects of altered nutritional states on endocrine function. Reproductive disorders and diabetes mellitus are dealt with in greater depth in Chapters 18 and 38.

GROWTH HORMONE
Metabolic Effects

The combined effects of growth hormone on intermediary metabolism are anabolic.[1] Administering human growth hormone to animals stimulates amino acid uptake by tissues and protein synthesis. Although acute administration of human growth hormone in humans causes nitrogen and phosphorus retention in excess of that required for rapid growth, prolonged administration gradually returns nitrogen excretion to normal.[2] Augmented fat breakdown, as evidenced by the increased mobilization of free fatty acids from adipose tissue, helps to provide energy for growth hormone-stimulated protein synthesis. Body protein reserves are preserved because the need for gluconeogenesis is limited when free fatty acids and ketone bodies are provided as substrates for energy. Optimum protein synthesis in animals also requires insulin.[3]

Hyperinsulinemia results from excessive growth hormone secretion or administration.[3] This may be due to both indirect and direct effects on pancreatic beta-cell secretion in addition to resistance to the blood sugar–lowering action of insulin. The insulin resistance may be caused by a specific effect of growth hormone on glucose transport, by a free fatty acid–mediated inhibition of glucose uptake, or both.

Syndromes of Growth Hormone Excess

The most striking pathologic and clinical features of acromegaly are caused by the effects of excess human growth hormone on bone and cartilage. Growth hormone hypersecretion before puberty results in increased bone length as well as width. Excessive hormone secretion beginning after puberty leads to marked periosteal overgrowth of bone, particularly in the acral parts—the head, ears, and nose, the hands, and the feet. Patients sometimes need a greater hat and ring size and progressively increasing shoe sizes. Changes in the skull account for striking facial changes. Enlargement of the mandible changes the bite, since the lower teeth extend well beyond the upper ones. The teeth also become widely separated. Cartilaginous overgrowth involves the nose and ears, accounting for part of their enlargement. The femur, tibia, and fibula become bowed because of increased length. The ribs and clavicle thicken and lengthen. Estimates of actual skeletal weight suggest only a slight increment compared to that occurring in normal subjects. Despite increased calcium absorption, there is negative calcium balance. Osteoporosis also can occur in acromegaly not complicated by other endocrine abnormalities.

Many of the classic features of acromegaly are due as much to soft tissue thickening as to bony overgrowth.[4] X-ray films and measurements of skinfold thickness confirm the increased soft tissue thickening. The subcutaneous tissues thicken as fat is replaced with noninflammatory connective tissue that is morphologically and chemically normal. Isotopic studies indicate other significant alterations in body composition.[2] There is an increase in total body water with a greater increase in extracellular than in intracellular water. Exchangeable body sodium and potassium increase in the acromegalic patient; however, the exchangeable body potassium is less than normal in terms of body weight. Body cell mass is normal relative to body weight, as is body fat. The increase in supportive tissue is greater than that of metabolically active tissue. Although body composition studies suggest enhanced nitrogen retention, long-term effects of excessive growth hormone on nitrogen balance are not known.

Another anabolic effect of excessive growth hormone is visceromegaly.[5] The lungs, liver, stomach, intestines, and kidney may be two to five times the normal size and weight. Enlargement of the liver and spleen usually may be explained by a second disease.

The diabetogenic and insulinogenic properties of growth hormone have been alluded to previously.[1] A sufficiently large dose of growth hormone will impair glucose tolerance despite hyperinsulinemia, since growth hormone can produce peripheral resistance to insulin. Diabetes mellitus occurs in 25% to 30% of patients with acromegaly. In many other acromegalics with normal blood sugar concentrations, plasma insulin concentrations are elevated markedly, especially after glucose ingestion. The insulin response in the nondiabetic acromegalic is prompt and exaggerated whereas in the diabetic acromegalic it is delayed and retarded.

The raised basal metabolic rate, palpable enlargement of the thyroid, and increased sweating may lead to a diagnosis of hyperthyroidism,[2] although thyroid function test results are normal. Uptake of ^{131}I by the thyroid and serum PBI values are usually normal, with plasma thyrotropic hormone values normal or low. The increased basal metabolic rate may be due to an underestimate of body surface area from height-weight tables. When oxygen consumption is related to exchangeable body potassium, the patient's observed value is greater than normal, indicating an increase in basal metabolic rate.

Diagnosis. Physical findings in acromegaly are usually characteristic, but confirmation is based on measurement of growth hormone levels. Basal levels generally exceed normal (7 ng/ml) and are not suppressed by glucose administration. Somatomedin C levels are unequivocally elevated. Computed tomography generally confirms the presence of a pituitary tumor.

Treatment. The source of excessive growth hormone is generally a pituitary adenoma. In about 70% of cases, surgical removal is successful. Many physicians now advocate selective removal of the adenoma by the transsphenoidal approach, leaving the remaining pituitary intact.* Conventional radiotherapy also has a success rate of 60% to 70%, but growth hormone levels may not return to normal for 5 years or more after radiation therapy. High-intensity radiotherapy with proton or neutron beams provides rapid but nonselective pituitary destruction. Medical therapy with large doses of bromocriptine appears promising but does not provide a permanent cure. Apart from appropriate dietary management of glucose intolerance, no specific nutritional management is needed.

Syndromes of Growth Hormone Deficiency

The classic symptom of hypopituitarism in children is short stature, but short stature may be caused by a number of other factors, including malnutrition. Only about 10% of the cases of short stature are related to pituitary growth hormone deficiency.[5] The effects of growth hormone deficiency are greater and more prolonged than other causes of short stature in children. Pituitary dwarfs are generally three to four standard deviations below mean height for age, and obesity is common. Skinfold thickness greater than the 50th percentile for age indicates an increase in subcutaneous adipose tissue.[2] Standard texts divide pituitary dwarfism into two categories: those with growth hormone undetectable by radioimmunoassay (idiopathic hypopituitarism or organic hypopituitarism) and those with detectable but ineffective growth hormone (African pygmies, Laron dwarfs). Sexual ateliotic dwarfs have isolated growth hormone deficiency but normal thyroid function and reach sexual maturity. Retarded growth is not obvious until the first to third year, generally by age 5 years. In one third of the dwarfs, growth rate is normal

---

*This selective "adenomectomy" also is effective in about 70% of patients without damaging the adjacent normal gland.[6]

until late childhood. This type of dwarfism is due to suprasellar or intrasellar tumor. In untreated dwarfs bone age parallels height, both lagging behind chronologic age. There is a delay in epiphyseal maturation in children with hypopituitarism.

Growth hormone deficiency in children affects body composition in other ways as well.[7] Urinary excretion of creatinine and muscle cell size and number both indicate decreased muscle mass. The absolute number of muscle cells is significantly lower relative to age in hypopituitary dwarfs, although appropriate in relation to linear growth or lean body mass. In hypopituitary dwarfs the muscle cells are small for body size.

There are no metabolic manifestations of growth hormone deficiency in adults. Hypoglycemia may be a distressing and serious problem in children whose dwarfism is associated with either monotropic growth hormone deficiency or multiple anterior pituitary hormone deficiencies. Insulin hypersensitivity with insulinopenia may be caused by a lack of substrate for gluconeogenesis or impairment in amino acid mobilization.[8] A small group of hypopituitary dwarfs has normal insulin sensitivity with hyperinsulinism. Growth hormone–deficient patients also exhibit hypertriglyceridemia and hypercholesterolemia.

Diagnosis. Basal growth hormone levels are low and are not stimulated by hypoglycemia, arginine, or L-dopa. Somatomedin C levels are reduced. In the Laron* type of dwarf, somatomedin C is low despite increased serum levels of growth hormone.

Treatment. The ideal treatment for the child with growth hormone deficiency is the hormone itself. Growth deficiency clears in about 3 to 6 months, during which time the growth rate increases to an average of 7-8 cm/year but may approach 15-20 cm/year.[5]

Subcutaneous fat decreases once the linear growth rate increases in response to therapy.[7] Total body water, lean body mass, and extracellular and intracellular water increase in proportion to height whereas muscle mass increases at a faster rate than would be expected from the height gains.[9] The urinary excretion of creatinine, reflecting muscle mass, increases significantly after hormone treatment and is greater than in normal boys of similar height. Thus cellular growth is greater than linear growth. The increase in muscle mass suggests that growth hormone may affect the multiplication of muscle cells to a greater extent than it affects cells in the epiphyses of bones. Because growth hormone therapy itself returns body composition to normal, no specific dietary intervention is needed.

Somatomedins. Cartilage growth and other responses seen in growth hormone therapy are not stimulated directly by the hormone. Rather, growth hormone acts on the liver to promote synthesis of a substance or group of substances known as somatomedins. Originally called sulfation factors because they stimulated uptake of sulfate by cartilage, somatomedins now are known to be the mediators of many of growth hormone's activities.

The primary regulator of somatomedin synthesis appears to be growth hormone, and very low somatomedin levels are found after hypophysectomy and in most growth hormone–deficient dwarfs. Somatomedins also are reduced in Laron dwarfism, which is characterized by high growth hormone levels, tissue resistance to growth hormone, and lack of therapeutic response when growth hormone is administered. In acromegaly, somatomedin levels are generally high, as expected. Somatomedin generation is inhibited by glucocorticoids, perhaps accounting for the growth delay often seen in children with Cushing's disease or those treated with exogenous steroids.

Children with protein-energy malnutrition have low somatomedin levels and grow poorly in spite of normal or elevated growth hormone levels. It is not certain whether poor nutrition itself, or the accompanying low insulin levels, is responsible for the reduction in somatomedin. In any case these clinical observations, along with similar findings in animal studies, indicate that nutritional alteration may be a more important regulator of somatomedin activity than growth hormone is. Adequate caloric intake but inadequate protein appears to impair the ability of somatomedin to stimulate cartilaginous growth.[10] Interestingly, short but otherwise normal children also show a rise in somatomedin C levels after the injection of growth hormone.[11]

*Laron Z: Growth hormone resistance, Ann Clin Res **12:**269-277, 1980.

In view of the current availability of biosynthetic human growth hormone, there is now an ethical debate ongoing as to whether such therapy should be used in constitutionally short but healthy children.

THYROID HORMONE
Thyrotoxicosis (hyperthyroidism)

The most common forms of hyperthyroidism in the Western World are Graves' disease and toxic adenoma; however, in areas where goiter is endemic the most common cause may be toxic multinodular goiter. Thyroiditis can also be a cause of transient hyperthyroidism. The metabolic effects of thyrotoxicosis have important nutritional implications. Graves' disease (diffuse toxic goiter) has a fairly rapid onset and may affect children, adolescents, and adults of any age whereas the symptoms of toxic adenoma usually occur at a much slower rate in an older age group.

Many of the symptoms in persons with hyperthyroidism are related to the metabolic effects of excessive thyroid hormone.[12] Three out of four patients have a weight loss of 10 to 20 pounds despite a ravenous appetite. The weight loss results from an energy imbalance caused by increased oxygen consumption as measured by basal metabolic rate as well as increased energy cost of muscular work. Depending on the severity of thyrotoxicosis, the BMR may be double the standard in severe cases, 30% to 60% higher in moderately severe cases, or 10% to 30% higher in milder cases. Anorexia also may occur, especially in severe cases.[13]

The altered absorption of carbohydrate from the gut may activate or intensify diabetes. After a standard oral glucose load the patient with hyperthyroidism has an early and rapid rise in blood glucose concentration (as great as 200 mg/dl), which may be associated with glycosuria. In addition, hyperthyroidism increases the demand for insulin although the effectiveness of insulin on carbohydrate metabolism also is enhanced.

The levels of many lipids are depressed with hyperthyroidism. The balance of the increased synthesis and degradation of cholesterol results in a lower serum cholesterol concentration. The cholesterol-lowering action of excessive thyroid hormone may be due to the effects of malnutrition and weight loss. Another effect of thyroid hormone on cholesterol metabolism is the increased conversion of cholesterol to bile acids, with increased excretion in the bile. Plasma triglycerides, some of the lipoprotein fractions, and free tocopherol also are lowered with thyroid hormone. Nonesterified free fatty acids are increased in patients with thyrotoxicosis.

The excessive thyroid hormone accelerates protein metabolism, often producing clinical symptoms. Muscular symptoms vary from mild myasthenia to profound muscular weakness and atrophy.[12] Nitrogen balance may be normal or negative depending on whether the intake meets the demand of increased catabolism. The increased catabolism of protein and collagen causes an increase in the excretion of nitrogen and urinary hydroxyproline. Creatinuria also is seen in hyperthyroidism. Decreased creatine clearance results from a decreased ability of the muscles to use the creatine produced in the liver. The alterations in metabolism also result in altered needs for some of the vitamins in the hyperthyroid patient.[13]

The increased energy needs lead to an increased need for the B vitamins thiamine and riboflavin. The increase in protein metabolism leads to an increased need for vitamin B_6. The requirements for vitamin B_{12} are increased in experimental thyrotoxicosis, and lack of the B vitamins has been implicated as a cause of liver damage in hyperthyroidism. Although there is increased absorption of vitamin A and accelerated conversion of carotene to vitamin A, blood concentrations of vitamin A may be low because of increased needs.

The skeletal system often is affected in hyperthyroidism. Linear bone growth may be increased in children. Bone age may exceed chronologic age because of accelerated epiphyseal closure. X-ray films of the bones in adults frequently show evidence of decalcification from an increased rate of bone resorption. Treatment of hyperthyroidism restores bone density in younger patients but not in the elderly. Although fractures are uncommon, a chronically thyrotoxic post-menopausal woman may have a collapsed vertebra. Patients with hyperthyroidism extended over a period of years may have severe and premature osteoporosis.

Although the serum calcium concentration is usually normal, it may be elevated enough to produce nausea, vomiting, and weakness. The hypercalcemia leads to hypercalciuria, causing polydypsia and polyuria. The negative calcium balance sometimes can be corrected by administering calcium. Serum phosphorus concentration is generally normal rather than low, as in hyperparathyroidism. Adrenal steroid hormones also may correct the hypercalcemia. Phosphorus administration lowers the concentration of calcium in serum and urine to normal levels. Evidence suggests that abnormal calcium metabolism is due to a direct effect of the thyroid hormone on bone rather than to hyperparathyroidism; but hypomagnesemia, a characteristic of hyperthyroidism, may acutely stimulate the release of parathormone from the parathyroid glands (p. 258). As bone is rebuilt during treatment, the alkaline phosphatase value may remain elevated and the phosphorus concentration depressed. The serum calcium concentration will fall to normal only gradually.

Since blood volume is increased in hyperthyroidism, the hemoglobin and hematocrit are in the low normal range.[13] Normocytic anemia with hemoglobin values as low as 8 or 9 g/dl are occasionally seen in severe cases of thyrotoxicosis. These patients may show impaired iron utilization. The anemia is not responsive to hematinic therapy, but iron utilization returns to normal after control of hyperthyroidism.

Thyroid hormone appears to affect the gastrointestinal tract. The oral glucose tolerance curve may show an abnormally rapid rise and fall with resultant glycosuria. Bowel motility increases, resulting in decreased transit time and possible impairment of fat absorption, particularly with excessive intake of fat. The prominent symptom may be an increase in the frequency of stools, which are well formed. Although frank diarrhea is unusual, on occasion the increased bowel action progresses to diarrhea. Intestinal absorption of calcium is reduced in hyperthyroidism. The defect is probably in the distal portion of the small intestine and thus may be independent of the reductions in 1,25-dihydroxyvitamin D reported in thyrotoxicosis, since vitamin D acts in the proximal small intestine.[14]

Diagnosis. Even though Graves' disease may be diagnosed on the basis of clinical presentation (infiltrative ophthalmopathy, pretibial myxedema, symmetrically enlarged thyroid with a smooth surface), the diagnosis should be confirmed by determining thyroid hormone levels. Serum thyroid hormones are elevated in most cases.[15,16]

Treatment. Thyrotoxicosis may be treated surgically or medically (including use of radioactive iodine). Prior to surgical treatment, thyroid blocking drugs or beta-blocking agents are administered in an effort to make the patient euthyroid. During this time an attempt should be undertaken to improve nutritional status in patients who have lost weight by providing a high-calorie diet with adequate protein.[17] The increase in calories over normal needs depends on the elevation of metabolic rate, varying from 15%-25% above the normal allowance to 50%-75% above for severe cases. The total caloric need may be 4000 or 5000 kcal. Since in many cases there is a negative nitrogen balance, the protein content of the diet should be increased to 100 g. An increase in carbohydrate intake will spare the proteins and provide a source of easily assimilated food energy. All essential food nutrients should be supplied liberally in the diet and as supplements, particularly of the B vitamins, to meet the increased demand.

Thyrotoxicosis also can be treated medically, either by using propylthiouracil or methimazole (Tapazole) or by administering radioactive iodine. In both cases, return to the euthyroid state is gradual and nutritional management is similar to that described for the preoperative period.

After successful treatment of Graves' disease and hyperthyroidism, patients often experience increased appetite without the increased caloric needs, resulting in excessive weight gain. Thus the patient should be weighed regularly. If the weight reaches 120% of normal for height or an excessive gain occurs in those who were above normal weight for height prior to treatment, the patient should be counseled on weight control. For every pound of weight to be lost per week there should be a corresponding decrease in normal energy allowances of 500 kcal/day. Appropriate counseling has been shown to prevent weight gain in such patients.[18]

Hypothyroidism

A hypothyroid state may be caused by idiopathic, iatrogenic, or dietary factors. Causes associated with dietary habits induce biosynthetic defects in thyroid synthesis. In many parts of the world iodine deficiency is still the most common cause of hypothyroidism. Malnutrition causes low serum thyroid concentration. Generalized malnutrition has been shown[19] to aggravate any goitrogenic process. In such cases serum concentrations of amino acids fall, suggesting a down-regulation in protein metabolism. Goitrogens found in foods may act as antithyroid agents. In the United States, hypothyroidism is more likely to be idiopathic or due to therapy for hyperthyroidism.[20] Hypothyroidism also may result from iodide found in medicines formulated for patients with asthma. Hypothyroidism is most frequent after the fourth or fifth decade and is more common in women.

The lack of thyroid hormone alters energy metabolism.[2] There is a decrease in oxygen consumption as measured by basal metabolic rate. Decreased utilization of substrates results in lessened heat production, which leads to the cold intolerance commonly found in hypothyroid persons. The metabolic rate may fall between 30% and 45% below the standard with complete lack of thyroid hormone. In hypopituitarism the rate may be 50% below the standard.[13] The lethargy found in hypothyroid patients also leads to decreased energy expenditure from physical activity. Anorexia and decreased food intake compensate for the lowered energy needs. Therefore most persons with hypothyroidism lose weight in the initial stages and later gain only 10 to 20 pounds.

Protein digestion and amino acid absorption appear to be normal. Although protein balance is usually positive, there are defects in metabolism.[20] These are most obvious in hypothyroid children, who generally show retarded growth and weight from impaired synthesis of secreted, functional, and structural protein. Increased quantities of proteins such as albumin and lipoproteins can be found even though protein catabolism also is impaired. Since blood volume is reduced and plasma albumin concentrations are normal, the excess albumin is largely in the interstitial space.

Carbohydrate metabolism remains normal but glucose utilization is reduced.[20] Glucose absorption is slower, resulting in a glucose tolerance curve that is flat, probably because of delayed gastric emptying. Insulin responses differ depending on the method of glucose administration. The responses are appropriate for oral glucose but decreased if the glucose is administered intravenously. Thus intravenous glucose tolerance tests result in slower glucose utilization. The insulin requirements for diabetic patients may decrease because exogenous insulin is degraded more slowly.

Gastrointestinal function and structure alterations produce clinical gastrointestinal symptoms. The most frequent is a decrease in motility. Delayed gastric emptying and decreased intestinal motility cause nausea, vomiting, abdominal distention, and, quite frequently, constipation. Mucosal atrophy, lymphocytic infiltration, and mucinous infiltration of the bowel wall also are common. In some patients with idiopathic hypothyroidism or chronic autoimmune thyroiditis, pernicious anemia may develop. The gastric atrophy and achlorhydria frequently observed may lead to vitamin B_{12} and iron malabsorption.[13] The tongue is usually large and sometimes smooth as in pernicious anemia, but patients do not complain of soreness. When anemia is marked, the tongue may be pale, but more often it is red, in contrast to the pallid face.

When hypothyroidism is due to a primary defect in the thyroid gland, plasma cholesterol concentrations are elevated due to an imbalance in the steady state synthesis and destruction of cholesterol.[20] Decreases in cholesterol destruction and biliary excretion are more pronounced than is the decrease in cholesterol synthesis. Liver size and function are normal. Plasma triglyceride concentrations may be increased slightly and serum carotene concentrations frequently are elevated.

The mild anemia commonly found among patients with hypothyroidism may be attributable to a variety of factors alone or in combination. The bone marrow is depressed when there is a lack of thyroid hormone. Decreased oxygen demand in hypothyroidism causes diminished blood cell formation. Plasma and red cell iron turnover is decreased, and the bone marrow frequently is hypoplastic. If this is the sole cause of anemia, treatment with thyroid hormone will return the hemoglobin to normal. Blood loss from menorrhagia among hypothyroid women may lead to hypochromic microcytic anemia caused by iron deficiency. The decreased absorption of iron from gastric achlorhydria also may result in iron deficiency anemia. Hypochromic microcytic anemia will respond with iron alone, but optimum response occurs with thyroid and iron. Occasionally coincident pernicious anemia causes macrocytic anemia. Some hypothyroid patients who develop pernicious anemia no longer need parenteral B_{12} after treatment. Those who absorb oral B_{12} poorly are corrected by intrinsic factor, which may or may not need to be continued after thyroid therapy.

Diagnosis. Hypothyroidism is diagnosed by finding a low serum level of thyroxine. Because thyroxine is largely bound to serum proteins and the levels of these proteins are altered in many physiologic conditions (such as pregnancy) as well as in malnutrition and other disease states, it is necessary to obtain some measure of thyroxine binding proteins (e.g., the T_3 resin binding test) and use this value to correct the total thyroxine level. Alternatively, free thyroxine can be directly measured. In hypothyroidism resulting from primary failure of the thyroid gland, the diagnosis can be confirmed by finding an elevated serum level of thyroid-stimulating hormone (TSH). In hypothyroidism secondary to pituitary or hypothalamic failure, the TSH level is low.[21]

Treatment. Adequate replacement therapy with thyroid hormone reverses all the metabolic abnormalities of hypothyroidism, and no special diet is required. A patient who remains obese after the return of thyroid function tests to normal should be treated as if this were simple exogenous obesity. It is never acceptable to increase the dose of thyroid hormone to supraphysiologic level solely to achieve weight reduction; the adverse health consequences of the resulting thyrotoxicosis outweigh any benefits of weight reduction.

Several studies[22,23] have suggested that thyroid hormone administration is associated with negative calcium balance and loss of bone mineral content. It is not clear whether this is related to normal replacement doses or to doses that may be slightly excessive but without easily detectable clinical or laboratory signs of overdosage. In any case it has been suggested[24] that, because of the potential for bone mineral loss, all patients receiving thyroid replacement therapy be given supplemental calcium and vitamin D.

Soybeans and soybean-derived products may absorb thyroid hormone from the gastrointestinal tract and prevent its absorption. This may lead to an apparent failure to respond to thyroid replacement therapy. In most clinical settings, such heavy soybean consumption rarely occurs but it may be a problem in infants fed a soy-based formula.

Parathyroid Hormone (Parathormone)

The parathyroid glands play an essential role in calcium and phosphorus metabolism. It is now well established that a major function of parathormone (PTH) is to influence vitamin D metabolism. Another major mineral, magnesium, is itself an important regulator of parathyroid hormone secretion.

Parathormone secretion and synthesis both are regulated primarily by the concentration of ionized calcium in the blood. The hormone acts directly on bone and kidney, and it affects intestinal function indirectly through its influence on vitamin D metabolism; in bone, PTH increases the number and size of osteoclasts and may stimulate osteocytes to reabsorb calcium (this effect is to remove calcium from bone and to raise the serum calcium level); in the kidney, PTH increases the renal excretion of phosphate and the tubular reabsorption of calcium and magnesium (bicarbonate secretion also is enhanced, as is reabsorption of hydrogen ion and ammonia, which lead to the hyperchloremic metabolic acidosis commonly seen in hyperparathyroid states).

Another important function of PTH is to stimulate the hydroxylation, in the kidney, of 25-hydroxyvitamin D (25-OH-D) to 1,25-dihydroxyvitamin D (1,25-$(OH)_2$-D). Because 1,25-$(OH)_2$-D has 1000 to 5000 times the calcium mobilizing activity of vitamin D itself, this conversion may be responsible for many physiologic actions previously attributed directly to PTH.[25]

Vitamin D Metabolism

Vitamin D can be provided in the diet either as a substance naturally occurring in foods (animal and fish oils) or as a supplement in milk and other products. It may be ingested as either ergocalciferol (vitamin D_2) or cholecalciferol (vitamin D_3). In humans both forms have similar potency and share common metabolic pathways.[26] Vitamin D_3 also can be synthesized in the skin when adequate solar ultraviolet light is available. As noted, for full biologic activity vitamin D first must be metabolized to 25-OH-D in the liver and then to 1,25-$(OH)_2$-D in the kidney. The latter conversion is promoted by PTH and by low serum inorganic phosphate levels.

Vitamin D acts on the intestine to stimulate calcium absorption. Although this is usually accompanied by phosphate absorption, a separate small intestinal phosphate transport system is also activated by vitamin D. In bone, vitamin D mobilizes calcium from previously formed bone.

PTH also is needed for this to occur. Despite the fact that this may seem contrary to vitamin D's action in promoting bone calcification, it apparently is necessary for the elevation of extracellular calcium and phosphate concentrations and to permit mineralization of newly formed bone.[25] There is evidence that vitamin D also increases renal tubular reabsorption of calcium and phosphate, but these effects are minor and of uncertain homeostatic significance.

Magnesium

Parathormone secretion can be stimulated by acute lowering of the serum magnesium concentration. In clinical situations hypomagnesemia commonly is a chronic state, and PTH secretion is inappropriately low. Hypomagnesemia also appears to produce peripheral resistance to PTH.[27]

Hyperparathyroidism

Several clinical situations lead to increased amounts of circulating PTH. *Primary* hyperparathyroidism may be due to single or multiple benign parathyroid adenomas, hyperplasia of the four parathyroid glands, or parathyroid carcinoma. *Secondary* hyperparathyroidism is seen in vitamin D deficiency or states in which vitamin D metabolism is altered (e.g., liver or kidney disease, anticonvulsant therapy), in states of peripheral resistance to PTH (pseudohypoparathyroidism), and in hypocalcemia from causes other than hypoparathyroidism. *Tertiary* hyperparathyroidism occurs when PTH secretion remains increased after secondary hyperparathyroidism, especially that resulting from renal failure, has been treated (e.g., after renal transplantation). Occasionally nonparathyroid tumors are sources of ectopic PTH production.

Pathology. Most cases of hyperparathyroidism currently are discovered fortuitously when serum calcium is measured as part of routine screening blood tests. In such cases, symptoms are rare. The most common symptoms are weakness, fatigability, anorexia, constipation, and weight loss. Hypercalcemia and hypercalciuria impair the kidney's ability to concentrate urine, and polyuria results. Up to 50% of patients have nephrolithiasis, but many times the stones are asymptomatic. It is now rare in the United States to see extensive bone disease from hyperparathyroidism. The classic disease, osteitis fibrosa cystica, consists of bone demineralization, bone pain, bone cysts, and subperiosteal resorption of bone.

Diagnosis. Hyperparathyroidism usually is suspected when an elevated serum calcium concentration and hypophosphatemia are found. Elevated PTH concentrations usually confirm the diagnosis, eliminating most other causes of hypercalcemia. Appropriate studies to rule out ectopic PTH production and secondary hyperparathyroidism generally depend on the clinical presentation.

Treatment. Parathyroidectomy is usually the treatment of choice. After surgery, patients with extensive bone disease rapidly deposit calcium into demineralized bone. This "bone hunger" generally is treated by intravenous calcium or large oral doses of calcium carbonate. Hypomagnesemia may accompany the hyperparathyroid state and may need to be treated to correct postoperative hypocalcemia. If hypocalcemia lasts more than a week postoperatively, permanent hypoparathyroidism probably has resulted as a (sometimes unavoidable) complication of surgery and should be treated as described under "Hypoparathyroidism."

More patients with asymptomatic hyperparathyroidism are being diagnosed. The natural history of this disorder is not entirely understood. Some authorities feel that operative intervention may not be justified if the serum calcium concentration is within 1 mg/dl of normal. In such cases, treatment includes a low-calcium diet (less than 400 mg/da), forced hydration (3-4 liters/da), and a high salt intake (8-10 g/da). Phosphate supplementation (about 2 g/da) may reduce urine calcium, but at the risk of promoting ectopic tissue calcification. Thus rigorous medical management usually is advised only for persons with symptomatic hypercalcemia who are poor risks for surgical procedures.

Hypoparathyroidism

Spontaneous idiopathic hypoparathyroidism is relatively rare. Most often, hypoparathyroidism is due to intentional or inadvertent removal of, or damage to the vascular supply of, the parathyroid glands during thyroid or parathyroid surgery. As noted, chronic hypomagnesemia also leads to correctible hypoparathyroidism.

Pathology. The most common symptom is tetany. Thinning of the hair, coarse skin, dental hypoplasia, and cataracts also are common in longstanding disease. In idiopathic hypoparathyroidism, chronic cutaneous candidiasis is common. These patients often have circulating antibodies to parathyroid tissue and frequently have other autoimmune disorders (e.g., Addison's disease, Hashimoto's thyroiditis, pernicious anemia).

Diagnosis. Hypoparathyroidism usually is diagnosed by the presence of hypocalcemia, hyperphosphatemia, and low levels of PTH. Magnesium deficiency should be excluded.

Treatment. The therapeutic goal is to restore serum calcium levels to near-normal (>8.5 mg/dl) while keeping urine calcium under 4 mg/kg/day. Hyperphosphatemia should be controlled by a low-phosphorus diet, restricting meat and dairy products, and no vitamin D should be given until the serum phosphate level is normal. Vitamin D in supraphysiologic doses is needed by virtually all patients with hypoparathyroidism. The dose varies with patient age and size and disease severity, and also may depend on calcium intake. The usual starting dose in adults is 50,000 units daily. Because vitamin D acts rather slowly, dose changes should not be made more frequently than every few weeks and should be made in small increments (e.g., 100,000 units/

wk). Some resistant patients may require over 200,000 units/day.

Vitamin D preparations that act more rapidly (Table 17-1) sometimes are useful in that, if vitamin D toxicity results, it is of shorter duration and more easily managed. Recommended preparations and initial doses are dihydrotachysterol (Hytakerol), 0.75 mg/day; and 1,25-dihydroxycholecalciferol (calcitriol, Rocaltrol), 0.25 μg/day. Such preparations are substantially more expensive than other forms of vitamin D.

Calcium supplementation is also generally necessary, at a level of 1000 to 3000 mg/day. Calcium carbonate is the preferred preparation since it contains 40% calcium and therefore provides the most convenient dosage form. Calcium carbonate may (rarely) cause metabolic alkalosis, however, so in these cases either calcium lactate or calcium gluconate may be used (Table 17-2).

A low-phosphorus diet should be followed. This involves limiting the intake of foods high in phosphorus—liver, fish, poultry, eggs, milk, cheese, whole grain cereals, and nuts. Unless hyperphosphatemia is a problem, severe restriction of these items generally is not necessary.

Table 17-1 Vitamin D Preparations Useful in Treating Hypoparathyroidism

	Trade Name	Forms
Vitamin D$_2$ (ergocalciferol)	Deltalin	50,000 IU capsules
	Geltabs	50,000 IU capsules
	Drisdol	50,000 IU capsules
	Vitamin D (generic)	25,000-50,000 IU capsules
	Calciferol (generic)	50,000 IU tablets
Dihydrotachysterol	Hytakerol	0.125 mg capsules
	(Generic form)	0.125, 0.2, 4 mg tablets
Calcitriol	Rocaltrol	0.25, 0.5 μg capsules

Table 17-2 Calcium Preparations Useful in Treating Hypoparathyroidism

	Trade Name	Forms
Calcium carbonate (40% Ca^{+2})	Titralac	400 mg Ca^{+2}/5 ml
		170 mg Ca^{+2}/tablet
	Dicarbosil	500 mg Ca^{+2}/tablet
	Os-Cal	250 mg, 500 mg Ca^{+2}/tablet
	Tums	200 mg Ca^{+2}/tablet
Calcium lactate (13% Ca^{+2})	(Generic)	40 mg, 80 mg Ca^{+2}/tablet
Calcium gluconate (10% Ca^{+2})	(Generic)	45, 50, 60, 90, 100 mg Ca^{+2}/tablet

Adrenal Cortex

The adrenal cortex secretes three groups of hormones: mineralocorticoids, glucocorticoids, and androgens. These steroid hormones affect mineral balance, intermediary metabolism, and hence nutritional status. Diseases of the adrenal cortex, like most endocrine disorders, are primarily those of hormone overproduction or underproduction. Treatment consists of removing (when possible) the source of excess hormone or replacing the missing hormone. When this can be done satisfactorily, the diseases have no significant nutritional implications, and no special nutritional therapy is indicated. However, when treatment is not fully effective or takes substantial time to produce clinical improvement, it may be useful to direct one's attention to certain dietary principles as an adjunct to specific treatment. In some cases (for example, the therapeutic use of glucocorticoids [cortisone or prednisone]) an endocrinopathy is produced intentionally. Then proper nutritional management may be helpful in preventing or minimizing certain complications of therapy.

Mineralocorticoids

Mineralocorticoids are steroids that affect ion transport by epithelial cells, resulting in sodium conservation and potassium loss. The most important naturally occurring mineralocorticoid is aldosterone, followed by 11-deoxycorticosterone (DOC), 18-hydroxy-DOC, corticosterone, and cortisol.[28]

Mineralocorticoids and Salt Balance

Because of the physiologic importance of maintaining sodium, potassium, and water balance, multiple homeostatic mechanisms are responsible for this function. Mineralocorticoids are one such mechanism. Aldosterone secretion is controlled by three factors. The most important is the renin-angiotensin system. Both decreased circulating volume, as sensed by decreased pressure in the different renal arterioles, and decreased sodium load in the macula densa region of the distal tubule stimulate renin release. By activating angiotensin, renin stimulates aldosterone secretion. The serum potassium concentration also can affect aldosterone secretion; hyperkalemia increases aldosterone synthesis and release. ACTH also may be necessary for optimum aldosterone release.

Syndromes of Mineralocorticoid Excess

Increased aldosterone leads to increased tubular absorption of sodium and, in turn, to retention of sodium and water and expansion of extracellular volume. Normally this does not continue indefinitely. After about 250 to 400 mEq of excess sodium is retained, an "escape phenomenon" increases renal sodium excretion and establishes a new salt balance. The reason for this escape is unknown. Some authors postulate that the increased volume resulting from sodium retention stimulates secretion of an as yet unidentified natriuretic principle, which in turn stimulates sodium excretion. The escape prevents edema in persons subject to chronic aldosterone excess. Edema occurs only when the escape mechanism fails. Even when the escape occurs, and sodium and water balance are restored, potassium loss continues.

Endogenous oversecretion of aldosterone may be primary or secondary. Primary aldosteronism can be due to an adrenal adenoma, adrenal hyperplasia, or multiple microadenomas. Causes of secondary hyperaldosteronism include the following: malignant hypertension; renal vascular disease; renin-secreting tumors; edematous states associated with renal, cardiac, or hepatic disease; pregnancy; and medications containing estrogen. All of these are associated with hypokalemia. A diet low in sodium and high in potassium may correct hypokalemia, but it does nothing for the underlying condition. The low sodium intake facilitates potassium retention, presumably by limiting the amount of sodium available to the distal tubule for exchange with potassium.[29] However, potassium secretion usually remains high in the patient with excess aldosterone secretion and essentially equals potassium intake. Thus, very large intakes are needed to replace the potassium deficit. Ultimately, treatment must be aimed at the underlying disease, and dietary therapy is useful only during diagnosis and while awaiting definitive therapy.

Diagnosis. Patients usually present with a low serum potassium level. In contrast to hypokalemia caused by vomiting or diarrhea, urinary potassium levels are high despite the potassium deficit. The diagnosis is confirmed by demonstrating high serum or urine aldosterone with a suppressed level of plasma renin activity. This measurement should be made after serum potassium is normalized. The plasma renin activity should not be increased after volume depletion, which can be produced either by 3-5 days on a low-sodium diet (10 mEq/da) or by giving 80 mg of furosemide and maintaining an upright posture for 3 hours.

Treatment. A patient found to have a solitary adrenal adenoma is best treated surgically. Other causes of hyperaldosteronism may be treated with the aldosterone antagonist spironolactone along with, if necessary, the adjunctive dietary measures mentioned earlier.

Syndromes of Mineralocorticoid Deficiency

About one third of the patients with selective aldosterone deficiency also have diabetes. Neither the cause of the hypoaldosteronism nor the reason for its association with diabetes is known. On occasion, specific enzymatic blocks in aldosterone synthesis have been described, but most patients also are deficient in renin.

Diagnosis. The presenting symptom is hyperkalemia, which fails to stimulate aldosterone secretion. In diabetic patients, glucose-induced hyperkalemia also may appear.[30]

Treatment. Mineralocorticoid replacement with fludrocortisone acetate (Florinef) generally is indicated. Dietary therapy, such as potassium restriction, rarely is needed.

GLUCOCORTICOIDS

Steroid hormones that have a major effect on carbohydrate metabolism are called glucocorticoids. Four of the hormones naturally secreted by the adrenal gland—cortisol, cortisone, corticosterone, and 11-dehydrocorticosterone—have appreciable glucocorticoid activity. Cortisol is by far the most important of these in man. The synthetic steroids prednisone, prednisolone, methylprednisolone (Medrol), betamethasone (Celestone), dexamethasone (Decadron), triamcinolone (Aristocort), and fludrocortisone acetate (Florinef) all have glucocorticoid activity, although fludrocortisone is used primarily for its mineralocorticoid activity. In spite of the name glucocorticoid, these substances affect protein and fat metabolism as well as carbohydrate metabolism.

Effects of Glucocorticoids on Intermediary Metabolism and Nutritional Status

Carbohydrate metabolism. Glucocorticoids stimulate gluconeogenesis in a number of ways,

including increasing the transport of amino acids into liver cells, increasing the level of gluconeogenic enzymes within the liver (presumably by activating DNA transcription), and increasing mobilization of amino acids from muscle and other extrahepatic tissues. At the same time, glucocorticoids decrease the rate of glucose utilization by cells. The mechanism behind this is not known, but multiple factors may be involved. In pharmacologic quantities, cortisol impairs binding of insulin to its receptors. In contrast to the decreased insulin binding of obesity (with which hypercortisolism often is associated), the reduced binding of insulin is due not to a reduction in receptor number but to decreased receptor affinity.[31] Changes in glucose transport may precede measurable changes in insulin binding, and the binding changes may not fully explain the observed changes in transport, suggesting that glucocorticoids also may produce a postreceptor intracellular impairment in insulin-stimulated glucose metabolism.[32] The net effect of glucocorticoids on carbohydrate metabolism is to raise the plasma glucose level (although only rarely enough to cause diabetic symptoms, and then only if present in excessive quantities) and to increase liver glycogen stores.

Protein metabolism. Cortisol and other glucocorticoids reduce protein stores in virtually all cells except hepatocytes. This is a result of both decreased protein synthesis and increased catabolism. Amino acid transport into nonhepatic cells is decreased, while it is increased in liver cells. Plasma amino acid levels increase, and the liver may use these amino acids for synthesis of plasma proteins (e.g., albumin), for increased synthesis of liver proteins, and for gluconeogenesis. In effect, glucocorticoids mobilize amino acids from peripheral tissues, especially muscle, and facilitate their utilization by the liver.

Fat metabolism. Glucocorticoids weakly promote mobilization of fatty acids from adipose tissue and cause a slight increase in plasma fatty acids levels. Cortisol also appears to increase fatty acid oxidation. Thus utilization of fat reserves as a source of energy is facilitated by glucocorticoids. As will be discussed, excessive glucocorticoids can lead to increased fat accumulation, especially in certain parts of the body. This type of obesity may result from excessive stimulation of food intake, so fat is generated more rapidly than it is metabolized.

Permissive action of glucocorticoids. In physiologic quantities glucocorticoids may permit, rather than cause, many of the metabolic reactions to stress. For example, in contrast to normal animals, adrenalectomized animals fail to increase urinary nitrogen in response to surgical stress. When these animals are kept on constant maintenance doses of corticosteroids, their catabolic response to stress is appropriate.[33] This response depends on the presence of corticosteroids but not on an increase in their secretion. The mechanism for the permissive effect is not fully known, and multiple mechanisms may be present. These include modification of the actions of cyclic AMP (a second messenger of many hormones), other effects on hormones that work through cell surface receptors (glucagon epinephrine, growth hormone, ACTH), and alterations in enzymatic activity and transport processes.[34]

Other effects. In excessive quantities glucocorticoids may affect calcium metabolism, bone structure, and growth. It is not clear that these effects are important in normal physiology, however.

Syndromes of Glucocorticoid Excess

Glucocorticoid excess may result from either endogenous oversecretion or exogenous glucocorticoid taken in amounts beyond those needed for physiologic replacement. Metabolic consequences are similar regardless of cause. The general picture of glucocorticoid excess is called Cushing's syndrome. When it is specifically due to a pathologic increase in ACTH secretion by the pituitary, it is called Cushing's disease. Other causes of Cushing's syndrome include adrenal adenomas and (rarely) carcinomas and ectopic secretion of ACTH.

Diagnosis. The patient with Cushing's syndrome typically has truncal obesity, mild hirsutism, moderate hypertension, plethora, weakness, increased bruisability, and red or purple striae. Glucose intolerance and emotional changes also occur. The diagnosis is confirmed by demonstrating increased serum and/or urine cortisol. The major urinary metabolites of cortisol, 17-hydroxycorticosteroids (17-OHCS), also are increased. The major diagnostic problem is simple obesity, which increases cortisol production, thus elevating urinary cortisol and 17-OHCS levels. Plasma cortisol is usually normal, but isolated values may be high. Plasma and urine cortisol and 17-OHCS levels are suppressed by dexamethasone (0.5 mg q6h), in normal and obese persons, whereas in patients with Cushing's disease the levels usually are not suppressed by this dose (a so-called low-dose suppression test). The high-dose dexamethasone suppression test (2 mg q6h) will separate persons with Cushing's disease (whose cortisol secretion is suppressed on this dose) from those with other causes of Cushing's syndrome (whose cortisol levels are not suppressed on either high- or low-dose dexamethasone).* Measuring the plasma ACTH level will distinguish ectopic ACTH syndromes from adrenal neoplasms, the latter having suppressed ACTH secretion.

Pathology. Although hypercortisolism is associated with obesity, not all patients are obese, and extreme obesity is rare. The fat distribution is characteristic, with increased fat over the cheeks ("moon face"), increased supraclavicular fat pads, and an accentuation of the fat pad over the upper back ("buffalo hump"). The arms and legs are thin, possibly because of loss of muscle mass. In patients with carcinoma, both adrenal and ACTH-producing, the inanition accompanying larger tumors may cause weight loss rather than obesity. Hypokalemia may be the presenting symptom in such patients.

Effects of cortisol on carbohydrate, fat, and protein metabolism have been discussed. Growth may be retarded in children with Cushing's syndrome. Bone demineralization is common and may be due to inhibition of both protein matrix formation and vitamin D activity. Collagen formation is impaired, leading to easy bruising and impaired wound healing. The latter usually makes surgery on these patients difficult.

Therapy. In Cushing's disease, treatment often is directed at the pituitary. Hypophysectomy frequently is done, especially since microdissection techniques combined with a transsphenoidal approach have made it possible to remove an ACTH-producing adenoma while leaving other pituitary functions intact. The pituitary also may be treated by external irradiation or by the se-

---

*Some diagnostic confusion may result because the dexamethasone suppression test is also abnormal in depressive psychiatric illness. This abnormality may result from the vegetative disturbances of depression including loss of appetite and weight with subsequent nutritional deficiencies.[35]

rotonin antagonist cyproheptadine. Other forms of Cushing's syndrome are treated, when possible, by adrenalectomy. At times, however, the patient's general condition is such that this procedure carries a very high risk of major complications and death. In adrenal carcinoma and ectopic ACTH syndromes, total adrenalectomy often is not feasible. In these cases medical therapy can be used. Mitotane (*o,p'*-DDD) produces selective atrophy of the adrenal gland and interferes with cortisol synthesis. Aminoglutethimide also blocks cortisol formation, as does metyrapone.

Nutritional management. Because patients with Cushing's syndrome have excess body fat, it is tempting to institute weight reduction diets. This must be done cautiously because in hypercortisolism the caloric deficit is replaced not only from adipose tissue stores but also from functional protein. In fact, the increased body fat in the person with hypercortisolism is not accompanied by a proportional increase in body weight, since total protein mass actually is reduced.[2] The rate of protein degradation, although increased, is relatively constant and not affected by dietary protein. Thus a high-protein diet (>1 g/kg of body weight) may result in positive nitrogen balance, whether or not adequate calories are provided.[2] Such diets should be given to all persons with hypercortisolism, regardless of cause or method of treatment. Because such persons may wish to attempt severe caloric restriction to attain weight reduction, the reasons for a continued high-protein intake must be explained carefully.

As noted earlier, bone demineralization is common in chronic glucocorticoid excess. Although the mechanism behind this is not fully understood, most studies show decreased fractional and total intestinal calcium absorption with normal or increased urinary calcium. Glucocorticoids appear to impair conversion of vitamin D to 25-hydroxyvitamin D (25-OH-D); however, various studies have reported both normal and reduced serum 25-OH-D concentrations in persons chronically receiving supraphysiologic doses of glucocorticoids. Likewise, studies[36] have reported both normal and increased serum parathyroid hormone concentrations. It is not clear whether increased dietary calcium or vitamin D supplementation might be useful in treating patients with hypercortisolism. It seems prudent to ensure that dietary calcium be kept no lower than commonly accepted maintenance levels. Because a diet high in protein is being given, at least 800 to 1000 mg calcium/day should be provided. Some authors also suggest 50,000 units of vitamin D twice a week, if this does not cause hypercalciuria.

Syndromes of Glucocorticoid Deficiency

It is rare to see isolated glucocorticoid deficiency. The usual clinical picture is that of either primary adrenal insufficiency (Addison's disease), where both glucocorticoid and mineralocorticoid deficiency are present, or secondary adrenal insufficiency as a result of pituitary failure, in which case the presentation is that of panhypopituitarism. In most cases the nutritional consequences are the opposite of glucocorticoid excess. In addition, for unknown reasons, gastrointestinal symptoms such as anorexia, nausea, and diarrhea often occur in adrenal insufficiency. This leads to decreased nutrient intake. In general, most patients are in negative nitrogen balance if their weight is falling. Treatment with physiologic doses of glucocorticoids increases urinary nitrogen excretion[37]; but, because of increased food intake, protein balance improves.

Persons with Addison's disease do not tolerate salt restriction. Especially in warm weather, such patients should be encouraged to use salt liberally, even when on appropriate replacement therapy. At times of severe stress, increased salt intake by itself is not usually adequate, and extra glucocorticoid replacement must be taken. All patients with adrenal insufficiency should be instructed in these precautions and should wear proper identification necklaces or bracelets.

As previously noted, glucocorticoids are important in maintaining the plasma glucose concentration at normal levels during fasting. Some patients with adrenal insufficiency may be prone to fasting hypoglycemia. In the adequately diagnosed and treated patient this is rarely a problem, although long periods of fasting should be avoided. In the undiagnosed patient, who is often anorectic, hypoglycemia may be a presenting manifestation.

Diagnosis. The presenting signs and symptoms may be quite subtle, and the diagnosis should be suspected in any patient with hypotension, orthostatic hypotension, weakness in warm weather, anorexia or other unexplained gastrointestinal symptoms, and hyperpigmentation. Hyponatremia and hyperkalemia further suggest the diagnosis. A low plasma cortisol level in the morning (when cortisol is usually at its highest) is also suggestive, but failure to respond to injection of ACTH with increased plasma cortisol is needed to confirm the diagnosis. Other tests are needed to distinguish primary from secondary adrenal insufficiency.

Treatment. Replacement therapy usually is started with cortisone acetate (25 mg mornings and 12.5 mg evenings) or with prednisone (5 mg mornings and 2.5 mg evenings). Although both of these have some mineralocorticoid activity, most patients with primary adrenal insufficiency also need fludrocortisone (Florinef) in amounts from 0.05-0.2 mg daily. With proper hormonal replacement, no special dietary restrictions are needed and, as already noted, salt should be freely available.

ADRENAL ANDROGENS

The adrenal cortex secretes androgens in men and women. There are both overproduction and underproduction of adrenal androgens, but none have major nutritional implications. Large sex hormone–secreting adrenal carcinomas may cause general inanition similar to that produced by other tumors. In women, oversecretion of adrenal androgens may be responsible for some cases of hirsutism. Hyperandrogenism has been associated with obesity, whether or not hirsutism is present, and the clearance rate of androgens is increased in the obese.[38] Theoretically hirsutism could worsen if the obese hyperandrogenic woman loses weight, but there have been no clinical reports of this.

ADRENAL MEDULLA

The principal disorder of the adrenal medulla is the development of tumors that secrete the catecholamines epinephrine and/or norepinephrine. These tumors are called pheochromocytomas.

Catecholamines increase the rate of energy utilization and, as a result, increase heat production and oxygen consumption. They also mobilize stored fuels, both locally and systemically. At the local level, muscle glycogenolysis and brown fat lipolysis contribute substrate for use by the same or nearby cells; systemically stored fuels are released into the circulation for use by distant tissues.[39] In addition to stimulating glycogenolysis and lipolysis, catecholamines promote protein breakdown. Alpha-adrenergic stimulation inhibits insulin secretion whereas beta-adrenergic agents stimulate the release of both insulin and glucagon. The net effect of chronic excessive catecholamine secretion is a catabolic state, frequently aggravated by the anorexia common in patients with pheochromocytomas. Carbohydrate intolerance also may be present.

Diagnosis. Pheochromocytomas should be suspected in persons with hypertension, especially if it occurs at atypical ages, or in persons who have symptoms of hypermetabolism (often suggesting thyrotoxicosis) or a family history of pheochromocytomas or medullary thyroid carcinoma. In about half of all cases the hypertension will be episodic, with paroxysmal attacks of blanching, flushing, palpitations, or tachycardia. The diagnosis may be confirmed by demonstrating excess catecholamines in plasma or increased amounts of the catecholamine metabolites metanephrine, normetanephrine, or vanilmandelic acid (VMA) in the urine. Some methods for measuring VMA also detect other phenolic acids, so the urine collection may need to be preceded by a diet free of coffee, chocolate, vanilla, citrus fruits, and certain vegetables. With more specific assays, such diets are not necessary.

Treatment. If a surgically removable tumor can be identified, the disease is potentially curable, so surgery is the preferred treatment. Given the danger of hypertensive crises during surgery, the patient must be pretreated with an alpha-adrenergic blocking agent (phenoxybenzamine) and, if necessary, a beta-blocking agent (propranolol). During this time efforts should be made to improve nutritional status by providing a high-protein diet. If the patient is not a candidate for surgery or if an inoperable lesion is found, medical management and supportive nutritional care are continued indefinitely.

Paroxysmal attacks are sometimes precipitated by foods high in tyramine (e.g., Chianti wine, certain ripened cheeses including cheddar, Stilton, and Camembert). Patients whose tumors have not been removed should avoid such foods if they provoke symptoms. Alcohol has also been known to induce attacks.

Hypoglycemia

Hypoglycemia may be classified on a clinical basis or from a physiologic standpoint.[40] The clinical classification differentiates between patients who become hypoglycemic in a fasted state

---

HYPOGLYCEMIC STATES

Fasting Hypoglycemia

Liver disease
    Severe liver failure
    Glycogen storage diseases
Adrenal insufficiency
Ketotic hypoglycemia of childhood
Pituitary failure
Extrapancreatic neoplasms
Pancreatic beta-cell tumors
Ethanol
Chronic renal failure

Reactive Hypoglycemia

Functional ("reactive") type
Alimentary (postgastrectomy) type
Early diabetes
Hereditary fructose intolerance
Galactosemia
Erythroblastosis fetalis
Leucine-sensitive type

Drug-Induced Hypoglycemia

Insulin (surreptitious or accidental overdose)
Oral hypoglycemic agents

---

without external agents like drugs or toxins and those who are induced in a postprandial state by factors such as diet, exercise, or medication. The box gives a clinical classification of hypoglycemic states.

Normally the body maintains a circulating blood glucose concentration between 60 and 160 mg/dl (3.3-8.8 mM) during the fasted and fed states. Neural and hormonal factors are integrated to maintain the plasma glucose between these concentrations. If the circulating plasma glucose concentration decreases to values that deprive the central nervous system of glucose, a characteristic set of symptoms occurs—including those related to catecholamine release (palpitations, tremors, diaphoresis) and those related to neuroglycopenia (confusion, irritability, lethargy, seizures, loss of consciousness). The symptoms usually occur with plasma glucose values less than 50 mg/dl, although some individuals will not exhibit symptoms at values as low as 35 mg/dl.

Several factors influence glucose homeostasis. In a steady state the circulating glucose concentration depends on the input of glucose into circulation as well as the quantity being utilized.

Glucose in blood comes from absorption of the breakdown products of carbohydrates or from the liver. In fasted states glycogenolysis and gluconeogenesis occur in the liver to provide glucose to the circulating blood. For tissues such as muscle, the utilization of glucose depends on the amount of insulin available. By contrast, the brain utilizes glucose without any need for insulin. Thus the input of glucose into the circulation depends on the availability of glucose precursors and the capability of the liver to manufacture and release glucose. Inadequate precursor or defective machinery to manufacture glucose will result in hypoglycemia if utilization continues. Glucopenia also results when utilization is excessive or in any way exceeds the production rate. The ensuing discussion considers the causes of hypoglycemia from a physiologic perspective.

Diagnosis. Hypoglycemia is a clinical finding or symptom, not an etiologic diagnosis. Proper clinical evaluation requires that, first, the patient's symptoms be related to the occurrence of the hypoglycemia. Then, once this has been established, the specific cause of the hypoglycemia can be determined. To document hypoglycemia as the reason for the appearance of symptoms requires that three findings (called Whipple's triad) be demonstrated[41]: typical signs of hypoglycemia, plasma glucose levels in the hypoglycemic range, and amelioration of the condition when plasma glucose concentrations are restored to normal. Because many individuals may have plasma glucose levels below 50 mg/dl during a glucose tolerance test, current practice is to measure plasma glucose when symptoms occur on the patient's usual meal schedule.[42] This can be easily done by using the same home blood glucose test that diabetics use.

Once the symptoms have been related to hypoglycemia, determining the cause requires further testing. There is no such thing as an all-purpose "hypoglycemia diet"; specific dietary therapy depends on the etiology of the hypoglycemia.

Deficient Substrate Availability

Ketotic hypoglycemia of childhood presents with convulsions, hypoglycemia, and acetonuria, which occur after an overnight fast or during an acute illness. The symptoms usually occur in children between the ages of 18 months and

5 years who are mildly retarded in weight and height. Ketotic hypoglycemia is three times more common in boys than in girls and is also more common when the birth weight was low for gestational age. The hypoglycemia associated with ketonemia usually is outgrown by 8 or 9 years of age. The parent and child should be taught to recognize ketotic hypoglycemia. Acetonuria occurs prior to hypoglycemia and gives a warning signal. The urine should be tested for acetone whenever the child is ill, skips a meal, or is under stress. Ketotic hypoglycemia can be prevented by giving fruit juice, candy, or other high carbohydrate food when acetonuria develops. Frequent feedings of carbohydrate are encouraged, especially during illness. The daily diet should consist of frequent feedings of a high-protein high-caloric diet.[43]

Other causes of hypoglycemia from deficient substrate availability include chronic renal insufficiency and adrenocortical insufficiency. Spontaneous hypoglycemia in the presence of chronic renal failure occurs in both diabetics and nondiabetics. The hypoglycemia does not correlate with the severity of renal failure, however. The symptoms, which include a comatose state or lethargy, will respond immediately to intravenous glucose. The hypoglycemia of adrenocortical insufficiency rarely presents with symptoms except after periods of minimum starvation or during an illness that impairs chronic intake. Treatment with hydrocortisone readily reverses the lower fasting plasma glucose concentrations of patients with adrenal insufficiency. During acute situations, glucopenia can be corrected with parenteral glucose.

Failure of Glucose Production

Structural incompetency of the liver may interfere with glucose production. The liver is needed to maintain circulating glucose concentrations in both the basal state and during short-term fasts.[40] Common hepatic diseases rarely are associated with glucose values less than 50 mg/dl. Removal or destruction of 80% of the liver mass is necessary before disturbances in glucose homeostasis are apparent. Reduced glycogenolysis and gluconeogenesis cause the hypoglycemia that accompanies widespread destruction of the liver. The liver also has an impaired ability to form glycogen. This impaired ability to release glucose or form glycogen is documented by the

fasting glucose concentrations and elevated postprandial glucose values that decline gradually to low values within 4 to 5 hours of eating. Treatment of severe liver dysfunction necessitates maintenance of glucose levels until liver regeneration can occur.

The severity of hypoglycemia in glycogen storage disease depends on which enzyme is affected.[40] Glucose-6-phosphatase deficiency is the most commonly encountered glycogen-storage disorder. Affected children are short for their age and have protruding abdomens caused by liver enlargement. Values for fasting glucose are low-normal or low. Brief fasts result in ketonuria and metabolic acidosis. Impairment of glycogenesis and gluconeogenesis causes high plasma levels of lactate and pyruvate. The primary goal of therapy is to maintain glucose values that will prevent hypoglycemia and acidosis. For severe cases, feedings must be given every 3 or 4 hours continuously. Nocturnal intragastric tube glucose feedings have been found to accelerate growth and development. Supplementary oral sodium bicarbonate is given to combat the high blood lactate concentrations.

Gluconeogenesis in the liver is important for normal circulating levels of glucose after a short period of fasting. It requires integration of substrates, enzymatic components, and circulating hormones. Ethanol disrupts the process and can also potentiate the hypoglycemic effect of insulin. As a consequence, hypoglycemia may be induced by ingesting alcohol in the fasted state.[44] Children and nonalcoholic adults may show symptomatic hypoglycemia after large quantities of alcohol, but chronic alcoholics are the most vulnerable. The hypoglycemic action of alcohol also affects starved subjects, decompensated diabetics, and patients with thyrotoxicosis and adrenal insufficiency. In these persons a combination of factors causes hypoglycemia, including depleted glycogen stores, impaired gluconeogenesis, and ethanol metabolism. Very brief periods of food deprivation render some chronic alcoholics, infants, and children susceptible to ethanol-induced hypoglycemia.

The hypoglycemia resulting from ethanol abuse is indistinguishable from that resulting from other causes. Most of the patients are comatose and may demonstrate hypothermia, conjugate deviation of the eyes, extensor rigidity of the extremities, unilateral or bilateral Babinski reflexes, trismus, or convulsions. Glucose concentrations as low as 5 mg/dl have been reported. Intravenous glucose will produce an immediate response. To prevent coma from recurring, adequate carbohydrate is necessary. The reported mortality of 11% for adults and 25% for children necessitates prompt diagnosis and therapy.

Glucose Overutilization

Almost everyone who has undergone gastric surgery may manifest chemical hypoglycemia, known as alimentary hypoglycemia, after an oral glucose load.[40] Plasma glucose values are abnormally high within 35 to 65 minutes after a glucose challenge; glucose concentrations then fall precipitously 95 to 215 minutes after the challenge to values of less than 50 mg/dl. The proportion of patients with neuroglycopenic symptoms ranges from 5% to 50%. A rise in plasma insulin values parallels the increase in plasma glucose levels. The hypoglycemia is caused by the rapid gastric emptying that occurs after surgery. Recently an alimentary type of glucose tolerance curve has been described in the absence of previous gastrointestinal surgery or underlying organic gastrointestinal disease. The patients have a rapid gastric emptying and upper intestinal absorption of glucose.[44] A variety of methods has been used for treatment of alimentary hypoglycemia. Propranolol in 10 mg doses has been suggested but must be used cautiously since the defenses against hypoglycemia may be blocked. Diets low in carbohydrate, combined with anticholinergic agents, have been prescribed but success has varied. The diet for alimentary hypoglycemia includes frequent, small, high-protein and low-carbohydrate feedings. Refined sugars and excess liquids, except between meals, also should be avoided.

The most common cause of hypoglycemia among diabetics is the excessive administration of insulin and oral hypoglycemic agents, relative to food intake or exercise.[40] The total hypoglycemic effect of insulin and the sulfonylureas may be augmented by other agents, particularly in the presence of chronic liver and kidney failure and starvation. Agents that potentiate sulfonylureas include sulfonamides, coumadin, salicylates, phenylbutazone, probenecid, anabolic steroids, propranolol, clofibrate, monoamine oxidase inhibitors, guanethidine, alcohol, and methotrex-

ate. Combinations of these agents also may augment hypoglycemia; for example, alcohol and salicylates are exceptionally potent when combined with sulfonylureas. In diagnosing unexplained hypoglycemia in the nondiabetic, the physician always must consider factitious causes such as the surreptitious administration of insulin or sulfonylureas.

Drug-induced hypoglycemia should be considered in every unconscious patient.[44] The measurement of the blood sugar may help to exclude hypoglycemia as a complication of drug intoxication. If in doubt, a prudent procedure for the physician to follow is rapidly to check the plasma glucose using a reagent strip method and, if hypoglycemia is confirmed, to administer 50 cc of a 50% glucose solution intravenously followed by a 10% glucose infusion for one or more days, if needed. Prolonged hypoglycemia may result when there is impaired degradation of sulfonylurea or other drugs due to preexisting renal or hepatic disease. In this case intravenous glucose infusion is continued for 2 to 3 days to avoid relapse into hypoglycemia within the first 24 hours. Blood sugar levels should be monitored frequently during the first day. If the first liter of 10% glucose infused over the 6 hours fails to establish and maintain normoglycemia, 100 mg of cortisone sodium hemisuccinate may be added to each liter of glucose for as long as desired. The intravenous infusion of glucose should not be discontinued until a daily oral carbohydrate intake of 300 g or more has been established.

Postprandial hypoglycemia may be an early manifestation of maturity-onset diabetes.[40] The patients exhibit neuroglycopenic symptoms 3 to 5 hours after meals. The glucose tolerance curve may follow a typical diabetic pattern but show a paradoxically low blood sugar level of 50 mg/dl or less 3 to 5 hours after glucose ingestion. Insulin levels rise sluggishly but are excessive by 2 to 4 hours. These individuals tend to be obese and to have strong family histories of diabetes. Carbohydrate restriction, particularly of refined sugars, can prevent symptoms resulting from this type of reactive hypoglycemia.

Probably the most serious cause of hypoglycemia is spontaneous oversecretion of insulin by the pancreatic beta cells. This is usually due to the presence of a beta cell tumor, the so-called insulinoma, although (particularly in children) it may also be due to nesidioblastosis, a hyperplasia of the islets of Langerhans. Islet cell tumors sometimes occur in association with other endocrine neoplasms, especially those of the pituitary or parathyroid gland.

Islet cell tumors are diagnosed by the demonstration of continuing insulin secretion in the presence of hypoglycemia. Because the symptoms may be vague, diagnosis may be delayed for years. Most such patients discover that they feel better when they eat, so obesity is common. Treatment is surgical when possible. If the tumor cannot be removed, medical treatment with diazoxide may be undertaken. In malignant insulinomas, streptozocin is sometimes used. A diet with frequent feedings may provide useful adjunctive therapy.

Functional Hypoglycemia of Unknown Etiology

Idiopathic postprandial hypoglycemia has been termed reactive, functional, or vagotonic hypoglycemia.[40] Symptoms resembling insulin reactions with feelings of weakness, perspiration, yawning, sleepiness, palpitations, and nervousness occur 2 to 3 hours after meals, most commonly in the midmorning and midafternoon. Consciousness usually is preserved and recovery is spontaneous. Diagnosis requires that biochemical glycopenia correlate with the "true" glycopenic symptoms of hunger, sweating, palpitations, and irritability. Oral glucose tolerance tests for 5 to 6 hours establish the diagnosis. However, as noted previously, it may be more appropriate to use home glucose testing to see whether hypoglycemia actually occurs, and is related to the patient's symptoms, in everyday life.

Treatment. Various diets have been proposed for treating functional hypoglycemia, and there is not general agreement as to the distribution of macronutrients or micronutrients.[45] Some investigators recommend the inclusion of foods high in soluble fiber because of data suggesting that such foods prevent glycopenic symptoms. Treatment with a high-protein low-carbohydrate diet in frequent feedings should be tried initially. Education, reassurance, and a regimen that avoids simple sugars and uses starches and alternate sources of carbohydrate should be emphasized. The protein content of the regimen should be at least 70 to 130 g (15%-20% of calories) and the carbohydrate content no more than 40% to 45%

of calories. The carbohydrate content needs to be reduced to whatever level eliminates hypoglycemic symptoms. Fruits, vegetables, breads, cereals, and potatoes should make up the dietary carbohydrate. Concentrated sweets are digested and absorbed rapidly and stimulate insulin secretion. Therefore sugar, sweetened desserts, jellies, jams, honey, syrups, candy, sweetened fruits, fruits high in carbohydrates, and soft drinks should be omitted. The balance of the calories is alloted to fat. Levels of calcium and riboflavin may be very low because of the limited amount of milk permissible on a carbohydrate-restricted diet. It may be advisable to prescribe the necessary calcium and riboflavin as a supplement. Although both alcohol and caffeine are related to hypoglycemia, the need for restricting ingestion of these substances by persons with functional hypoglycemia has not been demonstrated. One approach is to begin treatment by eliminating alcohol and caffeine from the diet and, once symptomatic relief is obtained, gradually reintroducing them as long as symptoms do not recur.

OTHER DISORDERS WITH ENDOCRINE AND NUTRITIONAL IMPLICATIONS
Anorexia Nervosa

The basic features of anorexia nervosa are discussed in Chapter 26. To avoid confusion with other endocrine problems, a number of hormonal abnormalities frequently seen in anorexia should be recognized. Symptoms that may suggest endocrinopathies include low blood pressure, slow pulse, a small heart, and increased facial hair. Pubic hair is usually normal, but there may be atrophy of the breasts, uterus, and ovaries or of the testes.[46]

Luteinizing hormone (LH) levels are often low, but follicle-stimulating hormone (FSH) concentrations may be low or normal.[47] The basis of these findings appears to be of hypothalamic rather than anterior pituitary origin.[48] The endocrine abnormalities are reversible with improved nutrition and thus are probably due to malnutrition rather than to hypothalamic dysfunction.[49] Growth hormone levels are usually normal, which is inappropriate for a catabolic state. Prolactin is normal, as is thyroid function. Serum thyroxine levels must be interpreted carefully, since thyroxine-binding globulin may be depressed; nevertheless, the free thyroxine index should be normal. Triiodothyronine (T_3) may be low. Plasma cortisol is normal or increased, and diurnal variations may be abnormal. However, urinary 17-ketosteroids and 17-hydroxysteroids are often decreased. These findings appear to be due to a prolonged cortisol metabolic clearance rate rather than to abnormal secretion.[48]

Fasting blood sugar is usually normal or low whereas insulin levels are generally low. This suggests an increased sensitivity to insulin, which could be due to an increase in cellular insulin receptors.[50]

Carcinoid Syndrome

The carcinoid syndrome results from tumors, generally originating in the gastrointestinal tract, that secrete 5-hydroxytryptamine (5-HT). Typical symptoms include flushing and diarrhea. The diarrhea is due to increased motility rather than to malabsorption. However, malabsorption may occur and should be considered in the cachectic patient with carcinoid syndrome. Occasional patients will have pellagra-like skin lesions. These are thought to be due to a tryptophan deficiency arising from the tumor's using tryptophan for synthesis of 5-hydroxyindols. The skin lesions may respond to nicotinamide.[51]

EFFECTS OF NUTRITIONAL INADEQUACIES ON ENDOCRINE FUNCTION
Starvation

The normal response to starvation can be viewed as a continuum divided into three phases: the postabsorption state (6-12 hr after food intake), short-term starvation (3-7 da), and prolonged starvation (2 wk or longer).[52] Throughout this continuum the integrated endocrine-metabolic response strives to maintain normal glucose levels while providing the substrate requirements for specific tissues, particularly the brain. At the same time there is an attempt to minimize the losses of body protein.

Body fat provides the greatest source of body fuel, accounting for 80% of the total body fuel storage.[52] In the nonobese person 20% of the body weight is fat, with a caloric value of 130,000 to 140,000 kcal. This is sufficient to meet basal caloric needs for approximately 2 months. Within 6 to 12 hours after a meal, free fatty acids are mobilized from the triglycerides of adipose tissue to provide energy for the muscles, heart, and parenchymal tissue (kidney,

liver). Free fatty acid disposal occurs equally through three routes: oxidation to CO_2, synthesis of triglycerides, and conversion to ketone bodies (ketogenesis).

The major storage form of carbohydrate is glycogen, found in the liver (70 g) and in muscle (200 g). The circulating blood glucose contains 20 g of carbohydrate. Together these add up to an insignificant source of energy (1100 kcal), barely enough to provide basal needs for 1 day in an adult man, let alone the total energy needs for 1 day. Liver glycogen is an important source of glucose to meet the needs of the brain, particularly overnight. Liver glycogen is depleted within 18 to 24 hours after starvation begins, and the body must provide glucose from other sources.

The conversion of noncarbohydrate sources to glucose is known as gluconeogenesis. The principal precursors of glucose are amino acids, pyruvate, lactate, and glycerol. Pyruvate and lactate are breakdown products of muscle glycogen. Thus they represent recycled products of glucose rather than de novo synthesis. The amino acids come from the breakdown of visceral proteins and muscle protein. The major reservoir of body protein is muscle tissue, which weighs 10 kg and provides 40,000 kcal. Protein is the fuel that limits survival in starvation. Depletion of 30% to 50% of body protein is incompatible with survival. Death in starvation results from a loss of respiratory muscle function that leads to terminal pneumonia.

Insulin stimulates fuel storage by promoting glycogen synthesis, fat synthesis and storage, and protein synthesis.[52] In nonobese individuals circulating insulin falls from a peak value of 50-150 μU/ml at 1 hour postprandially to 5-20 μU/ml in the postabsorptive state. The fall is initiated by the postprandial drop in blood sugar. Changes in blood glucose of no more than 10 to 15 mg/100 ml are sufficient to cause insulin values to change by 50% or more. The fall in insulin reverses the process of fuel storage and leads to glycogenolysis, lipolysis and gluconeogenesis.

As serum insulin concentrations fall, fatty acid mobilization and utilization accelerate. Production of ketone bodies accelerates simultaneously through activation of the β-oxidative pathways. The catabolism of glycogen is stimulated. Protein synthetic processes decline while catabolic reactions of protein increase. The net result is mobilization of amino acids from the muscles.

Food intake or deprivation influences circulating levels of glucagon as well as insulin. There is an increase in glucagon levels in the basal postabsorptive state over that observed after ingestion of a carbohydrate meal. Inhibition of glucagon activity can result in a decrease in postabsorptive blood glucose of approximately 40 mg/dl over a 1-hour period. Thus glucagon is important in the liver's output of glucose from glycogenolysis. Another function of glucagon in starvation is to stimulate gluconeogenesis.

Brief fasting (3-7 da) produces acceleration of the gluconeogenic, lipolytic, and ketogenic processes that already have been stimulated at a less rapid rate in the postabsorptive state.[52] Key factors in enhancing gluconeogenesis and ketogenesis are glucagon and insulin. As starvation extends from 12 hours to 3 days or 1 week, there is a further drop in insulin and an increase in glucagon. The overall rate of gluconeogenesis increases 2 to 3 times above postabsorptive values and accounts for almost the entire output of glucose from the liver. (The liver glycogen is depleted within 18-24 hr after starvation begins.) To supply glucose precursors for gluconeogenesis, there is an increase in proteolysis and amino acid mobilization from the muscles. The nitrogen balance during this stage of starvation is markedly negative at the rate of 10-12 g/day, indicating a breakdown of 75-100 g of protein/day.

During starvation longer than 1 week, nitrogen losses decline markedly. If gluconeogenesis and proteolysis were to persist at the rates observed during early starvation, 30% to 50% of the total body protein would be lost within 4 to 6 weeks, well before body fat stores had been fully utilized. The rate of urinary nitrogen losses in prolonged fasting falls progressively to values as low as 3 g/day—equivalent to a loss of 20 g body protein. The nitrogenous end products change from predominantly urea to primarily ammonia.

A decline in the availability of amino acids from decreased protein breakdown in prolonged starvation causes hepatic glucose production to diminish from postabsorptive rates of 150-250 g/day to approximately 50 g/day.[52] In prolonged fasting the kidney produces an amount of glucose equivalent to that produced by the liver. The rate-limiting step is a marked decrease in muscle release of alanine. Thus prolonged starvation differs from early starvation, in which there is a rise in muscle alanine output. With the contribution of the kidney to gluconeogenesis, the total glucose production in prolonged fasting is 90 g/day, or half that observed in postabsorptive states. Adaptive changes in glucose consumption, particularly by the brain, occur, so hypoglycemia is averted. After 3 days of fasting, blood glucose values level off at 50 to 70 mg/dl. There is enhanced brain uptake of ketones with a corresponding decline in brain uptake of glucose. Thus ketone bodies become the major fuel for the brain in prolonged fasting. A variety of adaptive events occurs and the arterial concentration of ketones increases, allowing the preferential utilization of ketone bodies by the brain. Muscle uptake of ketones in prolonged fasting decreases by 75% as compared to the early fasting period. Between days 3 and 10 of starvation there is a rapid rise in the net rate of ketone reabsorption by the renal tubule, which decreases urinary ketone losses.

The metabolic regulation of the adaptive changes described for prolonged fasting is not entirely clear.[52] Insulin levels reach their lowest point within 7 to 10 days and remain at a low level. Therefore, further changes cannot be used as an explanation for the diminished gluconeogenesis and protein conservation in prolonged fasting. Recently it has been suggested that ketones, in addition to acting as a substrate for the brain, may act as the signal to muscle tissue that limits proteolysis and secondarily reduces availability to the liver of precursor (alanine) for gluconeogenesis.

A variety of other hormonal changes have been observed during starvation. In contrast to the metabolic role of insulin and glucagon in starvation, particularly short-term fasting, growth hormone and cortisol exert their effects through a permissive role. An increase in growth hormone values has been demonstrated in briefly fasting individuals. Although timing and magnitude are variable, in most cases the growth hormone values return to baseline within 5 to 10 days. A progressive decline in secretion of cortisol has been documented by measurements of urinary free cortisol.

Prenatal Malnutrition

Animal studies suggest that there are effects of prenatal malnutrition on the endocrine development of the progeny of malnourished rat dams.

Even if the offspring consume normal diets after birth, they grow less rapidly and have a reduced capacity for in vitro synthesis of growth hormone.[53] Exogenous growth hormone administration prevents the growth depression. In other studies rats that were malnourished prenatally and during weaning but had free access to optimum diet after weaning had increased plasma corticosteroid concentrations later in life, especially in response to stress. Another long-term change in endocrine function also has been reported in rats. When female offspring of malnourished rats were allowed to grow on an adequate diet, they produced progeny that were smaller at birth and suffered from decreased brain development. It has been suggested that this is attributable to suboptimal endocrine performance during the pregnancy of the second-generation rats.

Studies in rats indicate that both the amount of protein in the diet and the timing of the protein supplement is crucial for adequate reproductive behavior.[54] Below the critical level of protein in the diet, fetal death and resorption occur in a majority of the animals. Pair-fed controls had normal reproduction, which eliminated caloric restriction and other dietary differences as causes for reproductive failure. Resorption in rats on protein-free diets is prevented by transitory feeding or protein supplements for only 2 or 3 days after conception. In the complete absence of dietary protein, a combination of estrogen and progesterone will maintain the pregnancy.[55]

Protein-Energy Malnutrition

The effects of protein-energy malnutrition on hormonal changes depend upon the relative amounts of calorie and protein deprivation. Kwashiorkor, which is associated primarily with protein deficiency, commonly occurs in children aged 1 to 3 years. Marasmus, the result of an overall deficit of food intake, is found most commonly, but not exclusively, in children until 1 year of age. Practically, protein-energy malnutrition is a complex condition that presents as a spectrum between these two extremes. The hormonal responses depend on which of the two extremes is predominant.

Most studies of adults and children with protein-calorie malnutrition (PCM)[56,57] demonstrate high levels of immunoassayable growth hormone, which return to normal on nutritional therapy. Basal growth hormone concentrations are more likely to be normal in children at the marasmic end of the PCM spectrum. Some of the actions of growth hormone depend on somatomedin, which is decreased in protein-energy malnutrition.

Plasma insulin levels in protein-energy malnutrition usually are low.[53] There is conflicting evidence on the relative effects of kwashiorkor and marasmus on carbohydrate metabolism and the capacity to secrete insulin. A reduced capacity to remove intravenously administered glucose has been observed for kwashiorkor, while the rate of removal is often normal in marasmus. Both growth hormone and insulin levels in normal subjects respond to protein or amino acid administration. When patients with protein-energy malnutrition are given orally a mixture of essential amino acids, the growth hormone values decrease but the plasma insulin concentrations remain low. The altered carbohydrate metabolism seen in such patients continues long after rehabilitation is started. Glucagon concentrations are low to normal in most persons with PCM.[56]

As with growth hormone and carbohydrate metabolism, changes in adrenocortical metabolism depend on whether marasmus or kwashiorkor is being investigated.[53] An increased output of urinary steroids has been observed in marasmus but not in kwashiorkor. These results correspond to findings reported with plasma cortisol values. Generally cases of marasmus have been associated with increased plasma cortisol concentration, but in kwashiorkor there were no changes or moderate to extensive elevations. Preservation of the pituitary adrenal axis has been suggested as an explanation for these findings. Even though plasma cortisol values were elevated, they responded to ACTH stimulation and were depressed by dexamethasone. Cortisol production rates were normal but catabolism appeared to be reduced. The corticosteroid overactivity may be more than the total plasma values would indicate. The physiologically active form of cortisol is found free and the remainder (90%) is bound to albumin and transcortin, which may be reduced in PCM. Thus there is an increase in the free plasma cortisol. The proportions become normal when plasma proteins are restored following treatment.

The metabolism of aldosterone also has been

studied in patients with protein-energy malnutrition,[53] but the effects on metabolism depend upon whether kwashiorkor or marasmus is being considered. Aldosterone values in marasmic children were similar to those of age- or height/weight-matched controls, but the rate of aldosterone production was increased, suggesting that aldosterone turned over more rapidly. In kwashiorkor, aldosterone concentrations were increased despite a normal secretion rate, suggesting decreased catabolism.

Some patients with PCM have an elevated basal level of thyroid-stimulating hormone (TSH) and an exaggerated response to thyrotropin-releasing hormone (TRH). However, especially in marasmus, TSH may also be reduced.[56] Studies among children with PCM suggest that the conversion of thyroxine to triiodothyronine in the liver and elsewhere is impaired. Histologic investigations of the thyroid gland from patients who have died give contradictory results. Sometimes the thyroid glands have been normal; other times atrophy has been demonstrated. Since treatment restores normal metabolic rate and induces catch-up growth, the atrophy seen in the thyroid of malnourished children must be reversible.

In a great many types of severe illness, alterations in thyroid function are seen. Serum thyroxine (T_4) may be high or low, with triiodothyronine (T_3) usually low and reverse T_3 high. A large part of these thyroid alterations in "euthyroid sick" states are due to the caloric deprivation associated with such severe illness and can be reversed with nutritional therapy.[58,59]

Malnourished children also exhibit alterations in the hypothalamic-pituitary-gonadal axis. Malnourished children have delayed puberty, and malnourished adults amenorrhea or testicular failure. Unequal degrees of malnutrition and unequal dysfunctional effects have led to conflicting evidence regarding gonadotropin release. Severe PCM results in normal or decreased basal concentrations of LH and FSH. One study reported lower FSH and higher LH concentrations in age-matched controls with pubertal changes similar to those in normal boys occurring as weight, height, and lean body mass were attained.

A pituitary hypothalamic defect is suspected in very young children because with severe PCM these patients have poor LH response to LHRH.

By contrast, in adult men with PCM a primary testicular disorder is suspected because mean plasma LH is increased and declines during refeeding. Low plasma testosterone concentrations return to normal. As in children, some adults also have low plasma LH and FSH, suggesting a pituitary/hypothalamic disorder. A hypothalamic defect is substantiated because LHRH injection results in the normal responsiveness of the pituitary with FSH and LH response. After refeeding, hypothalamic and pituitary function returns in men with PCM but a primary gonadal failure is still evident with persistently low testosterone concentrations.[56]

Prolactin levels also are elevated in undernourished states. In lactating women this may serve to ensure milk production when food intake is limited, by preferentially channeling nutrients toward the breast. Improved nutrition reduces prolactin levels and may shorten postpartum infertility.[60]

Iodine

Goiter. An insufficient supply of dietary iodine leads to endemic goiter, one of the most frequent diseases of the endocrine system throughout the world. Some authors[61] state that endemic goiter exists in a population when more than 20% of preadolescent children have thyroids whose lobes are each larger than the distal phalanx of the subject's thumb. Others have suggested 10% of the whole population as the criterion. Iodine deficiency can be classified as in the box on p. 274.

Endemic goiter is one of the most extensive problems of malnutrition in several countries. An estimated 400 million people are presently at risk of iodine deficiency disorders.[62] Some of the major endemic areas are mountainous regions of the Andes, Himalayas, Alps, Greece, and the Middle East as well as the highlands of New Guinea. Endemic goiter also has been reported in nonmountainous areas such as Holland, the Uele region of Zaire, and the interior of Brazil. Endemic goiter existed in the Great Lakes area of the United States a few generations ago. All these areas have in common a low amount of environmental iodine and a low iodine content in the water. The daily urinary excretion of iodine in these regions is minimal—generally below 50 µg and in some cases as low as 20 µg. The Ten-State Nutrition Survey,[63] conducted in

---

IODINE DEFICIENCY DISEASE (IDD)

Grade I (mild)
  Goiter prevalence 5-20%
  Median urine iodine over 50 μg/g of creatinine
  Normal physical and mental development
  Can be controlled with iodized salt
  May disappear with economic development
Grade II (moderate)
  Goiter prevalence to 30%
  Median urine iodine of 25-50 μg/g of creatinine
  Some hypothyroidism
  Controlled with iodized salt or iodized oil
Grade III (severe)
  Goiter prevalence over 30%
  Median urine iodine under 25 μg/g of creatinine
  Endemic cretinism (prevalence 1-10%)
  Requires iodized oil to prevent CNS defects

Modified from Hetzel BS: In Medeiros-Neto G, et al, editors: Iodine deficiency disorders and congenital hypothyroidism, Sao Paulo, 1986, ACHÉ, pp 1-6.

---

the United States, found 3.1% of that population to have goiter. The daily excretion of iodine in the United States ranges between 240 and 700 μg[61] whereas in several European countries with no abnormal incidence of goiter, iodine excretion averages 60 to 100 μg/day.

Goiter prevalence is influenced by sex and age.[61] In severe endemic areas the disease may appear early but the prevalence increases dramatically as children reach puberty, when the peak incidence is observed. The prevalence is higher in girls than in boys, and the difference between the sexes becomes greater as adulthood is reached. Goiter has been found in several populations living in poor socioeconomic conditions. Its effects on general health—including mechanical complications (compression of vital organs of the neck), endocrine disorders, neoplastic alterations after a lifetime of increased growth and hyperfunction of the thyroid tissue, and cretinism—are seen at both extremes of thyroid function. Hyperthyroidism occurs especially in the presence of a large supply of iodine (Jod-Basedow syndrome). Hypothyroidism usually occurs in older women after many pregnancies and prolonged breast-feeding. The incidence of thyroid carcinoma is twice as high in areas where endemic goiter exists, and follicular and anaplastic tumors are twice as common in patients with iodine-deficient goiter as in patients with a normal thyroid.

Prior to being absorbed by the gastrointestinal tract, dietary iodine is converted to iodide.[64] After absorption the iodide is distributed within the extracellular fluid in unbound form. This free iodide is either taken up by the thyroid gland or excreted in the urine. There is no renal mechanism for conserving iodide. Consequently an osmotic diuresis (as in diabetes) increases the urinary iodide loss and lowers the plasma concentration. Conversely an impairment in renal function elevates plasma iodide values.

Since iodide is an important constituent of thyroxine, it plays an integral role in the synthesis of the biologically active forms, T_4 (thyroxine) and T_3 (3,5,3-triiodothyronine):

1. The first step in synthesis is the transport of iodide from the blood into the follicular cells of the thyroid gland by a concentrating mechanism. Aerobic processes aid this by providing metabolic energy. Patients with goiter have augmented iodide trapping, which increases the thyroid gland's accumulation of iodide, whatever the size of the environmental iodine supply. Thyroid uptake of ^{131}I may increase to 50% and in a few cases to 85% of the administered dose. The transport of iodide is inhibited by certain monovalent ions (perchlorate, thiocyanate, nitrate).[64] Some vegetables that are goitrogenic act through this mechanism.[63] Cabbage and similar species of vegetables (kale, brussels sprouts, cauliflower, turnips) contain thioglycosides, which are degraded to thiocyanate during digestion. Cassava contains cyanogenic glycosides that, when ingested, release cyanide, which subsequently is converted to thiocyanate. The seeds of *Brassica* (family Cruciferae) contain goitrin, which when ingested by dairy cattle becomes incorporated into the milk supply. (See box on p. 275.)

In addition to these foods, other substances have been implicated in the etiology of goiter. Bacterial products from shallow drinking water have been related to an increased incidence, as have disulfides of saturated and unsaturated hydrocarbons. Synthetic goitrogens include polychlorinated and polybrominated biphenyls, organochloride insecticides (DDT, DDD, dieldrin), the fungicide ethylenebis-

---

DIETARY GOITROGENS

Substances containing cyanogenic glycosides
    Almond seed
    Cassava
    Sorghum
    Maize
    Millet
Substances arising from thioglycosides that are metabolized to goitrin (5-ethenyl-2-oxazolidinethione), thiocyanate, or isothiocyanate
    Cabbage
    Kale
    Brussels sprouts
    Cauliflower
    Turnips
    Rutabaga
    Mustard
    Horseradish
Substances that may cause excess fecal loss of thyroxine
    Soybean

From data contained in DeGroot LJ, Stanbury JB: The thyroid and its diseases, New York, 1975, John Wiley & Sons Inc, pp 173-174.

dithiocarbamate (EBDC), sulfonamides, and tetracyclines. The significance of polychlorinated biphenyls and EBDC, however, as human goitrogens is not precisely known.

2. Inside the thyroid cell, iodide is converted to a higher oxidation state. All the subsequent reactions converting tyrosine residues to thyroid hormones occur within a thyroglobulin molecule. The active form of iodine reacts with the tyrosine molecules in the thyroglobulin to form mono- and diiodotyrosine residues. A coupling process involving the iodotyrosines yields the active hormones T_4 and T_3. The iodine content of thyroglobulin from normal human thyroid glands varies widely, depending in part on the iodine supply. Thyroglobulin is synthesized more rapidly when there is a lack of iodine. There is also reduced efficiency of iodothyronine synthesis in severe cases of hyperplasia induced by iodine deficiency.

3. Before thyroid hormones are secreted by the thyroid gland, proteolytic enzymes break down thyroglobulin into its constituent amino acids, including iodinated forms of tyrosine.[64] The free hormones T_4 and T_3 and free iodo-

tyrosines are released inside the follicular cells. An enzyme strips the iodine from the iodotoyrosines, releasing the iodide into the cell. The iodide then can be reutilized by the gland, and this recycling conserves iodine when the dietary supply is low.

4. Normally about 20 molecules of T_4 are secreted for every molecule of T_3,[64] but the ratio of T_4 to T_3 in the blood varies. The biologic activity of T_3 is about three times greater than that of T_4. Peripheral production of T_3 from T_4 also occurs in various tissues, including the liver and kidney. The conversion of T_4 in extrathyroidal sites accounts for approximately 80% of the total production of T_3. Any stress of severe systemic illness is associated with reversible inhibition of the process. Starvation and even short-term caloric restriction, especially of carbohydrates, promptly decrease the conversion of T_4 to T_3. More T_3 and less T_4 are formed and secreted proportionally when iodine is lacking. Thus the T_3/T_4 ratio is increased in longstanding hyperplasia of the thyroid gland resulting from severe iodine deficiency.

Thyrotropic hormone (TSH) is the most important regulator of the thyroid gland.[64] It is a peptide hormone secreted by the anterior pituitary. A lack of thyroid hormone stimulates TSH secretion. Thyrotropic hormone stimulates every step in the biosynthesis of thyroid hormones, from iodide transport into the thyroid cell to proteolysis of thyroglobulin. Metabolic alterations induced by iodine deficiency are mediated largely by an increase in TSH. Subjects living in areas where the iodine supply is severely reduced have increased mean serum TSH values. There is a large individual variation in the values and they may appear normal in many subjects. High serum concentrations also have been observed in populations without abnormal prevalence of goiter but with a definitely low iodine supply.[61]

Endemic goiter is distinguished from sporadic goiter on an epidemiologic basis.[61] When there is a dietary insufficiency of iodine, the protein-bound iodine and urinary iodine excretion are lowered and the radioiodine uptake is increased.[65] The ^{131}I thyroid uptake at 24 hours is greater than 50%, and urinary excretion of iodine is less than 50 μg/day. The T_4 serum concentrations are low, and the T_3 concentrations high.

The TSH levels may be high or normal. Occasionally there is an exaggerated response to thyrotropin-releasing hormone (TRH), a peptide secreted by the hypothalamus to cause secretion of TSH from the anterior pituitary. Laboratory tests must be supported by clinical and dietary history information because so many physiologic states and drugs produce similar trends.

Cretinism. Cretinism is a disease frequently associated with endemic goiter in infants and children.[61] It is the most severe complication of endemic goiter and affects 5% to 12% of the population in some communities of Equador, the Himalayas, and Zaire. The condition is characterized by a wide range of clinical abnormalities occurring singly or as a group. The dominant characteristics are mental retardation and biochemical signs related to impairment of the central nervous system and of thyroid function. Clinical signs observed in infants include unusually large birth size; subnormal temperature; lethargy; thick, dry, wrinkled, and sallow skin; enlarged tongue; thick lips; broad face; flat nose; spade-shaped, puffy hands; deaf mutism; and cerebral diplegia. Recognition of the syndrome in the first week of life is essential to minimize mental retardation. Cretinism results from a deficiency of thyroid hormone during fetal or early life. Besides prolonged iodine deficiency (especially in endemic goiter regions), other causes include anatomic dysgenesis of the thyroid gland and inborn errors of metabolism.

Regional differences result in extreme variability of the syndrome in children.[61] In 1908 McCarrison suggested distinguishing between the "neurologic" form and the "myxedematous" form.[61] The neurologic cretin has severe mental retardation and is characterized by outstanding neurologic anomalies. Most of these cretins are deaf; they are short in stature; and the thyroid gland is enlarged or nodular or both. Clinical examination reveals that these cases are euthyroid. Plasma PB[127]I or T_4 is low-normal or low; plasma TSH and TRH responses are increased. The myxedematous cretin is less retarded but demonstrates signs of congenital hypothyroidism, including dwarfism, thickened dry skin, puffiness of the face, sparseness of hair, and delayed sexual maturation. The thyroid gland usually is not enlarged. Radioiodine uptake by the thyroid is markedly reduced, especially when compared with the values observed in other subjects in the same areas. Plasma PBI concentrations are high and TSH values are extremely high, often exceeding 200µl/ml. Serum concentrations of T_4 and T_3 are low.

Prevention. The daily iodine requirement of adults with goiter is 50 to 75 µg or approximately 1 µg/kg of body weight.[66] The Food and Nutrition Board of the National Research Council suggests 150 µg for adolescents and adults to allow for an extra margin of safety and to meet increased demands that may be imposed by natural goitrogens.[66] Additional allowances of 25 and 50 µg for pregnant and lactating women, respectively, are suggested to meet the demands of the fetus and to allow for the extra iodine excreted in milk. A woman who is breast-feeding and has an adequate intake of dietary iodine will provide her infant with 30 µg or more of iodine in the milk.

Small to moderate increases in iodide intake (i.e., up to 1000 µg) cause no chemical effects in individuals with normal thyroids.[66] The acute effects of large doses of iodide in humans without hyperthyroidism include inhibition of thyroid hormone synthesis.[64] However, humans adapt to excessive iodide and then thyroid hormone synthesis proceeds unimpaired. In some individuals with a history of preexisting thyroid disorder, prolonged ingestion of iodide (200 mg/da for weeks to months) leads eventually to hypothyroidism and usually to some degree of thyroid enlargement. Any drug, such as antiasthmatic medication or iodopyrine, that contains iodine may cause iodide myxedema and/or goiter. Iodide-induced hypothyroidism usually is reversed upon withdrawal of the iodide. The cause of a form of simple goiter that affects 10% of the population along the coast of Northern Island in Japan has been traced to consumption of a specific seaweed with an extremely high iodine content.

It is not possible to estimate the daily intake of dietary iodine because the iodine content of a given food depends on the type of soil, animal feed, and method of processing.[66] Seafoods are the best and most consistent sources of iodine. The iodine content of dairy products and eggs depends on the composition of animal feed. Generally vegetable products are low in iodine. One slice of bread made by the continuous mix process may contain the daily requirement of iodine, but bread made by the batch process may contain very little. The use and consumption of iodized salt is another important variable. The average amount of salt added to the diet in the United States is about 3.4 g, which provides approximately 260 μg of iodine (76 μg/g salt). Many people add as much as 8 g of salt per day, which provides about 600 μg of iodine. The estimated mean intake of dietary iodine in the United States ranges between 64 and 677 μg per day.

Salt has been iodized successfully for 50 years.[61] Its efficacy in providing extra iodine in the diet has been confirmed in a large number of countries. The compound usually added to table and cooking salt is potassium iodide. Iodate may be preferred in humid environments since it is more stable. In some developing countries it has been difficult or impossible to distribute iodized salt. A single injection of slowly absorbable iodized oil has proved an effective prophylaxis in these areas.[61] From 0.2 to 2 ml of ethiodized oil (Ethiodol), containing 37% iodide, is given by intramuscular injection. Dosage depends on a patient's age and sex and the size of goiter. Injection markedly decreases goiter prevalence; normal thyroid function also appears to return as serum concentrations of T_4 and TSH become normal for several years.

Copper

Although the mechanisms are not understood thoroughly, studies in animals suggest that copper plays an important role in reproduction. Copper deficiency in rats and guinea pigs produces infertility. Furthermore, copper deficiency has a teratogenic effect in rats. In vitro bovine studies have shown that copper acts directly on the pituitary gland. The intravenous administration of copper in rabbits produces ovulation.

Intrauterine devices that contain copper consistently produce infertility in women when implanted in the cervical os.[67] Copper ions are thought to act as a contraceptive agent by preventing implantation of the ovum when tissues absorb the copper from an intrauterine device or by decreasing progesterone binding to the presumed endometrial receptors and thereby producing a local effect on ovulation.

Several investigators[67] have reported an effect of copper deficiency on steroidogenesis. The conversion of pregnenolone to progesterone requires a copper-dependent enzyme. It is hypothesized that copper depletion affects this step in the metabolism of cholesterol to progesterone, corticosterone, and cortisol. Hyperplasia of the adrenal cortex also has been observed in the copper-deficient cat, suggesting an increased production of ACTH. Serum T_4 responses to TRH have been found to be decreased in copper-deficient rats.[68]

Zinc

Zinc deficiency in humans has been reported to be associated with hypogonadism.[67] Both animal and human studies[69] show Leydig cell failure in conjunction with oligospermia. The effect on testicular function appears to be directly at the end organ level since the hypothalamic-pituitary axis is intact.[70] Testicular size may be reduced because of the need for zinc in cell division. Zinc is also required for the function of several testicular enzymes.

Most reports of zinc deficiency affecting human testicular development have involved interference with the absorption of zinc and/or abnormal medical conditions affecting zinc metabolism. Hypogonadism in Egyptian and Iranian dwarfs was associated with impaired absorption of zinc caused by the intake of phytate-rich bread. In the United States a boy with hypogonadism had been receiving penicillamine, which interfered with zinc absorption. Zinc deficiency appears to be related to decreased circulating androgen levels observed in men with sickle cell anemia. Treatment with zinc acetate (15 mg t.i.d.) has been useful in such patients.[70] Zinc deficiency has also been implicated in the gonadal dysfunction of uremic men on maintenance dialysis therapy.

A number of other hormonal abnormalities have been associated with zinc deficiency, although their clinical significance is not clear. Abnormal glucose tolerance is seen in animals; and in humans with insulin-dependent diabetes, serum zinc concentration is inversely correlated with the glycohemoglobin level.[71] Zinc at physiologic concentrations reduces pituitary prolactin secretion.[70]

Chromium

Chromium is an essential trace element for humans.[72] The earliest and most detectable feature of chromium deficiency in animals is abnormal glucose tolerance. Severe chromium deficiency in animals leads to a syndrome indistinguishable from mild diabetes mellitus, including glycosuria and fasting hyperglycemia.

Animal and human studies suggest that the role of chromium in improving glucose tolerance is mediated through the action of insulin. It appears to act as a catalyst for binding insulin to its specific receptor sites.[73] The active chromium compound in vivo is an organic low–molecular weight complex believed to contain (in addition to trivalent chromium) glycine, glutamic acid, cysteine, and nicotinic acid. This compound has been named glucose tolerance factor.

Therapeutic trials of dietary chromium supplementation in physiologic quantities document a human requirement for chromium and a human chromium deficiency. Supplementation trials[74-77] have been conducted among groups with impaired glucose tolerance, including persons with maturity-onset diabetes, middle-aged women, and the elderly. The studies showed improved glucose tolerance, reduced insulin response to glucose tolerance tests, and lowered serum cholesterol.

Inorganic forms of chromium are utilized less well than organic forms and require longer periods of supplementation, primarily because of their slow incorporation into glucose tolerance factor. The latter is the natural chromium compound that has outstanding insulin potentiating activity in vitro, is absorbed better than chromic chloride (in rats), is transported across the placenta, and has access to a body pool that is the source of the acute plasma increase (in humans) in response to insulin.[78] The best known source of chromium in the form of glucose tolerance factor is brewer's yeast.

REFERENCES

1. Merimee TJ: Growth hormone: secretion and action. In Degroot LJ, et al, editors: Endocrinology, vol. 1, New York, 1979, Grune & Stratton Inc, pp 123-132.
2. Kreisberg RA, et al: Nutrition and endocrine disease, Med Clin North Am 54:1473-1494, 1970.
3. Eisenstein AB, Singh SP: Hormonal control of nutrient metabolism. In Goodhart RS, Shils ME, editors: Modern nutrition in health and disease, Philadelphia, 1980, Lea & Febiger, pp 537-559.
4. Bondy PK, Felig P: Disorders of carbohydrate metabolism. In Bondy PK, Rosenberg LE, editors: Duncan's Diseases of metabolism, ed 7, Philadelphia, 1974, WB Saunders Co, pp 246-309.
5. Christy NP, Wanen MP: Disease syndromes of the hypothalamus and anterior pituitary. In DeGroot LJ, et al, editors: Endocrinology, vol. 1, New York, 1979, Grune & Stratton Inc, pp 215-252.
6. Serri O, et al: Acromegaly: biochemical assessment of cure after long term follow-up of transsphenoidal selective adenomectomy, J Clin Endocrinol Metab 61:1185-1189, 1985.
7. Cheek DB, et al: Body composition in endocrine disease before and after therapy. In Cheek DB, editor: Human growth: body composition, cell growth, energy, and intelligence, Philadelphia, 1968, Lea & Febiger, pp 198-206.
8. Hopwood NJ, et al: Hypoglycemia in hypopituitary children, Am J Dis Child 129:918-926, 1975.
9. Parra A, et al: Body composition in hypopituitary dwarfs before and during human growth hormone therapy, Metabolism 28:851-857, 1979.
10. Phillips LS, Vassilopoulou-Sellin R: Somatomedins, N Engl J Med 302:371-380, 438-446, 1980.
11. Van Vliet G, et al: Growth hormone treatment for short stature, N Engl J Med 309:1016-1022, 1983.
12. McKenzie JM, et al: Hyperthyroidism. In DeGroot LJ, et al, editors: Endocrinology, vol 1, New York, 1979, Grune & Stratton Inc. pp 429-459.
13. DeGroot LJ, Stanbury JB: The thyroid and its disease, New York, 1975, John Wiley & Sons Inc, pp 249-315, 405-471.
14. Haldimann B, et al: Intestinal calcium absorption in patients with hyperthyroidism, J Clin Endocrinol Metab 51:995-997, 1980.
15. Larsen PR: The thyroid. In Wyngaarden JB, Smith LH, editors: Cecil's Textbook of medicine, ed 16, Philadelphia, 1982, WB Saunders Co, pp 1201-1225.
16. Spaulding SW, Lippes H: Hyperthyroidism—causes, clinical features, and diagnosis. In Kaplan MM, Larsen PR, editors: Symposium on thyroid disease, Med Clin North Am 69:937-988, 1985.
17. Krause MV, Mahan LK: Food, nutrition, and diet therapy, ed 6, Philadelphia, 1979, WB Saunders Co, pp 544-552.
18. Alton S, O'Malley BP: Dietary intake in thyrotoxicosis before and after adequate carbimazole therapy; the impact of dietary advice, Clin Endocrinol 23:517-520, 1985.
19. Ingenbleek Y, et al: Nutritional significance of alterations in serum amino acid patterns in goitrous patients, Am J Clin Nutr 43:310-319, 1986.
20. Utiger RD: Hypothyroidism. In DeGroot LJ, et al, editors: Endocrinology, vol 1, New York, 1979, Grune & Stratton Inc, pp 471-488.
21. Sawin CT: Hypothyroidism, Med Clin North Am 69:989-1004, 1985.
22. Coindre JM, et al: Bone loss in hypothyroidism with hormone replacement: a histomorphometric study, Arch Intern Med 146:48-53, 1986.
23. Ross DS, et al: Prolonged suppression of the pituitary-thyroid axis with L-thyroxine treatment reduces bone density, Endocrinology, vol 118 (suppl 37), 1986 (abstract).
24. Perry HM 3rd: Thyroid replacement and osteoporosis (editorial), Arch Intern Med 146:41-42, 1986.
25. DeLuca HF: Vitamin D endocrinology, Ann Intern Med 85:367-377, 1976.
26. Hahn TJ: Parathyroid hormone, calcitonin, vitamin D, mineral, and bone: metabolism and disorders. In Mazzaferri EL, editor: Endocrinology, Garden City NJ, 1980, Medical Examination Publishing Co Inc, pp 425-558.
27. Weigmann T, Kaye M: Hypomagnesemic hypocalcemia, Arch Intern Med 137:953-955, 1977.

28. Liddle GW, Melmon KL: The adrenals. In Williams RH, editor: Textbook of endocrinology, ed 5, Philadelphia, 1974, WB Saunders Co, pp 233-322.

29. Nelson DH: The adrenal cortex: physiological function and disease, Philadelphia, 1980, WB Saunders Co, pp 210-239.

30. Cox M, et al: The defense against hyperkalemia: the roles of insulin and aldosterone, N Engl J Med 299:525-532, 1978.

31. Kahn CR, et al: Alterations in insulin binding induced by changes *in vivo* in the levels of glucocorticoids and growth hormone, Endocrinology 103:1054-1066, 1978.

32. Olefsky JM: Effect of dexamethasone on insulin binding, glucose transport and glucose oxidation of isolated rat adipocytes, J Clin Invest 56:1499-1508, 1975.

33. Ingle DJ: Some studies on the role of the adrenal cortex in organic metabolism, Ann NY Acad Sci 50:576-595, 1949.

34. Nelson DH: *op cit* (reference 29), pp 240-269.

35. Abou-Saleh MT: Dexamethasone suppression tests in psychiatry: Is there a place for an integrated hypothesis? Psychiatr Dev 3:275-306, 1985.

36. Hahn TJ, et al: Effects of short term glucocorticoid administration on intestinal calcium absorption and circulating vitamin D metabolite concentrations in man, J Clin Endocrinol Metab 52:111-115, 1981.

37. Thorn GW, et al: Advances in the diagnosis and treatment of adrenal insufficiency, Am J Med 10:595-611, 1951.

38. Rosenfield RL: Studies of the relation of plasma androgen levels to androgen action in women, J Steroid Biochem 6:695-702, 1975.

39. Young JB, Landsberg L: Catecholamines and the sympathoadrenal system: the regulation of metabolism. In Ingbar SH, editor: Contemporary endocrinology, vol 1, New York, Plenum Press Inc, 1979, pp 245-303.

40. Arky RA: Hypoglycemia. In DeGroot LJ, et al, editors: Endocrinology, vol 2, New York, 1979, Grune & Stratton Inc, pp 1099-1123.

41. Nelson RL: Hypoglycemia: fact or fiction? Mayo Clin Proc 60:844-850, 1985.

42. Feingold KR, et al: Endocrine disease. In Andreoli TE, et al, editors: Cecil's Essentials of medicine, Philadelphia, 1986, WB Saunders Co, pp 487-500.

43. Oliver J: Hypoglycemia. In Palmer S, Ekvall S, editors: Pediatric nutrition in developmental disorders, Springfield Ill, 1978, Charles C Thomas Publisher, pp 271-274.

44. Walfish PG: Hypoglycemia. In Zzrin C, et al, editors: Systematic endocrinology, ed 2, New York, 1979, Harper & Row Publishers Inc, pp 435-457.

45. Bell LS, et al: Dietary strategies in the treatment of reactive hypoglycemia, J Am Diet Assoc 85:1141-1143, 1985.

46. Danowski TS: Outline of endocrine gland syndromes, Baltimore, 1976, The Williams & Wilkins Co, pp 421-425.

47. Editorial: Anorexia nervosa: to investigate or to treat, Lancet 2:563-564, 1979.

48. Boyar RM, et al: Cortisol secretion and metabolism in anorexia nervosa, N Engl J Med 296:190-193, 1977.

49. Schwabe AD, et al: Anorexia nervosa, Ann Intern Med 94:371-381, 1981.

50. Wachslicht-Rodbard H, et al: Increased insulin binding to erythrocytes in anorexia nervosa, N Engl J Med 300:882-887, 1979.

51. Grahame-Smith DG: The carcinoid syndrome. In DeGroot LJ, et al, editors: Endocrinology, vol 3, New York, 1979, Grune & Stratton Inc, pp 1721-1731.

52. Felig P: Starvation. In DeGroot LJ, et al, editors: Endocrinology, vol 3, New York, 1979, Grune & Stratton Inc, pp 1927-1940.

53. Crim MC, Munro HN: Protein-energy malnutrition and endocrine function. In DeGroot LJ, et al, editors: Endocrinology, vol 3, New York, 1979, Grune & Stratton Inc, pp 1987-2000.

54. Berg BN: Maintenance of pregnancy in protein-deprived rats by transitory protein supplements during early gestation, J Nutr 92:66-70, 1967.

55. Nelson MM, Evans RM: Maintenance of pregnancy in the absence of dietary protein with estrone and progesterone, Endocrinology 55:543-549, 1954.

56. Becker DJ: The endocrine responses to protein calorie malnutrition, Ann Rev Nutr 3:187-212, 1983.

57. Pugliese MT, Lifshitz F: Endocrine adaptations to undernutrition, Clin Nutr 4:48, 1985.

58. Richmond DA, et al: Altered thyroid hormone levels in bacterial sepsis: the role of nutritional adequacy, Metabolism 29:936, 1980.

59. Kien CL, et al: Low serum reverse T_3 concentration in burned children; its relationship to nutritional state, Am J Clin Nutr 33:1215-1219, 1980.

60. Lunn PG, et al: The effect of improved nutrition on plasma prolactin concentrations and postpartum infertility in lactating Gambian women, Am J Clin Nutr 39:227-235, 1984.

61. Ermans AM: Endemic goiter and endemic cretinism. In DeGroot LJ, et al, editors: Endocrinology, vol 1, New York, 1979, Grune & Stratton Inc, pp 501-508.

62. Hetzel BS: The concept of iodine deficiency disorders. In Medeiros-Neto G, et al, editors: Iodine deficiency disorders and congenital hypothyroidism, Sao Paulo, 1986, ACHÉ, pp 1-6.

63. Health Services and Mental Health Administration, Center for Disease Control: Ten-State Nutrition Survey, 1968-1970, DHEW Publ, Washington DC, 1972, Department of Health, Education, and Welfare.

64. Cavalieri RR: Trace elements: iodine. In Goodhart RS, Shils ME, editors: Modern nutrition in health and disease, Philadelphia, 1980, Lea & Febiger, pp 395-407.

65. Sauberlich HE, et al: Laboratory tests for the assessment of nutritional status, Cleveland, 1974, CRC Press, pp 124-251.

66. Committee on Dietary Allowances, Food and Nutrition Board, National Research Council: Recommended dietary allowances, ed 9, Washington DC, 1980, National Academy of Sciences.

67. Henkin RI: Copper-zinc-hormone interrelationships. In Karcioglu ZA, Sarper RF, editors: Zinc and copper in medicine, Springfield Ill, 1980, Charles C Thomas Publisher, pp 126-159.

68. Allen DK, et al: Function of pituitary-thyroid axis in copper-deficient rats, J Nutr 112:2043-2046, 1982.

69. Abbasi AA, et al: Experimental zinc deficiency in man. Effect on testicular function, J Lab Clin Med 96:544-550, 1980.

70. Prasad AS: Clinical endocrinological and biochemical effects of zinc deficiency, J Clin Endocrinol Metab 14:567, 1985.

71. Hayes A, et al: Effect of zinc status on glycohemoglobin and serum triglycerides in persons with diabetes, Trace Elements Med **4:**57-60, 1987.

72. Mertz W: Chromium—an overview. In Shapcott D, Hubert J, editors: Chromium in nutrition and metabolism, New York, 1980, Elsevier/North Holland Inc, pp 1-14.

73. Mertz W: Effects and metabolism of glucose tolerance factor, Nutr Rev **33:**129-135, 1975.

74. Liu VK, et al: Effects of high-chromium yeast-extract supplementation on serum lipids, serum insulin, and glucose tolerance in older women, Fed Proc **34:**4509, 1977.

75. Offenbacher EG, Pi-Sunyer FX: Beneficial effect of chromium-rich yeast on glucose tolerance and blood lipids in elderly subjects, Diabetes **29:**919-925, 1980.

76. Kohrs MB, et al: Iron and chromium nutrition in the elderly. In Hemphill D, editor: Annual Conference on Trace Substances in Environmental Health, vol 18, Columbia, 1984, University of Missouri Press.

77. Elias AN, et al: Use of artificial beta cell (ABC) in the assessment of peripheral insulin sensitivity: effect of chromium supplementation in diabetic patients, Gen Pharmacol **15:**535-539, 1984.

78. Canfield W: Chromium, glucose tolerance, and serum cholesterol in adults. In Shapcott D, Hubert J, editors: Chromium in nutrition and metabolism, New York, 1980, Elsevier/North Holland Inc, pp 145-162.

CHAPTER 18
Reproductive System

José Villar
Natalie Kurinij
Howard N. Jacobson

DIABETES MELLITUS AND PREGNANCY

The pregnancy of diabetic women is a model of how comprehensive team care coupled with good glycemic control can lower the complication rates for mother and newborn. The perinatal mortality rate in insulin-dependent diabetics receiving optimum care has improved dramatically over the years.[1]

This reduction in perinatal mortality is largely attributable to the maintenance of maternal blood glucose at levels similar to those of normal pregnancy or within the physiologic range of 60 to 120 mg/dl. The best morbidity and mortality outcomes are found among infants born to diabetic mothers who maintain blood glucose levels at or below 100 mg/dl during pregnancy.[2,3]

Approximately 10,000 to 15,000 insulin-dependent diabetics[4] and 60,000 to 90,000 women diagnosed with gestational diabetes[5] deliver infants yearly in the United States. Both forms of diabetes mellitus, pregestational and gestational, complicate 1% to 2% of all pregnancies. Pregestational diabetes is usually a juvenile-onset insulin-dependent condition. In contrast, gestational diabetes typically occurs during the third trimester of pregnancy but abnormal blood glucose levels usually return to normal postpartum.[6] Obesity is very common in gestational diabetics and up to 60% of patients will develop permanent maturity-onset diabetes within 16 years of follow-up.[7] Weight reduction after delivery may be crucial to the long-term outcome for these patients.

In management of gestational diabetes during pregnancy, dietary changes alone may be sufficient to control blood glucose levels, since the maternal pancreas can produce insulin. If hyperglycemia persists, exogenous insulin may be required. Oral hyperglycemic agents should not be used, since questions remain about both their efficacy and their fetal and neonatal effects. Diet is important in managing both insulin-dependent and gestational diabetes, but the insulin-dependent diabetic must be much more careful about coordinating diet and activity level to avoid both hyperglycemia and insulin shock.[8,9]

Metabolic Adaptations in Pregnancy

Early pregnancy is an anabolic state resulting from increased secretion of estrogen and progesterone and from increased production by the beta-cells of insulin. Maternal blood glucose levels normally are lower during the first 20 weeks of gestation, because of the exaggerated insulin response. Hyperinsulinemia effects include increased tissue glycogen storage and peripheral glucose utilization as well as increased fat synthesis and storage.[10] In the second 20 weeks of gestation the transport of glucose and amino acids to the fetus and placenta rises, and mobilization of maternal fat stores occurs. Glucose tolerance decreases, and an insulin resistance is present. Liver glycogen stores become depleted as hepatic glucose production is increased. Although by the third trimester insulin concentrations are high, glucose utilization is retarded. This effect is a consequence of (1) increased insulin degradation by the greater concentrations of placental enzymes and (2) peripheral resistance to insulin binding caused by the placental lactogenic hormones progesterone and cortisol.

"Accelerated starvation" can occur in a fasted state during the third trimester because of the higher insulin and lower glucose levels.[11] Lipolysis leads to an increase in the circulation of free fatty acids and ketones. Metabolism in the fed state is also modified: the high plasma glucose levels tend to promote carbohydrate-induced triglyceridemia.[11] Alterations in circulating insulin in the fed and fasted states produce an overall lowering of plasma glucose and amino acid concentrations.[11]

Normal glucose metabolism is maintained in later pregnancy despite these hormonal changes by increased maternal secretion of insulin. Women who have marginal insulin reserves cannot respond efficiently to the challenges of pregnancy, and they will have abnormal glucose levels and will develop gestational diabetes. The maternal hyperglycemia produces fetal hyperglycemia and fetal reactive hyperinsulinemia, and the consequent increase in the fetus' nutrient deposits (fat) produces the macrosomic characteristics.

Diagnosis

Urinary glucose excretion increases markedly during normal pregnancy. Urinalysis therefore is not a useful screen for diabetes during pregnancy. Blood glucose levels can be determined postprandially, after an overnight fast, or during a glucose-tolerance test. In pregnancy the fasting glucose level is reduced, and it declines gradually as term approaches. Morning postprandial glucose is a reliable method for third-trimester screening and can be measured after the patient has had breakfast. Normal postbreakfast blood glucose levels in the third trimester[12,13] are shown in Table 18-1.

Gestational diabetes typically appears in the third trimester. O'Sullivan et al.[14] recommend a 50 g 1-hour oral glucose screening test at 24 to 28 weeks of gestation for all pregnant women over the age of 25 and for those with a clinical history suggestive of a diabetic predisposition. The American Diabetes Association[15] has taken a more conservative stand and recommends screening tests be done on all pregnant women. The cost effectiveness of universal screening has been questioned[16] because the diagnostic accuracy of screening patients aged 24 years or greater with a threshold value of 150 mg/dl is satisfactory.

Plasma glucose levels at 1 hour that are 140 mg/dl and higher[12] or 135 mg/dl and higher[17,18] indicate a need for the 3-hour oral glucose tolerance test. Leiken et al.[19] screened 2276 women for gestational diabetes using the 50 g carbohydrate load and found 16% with abnormal serum glucose values (>135 mg/dl). These women were subsequently challenged with a 100 g 3-hour oral glucose test, and 49% ($N = 179$) were determined to be nondiabetic. However, these women went on to deliver babies who were significantly larger than those of the 1879 women with normal screening values, suggesting that minor abnormalities in carbohydrate metabolism during pregnancy pose a risk for macrosomia.

Standards for 3-hour oral glucose tolerance tests during pregnancy have been debated for years; the criteria proposed in 1964 by O'Sullivan and Mahan appear to be the most useful and were adopted by the National Diabetes Data Group (NDDG)[20] in 1979. They are presented in Table 18-2.

Pregnant women at high risk of gestational

Table 18-1 Postbreakfast Blood Glucose Levels in Nondiabetic Ambulatory Women During the Last Trimester of Pregnancy

Hours after Breakfast	N	Blood Glucose (mg/100 ml)*	
		Mean ± SD	2 SD above Mean
½-1	54	81.6 ± 16.4	114.4
1-2	323	74.3 ± 15.2	104.7
2-3	166	68.6 ± 12.6	93.8
3-4	54	67.3 ± 12.5	92.3
>4, or fasting	77	65.9 ± 9.3	84.1

From Knopp R, et al: Carbohydrate and lipid metabolism in laboratory indices of nutritional status of pregnancy, Washington DC, 1978, National Research Council, National Academy of Sciences, p 35.

Diets consisted of 30 kcal/kg of ideal body weight with 1.5 to 2 g/kg of protein, and 40% of calories as fat. The amount taken at breakfast was unspecified.

*Somogyi-Nelson method.

diabetes should be screened on their first prenatal visit. The presence of any of the following signifies the need for a glucose tolerance test: (1) a family history of diabetes, (2) an obstetric history of stillbirth, large for date infants (4-5 kg at birth), unexplained perinatal death, prematurity, hydramnios, severe fetal abnormality, or caudal agenesis, (3) obesity (>20% expected weight for height), (4) fasting glycosuria, (5) acute hydramnios, (6) previous gestational diabetes, and (7) older maternal age or (8) parity of 5 or greater.

Postprandial glycosuria is not an indicator of abnormal glucose metabolism during pregnancy, but the presence of glucose in the urine after a fasting period does suggest the need for further diagnostic tests. Glycosylated hemoglobin (HbA$_1$), measured by ion exchange chromatography, has been determined to be a poor screen in early pregnancy for gestational diabetes.[21] However, the more recent assessment of HbA$_1$ by affinity chromatography between 10 and 15 weeks of gestation may be more sensitive.[22]

Complications

In general, all diabetic complications occur and may be more severe in pregnant patients— particularly cardiopathy, microvascular retiopathy, nephropathy, and infections (most frequently urinary, especially pyelonephritis, and candidal vaginitis). The incidence of hydramnios and preeclampsia is also greater. The placenta may be large, because of increased glycogen, lipid deposition, and edema in noncomplicated diabetics, or it may be small with infarcts in patients with vascular disease.

There is a higher rate of fetal intrauterine death, especially after 30 weeks of gestation, usually because of placental insufficiency, preeclampsia, or metabolic imbalance (e.g., maternal and fetal hypoglycemia or acidosis). Commonly fetuses are macrosomatic, with pancreatic beta-cell hypertrophy, consequent hyperinsulinism, and poor development of pancreatic alphacells. Fetal hyperinsulinemia can inhibit cortisol-induced lecithin synthesis. The resultant surfactant deficiency can lead to respiratory distress syndrome. The incidence of respiratory distress syndrome has decreased in recent years, however, because of strict metabolic control and delivery near term.[23]

Newborns of insulin-dependent diabetics have a rate of congenital anomalies two to three times greater than that in the nondiabetic population.[24] This may be due to poor diabetic control during organogenesis.[24,25] In light of the evidence that congenital malformations occur early in pregnancy and may be complicated by the metabolic disturbances of diabetes, strict diabetic control before conception is advised. Freinkel et al.[11] advocate that diabetic women contemplating pregnancy do so only when glycosylated hemoglobin levels are normal, indicating prolonged preconceptual metabolic control. Women with gestational diabetes do not have a rate of malformations in newborns different from that of the nondiabetic population.

Infants of diabetic mothers tend to be hypoglycemic in the immediate postnatal period because of the maternal hyperglycemia. Hypocal-

Table 18-2 Glucose Tolerance Test Results in Randomly Selected Pregnant Women (N = 752) After 100 g Oral Glucose

	Whole Blood Glucose (mg/100 ml)*			
	0 Hour	1 Hour	2 Hours	3 Hours
Mean ± SD	69.3 ± 10.4	103.6 ± 30.8	91.7 ± 25.8	79.4 ± 24
2 SD upper limit	90	165	143	127
O'Sullivan criteria†				
Whole blood	90	165	145	125
Plasma‡	103	188	165	143

From Knopp R, et al: Carbohydrate and lipid metabolism in laboratory indices of nutritional states of pregnancy, Washington, DC, 1978, National Research Council, National Academy of Sciences, p 35.

*Somogyi-Nelson method.

†Two or more elevated values constitute an abnormal test.

‡Plasma criteria are calculated from whole blood × 1.14.

cemia and hyperbilirubinemia occur less frequently if delivery occurs after 37 weeks of gestation.[26] Although an association has been reported between ketonuria and decreased intelligence quotient[27] as well as an increased incidence of cerebral palsy and seizure disorders,[28] these findings remain controversial.

Nutritional Management

The primary goals of diet modification for the pregnant diabetic are to meet the nutrient needs of both the mother and the fetus[8] and to achieve and maintain physiologic glucose homeostasis in the mother.[3] Many nonpregnant diabetic women achieve glycemic control through low-calorie diets, but these diets are incompatible with the nutritional needs of pregnancy. The nutritional recommendations for diabetics published by the American Diabetes Association in 1979 have been updated to emphasize high carbohydrate, high fiber diets with a low fat content.[29]

Energy, nutrient requirements, and recommended weight gain for pregnant diabetics are comparable to those for nondiabetic pregnant women. Intake should be 30 to 35 kcal/kg of body weight.[30] Regular meals and snacks are essential, and bedtime snacks may be critical because of the tendency toward overnight hypoglycemia and ketosis. A glass of milk and two graham crackers at bedtime can meet the need for an extra 25 g of carbohydrate. *Carbohydrates* should account for 55% to 60% of total calories.[29] Intake should be individualized to achieve optimum blood glucose and lipid levels and account for eating patterns. *High-fiber* diets have received increasing attention in the treatment of diabetes because they improve glycemic control and lower serum cholesterol and triglycerides.[31] A gradual doubling of fiber intake has been recommended; however, there are too few studies of fiber intake in pregnant diabetic women to advise for or against increased fiber intake during pregnancy.[29] Nevertheless, pregnant women appear to tolerate fiber well. Water-soluble fibers (e.g., guar gum) are more effective at lowering postprandial glycemia than are water-insoluble fibers such as those in wheat bran.[32] Dietary fiber is found in unrefined complex carbohydrates, such as whole grain breads and cereals, bran, fruits, and vegetables. The long-term effect of fiber on mineral and vitamin bioavailability must be considered.[31,33] *Protein* should constitute about 15% to 20% of the total caloric intake each

day.[30] The recommended protein allowance of 0.8 g/kg of body weight for adults should be increased in pregnancy by 30 g/day to provide sufficient protein for deposition in the uterus, breasts, and fetal and placental tissues and for the expanding blood volume. *Fat* intake should comprise less than 30% of calories and cholesterol intake should be less than 300 mg/day. The total calories from fat should be less than 10% from saturated fat, less than 10% from polyunsaturated fat, and the remaining 6% to 8% from monounsaturated fat. The addition of eicosapentaenoic acid is acceptable; however, more research is needed regarding its benefits.[29] Heavy use of *saccharin* should be discontinued during pregnancy, since saccharin crosses the placenta and its effects on the fetus are not fully understood.[34] *Aspartame* may be used during pregnancy within established safe levels.[34] *Salt* intake should not exceed 3 g/day, and the recommended level is approximately 1 g/1000 kcal.[29]

Insulin

In patients for whom insulin treatment is indicated, the dosage should control extreme fluctuations in blood sugar levels and should maintain those levels as close to normal range as possible. A minimum of two daily injections of insulin is recommended,[35,36] the first before breakfast and the second before dinner. To meet the increased insulin requirement during pregnancy, Jovanovic et al.[37] prefer three injections, one before breakfast, one before dinner, and one at bedtime. Insulin doses and composition of the mixture (NPH and regular insulin) are continually adjusted based on individual needs. Effective dosage adjustments and determining the number of injections per day require frequent interaction between patient and physician.[38]

Continuous subcutaneous insulin infusion has been used in the management of pregnant diabetics[39-41] and has produced excellent glycemic control. Insulin as miniboluses before a meal, or as a constant basal infusion otherwise, also has been delivered through a catheter needle to subcutaneous tissue in the abdomen.[38] Widespread use of the method is limited, however, because demands are placed on the patient in achieving proper pump usage, the pump is expensive, and complications often arise—such as nocturnal hypoglycemia, catheter obstruction, pump failure, and abscess formation at the infusion site.[38]

Self-Monitoring

Pregnant diabetic patients increasingly monitor their own blood glucose levels at home with a glucose reflectance meter. A drop of blood is smeared on the end of a glucose oxidase reagent test strip and is washed off 60 seconds later, and the darkened test strip placed in the reflectance meter. The values of blood sugar can be read directly from the meter and recorded by the patient. Blood sugar levels are monitored daily before each meal and at bedtime; in addition, on a weekly basis, blood sugar is monitored 1 hour after each meal.[38] Meter readings are reliable in the range of 100 to 300 mg/dl.[38] A Consensus Development Conference on Self-Monitoring of Blood Glucose (SMBG) held in 1986[42] indicated that SMBG is a valuable tool in the management of diabetics and addressed the need for greater quality control to ensure accurate and precise readings. North et al.[43] compared the precision and accuracy of a number of home monitors and found that the Accuchek bG and Glucoscan 2000 were the most accurate and precise. During pregnancy, self-monitoring improves diabetic control by providing instant feedback, which promotes dietary adherence.

Long-term control of blood glucose is generally assessed by the physician on a monthly basis by measuring glycosylated hemoglobin. The formation of glycohemoglobin occurs through an irreversible nonenzymatic reaction between blood glucose and hemoglobin. Glucose remains attached to hemoglobin for the life of the red blood cell (100–120 da). The amount of glycosylated hemoglobin formed reflects the time-averaged blood glucose levels for the preceding 2 to 3 months.[44,45]

Urine testing is not the ideal way to monitor diabetes control. The glomerular filtration rates increase in pregnancy, and nondiabetic women can also have glycosuria. If heavy glycosuria occurs, more carbohydrates must be added to the diet. However, urine is monitored for ketones (by assessing the first morning specimen each day and whenever preprandial glucose levels exceed 150 mg/dl) to prevent acidosis.

Dietary Plans

The American Diabetes Association and the American Dietetic Association have developed a food exchange system that enables the pregnant diabetic to translate her diet prescription into meaningful food choices and servings. Foods are divided into six categories: vegetables, fruits, breads, cereals, meats, and fat. Within a category, items may be exchanged for one another since all contain similar food values. Use of the exchange plan provides a balanced diet based on a particular caloric intake without having to count calories but rather choosing the appropriate number of exchanges from each of the food categories.

The exchange system has recently been modified[29] to emphasize high-carbohydrate high-fiber diets, nonfat or low-fat milk products, and leaner meat. To promote appropriate food choices, symbols are used to identify foods containing at least 3 g of fiber and those with 400 mg or more of sodium per serving. Diet therapy in minority patients should be individualized to include ethnic foods.

The glycemic index represents a physiologic blood glucose response to specific food items. Classification of foods by their ability to elevate blood glucose could aid in the management of diabetes. However, controversy exists[46,47] because simple carbohydrates have been found to elicit smaller blood glucose responses than complex carbohydrates. For example, legumes produce the smallest glycemic response whereas root vegetables and grains produce the greatest.

Factors such as the form in which a meal is eaten, the combining of meals, the methods of preparation, portion size, and the fiber and fat content of foods affect the glycemic response.[48] As an educational tool second to the exchange system, the glycemic index table can be used to identify starchy foods with a low glycemic potential that may be incorporated into the diet.

Pregnancy Monitoring and Delivery

Antenatal care for the diabetic mother should be performed at a high-risk obstetric unit by a maternal and fetal medicine specialist. Accurate assessment of the length of gestation and close fetal monitoring are required. Early ultrasound evaluation and fundal uterine height determinations should be performed throughout gestation. Additionally, fetal surveillance should be initiated between the thirty-fourth and thirty-eighth weeks of gestation depending on the woman's diabetic class. The patient should be hospitalized at 34 or 35 weeks, or at least 1 week before delivery if glucose control has been suboptimal. In the past, delivery was induced at 35 to 38 weeks, depending on the diabetic classification or obstetric history. With more sensitive methods of fetal monitoring, pregnancies can be managed individually (and generally less conservatively). The lecithin:sphingomyelin (L/S) ratio may be of limited value before week 38 of gestation in diabetic patients.[49] When evidence of fetal compromise or maternal complications indicates preterm delivery, the L/S ratio can provide some information. However, delivery before 36 weeks should be avoided unless necessary. Vaginal delivery at term with very close fetal monitoring is recommended. Prolonged labor or electronically and biochemically corroborated fetal distress is an indication for cesarean delivery.

PREGNANCY-INDUCED HYPERTENSION AND PREECLAMPSIA

Hypertension during pregnancy (BP above 140/90 mm Hg) alone or with proteinuria after week 20 of pregnancy is a frequent but poorly understood complication. A major complication, fortunately infrequent, is eclampsia, in which convulsions occur and death may ensue.

One of the first signs of preeclampsia is a sudden weight gain (more than 1 kg/wk or 3 kg/mo) that cannot be explained by a large increase in food intake. Hypertension follows, with intermittent and then consistent proteinuria followed by severe headaches and blurred vision. The pathophysiology of the disorder includes generalized vasospasm, with reduced circulation and substance exchange across the placenta.[50] Intrauterine growth retardation, fetal hypoxia, and in severe cases fetal death can be observed.

Preeclampsia is primarily a disease of primigravidas and occurs most frequently in women near the extremes of reproductive age (younger than 20 or over 35). Women in their second pregnancy who have had preeclampsia during their first gestation are also at higher risk of the syndrome, which is associated with low socioeconomic status, low levels of education, poor nutrition, and limited utilization of health care and sometimes with severe emotional stress. Increased caloric intake leading to a large weight gain does not predispose women to the disease.

Although nutritional factors have long been considered to be associated with the course and outcome of preeclampsia, their actual role in the etiology of the disease remains to be demonstrated. Three types of study have explored this association: *Retrospective* diet information has been collected from normal (controls) and preeclamptic patients, and the preeclamptics have been shown to consume less nutrients than their normal counterparts did. This might be expected since reduced dietary intake could just as well be a result of the disease as a cause of it. *Prospective* studies have followed a cohort of pregnant women, recording their intakes and attempting to relate these to subsequent appearance of the disease. However, this type of study has two problems: low-income groups, in which preeclampsia is more prevalent, generally receive prenatal care late in pregnancy, and the information consequently is not collected over a significantly long time; furthermore, the reliability and validity of the measurements of nutrient intake under these conditions are questionable. *Supplementation* appears to be the most appropriate method of exploring the association between nutrition and preeclampsia. A daily vitamin-mineral supplement is administered to a group of patients, and the incidence of preeclampsia is compared with that in a nonsupplemented (control/placebo) group.

In one supplementation study[53] the incidence of preeclampsia was successfully reduced by a vitamin-mineral tablet given to women daily from the twenty-fourth week of gestation onward. The incidence of preeclampsia was 14.6% in the nonsupplemented group compared to 4.8% in those who received the supplement.[52] The 118 pregnant women who had no supplementation also manifested higher mean systolic and diastolic pressures and a greater incidence of edema and albuminuria than did the 122 women who received the supplement.[53] The differences were statistically significant.

Table 18-3 gives a historical view of the results of the studies available to date. Despite these early findings, it is difficult to assign relative amounts of influence to each of the many nutritional variables encountered.

In contrast to these early results, more recent metabolic studies[56] have failed to demonstrate any significant difference in nitrogen intake or balance between women in whom pregnancy-induced hypertension developed and those in whom pressures remained normal. The role of fat also is controversial. Dietary studies[57] have suggested an association between higher total fat and fatty acid intake and toxemia. However, studies of pregnant rabbits deprived of essential

Table 18-3 Incidence of Preeclampsia in Nutritionally Supplemented Pregnant Women

Study	Type of Supplementation	Other Characteristics	Results
Tompkins, Wiehl[51]	Group 1: control ($N = 170$) Group 2: multivitamins; no information on composition ($N = 244$) Group 3: additional proteins (50 g/da); no other information ($N = 186$) Group 4: vitamins and proteins ($N = 160$)		Incidence of toxemia Group 1: 4.12% Group 2: 3.28% Group 3: 2.69% Group 4: 0.63%
Chandhuri[52]	Vitamin-mineral tablets Calcium: phosphate (0.25 mg/da) and gluconate (3 g/da)	Group 1: with poor prenatal care ($N = 200$) Group 2: with better prenatal care (beginning before 24 wk) ($N = 178$) Group 3: same as 2, plus vitamin-mineral tablets ($N = 164$)	Incidence of toxemia (moderate and severe) Group 1: 23% Group 2: 14.6% Group 3: 4.8%
Osofsky[53]	Group 1: nonsupplemented; intakes approximating or exceeding recommended daily allowances, except for calcium and iron; daily calcium, 673.2 mg ($N = 118$)	No difference between groups in age, socioeconomic status, parity, weeks of gestation at first visit, weight, arterial pressure at first visit	Nonsupplemented group had higher systolic and diastolic pressures, higher rise in systolic and diastolic pressures, and higher incidence of albuminuria All differences were statistically significant
	Group 2: protein-mineral supplementation (Meritene); significant differences from Group 1 in daily intakes of protein, calcium (1028.1 mg), phosphorus, and iron	Supplemented group averaged 11.1 prenatal examinations, nonsupplemented group 10.2	
Holmes[54]	Group 1: 60-70 g of protein daily Group 2: 110-120 g of protein daily Proteins given in meat, fish, eggs, milk, and milk products; all diets rich in green leafy vegetables and fruit juices; at least 1 qt of milk included in daily intake	All private patients with prenatal care	Incidence of toxemia Primipara: Group 1: 6.2% Group 2: 3.4% Multipara: Group 1: 3.4% Group 2: 1.7% ($N = 350$ for all groups)

Modified slightly from Belizán JM, Villar J: Possible role of calcium in the development of toxemia of pregnancy, Institute of Nutrition of Central America and Panama (INCAP), Division of Human Development. Internal document, Guatemala City, 1978.

fatty acids[58] have shown an increased sensitivity to angiotensin II, characteristic of toxemic patients. Although this is an attractive possibility given the relationship between essential fatty acids and prostaglandin production, more extensive work is needed before any practical consideration can be contemplated.

Calcium intake and calcium metabolism have been suggested also to be related to pregnancy-induced hypertension and blood pressure during pregnancy. The first epidemiologic observation[59,60] showed an inverse association between calcium intake and the incidence of eclampsia after adjusting for several confounding factors.

Several randomized controlled clinical trials with calcium supplementation have been conducted. In one,[61] healthy nonpregnant women of childbearing age receiving a daily 1 g supplement of elemental calcium had blood pressure values, after 10 weeks, that were significantly lower than those in a placebo group. In two others,[62,63] a dose-effect relationship was shown when their data were combined: groups with calcium supplementation of 1, 1.5, and 2 g per day had, at term, systolic blood pressure values that were 2.9,[63] 3.7,[62] and 8.5[63] mm Hg, respectively, lower than in corresponding placebo groups.

The prevention of preeclampsia or pregnancy-induced hypertension with calcium supplementation is less conclusive, although preliminary data appear to support this effect.[62,64,65] Interesting, and supporting the possible protective effect of high calcium intakes, is the fact that preeclamptic patients have lower urinary calcium excretion than normotensive controls.[66] Furthermore, it has been demonstrated[67] that patients with lower urinary calcium values have the largest blood pressure reductions with calcium supplementation.

Although this is a promising nutritional area, a large randomized clinical trial demonstrating reductions in the incidence of preeclampsia is required before supplementation with high calcium doses during pregnancy can be recommended. Pregnant women should be encouraged to reach at least the present calcium RDA (1200 mg/da) during gestation and their intakes should be monitored.[30]

Excessive weight gain has been reported more frequently among women with preeclampsia. True, preeclampsia can cause edema and it is easy to confuse the fluid weight with weight gained as a consequence of tissue deposit; but little evidence supports the concept that high weight gains cause preeclampsia. Nevertheless, because of the association of preeclampsia, edema, and weight gain, a low-calorie low-sodium diet has been erroneously recommended in the past as a preventive and therapeutic measure.

Diuretics also have been prescribed for severe cases of preeclampsia, although they have not been shown to be effective in treating this disease. The preventive role of diuretics in the development of preeclampsia has recently been evaluated.[68] A review of nine clinical trials showed significant reductions in high blood pressure among treated women, a well-known effect of these drugs, although no evidence was found of protection against perinatal mortality. Furthermore, the possible adverse effects of diuretics during a pregnancy have been clearly recognized.[69]

Thiazide diuretics and a low-carbohydrate (1200 kcal/da) weight-reducing diet had no effect on the incidence of preeclampsia in one study[70] and, in fact, they may have produced an excessive number of newborns below the 25th weight percentile. In another[71] there was an increase in fetal death rates when women lost 1 or more pounds per week, no matter whether they had low (<74 mm Hg) or high (>94) diastolic pressures and no matter their levels of proteinuria. Furthermore, restricting weight gains during pregnancy and using diuretics and low-sodium diets have interfered with placental circulation, thus mimicking in part the pathophysiology of preeclampsia itself.[72]

Thus there seems to be no sound reason for the recommendation of low-calorie low-sodium diets or the routine use of diuretics. Indeed, they have been shown to be potentially harmful. In clinical practice excessive weight gain without medical complications is an indication for only dietary counseling and not calorie or sodium restrictions.

To summarize, in the routine management of pregnancy, neither physiologic edema nor the edema associated with hypertension should be treated with diuretics or low-sodium diets. These therapies lower the maternal blood volume, reduce renal and placental circulation, and lead to an insufficient transfer of nutrients to the fetus. Only under the rare circumstances of severe chronic hypertension, renal disease, and congestive heart disease should diuretics be used in pregnancy, and in these cases potassium intake should also be monitored closely.

ANEMIA IN PREGNANCY

The normal physiologic anemia of pregnancy results from a greater relative increase in plasma volume over red cell mass. The hemodilution of red cells is seen in a hematocrit that drops from approximately 40% in the nonpregnant state to 33% in the last trimester of pregnancy.[73] Similarly, hemoglobin values fall by up to 2 g/dl.[74] The reduction of hemoglobin values, particularly during the second half of pregnancy, has been traditionally used as an indicator of anemia, and values below 10 g/dl are considered to be clearly abnormal. However, the effects of hemoglobin levels between 10 and 11 g/dl on maternal and fetal outcome are less clear. The most favorable outcomes seem to be associated with values between 11 and 12 g and a hematocrit of 33% to 35%. For black mothers the suggested values are about 1 g lower for hemoglobin and 3% lower for the hematocrit.[75]

Patients should be screened as early as possible, ideally during the first trimester, by the twenty-sixth to twenty-eighth week, and finally sometime prior to delivery. A postpartum test is recommended if blood loss during delivery was extensive. Screening during the prenatal period should include at least hemoglobin and hematocrit tests. Hb S testing is recommended for all black women, and a red cell folate assessment for patients with a hemoglobin count below 10 g/dl if folate deficiency is prevalent in the population from which the patient is drawn.

IRON DEFICIENCY ANEMIA

Ninety percent of the anemias found during pregnancy are iron deficiency anemias. Twenty percent of women in the United States enter pregnancy with low or depleted iron stores[76] and cannot meet the increased iron demands of pregnancy by diet alone. The iron requirements of pregnancy, approximately 600-800 mg of elemental iron, allow for expansion of the maternal red cell mass and fetal growth. Dietary intake over the course of pregnancy maximally provides 300-400 mg of iron. Absorption of iron increases during pregnancy,[77] from about 10% to almost 30% during the last trimester.[78] Women who enter pregnancy with low iron stores and who are not supplemented during pregnancy are at risk of exhausting their reserves and developing iron deficiency anemia.

The recommended daily dietary intake is 30 mg of supplemental iron throughout pregnancy.[79] This recommendation is based on the increased need for iron, particularly during the last two trimesters, and the inability of dietary iron or the existing iron stores of many women to meet the requirement. In women who are not iron depleted when iron supplementation is begun, 20 mg of supplementary iron per day may suffice.[79] The bioavailability of iron from prenatal multivitamin supplements should be determined, since other agents in the supplement (calcium, phosphate, zinc) can impair iron absorption.[79]

The efficacy of prophylactic iron treatment throughout pregnancy has been questioned, and it has been suggested that iron supplementation may be superfluous or harmful.[80,81] High hemoglobin (>13-14 g/dl) and hematocrit values (>35%-36%) have been associated with increased perinatal morbidity, low birth weight, and fetal death.[75,81] Also, intake of iron-folate supplements may compromise zinc absorption.[82] Bentley[83] suggests that women who present early in pregnancy with a serum ferritin concentration less than 50 μg/liter should be supplemented whereas women who present with a serum ferritin concentration greater than 80 μg/liter may not require routine prophylactic iron therapy throughout their pregnancy.

The possible consequences of iron deficiency anemia in pregnancy are hypothetically described as a depletion of iron stores leading to reduced hemoglobin synthesis and a compromised oxygen supply to the fetus, which may result in poor fetal development.[84] Conversely, a reduced hemoglobin synthesis may be compensated by increased maternal cardiac output, which, though it increases the workload on the maternal heart, augments blood flow to the placenta and thereby satisfies the oxygen needs of the fetus. Hypertrophy of the placenta in anemic mothers has been reported.[85]

Infants of anemic mothers have reduced iron stores in the first year of life.[86] An association between maternal iron deficiency and decreased birthweight,[87] prematurity,[88] and increased incidence of pica[87] has been reported, but these findings remain controversial.

A precise diagnosis of iron deficiency anemia

can be made using bone marrow examination. The method is costly, however, as well as time consuming and painful and is therefore out of the question for screening purposes. Hematocrit has some value but it produces 25% false-negative results. A reduced hemoglobin level in conjunction with red cells that are microcytic and hypochromic suggests severe iron deficiency anemia.

Plasma ferritin seems to be the most sensitive method for screening during pregnancy,[89] since it has been reported to correlate excellently well with body iron stores.[90,91] Plasma ferritin at a level of 1 μg/liter of plasma is equivalent to 8 μg of stored iron. A serum ferritin concentration below 40 μg/liter indicates compromised iron storage,[83] and values of less than 12 μg/liter are indicative of iron deficiency.[92] Depletion of iron stores is identified by serum ferritin levels below 12 μg/liter, which should be treated to avert the development of severe anemia.

Second to the depletion of iron stores as a cause of anemia is deficient erythropoiesis. This is characterized by normal hemoglobin levels but elevated red cell protoporphyrin and reduced transferrin saturation (<15%).

Ferritin levels can be elevated in hypochromic anemia secondary to infection, in which case serum iron is below 42 μg/100 liter; when the infection is treated, the hematologic values usually return to normal.[87] This effect appears to be attributable to an alteration in the bone marrow utilization of iron rather than to a true decline in body iron. Therefore urinary infection should be ruled out before iron therapy is instituted.[87]

Dietary iron is present in two forms: heme and nonheme. Heme iron is found in animal tissues, and 35% of the total is absorbed. Nonheme iron, from plant sources, is less available; only 10% to 20% of it is absorbed. Enhanced absorption of nonheme iron occurs with deteriorating iron status as well as with increased intakes of a meat factor (heme iron) and ascorbic acid. Decreased absorption of dietary nonheme iron occurs with consumption of antacids, phytates, bran, and tannic acid; therefore ingestation of these items should be limited.

Treatment of iron deficiency has two major goals: correction of the deficit and replenishment of the depleted iron reserves. Iron supplementation at a level of 30 mg/day during pregnancy

prevents the depletion of tissue stores and raises the hemoglobin concentration. Severe anemia in pregnancy has become less prevalent in developed countries, and large doses of parenteral iron or blood transfusion are rarely required.[83] Oral elemental iron (180-220 mg/da) should be sufficient to correct the deficiency and replenish stores in cases of iron deficiency anemia.

FOLATE DEFICIENCY ANEMIA

Folic acid deficiency in its most severe form leads to megaloblastic anemia, characterized by large immature red blood cells. In the United States megaloblastic anemia is rare. In developing countries, without routine folate supplementation, it has been reported to occur in about 3% of all single pregnancies[93] and about 20% of twin pregnancies.[94] Cases of megaloblastic anemia generally become evident in the last 4 weeks of pregnancy or shortly after delivery. Treatment during pregnancy is 5 mg of pteroylglutamic acid daily for several weeks.

In the United States low serum or low red cell folate levels have been reported in as many as 20% of pregnant women[95] and are especially prevalent in low-income populations.[96] The clinical significance of low serum folate levels remains debatable. Folate deficiency has been associated with abruptio placentae, spontaneous abortion, preeclampsia, and fetal malformation.[97-101] However, these findings remain controversial. Two reports[102,103] indicate that folate supplements (500 μg/dl) are associated with decreased incidence of small for date babies.

Low red cell folate levels also have been associated with fetal neural tube defects (NTDs);[101] however, a randomized trial of folate supplementation or placebo to women previously delivering an infant affected by NTDs was inconclusive.[104] Women with severe folate deficiency expressing as megaloblastic anemia do not appear to be at increased risk for NTDs.[105] Preconceptual vitamin supplementation of women at low risk does not appear to be justified; however, for high-risk women a daily multivitamin may be advised on the grounds of its being safe and possibly effective.[106]

The metabolic demands for folate increase during pregnancy because of increased maternal erythropoiesis and accelerated cell multiplication in placental and uterine tissues as well as fetal growth. Folate plays an important role in the transfer of one-carbon units in nucleic acid synthesis (i.e., the purine and phyrimidine bases of DNA) and acts as a coenzyme in intracellular reactions.

The recommended dietary intake for folate during pregnancy is 500 μg/dl, which cannot be met by diet alone.[107] The requirement is set to meet the needs of women with poor folate stores, no dietary intake of folate, and multiple pregnancy.[107] Green leafy vegetables, kidney, liver, and peanuts are major food sources of folic acid; however, cooking and storage processes can cause vegetables and meat to lose almost 90% of their folate activity.

Diagnosis of folate deficiency is most reliably made using red cell folate levels; neutrophils may also be hypersegmented (>5% with five lobes or more) as well as macrocytic, but normochromic red cells also can be present. Folate is incorporated into red blood cells, and a decrease in red cell folate is evidence of tissue depletion; moreover, red cell folate levels reflect folate status of the preceding several weeks. Bone marrow examination, although generally not necessary for diagnosis, shows megaloblastic maturation and enlargement of metamyelocytes. Increased serum iron, percent saturation of transferrin, and mean corpuscular volume (>110 fl [femtoliters]), with low white cell and platelet counts, are complementary evidence of the disease. If the patient is given an oral dose of histidine, the increase of formiminoglutamic acid (FIGLU) excretion is used as an indicator of folic acid deficiency. Serum folate decreases from the sixteenth week of pregnancy and is less reliable than red cell folate as an indicator of folate deficiency.

Special care should be taken with pregnant women being treated by anticonvulsant therapy. These patients have a tendency toward low folic acid levels, possibly because of reduced intestinal absorption and increased hepatic metabolism of folic acid.[108] The process appears to be dose-related, and it increases when barbiturates are added. Furthermore, pregnant epileptics can have more frequent seizures when they use phenytoin (Dilantin) and receive folate therapy, since folic acid reduces phenytoin blood levels.[108] Therefore these patients should be given folic acid supplementation only if marked deficiency is found.

PREPREGNANCY WEIGHT AND WEIGHT GAIN PROBLEMS

Both prepregnancy underweight and overweight, as well as the weight gained over pregnancy, are associated with fetal growth and pregnancy outcome. The definitions used to classify pregnant women as underweight or overweight are not totally clear or standardized, but the National Academy of Sciences[109] has prepared a useful set of guidelines for evaluating weight changes during pregnancy. Underweight is defined as prepregnancy weight 15% or more below the standard weight for height and age. Overweight is considered a prepregnancy weight that is 20% or more above the standard weight for height and age. The reference weights for height and age are routinely obtained from Metropolitan Life Insurance Company standards.

Women who enter pregnancy underweight are at increased risk of delivering a low–birthweight infant.[110-112] For underweight women who also have inadequate weight gain (<20 lb at term) the low birth weight rate approaches 50%[112] and the perinatal mortality rate can be as high at 155 per 1000 births.[113] A case-control study of 354 underweight women (<10% standard weight for height) matched on age, race, parity, and socioeconomic status to normal prepregnancy weight women[114] reported an increase in the incidence of anemia, premature rupture of membranes, and endometritis in the underweight group. Infants born to the group of underweight women were more often premature, were twice as likely to be of low birth weight, and had low 5-minute Apgar scores.[114] Regardless of adequate weight gain, underweight women who were anemic had a low birth weight rate of 17.4% compared to 3.6% among anemic women of normal weight. Infants of these mothers also showed inadequate growth (<25th percentile of weight for length at 1 yr) and delayed neurologic development at 1 year, which suggested that intrauterine damage has long-term effects.

Naeye[115] examined the effect of net pregnancy weight gain (weight gain minus weight of infant and placenta) on birth weight in women in the Perinatal Collaborative Project. Women with a prepregnancy weight of less than 96 pounds who had a weight gain of less than 13 pounds were at increased risk of delivering a low–birthweight infant. As pregnancy weight gain exceeded 13 pounds in this low–prepregnancy-weight group, birth weight increased. Conversely, pregnancy weight gain among women with a prepregnancy weight of 96 pounds or more only had a modest effect on birth weight.[115] The lowest perinatal mortality rate in underweight women is reported to be among those who gain at least 30 pounds during pregnancy.[113]

The effect of obesity on pregnancy outcome needs to be more thoroughly investigated. Early reports suggest that obesity contributes to complications of labor and delivery. However, a study of 279 obese women[116] found no increase in the need for oxytocin augmentation and primary cesarean sections. Moreover, obese women were similar to the normal-weight control group during the first and second stages of labor. The overweight women had a higher rate of oxytocin induction and repeated cesarean section than the controls, as could be expected given the elevated incidence of diabetes and hypertension in the overweight. Therefore, when associated pathologies are controlled, obesity itself should not increase the incidence of abnormalities during labor and delivery. In short, obese women without complications should have normal deliveries.

Obesity increases the incidence of very heavy newborns (>4 kg)[116-118] and post-term infants, and it reduces the number of small for gestational age and preterm newborns.[116] This effect is independent of the increased incidence, among obese women, of diabetes mellitus, which is associated with very heavy babies and macrosomia. In one report[116] a 31% incidence of large for date infants could not be explained by a 9% incidence of diabetes in the population studied. Furthermore, even after the exclusion of diabetic women, birth weight was associated with the degree of obesity among women who had a weight gain of at least 6 kg.

The extent and pattern of weight gain for the overweight woman remain controversial. The uncertainty is reflected in dietary recommendations[119]; some programs limit weight gain to about 12-15 pounds whereas others recommend that obese patients gain as much weight as normal-weight women. Edwards et al.[120] compared birth weight outcomes between women with a prepregnancy weight of 73 kg who gained 13.6 kg and those who gained only 5 kg during pregnancy. Lower weight gain resulted in a 2.3% increased incidence of low–birth-weight infants

and a 200 g difference in birth weights. Other evidence[113] indicates that overweight mothers with very low weight gain during gestation (<25% of optimum values) have a significant increase in infant perinatal mortality rates compared to overweight patients with normal weight gain.

The components of a normal pregnancy weight gain of 24 to 28 pounds are such that approximately 7.5 pounds resides in the fetus, 1 pound in the placenta, 2 pounds in the amniotic fluid, 3.5 pounds in the uterus, 3 pounds in breast tissue, 4 pounds in blood volume, and 4-8 pounds in maternal stores. Maternal stores are largely represented by fat deposition, although there is some increase in maternal lean body mass as well.

The pattern of weight gain during a pregnancy has been described as being minimal in the first 10 weeks. As the fetus grows in the second and third trimester, maternal weight increases. The rate of gain should be 2-4 pounds by the end of the first trimester and approximately 1 pound per week thereafter. Maternal weight gains can be charted on a grid.[121] Any sudden or dramatic shifts, particularly in the second trimester, may reflect excessive fluid retention and suggest a possible toxemia.

Naeye[113] indicates that weight gains (and the range of variation from them) associated with the best outcomes are as follows: normal prepregnancy weight, 27-pound gain recommended (range 80%-120%); underweight, 30-pound gain recommended (range 80%-120%); overweight, 15-pound gain recommended (range 24%-54%). Teenage mothers require individualized care to ensure that their dietary intake will be sufficient to promote adequate maternal growth and meet gestational needs. Aside from the actual number of pounds gained, the "quality" of the weight gain should be stressed; that is, it may be advisable to remind a woman that her increased intake of high calorie foods low in essential nutrients may increase weight but will not necessarily promote good nutritional status.

NUTRITIONAL SUPPLEMENTATION DURING PREGNANCY

Clinically the important question is whether nutritional intervention during pregnancy can overcome the negative outcome of poor pregnancy nutritional status. Several nutritional supplementation programs have been published in the last 10 years. Maternal supplementation during pregnancy has, in general, a positive effect on birth weight. The more malnourished the mother was before pregnancy, the greater the birth weight tends to increase.[122] Malnourished mothers in a hospital in India had an increase in birth weight up to 458 g when given food supplementation and bed rest.[123] However, the effect on birth weight on nutritional supplementation in well-nourished or moderately malnourished women is rather modest, with an average increase of less than 100 g.[122] Among chronically malnourished women the limiting nutrient related to reduced fetal growth has been suggested to be calories.[124] High protein supplementation among women with adequate protein intake has been reported to be associated with a small increase in preterm birth and neonatal mortality.[125]

Nutritional supplementation during pregnancy is also associated with a reduction of the incidence of low birth weight in developing[124,126] and developed[127] populations.

In an analysis of the Guatemalan study, Villar et al.[128] showed that the effect of supplementation during only one pregnancy is explained mainly by an increase in gestational age rather than an effect on fetal growth. The effect was statistically significant after controlling for interfering variables (e.g., other nutritional factors, morbidity, sociodemographic characteristics). Furthermore, the effect of nutritional supplementation on chronically yet moderately malnourished women during two consecutive pregnancies and the lactation period in between has been reported.[129] The adjusted mean birth weight of the second offspring of women with high supplementation during pregnancy and lactation (about 110 extra kcal/da) was up to 301 g greater than that of women with low supplementation. Women who were given high supplementation while lactating their first offspring and during the second pregnancy had babies up to 150 g heavier than in the reference group; those given high supplementation only during the second pregnancy had infants about 124 g heavier than in the reference group.[129]

On the basis of published studies, we can conclude that for women with acute malnutrition, food supplementation during pregnancy increases birth weight by about 230 g (as has been shown in Gambia during the wet season).[130]

However, chronically but moderately malnourished mothers benefit significantly from extra food (i.e., a 300 g increase in mean birth weight) if the period of treatment is long enough to meet their nutritional deficits.[129] An increase in birth weight of only 100 g can be expected if supplementation occurs solely during the present pregnancy.

EFFECTS OF MATERNAL ALCOHOL CONSUMPTION ON THE FETUS

It is reported[131,132] that alcohol abuse during pregnancy has detrimental effects on the fetus. The more dramatic consequence, fetal alcohol syndrome (FAS), is clearly associated with heavy or chronic alcoholism in the mother. Typical manifestations of FAS include microcephaly, micrognathia, microphthalmia, cardiac defects, prenatal and postnatal growth retardation, poor motor development, and mental retardation.[113] Despite several methodologic limitations, the data reported to date[133,134] strongly suggest a causal association between maternal alcohol abuse and FAS. Furthermore, craniofacial transformations similar to those found in FAS have been found in mice exposed to ethanol during a period corresponding to the third week in human pregnancy.[135] In one prospective study[131] infants of alcoholic mothers were at higher risk of intrauterine growth retardation (IUGR) and prematurity. Length, weight, and head circumference at birth were uniformly affected by maternal alcoholism; the infants' physical characteristics were those of proportionate IUGR.

Furthermore, available evidence suggests that moderate drinking is also associated with intrauterine growth retardation[136,137] as well as with an increased risk of spontaneous abortion.[138,139] Finally, although earlier reports[140,141] showed conflicting results as to the effect of moderate drinking on the incidence of congenital malformations, it now appears[142] that an average of one or two drinks per day does not increase the rate of malformations compared to what occurs among nondrinkers.

Long-Term Effects

Mental retardation and the absence of catchup growth are considered to be the most important and consistent long-term effect of FAS.[143] Furthermore, maternal alcohol abuse without FAS could be associated with disturbance of the infant's sleep-awake pattern by the third day of life, a decrease in total time spent sleeping, and more frequent major body movements.[144] Some of the alterations, particularly the motor and EEG changes, can persist up to 4-6 weeks.[145] Moreover, children of alcoholic mothers present problems of activity and attention regulation and experience persistent academic failure, even though their IQs may be within the normal range.[146]

To summarize, a long history of alcohol abuse before pregnancy and the drinking patterns during pregnancy are foci of concern. The clinician should make efforts to change the life-style, living patterns, and alcohol consumption of alcoholic women if at all possible. Alcohol abuse should be discouraged. Pregnant women must be informed of risks, and chronic alcoholics should be advised to defer pregnancy until their problem is controlled.

EFFECTS OF ORAL CONTRACEPTIVES ON NUTRITIONAL STATUS

Oral contraceptives (OCs) are the most popular birth control method. In the United States over 10 million women use one of the several types of hormonal contraceptives. They are also used by increasing numbers of women in developing countries.

In general, the OCs in use today are combinations of a synthetic estrogen and one of several progestogens taken everyday for 3 weeks with a 1-week interval when normal uterine bleeding appears. The most commonly used preparations include 30-35 μg of ethinyl estradiol (sometimes as little as 20 μg) per tablet and a variable concentration of progestin. The "phasic pills" include a low dose of progestin at the beginning with an increase in the dose later in the menstrual cycle. Oral contraceptives produce pseudopregnancy. Thus their nutritional effects can be qualitatively similar to those produced by gestation.

Weight Gain

Weight gain was one of the first side effects observed clinically when oral contraceptives with high estrogen content were used. The observed short-term weight loss after their use was stopped suggested a water retention effect. The present-day low-dose estrogen pill's effect on weight gain is minimal.

Protein, Lipid, and Carbohydrate Metabolism

Changes in protein metabolism produced by oral contraceptives are similar to those induced by pregnancy and are mediated by the effect of estrogens in the liver. Estrogens act on the endoplasmic reticulum, thereby altering the metabolism of proteins.[147] Doses higher than 50 μg/day can produce changes in plasma enzymes or bilirubin levels in healthy women.

In normal women, oral contraceptives increase plasma globulins, particularly hormone-binding globulins, but reduce plasma albumin and fasting levels of amino acids. During oral contraception an alpha-2 globulin that is present during pregnancy appears[148]; however, alpha-fetoprotein, though elevated during pregnancy, does not increase during use of oral contraceptives.[149] No additional effect appears when OCs are used by women whose diets are low in protein.

Oral contraceptives have been reported to increase the risk of deep vein thrombosis, pulmonary embolism, myocardial infarction, and cerebrovascular accidents (particularly among women who are over 35 years of age, heavy smokers, obese, or under treatment for hypertension, diabetes, or Type II hyperlipoproteinemia). Nevertheless, several of these reports had methodology problems[150] and the effects were generally attributed to high-dose OCs. It appears therefore that low-dose OC use is unlikely to be an independent risk factor for cardiovascular diseases among risk factor–free healthy women.

The estrogen components of modern low-dose oral contraceptives have very limited effect on LDL, HDL, HDL subfractions (HDL_2 and HDL_3), cholesterol, and triglyceride fractions. The progestogen components of the pill are associated with a reduction in HDL cholesterol and an increase in LDL cholesterol. Although triglyceride levels do not increase above the standard values in normal women, they can reach levels similar to those found in hypertriglyceridemia when patients who have elevated basal values or hyperinsulinemia are using OCs.[151]

Oral contraceptives containing estrogen-progestogen or progestogen preparations can induce a prolonged glucose tolerance test as well as increases in blood insulin levels.[147] They also can aggravate diabetes symptoms and induce apparent disease in high-risk women (those who are overweight and have a family history or previous evidence of abnormal carbohydrate metabolism). The changes in glucose metabolism produced by OCs are mediated by the progestogen component, through a reduction in the peripheral activity of insulin. A compensatory increase in insulin levels has been shown in women using norethindrone for a year.[152] Estrogens do not appear to have a great impact on glucose tolerance.

The glucose metabolic changes are considerably reduced when triphasic ethinyl estradiol–levonorgestrel formulations are used, because these compounds have about 40% less progestogen than do nonphasic pills. When OCs containing these compounds have been used, no changes in glucose tolerance tests were reported among women without risk factors, no aggravation of glucose tolerance tests has been observed among those with a history of gestational diabetes,[153] and no changes from pretreatment values have occurred in serum cholesterol or HDL-LDL levels.[153]

In short, levonorgestrel triphasic pills maintain both carbohydrate and lipid metabolisms within the normal range in studies with at least 1 year of follow-up. Whether the contraceptives used in the past increased the risk of developing diabetes later in life is not clear, but the data presently available show that this may not have been the case.

Vitamin and Mineral Metabolism

Oral contraceptive users often show biochemical evidence of low serum folate and low blood-cell folate levels, possibly because of an increased inhibition of folate polyglutamate absorption,[154] increased urinary excretion of folate,[155] or elevated folate transfer to the tissues from the plasma.[156] Although megaloblastic anemia following OC use is rare, there are groups of women at increased risk[151,157]: those with previous marginal folate intake, alcoholics, those with malabsorption syndromes, or those who become pregnant after recently taking oral contraceptives. A 35 μg/day increase in folate consumption should compensate for the additional requirements brought on by the use of OCs. However, for women with low serum levels or who have been receiving OC therapy for long periods, a folate increase of 100 μg/day may be advisable. These levels can be obtained by increasing dietary intake alone.

Oral contraceptives have the same effect on vitamin B_6 metabolism (as measured by xanthurenic acid excretion) that pregnancy has. The effect is partially mediated by the estrogen component, through simulation of the tryptophan oxygenase activity and inhibition of the pyridoxal phosphate–dependent enzymes but not the enzymes involved in the production of xanthurenic acid. Supplementation may be necessary only in a small group of patients who show vitamin B_6 deficiency associated with contraceptive-induced depression. For the rest of the women 1.5-5 mg/day of the vitamin has been shown to be sufficient.[158]

Plasma leukocyte and platelet vitamin C levels are reduced among OC users.[159] These levels may be mediated by the estrogen component of the pill and may be related to an elevation of serum copper and ceruloplasmin induced by pill use as well as by pregnancy.[160] Ceruloplasmin has an ascorbic acid oxidation activity that can be responsible for the effect. Pill users need an intake higher than the 55 mg/day recommended for nonpregnant women.

Several reports have suggested that riboflavin requirements may be higher among pill users. A recent literature review[161] found that six of ten papers published in the last few years have reported incidences of elevated riboflavin metabolism as measured by erythrocyte glutathione reductase or urinary riboflavin excretion. This effect may be aggravated if previous deficiency is present, as is often the case in malnourished populations.[162] However, when healthy patients were studied under metabolic conditions and dietary intake of riboflavin was controlled,[161] no significant effect of oral contraceptives on riboflavin status was observed.

Oral contraceptives can also reduce the requirements for some nutrients. Serum iron levels and serum iron binding capacity increase in patients taking the pill. There is no clear understanding of how the effect is produced, but OCs do reduce blood loss during menstruation and thus iron needs are lower and hemoglobin and hematocrit values are increased. The higher serum iron levels may be a metabolic effect of the progestogen component of the pill.

Vitamin A serum levels are also increased in pill users. This effect is mediated not by increased absorption but by an increased transfer of the vitamin from liver deposits to the serum.

Serum carotenoids have actually been found to be lower during OC use.[151] Increased serum vitamin A levels do not appear to increase the risk of congenital malformations in infants of women who become pregnant after discontinuing OCs. However, there may be a risk of liver depletion in women with marginal vitamin A intake, such as those who suffer protein-energy malnutrition or who are vegetarians.

Despite some suggestions, routine supplementation to otherwise healthy women taking oral contraceptives is not recommended. Instead, whenever possible, nutritional screening for high-risk patients, including dietary assessment and counseling, should be included in family-planning programs, especially in those provided to populations with marginal nutritional status.

CAFFEINE

Caffeine has been used in drinks and beverages for many years. It is naturally present in coffee, tea, and chocolate and in the kola nut extract used in cola drinks. Coffee usually has a higher concentration of caffeine (107 mg/serving) than any other beverages do (34-47 mg/serving for tea and colas).

In small animals caffeine has been associated with birth defects, fetal resorption, fetal death, and lower fetal weight.[163-165] Results varied, however, depending on the species and strain of test animal, the route of administration, and the duration of ingestion. Whether these results can be extrapolated to humans remains to be determined.

Several epidemiologic studies have published contradictory results. Some have shown an increased risk of low birth weight,[166,167] spontaneous abortion, stillbirth, preterm delivery,[168] and intrauterine growth retardation in term infants[169] for women with high caffeine consumption as compared to those with no caffeine consumption. Others[170,171] have not found any association, nor have there been any definitely recognizable defect patterns (like the fetal alcohol syndrome) or adverse influences on gestational age.

Although the evidence is limited and contradictory, any substance that crosses the placenta may be regarded as potentially hazardous, especially during the first trimester. A moderate intake of caffeine (about 2 cups of coffee per day) seems to be a safe level of intake.

REFERENCES

1. Gabbe SG: Management of diabetes mellitus in pregnancy, Am J Obstet Gynecol **153**:824-828, 1985.
2. National Diabetes Advisory Board, Public Health Service, Department of Health and Human Services: The prevention and treatment of five complications of diabetes, Publication (HHS) 83-8392, Atlanta, Ga, 1983, Centers for Disease Control.
3. Karlson K, Kjellner I: The outcome of diabetic pregnancies in relation to mother's blood sugar level, Am J Obstet Gynecol **112**:213-220, 1972.
4. Frienkel N, et al: Pregnancy in diabetes. In Ellenber M, Rifkin H, editors: Diabetes mellitus: theory and practice, New York, 1983, Medical Examination Publishing Co Inc.
5. Sepe SJ, et al: Gestational diabetes: incidence, maternal characteristics, and perinatal outcome, Diabetes **34**:13-16, 1985.
6. O'Sullivan JB: Gestational diabetes: Unsuspected, asymptomatic diabetes in pregnancy, N Engl J Med **264**:1082-1085, 1961.
7. Hoett JJ, Beard RW: Clinical perspectives in the care of the pregnant diabetic patient. In Pregnancy metabolism. diabetes, and the fetus, Ciba Found Symp **63**:283-300, 1978.
8. American Diabetes Association: Principles of nutrition and dietary recommendations for individuals with diabetes mellitus: 1979, Diabetes **28**:1027-1030, 1979.
9. Franz M: Nutritional management in diabetes and pregnancy, Diabetes Care **1**:264-270, 1978.
10. Hollingsworth DR: Maternal metabolism in normal pregnancy and pregnancy complicated by diabetes mellitus, Clin Obstet Gynecol **28**:457-472, 1985.
11. Freinkel N, et al: Care of the pregnant woman with insulin-dependent diabetes mellitus, N Engl J Med **313**:96-101, 1985.
12. Knopp R, et al: Carbohydrate and lipid metabolism in laboratory indices of nutritional status in pregnancy, Washington DC, 1978, National Research Council, National Academy of Sciences, p 35.
13. O'Sullivan JB, Mahan CM: Criteria for the oral glucose tolerance test in pregnancy, Diabetes **13**:278-285, 1980.
14. O'Sullivan JB, et al: Screening criteria for high-risk gestational diabetic patients, Am J Obstet Gynecol **116**:895-900, 1973.
15. American Diabetes Association Workshop—Conference on Gestational Diabetes: Summary and recommendations, Diabetes Care **3**:499-501, 1980.
16. Marquette GP, et al: Cost-effective criteria for glucose screening, Obstet Gynecol **66**:181-184, 1985.
17. Felig P, Coustan, D: Diabetes mellitus. In Burrow G, Ferris T, editors: Medical complications during pregnancy, Philadelphia, 1982, WB Saunders Co.
18. Carpenter MW, Coustan DR: Criteria for screening tests for gestational diabetes, Am J Obstet Gynecol **144**:768-773, 1982.
19. Leiken EL, et al: Normal glucose screening test in pregnancy: a risk factor for fetal macrosomia, Obstet Gynecol **69**:570-573, 1987.
20. National Diabetes Data Group: Classification and diagnosis of diabetes mellitus and other categories of glucose intolerance, Diabetes **28**:1039-1057, 1979.

21. Shah BD, et al: Comparison of glycohemoglobin determination and the one-hour oral glucose screen in the identification of gestational diabetes, Am J Obstet Gynecol **144**:774-777, 1982.

22. Morris MA, et al: Glycosylated hemoglobin: a sensitive indicator of gestational diabetes, Obstet Gynecol **68**:357-361, 1986.

23. Gabbe SG, et al: Current patterns of neonatal morbidity and mortality in infants of diabetic mothers, Diabetes Care **1**:335-339, 1978.

24. Mills JL, et al: Malformations in infants of diabetic mothers occur before the seventh gestational week: implications for treatment, Diabetes **28**:292-293, 1979.

25. Baker L, et al: Meticulous control of diabetes during organogenesis prevents congenital lumbosacral defects in rats, Diabetes **30**:955-959, 1981.

26. Soler NG, et al: Neonatal morbidity among infants of diabetic mothers, Diabetes Care **1**:340-350, 1978.

27. Stehbins JA, et al: Outcome at ages 1, 3, and 5 years of children born to diabetic women, Am J Obstet Gynecol **127**:408-413, 1977.

28. Yssing M: Long-term prognosis in children born to mothers diabetic when pregnant. In Camerini-Davalos RA, Cole HS, editors: Early diabetes in early life, New York, 1975, Academic Press Inc.

29. American Diabetes Association: Nutritional Recommendations and Principles for Individuals with Diabetes Mellitus: 1986, Diabetes Care **10**:126-132, 1987.

30. Committee on Dietary Allowances, Food and Nutrition Board, National Research Council: Recommended dietary allowances, ed 9, Washington DC, 1980, National Academy of Sciences.

31. Anderson JW, et al: Dietary fiber and diabetes: A comprehensive review and practical application, J Am Diet Assoc **87**:1189-1197, 1987.

32. Blackburn NA, et al: The mechanism of action of guar gum in improving glucose tolerance in man, Clin Sci **66**:329-336, 1984.

33. Kelsay JL: Effects of fiber on mineral and vitamin bioavailability. In Vahouny GV, Kritchevsky D, editors: Dietary fiber in health and disease, New York, 1982, Plenum Press Inc.

34. American Diabetes Association: Position statement: Use of noncaloric sweetner, Diabetes Care **10**(4):526, 1987.

35. Coustan DR, et al: Tight metabolic control of overt diabetes in pregnancy, Am J Med **68**:845-852, 1980.

36. Gabbe SG: Diabetes mellitus in pregnancy: Have all the problems been solved? Am J Med **70**:613-618, 1981.

37. Jovanovic L, et al: Feasibility of maintaining normal glucose profiles in insulin-dependent diabetic women, Am J Med **68**:105-112, 1980.

38. Blumenthal SA, Abdul-Karim RW: Diagnosis, classification, and metabolic management of diabetes in pregnancy: therapeutic impact on self-monitoring of blood glucose and of new methods of insulin delivery, Obstet Gynecol Surv **42**(10):593-604, 1987.

39. Edwards CQ, et al: Control of diabetes during pregnancy using continuous insulin infusion, West J Med **136**:249-251, 1982.

40. Potter JM, et al: The effect of continuous subcutaneous insulin infusion and conventional insulin regimens on 24-hour variations of blood glucose and intermediary metab-

41. Rudolf MC, et al: Efficacy of the insulin pump in the home treatment of pregnant diabetics, Diabetes **30**:891-895, 1981.

42. Consensus Development Panel: Consensus statement on self-monitoring of blood glucose, Diabetes Care **10**:95-99, 1987.

43. North DS, et al: Home monitors of blood glucose: comparison of precision and accuracy, Diabetes Care **10**:360-366, 1987.

44. Jovanovic L, Peterson CM: The clinical utility of glycosylated hemoglobin, Am J Med **70**:331-338, 1981.

45. Bunn HF: Nonenzymatic glycosylation of protein: relevance of diabetes, Am J Med **70**:325-330, 1981.

46. Jenkins DJ, et al: Glycemic index of foods: a physiological basis for carbohydrate exchange, Am J Clin Nutr **34**:362-366, 1981.

47. Jenkins DJ, et al: Rate of digestion of foods and postprandial glycaemia in normal and diabetic subjects, Br Med J **281**:14-17, 1980.

48. Beebe CA: Self−blood glucose monitoring: an adjunct to dietary and insulin management of the patient with diabetes, J Am Diet Assoc **87**:61-65, 1987.

49. Mueller-Hueboch E, et al: Lecithin/sphingomyelin ratio in amniotic fluid and its value for the prediction of neonatal respiratory distress syndrome in pregnant diabetic women, Am J Obstet Gynecol **130**:28-34, 1978.

50. Gant NF, Worley RJ: Hypertension in pregnancy: concepts and management, New York, 1980, Appleton-Century-Crofts.

51. Tompkins WT, Wiehl DG: Nutritional deficiencies as a causal factor in toxemia and premature labor, Am J Obstet Gynecol **62**:898-919, 1951.

52. Chandhuri SK: Effect of nutrient supplementation on the incidence of toxemia of pregnancy, J Obstet Gynecol (India) **19**:156, 1969.

53. Osofsky H: Relationship between prenatal medical and nutritional measures, pregnancy outcome, and early infant development in an urban poverty setting. I. The role of nutritional intake, Am J Obstet Gynecol **123**:682-690, 1975.

54. Holmes OM: Protein diet in pregnancy, West J Surg Obstet Gynecol **49**:56-60, 1941.

55. Belizán JM, Villar J: Possible role of calcium in the development of toxemia of pregnancy, Institute of Nutrition of Central America and Panama (INCAP), Division of Human Development. Internal document, Guatemala City, 1978.

56. Johnstone FD, et al: Nitrogen balance studies in human pregnancy, J Nurt **111**:1884-1893, 1981.

57. Chung R, et al: Diet related toxemia in pregnancy. I. Fat, fatty acids, and cholesterol, Am J Clin Nutr **32**:1902-1911, 1979.

58. O'Brien PM, Pipkin FB: The effects of prostaglandin precursors on vascular sensitivity to angiotensin II and on the kidney in the pregnant rabbit, Br J Pharmacol **65**:29-34, 1979.

59. Belizán JM, Villar J: The relationship between calcium intake and edema proteinuria and hypertension-gestosis: an hypothesis, Am J Clin Nutr **33**:2202-2210, 1980.

60. Villar J, et al: Epidemiologic observations on the rela-

tionship between calcium intake and eclampsia, Int J Gynaecol Obstet **21**:271-278, 1983.

61. Belizán JM, et al: Reduction of blood pressure with calcium supplementation in young adults, JAMA **249**:1161-1165, 1983.

62. Villar J, et al: Calcium supplementation reduces blood pressure during pregnancy: results from a randomized controlled clinical trial, Obstet Gynecol **70**:317-322, 1987.

63. Belizán JM, et al: Preliminary evidence of the effect of calcium supplementation on blood pressure in normal pregnant women, Am J Obstet Gynecol **146**:175-180, 1983.

64. Belizán JM, et al: The relationship between calcium intake and pregnancy-induced hypertension: up-to-date evidence, Am J Obstet Gynecol **158**:898-902, 1988.

65. Kawanaki N, et al: Effect of calcium supplementation on the vascular sensitivity to angiotensin II in pregnant women, Am J Obstet Gynecol **153**:576-582, 1985.

66. Tanfield PA, et al: Hypocalciuria in preeclampsia, N Engl J Med **316**:715-718, 1987.

67. Repke J, et al: Biochemical changes associated with calcium supplementation induced blood pressure reduction during pregnancy. In Proceedings of the 34th meeting of the Society Gynecologic Investigation, Atlanta, Ga, 1987.

68. Collins R, et al: Overview of randomized trials of diuretics in pregnancy, Br Med J **290**:17-23, 1985.

69. Hemminki E: Diuretics in pregnancy; a case study of worthless therapy, Soc Sci Med **18**:1011-1018, 1984.

70. Campbell DM, MacGillivray I: The effect of a low calorie diet on a thiazide diuretic on the incidence of preeclampsia and birthweight, Br J Obstet Gynaecol **82**:572-577, 1975.

71. Friedman EA, Neff RK: Pregnancy hypertension: a systematic evaluation of clinical diagnostic criteria, Littleton, Mass, 1977, PSG Publishing Co, p 159.

72. Gant NF, et al: The metabolic clearance rate of dehydroisoandrosterone sulfate. III. The effect of thiazide diuretics in normal and future preeclamptic pregnancies, Am J Obstet Gynecol **123**:159-163, 1975.

73. Hytten F: Blood volume changes in normal pregnancy, Clin Haematol **14**:3, 601-612, 1985.

74. Lind T, et al: Anaemia in pregnancy, (letter), Br Med J **1**:627, 1975.

75. Garn SM, et al: Hematological status and pregnancy outcomes, Am J Clin Nutr **34**:115-117, 1981.

76. Life Sciences Research Office: Assessment of the iron nutritional status of the United States population based on data collected in the third HANES, 1980-84, Bethesda Md, 1984, Federation of American Societies for Experimental Biology.

77. Svanberg B, et al: Absorption of supplemental iron during pregnancy—a longitudinal study with repeated bone marrow studies and absorption measurements, Acta Obstet Gynecol Scand **48**:87-108, 1975.

78. Hahn PG, et al: Iron metabolism in human pregnancy as studied with the radioactive isotope F⁵⁹, Am J Obstet Gynecol **61**:477-486, 1987.

79. Herbert V: Recommended dietary intakes (RDI) of iron in humans, Am J Clin Nutr **45**:679-686, 1987.

80. Hemminki E, Starfield B: Routine administration of iron and vitamins during pregnancy: review of controlled clinical trials, Br J Obstet Gynaecol **85**:404-410, 1978.

81. Koller O, et al: High haemoglobin levels during pregnancy and fetal risk, Int J Gynaecol Obstet **18**:53-56, 1980.

82. Simmer K, et al: Are iron-folate supplements harmful? Am J Clin Nutr **45**:122-125, 1987.

83. Bentley DP: Iron metabolism and anemia in pregnancy, Clin Haematol **13**(3):613-627, 1985.

84. Worthington-Roberts BS: Nutritional issues related to pregnancy. In Worthington-Roberts BS: Contemporary developments in nutrition, St. Louis, 1981, The CV Mosby Co.

85. Beischer NA, et al: Placental hypertrophy in severe pregnancy anemia, J Obstet Gynaecol Br Commonwlth **77**:398-409, 1970.

86. Lubin AH, et al: Effect of maternal iron status on the subsequent development of iron deficiency in the infant [abstract], J Pediatr **96**:1114, 1980.

87. Kitay DZ, Harbort RA: Iron and folic acid deficiency in pregnancy, Clin Perinatol **2**:255-273, 1975.

88. Scott JM: Anemia in pregnancy, Postgrad Med J **38**:202-213, 1962.

89. Romslo I, et al: Iron requirement in normal pregnancy as assessed by serum ferritin, serum transferrin saturation, and erythrocyte protoporphyrin determinations, Br J Obstet Gynaecol **90**:101-107, 1983.

90. Jacobs A, et al: Ferritin in the serum of normal subjects and patients with iron deficiency and iron overload, Br Med J **4**:206-208, 1972.

91. Lipschitz DA, et al: A clinical evaluation of serum ferritin as an index of iron stores, N Engl J Med **290**:1213-1220, 1974.

92. Worwood M: Serum ferritin. In Jacobs A, Worwood M, editors: Iron in biochemistry and medicine. II. New York, 1980, Academic Press Inc, pp 203-244.

93. Dawson D, et al: Prevention of megaloblastic anemia in pregnancy by folic acid, Lancet **2**:1015-1018, 1962.

94. MacKenzie A, Abbot J: Megaloblastic erythropoiesis in pregnancy, Br Med J **2**:1114-1116, 1960.

95. Herbert V, et al: Folic acid deficiency in the United States: folate assays in a prenatal clinic, Am J Obstet Gynecol **123**:175-179, 1975.

96. Bailey LB, et al: Folacin and iron status in low-income pregnant adolescents and mature women, Am J Clin Nutr **33**:1997-2001, 1980.

97. Hibbard ED, Smithells RW: Folic acid metabolism and human embryopathy, Lancet **1**:1254, 1965.

98. Gross R, et al: Adverse effects on infant development associated with maternal folic acid deficiency [abstract], Nutr Rep Int **10**:241, 1974.

99. Hibbard BM: Folates and the fetus, So Afr Med J **49**:1223-1226, 1975.

100. Dutta JP: Serum folic acid level in abortion [abstract], J Indian Med Assoc **69**:149, 1977.

101. Smithells RW, et al: Vitamin levels and neural tube defects, Arch Dis Child **51**:944-950, 1976.

102. Baumslag N, et al: Reduction of incidence of prematurity by folic acid supplementation in pregnancy, Br Med J **1**:16-17, 1970.

103. Iyengar L, Rajalakshmi K: Effect of folic acid supplement on birthweights of infants, Am J Obstet Gynecol **122**:332-336, 1975.

104. Laurence KM, et al: Double-blind randomized controlled trial of folate treatment before conception to prevent re-

currence of neural tube defects, Br Med J **282:**1509-1511, 1981.

105. Pritchard JA, et al: Infants of mothers with megaloblastic anemia due to folate deficiency, JAMA **211:**1982-1984, 1970.

106. Rhoads GG, Mills JL: Can vitamin supplements prevent neural tube defects? Current evidence and ongoing investigations, Clin Obstet Gynecol **29**(3):569-579, 1986.

107. Herbert V: Recommended dietary intakes (RDI) of folate in humans, Am J Clin Nutr **45:**661-670, 1987.

108. Strauss RG, Bernstein R: Folic acid and Dilantin antagonism in pregnancy, Obstet Gynecol **44:**345-348, 1974.

109. Committee on Nutrition of the Mother and Preschool Child, Food and Nutrition Board, National Research Council: Nutrition services in perinatal care, Washington DC, 1981, National Academy of Sciences.

110. Tompkins WT, Wiehl DG: Nutrition and nutritional deficiencies as related to the premature, Pediatr Clin North Am **1:**687-708, 1954.

111. Jacobson HN: Weight and weight gain in pregnancy, Clin Perinatol **2:**223-242, 1975.

112. Brown JE, et al: Influence of pregnancy weight gain on the size of infants born to underweight women, Obstet Gynecol **57:**13-17, 1981.

113. Naeye R: Weight and the outcome of pregnancy, Obstet Gynecol **135:**3-9, 1979.

114. Edwards L, et al: Pregnancy in the underweight woman. Course, outcome, and growth patterns of the infants, Am J Obstet Gynecol **135:**297-302, 1979.

115. Naeye RL: Nutritional/nonnutritional interactions that affect the outcome of pregnancy, Am J Clin Nutr **34:**727-731, 1981.

116. Gross T, et al: Obesity in pregnancy: risks and outcome, Obstet Gynecol **56:**446-450, 1980.

117. Harrison G, et al: Maternal obesity, weight gain in pregnancy and infant birth weight, Am J Obstet Gynecol **136:**411-412, 1980.

118. Papiernik E, et al: Nutrition in slim, normal and obese pregnant women.—In Dobbing J, editor: Maternal nutrition in pregnancy—eating for two, New York, 1981, Academic Press Inc, pp 71-81.

119. Standards for obstetric-gynecologic services, ed 1, Washington DC, 1982, American College of Obstetricians and Gynecologists.

120. Edwards LE, et al: Pregnancy in the underweight woman: course, outcome, and growth patterns of the infant, Am J Obstet Gynecol **135:**297-302, 1979.

121. Committee on Maternal Nutrition, Food and Nutrition Board, National Research Council: Maternal nutrition and the course of pregnancy, Washington DC, 1970, National Academy of Sciences.

122. Villar J, Gonzalez-Cossio T: Nutritional factors associated with low birth weight and short gestational age, Clin Nutr **5:**78-85, 1986.

123. Iyengar L: Urinary estrogen excretion in undernourished pregnant Indian women. Effect of dietary supplement on urinary estrogens and birth weight of infants, Am J Obstet Gynecol **102:**834-838, 1968.

124. Letchtig A, et al: Effect of food supplementation during pregnancy on birth weight, Pediatrics **56:**508-520, 1975.

125. Rush D, et al: A randomized controlled trial of prenatal nutritional supplementation in New York City, Pediatrics **65:**683-697, 1980.

126. Chaves A, Martinez C: The effect of maternal supplementation on infant development, Arch Latinoam Nutr **29**(suppl 1):143-153, 1979.

127. Kennedy ET, Kotelchick M: The effect of WIC supplemental feeding on birth weight: a case control analysis, Am J Clin Nutr **40:**579-585, 1984.

128. Villar J, et al: Differences in the epidemiology of prematurity and intrauterine growth retardation, Early Hum Dev **14:**307-320, 1986.

129. Villar J, Rivera J: Maternal nutritional supplementation and effect on birth weight, consecutive pregnancies and the interim lactation period: its effect on birth weight, Pediatrics **81:**51-57, 1988.

130. Prentice AM, et al: Prenatal dietary supplementation of African women and birth weight, Lancet **1:**489-491, 1983.

131. Oullette E, Rosett HL: The effect of maternal alcohol ingestion during pregnancy on offspring. In Moghissi K, Evans T, editors: Nutritional impacts on women, New York, 1977, Harper & Row Publishers.

132. Jones KL, et al: Pattern of malformation in offspring of chronic alcoholic mothers, Lancet **1:**1267-1271, 1973.

133. Olegard R, et al: Effect on the child of alcohol abuse during pregnancy, Acta Paediatr Scand **275**(suppl):112-127, 1979.

134. Hanson JW, et al: The effect of moderate alcohol consumption during pregnancy on fetal growth and morphogenesis, J Pediatr **92:**457-460, 1978.

135. Sulik K, et al: Fetal alcohol syndrome: embryogenesis in a mouse model, Science **214:**936-938, 1981.

136. Mills JL, et al: Maternal alcohol consumption and birthweight: How much drinking during pregnancy is safe? JAMA **252:**1875-1879, 1984.

137. Little RE: Moderate alcohol use during pregnancy and decreased infant birth weight, Am J Public Health **67:**1154-1156, 1977.

138. Harlap S, Shiono PH: Alcohol, smoking, and incidence of spontaneous abortions in the first and second trimester, Lancet **2:**173-176, 1980.

139. Kline J, et al: Drinking during pregnancy and spontaneous abortion, Lancet **2:**176-180, 1980.

140. Davis PJM, et al: Alcohol consumption in pregnancy: How much is safe? Arch Dis Child **57:**940-943, 1982.

141. Rosett HL, et al: Patterns of alcohol consumption and fetal development, Obstet Gynecol **61:**539-546, 1983.

142. Mills J, Graubard B: Is moderate drinking during pregnancy associated with an increased risk for malformations? Pediatrics **80:**309-314, 1987.

143. Clarren SK, Smith DW: The fetal alcohol syndrome, N Engl J Med **298:**1063-1067, 1978.

144. Rosett HL, et al: Effects of maternal drinking on neonate state regulation, Dev Med Child Neurol **21:**464-473, 1979.

145. Havlicek V, et al: EEG frequency spectrum characteristics of sleep states in infants of alcoholic mothers, Neuropaediatrie **8:**360-373, 1977.

146. Shaywitz S, et al: Behavior and learning difficulties in children of normal intelligence born to alcoholic mothers, J Pediatr **96:**978-982, 1980.

147. Belsey M: Hormonal contraception and nutrition. In Moghissi K, Evans T, editors: Nutritional impact on women, New York, 1977, Harper & Row Publishers, p 189.

148. Joseph JC, et al: Changes in plasma proteins during pregnancy, Ann Clin Lab Sci **8**:130-141, 1978.

149. Seppala M: Alpha-fetoprotein in women taking oral contraceptives, Int J Fertil **18**:206-208, 1973.

150. Realini JP, Goldzieher JW: Oral contraceptives and cardiovascular disease: a critique of the epidemiologic studies, Am J Obstet Gynecol **152**:729-798, 1985.

151. Aftergood L, Alfin-Slater B: Oral contraceptives and nutrient requirements. In Jelliffe DB, Jelliffe EFP, editors: Nutrition and growth. A comprehensive treatise, New York, 1979, Plenum Press Inc, p 382.

152. Spellocy WN, et al: Effects of norethindrone on carbohydrate and lipid metabolism, Obstet Gynecol **46**:460-563, 1975.

153. Skouby SO, et al: Triphasic oral contraception: metabolic effects in normal women and those with previous gestational diabetes, Am J Obstet Gynecol **153**:495-500, 1985.

154. Necheles TF, Synder LM: Malabsorption of folate polyglutamates associated with oral contraceptive therapy, N Engl J Med **282**:858-859, 1970.

155. Shojania AM: The effect of oral contraceptives on folate metabolism. III. Plasma clearance and urinary folate excretion, J Lab Clin Med **85**:185-190, 1975.

156. Stephens ME, et al: Oral contraceptives and folate metabolism, Clin Sci **42**:405-414, 1972.

157. Martinez O, Roe DA: Diet and contraceptive steroids (OCA) as determinants of folate status in pregnancy, Fed Proc **33**:715, 1974.

158. Bosse TR, Donald EA: The vitamin B_6 requirements in oral contraceptive users, Am J Clin Nutr **32**:1015-1023, 1979.

159. Briggs M, Briggs M: Vitamin C requirements and oral contraceptives, Nature **238**:277, 1972.

160. Crews MG, et al: Effects of oral contraceptive agents on copper and zinc balance in young women, Am J Clin Nutr **33**:1940-1945, 1980.

161. Roe D, et al: Factors affecting riboflavin requirements of oral contraceptive users and non-users, Am J Clin Nutr **35**:495-501, 1982.

162. Ahmed F, et al: Effect of oral contraceptive agents on vitamin nutrition status, Am J Clin Nutr **28**:606-615, 1975.

163. Collins TF: Review of reproduction and teratology studies of caffeine, FDA Drug Bull **7**:352-372, 1979.

164. Soyka LF: Effects of methylxanthines on the fetus, Clin Perinatol **6**:37-51, 1979.

165. Gilbert EF, Pistey WR: Effect on the offspring of repeated caffeine administration to pregnant rats, J Reprod Fertil **34**:495-499, 1979.

166. Mau G, Netter P: Are coffee and alcohol consumption risk factors in pregnancy? Geburtshilfe Frauenheilkd **34**:1018-1022, 1974.

167. Hogue CJ: Coffee in pregnancy (letter), Lancet **1**:554, 1981.

168. Weathersbee PS, et al: Caffeine and pregnancy: a retrospective survey, Postgrad Med **62**:64-69, 1977.

169. Martin T, Bracken M: The association between low birth weight and caffeine consumption during pregnancy, Am J Epidemiol **126**:813-821, 1987.

170. Berkowitz GS, et al: Effects of cigarette smoking, alcohol, coffee and tea consumption on preterm delivery, Early Hum Dev **7**:239-250, 1982.

171. Linn S, et al: No association between coffee consumption and adverse outcomes of pregnancy, N Engl J Med **306**:141-145, 1982.

CHAPTER 19

Nutrition and Skeletal Diseases

Lindsay H. Allen

STRUCTURE AND COMPOSITION OF BONE

Bone has two major functions, mechanical support and maintenance of normal mineral homeostasis. It is composed of bone cells, an organic matrix, and minerals deposited on the matrix. The bone cells are predominantly of three types. *Osteoblasts* are the bone-forming cells. They synthesize collagen, which constitutes approximately 90% of the bone matrix, and noncollagen "ground substance" containing glycoproteins. *Osteoclasts* are responsible for bone resorption. *Osteocytes,* the most most common type of bone cell, are probably osteoblasts trapped in bone that has become mineralized. These cells may function in the exchange of minerals between the extracellular fluid of bone and plasma.

Bone Matrix

Traditionally, research on metabolic bone diseases has focused on the mineral constituents of bone, partly because there are more easily measured and examined. However, a deficiency of one of several nutrients will result in abnormal collagen synthesis during bone development and subsequent poor bone mineralization. The formation of the fetal skeleton is largely determined by the deposition of mineral on collagen templates. The hydroxylation of lysine to form hydroxylysine, an important constituent of collagen, requires ascorbic acid. This explains the defective mineralization of scorbutic bone. Mature collagen fibers are composed of cross-linked collagen molecules. Some of these crosslinks are aldehyde derivatives of hydroxylysine or lysine residues produced by the action of a copper-dependent enzyme, lysyl oxidase. Thus defec-

tive collagen synthesis and osteoporosis occur in copper deficiency. Zinc is also required for the normal formation of bone matrix, and a deficiency affects the proliferation of both undifferentiated mesenchyme and the epiphyseal plate cartilage.

The noncollagenous proteins of bone are principally glycoproteins and proteoglycans. In addition, osteocalcin, a protein containing gamma-carboxyglutamic acid (GLA), has been identified. Vitamin D stimulates the synthesis of osteocalcin, and vitamin K is essential for the formation of GLA.

Some bone matrix is lost in osteoporosis, and vitamin D may have an effect on collagen cross-linking. Thus the maintenance of mineralization in adult bone also involves the integrity of the bone matrix.

Bone Mineral Constituents

The bones contain 99% of the body's calcium, 85% of the phosphorus, and 66% of the magnesium. The deposition of mineral on collagen does not occur until a few days after collagen has been formed. Following this it is deposited mainly as amorphous tricalcium phosphate, which slowly changes to crystals of hydroxyapatite ($Ca_{10}(PO_4)_6(OH)_2$).

Small amounts of other minerals can substitute in the crystal lattice. Fluoride improves crystal stability and has been investigated for use in therapy of osteoporosis. Ingestion of lead results in the accumulation of this mineral in bone, with subsequent toxic effects. Radium and radioactive isotopes of strontium cause a hazard by their accumulation and long-term retention in bone. Sodium, lithium, magnesium, copper, and zinc also become incorporated in the crystal lattice.

Bone Modeling and Remodeling

The bone cells are responsible for bone modeling during growth and for remodeling of adult

□ Scientific Contribution 1158, Storrs Agricultural Experiment Station, University of Connecticut, Storrs, Conn, 06268.

bone. During growth, bone elongation occurs by endochondral ossification of the epiphyseal plates whereas increase in width occurs by periosteal apposition and endosteal resorption.

Once growth has ceased, bone remains a dynamic tissue. It is continually being remodeled by "bone remodeling units."[1] In this process, resorption occurs prior to formation and is performed by groups of osteoclasts moving longitudinally through the bone cortex. New bone is then formed by osteoblasts in the same location. The resorptive phase lasts 1-3 weeks, but the subsequent formation may take over 3 months. The rate of bone turnover depends on the frequency with which new bone remodeling units are initiated and new bone is synthesized.

For adult bone mass to remain constant, resorption and formation must be coupled. The nature of this coupling is uncertain. However, the underlying defect in many cases of osteoporosis appears to be an excessive resorption of bone unaccompanied by an increased bone formation. The exchange of calcium resulting from bone remodeling is considerable, amounting to 400 mg/day.

Factors Affecting Bone Composition

Hormones are among the principal factors affecting bone composition. They not only control calcium and phosphorus metabolism but also affect bone turnover. Most of them affect both osteoblasts and osteoclasts. A list of the hormones known to affect bone metabolism and a summary of their effects are provided in Table 19-1. Greater detail of the mechanisms involved has been provided in Chapter 17.

The skeleton supplies calcium and phosphorus to the rest of the body when the absorption of these nutrients from the intestine is insufficient or when their excretion from the body is excessive. Phosphorus, sodium, and carbonate from bone can buffer excesses of acid in the diet. All these responses take priority over the structural functions of bone; thus growth, remodeling, and mineralization are impaired in deficiencies of calcium or phosphorus and in chronic acidosis.

Three hormones control the movements of calcium and phosphorus. Parathyroid hormone (parathormone) maintains serum calcium concentration by stimulating bone resorption, by increasing the renal reabsorption of filtered cal-

Table 19-1 Effect of Hormones on Bone Metabolism

Hormone	Effects
Vitamin D	Increases intestinal absorption of calcium and phosphorus
	Increases bone resorption
	Increases renal reabsorption of phosphate
Parathyroid hormone	Increases renal 1α-hydroxylase and 1,25-dihydroxyvitamin D (1,25-$(OH)_2$ D)
	Increases bone resorption
	Increases renal reabsorption of calcium
	Decreases renal reabsorption of phosphate
	Excess causes bone demineralization
Calcitonin	Decreases osteoclastic bone resorption
	Decreases renal reabsorption of phosphate
Growth hormone	Increases somatomedin synthesis, thereby stimulating cartilage and collagen synthesis
	Increases production of 1,25-$(OH)_2$ D and calcium absorption
	Excess causes gigantism and acromegaly
	Deficiency produces dwarfism in children
Thyroxine	Stimulates bone resorption
	Excess causes increased bone resorption
	Deficiency causes growth retardation in children and decreased bone turnover in adults
Insulin	Stimulates osteoblastic collagen synthesis
	Deficiency impairs growth and bone mass
Estrogens	Deficiency leads to increased bone resorption and osteoporosis
Testosterone	Deficiency leads to osteoporosis
Glucocorticoids	Excess (Cushing's syndrome) causes growth stunting, suppressed collagen synthesis, osteoporosis, decreased calcium absorption
	Adrenal androgens cause adolescent growth spurt
Prostaglandins	Prostaglandin E stimulates bone resorption

cium, and by stimulating the formation of 1,25-dihydroxyvitamin D, which increases intestinal calcium absorption. Parathormone also decreases the renal reabsorption of phosphorus and inhibits collagen synthesis, so the formation of new bone is limited.

Vitamin D is obtained either by synthesis of vitamin D_3 (cholecalciferol) in the skin or from dietary sources of vitamin D_2 or D_3. Cholecalciferol is converted in the liver to 25-hydroxyvitamin D, which is then converted in the kidney to 1,25-dihydroxyvitamin D. The latter form of the vitamin is the one that is active in stimulating intestinal calcium and phosphorus absorption and is therefore essential for bone growth and mineralization. However, if the diet is deficient in vitamin D, 1,25-dihydroxyvitamin D can stimulate bone resorption.

The roles of calcitonin in the maintenance of the skeleton are unclear. Calcitonin is secreted in response to high serum calcium levels, and it then inhibits bone resorption to control the hypercalcemia.

A deficiency or excess of parathormone and 1,25-dihydroxyvitamin D has marked effects on calcium regulation and bone mineralization. The levels of these hormones can be altered by the intake of calcium, phosphorus, and vitamin D. As shown in Table 19-1, many other hormones affect bone metabolism. Deficiencies or excesses of these result from abnormalities of the endocrine system and are less influenced by diet. Nevertheless, diseases in which the production or metabolism of these hormones is abnormal can have severe effects on the growth and modeling of developing bone and on the maintenance of bone structure and mineralization.

DIAGNOSIS OF METABOLIC BONE DISEASE

Metabolic bone disease is not usually suspected until clinical symptoms of rickets, osteoporosis, or osteomalacia are apparent. Confirmation of the disease by biochemical or clinical methods is sometimes difficult. An excellent scheme for the diagnosis of metabolic bone diseases has been provided by Smith.[2]

Biochemical tests include those for serum calcium and phosphorus, alkaline phosphatase, and vitamin D metabolites (Table 19-2). Serum calcium is aggressively defended by homeostatic mechanisms involving parathormone, 1,25-di-hydroxyvitamin D, and calcitonin. Normal levels are frequently found in the presence of metabolic bone disease. Low levels most commonly result from hypoalbuminemia, so the serum calcium should be corrected for variations in serum protein. Magnesium deficiency also produces hypocalcemia. Serum alkaline phosphatase is elevated in some, but not all, patients with rickets and osteomalacia. Ordinary chemical analyses show no consistent abnormalities in patients with osteoporosis, although preliminary studies[3] suggest that the urinary excretion of gamma-carboxyglutamic acid may be increased in this disease.

The assessment of bone mass is a major problem. Bone biopsy is an invasive and often painful procedure, although it can provide samples for direct determination of mineral density. If tetracyline labeling is also performed, turnover rate can be estimated. Biopsy allows differentiation between osteomalacia and osteoporosis. Radiologic assessment of vertebral body height or the cortical thickness of long bones is relatively simple but can detect only advanced demineralization. Photon absorptiometry[4] is more quantitative and is usually performed on the cortical bone in the forearm. However, ideally trabecular bone

Table 19-2 Diagnosis of Metabolic Bone Disease

	Signs and Symptoms
Rickets	Short stature
	Rachitic rosary, wrist and ankle widening, craniotabes, frontal bossing, bowing of lower extremities
	Low serum 25-OH vitamin D
	High serum alkaline phosphatase
	Low serum phosphorus
	High serum PTH
Osteomalacia	Decalcification of bone matrix, osteoid borders on trabeculae
	Looser's zones
	Low or normal serum calcium
	Secondary hyperparathyroidism
	High serum alkaline phosphatase
	Low serum 25-OH vitamin D
Osteoporosis	No consistent biochemical symptoms
	Loss of height, back pain, vertebral pain
	Loss of trabeculae in vertebrae and femoral neck
	Reduced cortical thickness in long bones, metacarpals, and phalanges

should also be evaluated (at the distal radius and lumbar vertebrae) since this bone turns over more rapidly and thus provides easier detection of the rate of loss and response to therapy.[5] Dual beam photon absorptiometry is needed for the assessment of mineralization of lumbar vertebrae because of the surrounding soft tissue mass.[5] The apparatus is expensive, however, and the measurement includes a large amount of cortical bone, especially in the spinous processes. Computed tomography can be used to assess relatively small selected areas of bone, but variations in the density of fatty and hematopoietic marrow can produce errors in the measurement of trabecular bone.[6] Neutron activation analysis[7] measures the calcium content of the whole body or of specific regions, but this is still an infrequently used procedure.

All these techniques are best used to follow the progress of individual patients or to compare populations, since there is considerable overlap between the values for normal individuals and those for patients with symptoms of bone loss.

NUTRITIONAL DISEASES OF DEVELOPING BONE
Rickets

Rickets usually results from vitamin D deficiency in infants and children. The incidence of this disease was very high in the United States prior to the supplementation of milk with vitamin D in the 1930s. Before that time, the majority of North American infants may have had some degree of rickets at the end of the winter during their first year of life.[8]

Rickets is now a relatively rare occurrence in the Western world, although it still occurs under certain conditions. Symptoms of this disease are shown in Table 19-2. Some of the factors predisposing an infant to rickets are listed as follows:

Vitamin D deficiency in the pregnant or lactating mother
Lack of vitamin D supplements
Lack of exposure to the sun
Vegetarian, especially vegan, diet
Pigmented skin
Twins
Avoidance of vitamin D–fortified milk
Protein-energy malnutrition
Malabsorption syndromes
Anticonvulsant therapy
Prematurity
Very low birth weight

The American Academy of Pediatrics[9] has taken the position that the antirachitic properties of breast milk seem adequate for normal term infants of well-nourished mothers; however, if the mothers' vitamin D intakes have been substandard, or if the infants have not benefited from ultraviolet exposure (because of dark skin or being shielded from the sun) "supplements of 400 IU of vitamin D daily may be indicated."

In spite of this recommendation, the need for vitamin D supplementation in full-term healthy infants of well-nourished mothers is still somewhat controversial. The content of 25-hydroxyvitamin D and 1,25-dihydroxyvitamin D in human milk is low; but antirachitic sterols constitute 25 IU/liter and 27 IU/liter, respectively, of human and bovine milk, and 25-hydroxyvitamin D comprises the majority of these sterols. The significance of this lies in the fact that the 25-hydroxy moiety is probably better utilized than vitamin D_3. Supplementation of healthy breast-fed babies has produced conflicting results. In one study[11] postnatal administration of 400 IU of 25-hydroxyvitamin D increased the bone mineral and serum levels of this vitamin at 12 weeks, but in another[12] the bone mineral was not affected. The long-term benefits of vitamin D supplements to breast-fed infants of well-nourished mothers remain to be determined. However, no doubt exists that mothers who are vitamin D deficient during pregnancy can produce rachitic infants and also there is a close correlation between the vitamin D status of the mother and that of her newborn during the first week of life.[13] It thus seems essential that these infants be supplemented.

Human milk apparently provides considerable protection against rickets, despite frequent reports of this disease in breast-fed infants. For example, several reports have shown a high incidence in Greece, South Africa, Ethiopia, and Nigeria. Although sunlight is plentiful in these countries, the custom of wrapping infants and keeping them indoors, plus the observance of purdah by their mothers, combines to prevent the synthesis of vitamin D in the infants' skin.[14] In Finland, where sunlight is scant in the winter, breast-feeding has been associated with low serum 25-hydroxyvitamin D levels in babies,[15] and the supplementation of lactating mothers with 1000 IU daily has not had a beneficial effect. The milk of vitamin D–deficient mothers is low in this vitamin; also protein-energy malnutrition and twinning tend to increase the incidence of rickets.

In the United States, cases are still reported as the result of vegetarianism,[17] low consumption of vitamin D-fortified milk or vitamin D supplements after weaning, and lack of exposure to sunlight.[18,19] The incidence is highest between 6 months and 5 years of age and is especially high at the end of winter or during spring of the first year of life. Infants with heavily pigmented skin are more susceptible; a reduced capacity for dermal synthesis of vitamin D may exist in this group, although increased circulating 1,25-dihydroxyvitamin D as a result of secondary hyperparathyroidism may compensate somewhat.[20] Gastrointestinal diseases in which the absorption of the vitamin is impaired can also produce rickets, as can anticonvulsant therapy. (See Chapter 12.)

In vitamin D deficiency a therapeutic response should be obtained by a daily dose of a few hundred units, but usually doses of 400 to 5000 IU/day are provided. A lack of response at these levels suggests that the rickets is not due to a simple deficiency of the vitamin.

Rickets in low–birth weight infants. Approximately 80% of the calcium in the fetal skeleton is acquired during the last trimester of pregnancy, and it is deposited at a rate of 125-175 mg/kg/day during the last 6 weeks. Very low–birth-weight (VLBW) infants cannot absorb sufficient calcium from breast milk or standard infant formulas to achieve the rate of calcium accretion that would have occurred in utero. Consequently, inadequate bone mineralization is common in this group. Given that breast milk provides 60-80 mg/kg of calcium daily and that 65% of this is absorbed, retention by the VLBW infant is only about 20% of the in utero rate. Most infant formulas and cow's milk contain more calcium, but absorption is just 30% from these sources, permitting 20% to 50% of the in utero rate of accretion. However, the in utero rate of calcium accumulation has been achieved by a specially developed formula.[21]

Alterations in vitamin D metabolism are also apparent in premature VLBW infants. In neonates with "rickets of prematurity," plasma 1,25-dihydroxycholecalciferol levels are markedly elevated, but supplements of vitamin D are needed to alleviate the rickets.[22] Concern has also been voiced[23] as to the need for phosphorus supplementation to prevent rickets in these infants. The use of a high-calcium formula resulted in more calcium absorption in the first 3 days of life.[24]

VLBW infants are frequently dependent on total parenteral nutrition (TPN) for their nourishment in the early postnatal period. Originally, intravenous intakes of 20-40 mg/kg/day of calcium and phosphorus were recommended for these infants. In 1976, however, it was shown that 50-100 mg/kg of calcium and 600 IU/day of vitamin D were sufficient to prevent onset of rickets in these infants when nourished predominantly by TPN.[25] Presumably the requirement is closer to the in utero rate of calcium accretion, 125-175 mg/kg/day. In addition, 600-800 IU/day of vitamin D has been recommended for VLBW infants receiving TPN, since their ability to hydroxylate vitamin D may be limited.

Copper deficiency. Osteopenia has been observed in infants with copper deficiency resulting from prematurity, inadequate copper content of infant formulas, TPN without copper supplementation, and severe malnutrition. The bones resemble those in scurvy (i.e., with osteoporosis, metaphyseal irregularities, and periosteal reactions).[26] Lysyl oxidase, which is involved in the cross-linkage of peptide chains in collagen, is a copper-containing enzyme. This may explain the effect of copper deficiency on bone, but alternative hypotheses[27] include an essential role for copper in ascorbic acid metabolism or a direct effect of copper in inhibiting bone resorption. Infants with Menkes' disease have many symptoms of copper deficiency,[28] for example, scurvy-like changes in the metaphyseal growth plates of long bones. The dramatic changes in copper metabolism that occur in Wilson's disease are associated with bone abnormalities such as osteoporosis, osteomalacia, rickets, arthritis, and osteochondritis. These are probably the result of disturbances in renal tubular function or excessive use of penicillamine therapy.

Copper concentrations in blood and synovial fluid are elevated with rheumatoid arthritis, perhaps as an adaptive response to retard bone resorption. Copper analogues of nonsteroidal antiinflammatory drugs are more effective than the parent compounds in treating this disease.[29]

Vitamin K deficiency. Up to 10% of the noncollagenous protein of bone consists of osteocalcin, a protein that contains three residues of gamma-carboxyglutamic acid (GLA) per molecule.[30] GLA is synthesized by a vitamin K–dependent microsomal system, which carboxylates the glutamyl residues. 1,25-Dihydroxyvitamin D stimulates osteocalcin synthesis.[31] The GLA enables osteocalcin to bind calcium. The function of osteocalcin is unclear, but it may inhibit hydroxyapatite crystallization and stimulate increased calcium release from bone.[32]

Warfarin derivatives (e.g., Coumadin), which are used as oral anticoagulants and rodenticides, inhibit the vitamin K–dependent carboxylation step. This may explain the high incidence of fetal bone malformations in women who take these anticoagulants early in pregnancy. The bones of infants born to such women have islands of calcification in the growth plate (which normally remains uncalcified) resembling the early stages of calcification that actually causes growth plate closure in warfarin-treated rats.[33] The plasma osteocalcin concentrations are elevated in diseases with high rates of bone turnover (e.g., Paget's disease of bone, hyperparathyroidism, renal failure, osteoporosis).[34]

Vitamin C deficiency. Scorbutic bone changes occur in ascorbic acid deficiency. A dietary deficiency of this vitamin occurs most frequently in infants at 6-15 months of age. In adults scurvy is now rare, but it sometimes occurs in alcoholics, diet faddists, and severely malnourished individuals. The histologic appearance of bones in infantile scurvy is quite different from that in rickets. There are obvious hemorrhages in the bone marrow and under the periosteum, where they stimulate the formation of reactive irregularly shaped new bone. Endochondral ossification is disrupted. These bone changes result from defective collagen synthesis; ascorbic acid is a cofactor for the enzyme collagen prolyl hydroxylase, which hydroxylates peptide-bound proline to hydroxyproline.

Osteomalacia

Estimates of the frequency of osteomalacia vary from "uncommon" to "25% of patients with bone loss and hip fractures." It can occur together with osteoporosis. Most cases arise secondary to surgery or other diseases in which vitamin D absorption or synthesis is impaired. The most common causes of osteomalacia are the following:

Dietary vitamin D deficiency
Lack of exposure to the sun
Reduced dermal synthesis of vitamin D in the elderly
Total parenteral nutrition

Gastrectomy, celiac disease, primary biliary cirrhosis, chronic renal disease, intestinal resection
Anticonvulsant therapy

Clinical symptoms of osteomalacia include diffuse bone pain, especially in the limbs and ribs. Vertebrae become more biconcave. The bone matrix is relatively decalcified, and biochemically there is a low serum calcium, secondary hyperparathyroidism, and an elevated serum alkaline phosphatase (Table 19-2).

Symptoms of dietary vitamin D deficiency are rare in adults but will occur if intake is below 70 IU/day (compared to the RDA of 400 IU/da). Large amounts of vitamin D are naturally present in fish oils and some fish. Other foods, such as eggs, cheese, animal liver, and butter, supply small amounts of the vitamin. In general, intake of the vitamin from usual foods is much lower than required, unless fortified milk (containing 400 IU/qt) is consumed. Vegetarians who consume no animal products, those individuals who avoid fatty foods, and those not drinking fortified milk will be at considerable risk of a dietary vitamin D deficiency.

A far more important source of vitamin D is ultraviolet radiation from the sun, which induces vitamin D_3 synthesis in the skin. Lack of sunlight or a tendency to remain indoors has been implicated in the higher incidence of bone fractures at the end of winter, osteomalacia in gastrectomy patients, and osteomalacia in Asian immigrants to Europe.[35] Furthermore, it has been established that the elderly have a marked decrease in their ability to synthesize vitamin D_3 in their skin.

The use of anticonvulsant drugs for epilepsy has resulted in rickets in infants[36] and osteomalacia in adults.[37] These drugs, including phenobarbital and phenytoin, stimulate the activity of hepatic cytochrome P-450 microsomal enzyme systems, leading to an accelerated degradation of 25-hydroxycholecalciferol. Consequently, serum levels of 25-hydroxyvitamin D are lower in individuals on anticonvulsant therapy,[38] with the lowest values found in blacks and those with limited vitamin D intakes or exposure to sunlight. Relatively large doses of vitamin D (2000-10,000 IU/day) are necessary to prevent osteomalacia during this therapy.

Many commonly used medications stimulate the activity of these hepatic microsomal enzymes and can induce vitamin D deficiency. These include tranquilizers, sedatives, muscle relaxants, and oral diabetic agents.

Osteomalacia and total parenteral nutrition. Historically, there has been little concern about appropriate calcium nutriture during TPN. However, more recently it has become apparent that long-term TPN frequently results in significant losses of skeletal mineral. Symptoms of osteomalacia can appear within a few months of starting TPN, even at intakes of calcium and vitamin D formerly assumed adequate to maintain calcium balance.

Two reports[39,40] have reawakened interest in the problem of calcium status during TPN. In these studies patients with severe bone pain were given 300-400 mg of calcium and 250-1000 IU of vitamin D daily. Bone biopsies revealed demineralization, absence of osteoblastic cells, and diffuse osteopenia and osteomalacia after 6-27 months. Serum levels of calcium, phosphorus, magnesium, bicarbonate, copper, zinc, albumin, parathormone, and 25-hydroxyvitamin D were normal, although serum alkaline phosphatase was frequently elevated. A later study[41] demonstrated reduced serum levels of 1,25-dihydroxyvitamin D. The most consistently abnormal finding was a markedly elevated urinary calcium, which exceeded the calcium intake of many of the patients. The reasons for this hypercalciuric response remain to be established but could include excessive intakes of vitamin D in the TPN solutions,[40] increased sensitivity to 1,25-dihydroxyvitamin D,[42] or amino acid and glucose stimulation of insulin release with subsequent inhibition of renal calcium reabsorption.[43,44] Aluminum contamination of casein hydrolysate in the TPN solutions has also been implicated as the problem,[45] but aluminum may simply accumulate in poorly mineralized bone, rather than being the cause of the demineralization.[46]

Osteoporosis

Osteoporosis is a disease commonly encountered in postmenopausal women, but it occurs to some extent in most elderly individuals. It has been estimated that one quarter of women over the age of 60 years have clinical symptoms of osteoporosis.

The term osteoporosis includes at least two separate clinical entities: Type I, postmenopausal osteoporosis or the "vertebral crush fracture" syndrome, usually occurs in women around 10-15 years after menopause. It is seen at sites where trabecular bone predominates (e.g., the lumbar vertebrae, distal radius, proximal femur, endosteal cortical bone in the forearm and metacarpals). The result is vertebral compression, lower back pain, loss of height, and "dowager's hump." Type II is senile osteoporosis, the incidence of which reaches a peak between 70 and 90 years of age in both men and women. Loss of trabecular and cortical bone occurs and is associated with an increased incidence of hip and wrist fractures.

Histologically there is a loss of bone matrix and bone mineral content, with the remaining bone relatively normally mineralized. There are no reliable biochemical tests that can be used to diagnose osteoporosis (Table 19-2). Urinary calcium, hydroxyproline, and gamma-carboxyglutamic acid may be slightly increased, and calcium absorption is often decreased.

Causes and complications of osteoporosis include the following:

Reduced estrogen secretion
Dietary calcium deficiency
Low bioavailability of dietary calcium (fiber, alcohol)
Reduced calcium absorption in elderly
Reduced ability to adapt to calcium deficiency in elderly
Immobilization
Gastrointestinal diseases (primary biliary cirrhosis, chronic obstructive jaundice, gastric surgery)

Estrogens and osteoporosis. Our understanding of the cause of osteoporosis is not yet complete, although there is basic agreement that the underlying defect is an excessive resorption of bone. The highest rates of resorption are seen in menopausal women with the lowest serum estrogen levels, which has led to the hypothesis that bone resorption is related to the fall in estrogen secretion that occurs at menopause. Balance studies in women[47] have shown that calcium absorption is reduced, urinary calcium increased, and calcium retention more negative between 42 and 47 years of age.[47]

Further evidence for a role of estrogen has been obtained by monitoring the biochemical events after estrogen administration to osteoporotic women. Following 6 months of estrogen treatment,[48] calcium absorption improved, serum parathormone decreased, and serum 1,25-dihydroxyvitamin D was higher. The sequence of events was hypothesized to occur in this manner: Estrogen slows down the excessive resorption of bone, subsequently lowering serum calcium and stimulating parathormone secretion and 1,25-dihydroxyvitamin D production. Higher levels of this vitamin D metabolite then promote calcium absorption by the intestine and reabsorption by the kidney. Alternatively, estrogen may produce its effect by acting on other factors regulating bone metabolism, such as calcitonin (which inhibits bone resorption) and prostaglandins.[49]

The role of dietary calcium intake. When calcium consumption is low, the synthesis of calcium-binding protein is stimulated and the efficiency of intestinal absorption is improved. Because this adaptive response occurs and because the effects of marginal deficits in calcium intake have been difficult to demonstrate, it is commonly assumed that inadequate calcium intakes are not important in the etiology of osteoporosis. More recent studies have demonstrated that this assumption is most likely incorrect.

The adult RDA for calcium is 800 mg/day.[50] In a Yugoslavian study[51] individuals who consumed an average of 400 mg/day had smaller amounts of bone than those who consumed an average of 900 mg/day. This difference was apparent by 30 years of age. In calcium balance studies,[52] most individuals are in a negative status if intake is less than 600 mg/day; thus it is reasonable to assume that skeletal demineralization must be the result. Loss of bone mineral from dietary calcium deficiency causes osteoporotic lesions in monkeys; and it is not unreasonable to conclude that an adequate calcium intake is important in preventing this disease in humans. Women who consumed milk frequently during childhood and adolescence had a higher postmenopausal bone density than did those who consumed milk rarely.[53]

The average calcium intake of North American adults is close to the RDA (800 mg/da). Inadequate intakes (about 500 mg/da) are consumed by the elderly and those who do not drink milk. In addition to the issue of consuming sufficient calcium, it is important to consider factors that affect calcium absorption and retention.[54] Dietary constituents that can severely reduce absorption include the uronic acids of dietary fiber, phytate and oxalate in plant foods, and alcohol. Inadequate absorption occurs in vitamin D deficiency. Dietary fat impairs absorption only in the presence of steatorrhea. Negative balance is induced by high protein intakes, because of an impairment in renal calcium reabsorption. The elderly generally absorb calcium less efficiently and cannot adapt as well to a dietary deficiency.[55]

Prevention and therapy. Prevention of osteoporosis rather than reversal is probably a more realistic objective. Estrogen therapy is effective in reducing postmenopausal bone loss, even if treatment is started as long as 10-15 years after menopause. Most patients receiving estrogens should be treated for at least 5 and possibly 10 to 15 years. Discontinuation leads to reappearance of bone resorption, and the degree of lasting beneficial effect remains controversial.[56] The effective dose is 0.625 mg of conjugated estrogens or 20-50 μg of ethinyl estradiol for 21-25 days per month, replaced by progestin for the last 10 days to reduce the risk of endometrial cancer. This therapy may lead to the restoration of menstrual bleeding and is contraindicated in patients with carcinoma of the breast or endometrium, severe fibrocystic breast disease, and hypertension or vascular disease. The suggestion has been made that estrogen therapy should be used in women who are at high risk for osteoporosis, considering factors such as frame size, bone mass, diet, ethnicity, activity level, disease, and endocrine function.[57]

Calcium supplements have been reported effective at restoring calcium balance in postmenopausal women. Premenopausal women can maintain calcium balance with an intake of 1000 mg/day whereas 1500 mg/day is required after menopause.[58,59] Since most women consume closer to 600 mg/day, supplements are needed to achieve the level of intake that maintains balance. Although harmful effects of higher calcium intakes have not been demonstrated, there is concern that calcium carbonate supplements may suppress bone renewal rates if intakes of 1500-2000 mg/day are given to older women. If the calcium is provided in the form of milk, it appears that bone remodeling is less severely suppressed.[60] In persons with alchlorhydria, calcium is much better absorbed from calcium citrate than from calcium carbonate.[61]

Research on the benefits of vitamin D supplements has produced somewhat conflicting results, but low serum levels of 25-hydroxycholecalciferol and 1,25-dihydroxycholecalciferol occur frequently in osteoporosis and may be at least partly responsible for the impairment of intestinal calcium absorption in this condition. In one study[62] supplements of 15,000 IU of vitamin D_2 per week for 2 years led to a reduced rate of cortical bone loss, with some patients actually regaining some mineral over this time. Administration of 40-50 µg/day of 25-hydroxycholecalciferol may increase serum levels of 1,25-dihydroxyvitamin D and stimulate calcium absorption in some patients.[63] However, approximately 50% of postmenopausal osteoporotics fail to respond, perhaps because of an impairment in the renal enzyme (25-hydroxyvitamin D–alpha-hydroxylase) that stimulates 1,25-dihydroxycholecalciferol synthesis.[64]

The level of 25-hydroxyvitamin D hydroxylase enzyme in most postmenopausal osteoporotic subjects demonstrates a normal responsiveness to parathyroid hormone.[65] Nevertheless, there is substantial evidence[66] that the conversion of 25-hydroxycholecalciferol to 1,25-dihydroxycholecalciferol is impaired: 0.5 µg/day supplements of 1,25-dihydroxycholecalciferol for 6-8 months restored calcium absorption to normal, changed calcium balance to positive, and decreased bone resorption. However, after 2 years of therapy bone resorption returned to pretreatment rates and calcium retention became more negative. In a 1-year trial[67] therapy with 1,25-dihydroxycholecalciferol plus estrogens and calcium was less effective in slowing bone loss than were either estrogens plus calcium or calcium supplements alone. Thus there is currently little evidence that 1,25-dihydroxycholecalciferol therapy is a useful long-term treatment, perhaps because of the bone-resorbing action of this metabolite.

Fluoride therapy decreased the rate of vertebral fracture occurrence in a year-long study.[68] Randomized controlled prospective trials of the effectiveness of fluoride treatment are needed. Many patients suffer gastrointestinal problems and arthralgias, but these symptoms may disappear at lower doses or over time. The usual treatment dose is 20-60 mg/day of fluoride, together with calcium and possibly vitamin D.

The most effective treatment, or combination of treatments, for osteoporosis probably varies with the individual being treated. For example, calcium supplements will be less beneficial in patients with an impaired ability to absorb calcium. Estrogen and/or 25-hydroxyvitamin D

therapy may be needed to improve absorption of the supplement. Finally, sufficient exercise and avoidance of excessive fiber and alcohol consumption may be useful preventive measures. Of interest are the observations[69,70] that severe physical exercise or anorexia nervosa leading to amenorrhea may cause premature osteoporosis. Smoking and alcohol consumption are risk factors for osteoporosis in men whereas obesity is protective.[71]

GASTROINTESTINAL DISEASES AND SURGERY

Gastrointestinal diseases generally affect calcium status and bone mineralization by altering the absorption of calcium and vitamin D as well as the synthesis of vitamin D metabolites. Consequently these diseases result in osteomalacia more frequently than in osteoporosis.

Hepatobiliary disorders (e.g., primary biliary cirrhosis,[72] chronic obstructive jaundice) are associated with a high incidence of both osteomalacia and osteoporosis. Reasons for this include bile salt deficiency, with subsequently poor fat and calcium absorption due to the formation of insoluble calcium "soaps." In biliary cirrhosis, malabsorption of vitamin D and low levels of plasma 25-hydroxyvitamin D have been documented. This disease responds better to 25-hydroxyvitamin D than to vitamin D_3 therapy, perhaps because of impaired ability of the liver to perform the hydroxylation step.

Bone demineralization has been shown to occur frequently in children with cystic fibrosis. The bone loss is most prevalent in older adolescent or preadolescent girls, so that rickets does not occur unless there is severe hepatic involvement.[73]

Celiac disease can produce rickets and osteomalacia. Even intravenous doses of vitamin D metabolites are of little use in treating this disease. The vitamin resistance may result from a lack of sufficient intestinal cell integrity to respond to vitamin D.

Gastric surgery frequently results in osteomalacia, although osteoporosis is sometimes seen. The pathogenesis is unknown. The absorption of vitamin D is relatively normal, and calcium absorption may be normal or even increased. There is no relationship between the severity of the disease and fecal fat, calcium, or vitamin D. Serum levels of 25-hydroxyvitamin

D are reduced whereas those of 1,25-dihydroxy-vitamin D may be raised as the result of a compensatory process to maintain adequate calcium absorption.[74] Poor dietary intakes of vitamin D and a tendency to stay indoors may be causative in the vitamin D deficiency.

Skeletal demineralization in chronic renal disease is well documented.[75] A number of alterations in calcium, phosphorus, and magnesium metabolism may be involved, including reduced calcium absorption and hyperparathyroidism. Low glomerular filtration rates ($<$15-25 ml/min) indicate that functional renal tissue is inadequate to synthesize sufficient 1,25-dihydroxyvitamin D. Large doses of vitamin D or 25-hydroxyvitamin D are therapeutic by a mass action effect.

Finally, intestinal bypass surgery for the treatment of obesity leads to osteomalacia, especially if a substantial portion of the ileum is removed.[76] Osteomalacia appears in one third of the patients who have undergone intestinal resection for conditions such as Crohn's disease.[77] Interestingly, the colon plays an important role in calcium absorption after small intestinal resection, so patients with intact colons remaining have little impairment of calcium uptake.[78]

TOXIC EFFECTS OF MINERAL EXCESSES

Several minerals can produce toxic effects on the skeleton by causing renal damage and subsequent alterations in vitamin D metabolism or by affecting collagen synthesis.

Cadmium toxicity may arise through industrial pollution. In addition, tobacco smoke contains large amounts of this nonessential mineral. Perhaps the best-known syndrome of cadmium toxicity is Itai-Itai disease, which appeared as a result of industrial pollution in an area of Japan. Clinical symptoms resemble those of osteomalacia and/or severe osteoporosis with pseudofractures. Cadmium inhibits the enzyme renal 25-hydroxyvitamin D–alpha-hydroxylase; thus 1,25-dihydroxyvitamin D synthesis is impaired and intestinal calcium absorption reduced.[79] It also inhibits the activity of the enzymes lysyl oxidase and proline oxidase, which are essential for collagen formation. Urinary proline is elevated. Treatment with large doses of vitamin D (20,000-100,000 IU/da) relieves the symptoms of many patients after several months.

Aluminum toxicity has been reported in industrial workers exposed to high levels of the mineral and in renal dialysis patients due to contamination of the dialysate. Symptoms include severe, symptomatic osteomalacia that is resistant to vitamin D treatment.[80] The complex action of aluminum includes effects on phosphate absorption, osteoblast function, and mineral deposition. It has been suggested[46] that, rather than being the cause of impaired mineralization, aluminum simply accumulates in renal osteodystrophy at sites of slow mineralization. The excessive use of aluminum phosphate gels in the treatment of renal disease reduces calcium and phosphorus absorption and produces osteomalacia.

Lithium has a variety of uses in medicine, including the treatment of psychiatric disorders and disturbances of water metabolism. It is also used as a sodium substitute in low-sodium diets. Because of its physiochemical similarity to calcium and magnesium, lithium is retained readily in bone. It may also interfere with the action of parathormone on bone. Chronic lithium therapy produces osteoporosis, especially in women.[81]

Lead poisoning among children is still a common medical problem in the United States. The lead is usually ingested in paint chips, especially where people live in substandard housing. Children with elevated blood lead levels frequently have low serum concentrations of 1,25-dihydroxyvitamin D, which are restored by chelation therapy.[82] Their long bones show transverse radiopaque lines at the growth plates, caused by abnormally condensed calcified cartilage and new bone. In adults, lead also impairs the renal tubular secretion of uric acid, resulting in hyperuricemia and acute attacks of gout.

The use of *fluoridated water* in hemodialysis baths has been associated with an increased incidence of osteomalacia, although this is controversial.[83] Industrial fluoride poisoning produces arthritis as well as pain and stiffness in the lumbar and cervical spine. Bone changes include diffuse osteosclerosis (hypermineralization) and multiple periosteal hyperostoses. In addition, regions of excessive bone resorption (as in osteoporosis) and unmineralized osteoid may occur.

REFERENCES

1. Parfitt AM: Quantum concept of bone remodeling and turnover: implication for the pathogenesis of osteoporosis, Calcif Tissue Int **28**:1-5, 1979.
2. Smith R: Diagnosis of metabolic bone disease. In Smith R, editor: Biochemical disorders of the skeleton, London, 1979, Butterworth & Co (Publishers) Ltd, pp 35-70.

3. Gunderg CM, et al: γ-Carboxyglutamic acid excretions as a marker for metabolic bone disease. In DeLuca HF, et al, editors: Osteoporosis: recent advances in pathogenesis and treatment, Baltimore, 1981, University Park Press, p 473.

4. Cameron JR, Sorenson J: Measurement of bone mineral in vivo: an improved method, Science 142:230-232, 1963.

5. Dunn WL, et al: Measurement of bone mineral content in human vertebrae and hip by dual photon absorptiometry, Radiology 136:485-487, 1980.

6. Cann CE, Genant HK: Precise measurement of vertebral mineral content using computed tomography, J Comput Assist Tomogr 6:216-217, 1982.

7. Harrison JE, et al: Bone mineral measurements of the central skeleton by in vivo neutron activation analysis for routine investigation of osteopenia, Invest Radiol 14:27-34, 1979.

8. Weick MT: A history of rickets in the United States, Am J Clin Nutr 20:1234-1241, 1967.

9. Committee on Nutrition, American Academy of Pediatrics: Vitamin and mineral supplement needs in normal children in the United States, Pediatrics 66:1015-1021, 1980.

10. Hollis BW, et al: Vitamin D and its metabolites in human and bovine milk, J Nutr 111:1240-1248, 1981.

11. Greer FR, et al: Bone mineral content and serum 25-hydroxyvitamin D concentration in breast-fed infants with and without supplemental vitamin D, J Pediatr 98:696-701, 1981.

12. Roberts CC, et al: Adequate bone mineralization in breast-fed infants, J Pediatr 99:192-196, 1981.

13. Markestad T, et al: Serum concentration of vitamin D metabolites in maternal and umbilical cord blood of Libyan and Norwegian women, Hum Nutr Clin Nutr 38(1):55-62, 1984.

14. Mumdziev N: Rachitis in children up to two years of age in Addis-Ababa and some peculiarities in its clinical picture, Folia Med 10:198-201, 1968.

15. Ala-Houhala M: 25-Hydroxyvitamin D levels during breast-feeding with or without maternal or infantile supplementation of vitamin D, J Pediatr Gastroenterol Nutr 4:220-226, 1985.

16. Robertson I: Survey of clinical rickets in the infant population in Cape Town, 1967-1968, S Afr Med J 43:1072-1076, 1969.

17. Dwyer JT, et al: Risk of nutritional rickets among vegetarian children, Am J Dis Child 133:134-140, 1979.

18. Edidin D, et al: Resurgence of nutritional rickets associated with breast-feeding and special dietary practices, Pediatrics 65:232-235, 1980.

19. Bachrach S, et al: An outbreak of vitamin D deficiency rickets in a susceptible population, Pediatrics 64:871-877, 1979.

20. Bell NH, et al: Evidence for alteration of the vitamin D–endocrine system in blacks, J Clin Invest 76:470-473, 1985.

21. Shenai JP, et al: Nutritional balance studies in very-low-birth-weight infants: enhanced nutrient retention rates by an experimental formula, Pediatrics 66:233-238, 1980.

22. Chesney RW, et al: Rickets of prematurity: supranormal levels of serum 1,25-dihydroxyvitamin D, Am J Dis Child 135:34-37, 1981.

23. Rowe JC, et al: Nutritional hypophosphatemic rickets in a premature infant fed breast milk, N Engl J Med 300:293-296, 1979.

24. Moya M, Domenech E: Role of calcium-phosphate ratio of milk formulae on calcium balance in low birth weight infants during the first three days of life, Pediatr Res 16:675-681, 1982.

25. Leape LL, Valaes T: Rickets in low birth weight infants receiving total parenteral nutrition, J Pediatr Surg 11:665-674, 1976.

26. Blumenthal I, et al: Fracture of the femur, fish odour, and copper deficiency in a preterm infant, Arch Dis Child 55:229-231, 1980.

27. Wilson T, et al: Inhibition of active bone resorption by copper, Calcif Tissue Int 33:35-39, 1981.

28. Menkes JH, et al: A sex-linked recessive disorder with retardation of growth, peculiar hair, and focal cerebral and cerebellar degeneration, Pediatrics 29:764-771, 1962.

29. Sorenson JPJ: Copper chelates as possible active forms of antiarthritic agents, J Med Chem 19:135-148, 1976.

30. Hauschka PV, et al: Vitamin K and mineralization, Trends Biochem Sci 3:75-78, 1978.

31. Price PA, Bankel SA: 1,25-Dihydroxyvitamin D₃ increases serum levels of the vitamin K–dependent bone protein, Biochem Biophys Res Commun 99:928-935, 1981.

32. Price PA, et al: Excessive mineralization with growth plate closure in rats on chronic warfarin treatment, Proc Natl Acad Sci USA 79:7734-7738, 1982.

33. Hall JG, et al: Maternal and fetal sequelae of anticoagulation during pregnancy, Am J Med 68:122-140, 1980.

34. Price PA, et al: New biochemical marker for metabolism: measurement by radioimmunoassay of bone GLA protein in the plasma of normal subjects and patients with bone disease, J Clin Invest 66:878-883, 1980.

35. Allen LH: The role of nutrition in the onset and treatment of metabolic bone disease. In Briggs GM, Weininger J, editors: Nutrition update series, New York, 1982, John Wiley Inc, pp 263-281.

36. Borgstedt AD, et al: Long-term administration of anti-epileptic drugs and the development of rickets, J Pediatr 81:9-15, 1972.

37. Dent CE, et al: Osteomalacia with long-term anticonvulsant therapy in epilepsy, Br Med J 4:69-72, 1970.

38. Hahn TJ, et al: Effect of chronic anticonvulsant therapy on serum 25-hydroxycalciferol levels in adults, N Engl J Med 287:900-904, 1972.

39. Klein GL, et al: Bone disease associated with total parenteral nutrition, Lancet 2:1041-1044, 1980.

40. Shike M, et al: Metabolic bone disease in patients receiving long-term total parenteral nutrition, Ann Intern Med 92:343-350, 1980.

41. Klein GL, et al: Reduced serum levels of 1,25-dihydroxyvitamin D during long-term total parenteral nutrition, Ann Intern Med 94:638-643, 1981.

42. Jeejeebhoy KN, et al: TPN bone disease at Toronto. In Coburn JW, Klein GL, editors: Metabolic bone disease in total parenteral nutrition, Baltimore, 1985, Urban & Schwarzenberg, pp 17-29.

43. Allen LH: Calcium nutrition during total parenteral alimentation, Clin Nutr Suppl Ser 2:18-22, 1983.

44. Bengoa JM, et al: Amino acid–induced hypercalciuria in patients on total parenteral nutrition, Am J Clin Nutr 38:264-269, 1983.

45. Ott SM, et al: Aluminum is associated with low bone formation in patients on chronic parenteral nutrition, Ann Intern Med 98:910-914, 1983.

46. Quarles LD, et al: Aluminum deposition at the osteoid-bone interface, J Clin Invest 75:1441-1447, 1985.

47. Heaney RP, et al: Calcium balance requirements in middle-aged women, Am J Clin Nutr **30**:1603-1611, 1978.
48. Gallagher JC, et al: Effect of estrogen on calcium absorption and serum vitamin D metabolites in postmenopausal osteoporosis, J Clin Endocrinol Metab **51**:1359-1364, 1980.
49. Raisz LG: Role of estrogen in the prevention and treatment of osteoporosis, Musc Skel Med **2**:25-33, 1985.
50. Committee on Dietary Allowances, Food and Nutrition Board, National Research Council: Recommended dietary allowances, ed 9, Washington DC, 1980, National Academy of Sciences.
51. Matkovic V, et al: Bone status and fracture rates in two regions of Yugoslavia, Am J Clin Nutr **92**:953-963, 1979.
52. Marshall DH, et al: Calcium, phosphorus, and magnesium requirement, Proc Nutr Soc **35**:163-173, 1976.
53. Sandler RB, et al: Postmenopausal bone density and milk consumption in childhood and adolescence, Am J Clin Nutr **42**:270-274, 1985.
54. Allen LH: Calcium bioavailability and absorption: a review, Am J Clin Nutr **35**:783-808, 1982.
55. Ireland P, Fordtran JS: Effect of dietary calcium and age on jejunal calcium absorption in humans studied by intestinal perfusion, J Clin Invest **52**:2672-2681, 1973.
56. Christiansen C, et al: Bone mass in postmenopausal women after withdrawal of oestrogen/gestagen replacement therapy, Lancet **1**:459-461, 1981.
57. Raisz L, Johannesson A: Pathogenesis, prevention, and therapy of osteoporosis, Am J Med **15**:267-274, 1985.
58. Recker RR, et al: Effect of estrogens and calcium carbonate on bone loss in postmenopausal women, Ann Intern Med **87**:649-655, 1977.
59. Heaney RP, et al: Menopausal changes in calcium balance performance, J Lab Clin Med **92**:953-963, 1978.
60. Recker RR, Heaney RP: The effect of milk supplements on calcium metabolism, bone metabolism, and calcium balance, Am J Clin Nutr **41**:254-263, 1985.
61. Recker RR: Calcium absorption and achlorhydria, N Engl J Med **313**:70-73, 1985.
62. Nordin BEC, et al: A prospective trial of the effect of vitamin D supplementation on metacarpal bone loss in elderly women, Am J Clin Nutr **42**:470-474, 1985.
63. Crilly RG, et al: The vitamin D metabolites in the pathogenesis and management of osteoporosis, Curr Med Res Opin **7**:337-341, 1981.
64. Terwekh JE, et al: Long-term 25-hydroxyvitamin D₃ therapy in postmenopausal osteoporosis: demonstration of responsive and nonresponsive subgroups, J Clin Endocrinol Metab **56**:410-413, 1983.
65. Riggs BL, et al: Assessment of 25-hydroxyvitamin D 1-α-hydroxylase reserve in postmenopausal osteoporosis by administration of parathyroid extract, J Clin Endocrinol Metab **53**:833-835, 1981.
66. Gallagher JC, et al: 1,25-Dihydroxyvitamin D₃: short- and long-term effects on bone and calcium metabolism in patients with postmenopausal osteoporosis, Proc Natl Acad Sci **79**:3325-3329, 1982.
67. Jensen GF, et al: Does 1,25(OH)₂D₃ accelerate spinal bone loss? A controlled therapeutic trial in 70-year-old women, Clin Orthop Rel Res **192**:215-221, 1985.
68. Riggs BL, et al: Effect of fluoride/calcium requirement on vertebral fracture occurrence in postmenopausal osteoporosis, N Engl J Med **306**:446-450, 1982.
69. Rigotti DA, et al: Osteoporosis in women with anorexia nervosa, N Engl J Med **311**:1601-1606, 1984.
70. Marcus R, et al: Menstrual function and bone mass in elite women distance runners, Ann Intern Med **102**:158-163, 1985.
71. Seeman BGO, et al: Risk factors for spinal osteoporosis in men, Am J Med **75**:977-983, 1983.
72. Kehayoglou AK, et al: Bone disease and calcium absorption in primary biliary cirrhosis with special reference to vitamin D therapy, Lancet **1**:715-719, 1968.
73. Mischler EH, et al: Demineralization in cystic fibrosis, Am J Dis Child **133**:632-635, 1979.
74. Nilas L, et al: Regulation of vitamin D and calcium metabolism after gastrectomy, Gut **26**:252-257, 1985.
75. Catto GRD: Renal bone disease, J R Coll Phys **11**:75-86, 1976.
76. Dano P, Christiansen C: Calcium absorption and bone mineral content following intestinal shunt operation for obesity. A comparison of three types of operation, Scand J Gastroenterol **9**:775-779, 1974.
77. Compston JE, et al: Osteomalacia after small-intestinal resection, Lancet **1**:9-12, 1978.
78. Hylander E, et al: The importance of the colon in calcium absorption following small-intestinal resection, Scand J Gastroenterol **15**:55-60, 1980.
79. Friberg L, Kjellstrom T: Cadmium. In Bronner F, Coburn JW, editors: Disorders of mineral metabolism, vol 1, New York, 1981, Academic Press Inc, pp 317-352.
80. Parkinson IS, et al: Fracturing dialysis encephalopathy. An epidemiological survey, Lancet **1**:406-409, 1979.
81. Christiansen C, et al: Osteopenia and dysregulation of divalent cations in lithium treated patients, Neuropsychobiology **1**:344-354, 1975.
82. Rosen JF, et al: Reduction in 1,25-dihydroxyvitamin D in children with increased lead absorption, N Engl J Med **302**:1129-1131, 1980.
83. Oreopoulos DG, et al: Fluoride and dialysis osteodystrophy: results of a double-blind study, Trans Am Soc Artif Intern Organs **20A**:203-208, 1974.

CHAPTER 20
The Mouth

Edward A. Sweeney

Many of the common oral diseases have a marked nutritional component to their etiology. In dental caries, the most common human chronic disease in developed countries, nutritional factors influence both susceptibility and resistance. Similarly, nutrition affects resistance and susceptibility to diseases of the periodontal tissue. Although most common oral diseases are not life-threatening, they accounted for over $19 billion spent on dental care in the United States in 1982[1] and thus represented a significant economic problem. They decrease the quality of life for many persons in terms of pain, cosmetic appearance, and masticatory function.

NORMAL TISSUES

The tissues of the oral cavity are subjected to a variety of thermal, physical, and chemical forces, and they are uniquely adapted for their environment. The cell turnover times of the oral soft tissues are among the most rapid in the body, ranging from 3 to 5 days for the tongue and oral mucosa.[2] This turnover, in part, accounts for the speed with which oral lesions can develop, as well as resolve when appropriate therapy is given.

Lips

The lips represent transitional tissue from the dry keratinized squamous epithelium of the facial skin to the moist mucosa of the oral cavity. The outer aspects of the lips lack the minor mucous salivary glands that line the oral mucosa and are more susceptible to dryness. Their red color comes from richly vascularized subjacent connective tissue.

Oral Mucosa

The mucosa that line most of the oral cavity contain hundreds of small simple mucous glands. In conjunction with the major salivary glands, these provide the moistened environment that permits the tissues to move against one another, facilitates the mastication of food and its formation into a bolus for swallowing, buffers undesirable chemicals, prevents colonization of pathogenic organisms, and provides other beneficial effects.

Tongue

The anterior two thirds of the tongue is covered by many fine filiform papillae composed of a connective-tissue core and a keratinized epithelium. A smaller number of fungiform papillae are scattered among the filiform. If the taller filiform papillae atrophy, a rich red vascular bed allows the fungiform papillae to appear more prominent, giving the tongue a strawberry appearance. Large circumvallate papillae are found in a U-shaped demarcation between the anterior two thirds and posterior one third of the tongue. Each circumvallate papilla is surrounded by a moatlike depression. On the inner walls of the depression, taste buds open into the moat and are bathed by secretions from small serous glands at the bottom of the moat (von Ebner's glands). Taste buds on the dorsal surface of the fungiform papillae and in the folds of foliate papillae, located on the dorsolateral surface of each side of the tongue, resemble the circumvallate. Other taste buds are scattered among the oropharynx, pharynx, and palate.

Taste Buds

Taste buds are important sensors from a nutritional standpoint, since they dictate much of what we eat and also serve a protective function in warning of potentially deleterious substances. Sweetness is associated with high-carbohydrate food items needed for energy and protein sparing. The taste for sweetness is present at birth and has been shown to be pleasant to newborns. The qualities of acid and bitter taste protect from potentially injurious substances. Most of the toxic plant alkaloids have a bitter, hence aversive, taste.

Both the taste buds and receptors in the olfactory epithelium markedly influence salivary gland flow and thus mastication and deglutition. Some studies even show that, by their response to the presence of food in the oral cavity, they influence the gastrointestinal secretion of various digestive enzymes as well. However, the tremendous complexity of the relationships among taste buds, olfactory epithelial cells, and temperature, pain, and tactile receptors in the selection of foods is beyond the scope of this discussion. Nevertheless, the importance of these factors should not be overlooked, especially when dealing with persons for whom sensory acuity has been reduced by sickness or aging.

Salivary Glands

The three major salivary glands are paired structures with ducts that open into the oral cavity. The parotid gland, which is serous in nature, empties into the mouth on the buccal mucosa opposite the maxillary permanent first molar. The submaxillary gland, which is both mucous and serous, drains into the anterior part of the floor of the mouth on the frenum lingual to the mandibular incisors. The sublingual gland is essentially mucous in nature and empties through the duct of the submandibular gland and through multiple openings on the ventral surface of the tongue, where it joins the oral mucosa. In addition to secreting saliva, these glands provide inorganic ions (e.g., calcium, phosphorous) in concentrations sufficient to facilitate enamel remineralization and reduce the potential for demineralization. A number of organic molecules also are secreted. Some have lubricating, enzymatic, or antimicrobial capabilities; the significance of others is unknown.

One of the secreted macromolecules, immunoglobulin A (IgA), has protective functions that are directed against the colonization of certain pathogenic organisms. Secretory IgA is a dimeric form of serum IgA but has a smaller protein (transport piece) bound to it that seems to prevent its rapid denaturation in the oral cavity.

There are also a number of degradative enzymes in saliva, most of which probably provide little molecular degradation in the adult but may have some digestive function in the young child. The salivary enzyme in greatest amount is am-

ylase, which may break down some starch in the oral cavity, particularly if the starch is not cleared rapidly by swallowing.

Periodontal Tissues

The periodontal tissues anchor the teeth in the jaws.[3]

Gingivae. The gums or gingivae are keratinized squamous epithelium that covers the subjacent connective tissue and alveolar bone and merges with the oral mucosa. These tissues are divided into the attached gingiva, which merges with the oral mucosa, and the free (marginal) gingiva, which surrounds the necks of the teeth and acts as a transition zone between the attached (fixed) gingiva and the tooth. At the base of the gingival sulcus, the junctional epithelium attaches the gum to the tooth at the cementoenamel junction. The gingival papillae have a connective-tissue core containing many collagen fibers that connect the gums to the cementum of the tooth and surrounding bone.

Alveolar bone. Beneath the gums and connective tissue is the spongy alveolar bone, in which the roots of the teeth lie. This bone is formed as teeth erupt and is partially lost when teeth exfoliate. The plates of the buccal and lingual surfaces are thin compact bone, as is the lining of the tooth socket, the lamina dura.

Periodontal ligament. Between the lamina dura and the root of the tooth lies the dense collagenous periodontal ligament, whose fibers insert (on one side) into bone and (on the other) into the cementum of the root surface. The fibers of the periodontal ligament act as shock absorbers spreading the large forces of mastication over a wide area.

Teeth

Besides alveolar bone, the three other oral hard tissues are enamel, dentin, and cementum.

Enamel. Enamel is the hardest and most highly mineralized substance in the body. It forms a cap of variable thickness over the tooth. It is formed by ameloblasts, which derive from an ectomesenchyme, probably of neural crest origin. Only 2% to 3% of the enamel is organic matter, and its crystals are 200 times larger than those found in bone.[4]

Dentin. The bulk of the tooth consists of dentin, a bonelike substance of mesodermal origin that surrounds the pulp cavity in the center of the tooth. Tiny extensions of the odontoblasts of the pulp chamber radiate out to the dentoenamel junction. These dentinal tubules become calcified as teeth wear or decay. When stimulated by wear or decay, the odontoblasts that line the pulp chamber can lay down secondary reparative dentin, which effectively removes the vital pulp from the source of the stress. Besides the odontoblasts, the pulp contains numerous blood vessels and nerves embedded in a collagenous matrix.[5]

Cementum. Lying on the surface of the root dentin is cementum, a bonelike mineral that is laid down by cementoblasts and into which the collagen fibers of the periodontal membrane insert.

• • •

The primordia of the primary teeth begin to calcify in utero during about the fourth month of gestation. At birth most of the crowns of the lower primary incisors are complete whereas the crowns of the upper incisors are about two third complete. The crowns of the primary canines and molars are not completely calcified until 6 months to 1 year of age.

Although the primordia of many of the permanent teeth are present before birth, crown calcification does not begin until after birth. Except for the third molars, the process is complete by age 8 to 9 years.[6]

Metabolic disturbances during the last trimester of gestation and the first few postnatal months may cause aberrations in crown formation of the primary teeth. The maternal-fetal relationship generally protects the developing tissues of the child but is not perfect, since severe metabolic disturbances (e.g., Rh incompatibility) often result in hypoplasia of developing teeth. If no metabolic problem exists, the calcification of prenatal tooth structure is far more perfect than that of early postnatal tooth structure. Severe protein restriction of pregnant rats has been shown to result in smaller teeth of the offspring and a greater caries susceptibility. The major limiting factor seems to be methionine. This has not been demonstrated in humans, probably because prenatal dental development is limited.

Birth is manifested dentally by a short period of arrested growth and calcification that can be seen microscopically as the neonatal line. The actual cause of this growth arrest is not known;

it may merely represent the transient metabolic readjustment of birth. However, the grossly evident hypoplastic neonatal lines seen in children in developing countries occur in association with low vitamin A stores and/or neonatal infection. Strangely, the prevalence of such lines in children recovering from severe protein-energy malnutrition was found in one study[7] to be three times that occurring in the general poorly nourished population. The suggestion has been made that the same familial and socioeconomic factors that predispose to severe protein-energy malnutrition in children operate in the neonatal period to produce enamel hypoplasia.

Growing teeth are quite susceptible to disturbances in normal metabolism associated with systemic infection. Although usually discernible only by microscopy, certain states may cause gross enamel hypoplasia. Disturbances in serum levels of calcium and phosphorus (i.e., hypophosphatemia, rickets, hypoparathyroidism) can disrupt tooth mineralization.

The permanent dentition may reflect metabolic disturbances occurring from about 6 months to 8 years of age when the individual teeth are being formed or calcifying.

DENTAL CARIES

Dental caries is a multifaceted chronic disease that has been a major problem in developed countries (and less of a problem in underdeveloped countries, where the diet is less conducive to the disease*). The basic lesion results from demineralization of the enamel by acids formed from sugars in microbial plaques or mats. The initial lesion involves subsurface dissolution of mineral. If the process is not reversed, the enamel becomes cavitated, creating a favorable anatomic niche for further bacterial growth, dissolution of enamel, and progression of the lesion into the dentin and toward the pulp.[8]

In older people with receding gums, the initial lesion may occur on the exposed cementum or dentin. These cemental carious lesions seem to be caused by a different bacterial flora from what exists in enamel lesions.

Enamel demineralization occurs intermittently when fermentable substrates are present

---

*This balance is changing as the overall decay rate in developed countries decreases and the rate in emerging nations that are adopting a more westernized diet increases.

for the microbial flora to metabolize to acid end products. The process may remain stationary when the flora lacks such substrates or it may reverse when the appropriate concentrations of inorganic ions are present to facilitate remineralization. The rate at which a lesion progresses depends on the balance between demineralization and remineralization as determined by the resistance of the enamel, the site on the tooth under attack, the frequency and form of fermentable carbohydrates consumed, and the quantity and quality of saliva.

Most carious lesions begin several months before they can be detected. As much as 50% of the enamel substance is lost before a lesion is visible by x-ray examination. Sites most commonly affected are the pits and fissures of the grinding surfaces and the smooth enamel of the crown, particularly the proximal surfaces. This distinction is especially important since systemic fluoride ingestion affects primarily the smooth surfaces, not the pits and fissures. Thus, by consuming fluoridated water throughout the period of dental development, a child benefits by having less dental decay (60% more or less), with 90% of this reduction in smooth surface decay, and 25% to 35% in decay of pits and fissures. Since smooth surface decay is the most difficult to detect and repair, this finding is especially significant.

Any discussion of a multifaceted disease such as dental caries is clarified by considering the various susceptibility and resistance factors in the agent, the host, and the environment.

Agent

Dental caries does not develop without appropriate bacteria. Germ-free caries-susceptible rats fed a highly cariogenic diet do not develop caries. Similarly, humans who have been maintained for long periods on antibiotic prophylaxis have a significantly reduced number of carious lesions. Although it is clear that microorganisms are needed to produce caries, it is less clear which ones bear the prime role in the initiation and progression of the lesions.[9]

Lactobacilli long were thought to play the predominant role in the disease process because of the numbers found in plaque accumulations on teeth and in saliva and because they are quite acidogenic and aciduric. Recent evidence indicates that *Streptococcus mutans* plays a more significant part, at least in initiating lesions. This organism synthesizes an extracellular polymer, glucan, from sucrose that is highly viscous and sticky and thus allows the *S. mutans* to stick to smooth surfaces of the teeth. Ordinarily these smooth surfaces are difficult to colonize because of the abrasive action of tongue and cheek and the presence of saliva. Once a lesion is established, the niche is available for a larger variety of acidogenic organisms. Pit and fissure sites, by their anatomic shape, do not seem to require adhesion as a prerequisite for establishing a cariogenic microbial plaque, since the depths of such areas offer their own protective environments.

The lactobacilli, *S. mutans,* and other acidogenic organisms can maintain a pH of 5.5 and below. At these values the hydroxyapatite crystals of the enamel begin to dissolve. In germfree rats that subsequently are monoinfected, various microorganisms are capable of eliciting smooth surface and fissure decay. Thus it may be impossible to pinpoint absolutely which microorganism is the prime offender. Some immunologic studies in rats and monkeys have shown caries-protective effects of vaccines directed against *S. mutans.* One issue is clear: the total numbers of acidogenic organisms increase in proportion to the provision of fermentable carbohydrate. As the amount and frequency of substrate are increased, so are the potential pathogens.

Host

Genetic factors. Frequently a parent ascribes severe dental decay in a child to heredity. The data supporting such a position, however, are weak. Although epidemiologic surveys of people from developing nations and remote areas of the world have supported the role of heredity in caries resistance, this was often due to the fact that the rate of dental caries in adults seemed low in comparison to that of adults from developed nations. It was thought that the gene pool of such groups produced teeth and an oral environment that were not conducive to dental decay. However, when these groups (e.g., Eskimos) began to consume refined flours and foods available at trading posts or when they moved en masse into an industrialized society, remarkable increases in dental caries occurred.[10] More recently studies of monozygotic and dizygotic twins[11] have shown a very small genetic component in decay resistance. The caries experience of identical twins is similar but does not parallel that of other siblings or of dizygotic twins of the same sex. Controlled animal studies indicate that selective inbreeding can produce strains of rodents susceptible or resistant to decay. The major differences between such strains seem to be in the shape of the fissures of the teeth and in the saliva.

The genetic influences at work in humans probably are similar. A further genetic influence may be in the size of teeth and jaws, since if the teeth are small, as in Down's syndrome, or the jaws large enough that spacing occurs proximal caries tends to be reduced because access to these areas facilitates both self-cleansing and personal oral hygiene.

Developmental factors. The earliest experimental studies of developmental influences on the teeth and gums were nutritional. Wolbach and Howe[12,13] indicated the need for vitamin A to maintain the functional secretory capacity of ameloblasts and for adequate ascorbic acid to promote proper functioning of the odontoblast in laying down dentin matrix. Vitamin D also was shown to be necessary to promote adequate mineralization of both enamel and dentin matrices. Others showed that gross deficiencies of calcium or phosphorus or of unbalanced calcium:phosphorus ratios had adverse effects on the mineralization of enamel and dentin.

These experimental nutritional imbalances are not likely to be found in human populations, and the epidemiologic evidence is inadequate to indicate any clear effect on caries susceptibility. However, the fact that such nutritional deficiencies or imbalances can alter the tissues of the host indicates the need to insure that the diet contains adequate amounts of these nutrients, especially during tooth development (i.e., through age 10 yr).

Experimental data[14] also indicate that borderline protein deficiency in rats can alter tooth size and shape as well as salivary gland size and saliva quantity and quality. Each of the changes increases caries susceptibility.

Diets with an increased density of calories from fat and protein result in a lower rate of decay, probably not only because of diminished sugars but also from physical factors favoring oral clearance.

Saliva may be the host's most important non-dental protective mechanism against dental caries. Changes in its quantity and perhaps in its inorganic ion or organic IgA or lysozyme composition may have deleterious effects on dentition. When major salivary glands are removed in animals[15] or humans, or when glands atrophy as a result of radiation therapy, the caries rate increases markedly.

Although borderline protein deficiency in rats has been shown to increase dental caries, human studies of protein-energy malnutrition do not show a clear relationship, perhaps because the economic conditions that dictate such malnutrition also militate against the consumption of high amounts of refined carbohydrate, particularly between meals. Some investigators[16] point to the paradox of a high rate of decay among children in many developing countries, where the prevalence of caries is very low in adult populations. The paradox has not been generally recognized because most nutritional surveys of such populations have not examined very young children. When young children have been examined, frequently the decay rate was very high, particularly in teeth formed during the neonatal period. Some other data[17] suggest an interplay of inadequate vitamin A stores and neonatal infection that may create hypoplastic defects of teeth, increasing their susceptibility to caries.

Deficiencies of the nutrients previously described may have some role in caries susceptibility, but the single nutrient associated unequivocally with increasing host resistance to decay is fluoride. Early in the twentieth century white mottling of teeth was associated with low rates of caries and with drinking water supplies. In the early 1930s the factor in water sources was found to be fluoride. Studies by Dean et al.[18] indicated that where the fluoride content was between 1 and 1.5 ppm fluoride helped prevent caries and enamel mottling was insignificant. The lowered decay rate persisted at least through middle age, when tooth loss from periodontal disease tended to obscure the data. The greatest reduction in decay was on the smooth surfaces of permanent teeth, particularly the anteriors. In addition to reducing the overall rate of decay by some 60%, fluoride resulted in lesions that were smaller and more easily restored. Thus far fewer teeth needed to be extracted because of pulpal involvement.

The ameloblast appears to be the most sensitive cell in humans to excess fluoride intake. In a temperate region, water containing more than 1.5 to 2 ppm of fluoride will alter ameloblast function and produce aberrations of crystal structure. The severity of mottling is a function of fluoride in excess of 2 ppm.

Studies in communities with fluoride contents greatly in excess of 1 ppm and in experimental animals showed no discernible physiologic effects at doses of less than 20 mg/day (1 liter of water of 1 ppm fluoride = 1 mg fluoride). At fluoride levels greater than 20 mg/day consumed over a number of years, skeletal fluorosis can result in osteoarthritis. This has been observed only in certain industrial and mining situations where cryolite dust has been a hazard and in certain areas in India.

In the middle 1940s clinical trials were begun in a number of cities. The natural fluoride content of the water supply was adjusted to 1.0 ppm or the equivalent concentration based on the mean annual temperature, which regulates water intake. The data after about 10 years showed the expected decrease in dental decay for teeth formed during the period of optimal fluoride intake. Teeth largely formed without adequate dietary fluoride benefited to some extent but not maximally. Although fluoride is deposited throughout the tooth during development, the major accretion occurs on the outer enamel surface after crown formation is complete and prior to eruption into the oral cavity. Undoubtedly, the enamel continues to accrete fluoride from food, water, toothpaste, and saliva after eruption, but the maximum benefit is achieved before the tooth erupts. The tooth probably is not fully mineralized when it erupts into the oral cavity. If it lacks the protective fluorhydroxyapatite crystal structure that resists the potentially destructive environmental influences of the mouth, it can decay readily before full maturity is achieved via the mineralization potential of saliva.

The mechanism by which fluoride protects against caries is not known for certain, but experimental data indicate a reduced acid solubility of the fluorhydroxyapatite crystal as compared to unsubstituted hydroxyapatite. Crystalographic studies have shown that the fluoride-substituted crystal is larger and more stable than the crystal without fluoride. Finally, remineralization is facilitated by the presence of fluoride ions in the surrounding medium. Thus, fluoride ions in the area of demineralization may shift the equilibrium toward more remineralization than if absent.[19]

There is confusion both on the part of the public and among some health professionals about administering substances containing fluoride. The benefits of toothpastes, rinses, and professionally applied topical fluoride treatments are equated with those derived from fluoridated water or a daily fluoride supplement during the critical periods of tooth development. Topical fluorides are effective in reducing dental decay by about 20% for fluoridated toothpastes and 40% to 50% for mouth rinses containing fluoride when used daily or weekly. However, topical fluoride agents are effective only when used regularly and do not lend themselves to mass public health programs. In addition to being less effective than systemic fluorides in reducing decay, topical fluoride agents are less cost effective. No procedure is more economical than water fluoridation, which approximates $0.25 to $1.00 per person per year. The effectiveness of highly concentrated topical fluoride vehicles is probably due more to a bactericidal action than to the suggested mechanism for systemic fluoride incorporation into tooth structure.[20]

Opponents of water fluoridation suggest that since very little of the water consumed by a community is drunk it would be more economical to provide fluoride pills. Aside from the fallacy of cost, however, such efforts usually are doomed to failure because of poor compliance. In addition, fluoride supplements of 0.5 mg/day given from birth through age 3 years have produced unnecessary mild mottling of the very early-forming parts of some permanent teeth.[21] For this reason the recommended daily supplements have been reduced to 0.25 mg of fluoride below age 2 years, 0.5 mg until age 3 years, and 1 mg after age 3 years.

Although the dental benefits from consuming optimally fluoridated water are well known and unequivocal, there is evidence that the skeletal acquisition of fluoride over a lifetime also benefits adults by reducing the prevalance of osteoporosis.

An early study of Bernstein et al.[22] suggested that older residents of two communities whose water supply contained 4.0 and 5.8 ppm of fluoride exhibited fewer instances of vertebral collapse detected radiographically than did comparable residents from three communities whose water contained from 0.15 to 0.3 ppm. A more recent confirmation of these findings comes from a study in Finland[23] of the incidence of femoral-neck fractures in two communities one of which had a water supply optimally fluoridated at 1.0 ppm and the other whose water contained only trace amounts of fluoride. The data indicated that the risks of fracture was 2.5 and 1.5 times greater for men and women, respectively, who lived in the low-fluoride communities.

Over 10 million Americans live in communities where the water naturally contains fluoride in optimum concentrations and another 100 million have had their water supplies adjusted to an optimum fluoride level; nevertheless, opposition to fluoridation persists. None of the objections have withstood the scrutiny of the courts, however, or of any reputable national or international health organization.

Environmental Factors

External. The external factors associated with dental caries are largely socioeconomic. A community's decision about water fluoridation is primarily a sociologic phenomenon. Whether young people have their own money to spend on between-meal cariogenic snacks is largely economic. A major factor in the relatively low caries rates of permanent teeth reported from developing nations is the lack of funds to purchase high–sugar content confections and the lack of places to buy such items. When money and the availability of such foods increase, so does the caries rate.

Other external environmental influences include familial attitudes toward dental health, sound nutrition, and the availability and utilization of dental care. For example, it appears that the removal of infected decayed tooth substance reduces the microbial burden on the teeth and the potential for gross infection of adjacent sound tooth surfaces.

A community that allows nonnutritious high–sugar content foods to be sold in schools during mealtime hours can expect greater potential for dental decay than one that chooses either to prohibit the sale of such items or to restrict the hours during which they can be purchased.

Oral. The oral environment is not a single ecologic entity. The biochemical conditions favoring decay may differ markedly in various parts of the mouth and even in various areas of a single tooth. The pH at the opening of salivary gland ducts differs markedly from that deep in the microbial plaque at the plaque-tooth interface. Within minutes fermentable sugars can cause the pH in dental plaque to drop to a level below that believed to initiate tooth dissolution. The rapid drop to a pH of 5.5 or less usually does not return to the normal value (about 7) for up to 30 minutes.

These pH values are modified by the buffering action of saliva and total salivary flow. If sufficient time occurs between pH drops, areas demineralized during the period of low pH can be remineralized when the pH returns to a more favorable level. If food containing sugar is not readily cleared from the oral cavity, the teeth are subject to decay for longer periods than if the numbers of acidogenic insults are restricted to regular mealtimes. Therefore, it is better to consume a soft drink containing 10% sugar in a short time than to sip it repeatedly over a longer period. Even though the pH drops with rapid consumption, it returns to nondetrimental levels in a half hour; by contrast, with slow sipping it stays below critical levels during the entire time of consumption and for a half hour afterwards.

The frequency of pH drops is also critical, since increased frequency results in longer periods of subcritical levels, severely limiting the time available for remineralization. These characteristics of decay potential were confirmed in a clinical trial conducted over two decades ago. Groups of institutionalized adults were fed supplemental cariogenic amounts of sugar either as a liquid and in bread at meals or as between-meal snacks and/or in a very sticky form. The decay rate of those consuming the supplements as an easily cleared liquid or at mealtimes was affected very little. Those who consumed the supplements between meals and in a very sticky form (toffees) had significantly greater decay than the control group. Sweet foods that are sucked for prolonged periods, such as lozenges and hard candies, have significant decay potential.

Little is known about the cariogenic hierarchy of foods as they are processed or manufactured, nor are all cariogenic foods necessarily manufactured. Foods such as dates, figs, and raisins can cause detrimental pH changes. Despite our current inability to assess the relative cariogenicity of every foodstuff, it seems reasonable to conclude that foods like fresh fruits, crisp vegetables, nuts, pizza, and cheese are preferable as snacks to candy, cake, and gum or lozenges containing sugar.

Federal Trade Commission efforts to promulgate a ruling with regard to the television advertising of highly sugared foods (e.g., some breakfast foods and candies) have elicited data on the relationship between eating presweetened breakfast foods and caries.[24] Not surprisingly, these studies failed to show an association with caries and the consumption of such items. The amount of sugar contained in a serving of presweetened breakfast food is small compared to a day's total sugar consumption and is not likely by itself to cause a significant increase in caries, especially if consumed at mealtime with milk added. However, if the presweetened food is consumed as a snack without milk, which aids in its oral clearance, it should be viewed as having significant cariogenic potential. Estimates that about 10% of presweetened cereals may be eaten in this manner are worrisome.

There is little evidence that starches pose a major cariogenic hazard, since salivary amylase has such a short time to degrade the starch to glucose in the oral cavity. There may be some cariogenic potential, however, with baking and cooking procedures that partially hydrolyze the starch molecule or with starches not easily cleared from deep occlusal fissures on the tooth.

Little reason exists to believe that replacement of sucrose by monosaccharides or disaccharides reduces dental decay appreciably, since most oral microorganisms can metabolize these molecules to acid end products. The use of sugar substitutes in creating food snacks with a lowered cariogenic potential has not been very rewarding, in part because of the difficulty of substituting for sucrose in cooking and baking recipes. Other problems (e.g., the reported carcinogenic potential of saccharin and cyclamates) also have limited the usefulness of sucrose substitution. Currently the dipeptide aspartame is being used in the food industry as a sucrose substitute, particularly in soft drinks. However, there is still controversy as to whether some persons exhibit a sensitivity to it. Reports of seizures and the possibility of elevated phenylalanine levels in individuals at risk have been reviewed by the Council on Scientific Affairs of the American Medical Asso-

ciation,[25] which considered that the consumption of aspartame by normal humans is ". . . safe and not associated with serious adverse health effects." The Council also stated that those who need to control their phenylalanine intake should handle aspartame as any other source of phenylalanine. Xylitol, a sugar alcohol, has been shown to be noncariogenic in humans when used in foods, but it has been implicated in the development of bladder stones and tumors in rats, thus precluding its use in the United States under current regulations. Other substances such as glycyrrhizin and the dihydroxychalcones derived from plant compounds currently also offer the potential for use.[26]

Young children bottle-fed or even breast-fed for prolonged periods have had rampant dental decay that seems to result from the fermentation of lactose.[27] Other host factors contribute to this problem, since the major damage occurs when the child falls asleep with a mouthful of milk. Salivation effectively ceases and tongue and swallowing activity decrease. Under these circumstances the oral microbiota can degrade the carbohydrate, producing acid that can decalcify tooth structure uninterruptedly for prolonged periods. The problem is not usually seen below age 15 months and is avoided easily by not allowing the child to go to sleep with a bottle filled with milk or other fermentable substances or with acid liquids such as juices and soft drinks. There is evidence suggesting that even breast-feeding on demand, if prolonged into the second year or longer, can produce this rampant decay. In developing countries, prolonged breast-feeding also may play a role in starting decay in hypoplastic areas of teeth among children whose primary maxillary incisors characteristically have deep linear hypoplastic grooves. These findings may explain in part the paradoxically high rate of decay seen in children from these countries, but they should not be interpreted as suggesting that breast-feeding be discouraged, particularly in developing nations.

PERIODONTAL DISEASE

In contrast to those associated with dental caries, the epidemiologic factors associated with periodontal disease are poorly understood. They are clearly multifaceted and microbial in nature, but the agent, host and environmental factors remain largely to be elucidated.[28]

Some forms of periodontal disease in the very young do not seem to have gingivitis as a major antecedent but represent a failure of the body's mechanisms to resist infection, as in chemotaxis of leukocytes.[29]

Gingivitis

Gingivitis, by far the most common of the periodontal pathoses, is due to the accumulation of bacterial plaque and metabolic products around the cervical area of the tooth and in the gingival sulcus. It is characterized by erythema, edema, and easily provoked hemorrhage of the gingival vessels. Before the gross manifestations are evident, histologic changes in the walls of the gingival sulci can be seen in as little as 2 to 4 days after normal oral hygiene is stopped. Large numbers of polymorphonuclear leukocytes migrate into the tissue and gingival sulcus. As much as 15% of the gingival collagen disappears and edema fluid and inflammatory cells occupy the available space.

Within a week most of the cells are lymphoid and as much as 60% of the gingival collagen is lost. The pathologic appearance of the lesion at this stage suggests that cellular hypersensitivity is a major contributor to these early lesions[30] Later, antigen-antibody complexes develop around blood vessels in the deeper tissues.

Many periodontists have argued that unresolved gingivitis leads to frank destruction of the peridontal ligament, bone loss, and periodontitis. In fact, most gingival lesions do not progress this way but remain as gingivitis for years. It is not known why the established gingival lesion becomes aggressive and begins to destroy the periodontium. Similarly, it is not possible to predict which gingival lesion will progress to a periodontitis and which will remain as a gingivitis.

Simple gingivitis has certain nutritional components, the amount of bacterial plaque associated with the disease depends on the quantity of fermentable carbohydrates consumed. Unlike the situation with dental caries, with gingivitis mechanical removal of the plaque deposits by brushing and flossing usually leads to a rapid reversal of the inflammation.

Vitamin C deficiency frequently is associated with simple gingivitis, but there is no evidence of a firm relationship.

Scurvy. In frank vitamin C deficiency, gingivitis is often a prominent feature. The gums usually are grossly edematous and hemorrhagic because of the loss of capillary integrity. In addition, the teeth become mobile from a loss of collagen fibers of the periodontal ligament, which anchors the tooth to the bony socket. The condition is not usually evident in areas where teeth have not erupted or have been extracted. If the deficiency is corrected before teeth become so loose that they are lost, the condition usually can be corrected rapidly. When oral hygiene is optimal, gingival signs of deficiency are minimal.

With the many sources of ascorbic acid in the normal diet, it is rare to see adult scurvy except under quite bizarre nutritional intakes. Occasional cases of infantile scurvy are seen when infants do not receive adequate supplemental vitamin C and are maintained on processed milk diets with little vitamin C content. Breast milk of healthy well-nourished mothers contains an adequate amount of vitamin C and the condition is not associated with breast-feeding of infants.

Periodontitis

Little is known about why a simple gingival lesion becomes aggressive and begins to destroy the bone and collagen of the periodontal apparatus. There is not much firm evidence that nutrition plays a major role in the disease process. Although some authors have suggested that imbalances of calcium, phosphorus, and vitamin D may be involved in the loss of integrity of the alveolar bone, few studies have confirmed this. Vitamin C is necessary in maintaining the integrity of the periodontal ligament and attachments. Monkey studies[31] suggest that deficiencies in the B vitamins may be involved in periodontitis, but the lesions produced do not resemble those of ordinary periodontitis and are more akin to the lesions of noma. They probably represent merely a generalized susceptibility of oral tissues to infection because systemic resistance is reduced by malnutrition or disease.

Although there is little that can be said about the role of nutrition in periodontitis, much can be said about the role of eating. Mastication maintains bony stimulation via the tensions exerted on the bone by the periodontal ligament. If periodontal or other oral surgery is necessary, adequate dietary intakes can be achieved for short periods with liquid nutritional preparations, but the patient should be returned as soon as possible to a solid diet using regular table food. Perfectly adequate substitutes for nutritional supplements can be prepared with a kitchen blender and a normal menu.

Acute Necrotizing Ulcerative Gingivitis

Acute necrotizing ulcerative gingivitis (or trench mouth) is moderately common in young adults who have a poor diet and are under acute psychologic stress. The organisms found in the deeper gingival tissues are fusiform bacilli and spirochetes, both of which normally occur in the mouth. The gums between the teeth become necrotic and slough, leaving painful ulcerated interdental areas. During the acute phase of the disease, bland foods are given to maintain adequate nutritive intake but avoid excessive pain.

The organisms found in the gingival tissues of a person with trench mouth seem to be the same as those found in the rapidly progressive gangrenous catastrophic lesion noma. This condition, which is not common, occurs in malnourished populations or immunosuppressed individuals. In most cases the initial lesion seems to originate around the tooth and then involve the deeper facial bones and soft tissues of the cheeks, lips, and surounding areas. Noma also occurs only in periods of major stress associated with protein-energy malnutrition.

The causes of ANUG and noma are not known, but both can be halted quickly by systemic antibiotics (penicillin). The rapid progress of both diseases usually leads to residual tissue damage and scarring.

NUTRITIONAL ABNORMALITIES OF OTHER ORAL TISSUES

Much of the classic nutritional literature dwells on the oral signs and symptoms of deficiencies in the B vitamins and iron. In reality there is great similarity in all the findings such as pain, erythema, atrophy, and superimposed infection. The cellular turnover of most of the oral epithelia is so rapid that the first signs of deficiencies that interfere with cell division or metabolism naturally occur in the oral cavity. Oral signs and symptoms of acute deficiency also are reversed rapidly with treatment.[32]

Usually the epithelium, such as lips and tongue, becomes atrophic and thin with little keratinization. This thinning allows the subjacent vasculature to be more readily apparent and hence the tissue appears redder. The thinning of the labial epithelium often leads to cracking of the commissural areas, producing an angular cheilitis or cheilosis. With repeated cracking and infection, the area can become permanently scarred. The tongue usually loses its filiform papillae, beginning at the tip and progressing posteriorly, allowing the fungiform and foliate papillae to be seen more readily. These papillae may swell, further accentuating the "strawberry" or "pebbled" appearance. Later, even these papillae can be lost, giving the smooth reddened atrophic appearance of many chronic deficiency states. There are no experimental data linking the loss of taste buds with a concomitant loss of taste function, but changes in taste sensation have been reported anecdotally.

Salivary gland swellings in humans have been associated with deficiencies of niacin, thiamine, and vitamin A. It is difficult to relate these nutrients specifically to the swellings, since such deficiencies seldom are found separate from a generalized malnutrition.[33] Realimentation of severely malnourished concentration camp survivors frequently has resulted in parotid gland swellings of an unknown cause.[34]

Deficiencies
Niacin

Niacin deficiency seems to have the clearest manifestations of all the individual vitamin deficiency states. The earliest symptom often is burning pain throughout the oral cavity. The tongue becomes red, swollen, and eventually smooth as the papillae atrophy. Patchy loss of epithelium on the tongue and gums produces raw, bleeding areas. Fissures of the commissural angles of the lips can result in fanlike scarring after an initial stage of maceration.

Riboflavin

The initial commissural changes—pallor becoming erythematous with maceration and fissuring—in riboflavin deficiency are followed rapidly by lingual changes that give the tongue a granular appearance. The magenta-colored tongue associated with this condition at a later stage is probably due to vascular dilation and stasis.[35] Pain is not as prominent a feature as in some other B-vitamin deficiencies.

Pyridoxine

Initial signs of pyridoxine deficiency include a scalding pain of the tongue that progresses to erythema and swelling of the tip. Shallow ulceration of the buccal mucosa and palate responds rapidly to replacement therapy. Cheilitis, if present, responds less readily to therapy.[36]

Folic Acid and Vitamin B₁₂

Deficiencies of folic acid and vitamin B_{12} also involve reddening of the lingual tip and the formation of small ulcers. The tongue eventually takes on a smooth shiny appearance, which may be red or pale depending on the degree of anemia. In vitamin B_{12} deficiency, lingual pain precedes other physical changes and is more prominent than in folic acid deficiency. Ulceration of the buccal mucosa and of the palatal and gingival epithelia, along with cheilitis, may ccur, but these lesions seem more prominent in folic acid deficiency. The painful ulcerated lesions are the same as those in patients receiving antifolate chemotherapeutic agents like methotrexate.

Iron

Iron deficiency can at times produce lingual changes—characterized by lingual pain, swelling, and pallor with subsequent surface atrophy and frequently cheilitis. These symptoms are found only rarely, however.[37] Iron deficiency also may interfere with pyridoxine metabolism, since this vitamin has been found to reverse many of the oral symptoms of iron deficiency.

Protein

Protein deficiency produces many of the tissue changes seen in deficiencies of the B vitamins and iron, but since it is usually part of generalized malnutrition its pure effect is difficult to distinguish from that of the more generalized condition.

Vitamin A

Descriptions of the effect of vitamin A deficiency on oral tissues are contradictory. If signs exist, they probably are attributable to aberrant salivary gland and taste bud function because of hyperkeratosis of ducts and taste pores.

Zinc

One study[38] indicated a possible relationship between zinc deficiency and dysfunctions of taste. The findings were tentative and controversial, however, and more work is needed before a definite relationship can be established.

Oral Cancer

Recently experimental evidence has accumulated indicating that some of the vitamin A–related compounds and also vitamin E may play a beneficial role in cancers of the hamster cheek pouch and tongue induced by 9,10,-dimethyl-1,2-benzanthracene (DMBA). Tongue tumor development was significantly delayed by the twice weekly oral provision of 13-*cis*-retinoic acid, and both the size and the invasiveness of tumors were diminished at the end of the experimental period.[39] Similar results were obtained in the cheek pouch made in a parallel experiment and also by the use of topically applied beta-carotene during various phases of initiation and proliferation of the chemically induced tumors.[40]

Vitamin E (alpha-tocopherol) supplementation in the same animal model evidenced fewer, less invasive, and smaller tumors that exhibited less surface necrosis than in unsupplemented controls.[41]

NUTRITIONAL GUIDELINES

Dietary recommendations for optimum oral health at any age do not differ significantly from those that apply to general health. These are achieved easily by the consumption of a well-balanced diet from each of the major food groupings.

For the young child developing and calcifying teeth, it is important that adequate amounts of calcium, phosphorus, and vitamins A and D be consumed and, if the communal water supply does not contain an optimum amount of fluoride, a supplement be given. Except for fluoride, the other necessary nutrients are readily available from grains, dairy products, fruits, and vegetables that should form a part of each child's diet. Occasionally the child with lactose intolerance may require additional amounts of items such as cheese or green vegetables to assure adequate calcium and phosphorus intakes.

The teenage years present problems in diet management generally and for oral health specifically since the teenager's snacking patterns may result in few full meals and many between-meal snacks. Teenagers should be counseled on the need to avoid snack items that are high in sugar content, and in a form not easily cleared from the mouth. Since the early teen years are when the newly erupted permanent premolars and molars are the most susceptible to decay because of their immaturity, it is critical to reduce the number of daily cariogenic insults to a minimum. The mere proscription of snacking is ineffective. The snacking pattern should make use of foods with low cariogenic potential (e.g., pizza, nuts, popcorn, hamburger, diet soft drinks). Provision of adequate iron intake for the teenage girl is also necessary, not only for adequate oral health but for general health as well.

Little attention has been given to dietary recommendations for good oral health in adults and senior citizens since it is assumed that they receive a well-balanced diet, in which mineral, vitamin, calorie, and protein content is adequate for the metabolic needs of the oral tissues. However, there are periods during which psychologic or metabolic stress may cause inadequate intakes or increased demand and special prescriptions may be necessary. The senior citizen who has lost a mate is at special risk of adopting an eating pattern of convenience that does not include adequate nutrients. Such a person is at risk for developing generalized deficiencies as well as specific oral signs.

Throughout life, but especially in the adult years, it is important to oral health that foods high in sugar content be consumed only at mealtimes and an adequate amount of fibrous foods be eaten, for they facilitate the removal of cariogens by their detersive action. Adults and elderly persons whose food may be soft and high in starch and sugar are at special risk for the development of dental caries on the roots of teeth because of gum recession.

With good oral hygiene, systemic fluoride, and fluoride dentifrices, there is no reason that the two major oral diseases, caries and periodontitis, cannot be virtually prevented.

REFERENCES

1. Bureau of Economic and Behavioral Research, American Dental Association: Dental statistics handbook, 1984-85, Chicago, 1984, The Association.
2. Cutright DE, Bauer H: Cell renewal in the oral mucosa and skin of the rat. I. Turnover time. Oral Surg **23**:249-259, 1967.
3. Williams RC, Zager NI: The periodontium. In Shaw JH, et al, editors: Textbook of oral biology, Philadelphia, 1978, WB Saunders Co, pp 255-276.
4. Garant PR: Microanatomy of the oral mineralized tissues. In Shaw JH, et al, editors: Textbook of oral biology, Philadelphia, 1978, WB Saunders Co, pp 181-225.
5. Cappuccino CC, Sheehan RF: The biology of the dental pulp. In Shaw JH, et al, editors: Textbook of oral biology, Philadelphia, 1978, WB Saunders Co, pp 226-254.
6. Moyers R, Kopel H: Facial growth and dentition. In Lowry GH, editor: Growth and development of children, ed 6, Chicago, 1973, Year Book Medical Publishers Inc, pp 354-384.
7. Sweeney EA, et al: The prevalence of linear hypoplasia of deciduous incisor teeth in malnourished children, Am J Clin Nutr **24**:800-803, 1970.
8. Shaw JH: Cariology: a definition, epidemiology, and etiology of dental caries. In Shaw JH, et al, editors: Textbook of oral biology, Philadelphia, 1978, WB Saunders Co, pp 955-974.
9. Gibbons RJ, van Houte J: Oral bacterial ecology. In Shaw JH, et al, editors: Textbook of oral biology, Philadelphia, 1978, WB Saunders Co, pp 684-705.
10. Barmes DE: Epidemiology of dental disease, J Clin Periodontol **4**:80-93, 1977.
11. Kent RL Jr, Moorrees CFA: Associations in interproximal caries prevalence from a longitudinal twin study, Proc Int Assoc Dent Res, Abstr 526, 1979.
12. Wolbach SB, Howe PR: Tissue changes following deprivation of fat soluble A vitamin, J Exp Med **42**:753-778, 1925.
13. Wolbach SB, Howe PR: The effect of the scorbutic state upon the production and maintenance of intercellular substances, Proc Soc Exp Biol Med **22**:400-402, 1925.
14. Shaw JH, Griffiths D: Dental abnormalities in rats attributable to protein deficiency during reproduction, J Nutr **80**:123-141, 1963.
15. Schwartz A, Shaw JH: Studies on the effect of selective desalivation on the dental caries experience of albino rats, J Dent Res **34**:239-247, 1955.
16. Russell AL: World epidemiology and oral health, In Kreshover SJ, McClure FJ, editors: Environmental variables in oral disease, Washington DC, 1966, American Association for the Advancement of Science, pp 21-39.
17. Sweeney EA, et al: Factors associated with linear hypoplasia of human deciduous incisors, J Dent Res **48**:1275-1279, 1969.
18. Dean HT, et al: Domestic water and dental caries. V. Additional studies of the relation of fluoride domestic waters to dental caries experience in 4,425 white children aged 12 to 14 years of 13 cities in 4 states, Public Health Rep **57**:1155-1179, 1942.
19. Shaw JH, Sweeney EA: Nutrition in relation to dental medicine. In Goodhart RS, Shils MF, editors: Modern nutrition in health and disease, Philadelphia, 1980, Lea & Febiger, pp 852-891.
20. Loesche WJ: Topical fluorides as an antibacterial agent, J Prev Dent **4**:21-25, 1977.
21. Aasenden R, Peebles TC: Effects of fluoride supplementation from birth on human deciduous and permanent teeth, Arch Oral Biol **19**:321-326, 1974.
22. Bernstein DS, et al: Prevalence of osteoporosis and high and low fluoride areas in North Dakota, JAMA **198**:499-504, 1966.
23. Simonen O, Laitinen O: Does fluoridation of drinking water prevent bone fragility and osteoporosis? Lancet **2**:432-434, 1985.
24. Glass RL, Fleisch S: Diet and dental caries; dental caries incidence and the consumption of ready-to-eat cereals, J Am Dent Assoc **88**:807-813, 1974.

25. Council on Scientific Affairs, American Medical Association: Aspartame: review of safety issues, JAMA **254:**400-402, 1985.

26. Scheinen A, et al: Final report on the effect of fructose and xylitol diets on the caries incidence in man, Acta Odontol Scand **33**(suppl 70):67-104, 1975.

27. Dilley FJ, et al: Prolonged nursing habit; a profile of patients and their families, J Dent Child **47:**102-108, 1980.

28. Page RC, Schroeder HE: Pathogenesis of inflammatory periodontal disease, Lab Invest **34:**235-249, 1976.

29. Horton JE, et al: A role for cell-mediated immunity in the pathogenesis of periodontal disease, J Periodontol **45:**351-360, 1974.

30. Chapman OD, Harris AE: Oral lesions associated with dietary deficiencies in monkeys, J Infect Dis **69:**7-17, 1941.

31. Tanner ACR, et al: A study of the bacteria associated with advancing periodontal disease in man, J Clin Periodontol **6:**278-307, 1979.

32. Driezen S: Oral indications of the deficiency states, Postgrad Med **49:**97-102, 1971.

33. Buchner A, Sreebny LM: Enlargement of salivary glands, Oral Surg **34:**209-222, 1972.

34. Sandstead HR, et al: Enlargement of the parotid gland in malnutrition, Am J Clin Nutr **3:**198-214, 1955.

35. Sydenstricker VP, et al: Ariboflavinosis with special reference to the ocular manifestations, South Med J **34:**165-170, 1941.

36. Vilter RW, et al: The effect of vitamin B_6 deficiency induced by desoxypyridoxine in human beings, J Lab Clin Med **42:**335-357, 1953.

37. Jacobs A, Cavill I: The oral lesions of iron deficiency anaemia; pyridoxine and riboflavin status, Br J Haematol **14:**291-295, 1968.

38. Atkin-Thor E, et al: Hypogeusia and zinc depletion in chronic dialysis patients, Am J Clin Nutr **31:**1948-1951, 1978.

39. Shklar G, et al: Retinoid inhibition of lingual carcinogenesis, Oral Surg **49:**325-332, 1980.

40. Shklar G, et al: Inhibition of hamster buccal pouch carcinogenesis by 13-cis-retinoic acid, Oral Surg **50:**45-52, 1980.

41. Odukoya O, et al: Retardation of experimental oral cancer of topical vitamin E, Nutr Cancer **6**(2):98-104, 1984.

CHAPTER 21
The Eye

David A. Newsome

People are highly interested in their eyes. This interest extends beyond the fear of blindness, which ranks second only to fear of cancer in the hierarchy of phobias shared by many Americans. It is not uncommon for the physician to be asked, "Is there anything I can do to help my eyes?" in addition to whatever medications or optical aids may have been prescribed. The answer is: Yes. This chapter provides specific information on nutrition as it relates to both the developing and the adult eye. Some simple recommendations that obstetricians, pediatricians, internists, family practitioners, nutritionists, and others may share with appropriate patients are offered based on current laboratory and clinical scientific knowledge.

Knowledge of nutritional influences on ocular development, structure, and function has increased significantly in the past decade. Notable advances have been made in elucidating prenatal nutritional influences on eye development, and nutritional management recently has been emphasized in the control of certain metabolic disorders that affect the eye. However, our understanding of the many ways in which the foods we eat affect our eyes remains incomplete. Increasing numbers of nutritional and nutrition-related diseases are recognized to have prominent ocular manifestations. As general dietary conditions have changed, diseases like scurvy have become less prevalent. In some cases the reasons for these trends are apparent; in others they remain mysterious. For example, attempts to relate the decreased incidence of tobacco-alcohol amblyopia in the United States over the past several decades to a decrease in pipe smoking have proved inconclusive.

The eye is composed of a number of highly specialized and in some cases unique tissues. It has been estimated to contain over 90% connective-tissue elements, with the remaining tissues being neural, muscular, and vascular. The eye is particularly avid in sequestering required nu-trients from the available pool. Several specific nutrients are required by the various ocular components. These special requirements are, of course, superimposed on general nutritional requirements similar to those of other bodily tissues. In the following sections, general and specific nutritional requirements are discussed as they apply to the eye in the prenatal stage and in infancy, childhood, and adulthood.

EYE DEVELOPMENT AND PRENATAL INFLUENCES

Useful visual function depends on an orderly and precisely controlled series of developmental events. The eye commands a disproportionately large share of cortical sensory representation. Its importance to the survival of the individual may also be reflected in its developmental vitality. Animal studies[1] have demonstrated that, with total food deprivation in newborn and prenatal animals, the eye continues to increase in size at a time when body weight actually falls. Measured against other organs in a state of complete deprivation, the rodent eye showed the greatest proportional increase in weight. More recent studies[2] have documented that this weight increase is due to true growth rather than to simple sequestration of water. Even severely malnourished children commonly have prominent and gleaming eyes.

The eye (like the central nervous system, with which it is embryologically, anatomically, and functionally connected) exhibits little postnatal growth in comparison to bones, for example. Thus prenatal nutritional influences affect the eye's structural development and differentiation more directly that they do its functional development.

PROTEINS AND AMINO ACIDS

Proteins are found in the anterior chamber fluid (aqueous) and in the vitreous. Indeed, the major protein component of the vitreous appears to be serum-derived proteins. Ocular tissues require the same eight essential amino acids as other tissues of the body do. Recent investigations[3] have shown a direct influence of dietary protein on raising intraocular pressure, especially retinal concentrations of amino acids such as tyrosine. L-Tyrosine is the precursor of the retinal neurotransmitter dopamine.[4]

Effects of Protein Deficiency

Animals with diets deficient in protein have shown a notable absence of major deleterious effects on eye development.[2] Observations of humans in underdeveloped countries where protein-energy malnutrition is common, as well as in prisoner-of-war camps, have shown similar results.[1] Isolated protein deficiency is uncommon in the United States, except in scattered pockets of extreme poverty and among occasional dietary faddists and certain elderly individuals with poor dietary habits. The major ocular effect directly attributable to a generalized protein deficiency is a change in the refractive state of the eye.

In one study of 110 severely malnourished (marasmic) children aged 1 to 24 months[5] there was a highly significant incidence of myopia when compared to a similar group of healthy controls. Repeated determinations of refractive error made in these malnourished infants during several months of nutritional repletion indicated that the myopic refractive error disappeared. The investigators saw no signs of clinical vitamin A deficiency in this group.

In an experimental dietary study[6] rabbits were fed a diet approximating that eaten by some human vegetarians. The young experimental animals received a green vegetable diet that consisted of a significant percentage of sucrose. The control animals received an unsugared diet. The animals that presumably were protein deficient from the substitution of a large amount of carbohydrate in the diet were significantly more myopic than were the control animals.

The association of other ocular changes with severe protein deficiency in humans is less certain. Several authors have reported night blindness with retinal edema in persons who have undergone starvation. However, because it is difficult to isolate protein deficiency in a human being whose diet is generally poor, a causal relationship cannot be confirmed.

Some observers have taken pains to differentiate protein-deficient night blindness from night blindness that responds to vitamin A. These cases should not be confused with the more recently reported night blindness and decreased retinal function in individuals with intestinal absorption problems.[7] In the latter cases difficulties with absorbing vitamin A and related compounds probably are the primary cause of the ocular problem. Studies in patients undergoing long-term parenteral nutrition[8] have indicated that depressed retinal function can be alleviated by taurine, an endogenously synthesized amino acid usually not thought dietarily essential. It has been suggested[9] that taurine in breast milk may help protect against retinopathy of prematurity.

Accelerated development of senile cataract has been associated with generalized protein deficiency,[10,11] but most reports of kwashiorkor do not describe cataractous or other significant eye changes. Many elderly individuals at risk of cataract consume inadequate protein. Clinicians should encourage such persons to consume adequate amount of protein.

Amino Acid Disorders

Among the large number of disorders of amino acid metabolism described in humans, few have recognized ocular manifestations. Within the past 5 years many advances have been made in understanding not only the basis of these amino acid disorders but also their management. Management usually consists of a highly structured diet that provides for good general nutrition while restricting or otherwise limiting a particular amino acid or group of amino acids. In some of these disorders the experience with dietary therapy remains limited. In others special diets have proved effective. Amino acid disorders with prominent ocular manifestations are listed in Table 21-1.

In addition to the major amino acid disorders, several rare manifestations of abnormal amino acid metabolism (including sulfite oxidase deficiency, maple syrup urine disease, hyperlysinemia, and the more prevalent phenylketonuria) all have been associated with ocular abnormalities, most commonly with cataract or lens dislocation. In at least a few cases dietary management has been helpful in alleviating ocular symptoms. The cataractous manifestations, once established, do not improve with dietary therapy.

Table 21-1 Disorders of Amino Acid Metabolism That Affect the Eye

	Amino Acids Involved	Clinical Features	Nutritional Management
Cystinosis[12-16]	Cystine, methionine	Autosomal recessive Severe form: rickets, progressive renal failure, retarded growth, tissue deposits, including eye Mild form: deposits in ocular tissue and elsewhere; eye deposits not visually important but of diagnostic help; peripheral pigmentary retinopathy	Vitamin C Vitamin D Phosphate Methionine restriction helpful but unpalatable; risk of malnutrition with severe restriction Topical cysteine has been used to remove corneal crystals
Homocystinuria[17-18]	Homocysteine, methionine (cystathionine synthase)	Recessive Mental retardation, seizures, skeletal deformation, hepatomegaly, characteristic facies Ocular findings: glaucoma, lens dislocation, pigmentary retinopathy	Vitamin B_6 (pyridoxine) Methionine restriction (as for cystinosis)
Tyrosinemia	Phenylalanine, tyrosine (p-hydroxyphenyl pyruvic acid–oxidase deficiency in hereditary form; tyrosine aminotransferase deficiency in sporadic)	Mental deficiency, renal deficiency and rickets, hepatosplenomegaly and cirrhosis Ocular findings: cataracts and corneal erosions/ulcers	Phenylalanine and tyrosine restriction
Hyperornithinemia[19-22]	Ornithine, arginine (ornithine aminotransferase deficiency)	Recessive Deficiency of mitochondrial matrix enzyme ornithine aminotransferase Major manifestation: gyrate atrophy of choroid and retina, which can produce blindness; also associated cataracts, myopia	Vitamin B_6 (pyridoxine) helpful in responsive patients; arginine restriction may be helpful but requires careful monitoring to avoid hyperammonemia

For this and other reasons, an ophthalmologist should be part of the medical team treating these complex problems.

A recently reported and rare amino acid vitamin B_{12} disorder has been associated with retinal degeneration.[23] Dietary ingestion of glutamate is known to produce the so-called "Chinese restaurant syndrome" in sensitive persons.[24] Glutamate, at least in dietary amounts, has not been linked to human ocular disease although it has been shown to cause retinal damage in animals.[25]

The complete group of essential amino acids must be bioavailable simultaneously for optimum performance of metabolically active tissues. This point is illustrated by an experiment[10] in which rats were found to develop cataracts with tryptophan deficiency. In the experimental group, cataract formation could be prevented by administering all the essential amino acids, including tryptophan, together. In another experimental group, however, the addition of the tryptophan considerably after the other esential amino acids did not reduce cataract formation. The interactions among vitamins A and E, other nutritional factors, and the amino acids must be considered carefully in planning for adequate nutrition and nutritional therapy.

CARBOHYDRATES

Many ocular tissues have high energy needs. These demands are met in great part by the simpler sugars supplied through dietary carbohydrate intake. Ocular energy needs are usually well supplied by the average United States diet. Moderate dietary carbohydrate intake in the otherwise healthy person is consistent with normal ocular functioning.

Effects of Carbohydrate Excess

Diets that contain excessive amounts of carbohydrate can produce ocular changes that interfere with vision. Pathologic conditions associated with excessive carbohydrate in the diet almost always involve cataractous changes. The one important exception is diabetic retinopathy, although cataracts do develop earlier and more frequently in diabetics than in the healthier nondiabetic population.

Sugar-related pathologic cataracts are initiated, at least in part, by the accumulation of one or another sugar within the lens tissue. To understand the pathophysiologic mechanisms at work, one must keep in mind a few basic facts about the nourishment of the anterior segment of the eye. Both the lens of the eye and the cornea are avascular. The lens derives its nourishment from the aqueous humor in which it is bathed. The aqueous humor, derived from the plasma, is elaborated via the ciliary epithelium. It contains serum proteins, vitamins, mineral components and simple carbohydrates, including glucose. The lens is permeable to all these constituents of the aqueous humor except some of the proteinaceous ones. When glucose is present in a high concentration in the blood and subsequently the aqueous humor, it accumulates in the lens. This causes immediate osmotic changes in the lens, directly affecting its refractive index and focusing properties and blurring the vision. Since this process usually is acute, diabetic patients frequently experience blurred vision "when their sugar is high" or prior to insulin administration. The disruptive effect of unusual sugar accumulation within the lens probably initiates the more chronic and permanently destructive changes that have been seen in both animals and humans. Certain animals develop cataracts when their diet contains an excessive amount of a particular carbohydrate.[26] In humans, however, ingestion of excessive amounts of glucose does not cause permanent cataractous change directly.[27]

The lens maintains its osmotic balance through a finely tuned sodium-potassium ATP pump system. This pump system, in turn, depends on glucose for energy. As mentioned, glucose diffuses into the lens. However, under conditions of usual glucose concentration in the aqueous humor, the rate of utilization appears to be similar to the rate of diffusion. Thus a high carbohydrate load or inadequate pancreatic function can cause glucose to accumulate in the lens. The bulk of glucose metabolism within the lens utilizes anaerobic glycolysis, with a smaller proportion using aerobic glycolysis. There is also a unique pathway of carbohydrate metabolism important to the lens: the sorbitol pathway.[26] When the glucose concentration is normal, the sorbitol pathway is inactive. Local hyperglycemia activates the sorbitol pathway and results in the conversion of glucose to sorbitol, a reaction catalyzed by aldose reductase. The sorbitol itself may be further converted to fructose via a polyol dehydrogenase pathway. Accumulation of sorbitol and fructose within the lens produces optical changes similar to those produced by glucose. Intensive work using animal models of sugar cataracts has led to the availability of aldose reductase inhibitors for clinical use.[28,29] Several commercial inhibitors are now being tested in multicenter clinical trials.[30,31] Other naturally occurring dietary constituents, the flavonoids, are potent aldose reductase inhibitors but have not yet been clinically tested.[32]

It is not uncommon for newly diagnosed diabetics to have become somewhat myopic or nearsighted prior to hypoglycemic treatment, and to become more hyperopic or farsighted after treatment has been underway for several days. In these cases the opacities of the anterior cortex of the lens stabilize following institution of therapy.

Not all lens-related changes in diabetics are transient. Diabetics often have typical senile cataract some years earlier than a similar population of nondiabetics. The variability of refractive error and the reversibility of milder lens changes are probably directly related to the change in osmotic pressure within the lens from accumulations of various sugars. Cataractous changes in diabetes progress at a pace directly related to the concentration of glucose in the aqueous humor, which is significantly affected by the concentration of glucose in the bloodstream and hence in the diet. Good control of a diabetic's blood sugar can minimize these changes.[27] It is not clear whether strict maintenance of the so-called normal blood sugar range reduces both the senile type of cataractous change and the posterior subcapsular-cortical cataract change that is typical of diabetics.[33]

One major unanswered question in the nutritional and metabolic management of diabetes concerns the relationship between the development and progression of diabetic retinopathy and the control of blood sugar.[34,35] Even diabetic patients who maintain strict control of their blood sugar levels are not free of the risk of diabetic retinopathy. Completely scientific studies of blood sugar control and the development of diabetic cataractous changes and other changes are extremely difficult to execute. However, the studies that have been done consistently demonstrate either a small beneficial effect of good control or no effect at all.[36-38] None of the studies shows a deleterious effect. Some investigators[39] claim that continuous subcutaneous insulin reduces diabetic retinopathy, but others[40] have discovered no positive and perhaps a slightly deleterious effect on retinopathy. Therefore it is prudent to advise diabetic patients to maintain good control, insofar as is practical, and, considering the clinical revolution in treating the ocular complications of diabetes,[41,42] to refer all diabetics with eye ground changes for a baseline evaluation.

Effects of Hypoglycemia

Abnormally low blood sugar, hypoglycemia, can produce lens changes in humans. Hypoglycemia also has been associated with the clouding of lenses in rats. In these animals, when glucose was pharmacologically blocked from utilization in the energy pathways of the lens, cataractlike changes resulted.[43] Cataractous changes also are common in human newborns with hypoglycemia. There may be associated findings, including optic atrophy and deterioration in the central nervous system. This problem is most frequently seen in low–birth-weight babies. The tendency toward severe hypoglycemic episodes in the newborn may be caused in part by maternal fasting around the time of delivery. This fasting raises insulin levels, lower carbohydrate stores, and sets the stage for the hypoglycemic episode. Although some cataractous changes may be reversed, at least in part, optic and central nervous system changes are irreversible.

Disorders of Galactose Metabolism

The two major disorders of galactose metabolism differ widely in severity as well as in the specific enzymes that are deficient.

The more severe form, galactosemia, is inherited as an autosomal recessive trait. The disease is due to a deficiency of galactose-1-phosphate uridyltransferase, which is involved in the metabolism of galactose to glucose. Laboratory studies utilizing human tissues and cell cultures have demonstrated that galactose-1-phosphate and dulcitol accumulate in the tissues of affected individuals. This accumulation produces pathologic changes, including cataract, failure to thrive, mental retardation, hepatosplenomegaly and aminoaciduria. Cataracts are extremely common.

The milder form of galactose metabolic defect involves a deficiency of the enzyme glactokinase. Patients deficient in this enzyme are frequently afflicted with cataracts but spared the more severe manifestations of galactosemia. In fact, one study[44] showed 15% of heterozygotes with a detectable deficiency of galactokinase. Another study of galactokinase concentrations in mothers of children with idiopathic cataracts[45] demonstrated maternal deficiency of the enzyme, although the children had normal enzyme concentrations.

For both of these entities, galactose restriction is the preferred treatment. One prime source of galactose is the lactose in milk. Commercial yogurt has a high content (about 25%) of utilizable galactose and, when it is the sole diet in rats, has been associated with congenital cataracts.[46] Strict avoidance of lactose and galactose, from the first days of life, can prevent cataract formation. The use of lactose-free formula therapy may slow or halt the progression of cataractous changes and, in some cases, produce a frank regression of the cataract.[47,48]

There have been rare reports of false-normal assays for galactosemia in newborns.[48,49] In an infant with cataracts, especially of the zonular type, vomiting, and failure to thrive, a normal Beutler spot test should be confirmed by quantitative chemistry and confounding factors such as transfusion of normal erythrocytes carrying galactose-1-phosphate uridyltransferase considered.[48]

Studies in an Indian population[50] have associated childhood episodes of severe dehydration from a cholera-type illness with a threefold to fourfold increased incidence of presenile cataract. A history of heat stroke further increased the risk of cataract. Both insults produce blood solute imbalances, including elevated urea, that may damage lens proteins.

Other Sugars

Animal studies have identified certain sugars other than those already discussed as experimentally important cataractogenic agents. Xylose (found in plants), galactose, arabinose, and, of course, glucose all have been shown to be cataractogenic in animals. They have been ranked in potency, with D-xylose being the most potent. Newborn and young animals are much more susceptible to the cataractogenic effects of these materials than are older animals. Certain of the changes are reversible.

Persons who have adopted diets consisting largely of milk products, including yogurt, may be at risk for developing galactose cataract changes. Such dietary patterns should be discouraged in pregnant women.

A study in Italy[51] showed that among regular milk drinkers those who could hydrolyze and absorb lactose and associated sugars efficiently were more likely than the nonabsorbers or inefficient absorbers to have cataracts. This observation suggests that the dietary use of sources of lactose-hydrolyzing enzymes such as yogurt[52] along with lactose-rich products such as milk could provide repeated galactose challenge to the lens and thus possibly promote cataract.

Treatment of Sugar Cataracts

No medical therapeutic agents are currently accepted for the retardation or prevention of cataracts. Laboratory studies,[53] however, have shown that in experimental animals vitamin E can ameliorate experimental galactose-induced cataracts. There is much interest in anticataract drugs, and the future development of useful agents is possible.

DIETARY FATS

Certain ocular tissues, particularly the sensory retina, which is a typical central neural tissue, have high lipid contents. However, the concentration of dietary fats does not often produce direct effects on the eye.

Dietary fat deficiency in humans has not been shown to affect the eye. In experimental animals deprived of essential fatty acids and dietary fats, reduced visual acuity and lipid and cholesterol crystal deposition in various ocular tissues have been reported.[54-56] Linoleic and arachidonic acids have been administered to cure signs of essential fatty acid deficiency in rats; they also improved the electroretinographic response in these animals.

In humans hyperlipoproteinemias have varying degrees of ocular manifestation. This group of disorders is related to a combination of heredity and environment. Disorders of lipid metabolism that are amenable to dietary as well as chemical management have various ocular manifestations, which are summarized in Table 21-2. Dietary management of the hyperlipoproteinemias appears to be safer than drug therapy. A few ocular side effects from some of the blood lipid–lowering drugs have been reported, primarily cataract formation.

A small group of uncommon hereditary diseases involving abnormalities of dietary fat metabolism has prominent ocular manifestations. The Bassen-Kornzweig syndrome (abetalipoproteinemia) is inherited as an autosomal recessive trait. Primary systemic characteristics of the syndrome include malabsorption, steatorrhea, ataxia, acanthocytosis, and cardiovascular disease at an early age. The ocular manifestations are dominated by a pigmentary retinal degeneration with anatomic features similar to those of retinitis pigmentosa. Retinal blood vessel narrowing, clumping of pigment in the retinal midperiphery, optic nerve pallor, abnormal visual fields, poor dark adaptation, and reduced electroretinographic responses are typical. One histologic difference between this disorder and typical retinitis pigmentosa is that in abetalipoproteinemia both rods and cones are lost early and outer nuclear layer changes are prominent.[57]

It is thought that the ocular manifestations of abetalipoproteinemia are related to the failure of vitamin A transport and to an associated functional vitamin E deficiency resulting from defective chylomicron formation.[58] Vitamin A deficiency is known to produce severe retinal changes in both humans and experimental animals (see "Vitamin A," p. 332). In some cases the administration of vitamin A parenterally has brought improvement in certain parameters of retinal function, including electroretinographic

Table 21-2 Hyperlipoproteinemias That Affect the Eye

	Ocular Effects	Nutritional Management

Type I: hyperchylomicronemia
  Lipoprotein lipase defi-
    ciency; juvenile onset of-
    ten
	Xanthomas
	Lipid keratopathy
	Lipemia retinalis
		Strictly limit fats
		No routine drug therapy

Type IIA: hypercholesterolemia
  Elevated low-density lipo-
    protein fraction
	Xanthomas
	Xanthelasma
	Arcus senilis
	Retinal cholesterol
		Limit cholesterol
		Drug therapy often (clofi-
		  brate; also cholestyr-
		  amine, colestipol, nico-
		  tinic acid)

Type IIB: hypercholesterolemia and hypertriglyceridemia	Xanthomas Arcus senilis	Limit weight Limit fats Drug therapy (clofibrate)

Type III: hypertriglyceridemia
  Elevated LDL and VLDL;
    may have elevated choles-
    terol also
	Schnyder's corneal dystrophy
	Lipemia retinalis	

Type IV: hypertriglyceridemia	Xanthomas
	Lipemia retinalis
		Limit weight
		Limit simple carbohydrates
		Drug therapy may be ef-
		  fective (clofibrate, nico-
		  tinic acid)

Type V: hyperchylomicronemia
  Increased VLDL; usually as-
    sociated with other dis-
    eases (e.g., diabetic ne-
    phrosis, alcoholism)
	Xanthomas
	Lipemia retinalis
		Limit weight
		Limit fats
		No one drug always effec-
		  tive (nicotinic acid, clo-
		  fibrate used)

responses.[59] Oral administration of vitamin A, along with large doses of vitamin E and dietary fat restriction, also slow the progression of retinal and neurologic disease.[60-62]

Another rare inherited disorder, familial hypobetalipoproteinemia, produces retinal changes similar to those just described for the Bassen-Kornzweig syndrome. Vitamin administration and dietary fat restriction have not proved as beneficial in this group of patients as in those with the Bassen-Kornzweig syndrome.

In Refsum's disease, phytanic acid alpha-hydroxylase is absent. Consequently phytanic and other fatty acids accumulate in tissues, especially those of the central and peripheral nervous systems, the heart, skin, and ear. Symptoms can appear at nearly any age and typically demonstrate periods of exacerbation and remission. Elevated serum phytanic acid confirms the diagnosis. Ocular findings, including pigmentary retinopathy and associated features, are vir-

tually identical to those of abetalipoproteinemia. Histologic studies[63] have revealed widespread deposition of lipids in the retinal layers as well as in other ocular tissues.

The cornerstone of management of Refsum's disease is the avoidance of foods rich in phytanic acid. In particular, fatty meats, seafood, many vegetables, nuts, and unskimmed dairy products must be avoided. Successful adherence to the restricted diet can ameliorate the general neurologic manifestations of the disease; however, little or no change in the pigmentary retinopathy has been reported.

VITAMIN A

Vitamin A has profound effects on nearly every tissue of the body. Epithelial structures are particularly influenced by and dependent on vitamin A, and the eye has many epithelial tissues. In addition, it has a special requirement for vitamin A, since the photosensitive pigment of the rod cells is a specialized form of the vitamin A molecule, retinol. Despite the enormous importance of vitamin A in maintaining the health of human tissues, the only role of vitamin A that is well understood is its visual function. The modified light-receptive form of vitamin A, 11-*cis*-retinol, is the sole photopigment of the rod system; it allows a person to see in very dim illumination. For this reason, night blindness is one of the earliest symptoms of vitamin A deficiency.

Biochemical data[64] indicate that vitamin A enchances glycoconjugate biosynthesis. The synthesized proteins are specialized cell products or are used in maintaining the integrity of the epithelial layer and may increase disease resistance, including resistance to herpes simplex.[65,66]

The profound importance of vitamin A in preserving normal ocular health and function is well illustrated by the pathologic changes termed "xerophthalmia," a word from the Greek that means dry eye. This condition is seldom seen in the United States, except in chronic alcoholics, in pockets of extreme poverty, and in individuals with intestinal malabsorption syndromes either from disease or following surgery. Keratomalacia can also be seen in persons on a self-instituted vitamin A–poor diet, such as strict vegetarians.[67]

In a child with vitamin A deficiency, often complicated by protein-energy malnutrition, the earliest sign of vitamin A deficiency is night blindness.[68] With a persistent lack of vitamin A, the conjunctiva begins to keratinize and take on a dry appearance. A foamy collection can appear near the limbus, termed Bitot's spot. In the absence of vitamin A, the normally unkeratinized corneal epithelium also keratinizes, giving the cornea a dry appearance. When this stage is reached, there is apparently a heightened susceptibility to infection and trauma. The further progression of the disease involves ulceration of the cornea with actual melting away of the front of the eye in the most severe forms. This last condition is termed keratomalacia. In milder forms of the disease, even up to superficial corneal ulceration, administering vitamin A can return the cornea to normal in 48 hours or less. Xerophthalmia usually afflicts children between 1 and 5 years of age and is made more likely by associated diarrheal disease[69] and measles.[70]

Children with cholestasis associated with deficiencies of vitamins A and E can show a variety of ocular and nervous disorders.[71] Vitamin repletion is an essential part of therapy.[72]

Vitamin A deficiency occasionally is seen in adults. Its usual manifestation is night blindness, a disorder much more common in earlier times. A fourteenth-century Dutch poet was probably referring to adult night blindness and its treatment with the lines:

> He who cannot see at night must eat the liver of the goat.
> Then he can see all right.[73]

Night blindness is so characteristic of vitamin A deficiency that field workers in countries where nutritional deficiencies are common use it as an indicator of the prevalence of vitamin A deficiency in the local community.[68] The relationship between vitamin A and night blindness also has been documented by sophisticated psychophysical measurements, including dark adaptometry and its effects on the retina as reflected in a diminished response to electroretinography. Recovery of functional performance has been demonstrated after vitamin A repletion.

Advances in gastrointestinal surgery for the treatment of various diseases have been accompanied by the recognition of nutritional deficiency–related states in some patients.[8,74] Many of these deficiencies involve vitamin A and related nutrients, and they have prominent ocular involvement, including night blindness.[74] Optic atrophy has also been reported.[75] Similar ocular problems caused by deficiency states have also been reported in association with Crohn's disease[76-78] and biliary cirrhosis.[79] Recognition of these conditions is important, since vitamin-nutrient repletion can be either ameliorative or curative.

In vitamin-deficient adults, especially chronic alcoholics, superficial corneal ulceration and other changes have been seen.[80]

Since ocular manifestations of vitamin A deficiency are rare in the United States and in many other countries, both professionals and the lay community tend to ignore the magnitude of the worldwide problem.[81,82] For example, in India alone an estimated 100,000 new cases of blindness resulting from vitamin A deficiency with malnutrition occur annually. In India, Guatamala, and other countries both governmental and private groups have started programs for the administration of vitamin A to children. If these programs could reach all children at risk, the problem might be virtually eliminated. Because of the dietary content of vitamin A and the β-carotenoids that are converted in the body to vitamin A, people in the United States and in other developed countries usually have adequate body stores of vitamin A. Vitamin A has no effect on progressive night blindness in individuals with eye diseases such as retinitis pigmentosa, and little effect in those with inherited disorders of lipid metabolism, such as the Bassen-Kornzweig syndrome.

Side Effects of Ocular Vitamin A Therapy

Vitamin A has been used successfully to reverse night blindness and other ocular complications of its deficiency state. The use of retinoids and related substances for acne or basal cell carcinoma has been associated with various ocular side effects, including anterior segment changes, anterior polar cataract, night blindness, and abnormal retinal function.[83-86] These compounds may interfere with retinol esterification and storage. Hypervitaminosis A can cause a papilledematous appearance of the optic nerve, and should be considered in the evaluation of patients with such findings.[87]

VITAMIN B

Ocular tissues require significant amounts of the B vitamins. Deficiencies affect not only the anterior tissues of the eye but also the retina and optic nerve. However, appropriate administration of B vitamins can prevent blindness in certain diseases.

Ocular manifestations of vitamin B deficiency include changes in the lids, cornea, conjunctiva, and lens. Angular blepharitis, consisting of redness, irritation, breaks in the skin, and crusting at the outer canthus, is a well-known manifestation of riboflavin deficiency and is often associated with angular stomatitis and conjunctivitis. The latter may have a bacterial infectious component. Experimental evidence from both animal and human studies indicates that riboflavin, nicotinic acid, and thiamine deficiencies, separately or together, may be associated with conjunctivitis and with lid swelling and crusting. Pyridoxine is the most important component in alleviating blepharitis in humans. Because of the strong possibility of an infectious component in

conjunctivitis, any therapy also must address this facet of the disease.

Various changes in the cornea, including serious superficial keratitis and corneal vascularization, have been reported in studies of animals deficient in the B vitamins. Sjögren's syndrome has been linked to vitamin B complex deficiency.[88] Controlled therapeutic trials of vitamin B administration have not been done. The relationship between corneal vascularization and vitamin B deficiency in humans is considerably less clear. Corneal vascularization and keratitis have been associated with major deficiencies of nicotinic acid as well as low levels of other B vitamins. Since pellagra probably results from a number of nutritional deficiencies, it is difficult to link these eye lesions specifically to deficiencies of the B vitamins.

The role of B vitamins in maintaining the health of the retina and particularly the optic nerve is far more certain. Visual loss in eyes that appear healthy has been associated for centuries with the B vitamin deficiency states pellagra and beriberi. The ocular manifestations have been termed nutritional amblyopia and nutritional retrobulbar neuropathy. Tobacco usage and alcohol consumption have been linked with these conditions over the past 150 years; hence the frequently used term tobacco-alcohol amblyopia. All these diseases are deficiency states (even tobacco-alcohol amblyopia, which has been demonstrated to be a nontoxic condition).[73] Since the rare optic neuropathy associated with vitamin B_{12} deficiency or pernicious anemia produces similar symptoms, the physician must rely on the results of blood tests in making a differential diagnosis.

Nutritional amblyopia manifests as a gradual decrease in central visual acuity with sparing of the peripheral fields. Visual acuity in the worst cases is usually 20/200 (6/60) or better. Color vision (particularly red-green) is impaired. Other anatomic findings frequently include temporal pallor of the optic nervehead and, rarely, retinal hemorrhage. If the pathologic condition has not been present long enough to cause actual optic atrophy, appropriate therapeutic intervention can improve visual acuity, visual field, and other visual functions.

Unlike Wernicke's encephalopathy, which is generally agreed to be caused by an acute lack of thiamine, the exact cause of nutritional amblyopia is unknown. Successful treatment seems to depend on the administration of B vitamins. Vitamin B_{12} (cyanocobalamin) administration alone results in general improvement. The concurrent administration of other B vitamins is also very helpful. For example, thiamine has been used therapeutically; however, better results were obtained when other B vitamins also were administered. Vision usually improves even if the patient continues to smoke and consume alcohol. Thus adequate improvement can be obtained by dietary means alone.[73]

VITAMIN E

Vitamin E produces significant benefits in maintaining eye health. Its antioxidant properties, positive interactions with vitamin A, promotion of epithelial health, and general stimulation of certain aspects of the immune system all are important.

Recent reports have described progressive ataxia and spinocerebellar signs with ocular changes in rare cases of primary vitamin E deficiency without[89] and with abnormalities of fat absorption.[90-92]

Vitamin E has been used as a therapeutic agent in infants with retrolental fibroplasia. Although the efficacy of vitamin E is still controversial,[93] it appears to be an effective adjunct in these patients.[94,95] Toxicity and severe, sometimes fatal, complications have accompanied intravenous or intramuscular use.[96,97]

One of the many possible etiologies in the development of senile cataracts is oxidation of the proteins of the lens. Work with an inbred rat strain prone to the development of cataracts has demonstrated that a diet rich in sunflower seeds virtually precluded cataract formation.[98] Sunflower kernels are a rich source of vitamin E as well as of fatty acids, such as linoleic, and selenium. The mechanism of the experimental effect is, however, unclear.

Increasing attention has focused on the possible deleterious interactions between light and the retina in promoting retinal degeneration. Oxidizing radicals may be created when light is focused intensely on the retinal tissue. The presence of antioxidants clearly could be protective in such a case. Monkeys kept on a vitamin E–deficient diet for over 2 years develop marked macular degeneration and disintegration of the lipoprotein outer segments of the rods and cones.[99] These changes were consistent with lipid peroxidation.

The exact role of vitamin E in the maintenance of ocular health and the prevention of certain age-related ocular diseases is not clear.[100] It is nonetheless reasonable to advise persons to supplement their diets with safely nontoxic amounts of vitamin E.

OTHER VITAMINS

Other vitamins are, of course, important for healthy ocular tissues; however, a few of them seem to have special effects on the eye. For example, vitamin C deficiency is associated with subconjunctival hemorrhages and infection of the conjunctiva, both changes of little consequence. Although orbital hemorrhage once was common in infants with vitamin C deficiency (scurvy), this problem is rarely seen today. Daily ingestion of vitamin C has been suggested as beneficial in reducing the formation of senile cataract[101,102] and macular degeneration.[103,104]

There is little evidence that vitamin D has any direct effects on the eye. Vitamin K has been shown to reduce retinal hemorrhages in newborns when it is administered to mothers very shortly before delivery.[105]

Although other vitamins do not necessarily have dramatic effects on ocular tissues, they probably play important roles in maintaining ocular health. It is clear from the interactions of vitamins A and E and of the B vitamins that the balance of nutritional components is the most important factor in maintaining good health. Thus a balanced diet or supplements that contain appropriate amounts of required vitamins are advisable, at least for some patients, perhaps especially the elderly.

MINERALS AND TRACE ELEMENTS

The trace element content of ocular tissues is among the highest of any of the tissues in the body. The reasons for the eye's avidity for trace elements such as copper and zinc is not known. It may be related to the importance of many of these elements as cofactors for various enzyme systems. As specialized neural tissues, the retina, its pigmented epithelium, and associated structures have very high metabolic rates. Calcium plays an intimate role in the visual cycle; zinc and copper are important enzymic cofactors, and their metabolism is interrelated.[106-108] It had long been thought that trace element deficiencies in humans were impossible because of the wide distribution of these elements in foods. Such deficiencies are well known in laboratory animals. They also occur in humans of all ages, especially the elderly and in those receiving long-term parenteral therapy or who have undergone major gastrointestinal surgery.[109,110] Older people who have inadequate dietary intakes may suffer from mineral and trace element deficiencies that are clinically difficult to detect.[111] Copper deficiency with neurophthalmic manifestations can be produced iatrogenically.[112] Copper therapy can be useful in Menkes' syndrome, an inherited disorder of copper metabolism with associated retinal degeneration[113,114]; but failure of copper infusion therapy has been reported.[115] The use of vitamin C therapy in Menkes' also has been questioned.[116]

Zinc supplementation has received increasing attention, as evidence for its key roles in ocular metabolism, especially retinal and retinal pigment epithelial function accumulate.[117-119] Because of potential harmful side effects of zinc overload,[120,121] however, its use must be viewed with caution. Zinc has been shown in one controlled double-blind study[122] to retard vision loss from macular degeneration.

Table 21-3 summarizes the current understanding of the effects of excesses or deficiencies of trace elements on ocular function. As with so many other nutritional factors, balance is important. For example, ingesting excessive amounts of selenium can produce overt toxicity, both ocular and systemic. Selenium seems to be necessary, at least in experimental animals, for retinal integrity.[127] Its use has been advocated in humans with macular degeneration.[128] No controlled prospective randomized studies supporting this use are available, however. Selenium overload has been associated with many toxic effects, including experimental cataract formation,[129] that may occur more readily in individuals with substandard protein nutrition.[130]

Table 21-3 Ocular Effects of Minerals and Trace Elements

	Deficiency or Excess	Effects
Calcium	Hypercalcemia Excessive dietary intake of Ca^{+2} and/or vitamin D Hyperparathyroidism Sarcoidosis Kidney disease	Crystalline deposits in conjunctiva and cornea (cataract shown to be associated with elevated calcium only in vitro[123])
	Hypocalcemia Neonatal tetany Renal disease	Cataractous deposits in conjunctiva and cornea
Phosphorus	Hypophosphatemia Vitamin D–resistant rickets Long-term parenteral maintenance	Deposits in conjunctiva and cornea Cataract Papilledema
Copper	Deficiency Menkes' syndrome[113,114] (treated in infancy with i.v. copper) Excess Wilson's disease (treated with penicillamine)	Retinal degeneration and cataract[124] Kayser-Fleischer ring Cataract
Iron	Deficiency	Retinal edema and hemorrhages Papilledema (sizes proportional to severity of anemia)
	Excess Primary and secondary hemochromatoses	Pigmented deposits in cornea (sometimes ringlike), conjunctiva, sclera
Zinc	Deficiency Chronic alcoholism Chronic pancreatitis Acrodermatitis enteropathica[125,126] (treated with oral zinc therapy)	Poor dark adaptation Corneal deposits

LIGHT AS A NUTRIENT

The importance of sunlight and the effects of light in the maintenance of general health of human beings are controversial.

Is light a nutrient? Light entering the eye not only produces vision but also modulates a neuroendocrine matrix that profoundly affects metabolism.[131,132] Like ordinary food, light is taken into the body, where it interacts with and is converted by tissues, notably the retina and the skin. Light-influenced metabolic products exert significant effects on the enzyme, hormonal, and neurotransmitter systems, and, ultimately, on growth and development.[133,134] Evidence[135] indicates that both the type (spectrum) and the quantity of light are important. Deficiencies in either portion of the spectrum or the quantity of light exposure seem to be associated with disease. In the United States, until about 1900, nearly everyone was routinely exposed to the broad spectrum of light from the sun. After the turn of the century the introduction of artificial lighting made it possible for working environments to ignore the sun's schedule. By 1980 considerably less than 10% of the working population in the United States performed their work in sunlight. Loss of, or decreased exposure to, many of the wavelengths contained in natural sunlight may have a profound influence on one's physical and emotional health.[136]

The interaction of sunlight with the skin is well understood.[137] When sunlight of the shorter wavelengths, in the near-ultraviolet region, strikes the skin, it is absorbed by elements in the skin. During this absorption a photochemical reaction is initiated that stimulates the production of vitamin D, which is crucial to the maintenance of normal calcium metabolism. After the industrial revolution, the occurrence of soft deformed bones (rickets) was virtually epidemic among children of industrial centers. This epidemic halted in the early 1900s when the discovery that the interaction of ultraviolet light with skin produces vitamin D and that a synthetic form of vitamin D could be added to milk, producing the same salutary effects as exposure to sunlight. In adults the major bone-related problem is osteoporosis, but the relationship between sunlight intake by skin and osteoporosis is not clear. The biologic efficacy of synthetic vitamin D in adults is debatable. It has been demonstrated that the preponderance of vitamin D detectable in the blood of adults who are receiving oral vitamin D supplementation continues to be the biosynthetically produced form. Although this finding could possibly be explained by poor absorption, there are studies that suggest the decreased bioeffectiveness of synthetic vitamin D.

The importance of adequate exposure to the vitamin D–producing spectrum of sunlight has been illustrated in observations of elderly people.[138] One group of 10 elderly men was exposed to ambient limited-spectrum fluorescent lighting. Ten men of similar age receiving the same diet were exposed to ambient lighting with a spectrum much closer to that of natural sunlight. During the winter months of the experiment, the group exposed to the limited-spectrum light demonstrated an approximately 25% decrease in calcium absorption. The group exposed to broad-spectrum lighting had a mean increase of calcium absorption of approximately 15%. Exposure to full-spectrum light thus seems to enhance normal calcium metabolism.

Light and the Eye

Striking evidence that humans are not evolutionarily divorced from other animals is provided by the pineal hormone melatonin. Melatonin is a low–molecular-weight hormone synthesized in the pineal gland and then released into the bloodstream. The human retina also synthesizes melatonin.

In nonhuman species the pineal regulates, largely through changes in melatonin levels, many important and diverse functions, such as reproduction and other circadian and seasonally rhythmic activities. The pineal reacts to ambient light levels as follows: When the sun rises and ambient light levels are raised, the synthesis and release of melatonin are sharply curtailed. After sunset, melatonin synthesis increases and blood levels of melatonin rise progressively to a nighttime peak. It is apparently this cyclic alteration in blood melatonin concentration that regulates many important functions.[136] The pineal "third eye" of animals lies on the superior aspect of the cranium, where it is closer to the effects of environmental light than is the human pineal. In humans the pineal is buried in the center of the central nervous system and therefore must receive information about ambient light changes indirectly.

One study[139] demonstrated conclusively that humans do respond to sunlight. A typical light-dark melatonin response was elicited in normal persons by exposing them to strong full-spectrum artificial lighting. The amount of light required to elicit the response was equivalent to what one would be exposed to when standing at a clean window in a mid-Atlantic state on a fair early spring day. Thus, although humans in industrialized countries have adapted to low levels of artificial illumination, they have retained responsiveness to natural sunlight. It should be stressed that the artificial light ordinarily encountered in offices does not elicit the normal sunlight effects on melatonin levels. This lack of effectiveness is certainly due to the intensity of the lighting, but may also be due to its spectrum.

Human beings can also exhibit seasonal rhythms attuned to the solar photoperiod, much as other animals do.[140] Studies in Finland have revealed that the peak time for conception in that country is in the summer months, June and July, when the photoperiod is the longest. It has been amply demonstrated in many nonhuman species that full-spectrum or sunlight exposure is necessary for normal maturation of the genitals and for reproduction.

Light exposure also seems to have important influences on mental status. More than 50 years ago the psychiatrist Kraepelin[141] crystallized his own and even earlier observations on variations in emotional status with the seasons:

Repeatedly I saw in these cases moodiness set in during autumn and pass over to excitement in spring "when the sap shoots in the trees," corresponding in a sense to the emotional changes which come over even healthy individuals at the changes of the seasons.

In an investigation of a seasonal manic depressive illness,[142] individuals with winter depression were exposed to a prolonged photoperiod by the daily addition of several hours of strong artificial lighting before dawn and after dusk. The early results were encouraging. A control group of patients was exposed to dim yellow light, which had no consistent or significant effects in improving their mental status. In fact, some patients rapidly deteriorated and had to be returned to bright full-spectrum light. Light therapy appears useful in persons with seasonal affective disorder[143,144] and also "jet lag."[145] These observations emphasize the importance of high-intensity full-spectrum light exposure in the maintenance of human health. Caution is required in advising patients who ask for clinical advice after having seen an article in the popular press advocating limited-spectrum colored lights as therapy for arthritis or other illnesses. It is possible that either no amelioration will be achieved or even harm may be done.

Phototherapy with short-wavelength light has long been used in newborn nurseries to speed the resolution of neonatal jaundice.[146] The application of eye protection for newborns undergoing this treatment is now routine. Light in the premature nursery has also been questioned as a contributing factor to retinopathy of prematurity.[147]

Recommendations

More scientifically based investigation of the effects of low-level partial-spectrum light on human health is needed. However, some simple measures can be recommended with confidence. Whenever possible, and within the limits of common sense and safety, sunlight or bright daylight should be allowed into working areas. A daily (lunchtime) brief walk outside is recommended, since even this short exposure to daylight may fulfill the body's requirement. Incandescent lighting, although more costly, has a broader spectrum than ordinary fluorescent lighting. Certain fluorescent lights are available that do have a more nearly full-spectrum emission, and these should be used where individuals are office-bound all day throughout the year. In certain occupations obtaining adequate sunlight is difficult, and artificial measures should be devised. For example, in the Soviet Union, coal miners are given daily exposures to small amounts of certain elements of sunlight to which they are otherwise not exposed. It is thought that this dosage of light may help combat black lung disease. In the U.S. Navy, submarine personnel who have been given small doses of full-spectrum light have had fewer routine illnesses and emotional problems than unexposed crew members have had. The harmful effects of *over*exposure to sunlight and ultraviolet are well known and generally avoidable.

SUMMARY

The human eye serves as a neuroendocrine organ that conveys information about the level of ambient sunlight to the pineal gland. This information is reflected in changes in the blood concentration of melatonin that may be related to a host of biologic rhythms and important biologic functions. Investigations from a variety of laboratories have implicated exposure to low-level artificial partial-spectrum illumination, coupled with lack of exposure to full-spectrum lighting, such as sunlight, in softening of bones, calcium loss, reduced fertility, reduced enzymatic activity, reduced immunologic defenses, fatigue, and decreased ability to perform complex mental tasks and tasks involving eye-muscular coordination. New findings demonstrate conclusively that humans can benefit from adequate full-spectrum sunlight and that bright full-spectrum lighting can have a helpful effect in certain mental illnesses and in persons deprived of ordinary light exposure. Much more scientifically based research in this area is needed; however, until further knowledge is available, it is reasonable to recommend that people obtain prudent and safe exposure to full-spectrum sun and indoor lighting on a regular basis.

REFERENCES

1. Jackson CM: The effects of inanition and malnutrition upon growth and structure, Philadelphia, 1925, P Blakiston Co.
2. McLaren DS: Growth and water content of the eyeball of the albino rat in protein deficiency, Br J Nutr 12:254-259, 1958.
3. Gibson CJ: Dietary control of retinal dopamine synthesis, Brain Res 382:195-198, 1986.
4. Dyer RS, et al: Dopamine depletion slows retinal transmission, Exp Neurol 71:326-340, 1981.
5. Halasa AH, McLaren DS: The refractive state of malnourished children, Arch Ophthalmol 71:827-831, 1964.
6. Gardiner PA, Macdonald I: Dietary intake and refractive errors: an experimental correlation [abstract], Proc Nutr Soc 17:20, 1958.
7. Toskes PP, et al: Non-diabetic retinal abnormalities in chronic pancreatitis, N Engl J Med 300:942-946, 1979.
8. Geggel HS, et al: Nutritional requirement for taurine in patients receiving long-term parenteral nutrition, N Engl J Med 312:142-146, 1985.
9. Johnson L, et al: Does breast milk–taurine protect against retinopathy of prematurity? [abstract], Pediatr Res 19:347A, 1985.
10. Schaeffer AJ, Murray JD: Tryptophan determination in cataracts due to deficiency or delayed supplementation of tryptophan, Arch Ophthalmol 43:202-216, 1950.
11. Ratnakar KS: Interaction of galactose and dietary protein deficiency on rat lens, Ophthalmic Res 17:344-348, 1985.
12. Garron LK: Cystinosis, Trans Am Acad Ophthalmol Otolaryngol 63:99-108, 1959.
13. Wong VG, et al: Alterations of pigment epithlium in cystinosis, Arch Ophthalmol 77:361-369, 1967.
14. Goldman H, et al: Adolescent cystinosis: comparisons with infantile and adult forms, Pediatrics 47:979-988, 1971.
15. Dodd MJ, et al: Adult cystinosis: a case report, Arch Ophthalmol 96:1054-1057, 1978.
16. Kaiser-Kupfer MI, et al: Removal of corneal crystals by topical cysteamine in nephropathic cystinosis, N Engl J Med 316:775-779, 1987.
17. Field CMB, et al: Homocystineuria: a new disorder of metabolism, Lisbon, 1962, Tenth International Congress of Pediatrics, p 274.
18. Francois J: Ocular manifestations in amino-acidopathies, Adv Ophthalmol 25:28-103, 1972.
19. Simell O, Takki K: Raised plasma-ornithine and gyrate atrophy of the choroid and retina, Lancet 1:1031-1033, 1973.
20. Shih VE, et al: Reduction of hyperornithinemia with a low protein, low arginine diet and pyridoxine in patients with a deficiency of ornithine-ketoacid transaminase (DKT) activity and gyrate atrophy of the choroid and retina, Clin Chim Acta 113:243-251, 1981.
21. Berson EL, et al: Ocular findings in patients with gyrate atrophy on pyridoxine and low-protein low-arginine diets, Ophthalmology 88:311-315, 1981.
22. Weleber RG, et al: Gyrate atrophy of the choroid and retina. Approaches to therapy, Int Ophthalmol 4:23-32, 1981.
23. Rych K: Retinal degeneration in vitamin B12 disorder associated with methylmalonic aciduria and sulfur amino acid abnormalities [letter], Am J Ophthalmol 99:217, 1985.
24. Hyndman AF: The effects of glutamate and Kainate on cell proliferation in retinal cultures, Invest Ophthalmol Vis Sci 25:558-563, 1984.
25. Sisk DR, et al: Behavioral recovery in albino rats with glutamate-damaged retinas, Invest Ophthalmol Vis Sci 25:1124-1128, 1984.
26. Van Heyningen R: The sorbitol pathway in the lens, Exp Eye Res 1:396-404, 1962.
27. Patterson JW: Development of diabetic cataracts, Am J Ophthalmol 35:68-72, 1952.
28. Varma SD, et al: Implications of aldose reductase in cataracts in human diabetes, Invest Ophthalmol Vis Sci 18:237-241, 1979.
29. Dvornik D, et al: Polyol accumulation in galactosemic and diabetic rats: control by an aldose reductase inhibitor, Science 182:1146, 1973.
30. Beyer-Mears A, Cruz E: Reversal of diabetic cataract by sorbinil, an aldose reductase inhibitor, Diabetes 34:15-21, 1985.
31. Dvornik D: Effect of Tolrestat on red blood cell sorbitol levels in patients with diabetes, Clin Pharmacol Ther 38:625-630, 1985.
32. Varma SD: Inhibition of aldose reductase by flavonoids: possible attenuation of diabetic complications, Prog Clin Biol Res 213:343-358, 1986.
33. Reaven GM, et al: Nutritional management of diabetes, Med Clin North Am 63:927-44, 1979.
34. Cahill G, et al: "Control" in diabetes, N Engl J Med 294:1004, 1976.
35. Ingelfinger F: Debate on diabetes, N Engl J Med 296:1228-1230, 1977.
36. Job D, et al: Effect of multiple daily insulin injections on the course of diabetic retinopathy, Diabetes 25:463-469, 1976.

37. Engerman R: Pathophysiology of diabetic retinopathy. Report of the National Commission on Diabetes, DHEW (NIH)76-1023, Washington DC, 1976, Government Printing Office, pp 194-195.

38. Tchobroutsky G: Relation of diabetic control to microvascular complications, Diabetologica 15:143-152, 1978.

39. Irsigler K, et al: Reversal of florid diabetic retinopathy [letter], Lancet 2:1068, 1979.

40. Lauritzen T, et al: Effect of 1 years of near-normal blood glucose levels on retinopathy in insulin-dependent diabetics, Lancet 1:200-204, 1983.

41. Diabetic Retinopathy Research Study Group: Photocoagulation treatment of proliferative diabetic retinopathy: clinical application of Diabetic Retinopathy Study findings (Report #8), Ophthalmology 88:583-600, 1981.

42. Early Treatment Diabetic Retinopathy Study Research Group: Photocoagulation for diabetic macular edema (Report 1), Arch Ophthalmol 103:1796-1806, 1985.

43. Greiner JV, Chylack LT Jr: Anatomy of the experimental "hypoglycemic" cataract in the rat lens, Ophthalmol Res 8:133-145, 1976.

44. Levy NS, et al: Galactokinase deficiency and cataracts, Am J Ophthalmol 74:41-48, 1972.

45. Harley JD, et al: Maternal enzymes of galactose metabolism and the inexplicable infantile cataract, Lancet 2:259-261, 1974.

46. Richter CP, Duke JR: Cataracts produced in rats by yogurt, Science 168:1372-1374, 1970.

47. Kador PF, Kinoshita JH: Diabetic and galactosemic cataracts, Ciba Found symp 106:110-131, 1984.

48. Weinberg DA, et al: False-normal assays for galactosemia in a neonate with cataracts, Am J Ophthalmol 100:342-343, 1985.

49. Beutler E, Gelbart T: Falsely normal value in fluorometric transferase screening of galactosemic blood. A cautionary note, Am J Clin Pathol 76:841, 1981.

50. Minassian DC, et al: Dehydrational crises from severe diarrhea or heatstroke and risk of cataract, Lancet 1:751-753, 1984.

51. Rinaldi E, et al: High frequency of lactose absorbers among adults with idiopathic senile and presenile cataract in a population with a high prevalence of primary adult lactose malabsorption, Lancet 1:355-357, 1984.

52. Kolars JC, et al: Yogurt—an autodigesting source of lactose, N Engl J Med 310:1-3, 1984.

53. Creighton MO, et al: Modeling cortical cataractogenesis. VII. Effects of vitamin E treatment on galactose-induced cataracts, Exp Eye Res 40:213-222, 1985.

54. Wheller TG, et al: Visual membranes: specificity of fatty acid precursors for the electrical response to illumination, Science 188:1312-1314, 1975.

55. Hayasaka S, et al: Corneal arcus in Japanese family with type IIa hyperlipoproteinemia, Jpn J Ophthalmol 28:254-258, 1984.

56. Kruth HS: Accumulation of unesterified cholesterol in limbal cornea and conjunctiva of rabbits fed a high-cholesterol diet. Detection with filipin, Atherosclerosis 63:1-6, 1987.

57. von Sallman L, et al: Ocular histopathologic changes in a case of abetalipoproteinemia, Doc Ophthalmol 26:451-460, 1967.

58. Brin MF, et al: Electrophysiologic features of abetalipoproteinemia: functional consequences of vitamin E deficiency, Neurology 36:669-673, 1986.

59. Gouras P, et al: Retinitis pigmentosa in abetalipoproteinemia: effects of vitamin A, Invest Ophthalmol 10:748-793, 1971.

60. Muller DPR, et al: Long term management of abetalipoproteinemia, Arch Dis Child 52:209-214, 1977.

61. Runge P, et al: Oral vitamin E supplements can prevent the retinopathy of abetalipoproteinemia, Br J Ophthalmol 70:166-173, 1986.

62. Muller DPR, Lloyd JK: Effect of large oral doses of vitamin E on the neurological sequelae of patients with abetalipoproteinemia, Ann NY Acad Sci 393:133-144, 1982.

63. Toussaint D, Davis P: An ocular pathologic study of Refsum's syndrome, Am J Ophthalmol 72:342-347, 1971.

64. Hassell JR, Newsome DA: Vitamin A induced alterations in corneal and conjunctival epithelial glycoprotein biosynthesis, Ann NY Acad Sci 359:358-365, 1981.

65. Smolin G, et al: Herpes simplex keratitis treatment with vitamin A, Arch Ophthalmol 97:2181-2183, 1979.

66. Sommer A: Vitamin A treatment for herpes keratitis [letter], Arch Ophthalmol 98:1656, 1980.

67. Olver J: Keratomalacia on a "healthy diet," Br J Ophthalmol 70:357-360, 1986.

68. Sommer A, et al: History of night blindness: a simple tool for xerophthalmia screening, Am J Clin Nutr 33:887-891, 1980.

69. Stoll BJ, et al: Night blindness and vitamin A deficiency in children attending a diarrheal disease hospital in Bangladesh, J Trop Pediatr 31:36-39, 1985.

70. Roa V, et al: Conjunctival goblet cells and mitotic rate in children with retinol deficiency and measles, Arch Ophthalmol 105:378-380, 1987.

71. Alvarez F, et al: Nervous and ocular disorders in children with cholestasis and vitamin A and E deficiencies, Hepatology 3:410-414, 1983.

72. Guggenheim MA, et al: Progressive neuromuscular disease in children with chronic cholestasis and vitamin E deficiency: diagnosis and treatment with alpha tocopherol, J Pediat 100:51-58, 1982.

73. Carroll FD: Nutritional amblyopia, Arch Ophthalmol 76:406-411, 1966.

74. Brown GC, et al: Reversible night blindness with intestinal bypass surgery, Am J Ophthalmol 89:776-779, 1980.

75. Haag JR, et al: Optic atrophy following jejunoileal bypass, J Clin Neuro Ophthalmol 5:9-15, 1985.

76. Davidson S, et al: Human nutrition and dietetics, New York, 1979, Churchill Livingstone Inc.

77. Haeussinger D, et al: Zinc and vitamin A deficiency in patients with Crohn's disease is correlated with activity but not with localization or extent of the disease, Hepatogastroenterology 32:34-38, 1985.

78. Iansek R, Edge CJ: Nutritional amblyopia in a patient with Crohn's disease, J Neurol Neurosurg Psychiatry 48:1307-1308, 1985.

79. Walt RP, et al: Vitamin A treatment for night blindness in primary biliary cirrhosis, Br Med J 288:1030-1031, 1984.

80. Powell SR: Nutritional disorders affecting the peripheral cornea, Int Ophthalmol Clin 26:137-146, 1986.

81. Sommer A, et al: Incidence, prevalence and scale of blinding malnutrition, Lancet **1**:407-408, 1981.

82. Olson JA: Vitamin A deficiency, Nutr Rev **44**:121-124, 1986.

83. Fraunfelder FT, et al: Adverse ocular reactions possibly associated with isotretinoin, Am J Ophthalmol **100**:535, 1985.

84. Herman DC, Dyer JA: Anterior subcapsular cataracts as a possible adverse ocular reaction to isotretinoin, Am J Ophthalmol **103**:236-237, 1987.

85. Weleber RG, et al: Abnormal retinal function associated with isotretinoin therapy for acne, Arch Ophthalmol **104**:831-837, 1986.

86. Kaiser-Kupfer MI, et al: Abnormal retinal function associated with fenretinide, a synthetic retinoid, Arch Ophthalmol **104**:69-70, 1986.

87. Marcus DF, et al: Optic disc findings in hypervitaminosis A, Ann Ophthalmol **17**:397-402, 1985.

88. Altamar Rios J: Sjogren's syndrome, a manifestation of vitamin B complex deficiency. Statistical study of 98 cases in 17 years, An Otorrinolaringol Ibero Am **12**:443-457, 1985.

89. Harding AE, et al: Spinocerebellar degeneration associated with a selective defect of vitamin E absorption, N Engl J Med **313**:32-35, 1985.

90. Muller DPR, et al: Vitamin E and neurological function, Lancet **1**:225-228, 1983.

91. Harding AE, et al: Spinocerebellar degeneration secondary to chronic intestinal malabsorption: a vitamin E deficiency syndrome, Ann Neurol **12**:419-424, 1982.

92. Larsen PD, et al: Vitamin E deficiency associated with vision loss and bulbar weakness, Ann Neurol **18**:725-772, 1985.

93. Kretzer FL, et al: Pathogenic mechanism of retinopathy of prematurity: a controversial explanation for the efficacy of oral and intramuscular vitamin E supplementation and cryotherapy, Bull NY Acad Med **61**:883-900, 1985.

94. Schaffer DB, et al: Vitamin E and retinopathy of prematurity. Follow up at one year, Ophthalmology **92**:1005-1011, 1985.

95. Phelps DL, et al: Tocopherol efficacy and safety for preventing retinopathy of prematurity: a randomized, controlled, double-masked trial, Pediatrics **79**:489-500, 1987.

96. Committee on the Fetus and Newborn: Vitamin E and the prevention of retinopathy of prematurity, Pediatrics **76**:315-316, 1985.

97. Rosenbaum AL, et al: Retinal hemorrhage in retinopathy of prematurity associated with tocopherol treatment, Ophthalmology **92**:1012-1014, 1985.

98. Hess HH, et al: Effects of sunflower seed supplements on reproduction and growth of RCS rats with hereditary retinal dystrophy, Lab Animal Sci **31**:482-488, 1981.

99. Hayes KC: Retinal degeneration in monkeys induced by deficiency of vitamin E or A, Invest Ophthalmol **13**:499-510, 1974.

100. Katz ML, et al: Lipofuscin accumulation resulting from senescence and vitamin E deficiency: spectral properties and tissue distribution, Mech Age Develop **25**:149-159, 1984.

101. Ringvold A, et al: Senile cataract and ascorbic acid loading, Acta Ophthalmol **63**:277-280, 1985.

102. Varma SD, et al: Light-induced damage to ocular lens cation pump: prevention by vitamin C, Proc Natl Acad Sci USA **76**:3504, 1979.

103. Organisciak DT, et al: The protective effect of ascorbate in retinal light damage of rats, Invest Ophthalmol Vis Sci **26**:1580, 1985.

104. Li ZY, et al: Amelioration of photic injury in rat retina by ascorbic acid: a histopathologic study, Invest Ophthalmol Vis Sci **26**:1589-1598, 1985.

105. Maumenee AE, et al: Factors influencing plasma prothrombin in the newborn infant. IV. The effect of antenatal administration of vitamin K on the incidence of retinal hemorrhage in the newborn, Bull Johns Hopkins Hosp **68**:158-168, 1941.

106. Kay RG: Zinc and copper in human nutrition, J Hum Natr **35**:25-36, 1981.

107. Russell RM, et al: Zinc and the special senses, Ann Intern Med **99**:227-239, 1983.

108. Fischer PW, et al: Effect of zinc supplementation on copper status in adult man, Am J Clin Nutr **40**:743-746, 1984.

109. Burch RE: Trace elements in human nutrition, Med Clin North Am **63**:1057-1068, 1979.

110. Golden MH: Trace elements. Potential importance in huaan nutrition with particular reference to zinc and vanadium, Br Med Bull **37**:31-36, 1981.

111. Pennington JAT, et al: Mineral content of foods and total diets: the selected minerals in foods survey 1982 to 1984, J Am Diet Assoc **86**:876-878, 1986.

112. Pall H: Copper chelation and the neuro-ophthalmic toxicity of desferrioxamine, Lancet **2**:1279, 1986.

113. Hart DB: Menkes syndrome: an updated review, J Am Acad Dermatol **9**:145-152, 1983.

114. Leone A, et al: Menkes' disease: abnormal metallothonein gene regulation in response to copper, Cell **40**:301-309, 1985.

115. Garnica AD: The failure of parenteral copper therapy in Menkes Kinky Hair syndrome, Eur J Pediatr **142**:98-102, 1984.

116. Ueki Y, et al: Menkes disease: Is vitamin C treatment effective? Brain Dev **7**:519-522, 1985.

117. Morrison SA, et al: Zinc deficiency: a cause of abnormal dark adaptation in cirrhotics, Am J Clin Nutr **31**:276-281, 1978.

118. Leure-DuPree AE, Bridges CD: Changes in retinal morphology and vitamin A metabolism as a consequence of decreased zinc availability, Retina **2**:294-302, 1982.

119. Newsome DA, Rothman R: Zinc uptake in vitro by human retinal pigment epithelium, Invest Ophthalmol Vis Sci **28**:1795-1799, 1987.

120. Crouse SF, et al: Zinc ingestion and lipoprotein values in sedentary and endurance-trained men, JAMA **252**:785-787, 1984.

121. Chandra RK: Excessive intake of zinc impairs immune responses, JAMA **252**:1443-1446, 1984.

122. Newsome DA, et al: Oral zinc in macular degeneration, Arch Ophthalmol **106**:192-198, 1988.

123. Hightower KR, Arnum R: Calcium induces opacities in cultural human lenses, Exp Eye Res **41**:565-568, 1985.

124. Sakano T, et al: A case of Menkes syndrome with cataracts, Eur J Pediatr **138**:357-358, 1981.

125. Matta CS, et al: Eye manifestations in acrodermatitis enteropathica, Arch Ophthalmol **93**:140-142, 1975.

126. Patek AJ, Haig C: The occurrence of abnormal dark adaptation and its relation to vitamin A metabolism in patients with cirrhosis of the liver, J Clin Invest **18**:609-616, 1939.

127. Amemiya T: Retinal changes in the selenium deficient rat, Int J Vitam Nutr Res **55**:233-237, 1985.

128. Weiter J, et al: Role of selenium in senile macular degeneration, Invest Ophthalmol Vis Sci **26**:58, 1985.

129. Shearer TR, Anderson RS: Histologic changes during selenite cataractogenesis: a light microscopy study, Exp Eye Res **40**:557-565, 1984.

130. Ostadalova I, Babick YA: Nutritional dependence of the incidence of selenite-induced cataracts in rats, Physiol Bohemoslov **33**:507-510, 1984.

131. Wurtman RJ: The pineal as a neuroendocrine transducer, Hosp Pract **15**:82-86, 1980.

132. Lewy AJ, et al: Melatonin secretion as a neurobiological "marker" and effects of light in humans, Psychopharmacol Bull. (In press, 1988.)

133. Dreyfus H: Enzymatic biosynthesis of ethanolamine- and choline-phosphoglycerides in retina during development. Effects of light stimulation, J Neurochem **31**:1157-1162, 1978.

134. Hug DH: Light activation of enzymes, Photochem Photobiol **32**:841-848, 1980.

135. Ozaki Y: Spectral power distribution of light sources affects growth and development of rats. Photochem Photobiol **29**:339-341, 1979.

136. Lewy AJ, et al: Manic-depressive patients may be supersensitive to light, Lancet **1**:383-384, 1981.

137. Fraser DR: Regulation of the metabolism of vitamin D, Physiol Rev **60**:551-613, 1980.

138. Lawson DE: Relative contributions of diet and sunlight to vitamin D state in the elderly, Br Med J **2**:303-305, 1979.

139. Lewy AJ, et al: Light suppresses melatonin secretion in humans, Science **210**:1267-1269, 1980.

140. Wurtman RJ, Ozaki Y: Physiological control of melatonin synthesis and secretion: mechanisms generating rhythms in melatonin, methoxytryptophol, and arginine vasotocin levels and effects of the pineal of endogenous catecholamines, the estrus cycle, and environmental lighting, J Neurol Transm (suppl)**13**:59-70, 1978.

141. Kraepelin E: In Robertson GM, editor: Manic-depressive insantiy and paranoia (translated by RM Barclay), Edinburgh, 1921, E & S Livingstone, p 280.

142. Rosenthal NE, Sack DA: Seasonal variation in affective disorders. In Wehr TA, Goodwin FK, editors: Biological rhythms in psychiatry, Pacific Grove Calif, 1982, Boxwood Press.

143. Rosenthal NE, et al: Seasonal affective disorder and phototherapy, Ann NY Acad Sci **453**:260-269, 1985.

144. Lewy AJ, Sack RL: Light therapy and psychiatry, Proc Soc Exp Biol Med **183**:11-18, 1986.

145. Weaver RA: Use of light to treat jet lag: differential effects of normal and bright artificial light on human circadian rhythms, Ann NY Acad Sci **453**:282-304, 1985.

146. Ennever JF: Phototherapy in a new light, Pediatr Clin North Am **33**:602-620, 1986.

147. Glass P, et al: Effect of bright light in the hospital nursery on the incidence of retinopathy of prematurity, N Engl J Med **313**:401-404, 1985.

CHAPTER 22
Diseases of the Skin

Kenneth H. Neldner

The skin is one of the less sensitive indicators of minor states of malnutrition, but it usually is affected by more profound or prolonged nutritional deficiencies. Because of its visibility, it is of considerable diagnostic value in relating cutaneous signs to multiple organ system effects.

Reliable clinical studies have been hampered because, except for controlled animal experiments, there are few instances in which a single nutrient deficiency exists. This makes it difficult to ascribe a specific syndrome of symptoms and signs to a given nutrient. In most individuals, malnutrition due to any cause will produce multiple protein-carbohydrate-fat-vitamin-mineral deficiencies. The focus of this chapter is the influence of nutrition on the skin.

The effects of malnutrition on the skin[1] will be discussed from the following perspectives: (1) general inanition, (2) vitamin deficiencies and excesses, (3) trace mineral deficiencies and excesses, (4) fatty acid deficiency, (5) obesity, (6) dermatologic disorders and the diet, and (7) drug-nutrient-skin interactions.

GENERAL INANITION

The consequences of general protein-energy starvation on adult skin are nonspecific in nature. There are few controlled studies in humans. In a classic study, Keyes[2] maintained 23 subjects on a generally balanced diet with 1570 calories daily for periods up to six months. After varying times and degrees of weight loss, the skin in these subjects was described as thin, inelastic, pallid, grayish in color, and "cold or dead" to the touch. Many of these changes were likened to those of more aged skin, but skin rashes or specific dermatologic disorders were not observed in any of the subjects.

Victims of famine, prisoners of war, patients with anorexia nervosa, and individuals with any prolonged wasting disease may show similar features of thin, dry, rough, and inelastic skin, resembling the skin of old age. Pigmentary changes with hyperpigmentation of the face are also common. Decreased growth rate of hair and nails with more rapid graying of hair also occurs in such individuals.

Starvation in children may take at least two different forms: marasmus and kwashiorkor.

1. In marasmus total inanition leads to suppressed growth and a multitude of systemic symptoms. The general catabolism of body tissue required for energy leads to wasting and results in a skin that is "too big" for the body. The subject develops a "monkey face" with deep perioral grooves and a generally dry, wrinkled, loose skin secondary to loss of subcutaneous fat.

2. In kwashiorkor the diet is lacking, both quantitatively and qualitatively, in protein but has adequate or even an excess of carbohydrate. It occurs most commonly in the weanling child ("sickness of the weanling") in underdeveloped countries where overall malnutrition is common. These potbellied children have major features of edema, retarded growth, moon facies, and hypoalbuminemia. Skin changes consist of hypopigmentation (more apparent in black children), beginning with circumoral pallor and later involving any area of the body. These may coexist with areas of hyperpigmentation, resulting in slightly raised dusky purple patches over pressure areas, which gradually darken and develop a waxy feel with sharp borders described as resembling enamel paint fixed to the skin. A generalized exfoliative dermatitis also has been observed, beginning with a fine desquamation and a mosaic or cracked appearance. Perlèche (angular stomatitis) is common, as are depigmented, sparse, and easily pulled out hairs with alternating light and dark bands (flag sign) corresponding to periods of better and poorer nutrition.

VITAMIN DEFICIENCIES AND EXCESSES

There are very few individuals with single or multiple vitamin deficiencies in the general population of the United States, where two or three reasonably balanced meals are eaten daily. Exceptions obviously occur in people who are malnourished because of extreme poverty or in those with anorexia and catabolic wasting secondary to illness. When deficiencies do occur, they are often multiple, making it difficult to ascribe a given symptom or cutaneous sign to a specific vitamin deficiency. Despite these problems, a number of cutaneous and mucous membrane manifestations have been associated with each of the vitamins.[1,3-5] These will be discussed; their major features are summarized in Table 22-1.

Water-Soluble Vitamins

Vitamin B₁ (thiamine). Thiamine deficiency appears to have the least distinctive cutaneous manifestations of all the B vitamins. It is similar

Table 22-1 Skin and Mucous Membrane Disorders Caused by Vitamin Deficiencies and Excesses

	Syndromes of Deficiency		Syndromes of Excess
	Skin	**Mucous Membranes**	**Skin and Mucous Membranes**
Water-Soluble Vitamins			
B₁ (thiamine)	None definite	Small vesicles on buccal mucosae, ventral tongue, palate (may resemble herpes simplex infection)	None known
B₂ (riboflavin)	Perlèche, angular blepharitis, genital ulcerations, nasolabial dermatitis	Glossitis with glossodynia, glossopyrosis, cheilitis, angular stomatitis (perlèche)	None known
B₃ (niacin)	Pellagra; photosensitivity reaction in exposed areas producing erythematous itchy rash on backs of hands; blisters, scaling, hard dry skin, and fissuring elsewhere; Casal's necklace; tryptophan deficiency may produce similar clinical picture	Glossitis, glossodynia, glossopyrosis; stomatitis with red atrophic and ulcerated oral mucosa; pellagrous vulvitis	None known; large doses cause flushing and tingling from vasodilating effect; niacinamide may be pruritogenic; acanthosis nigrans from prolonged or excessive doses
B₆ (pyridoxine)	Seborrheic dermatitis-like facial lesions and perlèche	Glossitis with magenta-colored tongue, glossopyrosis, perlèche	None known
B₁₂ (cyanocobalamin)	Hyperpigmentation of hands and feet; lemon-yellow pallor in pernicious anemia; vegetarians may have vitamin B₁₂ deficiency	Glossitis with marked smooth atrophy of surface and edges of tongue; glossodynia, stomatitis, and oral mucosal ulcerations	None known
C (ascorbic acid)	Scurvy; begins with follicular hyperkeratosis on arms; later becomes generalized; and lesions hemorrhagic; impaired wound healing; skin bruising	Gingivitis, progressing to hemorrhagic glossitis, perlèche, aphthous ulcers, bleeding gums	None known; excess is excreted in urine and may give false-positive test for sugar
Folic acid (folacin)	Anemic pallor if associated with vitamin B₁₂ deficiency and pernicious anemia	Cheilosis, glossitis, pharyngitis, perirectal ulcerations	None known

to the other B vitamins in that it appears to play a role in preserving the normal integrity of the oral mucous membranes. Lesions attributed to thiamine deficiency include nonspecific buccal mucosal vesicles resembling the early stage of herpes simplex or aphthous stomatitis.

A pure thiamine deficiency is, no doubt, exceedingly rare and many oral lesions attributed to a lack of thiamine probably are unrelated in etiology. The major consequence of thiamine deficiency is beriberi, which is essentially without cutaneous manifestations.

Vitamin B₂ (riboflavin). Riboflavin deficiency produces severe systemic symptoms in experimental animals, but in humans the manifestations appear to be limited primarily to the skin and mucous membranes. The major features of human riboflavin deficiency include perlèche (angular stomatitis), glossitis with magenta discoloration, nasolabial dermatitis similar to that seen in seborrheic dermatitis, angular blepharitis, corneal vascularization, and genital lesions

Table 22-1 Skin and Mucous Membrane Disorders Caused by Vitamin Deficiencies and Excesses—cont'd

	Syndromes of Deficiency		Syndromes of Excess
	Skin	Mucous Membranes	Skin and Mucous Membranes
Water-Soluble Vitamins— cont'd			
Pantothenic acid	No deficiency syndromes known in humans; questionable role in utilization of copper for hair growth and melanin formation in animals	None known	None known
Biotin	Generalized exfoliative dermatitis in animals; seborrheic dermatitis-like rash in infants; dry flaky skin in adults	Papillary atrophy of the tongue	None known
Fat-Soluble Vitamins			
D	Rickets; no specific skin lesions; visible lesions include rachitic rosary (enlargement of costochondral junction), pigeon breast; enlargement of ankle, knee, and wrist joints	None known	Calcinosis cutis (metastatic calcification); nausea, vomiting, weight loss, polyuria, nocturia
E (alphatocopherol)	None known; many claims made but none proved	None known	None known; questionable interference with vitamin K activity
A (retinol)	Dry wrinkled skin; eyes develop xerosis of conjunctivae and corneas, keratomalacia, Bitot's spots; hyperkeratosis of skin, follicular hyperkeratosis (phrynoderma), "permanent gooseflesh"	Keratinizing metaplasia of salivary glands producing dry mouth (xerostomia)	Fissures of lips, dry scaly desquamation of skin, alopecia, hyperpigmentation; coarse skin with pruritus; beta-carotene (vitamin A precursor) causes generalized yellowing of skin
K	Ecchymoses and larger cutaneous hemorrhages; may resemble scurvy and thrombocytopenia	None known	None known

consisting of eczematous, lichenified, and exudative dermatitis. None of these signs are pathognomonic of riboflavin deficiency but may be associated with other dermatologic disorders.

Riboflavin deficiency also has been called pellagra sine pellagra and the orooculogenital syndrome. Both terms are misleading, particularly the latter, which also is used as a synonym for Behçet's syndrome; however, Behçet's has no known relationship to riboflavin. Plummer-Vinson syndrome (sideropenic anemia) may have an associated riboflavin deficiency.

Vitamin B₃ (niacin, nicotinic acid). Pellagra is the most common manifestation of gross nicotinic acid deficiency, although other B vitamin and tryptophan deficiencies usually contribute to the syndrome. The disease was once a common worldwide problem, but fortification of wheat flour with nicotinic acid and the ready availability of multiple vitamins have virtually eradicated the disease. Pellagra also may occur in chronic alcoholics and certain food faddists.

The classic triad of dermatitis, diarrhea, and dementia may be incomplete. Photosensitivity, a major feature of the dermatitis, causes the rash to be concentrated in the sun-exposed areas of the face, neck, hands, and arms. The rash begins with erythema, soon followed by vesicles, bullae, crusting, and a chronic eczematous dermatitis that commonly extends as a broad band or collar around the neck (Casal's necklace). Thickened lichenified skin and hyperpigmentation gradually replace the eczematous phase. Sebaceous gland follicular orifices become plugged. Mucous membrane changes of glossitis and perlèche are variable and thought to be related more to other B vitamin deficiencies than to a lack of nicotinic acid.

Nicotinic acid administration will cure the disease, but parts of the syndrome may be related to a lack of other B vitamins. Therefore it is recommended that the diet be supplemented with the entire B-complex group.

Hartnup's disease is a rare hereditary disorder whose skin lesions mimic those of pellagra in all respects. It is caused by an inborn error of tryptophan metabolism and has additional features of transient cerebellar ataxia and moderate mental deficiency.

Nicotinic acid has been used to treat hyperlipidemia, but it causes flushing and itching. The amide derivative (niacinamide) has no effect on lipids and causes no vasodilating (flushing) reaction. Niacinamide is commonly present in multiple vitamin preparations and may cause chronic pruritus in some persons taking large doses of multivitamin preparations.

Vitamin B₆ (pyridoxine). The known manifestations of pyridoxine deficiency overlap those of the other B vitamin deficiency states. Pyridoxine deficiency has been induced experimentally in humans by administering a specific antagonist, 4-deoxypyridoxine. The cutaneous response included glossitis, angular stomatitis, a seborrheic dermatitis–like rash on the face and intertriginous areas, plus a pellagra-like hyperpigmentation of the extremities. Pyridoxine deficiency has been observed in patients with convulsive disorders and various types of anemia and in those receiving isoniazid therapy.

Vitamin B₁₂ (cyanocobalamin). Vitamin B₁₂ deficiency, when severe enough to produce pernicious anemia, will usually have a cutaneous component. The skin takes on a lemon-yellow pallor, except for the hands and feet, where hyperpigmentation is common. Oral lesions may occur with stomatitis, glossitis, and glossodynia. A smooth atrophy of the dorsal and lateral surface of the tongue is considered a somewhat more specific sign of pernicious anemia.

It should be reemphasized that a number of dermatologic disorders, such as pemphigus, lichen planus, aphthous stomatitis, Behçet's syndrome, erythema multiforme, and drug eruptions, all commonly have oral lesions with no known relationship to B vitamin deficiencies. Patients with chronic oral lesions therefore deserve the benefit of complete medical evaluation to rule out other possibilities.

Vitamin C (ascorbic acid). Vitamin C deficiency severe enough to produce clinical scurvy has cutaneous manifestations that are diagnostic. Ascorbate (particularly L-ascorbate) has a profound effect on collagen synthesis. It is absolutely necessary for the hydroxylation of proline to hydroxyproline. In experimental in vitro systems ascorbate also markedly stimulates collagen synthesis. In ascorbic acid deficiency the lack of hydroxyproline impairs the stability of the collagen triple helix, with secondary effects on collagenous structures of the body. One manifestation of this is weakened blood vessels, which in cutaneous sites allow leakage of erythrocytes and production of hemorrhagic lesions characterizing the deficiency state.

The earliest cutaneous lesions consist of follicular hyperkeratosis on the posterolateral aspect of the upper arms resembling keratosis pilaris in appearance and location. The process gradually extends to become nearly generalized and the follicular lesions gradually take on hemorrhagic qualities, initially with erythema, then assuming a dusky purple color, and finally becoming frankly hemorrhagic. The worst lesions occur on the legs, where they may mimic those of palpable purpura or superficial thrombophlebitis.

Oral lesions are also characteristic, beginning with gingivitis and bleeding, progressing to extremely tender, swollen, and necrotic gums. Painful aphthous ulcers of the buccal mucosa complicate the later stages of scurvy.

Folic acid (folacin). Folic acid is found abundantly in vegetable and animal foods, either free or conjugated with glutamic acid. Deficiencies are rare but nevertheless are possible through decreased intake or malabsorption. The major consequence of folic acid deficiency is megaloblastic anemia. If concurrent with vitamin B_{12} deficiency, the full syndrome of pernicious anemia evolves.

In addition to anemia, folic acid deficiency produces cheilosis, glossitis, pharyngitis, perirectal ulcerations, and diarrhea. Individuals with malabsorption syndromes or who have undergone total gastrectomies are possible candidates for folic acid deficiency.

In individuals with pernicious anemia, ingestion of more than 100 μg of folic acid per day may mask the hematologic component of the disease while allowing the neurologic manifestations to progress, undiagnosed and unchecked.

Pantothenic acid. Pantothenic acid is an essential vitamin for humans but is so widely distributed in nature that deficiency syndromes are exceedingly rare. The vitamin is a constituent of coenzyme A and therefore required for energy metabolism in many biochemical reactions.

Experimental pantothenic acid deficiency in rats produces growth failure, impaired reproduction, adrenocortical hypofunction, and graying of black hair. Despite claims to the contrary, pantothenic acid does not prevent or reverse graying of human hair.

Biotin. Biotin is a water-soluble vitamin widely distributed in nature. It seldom is involved in clinically apparent deficiency syndromes because it also is synthesized in the gut by intestinal bacteria. Yet biotin deficiency is of some clinical interest because of the antibiotin factor (avidin) present in raw egg white. Avidin binds to biotin and prevents its absorption. Apparently certain food faddists have eaten diets high in raw egg white (at least 30% of total caloric intake must be derived from raw egg white) and in these persons a biotin deficiency has developed.

Experimental biotin deficiency in rats causes a dry scaliness of the skin and an eczematous rash in addition to alopecia, most prominent around the eyes, resulting in so-called spectacle eyes. Experimental biotin deficiency in humans also produces a grayish discolored, dry, flaky, and scaly skin besides papillary atrophy of the tongue, anorexia, nausea, insomnia, muscle pains, and elevated serum cholesterol. Severe seborrheic dermatitis in infants (Leiner's disease) has been at least partially responsive to biotin therapy, although adult seborrheic dermatitis is not improved by similar therapy.

There have been reports[3] of a biotin-responsive form of immunodeficiency in children who had total alopecia as one of the manifestations. Biotin is required for many carboxylation reactions in normal physiology. A deficiency of biotin may be suggested by the finding of increased urinary excretion of 3-hydroxyisovaleric acid, indicating a carboxylase deficiency.

Fat-Soluble Vitamins

Vitamin A (retinol). Vitamin A is required for normal growth and development, reproduction, epithelial differentiation, and vision. It is fat-soluble and found only in the animal kingdom, although the provitamin carotenoids (particularly beta-carotene) occur in many plants. Vitamin A aldehyde (retinol) plays an essential role in dark adaptation and night vision. The normal function of retinol is zinc-dependent. Experimental vitamin A deficiency in animals causes congenital malformations, growth failure, destructive corneal and conjunctival lesions, skin rashes, and death.

Humans generally have good bodily stores of vitamin A, so deficiency is uncommon unless there is prolonged deprivation of the vitamin through chronic steatorrhea with impaired fat absorption, pancreatic and biliary tract disease, sprue, or colitis.

Rough dry scaly skin (xerosis) is the major cutaneous manifestation of human vitamin A deficiency. The roughness is due to a follicular reaction called phrynoderma that was formerly considered to be diagnostic of vitamin A deficiency. A similar reaction has been seen in some vitamin B complex and fatty acid deficiency states indistinguishable from that occurring in vitamin A deficiency.

The eye is similarly affected, producing xerosis conjunctivae et corneae (Bitot's spots) and keratomalacia in addition to the gradually worsening symptoms of impaired dark adaptation.

Contrary to the situation with most water-soluble vitamins, excessive vitamin A in the diet is toxic.[6] Acute vitamin A intoxication seldom is encountered; but large doses (in excess of 1 million units daily, especially if given intravenously) produce drowsiness, anorexia, and desquamation of skin.

Chronic vitamin A intoxication is more common in patients taking large oral doses as part of multiple vitamin preparations obtained from nonprescription sources. Fatigue is one of the earliest signs of overdose, followed by bone pains, alopecia, generalized pruritus with erythema, and widespread desquamation. If alowed to progress, additional findings of nausea, vomiting, abdominal pain, hepatosplenomegaly, headache, dry rough and coarse skin with hyperpigmentation, dry lips, and increased intracranial pressure with symptoms suggesting brain tumor or meningitis may occur.

The dose required for chronic toxicity varies. The RDA for vitamin A is 400 IU/day during the first year of life, rising gradually to 5000 IU daily (1000 µg retinal equivalents) in adolescents and adults. Normal plasma levels are in the range of 50-150 IU/dl. In general, 20 times the RDA, or doses in the range of 100,000 IU daily, will produce toxicity if taken for many weeks or months. One million units daily usually will elicit toxic manifestations within 2 to 3 weeks.

Carotenoderma is yellow discoloration of the skin resulting from excessive ingestion of carotene, the precursor of vitamin A. Eating too many carrots is the most common cause. The yellow carotenoids are partly excreted through the sweat and they then become absorbed in the horny layer (stratum corneum) of the skin. Areas with the thickest stratum corneum, such as the palms and soles, are the first to become yellow,

followed by areas of increased perspiration, particularly the face. This uneven distribution, plus the lack of involvement of the mucous membranes and sclera, helps to distinguish carotenoderma from jaundice. Infants and children manifest carotenoderma more readily than adults do. The diagnosis may be confirmed by measuring the serum carotene level.

The normal serum carotene concentration in healthy adults is 40 to 150 µg/dl, and it rises rapidly if large quantities of carrots are eaten or if an individual is taking beta-carotene capsules as a treatment for erythropoietic protoporphyria.[7] Beta-carotene supplies the basic raw materials for vitamin A synthesis; however, serum vitamin A levels are not elevated by beta-carotene therapy.

Beta-carotene, taken in recommended doses of 30-300 µg daily, has very low toxicity. It does induce yellow discoloration of the skin, and it affords photoprotection in one type of porphyria (erythropoietic protoporphyria) but not in other types or in normal individuals. Therefore it has no value as a natural sunscreen for the general population.

In the past decade there has been an explosion of interest in the synthetic analogues of vitamin A; consequently new drugs with exaggerated effects on one or another of the basic biologic functions of natural vitamin A have been produced.

An all-*trans* form of retinoic acid (tretinoin [Retin-A]) was the first to be synthesized for the topical treatment of acne. Its effect on epithelial differentiation helped to prevent follicular hyperkeratinization and plugging, one of the basic etiologic mechanisms in acne. Retin-A has recently received great, though perhaps somewhat magnified, claims* of being able to reverse skin damage caused by prolonged sun exposure, particularly wrinkling and solar lentigos. The cream must be applied daily and used with a sunscreen lotion because tretinoin is itself a mild photosensitizer. The long-term effects of topical retinoids and the reversibility of their antiwrinkling effects are unknown.

A second-generation analogue (isotretinoin, 13-*cis*-retinoic acid [Accutane]) was next to be

---

*Weiss JS, et al: Topical tretinoin improves photoaged skin, JAMA **259**:527-532, 1988.

synthesized for oral administration and was found to have a much greater effect on epithelial keratinization, besides causing a reduction in sebaceous production. It has become the most effective drug available in the management of acne. Unexpected adverse effects have shown the drug to be a potent teratogen, however, and to cause elevations in serum triglyceride levels as well as dry, scaly, itchy skin, hyperostoses, and possible premature closure of epiphyses in growing adolescents.

A third-generation analogue (etretinate [Tegison]) has less effect on acne but greater inhibition of hyperkeratinization of skin, so it has been of value in the management of disorders such as psoriasis, icthyosis, and eczema. It has all the side effects of the previous synthetic derivatives but is even more teratogenic. Thus most physicians consider it to be contraindicated in women of childbearing years.

Research into fourth- and fifth-generation analogues of vitamin A is actively ongoing. Many of these are thought to have an anticarcinogenic effect and are being studied for possible future roles in the field of oncology.[8]

Vitamin D. One natural and important source of vitamin D for human physiology is the skin. The epidermis has the ability to convert provitamin D_3 (7-dehydrocholesterol) to previtamin D_3 through the action of ultraviolet light in the range of 290 to 305 nm. Previtamin D_3 is transported to the liver and thence to the kidney for two important hydroxylation steps that convert it to the metabolically active form $(1,25(OH)_2\text{-}D_3)$. Most foods contain only small amounts of vitamin D, but oral intake is usually not a critical factor as long as the skin has some ultraviolet light exposure. Generous quantities of the vitamin are stored in the liver.

Vitamin D is essential for calcium absorption from the gut. Hypovitaminosis D or rickets in children (osteomalacia in adults) is quite rare. It is more common in northern colder climates, where sun exposure is limited, and in dark-skinned people and those who almost totally avoid the sun. There are few if any cutaneous signs of rickets, although the underlying skeletal defects (rachitic rosary, frontal bossing, pigeon breast) are visible externally.

Reports of children with vitamin D–resistant rickets have appeared in which the deficiency led to complete and persistent alopecia in addition to the usual orthopedic and radiographic signs of active rickets. This evidence suggests a possible role for vitamin D in normal hair growth, but if such a requirement does exist its mechanisms are unknown.

Vitamin D in excess may be toxic. The signs and symptoms are essentially those of hypercalcemia: anorexia, nausea, weight loss, weakness, polyuria, polydipsia, mental depression, and calcific keratitis. Sensitivity to hypercalcemia appears to vary. If the blood calcium level rises to very high levels, metastatic calcification of the skin may occur, with large dermal deposits of amorphous calcium producing massive erythematous, ulcerated, and necrotic lesions. The RDA for vitamin D is 400 IU/day (10 μg of cholecalciferol). A daily dose of 50,000 units of vitamin D may be toxic for some very sensitive individuals. Other causes of hypervitaminosis D include drinking large quantities of vitamin D–fortified milk and excessive administration of vitamin D in actual or presumed vitamin D deficiency. Advocates of megavitamin consumption may come dangerously close to ingesting toxic doses.

Vitamin E (alpha-tocopherol). In adults deficiency of vitamin E is extremely rare. However, in infants a hemolytic anemia and a seborrheic dermatitis–like rash can develop, particularly if the infants are fed formulas containing over 20% of the fat as linoleic acid. Most of the signs disappear spontaneously without specific therapy if given sufficient time, perhaps because of changes in the intestinal synthesis of alpha-tocopherol.

Vitamin E has been heralded as an antiaging vitamin and a cureall for many skin diseases. It also has been applied topically as a treatment for almost every dermatologic disorder, with sporadic anecdotal reports of success. There is little or no evidence to support any of these claims for vitamin E, however, other than its known properties as a natural antioxidant. In fact, its topical application often aggravates eczematous rashes.

Vitamin K. This fat-soluble vitamin is required for the hepatic synthesis of prothrombin (Factor II), proconvertin (Factor VII), and Stuart and Christmas factors. It is synthesized by the intestinal flora shortly after birth, and thus natural deficiency beyond the neonatal period is extremely rare. Hemorrhagic disease of the newborn, caused by a deficiency of these blood factors, is characterized by hypoprothrombinemia, increased bleeding time, hemorrhage into the skin and gastrointestinal tract, and a severe mycrocytic hypochromic anemia.[9] Since vitamin K_1 has been given routinely to newborns, this disorder no longer exists.

Infants, particularly neonates, receiving long-term broad-spectrum antibiotics are theoretically at risk of vitamin K deficiency if sufficient intestinal flora is destroyed. Clinical examples of such complications are, however, extremely rare. Prolonged diarrhea, steatorrhea, pancreatic failure, or chronic treatment of constipation with mineral oil may interfere with absorption of this fat-soluble vitamin and, in severe cases, produce vitamin K deficiency.

Coumarin anticoagulant therapy is the most common cause of this deficiency. Rarely, large doses of salicylates may have a similar effect. The deficiency is corrected easily with intramuscular vitamin K_3 (menadione) (10 mg) or intravenous vitamin K_1 (phytonadione or phylloquinone). Intravenous vitamin K_1, however, can be hazardous: deaths have occurred following injection at rates greater than 1 mg/minute.

TRACE MINERAL DEFICIENCIES AND EXCESSES

Nutritional aspects of mineral deficiencies are reviewed in Chapter 34. Most disorders of trace element metabolism have more or less specific cutaneous manifestations, although systemic features often are clinically more apparent. The cutaneous manifestations of zinc deficiency are perhaps the most dramatic and specific and frequently allow the diagnosis to be made, or strongly suspected, on the basis of cutaneous findings alone.

Zinc

Zinc is utilized over a broad range of biologic functions—for example, it is incorporated into nucleic acids, it regulates enzyme activity, it stabilizes cell membranes and ribosomes, and it is found in zinc metalloenzymes. There are now more than 100 known zinc metalloenzymes, which function in all phases of protein, carbohydrate, and fat metabolism.

Although it has been known for years that zinc is essential for normal growth and development in animals, the fact that only trace amounts are required plus the ubiquity of the element in nature led to the belief that human zinc deficiency was highly unlikely if not impossible. This concept was disproved in the early 1960s by Prasad et al.[10] They reported a syndrome of dermatitis, growth failure, emotional instability, and hypogonadism in rural Iranian and Egyptian dwarfs whose diets were low in zinc and whose bread contained large amounts of phytates (which are known chelators of zinc).

Acrodermatitis enteropathica. All doubts about possible human zinc deficiency were dispelled when the hereditary disorder acrodermatitis enteropathica was shown to be caused by decreased serum zinc levels resulting from a failure to absorb zinc from the gut.[11] Infants with this hereditary disorder had a characteristic dermatitis in an acral distribution (face, hands, anogenital areas, feet; hence *acro*dermatitis) consisting of an eczematous rash with secondary vesicular, bullous, and pustular lesions that became infected with bacteria and yeast. Other major manifestations included diarrhea, alopecia, growth failure, hypoguesia, anorexia, and emotional instability. The entire syndrome was rapidly and dramatically reversed by simple oral supplementation with zinc in doses of three to four times the daily RDA.[12]

The recommended daily allowances for zinc in adults and children over 10 years of age are 15 mg. In infants 3-5 mg is required whereas children 1 to 10 years of age require 10 mg. In acrodermatitis enteropathica a dose of 50-75 mg Zn^{+2} is adequate and must be continued for life. Plasma levels should be checked from time to time to maintain the zinc concentration within the normal range of 70 to 110 µg/dl. Zinc is commercially available in several forms—the sulfate, gluconate, acetate, oxide, and amino acid–chelated. Furthermore, it may be formulated as a heptahydrate (7 $H_2O \cdot ZnSO_4$), a monohydrate (1 $H_2O \cdot ZnSO_4$), or other form. For this reason it is important to know the amount of elemental zinc in each preparation and to prescribe the desired amount based on the actual zinc content. (For example, 7 $H_2O \cdot ZnSO_4$ in a 220 mg capsule contains 44 mg of elemental Zn.)

Induced or conditioned deficiency. Improved methods of measuring trace elements in tissues and fluids by atomic absorption spectrophotometry have shown that zinc deficiency is more common than previously recognized. The symptoms and signs of induced or conditioned zinc deficiency are essentially those of acrodermatitis enteropathica, in both their clinical presentation and in their response to zinc therapy.[13] The major early signs of conditioned zinc deficiency include acral dermatitis with the facial component resembling seborrheic dermatitis, anorexia, hypogeusia, diarrhea (variable), alopecia, secondary cutaneous infection with bacteria and yeast, and emotional instability. These signs are so distinctive and characteristic that a "zinc deficiency rash" may usually be diagnosed clinically by physicians with a modicum of expertise in this area.

Although zinc concentration can be measured in any biologic tissue or fluid, the diagnosis of a deficiency is most reliable from the plasma or serum level. Attempts to correlate total-body zinc nutriture with urinary excretion rates and hair zinc concentration have been studied extensively but found to be less sensitive than blood level as an index. Blood concentration may not always be an accurate measure of total zinc nutriture, but until better biologic parameters are discovered it is the most reliable. Avoidance of trace element contamination is crucial in collecting specimens and in their laboratory mesurement. Acid-washed glassware and tubes with plastic stoppers (rubber stoppers contain zinc) are essential for collecting and storing specimens. A competent trace element laboratory also is essential for accurate and reproducible results.

The RDA of 15 mg zinc daily is met almost exactly by the average American diet. This narrow margin between requirements and intake sets the stage for potential zinc deficiency during extended dietary deprivation. Body stores provide adequate quantities for short-term deficits, but after 4 to 6 weeks of severe dietary deprivation, early manifestations of zinc deficiency can be expected, often with cutaneous signs.

Foods rich in zinc are meats, shellfish, and herring. Cereal grains contain phytates, which are natural chelators of zinc and may prevent absorption of zinc from the gut.

Overdose and toxicity. The ready availability of zinc preparations in health food stores and the incorporation of zinc and other trace elements into multiple vitamin-mineral preparations provide an opportunity for potential overdose and toxicity. The use of zinc in higher pharmacologic doses for treating various disorders also has demonstrated the toxic potential of zinc overdose. Modest zinc overdose is corrected by normal homeostatic mechanisms, but severe or prolonged overdoses raise the plasma concentrations to high levels and gradually induce adverse effects.

Gastric irritation and nausea, with or without mild gastric bleeding, are common. Anemia may gradually develop secondary to bleeding and/or hypocupremia. Zinc and copper are mutually antagonistic in that prolonged hyperzincemia leads to hypocupremia (and vice versa).[14] One of the consequences of hypocupremia is neutropenia and an intractable anemia that becomes unresponsive to iron therapy. Zinc smelter workers contract so-called metal fume fever with major manifestations of fever, chills, gastroenteritis, and pulmonary symptoms. Studies have shown that moderately high doses of oral zinc (160 mg of elemental Zn daily) for periods of 5 weeks lower the high-density-lipoprotein (HDL) cholesterol concentration to 25% below baseline values. This drop is followed by a gradual return to pre−zinc therapy levels after stopping the medication, which suggests that prolonged zinc therapy at this level may be atherogenic in humans. One relatively recent study* has shown that lower doses (50 mg of elemental Zn per day) had no effect on any of the plasma lipid fractions.

Thus fad zinc supplements should not be encouraged in healthy individuals with normal diets and normal plasma zinc levels. Those taking zinc supplements above 10-15 mg of elemental zinc daily should have plasma zinc and copper levels checked every 1 to 4 months depending on the dosage level. Patients on higher doses also should be followed with a hemogram (WBC, RBC, hemoglobin, hematocrit) and stool examination for occult blood.

Copper

The biologic function of copper is to serve as an essential constituent of copper metalloenzymes, notably those required for oxidative metabolism (including cytochrome oxidase). Copper amine oxidases are essential for cross-linking collagen and in elastin synthesis. Tyrosinase is

---

*Crouse SF, et al: Zinc ingestion and lipoprotein values in sedentary and endurance-trained men, JAMA **252:**785-787, 1984.

a copper metalloenzyme required for melanin synthesis.

Deficiency. As with zinc, until recently copper deficiency in humans was believed to be impossible because of the trace amounts required and the ready availability of the element in food and water. Foods rich in copper include meat, eggs, and nuts. Copper pipes add the mineral to drinking water. However, copper deficiency now is recognized in animals and in a variety of human conditions.[15]

The recommended copper intake is 2 to 3 mg/day for adults and 0.08 mg/kg/day for the average full-term infant. Premature infants need an estimated 200 to 500 μg/day. Infants normally are born with liver stores of copper sufficient to last several months, until a varied diet provides for continuing needs. Premature infants with proportionally small livers may have low bodily stores of copper and may become deficient, especially if fed exclusively on cow's milk.[16] Cow's milk is lower in copper content (≤100 μg/liter) than is breast milk (200-400 μg/liter). Most infant formulas provide 60 μg/100 kcal, which is sufficient for normal infants but may be inadequate for very small premature infants.

Symptoms of copper deficiency include neutropenia, hypochromic anemia that is unresponsive to iron therapy, and osteoporosis. Patients of any age receiving long-term total parenteral nutrition or those suffering from chronic malnutrition, prolonged diarrhea, or malabsorption disorders of medical or surgical etiology are at risk for copper deficiency. Prolonged high-dose zinc therapy also has been shown to induce copper deficiency due to the antagonistic relationship between zinc and copper.[14]

Studies of the relationship between iron utilization and cooper deficiency have shed light on the multifunctional role of the copper-transport protein ceruloplasmin. Patients with copper deficiency have low serum copper levels and extremely low ceruloplasmin levels. Besides copper transport, ceruloplasmin is required for (1) normal gastrointestinal absorption of iron, (2) the flow of iron from reticuloendothelial cells to plasma, (3) movement of iron out of the liver parenchymal cells, and (4) heme synthesis within the normoblast. Thus the anemia of copper deficiency requires both copper and iron for successful therapy.[17]

Menkes' syndrome. The cutaneous features of copper deficiency are limited primarily to the hair. Menkes' steely hair syndrome is a hereditary disorder of copper deficiency secondary to impaired copper metabolism. Supplemental oral or intravenous copper does not cure the disorder. Some currently unknown abnormality in metallothioneine function is believed to be the cause, despite the normal or even increased amounts of metallothioneine present. Children with Menkes' syndrome have developmental regression, seizures, temperature instability, arterial intimal disease, and scorbutic bone changes, in addition to alopecia with a specific structural defect in the hair shaft called pili torti.[18]

Toxicity. Copper toxicity occurs in Wilson's disease, in which a heritable defect in ceruloplasmin interferes with normal copper transport and leads to large accumulations in the liver. Subsequent cirrhosis and episodes of liver necrosis result in massive release of copper into the circulation. Major manifestations include Kayser-Fleischer corneal rings in the eyes, central nervous system involvement with choreic tremors, dysarthria, a multiple sclerosis–like syndrome, proteinuria, and hematuria. Penicillamine chelates excessive circulating copper and facilitates its urinary excretion, thereby providing palliative therapy. Patients receiving penicillamine for this or any other condition are susceptible to zinc deficiency.

Nickel

Nickel is an essential trace element whose physiologic role is not well established. At least one function appears to exist in nickel metalloenzymes such as ureases. The average daily dietary intake by American adults is 0.3 to 0.6 mg, of which 5% to 10% is absorbed from the gut; the remainder is excreted in the feces. The average normal blood level of nickel is approximately 2 μg/liter of plasma.

Deficiency. Nickel deficiency has been documented experimentally in rats, in which it retarded growth and decreased liver phospholipids and total lipids. Nickel deficiency has not been demonstrated conclusively in humans.

Contact dermatitis. There is among dermatologists considerable interest in nickel because it is a common cause for allergic contact dermatitis through exposure to metallic objects containing nickel. It is the most potent allergen of all the trace elements, accounting for more contact dermatitis than all the other metals combined.

Dyshidrotic eczema (pompholyx) is a rash limited to the hands and feet that is more common in nickel-sensitive individuals. Attempts have been made to correlate its exacerbation with dietary nickel intake and nickel supplementation in the form of nickel sulfate tablets (2.5 mg). In one study[19] 60% of 17 patients with nickel allergy and dyshidrotic eczema experienced a flare-up after taking a single nickel sulfate tablet. In dietary restriction experiments, about half the patients either cleared completely or improved within 2 weeks of beginning a diet low in nickel. These studies require verification with larger numbers of patients before a specific nickel dermatitis can be confirmed.

Carcinogenic effects and toxicity. Preliminary evidence suggests that prolonged nickel exposure in refinery workers may be carcinogenic, particularly for nasal sinus, pharyngeal, lung, and renal carcinomas. Again, however, these studies require confirmation. In animal experiments, nickel excess is teratogenic, with ocular specificity in rats.

Chromium

The average American diet contains 60 μg of chromium per day. An intake of 50 to 200 μg/day is suggested for adults. Brewer's yeast, meat products, cheese, whole grains, and condiments are good sources of chromium.

Deficiency. No specific deficiency syndromes have been described for this essential nutrient. Animal studies indicate possible roles in glucose metabolism and diabetes mellitus. Rats or monkeys maintained on low-chromium diets develop elevated blood glucose and lipid levels that are normalized with inorganic chromium salts.

Although chromium deficiency has not been demonstrated in the adult American diabetic population,[20] a chromium-responsive diabetes, characterized by weight loss and an encephalopathy-like confusional state, has been reported[21] in patients being maintained on long-term total parenteral nutrition. The action of chromium is associated with that of insulin through a chromium–nicotinic acid complex called glucose tolerance factor, which facilitates insulin's reaction with receptor sites on insulin-sensitive tissues. Poor weight gain in malnourished infants also has been linked to chromium deficiency.[22]

Toxicity and contact dermatitis. Chromium toxicity is caused by occupational exposure to dust and fumes or inadvertent contact with the skin. Inhaling chromium causes ulcerations of the nasal septum and chronic bronchitis, in which a carcinogenic effect on the lung has been postulated. In prevalence, allergic contact dermatitis caused by hexavalent chromium is second only to that caused by nickel; however, the development and course of the allergy do not appear to be influenced by dietary chromium intake.

Iodine

Iodine deficiency is one of many causes of goiter and hypothyroidism. The classic cutaneous manifestations of cold dry skin with sparse hair, decreased perspiration, and frank myxedema are well-known diagnostic criteria for hypothyroidism.

Toxicity. Iodine or iodide toxicity is of more interest to dermatologists. Iododerma (the multiple nodular, ulcerating, pustular, or fungating lesions on the skin of susceptible individuals following long-term ingestion of iodides) usually occurs after the patient has taken excessive iodine in expectorants or other medications or has eaten kelp as a dietary supplement. Kelp provides a rich source of iodides but has caused such marked flare-ups of acne in susceptible persons that the diagnosis of "kelp acne" has been coined.

Magnesium

Magnesium is known to be an essential trace element, but only in recent years has a deficiency syndrome been recognized with several possible clinical symptoms. These include neuromuscular excitability, smooth muscle hyperactivity, Bartter's syndrome (renal hyperplasia with hyperaldosteronism and hypokalemia), mitral valve prolapse, and increased responsiveness to histamine.[23]

Mast cells contain histamine and are normally present in the skin in small numbers, but they increase markedly in some skin diseases. An effect on their function has been demonstrated in rats,[24] in which magnesium depletion caused degranulation of the duodenal mucosal mast cells. There was an associated fourfold to fivefold rise in blood histamine levels, with return to normal after 2 to 3 weeks of magnesium repletion. Since histamine is a known mediator of cutaneous inflammation and is involved in the production of urticaria, some role for magnesium in chronic urticaria could be postulated; however, none has been proved.

Magnesium is concentrated selectively in mammalian cells and, next to potassium, is the predominant cation. It is an essential component of many enzymes. Hypomagnesemia has been observed in kwashiorkor and chronic alcoholism but is of questionable significance. Neuromuscular disturbances have been associated with magnesium deficiency but, again, the etiologic correlation is doubtful.[25]

The RDA for magnesium (300 mg/da for women, 350 for men) is easily supplied in the average diet.

FATTY ACID DEFICIENCY

Two unsaturated fatty acids, linoleic and linolenic, are essential dietary nutrients. The body can synthesize arachidonic acid from either of them. Fatty acid deficiency is of great theoretical interest because arachidonic acid is the precursor of the prostaglandins (via the cyclooxygenase pathway) and of leukotrienes (through the lipoxygenase pathway).[26] Prostaglandins and leukotrienes contain many subgroups, most of which are potent mediators of inflammation and are present in the epidermis. Epidermal irritation or stimulation releases them, causing erythema, DNA synthesis, epidermal proliferation, vasodilation, and chemotaxis of inflammatory cells. A deficiency of arachidonic acid can have adverse effects on these natural responses to injury or to normal epidermal physiology.

Arachidonic acid is present in large quantities in red meat, and linoleic acid is also present in animal fats and vegetable oils, making essential fatty acid deficiency virtually unknown in normal adults. A syndrome of fatty acid deficiency has been described in malnourished children and experimental fatty acid deficiency is induced easily in animals.[27] The major cutaneous features are a dry scaly rash in which the epidermis is hyperproliferative and hyperkeratotic, suggesting a role for the essential fatty acids in keratinization. In linoleic acid deficiency, plasma levels of linoleic acid fall to very low values and an abnormal metabolite, 5,8,11-eicosatrienoic acid, appears in the plasma. It is believed to be derived from oleic acid as a replacement for arachidonic acid, which no longer can be synthesized because of the absence of linoleic acid. It is further postu-

lated that this abnormal metabolite replaces arachidonic acid in cell membranes and in the epidermis, where it functions in an abnormal and incomplete manner. It is, however, not known whether the presence of 5,8,11-eicosatrienoic acid in the plasma is a specific indication of essential fatty acid deficiency. Topical application of sunflower seed oil has been shown to allow sufficient percutaneous absorption of essential fatty acids to correct the condition.

Individuals with severe malabsorption disorders are at risk of fatty acid deficiency, as are infants fed formulas low in lipids. Patients receiving total parenteral nutrition without added lipids for extended periods also may have fatty acid deficiency.

OBESITY

Rapid weight gain in children or adults, with its attendant pull on the skin, causes stretch marks (striae distensae) in and around the axillae, groin, and lower abdomen. These stretch marks are identical in appearance and prognosis to those of pregnancy (striae gravidarum). Once formed, they gradually lose their purple discoloration but otherwise remain for the life of the individual.

Intertrigo is a common skin problem of obese persons. The incubator effect in the intertriginous areas provides an ideal locale for the growth of bacteria, yeast, and other fungi. Diabetics are particularly prone to such infections. The enlarged intertriginous areas in obesity are also subject to increased mechanical irritation and maceration from rubbing and friction. Persons allergic to such items as clothing dyes, antiperspirants, soap, or lotions are more likely to have severe reactions in the intertriginous sites. Local treatment for any of the problems of the intertriginous areas is only palliative until weight reduction is achieved.

Acanthosis nigricans, a rare skin disorder consisting of velvety brown plaques most commonly appearing in the axillae, may occur in various flexural sites.[28] The disorder is seen in prepubertal children, in whom it is of doubtful significance. In older children and adults it is often associated with obesity, Stein-Leventhal syndrome, pituitary adenoma, cirrhosis, and the use of drugs (particularly stilbesterol, nicotinic acid, and corticosteroids). In nonobese persons it may be a cutaneous sign of an internal malignancy, most commonly adenocarcinoma of the gastrointestinal tract, although other carcinomas and lymphomas have been reported. Thus the finding of acanthosis nigricans in other than children or obese adults requires a thorough search for malignancy.

DERMATOLOGIC DISORDERS AND THE DIET

Several dermatologic disorders are either caused by or aggravated by dietary factors. The most obvious is the allergic reaction of foods causing urticaria of an acute or chronic nature. Although a detailed discussion of food allergy is beyond the scope of this text, in general, any food or drink can trigger an allergic reaction in a susceptible individual.

Eczema

Atopic dermatitis is a form of eczema that usually begins in infancy and is associated with a hereditary predisposition toward hay fever, allergic rhinitis, and asthma. The basic defect is unknown but complex interactions with immune factors (particularly IgE) and external triggering agents such as dry skin, exposure to irritants, secondary infection, and emotional stress are intermingled in poorly understood ways.

Possible aggravation by dietary factors or frank food allergies has been the subject of controversy. Basic nutrients such as milk, wheat, egg, and citrus fruits have been implicated, based largely on a positive response to allergy scratch testing procedures. Such tests are difficult to interpret and are often examples of false positive responses to any foreign protein scratched into the skin. Rigorous elimination diets are seldom of value in atopic dermatitis although temporary food intolerance, particularly to new foods introduced into the diet, may cause mild to moderate aggravation of the dermatitis. In most instances, an observant parent will be able to identify an aggravating food if such does exist. Temporary elimination of a suspected food is usually adequate, since permanent food allergy seldom has its origin in infancy.

Acne

The role of diet in acne remains the subject of controversy. Many dermatologists believe that dietary factors have no effect on the course of acne, although many acne sufferers readily recognize that certain foods or drinks aggravate their condition. Those most commonly implicated are chocolate, cola drinks, iodides, and excessive ingestion of dairy products or highly seasoned foods. No doubt, great individual variation is the rule, thereby adding to the confusion and controversy. Patients with persistent acne who are responding poorly to conventional therapy should make an effort to eliminate or greatly reduce their intake of the aforementioned nutrients. There appears to be no age-dependent relationship, although adults with acne extending well beyond the adolescent years often have one or more aggravating factors in their diets.

Dermatitis Herpetiformis and Iododerma

Dermatitis herpetiformis is a rare blistering disease of unknown etiology that causes intense itching and discomfort. It is known to be aggravated by foods rich in iodides and wheat flour gluten. Gluten sensitivity is believed to exist in this disease as it does in celiac disease.

An exquisite iodide sensitivity exists with localized pustular and furunculoid skin lesions (iododerma) as a result of either taking medications containing iodides or eating foods rich in iodide. Bromides produce similar reactions when medications and foods rich in them are ingested.

DRUG-NUTRIENT-SKIN INTERACTIONS

Drugs may interact with specific nutrients and cause a nutritional deficit. Specific examples include isoniazid (isonicotinic acid hydrazide, INH) interference with pyridoxine (vitamin B_6) metabolism. The result is a pellagra-like skin rash and other signs of pyridoxine deficiency. Penicillamine is a potent chelator of copper and zinc plus other heavy metals. It has been reported to induce a zinc deficiency dermatitis. Phenytoin interferes with vitamin D metabolism in the liver and may produce a deficiency of that vitamin. The antimetabolite drugs for cancer therapy (particularly 5-fluorouracil and methotrexate, as they interfere with uracil and folic acid metabolism, respectively) may produce severe oral ulcerations, stomatitis and gastrointestinal ulceration, and bleeding among many other adverse systemic effects.

REFERENCES

1. Fitzpatrick TB, et al, editors: Dermatology in general medicine, New York, 1979, McGraw-Hill Book Co.
2. Keyes A: The biology of human starvation, Minneapolis, 1950, University of Minnesota Press.
3. Goldsmith LA: Vitamins and alopecia, Arch Dermatol **116**:1135-1136, 1980.
4. Krause MU, Mahan LK, editors: Food, nutrition, and diet therapy, Philadelphia, 1979, WB Saunders Co.
5. Schneider HA, et al, editors: Nutritional support of medical practice, New York, 1977, Harper & Row Publishers.
6. DiBenedetto RJ: Chronic hypervitaminosis A in an adult, JAMA **201**:700-702, 1967.
7. Poh-Fitzpatrick MB: Erythropoietic protoporphyria, Int J Dermatol **17**:359-369, 1978.
8. Dicken CH: Retinoids; a review, J Am Acad Dermatol **11**:541-552, 1984.
9. Frick PG, et al: Dose response and minimal daily requirements for vitamin K in man, J Appl Physiol **23**:387-389, 1967.
10. Prasad AS, et al: Zinc metabolism in normals and patients with a syndrome of iron deficiency anemia, hypogonadism, and dwarfism, J Lab Clin Med **61**:537-549, 1963.
11. Moynahan EJ, Barnes PM: Zinc deficiency and a synthetic diet for lactose intolerance, Lancet **1**:676-678, 1973.
12. Neldner KH, Hambidge KM: Zinc therapy of acrodermatitis enteropathica, N Engl J Med **292**:879-882, 1975.
13. Sandstead HH, et al: Conditional zinc deficiencies. In Prasad AS, editor: Trace elements in human health and disease. Vol 1. Zinc and copper, New York, 1976, Academic Press Inc, pp 33-49.
14. Prasad AS, et al: Hypocupremia induced by zinc therapy in adults, JAMA **240**:2166-2168, 1978.
15. Graham GG, Cordano A: Copper deficiency in human subjects. In Prasad AS, editor: Trace elements in human health and disease. Vol 1. Zinc and copper, New York, 1976, Academic Press Inc, pp 363-372.
16. Alexander EW: Copper metabolism in children, Arch Dis Child **49**:589-590, 1974.
17. Lee GR, et al: Role of copper in iron metabolism and heme biosynthesis. In Prasad AS, editor: Trace elements in human health and disease. Vol 1. Zinc and copper, New York, 1976, Academic Press Inc, pp 373-390.
18. Danks DM, et al: Menkes's kinky hair syndrome: an inherited defect in copper absorption with widespread effects, Pediatrics **50**:188-201, 1972.
19. Kaaber K, et al: Low nickel diet in the treatment of patients with chronic nickel dermatitis, Br J Dermatol **98**:197-201, 1978.
20. Rabinowitz MB, et al: Comparison of chromium status in diabetic and normal man, Metabolism **29**:355-360, 1980.
21. Freund H, et al: Chromium deficiency during total parenteral nutrition, JAMA **241**:496-498, 1979.
22. Hambidge KM: Chromium nutrition in man, Am J Clin Nutr **27**:505-510, 1974.
23. Halpern MJ, Durlach J, editors: Magnesium deficiency. Pathophysiology and treatment implications, Basel, 1985, S Karger AG.
24. Kraeuter SL, Schwartz R: Blood and mast cell histamine levels in magnesium-deficient rats, J Nutr **110**:851-855, 1980.
25. Caldwell JL, Goddard DR: Studies on protein-calorie malnutrition. I. Chemical evidence for magnesium deficiency, N Engl J Med **276**:533-535, 1967.
26. Voorhees JJ: Leukotrienes and other lipoxygenase products in the pathogenesis and therapy of psoriasis and other dermatoses, Arch Dermatol **119**:541-547, 1983.
27. Wene JD, et al: The development of essential fatty acid deficiency in healthy men fed fat-free diets intravenously and orally, J Clin Invest **56**:127-134, 1975.
28. Curth HO: Classification of acanthosis nigricans, Int J Dermatol **15**:592-593, 1976.

V

SPECIFIC DISEASE STATES AND NUTRITIONAL MANAGEMENT

CHAPTER 23
Infection

William R. Beisel

Infectious illnesses stimulate a complex array of metabolic and nutritional responses that support generalized and antigen-specific immunologic defensive mechanisms and help meet the broad demands of body cells for the increased quantities of energy-generating substrates needed during periods of fever, infection-induced stress, and tissue repair.[1]

The magnitude and type of nutritional losses caused by an infection reflect both the severity and the duration of an illness. Nutritional losses also are influenced by the generalized or localized nature of a given infectious process; by the age, sex, and premorbid nutritional status of the patient; and by the possible presence of underlying or complicating medical or surgical conditions.

Despite the complexity of the interrelated biochemical, metabolic, endocrine, and nutritional responses to infection, these responses develop and eventually regress in an orderly predictable sequence that appears to be related to the evolving phases of the infectious process. An improved understanding of the fundamental cellular response mechanisms at play during the course of an infection should allow the thoughtful physician to anticipate probable nutritional deficits and plan the most appropriate measures for supportive care.

IDENTIFICATION OF NUTRIENT NEEDS

In attempting to define nutrient needs of a patient who suffers from an infectious illness, it is necessary for the physician to know which nutrients are influenced by the disease process. Two broad types of nutrient losses have been identified: absolute and functional:

Absolute (direct losses) ("wastage")
Following negative metabolic balances
From diarrhea, vomiting, sweating, bleeding
Via exudates, sputum, eschars, etc.
Through drainage tubes, dialysis, blood sampling, other therapeutic procedures

Functional
Due to increased metabolic utilization of specific nutrients, with depletion of bodily storage depots
Because of diversion of nutrients into different metabolic pathways
Following sequestration of nutrients in relatively inaccessible forms
Use of host nutrients for microbial replication

Absolute Nutrient Losses

The most conspicuous nutritional consequence of an infectious illness is an absolute (i.e., measurable) loss of body constituents.[1] This is reflected clinically by a loss of body weight and muscle tone, and by the progressive wastage of muscle mass and body fat. These losses are associated with negative body balances of the principal intracellular elements during generalized infections, including nitrogen, potassium, magnesium, phosphorus, zinc, and sulfur.[1,2] Absolute losses of nitrogen may vary from 20 to 90 g, with the losses of other intracellular elements being proportional to those of nitrogen.[2] If an infection is characterized by massive diarrhea and vomiting, absolute losses of body water, sodium, and chloride may become life-threatening. Diarrhea-induced fecal losses of bicarbonate and potassium ions may induce additional problems in acid-base balance. Some infections also cause absolute losses of body protein and red blood cells via exudates, sputum, eschars, or the therapeutic procedures required for their treatment (e.g., drains, dialysis, blood sampling).

Functional Nutrient Losses

In addition to the absolute or direct losses of body nutrients, several functional forms of nutrient loss must be anticipated. Functional losses are defined as the within-body losses of nutrients caused by infection-induced metabolic or pathophysiologic responses. These functional loss categories include an increased utilization, diversion, or temporary sequestration of nutrients.

Functional losses may progress to absolute losses.

One example is the metabolic rate increase of about 7% for each degree Fahrenheit rise in body temperature. Since these extra energy requirements typically are met through accelerated cellular utilization of carbohydrate, the rate of gluconeogenesis also must be increased. This process diverts both essential and nonessential amino acids from other uses, and, together with accelerated ureagenesis, helps to account for some of the direct losses of body nitrogen. Sizable amounts of tryptophan may be diverted into the kynurenine pathway during some infections, especially typhoid fever, and tryptophan metabolites then appear in the urine as diazo reactants. Increased metabolic utilization of vitamins also must be anticipated during infections.[1]

Another of the functional forms of nutrient loss during infection occurs as a redistribution of certain body electrolytes and minerals. Iron and zinc are sequestered rapidly in storage forms by hepatic cells; in contrast, copper is secreted by the liver as a component of ceruloplasmin. In infections of marked severity, sodium may be reduced in extracellular fluids and may accumulate within body cells. The replication of microorganisms in the host leads to further depletion of nutrients. These losses can be sizable, especially with massive growth of parasites.

Control Mechanisms Leading to Nutrient Losses

It is now recognized that the loss of numerous body nutrients during the febrile phase of acute infectious illnesses is a consequence of the multiple metabolic and physiologic responses of the body during the acute phase of illness. These acute phase responses include fever, accelerated cellular metabolism, anorexia, myalgia, muscle protein breakdown, leukocytosis (often), synthesis of many new proteins needed by the body to control the infection, production of many hormones, sequestration of certain trace elements, heightened degradation of amino acids and vitamins, and a stimulation of immune system functions.

Acute phase responses are all triggered, directly or indirectly, by the monokine interleukin-1,[3] which is released by macrophages, monocytes, and other body cells whenever they become activated. After its release, interleukin-1 acts in the manner of a hormone, stimulating responses of certain cells that lead, in turn, to the diverse phenomena characterizing the acute phase responses. Activation of interleukin-1—secreting cells may be initiated by phagocytosis or by contact with any of a number of different stimuli, including endotoxin, antigen-antibody complexes, nucleotides, and other single molecules. Another monokine that appears to act synergistically with interleukin-1 is tumor necrosis factor (cachectin), released in response to a gram-negative endotoxin.

INFECTION-INDUCED ANOREXIA

Acute febrile illnesses generally are accompanied by anorexia, nausea, and sometimes vomiting. These gastrointestinal symptoms appear to be triggered by the action of interleukin-1 at some yet undetermined site in the central nervous system. It remains uncertain whether infection-induced anorexia serves the host in a purposeful manner and therefore should be classified as a generalized defensive measure.[4]

Consequences of Anorexia

Anorexia reduces the intake of food appreciably, even to the point of total abstinence during days of high fever. The diminished intake contributes to negative balances of body nutrients during the fever. However, the febrile losses of body nutrients are far greater than can be accounted for by the anorexia. Hypermetabolic consequences of fever appear to inhibit the homeostatic mechanisms normally used by the body as nitrogen-sparing devices during periods of uncomplicated starvation and semistarvation.

Other Gastrointestinal Functions

In addition to anorexia and disturbed gut motility, generalized infections alter rates of intestinal mucosal cell replication and maturation, and some (e.g., measles) can cause protein-losing enteropathy.

Pathogenic enteric microorganisms may cause lesions within the mucosa, intestinal wall, and lymphatics that interfere with absorptive functions. Parasites also can cause intestinal losses of blood cells and protein. If their total mass becomes sufficiently great, parasites compete with mucosal cells for dietary nutrients. Alterations in the number, composition, and location of intestinal microflora can result fom antibiotics or purgative therapy. All these changes, along with the effects of microbial enterotoxins, may interfere with nutrient absorption.

NUTRITIONAL RESPONSES TO INFECTIOUS ILLNESSES

When virulent microorganisms penetrate host defenses, a sequence of nutritonally important events evolves in a relatively predictable manner. Nutritional costs of illness are related to the severity and duration of the illness, the occurrence of certain complications, or the localization of infection in a single organ system. Although the type of infecting microorganism will influence the nutritional response to some degree, the overall patterns of nutritional loss are quite similar, or stereotyped, despite organism-to-organism differences.[2]

Acute Febrile Illnesses

The variety of nutritional responses during a generalized infection is broad enough to include most major metabolic pathways of body cells. Alterations may occur in rates of protein synthesis and degradation; in the metabolic processing of individual amino acids and other nutrients, including electrolytes, minerals, trace elements, and vitamins; and in the production and utilization of cellular energy. Many of these responses are regulated by interleukin-1, hormones, or other biologically active substances released from body cells.

Pituitary Hormones

ACTH—Increased immediately before and during fever

GH—Variable increase immediately before and during fever; exaggerated secretion after intravenous glucose

TSH—Delayed increase, with overshoot (secondary to thyrotropin-releasing factor changes)

ADH—Secretion increased; may become inappropriate

Adrenocortical Hormones

Glucocorticoids—Short-lived twofold to fivefold increase in secretion; loss of circadian periodicity in plasma; impaired secretion in chronic infections; absent secretion after adrenopathy; supernormal plasma values in septic shock

Mineralocorticoids—Increased during fever

Adrenal androgens—Modest increase during fever

Adrenomedullary Hormones—Increased during septic shock; minimal increase in some other infections

Thyroid Hormones

PBI—Febrile period decline, followed by rebound; altered binding protein affinity

T_4—Acceleration of hepatic metabolic disposal during fever; greater conversion to rT_3; accelerated use by neutrophils

T_3—Acceleration of hepatic metabolic disposal during fever

Pancreatic Hormones

Insulin—Higher than expected for comparable degree of starvation; enhanced secretion after intravenous glucose; slowed rate of clearance

Glucagon—Increased secretion during fever

Other Hormones

Inadequate data to define responses of gonadal steroids and gonadotropins and parathyroid and neuroendocrine-gut peptide hormones

The responses also are influenced by the presence of fever (which is triggered by the direct action of interleukin-1, cachectin, or Type I interferon on the temperature regulating center in the hypothalamus), the availability of key nutrients derived from body stores or from the diet, and any nutrient losses caused directly by microorganism uptake.

Catabolic losses. Sharply negative balances of body nitrogen begin soon after the onset of fever (see Chapter 3). Nitrogen losses via the urine exceed dietary intake values, and occur in the forms of urea, ammonia, creatinine, alpha-amino nitrogen, and sometimes of creatine, diazo reactants, and uric acid.[2] An increased excretion of 3-methylhistidine indicates that a major portion of lost nitrogen is derived from protein components of skeletal muscle. Nitrogen also may be lost in sweat, but fecal losses generally do not increase unless diarrhea is present.

The patterns of nitrogen loss typify the proportional losses of other principal intracellular elements. During periods of rising fever, hyperventilation-induced respiratory alkalosis leads to a transient decrease in urinary phosphate loss; but thereafter, phosphate losses reflect those of nitrogen. Calcium, however, is not generally lost unless muscle paralysis supervenes, as in poliomyelitis. In a paralytic infection, prolonged loss of body calcium, ascribed to disuse atrophy of bone, is accompanied by phosphate losses from bone as well as from muscle.

Fluid and electrolyte losses. In most forms of infection the major extracellular electrolytes, sodium and chloride, are influenced more by hormonal events than by changes in dietary intake. However, infection-induced changes in salt and water homeostasis can reach life-threatening extremes at either end of the spectrum (i.e., severe dehydration or fluid overload).

A brief period at the onset of a generalized

symptomatic infection may be accompanied by an increased urinary excretion of sodium and chloride. Salt also will be lost via sweat if diaphoresis is an important component of an infection.

If diarrhea occurs, direct fecal losses of sodium, chloride, bicarbonate, and potassium result. Body losses of chloride and hydrogen ions also can be sizable if vomiting becomes excessive during an infection.

Despite these possibilities for acute losses of body salt, most severe generalized infections lead to saline and water retention. Initial brief renal losses do not persist. Rather, within a day or so after the onset of fever, the kidney begins to retain sodium and chloride. This renal conservation of electrolytes is brought about, in part, by increased secretion of adrenal mineralocorticoids. Retention of salt often is accompanied by retention of body water, sometimes to the point of dilutional hyponatremia. With a successful cure of a severe illness, excess accumulated body water typically is lost by diuresis in early convalescence.[1]

Severe retention of body water, especially during central nervous system infection, now has been widely ascribed to an inappropriate secretion of antidiuretic hormone from the posterior pituitary gland.[5] In addition, in some severe infections, membrane transport functions of cells are disturbed in a manner that allows sodium to accumulate intracellularly.

Acid/base balance. Pathogenic mechanisms that come into play during various infections can lead to metabolic alkalosis or acidosis, to respiratory alkalosis or acidosis, or to complex admixtures of these perturbations.

The onset of fever typically is accompanied by tachypnea and accelerated respiratory gas exchange, an exaggerated loss of CO_2, and a state of uncompensated respiratory alkalosis. Alkalosis may persist as long as febrile tachypnea lasts and gas exchange within the alveoli remains unimpeded. Conversely, infections that cause pulmonary consolidation can impair CO_2 exchange and lead to respiratory acidosis. Respiratory acidosis also develops if pulmonary musculature no longer can function effectively, as in poliomyelitis or tetanus.

Metabolic acidosis is seen whenever an infectious disease becomes extremely severe. With hypotension, vascular stasis, and cellular anoxia during gram-negative sepsis, for example, the generation of lactic and other metabolic acids exceeds the capacity of the body's buffering systems.

Diarrheal diseases can be accompanied by two additional forms of metabolic acid-base derangement. (1) Diarrhea characterized by extremely high-volume stool losses, as in Asiatic cholera, causes an excessive loss of bicarbonate in the stool with a resultant decline in blood pH. Bicarbonate is secreted actively in the lower ileum and cannot be reabsorbed completely by the colonic mucosa if there are high-volume losses of watery stool. (2) Diarrhea characterized by only low-volume stool losses tends to be associated with an exaggerated loss of fecal potassium rather than bicarbonate. If fecal potassium losses persist chronically over a long period or occur rapidly during massive acute diarrhea, bodily stores can be severely depleted. Loss of cellular potassium leads to metabolic alkalosis.

Trace element nutrition. Plasma concentrations of iron and zinc decline abruptly with the onset of fever. These phenomena are due to an accelerated uptake by the liver of both iron and zinc. The iron accumulates in granules as hemosiderin or ferritin complexes. Iron is not released readily from these storage forms as long as infection persists. The abrupt decline in plasma iron is most marked in pyogenic bacterial infection, but has been noted in viral infections as well. The movement of iron into the liver initially is not accompanied by a reduction in plasma iron-binding capacity; as a result, the percentage of unbound plasma transferrin increases. This increase in unsaturated transferrin is thought to be of positive benefit as a host defensive mechanism, for it minimizes the availability of iron needed to permit replication of some types of invading microorganisms.[1] Accumulation of iron in storage depots is accompanied by an increase in plasma ferritin values; this increase has diagnostic value and differentiates infection-induced changes in iron metabolism from iron-deficiency anemia, where plasma ferritin values are low.

The decline of plasma zinc is not as marked as that of iron, but, like iron, zinc also is taken up by the liver. The liver normally does not have an ability to store zinc; however, acute infectious or inflammatory processes activate phagocytic cells to release interleukin-1,[6,7] which, in turn, stimulates hepatocytes to initiate a rapid synthesis of metallothioneine proteins. The newly formed hepatic metallothioneines, with their unusually large number of sulfhydryl groups per molecule, are able to bind large quantities of zinc and to retain this element within the liver until the infectious process if terminated.

In addition to the redistribution of zinc within the body, overall zinc balances become negative because of a combination of factors, including reduced dietary zinc intake and increased losses via the urine and possibly via the feces and sweat as well. During acute infectious hepatitis there is an unusually large loss of zinc via the urine. This has been ascribed to an increase in the percentage of plasma zinc that is bound in the form of a microligand to the amino acids, histidine and cysteine. The small size of these zinc microligands permits them to pass through the renal glomerulus.

Plasma concentrations of copper begin to increase shortly after the onset of fever. This is the result of accelerated hepatic synthesis of ceruloplasmin, the copper-binding protein of plasma. Ceruloplasmin values remain elevated during infection and then begin a gradual return to normal with the onset of convalescence.

Vitamin metabolism. Plasma concentrations of some of the vitamins may decline during acute infections; negative balances of nitrogen may be accompanied by an increased urinary loss of riboflavin.[1] B vitamins, folate, and ascorbic acid all participate in the heightened cellular metabolism seen whenever phagocytic cells become activated. The B vitamins also participate in the replication and functional activities of lymphoid series cells. The rapid production of adrenocortical hormones during infection causes the vitamin C content of the adrenal gland to decline abruptly. Vitamins A and E also appear to be of value in maintaining the competence of normal host defense measures.[1]

The intestinal absorption of fat-soluble vitamins and folate may be impaired during enteric infections or parasitic infestations. Parasites with a large bulk, such as tapeworms, may take up enough B vitamins from intestinal lumen fluids to produce deficiency states in the host.

Although little is known yet about alterations of vitamin metabolism at the molecular level, severe acute infections can, on occasion, precipitate acute avitaminoses, including scurvy, beri-

beri, pellagra, and night blindness.

Protein metabolism. Acute infections trigger a unique admixture of concomitantly accelerated anabolic and catabolic effects on protein metabolism.[1] The contractile proteins of skeletal muscle and other proteins of somatic tissues in normally nourished persons appear to provide an available pool of labile body nitrogen. The accelerated catabolism of these proteins during acute infection is stimulated by interleukin-1, and this process generates free amino acids for use in the synthesis of other kinds of protein or for diversion into energy-yielding processes. Anabolic responses are summarized as:

Production of New Body Cells
Phagocyotosis, cell-mediated immunity, antibody synthesis, repair of structural damage, and intestinal nutrient absorption

Production of Additional Intracellular Components
Nucleic acids, ribosomes, enzymes, endoplasmic reticulum, metallothioneines, etc.

Production of Endogenous Substances for Secretion by Cells
Antimicrobial factors (e.g., interferon, lysozyme, transfer factor)
Immunoglobulins
Components of the coagulation, kinin, and complement systems
Hormones
Acute phase reactant serum glycoproteins
Endogenous mediators of
    Granulocytopoiesis
    Local inflammatory response
    Fever
    Trace element responses
    Altered lipid metabolism
    Lymphocyte, monocyte, and macrophage activation
    Hypersensitivity reactions

Liver cells take up free amino acids at an accelerated rate during acute infections, again as a direct response to interleukin-1. The affinity of the liver for amino acids is sufficiently great during early infections that their uptake exceeds their rate of release from degraded body proteins. This causes the concentrations of most free amino acids in plasma to decline. Amino acids entering the liver are used for the accelerated de novo synthesis of hepatic proteins or for gluconeogenesis. On the other hand, neither tryptophan nor phenylalanine can be utilized as rapidly as they are released during the catabolism of somatic proteins. Tryptophan excesses in plasma appear to be managed within the liver by shunting tryptophan into either the serotonin or kynurenine pathways. Excess phenylalanine accumulates for a time within the plasma in coincidence with an accelerated utilization of tyrosine. Thus the plasma phenylalanine:tyrosine ratio increases during acute infectious illnesses. In infections of overwhelming severity, the liver no longer can take up and metabolize free amino acids as rapidly as they are released, and a preterminal period of hyperaminoacidemia may develop.

Every host defensive measure utlimately depends upon the ability of body cells to synthesize new proteins. Protein anabolism is important for the production of new phagocytes, lymphocytes, and antibody-producing plasma cells. Interaction of neutrophils and macrophages with microbial pathogens or necrotic debris leads to the synthesis and release into plasma of cellular proteins, including lactoferrin, lysozyme, interleukin-1, and other mediators.[6,7] The lymphocytes produce proteins such as interferon and the lymphokines. Fibroblasts produce cold-insoluble globulin; endocrine organs secrete polypeptide hormones in increased amounts, including ACTH, growth hormone, insulin, and glucagon.

At the same time, the liver accelerates its synthesis of many proteins while slowing the production of albumin and transferrin. The accelerated or de novo synthesis of hepatic proteins stimulated by interleukin-1 includes a number of enzymes, metallothioneines, complement, kinin, coagulation system components, lipoproteins, and acute-phase reactant plasma proteins. The latter group includes haptoglobin, alpha$_1$-antitrypsin, C-reactive protein, alpha$_1$-acid glycoprotein (orosomucoid), ceruloplasmin, and fibrinogen.[1,6]

Carbohydrate metabolism. During periods of febrile illness the additional metabolizable energy needed by body cells is provided largely by glucose.[8] Hormonal mechanisms and substrate availability contribute to an increased hepatic output of glucose. Although some glucose is derived from glycogen, most comes from gluconeogenesis. Recycled lactate and gluconeogenic amino acids (alanine and glycine) are the principal substrates used by the liver; pyruvate and glycerol also contribute.

If the ability of the body to sustain the increased rate of glucose production should fail, hypoglycemia may emerge as an important clinical problem. Infection-induced hypoglycemia generally results from one of two pathogenic mechanisms: a diminished availability of substrate or a failure of hepatocellular competency. Hypoglycemia in septic newborn infants generally is due to a lack of substrate, while the hypoglycemia associated with severe hepatitis illustrates the breakdown of cellular gluconeogenic mechanisms.[1,8]

Lipid metabolism. Changes in lipid metabolism during the course of infection are far more difficult to understand than are those of carbohydrate and protein.[1,8] Plasma cholesterol values increase in some infections and decrease in others. Free fatty acids, which are transported in plasma through their binding to albumin, generally are reduced in concentration. Triglycerides, however, may accumulate in plasma in amounts sufficient to give it a creamy appearance. Such hyperlipidemia is most characteristic in severe gram-negative sepsis. Hypertriglyceridemia results from an increase in hepatic synthesis in combination with diminished activity of lipolytic enzymes in peripheral tissues. Some of these responses result from the actions of cachectin (also known as tumor necrosis factor) in inhibiting lipoprotein lipases. Like interleukin-1, cachectin is released from activated monocytes and macrophages.

The metabolic needs for extra energy during periods of acute fever largely are met by the oxidation of glucose and branched-chain amino acids. In contrast, fat depots do not appear to contribute more energy substrates than they generally yield under basal fasting conditions.

The hepatic conversion of free fatty acids to ketone bodies within the liver contributes importantly to body energy needs during periods of simple starvation. This mechanism normally "spares" or conserves body proteins during starvation. However, the capacity of the liver to synthesize ketones is not utilized fully during acute infectious illnesses.[8] The mechanisms responsible for inhibition of ketogenesis during infection are not known fully, but since pancreatic insulin secretion increases during fever, the antiketogenic effects of insulin may play a role. The lipogenic effects of insulin also may contribute to enhanced hepatic synthesis of fatty acids. This increase in the production of fatty acids also helps to explain the development of fatty metamorphosis of liver cells during severe acute infections.

Subacute and Chronic Infections

If an infectious process becomes subacute or chronic, metabolic functions of the body tend to reach new equilibrium settings. Concentrations of plasma albumin and transferrin begin to decline. In some subacute infections, iron concentrations in plasma may increase to values greater than normal. This has been noted during the second and third weeks of hepatitis and during late stages of typhoid fever.

The adrenocortical production of glucocorticoid and ketosteroid hormones often declines into a subnormal range. The labile pool of body nitrogen is depleted progressively and nitrogen balance enters into a precarious new steady state, but at a cachectic level. Body fat depots also become depleted slowly, and generalized protein-energy malnutrition may ensue. A similar state can emerge as a last result of a series of closely spaced acute infections. This gives rise to the concept that infection and malnutrition may interact to produce a vicious cycle or downhill spiral.[1] In this regard it is unusual for chronic severe malnutrition to exist in the absence of a superimposed or coexisting infectious complication.

Chronic infections accompanied by protein-energy malnutrition also are characterized by impairment of host defensive mechanisms and immune system competence. Functional anergy of nutritional origin involves both the cellular and the humoral arms of the immune system, but, fortunately, this defect generally can be reversed by correcting the nutritional deficits and curing the infection.

Patients subjected to severe starvation or protein-energy malnutrition may not manifest the expected typical signs of infection. They may be unable to mount a fever, produce a leukocytic or inflammatory response, or generate a granulomatous reaction. For these reasons the nutritional rehabilitation of a severely malnourished patient may allow a clinically nonapparent infection to emerge. A refeeding program thus may become complicated by the sudden appearance of a life-threatening infectious illness.[4]

The Convalescent Period

When acute infectious illnesses terminate uneventfully, negative nitrogen balances are reversed promptly. Thus, body nutrient stores generally reach their lowest levels within several days after fever has subsided. Anorexia disappears at the same time as fever in most patients, and appetite is regained. The body then begins to replenish its depleted nutritional stores, although full nutritional recovery may require many weeks. It seems desirable to utilize the early convalescent period following an acute illness to speed up the repletion of lost body nutrients by providing patients with increased quantities of highly nutritious food. Hyperphagia may stimulate convalescent children to consume about twice their normal daily intake of food until catch-up weight gain restores their weight:height ratios to normal.

On the basis of both metabolic balance studies and measurements of host defensive capabilities (e.g., phagocytosis),[1,2] patients seem highly susceptible to a superimposed new infection during the early stages of convalescence. A secondary infection acquired at that critical time may block nutritional recovery and lead instead to an additional depletion of body nutrients.

SPECIFIC RECOMMENDATIONS

Far too little is known about optimum techniques for using nutrient therapy as a key supportive measure in the management of infectious disease. The objectives of nutrient management should be to support physiological host defense mechanisms and to optimize the ability of the host to recover from illness. This will shorten convalescence and minimize the likelihood of a superimposed secondary infection.

In most acute infectious diseases that develop in a well-nourished person, the illness is relatively brief and the potential value of nutrient supportive therapy considerably less than the more pressing need to identify the causative microorganism without delay and initiate appropriate antimicrobial therapy quickly. Dietary measures thus should be used in support of the selected regimen of antimicrobial drugs.

In many of the common brief infectious illnesses (e.g., the respiratory viral diseases) effective antimicrobial therapy is not generally available, but the infection is likely to be short-lived and relatively mild. Any nutrients consumed during the illness will minimize the anticipated losses of body components. Since cumulative nutrient losses incurred during a mild, self-limited viral infection may not be fully reconstituted until after several weeks of convalescence, emphasis should be placed on providing additional nutrient support during the latter period.

In some acute infectious diseases, especially those associated with severe diarrhea, the need to provide immediate nutrient support in the form of fluid and electrolyte replacement therapy takes precedence over other forms of therapy. In occasional infections, oxygen may become a critical nutrient that must be supplied without delay.

Control of Fever

The duration and severity of fever influence the magnitude of both absolute and functional losses of body nutrients. Lessening of fever by antipyretic drugs and by direct physical methods minimizes the increased nutritional needs associated with a hypermetabolic state. Control of fever also reduces dermal losses of nutrients via sweat.

Modest elevations of body temperature provide positive benefit during some experimental infections in laboratory animals. Fever also may help to control a few infections in humans (e.g., central nervous system syphilis, localized chronic gonococcal infections). However, high fever can be dangerous, and, at best, its putative benefits do not outweigh those of an effective antibiotic. Accordingly, the control of fever has positive nutritional value, and the nutritional impact of fever must be taken into account when calculating daily needs for dietary energy and protein.

Estimation of Energy Requirements

The caloric needs of a patient with an infectious illness include the normal basal dietary allowance plus extra amounts needed because of fever. The extra daily requirements can be calculated according to the amount of fever (7% increase for each degree Fahrenheit of elevation).

Thus a 27-year-old man weighing 65 kg, who ordinarily requires an energy intake of 2500 kcal, with a body temperature 3° F above normal, would require 2500 kcal plus 3 times 7% of 2500 kcal. This amounts to 2500 plus 525 kcal, or 3025 kcal/day. Alternatively, a febrile adult arbitrarily could be given 30 to 40 kcal/kg/day; a child, 100 to 150 kcal/kg/day; and an infant, 200 kcal/kg/day as desirable total energy intakes. Although these calculated additions will likely minimize illness-induced body losses,

their overall effectiveness in individual patients can be evaluated best by measuring total body weight losses in early convalescence. If the sick patient cannot consume these calculated quantities of food, cumulative decrements should be corrected during early convalescence. In children, the objective should be to achieve "catch-up" growth in both height and weight.

The adequacy of energy intake during an extended illness also can be determined by changes in body weight. However, a loss of tissue mass may be masked by the tendency for febrile patients to retain salt and water. The true loss of body weight may not become apparent until early convalescence, when postfebrile diuresis causes excessive fluid to be excreted. In some societies it is customary to restrict feedings in convalescent children to diluted gruels. Such a practice is unwise; catch-up can be achieved best by offering diets with an energy and protein content about twice the normal during convalescence.

Protein Requirements

Despite the importance of the protein-synthesizing capabilities of individual cells, the body will sacrifice amino acids through functional diversions to provide for total energy needs. Thus the protein requirements of a febrile patient will depend in part on the availability of sufficient dietary energy input. It usually is possible to reduce excessive losses of body nitrogen in febrile patients by increasing energy intake.

If energy intake is inadequate, amino acids derived from dietary-protein or existing body pools are diverted to meet needs for energy rather than for incorporation into the structure of new proteins or for other metabolic uses unique for each amino acid. Since additional metabolic energy must be expended to deaminate the amino acids used for carbohydrate synthesis, the use of amino acids for calorigenesis is doubly wasteful.

Exact protein requirements have not been determined during fever. However, the nitrogen intake should be increased, if possible, to about 1.5 g/kg/day for febrile adults and 3 g/kg/day for febrile children. The nitrogen source should include a balanced supply of essential amino acids.[1]

Several simple alternative methods are available for estimating protein requirements. Urea nitrogen assays can be performed by most clinical laboratories on 24-hour urine specimens. A daily urea nitrogen excretion value plus 4 g (2 g for nonurea nitrogen in urine, 2 g for stool nitrogen) provides a reasonable estimate of nitrogen loss. If this value is compared with an estimate of nitrogen intake based on food table values, a rough approximation of nitrogen balance can be obtained.

Acid-Base Stabilization

The clinician must be aware of possible changes in acid-base equilibrium to determine the need for corrective therapy during illness or replacement therapy during convalescence. Metabolic acidosis during severe diarrhea can be treated by adding bicarbonate or lactate to replacement fluid infusions. Such treatment should be continued until the urine pH becomes alkaline. If potassium losses are great, vacuolar degeneration of body cells may develop, especially in the renal tubules. Hypokalemic metabolic alkalosis can persist for many months unless treated. The development of hypokalemic nephropathy and metabolic alkalosis can be prevented by replacement therapy with potassium, using commercial solutions to provide 20 to 35 mEq of potassium per liter during severe diarrhea. Any residual or chronic deficit then should be corrected with high-potassium foods given during the convalescent period.

Electrolyte and Water Requirements

An infectious process may lead to death from divergent types of fluid imbalance, which range from severe overload to severe dehydration. Direct losses of salt and water occur in diseases accompanied by massive or protracted diarrhea, vomiting, or marked diaphoresis. In the absence of such direct losses, the body usually retains fluid and electrolytes. With severe illness, sodium may accumulate within poorly functioning cells. Water retention due to inappropriate antidiuretic hormone secretion will increase the severity of hyponatremia. Appropriate therapy in the latter types of salt and water derangements requires a careful restriction of fluid and electrolyte intake.[5] Thus a patient with infectious illness may, on the one hand, have an emergency need for electrolyte replacement or, on the other, be seriously harmed by fluid and electrolyte administration.

Dehydration problems. In massive diarrhea the watery stools are virtually isosmotic with plasma. Because stool losses are isosmotic, water does not move from body cells to maintain the extracellular volume, and an immediate threat to life may arise from depletion of circulatory volume. The extent of body dehydration can be assessed by clinical signs, together with high hematocrit values and increased concentrations of total plasma proteins in relation to plasma water. This type of dehydration increases the specific gravity of both whole blood and plasma. Because plasma proteins can undergo a twofold increase in concentration during severe cholera, measured sodium and chloride concentrations may appear to be diminished if they are calculated and expressed conventionally, on the basis of whole plasma values. Electrolyte concentrations in plasma water of such dehydrated patients must be recalculated to reflect the high protein concentration and diminished amount of water present in the plasma.

Isosmotic dehydration from massive diarrhea should be corrected by the use of isotonic replacement fluids, given rapidly to correct shock and return hematocrit and plasma protein concentrations to normal. After initial rehydration, homeostasis is maintained by infusing intravenous solutions at a rate to match measured hourly stool volume losses. Alternatively, both rehydration (in mild to moderate dehydration) and maintenance fluids can be given orally by using solutions containing electrolytes (Na^+, Cl^-, K^+, HCO_3^-) and glucose. Potassium deficiency can be made up by mouth or by fluids containing potassium.

Overhydration problems. Dehydration is not usually a problem in generalized infectious diseases that do not include diarrhea or repeated vomiting. Rather, the onset of fever typically is accompanied by increased secretion of aldosterone and antidiuretic hormone. Acting in concert on the distal renal tubule, these hormones cause the kidney to retain both salt and water. Sodium and chloride may virtually disappear from the urine, and urine volume may be reduced sharply.

If the secretion of antidiuretic hormone persists in an inappropriate fashion, body water is retained even in the presence of declining plasma concentrations of both sodium and chloride.[5] Because of the retention of salt and water in many infectious illnesses, it is generally unwise to administer saline. Furthermore, if chronic metabolic acidosis develops, variable amounts of sodium may accumulate within the body cells. The sequestration of sodium within body cells is evidence of severe illness and is not easily reversed. The unwise intravenous administration of saline in an attempt to correct depressed plasma sodium concentrations in such patients may have serious consequences, such as cerebral edema or congestive heart failure.

Severe hyponatremia that cannot be explained by direct sodium losses should be managed by restricting salt and water intake until after the infectious process is controlled and plasma sodium concentrations begins to increase.[1,5] This type of hyponatremia is most common in the aged, or in children with central nervous system infections, Rocky Mountain spotted fever, or other severe generalized infections. In the presence of hyponatremia, daily fluid intake should be restricted. Body weight, urinary specific gravity and volume, and plasma and urine values for sodium and osmolality should be measured each day; central venous pressures may need to be followed in some patients. Only after urinary specific gravity begins to decline and the daily urine volume increases can fluid intake be liberalized.

Mineral and Trace Element Requirements

Little direct information is available about the need to employ minerals or trace elements as therapeutic agents.[8] For the present, the wisest course of action would seem to demand that natural foodstuffs be given, if possible, during illness and certainly during early convalescence.

Magnesium concentrations in serum may decline somewhat as the result of retention of body water. Negative balances of magnesium occur in close proportion to negative balances of nitrogen. Little has been said concerning the use of magnesium supplements in infectious illness, but they may be needed if there is a prolonged negative balance of this element.

The responses of calcium metabolism during most acute infectious illness are quite subtle and difficult to document with accuracy. There appears to be an influx of calcium into body cells whenever interleukin-1 acts on the cell surface membranes to cause an intracellular release of arachidonic acid from cell membrane phospholipids.[7] The actions of calmodulin may also be involved in this influx of calcium.

It may be possible to ascribe a slight lowering of plasma calcium concentrations during infection to hemodilution. These subtle changes are not usually accompanied by a loss of calcium from the body. However, the bodily balances of calcium and other bone minerals may become negative if an infectious disease causes prolonged immobilization or paralysis. Calcium accumulates in devitalized tissues, and the tendency for granulomatous tubercular lesions to become calcified is well known. On the one hand, a high calcium intake can be employed in the preantibiotic management of tuberculosis, but there is little to suggest that it will help arrest the disease. On the other hand, hypercalcemia can develop in tuberculous patients because of a sarcoidosis-like hypersensitivity to vitamin D. If this occurs, vitamin D and calcium intakes both must be controlled carefully to avoid hypercalcemia.

Unusually low serum concentrations of inorganic phosphate have been reported in patients with gram-negative sepsis and in Reye's syndrome.[8] Reduced plasma phosphate concentrations may serve as a possible diagnostic indicator of sepsis. Plasma phosphate values also decline rapidly but transiently during the early stages of fever, apparently as a secondary manifestation of respiratory alkalosis. Hypophosphatemia during an acute rise in body temperature is accompanied by the virtual disappearance of phosphate from urine and sweat. These changes occur too rapidly to be accounted for by parathyroid gland responses.

Organic phosphate moieties and high energy phosphate bonds undoubtedly contribute at the cellular level to host responses to infection. It is not known how these changes influence the outcome of an infection, and there is no direct evidence that the administration of phosphate as a single nutrient would be of clinical importance.

Iron metabolism is markedly altered by infection.[8] The initial acute decline in plasma iron occurs without appreciable changes in plasma iron-binding capacity. If an infectious process becomes chronic, plasma iron values remain low and iron-binding capacity begins to decline slowly. This infection-induced sequestration of iron in tissue stores, together with a tendency for red blood cell survival to be shorter, can give rise to the so-called anemia of infection.

During chronic infections the administration of iron by either oral or parenteral routes is ineffective in reversing the anemia of infection. If parenteral iron therapy is given while an infectious process remains active, the administered iron also becomes sequestered in storage forms. Liver extract, the folates, and vitamin B_{12} are similarly without value in reversing anemia of infection.

Furthermore, if iron therapy is given to children with kwashiorkor or protein-energy malnutrition, it can have unexpected consequences. The administered iron may saturate the low iron-binding capacity of protein-malnourished children. The presence of saturated transferrin in plasma increases the availability of iron to aerobic and facultative bacterial pathogens. The bacteria then may proliferate rapidly and overwhelm the impaired host defensive mechanisms of the malnourished child. Thus, if total plasma iron-binding capacity is depressed in a malnourished patient, iron therapy should be delayed until after protein repletion measures have restored plasma iron-binding capacity to near-normal values.

Like iron, serum zinc moves rapidly from plasma into the liver during the early stages of most infectious illnesses.[8] This response may be of positive value in terms of host survival, for neutrophilic phagocytosis is enhanced at zinc concentrations slightly lower than those of normal plasma. In addition, as illness progresses, zinc balances can become negative as a result of diminished dietary intake of the metal along with increased losses in urine, feces, and sweat. No data exist to document any potential therapeutic value of excess zinc administration during acute infections. Since bodily losses of zinc are to be anticipated, foods with a high content of zinc are of value for use during convalescence.

Vitamin Requirements

Despite the paucity of detailed information concerning the rate of utilization or metabolic fate of vitamins in body stores during infection, there can be no doubt that vitamins contribute to the competency of various host responses. Antimicrobial drugs also can influence vitamin metabolism. Isoniazid, for example, has been thought to induce peripheral neuropathy in some tuberculous patients by causing a deficiency of vitamin B_6. Pyridoxine supplementation therefore has been suggested for patients taking isoniazid.

Based on evidence presently available, practicing physicians should employ vitamins in normally recommended doses during a brief infectious illness or should increase doses onefold or twofold during more protracted illnesses to cover the increase in vitamin metabolism (or excretion) during hypermetabolic states. Scientific evidence to justify megavitamin therapy in the treatment or prevention of infectious illnesses does not exist.

MODE OF MEETING REQUIREMENTS

Infectious disease is the most common form of illness to afflict mankind. Most humans experience numerous bouts of infection during a lifetime. Secondary infections can develop to complicate therapy during virtually every other form of illness.

There are relatively few instances in clinical medicine when nutritional modalities of therapy are of specific and direct importance to the management of an immediate life-threatening infection. However, these situations must be recognized quickly and treated effectively when they occur. Perhaps the best example of such an emergency requirement is the need to correct the massive loss of body fluids and electrolytes that occurs during fulminant diarrhea. Acute nutritional imbalances also may occur in infections that damage key body cells, deplete key nutrient stores, or allow toxic metabolites to accumulate. If severe, infectious hepatitis may produce hypoglycemia or hepatic failure. Severe hypoglycemia is also a common danger in neonatal infants with sepsis. Life-threatening hypoglycemic shock can be suspected through clinical signs, diagnosed by blood glucose analysis, and corrected with glucose infusions.

In contrast to the preceding infections, which require rapid nutritional intervention, most other acute illnesses can be managed without aggressive nutritional therapy. Anorexia, often compounded by overt nausea and vomiting, is a common nutritional problem. Few febrile patients are able to maintain a normal oral intake of fluids, calories, protein, and other nutrients. This problem cannot be eliminated by merely writing orders for a properly calculated dietary intake or by instructing a sick patient to eat the quantities and varieties of foods calculated to meet nutritional needs. Kindly and purposeful encouragement by family members or an attentive nursing staff also may be ineffective. Forced feeding of a severely nauseated patient is unwise. However, a sick patient should be offered soft or liquid foods of high nutrient value. When marked anorexia and nausea severely restrict food intake, some of the deficits can be minimized by using conventional intravenous fluids to maintain fluid and electrolyte balance and to supply some nutrients. Any nutritional deficit incurred during a brief and self-limited or easily treated infection should be corrected by a well-managed program of convalescent-period refeeding. The postillness aspect of nutritional support too often is ignored.

If an infection becomes protracted or occurs as a complication of some other severe disease process, more aggressive nutritional support should be considered during the illness.

Most of the common infectious diseases can be managed by the family members in the home. Hospital-based management will be required for diseases of great severity, including those that require the frequent parenteral administration of antimicrobial drugs.

The most difficult forms of infection seen in modern medical centers occur as secondary complications of other medical or surgical conditions. Many of these infections are due to opportunistic organisms that respond poorly to available antibiotic drugs. Since infections originating in modern hospitals usually occur in patients whose nutritional status already is compromised, considerable effort may be required to reconstitute nutrient stores and build up bodily defensive measures.

Alimentation techniques developed to meet the unusually large nutritional requirements of severely burned or traumatized patients now allow surgeons to provide sufficient nutrients to meet high energy needs associated with hypermetabolic illnesses. This may be accomplished by infusions of nutrients into large central veins or by using a constant-drip gavage of a chemically defined diet. Gavage is accomplished through thin-walled nasogastric catheters to provide balanced free amino acid and carbohydrate mixtures. When given at proper concentrations and rates, these mixtures can be absorbed fully in the upper intestine with a minimum of digestive work; therefore gavage can be used in patients with lower intestinal lesions. Gut mobility and nutrient absorption may be severely impaired in a nauseated patient. Thus aggressive enteral

infusion techniques carry certain risks that must be balanced against their potential benefits.

Because of the need to infuse hypertonic solutions via chronically implanted central venous catheters, total parenteral alimentation is not without danger. Microorganisms can gain access to the body through or around the catheters and thrombus formation can occur. Hyperosmolality of the infused nutrient solutions can initiate an osmotic diuresis with dehydration and may cause impaired function of phagocytic cells. Severe hypophosphatemia can develop in patients receiving total parenteral alimentation; this reduces leukocytic ATP content and depresses the chemotactic, phagocytic, and bactericidal activities of granulocytes. Fluid overload also must be avoided. Intravenous alimentation fluids with a high glucose content were found to increase mortality rates appreciably in monkeys during experimental bacterial and viral illnesses associated with hepatocellular damage.

In patients whose nutritional stores have been depleted by severe disease or complex surgical problems, secondary sepsis is a relatively common complication. It is generally difficult, if not impossible, to control or eliminate the septic process by using the normally appropriate and effective antibiotic. In contrast, if supported by alimentation techniques to provide adequate nutritional intake, some patients then are able to become free of fever, to clear their blood and tissues of the invading microorganisms, and to heal their surgical lesions. The correction of nutritional deficiencies in patients with severe septic complications appears to permit host defensive mechanisms to regain their functional adequacy.

Despite the potential dangers of aggressive forms of nutritional therapy, patients with severe gram-negative bacterial sepsis or longstanding infectious processes may benefit by their usage. Life-threatening septic processes from opportunistic microorganisms often can be eliminated if appropriate antimicrobial therapy is supplemented by vigorous nutritional measures. Such demonstrations are highly instructive, for they point out the value of nutritional therapy in an unequivocal manner. However, this form of nutritional support has not been studied adequately in life-threatening acute hemorrhagic viral infections, and the dangers could outweigh any potential advantages.

CONVALESCENT PERIOD THERAPY

Infection-induced depletions of body nutrients are reversible, but complete restitution of nutritional losses that result from mild self-limited infections of relatively brief duration may require several weeks if food intake is not increased. Thus it becomes important to provide an optimum nutrient intake during convalescence from an infection.

With the cessation of fever and anorexia, the early convalescent period represents a "nutritional window" that should be used to restore earlier losses. Some patients become hyperphagic during early convalescence, making the replacement of nutrients an easy task if the diet is properly constituted. In nutritionally depleted children the nutritional aim should be to obtain catch-up growth. Since the mother has a key role in achieving this objective, she should be instructed about the needs for providing increased quantities of highly nutritious foods for a period of several weeks after recovery from an infection.

The temporary presence of nutritional deficits in early convalescence predisposes a patient to secondary infections by weakening resistance mechanisms. Body nutrient stores and the functional capabilities of host defensive mechanisms are at a low point in the days immediately after fever has abated. This problem is greatest in infants and small children whose nutritional requirements for growth are superimposed on other nutritional needs. Thus, in the growing child, an infection often creates nutritional deficits that lead to new problems with secondary infections.

Such synergistic cycles are the rule rather than the exception in children who suffer from preexisting deficits of protein, calories, or both. Nutritional therapy in early convalescence may be life-saving by reversing the cycle of infection, further malnutrition, and reinfection.

Because chronic malnutrition so commonly is associated with the occurrence of infectious diseases, refeeding programs should be conducted with a high degree of suspicion that a subclinical or smoldering infectious process may become activated. The nutritionist should be alert to the possible need to initiate prompt antimicrobial therapy for any such reemergent infection that occurs during a refeeding program.

REFERENCES

1. Beisel WR, et al: Proceedings of a workshop: Impact of infection on nutritional status of the host, Am J Clin Nutr **30:**1203-1371, 1449-1566, 1977.
2. Beisel WR, et al: Metabolic effects of intracellular infection in man, Ann Intern Med **67:**744-779, 1967.
3. Kluger MJ, et al: The physiologic, metabolic, and immunologic actions of interleukin-1, New York, 1985, Alan R Liss Inc.
4. Murray MJ, Murray AB: Anorexia of infection as a mechanism of host defense, Am J Clin Nutr **32:**593-596, 1979.
5. Kaplan SL, Feigin RD: The syndrome of inappropriate secretion of antidiuretic hormone in children with bacterial meningitis, J Pediatr **92:**758-761, 1978.
6. Kampschmidt RFP: Metabolic alterations elicited by endogenous pyrogens. In Lipton JM, editor: Fever, New York, 1980, Raven Press, pp 49-56.
7. Beisel WR, Wannemacher RW Jr: Gluconeogeneisis, unreagenesis, and ketogenesis during sepsis, J Parenter Enter Nutr **4:**277-285, 1980.
8. Beisel WR: Trace elements in infectious processes, Med Clin North Am **60:**831-849, 1976.

CHAPTER 24
Surgery and Burns

Cleon W. Goodwin
Douglas W. Wilmore

The stress of surgical operations and major trauma, including burns, initiates metabolic and hormonal responses that alter nutritional needs and requires specific supportive measures if repair and recovery are to occur. These alterations of body homeostasis are primarily catabolic in nature and manifested as increased metabolic rate, erosion of body mass, loss of nitrogen in the urine, and abnormalities of carbohydrate metabolism. Skeletal trauma results in severe muscle wasting, and injury initiates a series of catabolic processes. The intensity of the increased catabolism is proportional to the extent and duration of injury. Elective surgical procedures elicit a modest increase in metabolic expenditure and nitrogen loss, while following major trauma and large burns metabolic expenditure and nitrogen loss may exceed twice normal[1] (Fig. 24-1).

A spectrum of nutritional problems is encountered in patients sustaining major injuries or undergoing surgical procedures. Patients may be debilitated and malnourished because of chronic intermittent intestinal obstruction, gastrointestinal fistulas, inflammatory bowel disease, ischemic bowel disease, cancer, and chronic liver disease. As such, the quantity and quality of dietary protein before injury influence the endogenous protein pool, and previously malnourished patients exhibit an attenuated catabolic response to surgical stress as reflected by unexpectedly small nitrogen losses.[2] Conversely, previously healthy patients in whom acute surgical illnesses develop are well nourished and rapidly lose large quantities of nitrogen when unable to eat within 2 to 4 weeks. Women, with proportionally greater body fat and decreased lean body mass, manifest less of a catabolic response to injury and stress than do men of the same age and weight. Repeated stress without intervals of repletion of body mass result in a diminution of nitrogen excreted with each catabolic episode.

METABOLIC RESPONSE TO INJURY

The response to injury and acute illness has been described by Cuthbertson and Tilstone[3] as essentially biphasic. During the initial "ebb" phase, physiologic responses to hormonal discharge are depressed and manifested as circulatory instability and poor tissue perfusion. Metabolic reactions appear diminished. The ebb phase lasts a variable time, usually 3 to 5 days, but can be shortened by vigorous restoration of blood volume and ensurance of adequate oxygenation. Following adequate resuscitative measures the ebb phase gives way to the more prolonged "flow" phase, during which metabolic reactions increase. Total body blood flow and oxygen utilization rise above levels existing before injury. Such metabolic and physiologic alterations apparently are necessary to provide substrate for tissue repair.

The injured patient's homeostatic response following resuscitation may be partitioned further into four phases, each of which requires its own nutritional approach.[4]

1. The first phase of recovery following restitution of adequate tissue perfusion is manifested by a *marked catabolic response* and is associated with the onset of hypermetabolism and complex changes in intermediary metabolism. For moderate-sized operations and injuries, this period lasts 3 to 7 days but it may extend for many weeks in patients with large thermal injuries and sepsis. During this phase, lethal losses of protein mass can occur. Since death usually follows the rapid loss of more than one third of body protein, nutritional support is directed toward maintaining body weight and tissue protein. During this period the patient is usually anorectic or may

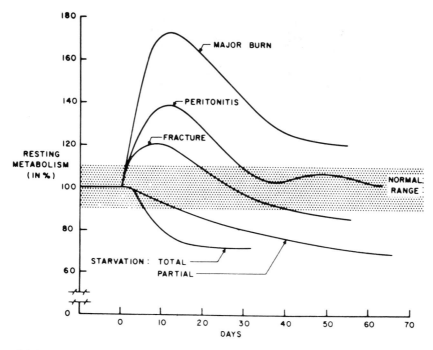

Figure 24-1 Alterations in resting metabolism following injury and starvation. The metabolic response to uncomplicated elective surgery is minimal and often does not exceed the normal range.

have a nonfunctioning gastrointestinal tract, and sophisticated carefully supervised nutritional support is necessary.

2. A few days to several weeks following surgery or other injury, the patient reaches a *turning point* and begins to feel better. Catabolic responses peak and begin to recede.

3. The patient then enters an *anabolic phase*. Spontaneous caloric intake increases as the patient becomes more active. A positive nitrogen balance appears and is reflected by a gain in muscle mass and muscle strength. This phase continues for 2 to 5 weeks depending on the duration of the previous catabolic response. Increased nutritional support at this time is better tolerated and is directed not only toward fulfilling maintenance requirements but also toward weight gain.

4. With the onset of the *fat gain phase* the patient's body composition begins to return to normal. Although this usually occurs after discharge from the hospital, patients with such extensive injuries as large burns may remain hospitalized while awaiting completion of essential reconstructive procedures.

For a few patients the fat gain phase may precede the anabolic muscle gain phase, particularly if the patient is immobilized by skeletal traction or air-fluidized beds. Vigorous caloric support at this time results in rapid and at times prodigious gains of body fat, while muscles may remain atrophic because of inactivity. This situation often occurs inadvertently when previously required maintenance levels of nutritional support are continued during the latter portion of the convalescent phase, a time when metabolic requirements diminish rapidly.

Although alterations in metabolic processes following surgical procedures and other trauma have been described, those following massive thermal injury have been studied most extensively and provide the archetypal illustration of the maximum response to injury. More limited injury and uncomplicated surgery evoke an attenuated version of this response. These changes manifest themselves primarily as hypermetabolism, negative nitrogen balance, and altered glucose flow. These alterations affect the total organism, regional beds, and cellular processes.

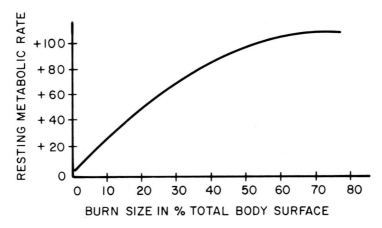

Figure 24-2 When demonstrated by a quantifiable injury (e.g., burns), the change in metabolic rate can be seen to be directly proportional to the extent of the injury.

Hypermetabolism

Following resuscitation, metabolic rate rises and is accompanied by an increase in total body oxygen consumption, which is proportional to the extent of injury (Fig. 24-2). This increase varies with time postinjury and may reach more than twice the levels encountered in uninjured persons before declining in a curvilinear fashion as the underlying pathologic process resolves.[5,6] Total body blood flow (cardiac index) increases with the rise of oxygen consumption, approaches a plateau that may exceed two to three times the level in uninjured individuals, and declines as the patient recovers.[7,8]

Regional blood flow to the viscera likewise increases, although its fraction of the total flow remains unchanged or only slightly increased.[9] Similarly, visceral oxygen utilization, although increased, maintains an unchanged or slightly elevated fraction of total body oxygen consumption. By contrast, blood flow to the wound or area of injury is markedly exaggerated in relation to total body blood flow. In studies of patients with leg burns,[10] blood flow to the injured extremity increased as burn wound size increased. However, blood flow to the underlying muscle was normal, indicating that the entire increment in extremity flow was directed to the overlying wound.[11] At the same time, oxygen consumption by the wound-bearing extremity was insignificantly elevated above that of the minimally injured extremity, suggesting that the wound utilizes primarily anaerobic intermediary mechanisms.

With marked hypermetabolism, heat production is elevated, and such patients usually exhibit elevated core and skin temperatures and higher core to skin heat transfer coefficients.[6] Although the precise signals that initiate the hypermetabolic response remain undefined, evidence points indirectly to the participation of the central nervous system. Central thermoregulation appears to be altered, especially in burned patients, with an upward shift of the temperature of maximal comfort and least metabolic expenditure. These patients seem to be internally warm and not externally cold.[12] Attempts to dampen the hypermetabolic response by externally heating injured patients do not decrease the metabolic rate. The Q_{10} effect of hyperpyrexia accounts for only a modest fraction of postinjury hypermetabolism, and the augmented heat production following injury is a consequence of an elevated metabolic state, not of increased thermoregulatory drives.[13] Only a small fraction of the hypermetabolic response can be ascribed to the endogenous specific dynamic action of accelerated protein breakdown.[14]

Catecholamines appear to be among the major mediators of the hypermetabolic response to injury.[6,15] Adrenergic activity, as measured by urinary catecholamine excretion, is related to the extent of burn injury and to oxygen consumption (Fig. 24-3). Adrenergic blockade of beta, but not alpha, receptors blunts many of the physiologic alterations of hypermetabolism, including the rises in metabolic rate, ventilation, and pulse and the serum levels of free fatty acids. Con-

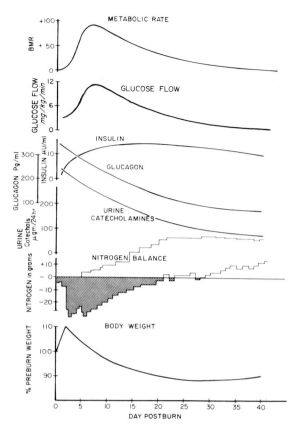

Figure 24-3 The increase in hepatic glucose production parallels the hypermetabolic response. Accelerated gluconeogenesis and negative nitrogen balance are associated with an increased glucagon:insulin molar ratio. As this ratio returns to normal and urine catecholamine excretion falls, nitrogen balance becomes positive and body weight stabilizes.

versely, many of the metabolic changes in injured patients can be reproduced by administering exogenous catecholamines to normal subjects.

Other hormones have been implicated in the hypermetabolic response, but all seem to facilitate the dominant action of catecholamines. Increased thyroid hormone activity is not the mediator of the increased metabolic rate observed in patients with complications following major surgery or with large burns. Depressed levels of triiodothyronine (T_3) and thyroxine (T_4) and elevated reverse T_3, a metabolically inactive thyroid hormone, have been found; however, unbound metabolically active forms of T_3 and T_4 are normal in the stable hypermetabolic injured patient and fall only when the patient deteriorates clinically.[16] That adequate thyroid function may be necessary to facilitate physiologic adaptation of the seriously injured patient to postinjury met-

abolic demands is demonstrated by the apparent relationship between the plasma levels of T_3 and catecholamines during the catabolic phase in severely burned patients.[17] Blood concentrations of human growth hormone, ACTH, and glucocorticoids are increased after injury and contribute to the subsequent metabolic sequelae, but these hormones play primarily permissive roles to the major effect of catecholamines.[18]

Negative Nitrogen Balance

Nitrogen loss increases following surgery and major injury, and 80% to 90% of the nitrogen appears in the urine as urea, which may exceed 40 g/day in alimented patients with severe burns. A small fraction of nitrogen is excreted as creatinine, ammonia, and uric acid, but their proportion may increase with prolonged starvation. Unless diarrhea is present, the gastrointestinal tract contributes less than 2 g/day. Skin losses are small unless the patient has a large thermal injury; in such cases, the exudate from the burn wound can account for 20% to 25% of total daily nitrogen loss. Nitrogen balance, the algebraic difference between nitrogen intake and nitrogen loss, reflects the status of lean body mass.

Although the extent of nitrogen loss is proportional to the postinjury increase in energy expenditure and follows its time course, the nitrogen-containing lean body mass is not the major source of metabolic fuel oxidized for energy. Over a range of metabolic responses varying from that of normal uninjured subjects to severely traumatized or burned patients, body protein contributes a constant 15% to 20% of the energy required to meet metabolic needs.[1] However, this constant daily nitrogen loss in patients not receiving nutritional support can result in substantial erosion of body protein stores and severe metabolic derangements. In the absence of exogenously ministered calories, lipid stores are the major source of energy for meeting metabolic requirements. Visceral proteins are quite labile and rapidly exhausted. Skeletal muscle is the primary source of nitrogen lost in the urine, and muscle proteolysis is reflected by increased excretion of creatinine and 3-methylhistidine. Depleted patients with muscle wasting lose less nitrogen following injury than do similar well-nourished individuals.

Alterations in nitrogen economy in regional organ beds are reflected by the changes in nitrogen transfer as amino acids. Following major injury amino acids, principally glutamine and alanine from skeletal muscle, are released in increased quantities into the circulation.[19] Glutamine is the most abundant free intracellular amino acid in the body, and increased catabolism is associated with a marked decline in the skeletal muscle content of glutamine. The small bowel demonstrates a net uptake of glutamine, which is associated with an increase in small bowel mucosal weight, DNA content, and villus height.[20] This increase in mucosal mass of the small intestine may improve small bowel function and facilitates the introduction of enteral nutrition. Concurrently the liver extracts larger quantities of the glucogenic amino acids, primarily alanine, glycine, and tyrosine, for gluconeogenesis.[9] Alanine appears to act as a carrier of nitrogen from muscle to the liver and is derived primarily from the transamination of pyruvate or directly from proteolysis. Alanine production allows increased oxidation of the branched-chain amino acids leucine, isoleucine, and valine, which yield, respectively, an additional 42, 43, and 32 ATP moles of amino acid for muscle energy utilization.[21]

Insulin plays a prime role in the regulation of protein metabolism (Fig. 24-3). It is an anabolic hormone, and changes in its plasma levels are associated with muscle amino acid uptake (elevated insulin concentration) or release (depressed insulin concentration). Glucagon initiates responses opposite those of insulin. Although it does not affect peripheral release of amino acids (as a reflection of proteolysis), glucagon increases liver uptake of glucogenic amino acids by accelerating hepatic gluconeogenesis. In severely injured and other critically ill patients, glucagon levels are elevated, even in the face of glucose administration and hyperglycemia. Insulin levels concomitantly are reduced relative to glucose levels, and the molar ratio of insulin to glucagon also is often markedly reduced.[22]

The depressed insulin:glucagon ratio reflects a catabolic state characterized by increased proteolysis and gluconeogenesis. Plasma glucagon levels accurately predict the metabolic rate in critically ill patients, suggesting that glucagon independently contributes a portion of the hormonal stimulus for the hypermetabolic response.[23] Catecholamines may modulate this hormonal response by actively influencing the activity of the pancreatic islet cells.

Altered Glucose Flow

Hyperglycemia often is observed following a complicated surgical procedure or major injury and is accentuated if resuscitation fluids contain glucose. This glucose intolerance has been labeled diabetes of injury or burn stress pseudo-diabetes. During the ebb, or shock, phase of injury, fasting blood glucose concentration and total body glucose frequently are elevated. Glucose flow, or turnover, is elevated only slightly, and hyperglycemia during this period is caused mainly by decreased peripheral tissue utilization of glucose.[24] On the third to the fifth days after injury, the patient enters the flow phase of the classic injury response (Fig. 24-3). Although hyperglycemia persists, glucose flow is elevated markedly.[25,26] At this time the hyperglycemia re-

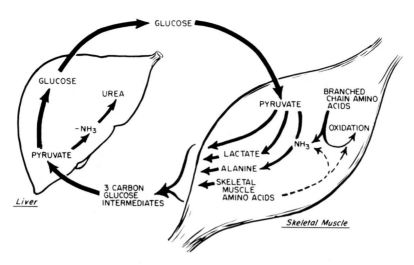

Figure 24-4 Skeletal muscle provides glucogenic amino acids as a three-carbon source for increased hepatic gluconeogenesis. Another source of three-carbon precursors in injured patients is the wound, not illustrated in this schematic.

sults from increased hepatic glucose production, not from decreased peripheral utilization, which has returned to preinjury levels.[27]

The major sources of three-carbon precursors for new glucose production by the liver are skeletal muscle and the wound. The wound utilizes glucose by anaerobic glycolytic pathways, producing large amounts of lactate as an end product. It fulfills its high glucose requirements by the high glucose delivery rates from the enhanced circulation to the wound. Glucose uptake by an injured extremity may exceed 10 times that by the contralateral uninjured extremity.[8] Skeletal muscle protein is the major source of increased amino acid delivery, mainly of alanine, from peripheral regional beds into the central circulation.

In the liver, lactate is extracted and utilized for new glucose production by the Cori cycle (Fig. 24-4). Concomitantly alanine and the other glucogenic amino acids contribute to the increased gluconeogenesis during injury.[9,28] Increased ureagenesis parallels the rise in glucose output. Peripheral amino acids and lactate from the wound account for approximately half to two thirds of new glucose produced by the liver. Gluconeogenesis is a process that requires energy, and oxidation of fatty acids provides a large portion of this energy, with heat as a byproduct.

Insulin also plays a major role in the regulation of glucose metabolism. Fasting insulin levels may be within normal ranges during both ebb and flow phases. Immediately following injury the effective insulin activity in relation to glucose concentration (and the insulinogenic index) is decreased. As hypermetabolism develops, insulin response to glucose returns to normal.[27] However, glucagon is markedly elevated at this time of increased metabolic response, and the depressed insulin:glucagon molar ratio stimulates gluconeogenesis. The elevated levels of the catecholamines inhibit glycogenesis, primarily through beta-adrenergic mechanisms, and stimulate new glucose production.[29]

Since glucose obtained by gluconeogenic pathways is ultimately derived from protein stores, depletion of body protein during periods of starvation leads to energy deficits and malfunctioning of glucose-dependent energetic processes at the cellular level. Active transport mechanisms responsible for maintaining transmembrane ionic gradients in erythrocytes are deranged in catabolic thermally injured patients.[30] The normal sodium and potassium gradients in red blood cells can be reversed by providing these injured patients with high caloric levels of carbohydrate (glucose). Hepatic clearance of indocyanine green, an energy-dependent active transport process, is decreased in severely injured patients when energy normally supplied as glucose is replaced by an isocaloric glucose-free source.[31] Glucose-insulin solutions correct the "sick cell syndrome" in burned patients, who exhibit a prompt natriuresis and nonosmotic diuresis when metabolic requirements for energy are met by glucose.[24]

Weight Loss

Change in body weight is the most easily recognized and quantified index of metabolic balance. Weight loss most often is associated with catabolic illnesses and injury, and its magnitude and duration are related directly to the extent of injury.[32] Approximately half the tissue loss is from fat stores and half from lean body tissues. Weight loss is not obligatory and can be reversed with vigorous nutritional support. Weight loss is associated with diminished physiologic function, and a rapid loss of 40% to 50% of body weight (equivalent to one fourth to one third of body protein mass) is usually fatal.

SUMMARY OF METABOLIC CHANGES

The increased total body oxygen consumption following serious injury and surgery with complications is a generalized systemic response that is characterized by increased requirements for biosynthesis, transport work, and body activity and is directed toward restoring homeostasis and healing injured tissue. Although fat oxidation

serves as the major source of energy (as evidenced by typical respiratory quotients of 0.70 to 0.75 in postabsorptive injured subjects), certain regional tissue beds can utilize only glucose as the primary metabolic fuel (Fig. 24-5). Ketone body formation is severely depressed or even prevented in hypermetabolic patients, largely because of the effects of cortisol, glucagon, and the catecholamines.[33] The brain continues to utilize glucose following injury and may have a reduced ability to utilize ketone bodies in such patients. The kidney and the cellular elements of the blood also utilize glucose. However, the wound has by far the largest obligatory requirement for glucose, which is metabolized by anaerobic pathways to lactate. The inefficient utilization of energy by the wound is compensated by increased wound blood flow, which ensures adequate delivery of substrate. Lactate produced by the wound and glucogenic amino acids derived from body protein breakdown are utilized by the liver to manufacture new glucose. In the absence of exogenously derived glucose, proteolysis (primarily from muscle) is required to meet glucose deficits arising from the complete oxidation of glucose by the brain, kidney, and cellular elements of the blood. Even then, the preferential direction of glucose

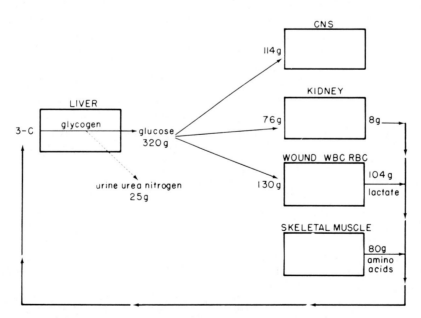

Figure 24-5 Twenty-four hour flux of six- and three-carbon units in a fasting injured metabolic patient. Lactate from the wound and amino acids from protein breakdown account for approximately half the carbon units used by the liver to maintain its daily glucose output; the brain and kidney represent the major routes of glucose loss from the body.

to the wound can produce energy deficits at the cellular level, with measurable alterations in important transport processes.

NUTRITIONAL IMPLICATIONS OF THE POSTINJURY METABOLIC RESPONSE
Increased Energy Requirements for Preservation of Lean Body Mass

Unlike starvation, injury (including surgery) increases energy requirements and accentuates nitrogen loss. Nitrogen balance appears to be more sensitive to minor stress, since uncomplicated elective surgery causes little or no increase in metabolic rate and caloric requirements while promoting a negative nitrogen balance. Starvation added to injury, exemplified by the maintenance of postoperative patients on saline infusions, accentuates negative nitrogen balance and erosion of lean body mass. Energy requirements and nitrogen loss parallel energy expenditure and are determined by the severity of injury. To preserve body integrity following injury, increased quantities of calories and nitrogen are necessary.

The provision of calories and nitrogen by a variety of modalities decreases negative nitrogen balance and preserves body protein. Food intake per se exerts a minimal effect on energy production, and the specific dynamic action of ingested nutrients is decreased in critically ill patients. Even small quantities of nonprotein calories ameliorate the negative nitrogen balance and eliminate the ketosis following illness and depressed energy intake. In such cases, nonprotein calories appear to spare protein by diminishing, but not eliminating, breakdown and nitrogen loss. The administration of 10% glucose solution containing 10 to 14 g of nitrogen as amino acids further improves nitrogen balance when compared to 5% dextrose alone. Increases of nonprotein calories (up to 600-700 g of glucose/da) to adults improve nitrogen equilibrium by decreasing loss; higher doses of calories without added nitrogen do not affect nitrogen excretion.

Increased Nitrogen Requirements

Visceral protein is the most easily mobilized source of nitrogen following starvation or injury.[34] Without nutritional support, these proteins are soon exhausted and are the major contributors to the early increased loss of nitrogen fol-lowing significant injury. If a patient is nutritionally depleted by chronic illness before injury or major surgery, visceral protein stores are depleted and the patient manifests an attenuated negative nitrogen balance. Malnutrition sufficient to cause skeletal muscle atrophy, especially if treated with a high-carbohydrate protein-free diet, causes dysfunction of metabolically active organs. When the liver is deprived of amino acids essential for enzyme synthesis and transport processes, including apoprotein transport function, lipids accumulate and are deposited in the hepatic parenchyma. This occurs frequently in critically ill patients maintained on nitrogen-free hypertonic glucose intravenous solutions.

The intake of nitrogen alone spares protein and improves nitrogen balance after injury. The addition of nonprotein calories to the source of nitrogen further improves nitrogen balance and enables more calories to be utilized for the restoration of nitrogen equilibrium. Energy and protein cooperatively contribute to this improvement in protein economy. Following parenteral administration, nitrogen balance on a fixed protein diet is determined by energy content; conversely, on a fixed energy diet, nitrogen content determines nitrogen balance[35] (Fig. 24-6). Similar enteral diets also demonstrate this interaction between nitrogen and nonprotein calories in nonstressed individuals.[36]

The addition of glucose to a previously carbohydrate-free protein diet causes enhanced amino acid incorporation into protein with no change in the rate of protein breakdown.[37] Following injury the individual effects of glucose and amino acids on nitrogen equilibrium appear to operate by at least two different mechanisms.[38] Amino acid administration accelerates synthesis of visceral and muscle protein without affecting the rate of protein breakdown. Glucose depresses whole body protein breakdown and decreases the total amino acid pool, exerting little effect on protein synthesis. Both mechanisms improve nitrogen balance, and both glucose and nitrogen should be components of the nutritional regimen for severely injured, catabolic patients. Glucose-free amino acid solutions have been proposed[39,40] as "protein-sparing therapy" for postoperative patients. The use of amino acids alone does spare protein in most patients, but the effect is most pronounced in nutritionally depleted patients ex-

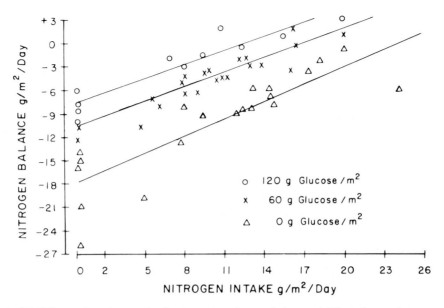

Figure 24-6 Increasing nitrogen intake promotes nitrogen balance. Adding glucose improves the nitrogen balance for each level of nitrogen intake.

From McDougall WS, et al: Surg Gynecol Obstet **145:**408-414, 1977.

hibiting little or no hypermetabolic response to illness. In general, this technique does not result in nitrogen equilibrium or positive nitrogen balance, and most of the administered amino acid is catabolized and excreted as urea. The protein-sparing effect of isotonic solutions of amino acids is related not to the degree of endogenous fat mobilization but to the metabolic effects of the amino acids alone.[41,42] The inclusion of glucose in amino acid solutions further decreases protein catabolism and increases nitrogen retention to a larger degree than either component does when used alone.[43,44] Initial studies[45] in animal models suggest that the utilization of branched-chain amino acid solutions following major surgery and trauma leads to improved nitrogen conservation and decreased muscle catabolism.

In the assessment of the minimum quantity of nitrogen necessary for nitrogen equilibrium, the nitrogen–to–total energy intake (nitrogen: calorie ratio) (g/kcal) in critically ill patients has been shown to be decreased from that in normal subjects.[46] Thus an injured hypermetabolic patient has an effective nitrogen:calorie ratio between 1:100 and 1:200, with an optimum of around 1:150 when activity is allowed. The ratio for a healthy individual or a minimally injured

patient eating a normal diet is around 1:350 whereas that for a severely hypermetabolic patient may approach 1:100. Therefore, if lean body mass is to be preserved, the inefficient utilization of administered protein by injured patients dictates that diets be high in nitrogen. However, with diets containing increased quantities of nitrogen, serum levels of urea and creatinine can rise in an alarming fashion, forcing a reduction in the nitrogen:calorie ratio of the nutrition formulas.

After routine elective surgical procedures on previously well-nourished patients in whom a rapid return to adequate oral alimentation is expected, 5% to 10% dextrose solutions with appropriate electrolytes are sufficient to maintain hydration and prevent ketosis. Solutions containing amino acids currently are more expensive and, although attractive for their metabolic effects, offer no practical advantages over glucose solutions in this clinical setting. When long-term nutritional support is expected, especially in cases of preexisting malnutrition and debilitation, sources containing both carbohydrate and nitrogen should be considered. Planning for any surgical procedure is such patients should include the potential placement of a central venous catheter or an enteral feeding tube.

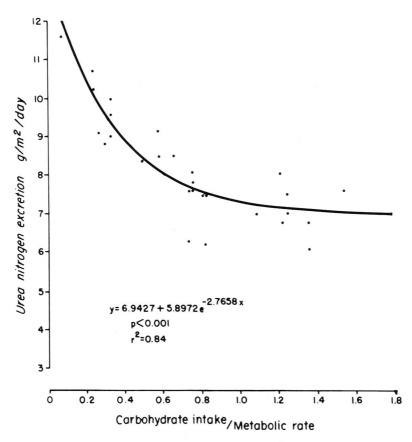

Figure 24-7 Progressive substitution of carbohydrate for fat as the source of nonprotein calories minimizes nitrogen loss.

From Long JM, et al: Ann Surg **185:**417-422, 1977.

Glucose Versus Fat as the Source of Nonprotein Calories

An increase in energy intake improves nitrogen retention and nitrogen balance in catabolic patients. In general, carbohydrate and fat can be used interchangeably as effective nonprotein caloric sources during adequate protein feeding. However, as the hypermetabolic response becomes pronounced, carbohydrate is more effective in sparing body protein than fat when each food source is used alone.[47] If fat alone is administered parenterally as a long-chain triglyceride emulsion, the reduced nitrogen excretion is accounted for by the glycerol in the emulsion.[48] The glycerol is incorporated into glucose by the three- to six-carbon cycle in the liver. Studies[49] have shown that emulsions of medium-chain triglycerides, in contrast to long-chain triglycerides, are much more effective in maintaining lean body mass. The medium-chain triglycerides demonstrate more rapid elimination kinetics, increased ketone production, and a greater lack of fatty deposition in the tissues.

In severely hypermetabolic patients receiving constant doses of amino acids ($11.7g/m^2/da$),[50] carbohydrate decreased nitrogen excretion, but equicaloric doses of fat (as lipid emulsions) failed to exert a similar effect (Fig. 24-7). The small improvement in nitrogen balance was due to the free glycerol present in the emulsion. The administration of insulin to this group of patients further decreased nitrogen loss. Conversely, in chronically ill starvation-adapted patients and in depleted surgical patients,[51-53] fat and carbohydrate combined with protein produced equal improvements in nitrogen balance. In contrast to the response of starvation-adapted patients, the signals in hypermetabolic patients that increase gluconeogenesis override the ability to adapt to starvation by decreasing nitrogen excretion, reducing energy expenditure, and utilizing lipid substrates.

Most surgical patients fall between the extremes of the chronically ill semistarved patient and the severely injured hypermetabolic patient and demonstrate varying abilities to utilize fat as a metabolic fuel. Following uncomplicated major surgical procedures one fourth to one half of caloric needs can be met by fat sources (while maintaining nitrogen:calorie ratios around 1:50). In critically ill patients, however, carbohydrate should provide the major source of energy and fat is utilized to provide essential fatty acids. Later, as such patients recover and the intensity of the stress decreases, fat can be used in increasing quantities to aid weight gain and restoration of body fat stores.

Vitamins

Although adequate vitamin intake in patients with functioning gastrointestinal tracts ordinarily is ensured by a normal well-planned diet with or without supplements, vitamin deficiencies frequently develop in severely injured and postoperative patients. The fat-soluble vitamins (A, D, E, and K) are stored in limited amounts and can become depleted with prolonged parenteral feeding or as a result of fat malabsorption. The water-soluble vitamins (B complex and C) are not stored in appreciable amounts and are depleted rapidly. Daily requirements can be met by a variety of enteral or parenteral preparations. Care must be taken to ensure that all vitamins are included, since most formulations are deficient in specific vitamins. Excessive doses of vitamins A and D produce toxic symptoms, and monitoring of serum levels is misleading if the concentration of the carrier proteins of these vitamins is decreased (as commonly occurs in critically ill patients). Requirements for ascorbic acid, niacin, thiamine, and riboflavin are said to be increased following injury and stress, but the clinical data are conflicting. The precise requirements for vitamins following surgery or trauma are not known, and until accurate balance data are available, it is prudent to administer fat-soluble vitamins at or near RDA dosages and water-soluble vitamins at approximately twice these levels.

Minerals

The major minerals—sodium, potassium, chloride, calcium, phosphorous, and magne-

sium—are essential for support of nutrition and other physiologic functions in severely ill patients. The adequacy of these minerals is determined by frequent monitoring of blood concentrations and urinary losses. Abnormal losses from other avenues (e.g., fistulas) also must be measured. Unique requirements for specific disease processes and the nutritional consequences of associated imbalances are discussed below and in accompanying chapters. These minerals usually are provided in sufficient quantities by most oral diets and feeding formulas; deficiencies occur most often after parenteral therapy. Potassium moves intracellularly with glucose and amino acids and is retained in a ratio of 3 mEq of potassium for each gram of nitrogen synthesized as protein. Hypophosphatemia commonly accompanies long-term intravenous therapy and is associated with potentially severe disruption of muscle, nervous, respiratory, and erythrocyte oxygen transport function.[54] Increased quantities of phosphorus are needed when glucose intake is increased; when glucose infusion is decreased rapidly, marked hyperphosphatemia can occur if phosphorus supplementation is not concomitantly decreased. Approximately 20 to 25 mEq of phosphorus is needed for each 1000 kcal administered.[55]

Iron deficiency is treated best with packed red blood cells, not by parenteral iron preparation. Requirements for zinc, copper, manganese, and chromium may be increased following prolonged critical illness, especially if the patient has large abnormal losses from the gastrointestinal tract. Symptoms of deficiency occur only after many months of illness. Periodic measurements of serum concentrations provide the best guide to replacement dosages. Certain trace elements, such as selenium, produce toxic symptoms and are apt to occur in patients with renal insufficiency.

NUTRITIONAL ASSESSMENT

Nutritional assessment includes a thorough history and physical examination not only when the patient first presents for evaluation but also on a regular basis thereafter. A deviation of actual weight from ideal weight and a recent weight change, especially if rapid and varying more than 10% from customary weight, indicate potential malnutrition and demand more extensive evaluation. However, edema may mask weight loss in severely debilitated patients. Food fads and specific nutritional deficiencies often can be detected by a careful review of daily food intake. A number of individual laboratory studies, including serum albumin, transferrin, hemoglobin, retinol-binding protein, and prealbumin, correlate roughly with nutritional adequacy.

Anthropometric measurements find their greatest utility in preoperative evaluation. Certain extremity measurements, such as triceps skinfold thickness and arm muscle circumference, may not be possible in patients with large thermal burns or amputations. Such measurements must be carefully related to the age and sex of the patient. Creatinine/height index is a sensitive indicator of protein-energy nutrition and appears to be one of the most accurate predictors of total body protein.[56]

Immune system dysfunction can result from both single and multiple nutrient deficiencies or excesses, alone or in combination with protein-calorie malnutrition.[57] A variety of laboratory studies (most commonly, total lymphocyte count, delayed skin sensitivity to recall antigens, T and B cell differentiation, and global leukocyte bactericidal activity) are employed to evaluate different aspects of the immune response.[58] An accurate predictor of postoperative morbidity and mortality is multiple regression analysis of a battery of laboratory determinations and anthropometric measurements.[59]

Metabolic requirements following surgery or injury are serially assessed by the daily measurements of weight, caloric intake, and nitrogen balance. These three convenient parameters provide an accurate appraisal of the metabolic response to injury, energy expenditure caused by the injury, caloric requirements, and the adequacy of nutritional support.[60] Indirect calorimetry occasionally is useful for explaining continued weight loss in patients who exhibit an unanticipated intense hypermetabolic response following injury. Body composition studies by isotope dilution techniques or whole body neutron activation analysis are utilized primarily as research tools.

PATIENT CARE CONSIDERATIONS
Minimization of Afferent Stimuli

Metabolic expenditure can be minimized by blunting a variety of noxious stimuli. Critically ill patients, especially children, who have a body surface area disproportionately large for body mass, and the elderly, have more difficulty maintaining body temperature in thermally diverse conditions. Because of an apparent change in

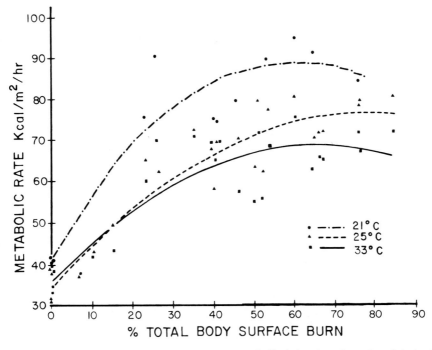

Figure 24-8 The resting metabolic rate of hypermetabolic injured patients is minimized in a thermal neutral environment. Progressive cooling drives the metabolic rate and increases energy expenditure.

hypothalamic set point, severely injured patients will choose higher ambient temperatures for comfort. As these temperatures approach thermal neutrality, resting metabolic expenditure and corresponding energy requirements decrease[61] (Fig. 24-8). Conversely, a cold environment imposes added stress and may exhaust the physiologic reserves of patients who exhibit a marked hypermetabolic response to injury. Since warming minimizes metabolic expenditure, thermal blankets, radiation reflectors, and heat lamps are utilized when necessary to maintain the patient's temperature above 37° C.

Although wound management, physical therapy, and nursing procedures are essential elements of patient care, they often cause pain and anxiety. Adequate analgesia diminishes fear and promotes patient cooperation. Unrelieved pain may heighten metabolic expenditure, and controlled administration of narcotics (morphine) will cause a moderate decrease in metabolic rate.[62] In addition, analgesics and sedatives allow the patient to sleep, and nursing schedules should provide uninterrupted periods for rest.

Hypovolemia, dehydration, and sepsis are potent stimuli for catecholamine secretion, and appropriate volume replacement and antibiotic administration should be employed expeditiously as indicated.

Maintenance of Muscle Mass

Lack of activity promotes muscle wasting and atrophy. Exercise can reverse this process and increase nitrogen incorporation into muscle protein. Vigorous physical therapy promotes maintenance of muscle protein mass, and supervised activity can and should be provided on a daily basis to almost all patients requiring prolonged hospitalization. Although the use of skeletal traction and air-fluidized beds encourages immobility, it predisposes to breakdown of lean body mass. Patients being treated by these modalities often can carry out simple isometric exercises and should be encouraged to do so.

Anabolic Hormones

Human growth hormone is a potent stimulus to growth and nitrogen storage. When adequate calories and nitrogen are provided in the diet, the administration of human growth hormone to injured patients further increases nitrogen retention.[63] Nitrogen storage is reflected by increased retention of potassium, phosphorus, and amino acids. The effects of human growth hormone apparently are mediated by alterations of carbohydrate metabolism in the presence of augmented insulin production.

Wound Management

Meticulous surgical techniques, adequate debridement, drainage of localized infection, and timely wound closure minimize the extent of tissue injury, accelerate healing, and diminish the often large metabolic requirements of the wound. Repeated operative interventions may be necessary to remove necrotic tissue, drain infection, and divert sources of contamination.

NUTRITIONAL ASPECTS OF SURGICAL PROCEDURES
Elective Abdominal Surgery

Most elective surgical procedures are performed on patients who have maintained reasonable nutritional habits. Although these patients have symptoms, from the effects of local disease, those requiring cholecystectomy for cholelithiasis or colon resection for chronic diverticulitis usually present with minimum weight loss and no signs of specific nutritional deficiencies. Rather, with them the major management problem is fluid and electrolyte balance, and the largest weight loss during an uneventful hospitalization often occurs because of preoperative bowel preparations and cessation of intake on the night before surgery. Postoperatively, patients undergoing abdominal surgery usually are treated with nasogastric intubation to prevent abdominal distension during the period of postoperative ileus. Effective gastrointestinal function, as reflected by audible bowel sounds and flatus, returns 2 to 7 days after surgery, and oral intake subsequently is reinstituted. Such patients, in whom no complications are foreseen and for whom resumption of oral intake is expected within 10 days of operation, should be supported with hypocaloric infusions to prevent ketosis and minimize protein breakdown.

Long-term nutritional support is indicated for the debilitated patient whose disease eventually will require surgical management. However, 1 week of preoperative hypercaloric feeding adds mostly water to the patient's body mass. At least 1 month of hyperalimentation usually is needed to effect a concrete improvement in nitrogen balance and lean body mass. Such patients should continue to be supported postoperatively until normal function has returned and the patient is able to meet his or her nutritional requirements by ordinary means. Since small bowel activity following surgery is usually maintained in spite of gastric and colon ileus, early postoperative feeding can be instituted conveniently by catheter jejunostomy.[64,65]

Head and Neck Surgery

Partial or total glossectomy, with or without mandibulectomy, interferes with mastication and swallowing, and attempts at oral feeding may contribute to pulmonary aspiration. If such patients cannot swallow, tube feeding may be utilized until they are able to adapt to safe oral feeding. Not infrequently permanent tube feeding will be necessary and patients may be able intermittently to intubate themselves for meals without discomfort. However, for most patients requiring a long-term feeding tube, permanent gastrostomy is the most convenient and easily maintained method. Commercially prepared complete liquid formulas are available and are no more expensive than homemade blenderized diets; and they are not subject to bacterial contamination when used properly. Advice from a dietitian experienced in dealing with these patients often will forestall nutritional inadequacies, which are related in part to an extensive psychologic overlay.

Esophageal Resection

As is the case with diseases necessitating head and neck surgery, cancer often necessitates esophageal resection, with its attendant systemic nutritional impact. Esophageal resection induces fat malabsorption by an as yet undefined mechanism. The cause is probably bilateral vagotomy, which almost always is a part of the surgical procedure.[66] Other postvagotomy sequelae include diarrhea and gastric stasis, which necessitate a concomitant drainage procedure. Carbohydrate absorption is unaffected. The use of medium-chain triglycerides is helpful in decreasing steatorrhea.

Gastric Resection

The nutritional complications following gastric resection are proportional to the extent of the procedure and include steatorrhea, afferent loop syndrome, long-term vitamin and mineral deficiencies, dumping, and hypoglycemia. Weight loss is frequent, especially after total or near total gastrectomy, and is caused by a decrease in caloric intake. The patient experiences early satiety because of the smaller stomach reservoir and may eat only small amounts for fear of having unpleasant postprandial symptoms.

Steatorrhea is a manifestation of fat malabsorption and causes weight loss and diarrhea. As with esophageal resection, the etiology of fat malabsorption is not known. Although many patients with gastric resection also undergo bilateral vagotomy, some do not and yet still have steatorrhea. Bowel transit is usually normal. Appropriate dietary manipulation can alleviate moderate symptoms of fat malabsorption. If dietary management is unsuccessful, the use of pancreatic enzymes or medium-chain triglycerides often alleviates these unpleasant side effects.

Anemia may develop several months to a few years after partial gastrectomy and probably arises from poor food intake and from chronic low-grade blood loss associated with gastritis or gastrojejunitis. Malabsorption of iron, although a suggested cause, has not been demonstrated consistently, and this anemia responds to oral iron administration. Loss of intrinsic factor accompanying gastric mucosal atrophy and achlorhydria or following total gastrectomy leads to vitamin B_{12} deficiency. Megaloblastic anemia develops late, if at all, and may also be a consequence of folic acid deficiency. Therefore patients who have undergone gastric resection should be given iron, vitamin B_{12}, and folic acid supplements. Calcium malabsorption is usually mild, accompanies fat malabsorption, and is treated with calcium and vitamin D supplements. Similar vitamin and mineral deficiencies can develop because of stasis in the afferent loop of an associated gastrojejunostomy. Antibiotics may be administered in either prolonged low dosages or in intermittent short courses for control of bacterial overgrowth in the afferent loop.

The most disturbing dietary sequela of gastric resective surgery is the dumping syndrome. Within 10 to 15 minutes of ingesting a meal, the patient experiences abdominal fullness and distention, rapidly followed by tachycardia, pallor, tachypnea, sweating, weakness, and even syncope. Clinical studies have documented rapid alterations of intravascular blood volume and erratic fluctuations of blood glucose during an attack, but a number of neuroendocrine mechanisms also apparently are involved. The dumping syndrome is a separate clinical entity from postprandial hypoglycemia. Although similar in character to those of dumping syndrome, the symptoms of hypoglycemia occur 2 to 3 hours after eating. Both are precipitated by high-carbohydrate meals taken in large quantities. Nutritional therapy is directed at limiting carbohydrate intake and encouraging high-protein high-fat diets (if the patient is not malabsorbing fat). Since these patients often are malnourished because of longstanding symptoms, 2000 to 3500 kcal/day is required for nutritional repletion. Small meals taken at 2-to-3-hour intervals with reduced fluids help attenuate symptoms. If dietary manipulation fails, the patient may require further surgery.

Intestinal Resection

The small intestine has a large adaptive capacity, and resection of small segments rarely causes nutritional disorders. Except for vitamin B_{12}, which is absorbed only in the ileum, all nutrients are absorbed most efficiently in the proximal small bowel. When large portions of the jejunum are resected, the ileum adapts quickly to the new absorptive load. However, if the entire terminal ileum is removed, vitamin B_{12} and conjugated bile salts fail to be absorbed. Vitamin B_{12} deficiency is prevented easily by monthly parenteral administration of the vitamin (50 μg/mo). Diarrhea occurs when unabsorbed bile salts enter the colon and may be massive if the ileocaecal valve is removed with the terminal ileum. The diarrheal fluid contains high concentrations of sodium, potassium, and bicarbonate; and severe electrolyte depletion and hypovolemia may develop. Cholestyramine binds bile salts and may be utilized to treat this form of diarrhea.

Without bile salts, micelle formation is depressed and fat malabsorption and steatorrhea occur. The fat-soluble vitamins (A, D, E, and K) also are malabsorbed and are required in increased amounts. Vitamin K is available in a water-soluble preparation and is administered most reliably in this form. Patients who have had ileal resection should utilize diets low in long-chain fats and high in medium-chain triglycerides, which are absorbed directly into the portal

circulation. Polyunsaturated fats are added as a source of essential fatty acids. Because unabsorbed long-chain fatty acids concentrate in the bowel and bind calcium, insufficient luminal calcium is available to prevent oxalate absorption from the intestine; thus hyperoxaluria and renal stones often develop in patients with ileal resection. Such patients are managed with calcium supplements (up to 4 g/da) and a restricted oxalate diet (50 mg/da) low in saturated fats and high in polyunsaturated fats. Aluminum hydroxide binds oxalate and decreases its absorption, and daily administration (6-12 g/da) provides good prophylaxis against oxalate stone formation.[67]

Bowel infarction following midgut volvulus or superior mesenteric artery occlusion may necessitate massive resection of the small intestine. The metabolic and nutritonal consequences of massive small bowel resection are extensive. The bile salt pool is lost through the colon and fat malabsorption ensues, as just described. The incidence of cholelithiasis is increased, and some centers actually perform a prophylactic cholecystectomy at the time of bowel resection. No dietary manipulation alters the incidence of gallstones. Hyperoxaluria and renal lithiasis commonly occur but can be prevented by the previously described dietary and pharmacologic therapy. A colectomy rarely is required to eliminate the absorptive interface for oxalate. Gastric secretory volume, as well as gastric acid, may increase considerably following massive resection, and the large volume of gastric juice is passed into what little small intestine remains, causing explosive diarrhea.[68] Acid may decrease nutrient absorption both by a direct mucosal effect and by acid inactivation of digestive enzymes. The high levels of acid may result in the formation of a frank ulcer. This hypersecretion probably is mediated by increased gastrin production, which may occur in the absence of a small bowel inhibitory factor.[69] Antacids and cimetidine effectively control the gastric hypersecretion and its complications.

Special nutritional support procedures are necessary in almost all patients with less than 40 to 50 cm of small bowel. Loss of the ileocecal valve intensifies feeding difficulties. Although total parenteral nutrition is theoretically an effective way to treat all these patients, most patients with more than 10 cm of jejunum eventually are able to utilize enteral methods in some fashion. In the interim, prolonged parenteral support is an obvious necessity and should begin soon after surgery. While the patient is being supported parenterally, a regimen is planned carefully to increase the absorptive capacity of the remaining bowel. Initially, nothing is administered by mouth except antacids for control of gastric secretion and acidity and opiates for diarrhea. After these are controlled, an isotonic dextrose-salt solution is infused continuously into the gut through a small nasal tube or gastrostomy. As increasing tonicity becomes better tolerated, the salt solution gradually is replaced by an elemental diet. This transition may require many months, and the rate of simultaneous parenteral infusion is reduced as the enteral infusion is increased to prevent fluid overload. The remaining bowel becomes hyperplastic and increases in length, an effect that may be enhanced by the introduction of nutrients into the gut.[70,71] Eventually parenteral nutrition may be replaced entirely by oral feedings, which should be advanced to a high-protein solid diet if possible. Depending on the length of remaining bowel, some patients require intermittent parenteral support and permanent defined-formula diets.

Jejunoileal Bypass for Obesity

Jejunoileal bypass performed for the treatment of morbid obesity results in permanent protein-energy malnutrition. Although it is now rarely used, familiarity with its associated metabolic derangements is essential since many patients who have undergone this procedure continue to seek treatment. Morphologic changes characteristic of hepatic steatosis and cirrhosis occur in 80% to 90% of these patients and appear to be permanent.[72,73] The intensity of these morphologic alterations depends on the amount of bypassed bowel and resulting weight loss but is not correlated with clinical liver failure. High-protein diets that include orally administered amino acids do not reverse this histologic picture.

Many of the metabolic complications are similar to those occurring in patients with small bowel resection. Renal oxalate stones are prevented by decreasing dietary intake of oxalate and by administering aluminum hydroxide. Calcium and magnesium supplements should be provided, and calcium binding in the intestinal lumen is diminished by restricting consumption of saturated fats. Steatorrhea is alleviated by using medium-chain triglycerides as a lipid source. However, medium-chain triglycerides may cause ketosis and metabolic acidosis if the patient is experiencing severe diarrhea. Whereas iron deficiency with anemia is unusual and is easily treated by iron supplements, vitamin B_{12} deficiency can readily occur because of decreased ileal absorption and bacterial overgrowth, and monthly vitamin B_{12} supplements are required. Multiple vitamin deficiencies are prevented by daily multivitamin supplements. Potassium losses are particularly high in bypassed patients, who require 30 to 60 mEq/day. Refractory diarrhea is usually a manifestation of fat or lactose intolerance and is treated best by avoiding the offending food items in the diet.

Pancreatectomy

Nutritonal problems following pancreatectomy arise from the absence of digestive enzymes and the fecal loss of fat, proteins, vitamins, and minerals. Many patients requiring pancreatic resection have cancer or chronic pancreatitis and are severely cachectic before surgery. Proximal or total pancreatectomy usually necessitates partial gastrectomy, with its attendant nutritional complications. In addition to total pancreatectomy, proximal resection with implantation of the tail in the jejunum also is associated with a high incidence of exocrine insufficiency, which is treated by pancreatic extracts administered with meals and at regular intervals between meals. Medium-chain triglycerides are absorbed without need for pancreatic enzymes and provide a convenient source of calories. Antacids and cimetidine may be utilized to decrease inactivation of pancreatic enzymes by gastric acid.[74] Vitamin B_{12} absorption is diminished following pancreatectomy and is facilitated by ingestion of pancreatic extract and vitamin B_{12} supplements. Total pancreatectomy results in diabetes mellitus, and while small amounts of insulin are required, control of blood sugar often is extremely difficult.

Gastrointestinal Fistulas

Fluid and electrolyte deficits are replaced as indicated by measured fluid losses and analysis of the chemical content of blood and fistula effluent. The composition of the drainage is variable and depends on the location of the fistula.

In earlier years mortality accompanying fistula formation exceeded 50% and was related to fluid and electrolyte imbalance, infections, and malnutrition. With increased emphasis on nutrition, mortality has fallen below 10%. Total parenteral alimentation, by improving nutrition and decreasing secretions, promotes spontaneous closure of fistulas and improves survival following surgical closure.[75-77] Longer fistulous tracts are most apt to close spontaneously and do so by 4 to 6 weeks. After this period, if they have not closed spontaneously, surgical closure is indicated and is tolerated better because of the patient's improved nutritional status. Experimental studies[78,79] have demonstrated that gastric and pancreatic secretions are reduced effectively by enteral elemental diets. Enteral feeding with defined-formula diets can be as successful in accomplishing fistula closure.[80] For patients with gastric and duodenal fistulas, placement of a feeding tube into the jejunum distal to the fistula allows maximum infusion of calories and nitrogen while minimizing drainage and attendant fluid and electrolyte imbalances.

NUTRITIONAL ASPECTS OF MASSIVE BURNS

Like other critically ill patients, those with massive thermal injuries (greater than 30% of the body surface) have increased nutritional requirements that are proportional to the degree of injury. Such patients require long-term nutritional support, and a complete feeding program should be integrated into their total care plans from the onset of injury. In particular, burned patients often require multiple surgical procedures for debridement and wound closure, and with the usual preoperative preparation and postoperative recovery, whole 24-hour periods may pass with no nutritional intake. Therefore operative treatment should be so planned that a general anesthetic is used only for major procedures. Local debridements and dressing changes can be accomplished with parenteral narcotic analgesia without interrupting feeding schedules for more than a few hours.

A number of factors may modify the estimation of nutritional needs in the burned patient. The preinjury nutritional status must be taken into account when determining caloric requirements. Debilitation with marked weight loss reduces the patient's ability to survive a large burn,

and this protein-energy deficit, in addition to that produced by the injury, must be corrected. Diabetes mellitus, whether longstanding or unmasked by the injury, may not only alter the patient's nutritional requirements but also exacerbate the difficulties of administering the required nutrients. Concomitant injury, such as long-bone fractures, may amplify the metabolic response and subsequent need for calories. Sepsis, a frequent postinjury complication, impairs glucose tolerance and alters hepatic gluconeogenesis in extensively burned patients and makes assimilation of exogenously administered glucose and amino acids difficult.

A number of methods are available for estimating calorie and nitrogen needs. Based on a comparison of percentage weight change with daily caloric intake for adult patients with a wide range of burn sizes, ideal daily caloric intake can be predicted closely by the formula[81]

25 kcal/kg of Body weight +
40 kcal % of Body surface burned

Daily calorie and nitrogen requirements for patients with extensive burns may be estimated conveniently by the following rules of thumb: caloric requirements equal 2000 to 2200 kcal/m² of body surface, and nitrogen requirements equal 15 g (12-18 g)/m² of body surface.[82] More accurate estimates can be obtained from nomograms that relate degree of weight loss, change in metabolic activity, preferred nitrogen to calorie ratio, as well as body weight and burn size.[83] For difficult to manage patients, periodic measurement of metabolic rate by indirect calorimetry is helpful. Most patients who are burned accidentally are healthy before the injury and exhibit no evidence of nutritional depletion. For such patients the goal of nutritional support is to provide enough calories to meet energy expenditure and maintain lean body mass. Supranormal dietary intake, although achievable in burned patients, leads to lipogenesis, a metabolically expensive and potentially hazardous condition. Specific nutritional requirements for patients with massive burns parallel those just outlined for any hypermetabolic critically injured patient.

No attempt is made to meet the predicted nutritional requirements of acutely burned patients during the period of resuscitation and hemodynamic stabilization. Resuscitation is carried out by glucose-free balanced electrolyte solutions. The infusion of glucose at this time results in marked hyperglycemia. Most of the infused fluid is lost into the injured tissues, and the resulting edema is reflected by weight gains of 10% to 20% of preinjury weight by the end of the first postburn day. Ileus develops soon after injury and precludes use of the gastrointestinal tract for either resuscitation or feeding. After 48 to 72 hours, tissue fluid begins to be reabsorbed and excreted, and the patient usually returns to preinjury weight by the seventh to tenth postburn day. Adequate bowel function returns at varying times during the first postburn week, and oral intake of fluid and calories then is begun.

When instituting nutritional support at this time, it is important to give priority to the enteral route as fully as possible. High-carbohydrate high-protein diets are planned individually to allow accurate quantitation of food consumed and to include adequate multivitamins and polyunsaturated fat. Since burned patients seldom eat more of their planned meals after injury than they consumed before injury, almost half their caloric requirements remain unsatisfied. High-calorie high-protein drinks fed between meals and throughout the night can make up for this energy deficit and, in patients with extensive burns, are often the major form of nutritional support during the early weeks following injury.

Tube feedings are necessary in certain patients to meet minimum nutritional requirements. This technique is particularly useful for infants and for patients with severe facial burns and tracheostomies. A variety of low-bulk defined formula solutions is available and can be administered through small feeding tubes. Mild diarrhea frequently occurs and is easily treated in most cases by adding paregoric to the mixture. By combining tube feedings with normal oral intake when possible, complete enteral support is feasible in institutions with multidisciplinary resources.[84]

In some patients, oral intake and tube feedings are inadequate or even precluded by associated injuries or complications and parenteral support is indicated. This technique is particularly useful in patients with burns over more than 40% of the body surface, in whom it is difficult or impossible to meet the entire nutritional requirements by enteral methods alone. Since evaporative water loss is large in burned patients

$$\text{Predicted evaporative water loss (ml/hr)} = 25 +$$
$$\text{Percentage of body surface burned} \times$$
$$\text{Body surface area (m}^2)$$

more dilute carbohydrate–amino acid mixtures may satisfy daily nutritional requirements. These solutions often are administered through central venous catheters. Because of the high risk of infection in burned patients, catheters must be changed every 48 to 72 hours.[85] The catheter tip should terminate in the superior vena cava, since intrusion into the atrium or ventricle is associated with a high incidence of endocarditis.[86]

REFERENCES

1. Duke JH, et al: Contribution of protein to caloric expenditure following injury, Surgery **68**:168-174, 1970.
2. Johnston IDA: The role of the endocrine glands in the metabolic response to operation, Br J Surg **54**:438-441, 1967.
3. Cuthbertson DP, Tilstone WJ: Metabolism during the post-injury period. In Advances in clinical chemistry, vol 12, New York, 1969, Academic Press Inc, pp 1-55.
4. Moore FD: Metabolic care of the surgical patient, Philadelphia, 1959, WB Saunders Co, pp 27-48.
5. Gump FE, Kinney JM: Energy balance and weight loss in burned patients, Arch Surg **103**:442-448, 1971.
6. Wilmore DW, et al: Catecholamines: mediator of the hypermetabolic response to thermal injury, Ann Surg **180**:653-669, 1974.
7. Gump FE, et al: Blood flow and oxygen consumption in patients with severe burns, Surg Gynecol Obstet **130**:23-28, 1970.
8. Wilmore DW, et al: Influence of the burn wound on local and systemic responses to injury, Ann Surg **186**:444-458, 1977.
9. Wilmore DW, et al: Effect of injury and infection on visceral metabolism and circulation, Ann Surg **192**:491-504, 1980.
10. Aulick LH, et al: Influence of the burn wound on peripheral circulation in thermally injured patients, Am J Physiol **233**:H520-H526, 1977.
11. Aulick LH, et al: Muscle blood flow following thermal injury, Ann Surg **188**:778-782, 1978.
12. Wilmore DW, et al: Alterations in hypothalamic function following thermal injury, J Trauma **15**:697-703, 1975.
13. Aulick LH, et al: The relative significance of thermal and metabolic demands on burn hypermetabolism, J Trauma **19**:559-566, 1979.
14. Gusberg RJ, et al: Can protein breakdown explain the increased calorie expenditure in injury and sepsis? Surg Forum **24**:79-81, 1973.
15. Harrison TS, et al: Relationship of increased oxygen consumption to catecholamine excretion in thermal burns, Ann Surg **165**:169-172, 1967.
16. Becker RA, et al: Free T_4, free T_3, and reverse T_3 in critically ill, thermally injured patients, J Trauma **20**:713-721, 1980.
17. Becker RA, et al: Plasma norepinephrine, epinephrine, and thyroid hormone interactions in severely burned patients, Arch Surg **115**:439-443, 1980.

18. Vaughn GM, et al: Cortisol and corticotropin in burned patients, J Trauma **22**:263-273, 1982.

19. Aulick LH, Wilmore DW: Increased peripheral amino acid release following burn injury, Surgery **85**:560-565, 1979.

20. Hwang TL, et al: Preservation of small bowel mucosa using glutamine-enriched parenteral nutrition, Surg Forum **37**:56-58, 1986.

21. Odessey R, et al: Origin and possible significance of alanine production by skeletal muscle, J Biol Chem **23**:7623-7629, 1974.

22. Wilmore DW, et al: Hyperglucagonaemia after burns, Lancet **1**:73-75, 1974.

23. Vaughn GM, et al: Nonthyroidal control of metabolism after burn injury: possible role of glucagon, Metabolism **34**:637-641, 1985.

24. Allison SF, et al: Intravenous glucose-tolerance, insulin, and free-fatty-acid levels in burned patients, Lancet **2**:1113-1116, 1968.

25. Long CL, et al: Carbohydrate metabolism in man: effect of elective operations and major injury, J Appl Physiol **31**:110-116, 1971.

26. Wilmore DW, et al: Impaired glucose flow in burned patients with gram-negative sepsis, Surg Gynecol Obstet **143**:720-724, 1976.

27. Wilmore DW, et al: Insulin response to glucose in hypermetabolic burn patients, Ann Surg **183**:314-320, 1976.

28. Gump FE, et al: The significance of altered gluconeogenesis in surgical catabolism. J Trauma **15**:704-713, 1975.

29. Rizza RA, et al: Adrenergic mechanisms for the effects of epinephrine on glucose production and clearance in man, J Clin Invest **65**:682-689, 1980.

30. Curreri PW, et al: Intracellular cation alterations following major trauma: effect of supranormal caloric intake, J Trauma **11**:390-396, 1971.

31. McDougal WS, et al: Glucose-dependent hepatic membrane transport in nonbacteremic and bacteremic thermally injured patients, J Surg Res **22**:697-708, 1977.

32. Newsome TW, et al: Weight loss following thermal injury, Ann Surg **178**:215-217, 1973.

33. Watters JM, Wilmore DW: Role of catabolic hormones in the hypoketonemia of injury, Br J Surg **73**:108-110, 1986.

34. Vinnars E, et al: Influence of the postoperative state on the intracellular free amino acids in human muscle tissue, Ann Surg **182**:665-671, 1975.

35. McDougal WS, et al: Effect of intravenous near isosmotic nutrient infusions on nitrogen balance in critically ill injured patients, Surg Gynecol Obstet **145**:408-414, 1977.

36. Fitzpatrick GF, et al: Nitrogen sparing by carbohydrate in man: intermittent or continuous enteral compared with continuous parenteral glucose, Surgery **78**:105-113, 1975.

37. Sim AJW, et al: Glucose promotes whole-body protein synthesis from infused amino acids in fasting man, Lancet **1**:68-71, 1979.

38. Moldawer LL, et al: In vivo demonstration of nitrogen-sparing mechanisms for glucose and amino acids in the injured rat, Metabolism **29**:173-180, 1980.

39. Blackburn GL, et al: Protein sparing therapy during periods of starvation with sepsis or trauma, Ann Surg **177**:588-594, 1973.

40. Schulte WJ, et al: Positive nitrogen balance using isotonic crystalline amino acid solution, Arch Surg **110**:914-915, 1975.

41. Greenberg GR, et al: Protein-sparing therapy in postoperative patients, N Engl J Med **294**:1411-1416, 1976.

42. Felig P: Intravenous nutrition: fact and fancy, N Engl J Med **294**:1455-1456, 1976.

43. Wolfe BM, et al: Substrate interaction in intravenous feeding: comparative effects of carbohydrate and fat on amino acid utilization in fasting man, Ann Surg **186**:518-540, 1977.

44. Elwyn DH, et al: Protein and energy sparing of glucose added in hypocaloric amounts to peripheral infusions of amino acids, Metabolism **27**:325-331, 1978.

45. Freund H, et al: The role of the branched-chain amino acids in decreasing muscle catabolism in vivo, Surgery **83**:611-618, 1978.

46. Long CL, et al: Parenteral nutrition in the septic patient: Nitrogen balance, limiting plasma amino acids, and calorie to nitrogen ratios, Am J Clin Nutr **29**:380-391, 1976.

47. Gottschlick MM, Alexander JW: Fat kinetics and recommended dietary intake in burns, J Parenter Enter Nutr **11**:80-85, 1987.

48. Brennan MF, et al: Glycerol: major contributor to the short-term protein sparing effect of fat emulsions in normal man, Ann Surg **182**:386-394, 1975.

49. Cotter R, et al: A metabolic comparison of five long-chain triglyceride lipid emulsion (LCT) and various medium-chain triglyceride (MCT)-LCT combination emulsions in dogs, Am J Clin Nutr **45**:927-939, 1987.

50. Long JM, et al: Effect of carbohydrate and fat intake on nitrogen excretion during total intravenous feeding, Ann Surg **185**:417-422, 1977.

51. Jeejeebhoy KN, et al: Metabolic studies in total parenteral nutrition with lipid in man, J Clin Invest **57**:125-136, 1976.

52. Gazzaniga AB, et al: Nitrogen balance in patients receiving either fat or carbohydrate for total intravenous nutrition, Ann Surg **182**:163-168, 1975.

53. Elwyn DH, et al: Some metabolic effects of fat infusions in depleted patients, Metabolism **29**:125-132, 1980.

54. Knochel JP: The pathophysiology and clinical characteristics of severe hypophosphatemia, Arch Intern Med **137**:203-220, 1977.

55. Sheldon GF, Grzyb S: Phosphate depletion and repletion: relation to parenteral nutrition and oxygen transport, Ann Surg **182**:683-689, 1975.

56. Bistrian BR, et al: Therapeutic index of nutritional depletion in hospitalized patients, Surg Gynecol Obstet **141**:512-516, 1975.

57. Beisel WR, et al: Single-nutrient effects on immunologic function, JAMA **254**:53-58, 1981.

58. Garre MA, et al: Current concepts in immunoderangements due to undernutrition, J Parenter Enter Nutr **11**:309-313, 1987.

59. Mullen JL, et al: Prediction of operative morbidity and mortality by preoperative nutritional assessment, Surg Forum **30**:81-82, 1979.

60. Kinney JM, et al: Tissue composition of weight loss in surgical patients, Ann Surg **168**:459-474, 1968.

61. Wilmore DW, et al: Anabolic effects of human growth hormone and high caloric feeding following thermal injury, Surg Gynecol Obstet **138**:875-884, 1974.

62. Wilmore DW, et al: Effect of ambient temperature on heat production and heat loss in burn patients, J Appl Physiol **38**:593-597, 1975.

63. Taylor JW, et al: The effect of central nervous system narcosis on the sympathetic response to stress, J Surg Res **20:**313-320, 1976.

64. Editorial: Postoperative ileus, Lancet **2:**1186-1187, 1978.

65. Page CP, et al: Continual catheter administration of an elemental diet, Surg Gynecol Obstet **142:**184-188, 1976.

66. Shils ME: The esophagus, the vagi, and fat absorption, Surg Gynecol Obstet **132:**709-715, 1971.

67. Earnest DL: Perspectives on incidence, etiology, and treatment of enteric hyperoxaluria, Am J Clin Nutr **30:**72-75, 1977.

68. Osborne MP, et al: Massive bowel resection and gastric hypersecretion, Am J Surg **114:**393-397, 1967.

69. Straus E, et al: Hypersecretion of gastrin associated with the short bowel syndrome, Gastroenterology **66:**175-180, 1974.

70. Bury KD: Carbohydrate digestion and absorption after massive resection of the small intestine, Surg Gynecol Obstet **135:**177-187, 1972.

71. Sheflan M, et al: Intestinal adaptation after extensive resection of the small intestine and prolonged administration of parenteral nutrition, Surg Gynecol Obstet **143:**757-762, 1976.

72. Kroyer JM, Talbert WM Jr: Morphologic liver changes in intestinal bypass patients, Am J Surg **139:**855-859, 1980.

73. Peters RL: Patterns of hepatic morphology in jejunoileal bypass patients, Am J Clin Nutr **30:**53-57, 1977.

74. Morishita R, et al: Effect of pancreatin on vitamin B_{12} malabsorption in patients with total pancreatectomy, Digestion **11:**240-248, 1974.

75. MacFadyen BV Jr, et al: Management of gastrointestinal fistulas with parenteral hyperalimentation, Surgery **74:**100-105, 1973.

76. Reber HA, et al: Management of external gastrointestinal fistulas, Ann Surg **188:**460-467, 1978.

77. Hamilton RF, et al: Effects of parenteral hyperalimentation on upper gastrointestinal tract secretions, Arch Surg **102:**348-352, 1971.

78. Rivilis J, et al: Effect of an elemental diet on gastric secretion, Ann Surg **179:**226-229, 1974.

79. McArdle AH, et al: Effect of elemental diet on pancreatic secretion, Am J Surg **128:**690-692, 1974.

80. Voitk AJ, et al: Elemental diet in the treatment of fistulas of the alimentary tract, Surg Gynecol Obstet **137:**68-72, 1973.

81. Curreri PW, et al: Dietary requirements of patients with major burns, J Am Diet Assoc **65:**415-417, 1974.

82. Wilmore DW: Nutrition and metabolism following thermal injury, Clin Plast Surg **1:**603-619, 1974.

83. Wilmore DW: The metabolic management of the critically ill, New York, 1977, Plenum Press Inc, pp 171-233.

84. Larkin JM, Moylan JA: Complete enteral support of thermally injured patients, Am J Surg **131:**722-724, 1976.

85. Pruitt BA Jr, et al: Diagnosis and treatment of cannula-related intravenous sepsis in burn patients, Ann Surg **191:**546-554, 1980.

86. Sasaka TM, et al: The relationship of central venous and pulmonary artery catheter position to acute right-sided endocarditis in severe thermal injury, J Trauma **19:**740-743, 1979.

CHAPTER 25
Cancer

M.J. Bunk
Lloyd S. Schloen
Richard S. Rivlin

Complex interrelationships now are recognized among nutrition, physical activity, lifestyle, and the development of various organsite cancers. The precise mechanisms underlying these connections as well as the nature of direct cause-effect relationships are the subjects of intense scientific investigation. The role of dietary practices in carcinogenesis is not understood completely, nor are there predictable nutritional means for altering host metabolism during chemotherapy to achieve optimum therapeutic results. Consequently, in cancer patient care, the clinician's interest in nutrition has been at best secondary.

The increasing attention being paid to nutrition and cancer has led to considerable advances in four general areas: the role of diet in influencing risk of tumor development, the effects of cancer on host metabolism, the effects of chemotherapy on the patient's nutritional status, and nutritional management of patients with cancer. By focusing on these four areas, this chapter provides an overview of the clinical nutritional management of cancer patients.

NUTRITION AND TUMOR DEVELOPMENT

Data from controlled animal studies have demonstrated clearly that nutrition influences tumor development in many organ systems. In humans previous investigations have focused on biochemical changes in nutrients, changes in intestinal flora produced by nutrients or additives, and clinical trials of the ability of single nutrients

☐ Supported by Research Grants 5P01 CA 29502 and CA 08748, by Nutritional Research Training Grant 5T32 CA 09427 from the National Institutes of Health, and by grants from the following: American Cancer Society, Stella and Charles Guttman Foundation, William H. Donner Foundation, General Foods Fund.

to prevent malignant disease. Efforts have also been made to assess the mutagenic or carcinogenic potential of nutrients and food additives. Epidemiologic research, moreover, has elucidated possible associations between dietary practices and cancer prevalence.

Nutritional Intake and Tumors in Animals

In 1914 Rous[1] provided the first evidence that reduction of caloric intake inhibits the development and growth of spontaneous and transplanted tumors in mice, and in 1940 Tannenbaum[2] confirmed these observations in rats. Subsequent studies[3] have revealed that caloric intake rather than dietary composition is the prime determinant in spontaneous tumor development and that caloric restriction early in life is critical for prevention of subsequent tumor development in laboratory animals.

To elucidate the mechanisms for the effect of caloric restriction on tumor development, Fernandes et al.[4] explored the influence of nutritional status on the immune system of tumor-bearing animals and those with congenital autoimmune syndromes. These studies were prompted by the long-observed relationships among malnutrition, infectious disease, and immunodeficiency in populations of developing countries.

Initial observations in mice[4,5] indicated that, while reducing the level of tumor-enhancing antibody, caloric restriction maintains or enhances cell-mediated immunity to tumor heterografts. The studies were extended to animals that develop spontaneous mammary tumors, hepatomas, and lymphoproliferative diseases, including leukemia and sarcoma, and to those that develop autoimmune degenerative diseases. Reduction of caloric intake by one third to one half at weaning prevented spontaneous tumors from developing and as much as doubled the life-span of these animals.[4] Caloric reduction was associated with maintenance of cell-mediated immunity, suppressor cell activity, and thymus size and serum thymus hormones, but with development of far fewer circulating immune complexes.

The proportion of carbohydrates and proteins in the diet did not influence tumor incidence or immune reactivity as greatly as did caloric intake; however, increases in the proportion of fat intake relative to total calories did prevent the reduction of mammary tumor incidence and appearance of autoimmune syndromes. In some animals the type of fat consumed did not seem to matter a great deal; in others, unsaturated lipid produced greater disorganization of the immune system than did saturated fat. There is now widespread agreement that unsaturated fat may serve as a tumor promoter, perhaps by this mechanism.

These experimental observations should be borne in mind when considering human epidemiologic findings regarding nutrition and cancer. Other specific nutrients (including essential amino acids, zinc, iron, and vitamins A, C, and E) have been shown to influence immune competence and tumor incidence in laboratory animals.

Nutrients that Modify Chemical Carcinogens

It is now widely believed that chemical carcinogens are responsible for a sizable proportion of human cancers, although few chemicals have been implicated directly as causing specific cancers. Studies in experimental animals[6] have revealed that chemical carcinogens can be modified and their conversion to active forms prevented by specific means. Carcinogens may be activated at almost any point in their absorption and metabolism, for example, by microbial action in the gut or by microsomal enzyme action in the liver.

Microsomal oxidase inducers. The relative proportions of major dietary constituents can alter the activity of the enzymes involved in these processes, conceivably inhibiting them.[7] Conversely, microsomal oxidases of the small intestine and lung in experimental animals can be induced by dietary factors, thus protecting the host against chemical carcinogens that enter by these routes.[6,8] Various indoles isolated from the Brassicaceae family of vegetables, includ-

ing brussels sprouts, broccoli, and cabbage, are powerful inducers of microsomal oxidases. Other as yet unidentified inducers of these enzymes protect against carcinogenesis through polycyclic hydrocarbons, flavones, barbiturates, and phenothiazines.

Antioxidants. Food constituents also may inhibit carcinogenesis by preventing oxidation, thereby inactivating the reactive species of carcinogens, or by preventing carcinogen-induced oxidation of substrates. Vitamin E has been proposed as such a natural antioxidant.[7] Butylated hydroxyanisole (BHA), butylated hydroxytoluene (BHT), and certain nonphenolic antioxidants inhibit carcinogenesis under controlled conditions in rats and mice.[7] Since BHA is used extensively as a food preservative, it may inhibit carcinogenesis caused by long-term carcinogen exposure, but additional research is needed to evaluate the safety and efficacy of these compounds.

Nitrites. The effects of nitrites and the potential role of ascorbic acid in preventing the formation of nitrosamines are of special interest. Nitrites commonly are used as preservatives in meat and vegetable products, at levels of about 100-150 ppm. Nitrites and amines occur in cigarette smoke, polluted air, and drinking water and are formed by oral bacteria following ingestion of food containing nitrate.[9] In the acid conditions of the stomach nitrites interact with secondary and tertiary amines to form nitrosamines, having the general formula

$$\begin{array}{c} R_1 \\ \diagdown \\ N-N=O \\ \diagup \\ R_2 \end{array}$$

This interaction also is catalyzed by commonly ingested materials such as formaldehyde, thiocyanate, coffee phenols, and tannins. Some 75 of the 100 members of the nitrosamine class that have been tested have been found to be carcinogenic in laboratory animals.[9]

Alkylnitrosamines and alkylureido compounds formed in the stomach through reaction with nitrates are carcinogenic to the stomach and other organs, including the colon.[10] Although the amount of nitrosamine in each source is relatively small, the many sources of nitrosamines in their entirety potentially could result in a surprisingly enhanced risk for an individual. Table

Table 25-1 Potential Daily Human Nitrosamine Exposure

Source	Possible Nitrosamine Delivered (mg)	
	Dimethyl-nitrosamine	Nitroso-pyrrolidine
Breakfast		
Bacon (4 oz)	0.4	4.4
Ten percent of fumes from 1 lb bacon	0.7	3.6
Luncheon sandwich		
Lunch meat (ham, tongue, salami) (4 oz)	2.8	
Smoked cheese (2 oz)	0.2	
Snack		
Frankfurters (4 oz)	2.8	
Cocktail hors d'oeuvres		
Sausage (2 oz)	2.8	2.8
Dinner		
Fish (300 g) containing dimethylamine	3.3*	
Cigarettes (20)	2.0	1.0
Urban air	14.0	
TOTAL	29.0	11.8

From Mirvish SS: J Toxicol Environ Health 2:1267-1277, 1977.
*Dimethylnitrosamine formed by nitrosation of dimethylamine in the stomach, as estimated by Mirvish.

25-1 indicates that 40.8 g of two types of nitrosamine (dimethylnitrosamine and nitrosopyrrolidine) could accumulate in a person in 1 day. The table is weighted toward foods that contain certain nitrosamines, but it minimizes the likely presence of other equally carcinogenic nitrosamines, the acceleration of nitrosation by the gastric and oral milieux, and the contribution of natural, pharmaceutical, and manufactured substances that contain or induce the formation of nitrosamines. Saliva itself contains large amounts of nitrites, formed by bacterial nitrate reductase.

The apparent inconsistencies between cancer incidence data and the evident carcinogenicity of nitrosamines and other environmental substances possibly may be explained by analyzing carcinogenesis at the fetal stage. Although the level of environmental dimethylnitrosamines may not cause tumors in a single generation of mice, constant exposure to this level of carcinogen for at least two generations does significantly increase tumor incidence.[11] Transplacental exposure to carcinogens may be required, and results of such exposure in human populations might not be evident over a 40-year study period, during which many new chemicals have been introduced.[10] Although the evidence for nitrite-induced carcinogenesis in animals and in vitro systems is compelling, direct evidence for a cause-effect relationship in humans must be obtained.

Ascorbic acid. Under certain conditions ascorbic acid appears to prevent nitrites from reacting with amines to form nitrosamines and nitrosamides.[10,12] Ascorbic acid has been shown to inhibit induction of tumors by nitrosamines in rats.[12] Lettuce and other green vegetables have similar protective effects, but observations about vitamin E in green vegetables[13] have not been supported by corresponding data in vitro.[7,10] Available evidence about the inhibitory effects of ascorbate on nitrosamine and nitrosamide formation from nitrite under gastric conditions suggests that vitamin C perhaps should be consumed at each meal, since its effects are short-lived. Foods containing vitamin C may be adequate for this purpose.

Vitamin A. Studies in vitamin A–deficient animals show greater susceptibility to epithelioid cancers of the colon, lung, bladder, and other organs in the presence of carcinogens. The effectiveness of topically and systemically administered vitamin A in experimental animals is limited by its toxicity and by the fact that the liver sequesters most of the vitamin before sufficient levels are reached in epidermal tissues. Preliminary animal studies indicate that synthetic analogues of vitamin A (retinoids) may prevent certain kinds of chemical-induced cancers.[14] The toxicity of vitamin A in large doses has prevented its widespread use as an antitumor agent in the United States; but in Germany and Austria vitamin A emulsions, often combined with radiation treatment, have been used for over a decade. Clinical trials of several retinoids currently are underway.[7] Because of the role of vitamin A in epithelial cell differentiation and metabolic processes, it appears that the amounts required to delay or prevent carcinogenesis may be much greater than those required only to prevent deficiency.[10]

Selenium. In some parts of the United States where the soil concentrations and blood levels of selenium are low, increased prevalence of certain cancers has been suggested by several reports.[15-17] Moreover, in experimental animals selenium derivatives may protect against various organsite cancers.[18,19] Several selenium-intervention experiments are presently underway both in the United States and in China and should indicate whether enhanced selenium status can decrease the cancer risk in humans. Selenium in large amounts may be toxic and is not recommended for routine use.

Other nutrients. Other nutrients also have been shown to influence the effects of carcinogens. Riboflavin, the precursor for the flavin coenzyme FAD, has been shown to inhibit carcinogenesis by butter yellow (*p*-dimethylaminoazobenzene) under certain circumstances. Riboflavin deficiency, however, seems to inhibit the growth of certain transplantable tumors.[20,21] In view of these findings, and the fact that phenothiazine derivatives interfere with riboflavin utilization,[22] it is important that the immunologic consequences of riboflavin deficiency be analyzed thoroughly.

In treating experimental animals with large doses of such nutrients as vitamins A and C, selenium, and riboflavin, the effects observed may be pharmacologic rather than nutritional. Caution should be exercised when extrapolating these results to dietary recommendations for patients.

Nutritional Epidemiology of Cancer

Growing evidence of the association between certain dietary practices and cancer prevalence,[23,24] improved understanding of chemical carcinogenesis,[25] and new perspectives on the role of nutrition in modifying immune and hormonal responses[26] make it appropriate for the clinician to begin to advise patients and their families about dietary practices most likely to delay and/or prevent cancer. Such recommendations should be based on information currently available, should not be given as absolute commandments, and should be modified as new information is obtained from advances in research.

Some authors[10] suggest that as many as 90% of all cancers may be environmentally caused and that as many as 50% may be associated with diet. These views are based on epidemiologic studies that relate specific diets to the risk of cancer at particular sites in a given population. Variations in cancer prevalence among different populations and geographic areas, changes in the prevalence of a particular cancer over time, and results of experimental studies conducted both in vitro and in vivo all suggest the importance of dietary factors; however, they do not prove conclusively that such factors are the etiologic agents.

In declining order of the weight of evidence, dietary factors are thought to play significant roles in the incidence of cancers of the colon, breast, stomach, and prostate. The incidence of these tumors does not appear to be correlated closely with increased industrialization or environmental pollution over the last 40 years in the United States or in Japan.[27] Furthermore, westernization of the Japanese diet and migration of Japanese to Hawaii and the continental United States suggest that dietary practices may be more important etiologic factors for these cancers. Genetic factors also may affect susceptibility to malignancy, especially malignancies associated with diet, as has been shown for colon cancer.[28] In our opinion more information is needed before the relative influence of all factors dietary and otherwise can be assessed quantitatively, but the weight of evidence implicating specific dietary components cannot be ignored.

Colon, breast, and prostate cancers. In Japan the prevalences of all three organsite cancers, colon, breast, and prostate, are low compared to the U.S. prevalences, although they are increasing, perhaps as a result of the growing westernization of the Japanese diet.[27] Since both the United States and Japan have long been highly industrialized societies, industrial pollution does not appear to be closely associated with the changing patterns of these malignancies.[10]

The risk of colon cancer increases with the first generation migrating from Japan (a low-risk area) to the United States (a high-risk area),[10,25] but breast cancer in migrant Japanese tends to increase only in the second generation.[28] One possible explanation for these findings may be that colon cells differentiate and incorporate thymidine throughout life[29] whereas similar processes take place in breast tissue primarily during puberty or pregnancy.[30] Thus each tissue may be differentially susceptible to carcinogens. This concept is supported by a study of the population exposed to radiation in Hiroshima. Exposed Japanese women in the 10-to-19-year age group were four times as likely to develop breast cancer as were older women.[31] According to these views, carcinogenic effects of diet on breast tissue would be most likely during critical periods but colon tissue would be susceptible throughout the individual's lifetime.

It has been suggested[32] that bile acids may be important agents in colon cancer. Experiments have shown that diets with either 20% saturated or 20% unsaturated fats produce the same high incidence of colon cancer in rats in the presence of carcinogens.[2] Both human and animal subjects fed a high-fat diet excrete more total bile acids and particularly more secondary bile acids than do those fed a 5% lipid diet.[10] Secondary bile acids, which are generated from primary bile acids by the action of intestinal microorganisms, but not cholesterol or neutral sterols, are thought to have promoting activity in the presence of colon carcinogens.

The suggestion that charcoal broiling of meat or fish may produce mutagenic activity for *Salmonella typhimurium*[33] indicates that carcinogens in cooked meat may influence development of colon cancer. The length of time meat is cooked at temperatures above 100° C is directly related to the amount of mutagenic activity.[34] Pyrolysis of tryptophan in meat yields arylamines, including *o*-methyl-arylamines, capable of inducing tumors in the liver, subcutaneous bladder, colon, and breast.[35] Other mutagens and carcinogens currently are being identified in cooked fish and meat.[36] The potential hazard that charcoal broiling may represent for the general population deserves further definition.

Fiber, such as that found in wheat bran and vegetables, has been shown to inhibit colon carcinogenesis in animals although the precise mechanisms have not been elucidated. Fiber may dilute the bile acids and shorten transit time, thereby reducing the intervals during which carcinogens can act on gut mucosa.[37] In Finland and Utah high-fiber intakes, coupled with high-fat diets, have been found to produce stool bile acid concentrations similar to those found in populations consuming low-fat diets.[10]

Fat intake also is associated with the increased prevalance of human breast and prostate cancers, but the mechanisms are unclear. Both hormonal and immunologic mechanisms are thought to play roles in breast cancer. In mice prone to virus-induced mammary adenocarcinoma, reduced caloric intake has prevented viral replication but has not interfered with normal breast tissue development. Adding 20% fat to the low-calorie (10 kcal/da) diet increases viral reproduction and the incidence of precancerous lesions and spontaneous breast tumors.[4]

Analyses of hormonal patterns in women at high risk of breast cancer[28] have linked dietary fat to changes in hormone patterns. Known hormone-associated risk factors in breast cancer include first pregnancy after age 30 years, early menarche, and late menopause. It has been suggested[38] that diet may influence these hormonally related risk factors. Urinary estrogens, androgens, and estriol:estradiol ratios also have been associated with human mammary tumors.[10,28] Estrogen receptors appear to modulate the growth of normal and neoplastic breast tissue[39]; the development of such receptors possibly could be influenced by diet as well. Further research is needed to clarify these points.

It is well known that experimental mammary tumors are prolactin-dependent.[26] Higher diurnal prolactin peaks have been observed in human volunteers ingesting a high-fat diet[40]; however, the association of disturbances in prolactin secretion with the development of human breast cancer has been difficult to demonstrate definitively. Animal data suggest an association between fat and breast carcinogenesis, but it is not known which immunologic or endocrine mechanisms mediate the observed effects. At present there is some controversy as to whether dietary fat or dietary calories are the more crucial factor in carcinogenesis. The findings (by Frisch et al.[41]) that breast and reproductive tract cancers have lower prevalence rates in women with a lifetime exercise habit pattern than in sedentary controls and that exercising women are leaner than nonexercising women suggest that body composition may be a crucial determinant of cancer risk.

Stomach cancer. In the last 50 years the incidence of stomach cancer in the United States has dropped from about 27 to 5 per 100,000. Stomach tumors appear to be influenced by the action of nitrosamines and possibly by the inhibiting action of vitamin C on nitrosamine formation. The risk factors for gastric cancer include a diet with limited protein, micronutrients, and vitamins A, C, and E; a diet containing mostly foods that are pickled, heavily salted, or grown in high-nitrate soils; and the consumption of water with high levels of nitrate.[10,27,42]

The Prudent Diet

Although the precise mechanisms by which diet can influence the development of certain human malignancies are not yet defined, it is evident that certain dietary practices, (e.g., excessive fat consumption) associated with cancer, cardiovascular disease, degenerative diseases of aging, and disorganization of the immune system.[4] Therefore physicians should consider recommending the "prudent diet" to patients and their families. Following these guidelines may minimize the effects of other risk factors such as genetic predisposition.

1. Avoid excessive alcohol consumption (especially in conjunction with tobacco use).
2. Avoid tobacco products.
3. Maintain ideal weight for sex, height, and age.
4. Restrict total fat intake of all kinds.
5. Get regular exercise.
6. Restrict fatty meat consumption (although to what extent is not established).
7. Consume adequate fiber to increase stool volume.
8. Avoid foods high in nitrate or grown in soils or water high in nitrate. (Excessive consumption of nitrates and heavily salted or pickled foods also should be avoided.*)
9. Consume foods containing ascorbic acid with meals, particularly if meals contain abundant nitrites.
10. Avoid regular consumption of charred foods (and in particular overcooked meats and fish).

These guidelines should be regarded as general suggestions that may minimize the effects of other predisposing factors, and not as established rules.

METABOLIC EFFECTS OF MALIGNANCY

An understanding of the important aspects of host-tumor metabolism is essential to appropriate nutritional management of cancer patients and to optimum antitumor therapy. One result of the host-tumor imbalance is cachexia, the state of malnutrition and wasting that frequently accompanies cancer and often is the most devastating aspect of the disease. Cachexia usually is characterized by anorexia, early satiety, weight loss,

and weakness. The cancer itself appears to initiate and maintain the cachetic state, but the mechanisms of this relationship are poorly understood. Removal or control of the tumor may reverse the syndrome entirely.[43]

The clinical manifestations of cachexia may not necessarily relate to the size, histology, site, or extent of the tumor; in some patients small tumors may initiate cachexia whereas in others terminal metastatic disease may not produce inordinate nutritional problems.[44] Furthermore, cachexia often develops without evidence of malabsorption or hypercatabolism resulting from infection or following surgery.

Anorexia

Although anorexia is a frequent problem in cancer patients, it is not certain whether it is a cause or an effect of cachexia. Several models have been proposed to explain the cues and control mechanisms in anorexia.[45] A mathematical model proposes a gating, motivational, and excitatory role for chemoreceptors in the ingestive apparatus and an inhibitory role for ingested substances that accumulate in the intestine.[46] Both components of this system would be integrated by the central nervous system. The model is based on observations in experimental animals and is supported by some normal human and cancer patient data.

Alterations in the central nervous system also may be pertinent to the development of anorexia. The hypothalamus influences ingestive behavior through two types of catecholamine mechanisms[46,47]: the alpha-adrenergic mechanism increases hunger; the beta-adrenergic and dopaminergic receptors tend to suppress it. Drugs and hormones may stimulate the second mechanism in anorexia. Glucagon, glucose, lactic acid, and imbalances of free fatty acids and amino acids may influence eating behavior, but the interrelationships are complex and not yet fully understood.

Abnormalities in taste and smell may possibly contribute to anorexia, although they also are poorly understood and have not been observed uniformly. Elevated recognition thresholds for sweet and lowered thresholds for bitter stimuli have been correlated in some instances with cancer patients' reported aversion to meat (urea).[45,48] Serum zinc levels may be lowered in cancer patients because of malnutrition, malabsorption, inflammation, increased excretion, etc. or be-

---

*In practice it may be difficult to reduce the nitrite load in the gastrointestinal tract because bacteria in the mouth and intestine readily convert dietary nitrates to nitrites by means of the enzyme nitrate reductase.

cause of the cancer itself. Since zinc is needed to maintain oral taste receptors, zinc supplements may be helpful in certain depleted patients; further research is needed to explore this approach.

Studies[49] have suggested that changes in taste or smell preference (e.g., finding odors of meat offensive, food aversions associated with side effects of chemotherapy) may influence feeding behavior. Patients with cancer tend to prefer slightly sweet rather than very sweet items. This critical subject requires clarification and further investigation and may provide promising approaches to increasing dietary intake in sick cancer patients.[50] In any case, altered perceptions of foods often cause decreased enjoyment in eating as well as changes in a person's eating patterns.[50]

Anorexia in cancer may also arise from inhibitory signals from the gastrointestinal tract.[45] Abnormalities of taste conceivably could reduce gastric secretions, leading to delayed digestion and a prolonged sense of satiety. Atrophy of the small intestinal mucosa[51] and wasting of the musculature of the stomach wall also could contribute to the inability of cancer patients to derive maximum benefit from the nutrients ingested.

Some of the metabolic features of cachexia also may contribute to anorexia. These include reduced insulin response (insulin normally increases appetite), increased metabolic activity of the liver (including firing of hepatic glucoreceptors to decrease appetite), and elevated serum lactic acid.[45] The psychologic attributes of anorexia are significantly affected by taste and by negative emotional sequelae of treatment or progressive disease.[52]

Several simple strategies may help patients overcome anorexia and thereby improve oral intake. Patients who reject meat because of its odor can obtain protein from vegetables and dairy sources or be served meats at room temperature or below. Oral feedings should be of high caloric density, since patients may reach satiety early. Another suggestion is that major calories be consumed early in the day, since the patient may become nauseated or anorectic later in the day as a result of chemotherapy. Greater use should be made of ethnic foods in patients who are used to consuming them.

Cachexia

The effects of starvation and cachexia are generally similar, but the metabolic character and complications of cancer cachexia may be peculiar to it because of the nature of the disease. The same tissues and organs deteriorate in starvation and in cancer, except for the liver, which may gain in absolute dry weight in some patients with cancer.[53] The negative caloric balance in cachectic cancer patients can arise from reduced intake because of anorexia, impaired digestion and absorption, external nutrient loss, host-tumor competition for energy and nutrients, increased energy loss by the host, and other mechanisms.[43] It is likely that cancer cachexia is caused at least in part by tumor-mediated changes in energy metabolism, as evidenced by a disorganization of carbohydrate, lipid, and protein metabolism and altered vitamin, mineral, acid-base, and electrolyte balance.[54]

Energy metabolism. Cancer cachexia may be characterized by increased energy expenditure by the host. This phenomenon has been observed even in experimental tumor transplantation when the total tumor cell burden was relatively low.[45] The basal metabolic rate in some cancer patients is elevated even when caloric intake is decreased. About one third of the elevated energy output under these circumstances is estimated to be due to maintained or increased protein turnover.[54,55] Clearer perspectives on the disorganization of normal energy metabolism may come from studies of individual metabolic substrate classes. Nevertheless, so-called "tumor hypermetabolism" probably occurs in only a small proportion of patients with cancer.

Carbohydrates. The hallmark of cancer cachexia has been said to be disturbances in the metabolic cycle known as the Cori cycle in tumor and host, in which lactate produced by the tumor is recycled in the host via gluconeogenesis, at great energy expense to the host, and the glucose produced is utilized in turn by the tumor. Warburg[56] originally observed that tumors carry on primarily anaerobic metabolism and the end product is lactate.

Although systemic lactic acidosis has been reported in some instances, the majority of cancer patients do not demonstrate elevated lactic acid blood levels.[44] These levels remain normal, probably because the lactic acid is consumed completely by gluconeogenic activity, which may be elevated twofold to threefold in cancer patients who undergo weight loss.[57]

The Cori cycle results in a net energy loss to the host of 8 mol of ATP: 6 mol are required to produce glucose from 2 mol of lactate and 2 mol are used by the tumor to produce the subsequent mole of glucose. Had the 2 mol of lactate proceeded through the normal Krebs cycle, 30 mol of ATP would have been formed. It has been hypothesized that the increased tumor-derived lactate induces elevated gluconeogenesis and Cori cycling, and that this may account for the energy strain on the host and may contribute to malignant cachexia.[57]

Hydrazine sulfate has been administered in rats to interrupt gluconeogenesis, shift the energy balance to favor the host, and thus produce a metabolic antitumor effect.[58] Although this strategy did inhibit sarcomas in rats, it also resulted in greater weight loss than in the controls. Moreover, hydrazine sulfate has failed to show major antitumor or nutritional benefits in patients with progressive cancer. These observations, plus the argument that Krebs cycle oxidation of 15% of total tumor lactate produces sufficient energy to balance the net energy lost in Cori cycling of the remaining lactate, make it uncertain whether Cori cycle activity contributes significantly to cachectic weight loss. Thus the possible role of the Cori cycle in cachexia remains a subject of controversy and is not universally accepted by investigators as being major.

Some cancer patients tend to have diabetic glucose tolerance and insensitivity to exogenous insulin. In these patients fasting blood glucose may be the same as in controls, but intravenously administered glucose tends to be cleared more slowly.[43,44] These observations correlate with the presence of tumor alone.[44] Despite this apparent insulin resistance, insulin receptors on circulating monocytes in cancer patients tend to be normal, in contrast to findings associated with glucose intolerance in obesity. Such receptors may be diminished in fat and liver cells of cancer patients. However, loss of major amounts of weight, poor dietary intake, liver metastases, malabsorption, and other factors may favor the development of hypoglycemia in patients with cancer.

Lipid metabolism. In tumor development, as in starvation or diabetes, the primary mobilization of free fatty acids from adipose tissue begins very early in animal studies.[59] The rapid reduction in total body fat in cancer patients generally correlates with elevated caloric expenditure in fatty acid metabolism.[44] Fatty acids are utilized by the liver, kidney cortex, and cardiac and skel-

etal muscle; the ketone bodies of fatty acid oxidation also are used by the brain during prolonged fasting. Some of the fat breakdown in cancer patients is likely to result from the release of glucagon, norepinephrine, ACTH, and growth hormone, which may be expected in response to the stress of the tumor and its related therapy. In a fasting state, fat breakdown is also facilitated by the lack of insulin secretion; or in cancer a possible lack or alteration of insulin receptors in appropriate tissues may be postulated.

There is some question whether fasting cachetic cancer patients exhibit significantly elevated free fatty acid levels in blood. Under basal conditions, the same rates of glucose and free fatty acid oxidation have been observed in cancer patients and in controls.[60] After glucose administration, fatty acid oxidation was suppressed less well in cancer patients and their Krebs cycle activity was not stimulated. Some authors[44] attribute this apparent inability to achieve fatty acid homeostasis to altered insulin function, others[61] to a postulated tumor-derived lipolytic substances. Clearly it is an area that deserves more attention.

Proteins. Free amino acids from either endogenous or dietary sources provide an additional reserve of gluconeogenic precursors for glucose production, as well as a source of nitrogen. In brief fasting this process supplies the brain and other tissues with glucose. With more prolonged fasting in normal subjects, skeletal muscle protein catabolism is reduced and fatty acids become the major source of energy.

In the cancer patient, however, skeletal muscle protein and visceral smooth muscle are lost because of increased protein catabolism.[43,51] Increased muscle protein breakdown may be observed even in a diet with adequate amino acid content and calories.[62]

Frequently there is negative nitrogen balance. Despite a nitrogen intake that appear to be adequate for both tumor and host, the host may tend to lose nitrogen. Total blood amino acid nitrogen in cancer patients may be elevated, despite decreased protein intake and in direct contrast to the low blood amino acid levels generally observed in long-starved individuals.[43,62]

The precise causes of these complex changes are uncertain. The simple explanation that increased lactate prompts heightened gluconeogenesis and that this precipitates increased protein catabolism is not sufficient. Indeed, it has been observed that a defect in the 40S component* of ribosomes occurs in tumor-bearing rats, and this may contribute to the impaired protein biosynthesis.[63] Whatever the mechanism, accelerated protein breakdown occurs regularly in cancer patients and is difficult to prevent by therapeutic means.

Conclusions

It is evident from the extensive research in this area that the mere presence of a tumor may affect host metabolism adversely. Tumors alter or induce the activity of pertinent enzyme systems, among them tumor-derived lipolytic substances and novel proteins and peptides. The malnutrition induced by cancer and/or its treatment can alter the blood and tissue levels of several minerals and vitamins, and these changes in turn can alter intermediary metabolism significantly. Finally, futile enzymatic cycles and abnormalities in ion pumping and in the rates of protein metabolism account for a considerable proportion of the host's energy expense and the failure of normal metabolic regulation.[54] The suggestion[64] that obesity may be related to low energy expenditure at the ion pump level lends credence to this rationale, but these findings require confirmation.

The most predictable means of correcting the metabolic abnormalities associated with malignancy is to remove the primary lesion. Otherwise, the effectiveness of other kinds of intervention may be less than optimal in the long run. The obvious need to intervene nutritionally in patients with advanced disease points to the importance of continued research in this area.

NUTRITIONAL EFFECTS OF CANCER THERAPY

In addition to the metabolic changes that accompany cancer, local effects of the tumor or its metastases can interfere directly with the patient's nutritional status. The variety and causes of localized nutritional problems produced by various forms of cancer are summarized as follows[65]:

Malnutrition secondary to persistent anorexia
Malnutrition associated with impaired food intake secondary to obstruction

Malabsorption associated with
  Deficiency of pancreatic enzymes or bile salts
  Infiltration of small bowel by neoplasms (e.g., lymphoma, carcinoma)
  Fistulous bypass of small bowel
  Gastric hypersecretion inhibiting pancreatic enzymes (in Zollinger-Ellison syndrome)
Protein-losing enteropathy (as with gastric carcinoma, lymphoma, or lymphatic obstruction)
Electrolyte and fluid balance disturbances associated with
  Persistent vomiting in obstruction
  Vomiting secondary to increased intracranial pressure from tumors
  Small bowel fluid losses from fistula
  Diarrhea associated with hormone-secreting tumors (e.g., carcinoid syndrome, Zollinger-Ellison syndrome, Verner-Morrison syndrome) and villous adenoma of colon
  Inappropriate antidiuretic hormone secretion with certain tumors
  Hyperadrenalism secondary to excessive corticotropin or corticosteroid production by tumors
  Hypercalcemia secondary to ectopic parathyroid hormone–like agents

The clinician must evaluate nutritional status before and after therapy and monitor the nutritional sequelae of local problems induced by cancer and its therapy. Only then will nutritional intervention be more than just a passive measure. One of the most common causes of malnutrition is direct interference with food intake by obstruction of the gastrointestinal tract. Surgery or other treatment obviously is required, and intravenous alimentation or tube feeding distal to the obstruction may be necessary.

The treatment of cancer has become increasingly multidisciplinary. Surgical intervention often accompanies radiation or chemotherapy or a combination of the two. Each of the three major types of treatment has its own nutritional side effects and complications.

Radiotherapy

Table 25-2 summarizes the major nutritional problems induced by radiotherapy. Since the effects of radiotherapy may persist for years, attention must be paid to the minimum doses tolerated by particular organs.[66] Radiotherapy can depress immune competence for as long as 10 years. It is not clear whether nutritional intervention can reverse such effects.

Radiotherapy to the central nervous system

---

*The nuclear protein fraction that settles with a sedimentation velocity of 40×10^{-13} second (or 40 svedbergs) during ultracentrifugation.

Table 25-2 Localized Effects of
Radiotherapy Leading to Nutritional
Alterations

Area	Effect	
	Acute	Chronic
Central nervous system	Nausea	
Head/neck	Sore throat	Ulcer
	Dysphagia	Xerostomia
	Xerostomia	Dental caries
	Mucositis	Osteoradionecrosis
	Anorexia	
	Altered smell	Trismus
	Loss of taste	Altered taste
Thorax	Dysphagia	Fibrosis
		Stenosis
		Fistula
Abdomen/pelvis	Anorexia	Ulcer
	Nausea	Malabsorption
	Vomiting	Diarrhea
	Diarrhea	Chronic enteritis
	Acute enteritis	Chronic colitis
	Acute colitis	

From Donaldson SS, Lenon RA: Cancer **43:**2036-2052, 1979.

may result in cerebral edema, which exacerbates the headache, nausea, and vomiting often produced by tumors in that area. Dexamethasone may reduce cerebral edema and the focal signs associated with increased intracranial pressure from brain tumors.[67] Corticosteroids, combined with radiotherapy, may relieve the symptoms of severe neurologic disease[68] and, when administered prophylactically, can prevent nausea and vomiting from cerebral edema when a high dose per unit of radiation is given.[67] However, when corticosteroids in high doses are continued for a prolonged period, hyperglycemia, hypertension, hypercalciuria, peripheral edema, and other well-known complications may result.

The symptoms resulting from radiotherapy to the oral cavity may be reversible or remain progressive and chronic. Denudation of the oral epithelium after acute radiation can cause pseudomembranous bleeding, superficial ulceration, or even chronic ulcers, with obvious consequences for oral intake. The sense of taste is lost rapidly. It may take as long as 60-120 days for taste thresholds to return to normal,[69] and much longer for full return of taste sensations. Salivary gland function also declines following radiation,

and the saliva becomes thick, viscous, more acidic, and of varied composition. Acinar cell damage is indicated by an increase in salivary amylase within hours of a single fraction of 100 rads.[66]

The rate at which salivary function is recovered varies with the individual, the therapy, and the presence of tumor; but even severe effects generally are reversed eventually. The change in salivary function is believed to be a factor in the increased prevalence of dental caries that occurs as a late complication in cancer patients who have received radiation. The combined effects of external radiation on taste, mucous membranes, salivary glands, and teeth clearly may limit oral intake and potentially may cause severe nutritional problems.

Radiation to the lung, mediastinum, or esophagus may cause dysphagia (resulting from irritation of the mucosa in the pharynx and esophagus) and secondary infection. The epithelium of these structures has moderate radiosensitivity, but the diseased esophagus has a lower radiation tolerance. Symptoms may persist throughout treatment and for several weeks thereafter. Late radiation effects (stenosis, ulceration, perforation) have important nutritional implications.

The stomach appears to tolerate radiotherapy relatively well. Low doses may cause nonspecific nausea, but generally no long-term nutritional problems result. High doses have been associated with ulcers that do not respond to conventional treatment and may require partial gastrectomy.[66]

Nausea, vomiting, and diarrhea may occur following small or large bowel radiation. Damage to the small intestine may interfere with the absorption of fats, glucose, proteins, and electrolytes.[66,70] Alterations in gastrointestinal tract flora may be responsible in part for intestinal radiation injury, since tissue damage provides opportunities for microbial infection. Generally, however, the symptoms disappear when therapy is stopped.[65] Late radiation effects may occur within approximately 1 year but sometimes as long as 10 years after irradiation; these include flattening or ulceration of the mucosa, telangiectasia, fibrosis, endarteritis of small vessels, and bowel stenosis.[65] If significant bowel obstruction occurs, surgery will be necessary. Procrastination only increases the surgical risks later. Patients with previous bowel resection plus radiation damage are more difficult to manage than those with bowel resection alone. Therefore each patient's status must be monitored carefully and addressed nutritionally.

Chemotherapy

Nearly all chemotherapeutic agents adversely affect dietary intake and nutritional status; and there is some evidence that nutritional status can influence the results of chemotherapy, although more research on this important subject needs to be undertaken. The nutritionally relevant effects of selected chemotherapeutic agents are summarized in Table 25-3. The sometimes severe gastrointestinal symptoms that result from chemotherapy generally are not prolonged after therapy is stopped.[66] Among the combined drug regimens currently in use, those that include high doses of vinblastine, cisplatin, and bleomycin may produce some of the most severe gastroin-

testinal toxicity, but intravenous alimentation has the capability of maintaining nutritional status.[71]

Combined Radiation and Chemotherapy

There is little information about the nutritional impact of combined radiation and chemotherapy, despite the fact that such combined approaches are used increasingly. Radiation-induced skin and mucosal reactions have been noted when actinomycin-D, Adriamycin (doxorubicin), methotrexate, bleomycin, and/or hydroxyurea were used concurrently.[66] "Recall phenomena" for latent radiation effects on gastrointestinal mucosa and oral intake have been observed when actinomycin-D and Adriamycin were given. These two agents may be true sensitizers with radiation, but the remainder of the chemotherapeutic drugs probably exert only additive effects with those of radiation.[72]

Various commonly used drugs produce radia-

Table 25-3 Gastrointestinal Effects of Chemotherapeutic Agents

	Agent	Clinical Course
Anorexia, nausea, vomiting	Nitrogen mustard	Severe but rarely prolonged
	cis-Diaminedichloro-platinum (cisplatin)	Severe with short infusions; less so with 24-hour infusion
	Hexamethylmelamine	Frequently necessitates termination of continuous oral therapy
	Streptozotocin	Severe; courses usually given weekly
	Adriamycin-cyclophosphamide	More severe in combination than with either agent given singly
Mucositis	5-Fluorouracil	Common endpoint for loading courses; high mortality if diarrhea appears
	Methotrexate	Similar to 5-FU; with both agents radiation increases severity
	Vinblastine	May be accompanied by ileus, especially with high dose schedules
	Bleomycin	May be severe; severity increases with high doses, which prolong the mucositis; effect also may be prolonged with radiation or high-dose vinblastine
	Actinomycin-D	May be severe; enhanced with radiation
	Adriamycin (doxorubicin)	Severe; enhanced with radiation
Ileus	Vincristine	Usually preventable with stool softeners and laxatives
	Vinblastine	As with vincristine; ileus rarely a problem with conventional low doses
Other toxicities	Mithramycin	Hepatocellular damage occurs
	Asparaginase	Loss of massive amounts of body weight has been reported; hepatic dysfunction, pancreatitis
	Methotrexate	Cirrhosis

Modified slightly from Donaldson SS, Lenon RA: Cancer **43**:2036-2052, 1979.

tion sensitization in the esophagus, and Adriamycin and daunorubicin have produced esophageal stricture when given with radiation. Damage to other parts of the gastrointestinal tract may be increased, particularly with actinomycin D, Adriamycin, and 5-fluorouracil.[66]

Surgery

Although the nutritional effects of surgery are not peculiar to cancer patients, the kinds of surgery used in cancer (e.g., head and neck resection, total esophagectomy, total gastrectomy, colostomy) may present their own special nutritional problems. These are summarized in Table 25-4.

Glossectomy or mandibulectomy interferes with chewing and swallowing. Oral intake may be possible with laryngectomy or with training; otherwise, oral tube feeding through another access route is required. If the patient cannot overcome the psychologic difficulties and associated throat irritation resulting from an indwelling tube, the tube must be inserted by esophagostomy or gastrostomy.[65]

Esophagectomy may present problems in fat malabsorption, gastric stasis, and diarrhea that appear to be due to the accompanying bilateral vagotomy, but the causes of intestinal sequelae are unclear.[73] Carbohydrate absorption generally is not affected. If medium-chain triglycerides are utilized as the major fat calorie source, steatorrhea can be minimized, because these fats are absorbed directly by the intestine and do not require chylomicron formation.[65,71]

The clinical problems associated with gastrectomy generally are proportional to the extent of the resection. Aside from concern about the dumping syndrome, hypoglycemia, steatorrhea, afferent loop syndrome, and loss of intrinsic factor, the clinician also should be alert to possible vitamin and mineral deficiencies.[65] These tend to develop slowly and are often poorly recognized by health professionals, especially in older patients receiving drugs.[74]

Malabsorption is the most obvious problem resulting from small bowel resection. The remaining portions of the small intestine can adapt; thus, with the exception of vitamin B_{12}, virtually all nutrients are absorbed efficiently by the proximal bowel.[65] Even if the entire jejunum is resected, the ileum generally can absorb nutrients sufficiently well if proper nutritional intake is

Table 25-4 Nutritional Implications of Surgery in Cancer

Treatment	Implication
Radical resection of oropharyngeal area	Chewing and swallowing difficulties; tube feeding may be required
Esophagectomy and esophageal reconstruction	Gastric stasis and hypochlorhydria secondary to vagotomy
	Steatorrhea
	Diarrhea
Gastrectomy (high subtotal or total)	Dumping syndrome
	Malabsorption
	Achlorhydria and lack of intrinsic factor
	Hypoglycemia
Jejunal resection	Decreased efficiency of absorption of many nutrients
Ileal resection	Vitamin B_{12} deficiency
	Bile salt losses with diarrhea
	Hyperoxaluria, renal oxalate stones
Massive bowel resection	Life-threatening malabsorption
	Malnutrition
	Metabolic acidosis
	Gastric hypersecretion
Ileostomy and colostomy	Complications of salt and water balance
Pancreatectomy	Malabsorption
	Diabetes mellitus
	Fistula
Major hepatic resection (postoperative)	Hypoalbuminemia
	Hypoglycemia

Modified from Shils ME: Med Clin North Am **63**(5):1027-1039, 1979.

maintained. Intramuscular vitamin B_{12}, at 100 µg/month, will certainly overcome any deficiency associated with intestinal resection. This is also true if the jejunum remains intact and only the ileum is removed; in that instance virtually all nutrients but vitamin B_{12} can be absorbed efficiently in the proximal bowel. After resection of the terminal ileum, conjugated bile salts are absorbed poorly, resulting in their increased fecal loss, steatorrhea, and subsequently reduced fat absorption. The recommended approach is to increase the proportion of medium-chain fatty acids as a fat source and to administer water-soluble forms of the fat-soluble vitamins, including vitamin K.[65]

An additional consequence of ileal resection is hyperoxaluria and the possible formation of renal stones. The normal binding of oxalate with calcium, leading to the formation of calcium oxalate in the small intestine, may be limited by the lack of free Ca^{+2}, which becomes bound to unabsorbed fatty acids in the intestinal lumen. The freely absorbed oxalate then is transported to the kidney, where it may produce nephrolithiasis. Reduced fat intake and addition of calcium supplements may minimize renal injury.[65]

Massive resection of the small bowel presents serious permanent problems in maintaining both adequate nutritional status and water and electrolyte balance. Damage to the remaining bowel by radiation, or damage to the ileocecal valve, exacerbates these difficulties. Comprehensive nutritional management may mean the difference between an unfortunate and a successful outcome.

NUTRITIONAL MANAGEMENT OF THE CANCER PATIENT

The nutritional and metabolic deterioration that often accompanies malignant disease may result from the presence of the tumor, the effects of treatment, and the psychologic factors related to the real or assumed existence of cancer. The clinical manifestations of malnutrition, in turn, complicate the clinical course and choice of treatment. Yet malnutrition need not be an inevitable outcome in cancer. Careful attention to the patient's nutritional problems and to the expected and actual nutritional results of therapy combined with nutritional intervention and support can prevent or reverse malnutrition and possibly improve the therapeutic outcome.[75]

Concern for the patient's status should begin with planning for initial treatment and should continue through the expected long-term survival of the patient. For example, preventive dentistry is best practiced before the onset of chemotherapy or radiation to the head and neck. Teeth, gums, and mucous membranes should be in optimum condition prior to the ordeal of cancer treatment. The patient's nutritional status should be monitored periodically to detect potential problems and prevent unnecessary deterioration. It is easier to maintain good nutritional status than to rehabilitate a malnourished patient. Malnutrition must be detected early, and patients at risk must be identified early.

Goals of Nutritional Therapy

Depending on its purpose or expected outcome, nutritional therapy may be supportive, adjunctive, or definitive.[75] Supportive therapy is the type required to improve the patient's nutritional status so the risks of surgical intervention, chemotherapy, or radiation therapy will be minimized. Adjunctive nutritional therapy is aimed at maintaining the patient's strength and immune responsiveness during therapy and thereby possibly improving the outcome. Definitive nutritional therapy includes short- or long-term measures required to ensure survival, for example, as a result of major bowel resection or radiation enteritis. All three approaches should be available to each cancer patient. Since persons with cancer increasingly are undergoing long-term treatment (frequently as outpatients), such therapy can and should be instituted.

Nutritional Support and Tolerance to Therapy

Total parenteral nutrition allows patients to maintain nutritional status when they are unable to eat or when their oral intake is otherwise inadequate. Nutritional support also has been shown to improve immune status and reduce susceptibility to infection,[66,76] but more controlled studies are needed to establish this point definitively.

Significant advances have been made in the use of defined-formula diets for patients undergoing radiotherapy or chemotherapy. In such diets specific constituents are modified to control nutritional side effects of therapy. For example, a gluten-free, milk-free, low-fat, low-residue diet has been effective in children with partial to complete obstruction from radiation enteritis.[77] The rationale is to limit gluten and milk products when there is gluten sensitivity and loss of intestinal villi containing lactase, to limit fat when there is lymphatic dilation, and to limit residue to prevent exacerbation of mechanical obstruction. When this dietary approach is used preventively during radiotherapy, prevalence of severe or delayed enteritis may be diminished. The efficacy of other formula diets in preventing radiation-induced side effects currently is being studied.

When, after thorough evaluation of clinical status, it is evident that the patient cannot take oral or tube feeding in adequate amounts, partial and total parenteral nutrition can be very effective.[65,75,76] Wider application of these techniques could reduce the mortality from cancer and the morbidity from antitumor treatments. Since parenteral nutrition is more expensive and involves greater risks than tube feeding, the latter approach should be explored thoroughly first. Parenteral nutrition should be administered only by personnel trained in this approach. Peripheral parenteral nutrition allows some caloric intake through an ordinary peripheral vein, is simpler than total parenteral nutrition, and is appropriate for short-term nutritional support, particularly when oral intake has not been stopped completely but cannot fully meet all the metabolic needs.

The role of nutritional therapy in cancer has been the subject of much research and discussion. In considering general nutritional support or in administering specific nutrients like zinc, there is concern that the tumor rather than the host will derive greater benefit. There are two issues involved. (1) Even if the tumor were to grow, the benefits to the patient in terms of improvement of general and immunologic status, prevention or amelioration of side effects of therapy, and ability to continue in therapy should probably outweigh this concern. Furthermore, several observers have found that tumor growth is not out of proportion to host increases in weight. (2) Since the efficacy of chemotherapy and radiotherapy depends on continuing tumor cell division, enhancing tumor growth through nutritional manipulation should facilitate therapy. Some physicians[77] deliberately infuse glucose in an attempt to promote tumor growth

before treatment by combined radiation and chemotherapy. Well-nourished animals have responded better to radiation therapy than have poorly nourished controls.[66] Such evidence supports the view that aggressive nutritional support should accompany any antitumor therapy regimen but that aggressive nutritional support should not be given unless there is a definite plan for cancer treatment.

With further research it may be possible to design specific nutritional interventions for each specific treatment modality. Evidence to support this approach is now accumulating.[78] Nutritional principles already are being utilized in antimetabolite therapy. Treatment with the antimetabolite methotrexate is followed by its metabolite, 5-formyltetrahydrofolate (leucovorin), a reduced stable form of folic acid. Nutritional supplementation may be used more generally to ensure the efficacy of such antimetabolites. For example, amino acid or folate deficiencies cause suboptimum therapeutic results for 5-fluorouracil (5-FU) or methotrexate but can be reversed by good nutrition.[78] Research is underway to determine whether dietary supplementation by leucovorin will improve the effectiveness of 5-FU, since it requires the folate coenzyme 5,10-methylene tetrahydrofolate to bind and inhibit thymidylate synthase. Greater awareness of host and tumor metabolism, coupled with a better knowledge of the biochemical pharmacology of particular drugs, should make it possible to tailor aggressive nutritional-metabolic approaches more specifically to cancer therapy.

REFERENCES

1. Rous P: The influence of diet upon transplanted and spontaneous mouse tumors, J Exp Med **20**:433-451, 1914.
2. Tannenbaum A: The initiation and growth of tumors, introduction. I. Effects of underfeeding, Am J Cancer **38**:335-350, 1940.
3. Ross MN, Bras G: Tumor incidence patterns and nutrition in the rat, J Nutr **87**:245-261, 1965.
4. Fernandes G, et al: Nutrition, immunity, and cancer, a review. III. Effects of diet on the diseases of aging, Clin Bull **9**(3):91-106, 1979.
5. Jose DG, Good RA: Absence of enhancing antibody in cell-mediated immunity to tumor heterografts in protein-deficient rats, Nature **231**:323-325, 1971.
6. Wattenberg JH: Inhibitors of chemical carcinogenesis, Adv Cancer Res **26**:197-219, 1978.
7. Shils ME: Diet and nutrition as modifying factors in tumor development, Med Clin North Am **63**(5):1027-1039, 1979.
8. Wattenberg JH: Inhibition of carcinogenic and toxic effects of polycycle hydrocarbons and ethoxyquin. J Natl Cancer Inst **48**:1425-36, 1972.

9. Wolff IA, Wasserman AE: Nitrates, nitrites and nitrosamines, Science **177:**15-18, 1972.

10. Weisburger JH, et al: Nutrition and cancer: on the mechanisms bearing on causes of cancer of the colon, breast, prostate and stomach, Bull NY Acad Med **56:**673-696, 1980.

11. Anderson LM, et al: Lung tumorigenesis in mice after chronic exposure in early life to a low dose of dimethylnitrosamine, J Natl Cancer Inst **62:**1553-1555, 1979.

12. Mirvish SS: N-nitroso compounds: their chemical and in vivo formation and possible importance as environmental carcinogens, J Toxicol Environ Health **2:**1267-1277, 1977.

13. Correa P, et al: A model for gastric cancer epidemiology, Lancet **2:**58-60, 1975.

14. Sporn MB, et al: Prevention of chemical carcinogenesis by vitamin A and its synthetic analogues (retinoids), Fed Proc **35:**1332-1338, 1976.

15. Shamberger RJ, Frost DV: Possible protective effect of selenium against human cancer, Can Med Assoc J **100:**682-687, 1969.

16. Allaway WH, et al: Selenium, molybdenum, and vanadium in human blood, Arch Environ Health **16:**342-348, 1968.

17. Clark, LC: The epidemiology of selenium and cancer, Fed Proc **44:**2584-2589, 1985.

18. Jacobs MM, et al: Inhibitory effects of selenium on 1,2-dimethylhydrazine and methylazoxy-methanol acetate induction of colon tumors, Cancer Lett **2:**133-138, 1977.

19. Thompson HJ, et al: Effect of combined selenium and retinyl acetate treatment on mammary carcinogenesis, Cancer Res **41:**1413-1416, 1981.

20. Rivlin RS: Hormones, drugs and riboflavin, Nutr Rev **37:**241-246, 1979.

21. Rivlin RS, et al: Nutrition and cancer: combined clinical and basic science seminar, Am J Med **75:**843-854, 1983.

22. Pinto J, et al: Inhibition of riboflavin metabolism in rat tissues by chlorpromazine, imipramine and amitriptyline, J Clin Invest **67:**1500-1506, 1981.

23. Higginson J, Muir CS: Epidemiology of cancer. In Holland JF, Frei E III, editors: Cancer medicine, ed 2, Philadelphia, 1982 Lea & Febiger, pp 257-327.

24. Wynder EL: Dietary habits and cancer epidemiology, Cancer **43:**1955-1961, 1979.

25. Weisburger JH, Williams GM: Chemical carcinogenesis. In Donll J, et al, editors: Toxicology: the basic science of poisons, New York, 1979, The MacMillan Co, pp 84-138.

26. Furth J: Hormones as etiological agents in neoplasia. In Becker FF editor: Cancer: a comprehensive treatise, vol 1, New York, 1975, Plenum Press Inc, pp 75-120.

27. Wynder EL, Hirayama T: Comparative epidemiology of cancers in the United States and Japan, Prev Med **6:**567-594, 1977.

28. McMahon B, et al: Etiology of human breast cancer: a review, J Natl Cancer Inst **50:**21-42, 1973.

29. Lipkin M: Memorial Hospital registry of population groups at high risk for cancer of the large intestine: development of risk factor profiles. In Pottes J, et al, editors: Genetics and heterogeneity in gastrointestinal disorders, New York, 1981, Academic Press Inc, pp 357-375.

30. Meyer JS: Cell proliferation in normal human breast ducts, dibroadenomas, and other ductal hyperplasias measured by nuclear labeling with tritiated thymidine: effect of menstrual phase, age and oral contraceptive hormones, Hum Pathol **8:**67-81, 1977.

31. McGregor DN, et al: Breast cancer incidence among atomic bomb survivors, Hiroshima and Nagasaki, 1950-69, J Natl Cancer Inst **59:**799-811, 1977.

32. Reddy BS, et al: Nutrition and its relationship to cancer, Adv Cancer Res **32:**237-245, 1980.

33. Sugimura T, et al: Mutagen-carcinogens in food, with special reference to highly mutagenic products in broiled foods. In Hiatt M, et al, editors: Origins of human cancer, Cold Spring Harbor NY, 1977, Cold Spring Harbor Laboratories, pp 1561-1577.

34. Spingarn NE, Weisberger JH: Formation of mutagens in cooked foods. I. Beef, Cancer Lett **7:**259-264, 1979.

35. Weisberger JH, Williams GM: Chemical carcinogenesis. In Holland JF, Frei E III, editors: Cancer medicine, ed 2, Philadelphia, 1982, Lea & Febiger, pp 42-95.

36. Spingarn NE, et al: Formation of mutagens in cooked foods. III. Isolation of a potent mutagen from beef, Cancer Lett **9:**177-183, 1980.

37. Eastwood MA, Kay RM: An hypothesis for the action of dietary fiber along the gastrointestinal tract, Am J Clin Nutr **32:**364-367, 1979.

38. Gray GE, et al: Breast cancer incidence and mortality rates in different countries in relation to known risk factors and dietary practices, Br J Cancer **39:**1-7, 1979.

39. Sherman MR, Miller MK: Fractionation of diverse steroid-binding proteins: basic and clinical applications. In Menon KMJ, Reel RR, editors: Steroid hormone action and cancer, New York, 1976, Plenum Press Inc, pp 51-67.

40. Hill P, Wynder EL: Diet and prolactin release, Lancet **2:**806-807, 1976.

41. Frisch RE, et al: Lower prevalence of breast cancer and cancers of the reproductive system among former college athletes compared to non-athletes, Br J Cancer **52:**885-891, 1985.

42. Weisberger JM, et al: Induction of cancer of the glandular stomach by an extract of nitrite-treated fish, J Natl Cancer Inst **64:**163-167, 1980.

43. Theologides A: Cancer cachexia, Cancer **43:**2004-2012, 1979.

44. Schein PS, et al: Cachexia of malignancy: potential role of insulin in nutritional management, Cancer **43:**2070-2076, 1979.

45. DeWys WD: Anorexia as a general effect of cancer, Cancer **43:**2013-2019, 1979.

46. Davis JD, Levine MW: A model for the control of ingestion, Psychol Rev **84:**379-412, 1977.

47. Leibowitz SF: Brain catecholaminergic mechanisms for control of hunger. In Niven D, et al, editors: Hunger: basic mechanisms and clinical implications, New York, 1976, Raven Press, pp 1-18.

48. DeWys WD, Walters K: Abnormalities of taste sensation in cancer patients, Cancer **36:**1888-1896, 1975.

49. Nielson SS, et al: Influence of food odors on food aversions and preferences with cancer, Am J Clin Nutr **11:**2253-2261, 1980.

50. Ferris AM, et al: Nutrition and taste and smell deficits: a risk factor or an adjustment? In Meiselman HL, Rivlin RS, editors: Clinical measurement of taste and smell, New York, 1986, The MacMillan Co, pp 264-278.

51. Barry RE: Malignancy, weight loss, and the small intestine mucosa, Gut **15:**562-570, 1974.

52. Bernstein IL, Sigmundi RA: Tumor anorexia: a learned food aversion? Science **209:**416-418, 1980.

53. Theologides A, Pegelow CH: Liver weight changes during distant growth of transplanted tumor, Proc Soc Exp Biol Med **134**:1104-1108, 1970.

54. Young VR: Energy metabolism and requirements in the cancer patient, Cancer Res **37**:2336-2347, 1977.

55. Waterhouse C: How tumors affect host metabolism, Ann NY Acad Sci **230**:86-93, 1974.

56. Warburg O: The metabolism of tumors, London, 1930, Constable & Co Ltd.

57. Holroyde CP, et al: Altered glucose metabolism in metastatic carcinoma, Cancer Res **35**:3710-3714, 1975.

58. Gold J: Cancer cachexia and gluconeogenesis, Ann NY Acad Sci **230**:103-110, 1974.

59. Kraclovic RC, et al: Studies of the mechanism of carcass fat depletion in experimental cancer, Eur J Cancer **13**:1071-1079, 1977.

60. Waterhouse C, Kemperman JM: Carbohydrate metabolism in subjects with cancer, Cancer Res **31**:1273-1278, 1971.

61. Liebelt RA, et al: Lipid mobilization and food intake in experimentally obese mice bearing transplanted tumors, Proc Soc Exp Biol Med **138**:482-490, 1971.

62. Stein TP, et al: Tumor-caused changes in host protein synthesis under different dietary situations, Cancer Res **36**:3926-3940, 1976.

63. Clark CM, Goodlad GAJ: Muscle protein biosynthesis in the tumor bearing rat: a defect in the post initiation stage of translation, Biochim Biophys Acta **318**:230-240, 1975.

64. De Luise M, et al: Reduced activity of the red-cell sodium-potassium pump in human obesity, N Engl J Med **303**:1017-1022, 1980.

65. Shils ME: Nutritional problems induced by cancer, Med Clin North Am **63**:1009-1025, 1979.

66. Donaldson SS, Lenon RA: Alterations of nutritional status: impact of chemotherapy and radiation, Cancer **43**:2036-2052, 1979.

67. Fishman RA: Brain edema, N Engl J Med **293**:706-711, 1975.

68. Hendrickson FR: Radiation therapy of metastatic tumors, Semin Oncol **2**:43-46, 1975.

69. Conger AD: Loss and recovery of taste acuity in patients irradiated to the oral cavity, Radiat Res **53**:338-347, 1973.

70. Duncan W, Leonard JC: The malabsorption syndrome following radiation therapy, Q J Med **34**:319-329, 1965.

71. Dudrick S: Summary of the informal discussion of nutritional management, Cancer Res **37**:2462-2468, 1977.

72. Phillips TL, Fu KK: The interaction of drug and radiation effects on normal tissues, Int J Radiat Oncol Biol Phys **4**:59-64, 1978.

73. Shils ME: The esophagus, the vagi, and fat absorption, Surg Gynecol Obstet **132**:709-716, 1971.

74. Roe DA, editor: Drugs and nutrition in the geriatric patient. Vol 7. Contemporary issues in clinical nutrition, New York, 1984, Churchill-Livingstone Inc, pp 105-120.

75. Shils ME: Principles of nutritional therapy, Cancer **43**:2093-2102, 1979.

76. Copeland EM, et al: Nutrition as an adjunct to cancer treatment in the adult, Cancer Res **37**:2451-2456, 1977.

77. Donaldson SS, et al: Radiation enteritis in children: a retrospective review, clinicopathologic correlation, and dietary management, Cancer **35**:1167-1178, 1975.

78. Bertino JR: Nutrients, vitamins, and minerals as therapy, Cancer **43**:2137-2142, 1979.

CHAPTER 26
Anorexia Nervosa

Arnold E. Andersen

Anorexia nervosa, a disorder of severe weight loss that occurs primarily in adolescent women, is associated with a variety of psychiatric and medical symptoms. It first was recognized almost three centuries ago but recently has increased greatly in incidence. Approximately 0.5% of adolescent women meet strict criteria for this syndrome, and another 5% may suffer from a milder subclinical form. The disorder is of interest to health professionals because of its seriousness and because of the interdisciplinary nature of its symptoms. Although the short-term mortality rate has decreased to less than 5%, many patients do not ever fully recover from it but remain chronically ill.

The etiology of anorexia nervosa is still uncertain and elusive. Why an individual goes against a profound physiologic drive to normal nutritional status and chooses instead self-induced starvation is not clear.

Anorexia frequently has been diagnosed by excluding medical or psychiatric diseases known to be associated with weight loss. However, rigorous and reliable criteria now have been formulated that allow a confident diagnosis of the disorder on the basis of its signs and symptoms rather than by exclusion. The essential features for the diagnosis are (1) self-induced starvation (a behavioral symptom), (2) fear that fatness will result from loss of control in eating (a psychologic symptom), and (3) alteration in reproductive hormone function (a physiologic symptom). The fact that the diagnosis is made by identifying symptoms rather than causes means that anorexia nervosa is a syndrome, a collection of signs and symptoms that follow a predictable course, rather than a disease with proved specific etiology.

Anorexia is of special interest to professional nutritionists, who often are called upon to prescribe diets to treat the weight loss. The recognition of anorexia nervosa can lead to a treatment more appropriate than a simple weight-gaining diet. The skill of a nutritionist is essential for all phases of inpatient treatment for anorexia nervosa as well as after discharge, to prevent relapse.

DIAGNOSIS OF ANOREXIA NERVOSA AND ITS VARIANTS

Two sets of distinctions should be considered in a discussion of the diagnosis of anorexia nervosa. The first is the difference between primary and secondary anorexias. The second is the difference between typical and atypical forms. It is important to distinguish among these variations because of the implications for treatment and outcome.

Primary and Typical Anorexia Nervosa

The essential features in the diagnosis of primary and typical anorexia are those formulated by Russell[1]: (1) self-induced starvation, (2) fear that loss of control of eating will lead to fatness despite being thin and of low weight, and (3) amenorrhea in women and loss of sexual drive and function in men. The criteria now used on the Phipps Psychiatric Service of the Johns Hopkins Hospital are those of the American Psychiatric Association's third edition of *Diagnostic and Statistical Manual (DSM III)*[2]:

Intense fear of becoming obese that does not diminish as weight loss progresses

Disturbance of body image (e.g., claiming to "feel fat" even when emaciated)

Loss of at least 25% of original body weight or, if under 18 years of age, loss from original body weight combined with projected weight gain (from growth charts) to make the 25%

Refusal to maintain body weight over the minimum normal for age and height

No known physical illness that would account for the weight loss

These are more quantitative criteria, but they are essentially the same psychopathologically. A proposal has been made to revise them. It would require not a loss of 25% of body weight but rather a refusal to maintain body weight above 85% of that appropriate for height and age. The proposed criteria would also add a requirement for at least 3 months of amenorrhea (although this would not adequately deal with men).

In making a diagnosis it is essential to use criteria that are positive to identify the disorder rather than only to exclude other medical or psychiatric disorders. Each patient should receive a thorough mental status examination. The superiority of this approach over the exclusionary approach has been proved in studies of patients at the National Institutes of Health. Of more than 35 patients diagnosed by rigorous clinical criteria as having anorexia nervosa, not one was found later to have any underlying psychiatric or medical disorder that would explain the weight loss.[3]

Among the beneficial results of accurate diagnosis are reduced morbidity from excessive medical testing and earlier treatment leading to improved outcome. In addition to lower mortality, a prompt and accurate diagnosis leads to decreased chronicity.

The diagnosis of anorexia should be considered in any adolescent who begins dieting and continues below a reasonable weight, especially when there is preoccupation with thoughts of food, fear of obesity, and perceptual distortion characterized by overestimation of body size. Although the syndrome is found most frequently in adolescent women, it also should be considered in adolescent men with similar symptoms. In the last decade, men increasingly have shared with women the emphasis on slimness through exercise and dietary restriction. Young men on high school or college wrestling teams are especially vulnerable to the development of eating disorders, as are teenagers with diabetes mellitus, who often manipulate insulin or diet to lose weight.

Secondary and Atypical Anorexia Nervosa

The term secondary anorexia is used for weight loss resulting from an identified medical or psychiatric disorder. The implication of this diagnosis is that the therapeutic approach should treat the underlying disorder rather than the anorexia itself. For example, successful treatment of depressive illness with antidepressants can correct the associated weight loss.

Among the differential diagnoses of medical disorders that cause weight loss are neurologic diseases (especially tumors of the hypothalamus), endocrine disorders (thyroid, adrenal, pituitary), malabsorption, and diabetes mellitus. Psychiatric disorders associated with weight loss include depression, obsessional states (globus hystericus), abuse of stimulant medications, and schizophrenia with delusions concerning food.

A number of atypical varieties of anorexia nervosa also should be considered.[4] For example, a patient may have all the essential features of the syndrome but be older at the time of onset than the criteria allow. Anorexia has been diagnosed in patients up to age 51 years at the Phipps Service. Thus, such a diagnosis should not be ruled out in those over 25 to 30 years on the basis of age alone. Alternatively, the subject may have lost less weight than the threshold amount specified in strict criteria. These discrepancies in no way affect the essential character of the disorder, which should be recognized and treated as anorexia nervosa. A more difficult problem occurs when an essential feature, such as the fear of obesity or fear of loss of control, is not discernible yet no satisfactory medical or psychiatric origin for weight loss can be found.

NUTRITIONAL PATHOPHYSIOLOGY

The major physiologic changes in anorexia nervosa are due to the effects of starvation. Most body systems are changed profoundly by the lowered weight. Some of the most significant and characteristic changes that accompany weight loss include lowered body mass; decreasing lipid stores, muscle bulk, and carbohydrate storage in the liver; and, at times, atrophy of cardiac muscle. In severe anorexia nervosa the patient appears cachectic, with prominent bone structure, sunken facial features, and the general appearance of a concentration camp victim or an individual terminally ill from a wasting disease. In contrast to such victims and terminally ill patients, anorectic individuals usually are alert and often excessively active. Up to 70% of patients with well-established anorexia show some degree of osteoporosis on dual-photon absorptiometry, a finding that has frightening implications for the future if one considers how many chronic dieters exist in the United States.

Temperature and Cardiac Changes

Temperature regulation is altered by a lowered core temperature and loss of the ability to regulate temperature in hot or cold environments.[5] Patients complain of being constantly cold and manifest acrocyanosis. They dress in multiple layers of clothing and cannot tolerate air conditioning or winter temperatures.

A profound bradycardia frequently is present. There are at least three mechanisms that account for the lowered pulse rate. Starvation results in lowered circulating norepinephrine levels and leads to decreased cardiac stimulation. For patients who overexercise as a means of weight loss, the exercise also contributes to bradycardia. Circulating thyroxine decreases and, in addition, the thyroid manufactures "reverse T_3," an ineffectively iodinated molecule. It has been speculated, but not proved, that in addition there is a direct central contribution to the bradycardia specific to anorexia nervosa. Hypotension usually is present, although it may not result in symptoms because of its gradual onset.

Malnutrition can affect cardiac function in a variety of ways. Structurally, severe starvation, especially in the presence of vitamin deficiency, may cause atrophy of cardiac muscle. Functional cardiac capacity (e.g., stroke volume) decreases. Ipecac-induced vomiting may be directly toxic to cardiac muscle.

Endocrine Changes

The endocrine changes in anorexia nervosa have been studied extensively and were demonstrated most clearly by Vigersky et al.[3] The most characteristic findings include (1) normal pituitary and peripheral endocrine response to stimulation, suggesting the absence of intrinsic pathology in the endocrine system, (2) increased growth hormone, especially when there is severe carbohydrate restriction, (3) decreased luteinizing hormone and follicle-stimulating hormone production, with step-by-step reversal of the normal stages of pubertal development, and (4) low-normal thyroxine levels, with the increased production of reverse T_3. In addition, Frisch[6] has demonstrated that diminished peripheral lipids play a role in reducing estrogen metabolism. She noted with statistical precision the relationship between weight and onset or restoration of menses for a given height (Fig. 26-1).

The clinical responses to these changes in endocrine function include amenorrhea, return to prepubertal body physique, and decrease in sex drive. The presence of lanugo hair, a fine downy hair characteristic of newborns, is frequently noted, but its significance is not known.

Gastrointestinal Function and Anemia

Intestinal function, especially motility, is reduced. Enzymes needed for the metabolism of lipids and lactose appear to be decreased. The subject frequently is constipated and complains of nonspecific gastrointestinal distress.

Patients with decreased intake of iron and vitamins may be anemic. There is no apparent decrease in the ability to combat viral infections, but there is some increase in susceptibility to less virulent organisms such as fungi.

Other Physiologic and Neurologic Symptoms

Many nonspecific systemic symptoms occur in anorexia—including weakness, fatigue, and loss of interest, especially when weight loss is severe. Most of these effects are due to starvation itself; and the question of whether there are specific physiologic changes unique to anorexia nervosa has not been settled. For a woman of average height, it appears that starvation symptoms become especially prominent at a weight below 90 pounds but may occur at higher weights when starvation is rapid or her pre-illness weight was in the obese range.

In addition to the direct effects of starvation, there are many secondary effects. These often are correlated with the method chosen to induce weight loss. For example, patients who vomit or use diuretics manifest hypokalemic alkalosis and sometimes fatal arrhythmias. Laxative or diuretic abuse may produce electrolyte disturbances as well. There is no evidence for a nearly 10% decrease in brain size as demonstrated by CT scan. Subjectively patients complain that mental concentration is diminished severely.

CLINICAL CHARACTERISTICS

The typical patient with anorexia nervosa is an adolescent girl who has begun dieting as a result of being slightly overweight, usually 5 to 15 pounds above the desired weight. She may diet because of criticism from friends or family

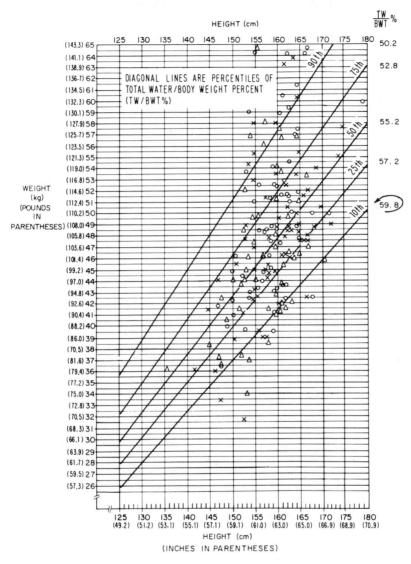

Figure 26-1 The minimum weight necessary for a particular height for onset of menstrual cycles is indicated by the 10th percentile diagonal line of total water/body weight percent *(59.8)* as it crosses the vertical height lines. Height growth of girls must be completed or approaching completion. For example, a 15-year-old girl whose completed height is 160 cm (63 in) should weigh at least 41.4 kg (91 lb) before menstrual cycles could be expected to start. Symbols are the height and weight at menarche of each of the 181 girls in the Berkeley Guidance Study (○); Child Research Council Study (×), and Harvard School of Public Health Study (△).

or because of her perception of being over her ideal weight. Whereas most individuals who diet plan to reach a chosen weight goal, patients with anorexia continue to lose. They often set their target weight lower and lower, reporting a sense of pleasure at each weighing when additional pounds are lost. They frequently develop perceptual distortions characterized by an inability to recognize their body's nutritional needs and by an overestimation of their bodily size. It is not uncommon for patients at 70 pounds to report that they still feel "a little bit hippy" or "still a little overweight."

Psychologic Profile

It is not possible in advance to distinguish exactly which individuals will proceed to set lower and lower weight goals, but there are a number of correlations to suggest that some groups in the population are especially predisposed to the syndrome. The premorbid personality of a patient in whom anorexia nervosa develops is frequently that of a perfectionist, self-critical, obsessional individual who is not psychologically insightful. Patients at times have been characterized as being the "perfect little girl" of the family, especially in terms of behavioral compliance. They are intellectually bright, sometimes in the 110 to 125 IQ range, but usually not exceptionally gifted. They excel at school especially before college-level work. In high school, they are frequently in the top quarter of their class. They complete homework assignments with great detail but are often lacking in creativity or abstract reasoning.

As weight is lost, their personality undergoes changes. They become more apathetic and anhedonic, unable to experience or express pleasure. They frequently become depressed and moody, at times being irritable, at other times seclusive. Anorectics frequently stop associating with friends and become more and more isolated.

Psychopathologically, anorexia nervosa does not fit any other category of psychiatric disease. It has been linked with obsessional disorders, depressive illness, or schizophrenia, but it is not a variant of any of these. When it recurs, it presents a clinical picture like its initial manifestation and does not transmute into other disorders. It is statistically correlated, however, with an increased incidence of affective disorder in the fathers of these patients.[7]

The anorectic individual frequently is a member of a family that is under stress from chronic marital disagreements, separation, or moves from one geographic location to another. Many, but not all, parents appear to have difficulty exercising appropriate parenting skills, especially in dealing with emotional expression and in striking an appropriate balance between support and responsibility.

Eating Behavior

Profound changes occur in eating behaviors. Most individuals restrict their food intake further and further, especially of high-calorie items. Food may be chopped into fine pieces and may be made unattractive with excessive condiments or unusual combinations. Some individuals go on binges, suggesting that hunger breaks through their fear of fatness and their pursuit of extreme thinness. They often begin to take meals by themselves.

A perplexing aspect of the syndrome is the tendency of these starved individuals to become more and more immersed in food preparation and insistent that individuals around them eat high-calorie foods. Patients report preoccupation with issues of food and weight, often to the exclusion of most other thoughts. Calories are counted with great precision.

Bulimia nervosa, a variant of anorexia nervosa, is characterized by episodes of overeating and vomiting in addition to weight loss.[8,9] These patients are usually somewhat older, are sometimes self-dramatizing rather than obsessional, may be married rather than single, and may have had the syndrome of overeating and vomiting with only moderate weight loss for a long time before bringing it to medical attention. Although patients who starve themselves often consider their symptoms a source of pride, individuals who binge and vomit invariably find their symptoms ego-dystonic. A small percentage of patients attempt suicide, suggesting the need for careful attention to the presence of depressive symptoms or despair.

Body Image Distortion

A peculiar feature of anorexia nervosa is the frequent presence of body image distortion.[10] The usual distortion is overestimation of body size despite intellectual awareness of starvation. A number of methods have been devised to test this symptom. Slade and Russell[11] used a set of pinpoints of light that could be moved apart in a darkened room until the patient indicated that the width of her face, shoulders, waist, and hips had been reached. Garfinkel and his group[12] used distortion lenses that allowed patients to identify their perceived sizes. Patients with anorexia may overestimate their size by 20% to 80%.

The origin of this symptom is not clear. It is not a delusion, because patients recognize that medically they are thin, although they *feel* overweight. This has been a source of confusion in the past, when the symptom was called psychotic. On Draw-A-Person-Testing, anorectic individuals portray themselves as larger than they actually are; but when asked to draw themselves as their doctors see them, they usually respond with a very thin image.

There is a practical significance to such perceptual distortion, for it drives weight lower and lower. Its presence *after* nutritional rehabilitation suggests an uncertain prognosis. It is extremely difficult for these individuals to perceive themselves as overweight and then continue to eat large prescribed meals. A measure of the strength of this perceptual distortion is the fact that it overrides admonitions, threats by family, and severe medical warnings about the dire consequences of starvation.

Several means have been considered for correcting these perceptual distortions, none of them wholly satisfactory. In general, the more normal a patient's personality is and the lower the perceptual distortion after nutritional rehabilitation, the better is the outlook. Attempts at confrontation have produced differing results. Some individuals who see themselves on videotape perceive their thinness and are shocked.[13] Others think they look normal. Some become demoralized and even suicidal. Confrontation is not recommended as a standard method of dealing with perceptual distortion. In general, indirect treatment to improve psychopathologic features and practice in choosing against the perceptual distortion are helpful. Cognitive-behavioral techniques have proved to be especially useful in dealing with irrational beliefs about body size.

Societal Factors

In addition to psychologic and behavioral factors, there is the general emphasis of our society on slimness as a model of the healthy and attractive person. In individuals without a confident sense of self-esteem, this comparison with unhealthily thin role models leads to imitation and weight loss. There is a demonstrated trend that, as the social class level rises, there is a decrease in average weight.[14]

As men become increasingly vulnerable to society's emphasis on slimness, and as jogging and other forms of exercise become more widespread, more men are demonstrating features of anorexia. They dip below critical body weights, which make them more vulnerable to the self-sustaining aspects of anorectic symptomatology. In contrast to women, who usually *feel* fat before dieting, more than half of the men in our experience in whom eating disorders developed were actually overweight before dieting, usually 25% to 35% above normal.

Clinical Presentation and Outcome

Anorexia nervosa presents to medical specialists in many forms. A gynecologist often is consulted because of the amenorrhea. Internists specializing in gastrointestinal disease or endocrinology may be consulted because of the similarities to thyroid disease or malabsorption. Neurologists often are consulted because of the possibility of hypothalamic tumor. Therefore health specialists should consider this disorder when examining young patients with weight loss and should include a mental status examination.

There are many patients who do not fit all aspects of the usual picture of the anorectic patient presented here. Anorexia nervosa may well be a final common state of heterogeneous disorders. Some individuals will have stronger biologic contributions whereas in others the psychodynamic or family issues may be predominant. At the present time clinicians should aim to understand the multiple factors that can cause this syndrome rather than rely on a single etiologic concept. This is especially important because conclusions about the origin of the disorder influence the kinds of treatment chosen.

The natural history of anorexia suggests a wide variety of possible outcomes. There are probably many individuals who have relatively brief and moderate weight loss with spontaneous recovery. Others sustain more substantial loss with only partial improvement. A smaller but significant percentage remains severely ill, with multiple hospitalizations; and finally, about 2%

to 5% die as a result of the disorder. These statistics are being improved as treatment methods become more sophisticated. (Older longer-term studies of outcome of chronically ill anorectics noted up to 19% mortality compared to controls over a 30-year follow-up.) When death occurs, it usually is the result of either starvation-related symptoms or suicide, both contributing about equally.

TREATMENT METHODS

There has been increasing agreement during the past decade that both nutritional rehabilitation and psychotherapy are essential for effective treatment.[15] The former practice of employing psychotherapy alone in the hope that weight would increase as conflicts resolved has not been proved effective. However, nutritional rehabilitation alone, especially behavioral therapy, results in no change in underlying psychopathology. Patients in behavioral therapy programs have a tendency to "eat their way out of the hospital." This then may lead to improvement in some patients but often results in individuals who remain in conflict and sometimes adopt the bingeing and vomiting sequence.

In any therapeutic approach it is absolutely essential not to assign blame to either the patient or the family. Frequently both have been told by various treatment facilities that one or the other is responsible for the disorder. It has not been confirmed that anorexia nervosa is the outcome of particular family practice. Attempting to attribute blame is a demoralizing and counterproductive technique.

In treating the anorectic patient a major decision must be made between hospitalization and outpatient management. In general, hospitalization is suggested when weight loss is severe, when outpatient treatment has not succeeded, when there are serious metabolic abnormalities such as hypokalemic alkalosis, when the patient is very depressed, and when the family is in crisis.

Inpatient Treatment

Inpatient rehabilitation is accomplished best in a very structured setting with 24-hour-a-day one-to-one nursing supervision. Patients require this supervision both because they tend to avoid eating or to eat inappropriately and because they are depressed and anxious. A team approach involving nutritionist, physician, psychologist, nursing staff, and social worker appears to produce the best results. The recommended sequence of treatment consists of (1) nutritional rehabilitation, (2) psychotherapy, (3) maintenance period, (4) follow-up.[16]

Nutritional rehabilitation. The dietitian or nutritionist is essential in all phases of treatment. The nutrition professional evaluates the patient's eating pattern and intake before hospitalization to identify the most probable nutritional and vitamin deficiencies. Diets for inpatients are structured with the advice of the nutritional expert, who understands that the individual has a variety of needs. The desire for rapid return to normal weight must be balanced by an appreciation of the medical symptoms that occur during rehabilitation. The most common complaints are those of nonspecific gastrointestinal distress and peripheral edema. Most gastrointestinal distress is mild and nonspecific and may be treated with encouragement, stool softeners, and at times a slightly reduced caloric intake. Patients who are extremely starved often do well by beginning with 1400 to 1600 kcal/day and by avoiding fats, dairy products, and concentrated sweets. This regimen may be increased gradually within several weeks to 3500 to 4000 kcal/day until a preselected weight range is reached.

The peripheral edema that accompanies refeeding is treated most effectively by decreasing salt intake, by encouraging elevation of the feet several times during the day, by using surgical hose when necessary, and at times by slowing the process of nutritional rehabilitation. A more serious complication is the occasional presence of gastric dilatation, a potentially life-threatening disorder that requires specialized medical techniques.

Nutritional rehabilitation should be predicated on an understanding of the patient's complex nutritional needs and on responding to them appropriately. It is possible to treat individuals promptly with adequate nutrition without resorting to tubes or parenteral hyperalimentation. Medication is seldom necessary and, when required, usually can be limited to small amounts of antianxiety agents. Occasionally, where depressive symptoms are severe and persist even after nutritional rehabilitation, an antidepressant may be helpful.

Psychotherapy. In the past, psychoanalytic

psychiatry has suggested the presence of a specific psychodynamic theme in all anorectic patients; present practice, however, suggests that psychotherapy should be individualized. The most common themes are fear of loss of control, an inner sense of lack of effectiveness, lack of individuation from the family, and fear of sexual development. Group therapy often is helpful in allowing patients to incorporate social feedback from others into their own perceptions. It is important that the family participate both in understanding the disorder and in identifying and treating aspects of family distress and ineffective functioning.

A major aspect of psychotherapy involves helping individuals identify their inner emotional states and deal directly with them rather than indirectly through the use of food. In anorectic patients, food becomes both the coinage of the limited pleasure they allow themselves and the means of treating dysphoric states. As anorectics become able to identify and deal more appropriately with inner emotions, they often become less centered about food.

Maintenance and follow-up. Once patients have returned to more optimum body weights and have accomplished what is possible in individual, group, and family therapy, the responsibility for choosing food and exercise should be returned to them gradually with professional encouragement and guidance.

Before patients are discharged, it is essential that they understand adequate nutrition and be able to choose foods appropriately, with emphasis on a balanced proportion of food groups rather than specific numbers of calories. It is helpful to have the patient practice eating at buffets and in fast food chains, since these are realities with which she will have to cope after discharge. A gradual reintroduction of responsibilities with close nursing and nutritional supervision is essential before discharge.

It is helpful to establish a weight range rather than a single weight goal for patients. This allows them to learn to negotiate within boundaries rather than always to be centering and hovering about a specific point. We often choose from Dr. Rose Frisch's charts the 25th or 50th percentile for weight plus or minus 3 pounds (Fig. 26-2). This range will permit the return of menstrual periods as the weight goal is achieved.[17] Most patients will not accept a weight goal greater than the 50th percentile, because they consider it excessive.

A small number of patients appear to recover completely from anorexia. A much larger proportion, perhaps 50%, improve substantially but are vulnerable to return of their symptoms at times of stress. If treatment is successful, however, they will be able to identify a return of fear of fatness and the pursuit of slimness as symptoms of a stress that needs to be identified and dealt with directly rather than indirectly. They learn both to distance themselves from their immediate urge to diet or occasionally binge or purge and to respond appropriately to the identified cause. About 25% or 30% of patients remain chronically ill with frequent hospitalizations. It is helpful for patients after discharge to have emergency coping plans when stressed beyond their capacity. Often eating remains a difficult chore for them after treatment but, with more and more practice and with development of normal personality and successful navigation of developmental tasks, their general eating behavior becomes more appropriate. The goals for treatment are summarized below.

1. Normal weight (25th to 50th percentile for height, ± 3 lb)*
2. Normal eating behavior
3. Psychologic and social maturity, including:
   (a) Understanding own temperament
   (b) Willingness to accept maturation and to take responsibility for own behaviors
   (c) Social skills appropriate to age
   (d) Assertive skills
4. No preoccupation with food or weight issues
5. Normal menses if female; normal sexual drive in males and females
6. Return to work or school with effective functioning
7. Satisfactory working relationships
8. Adequate self-esteem

Office and Outpatient Treatment

Outpatient treatment for anorexia nervosa sometimes is possible, especially where weight loss is mild, the individual's personality is not markedly abnormal, and the family is supportive and not extremely stressed. Some helpful techniques in outpatient treatment are as follows:

---

*See Fig. 26-1 for weight chart.

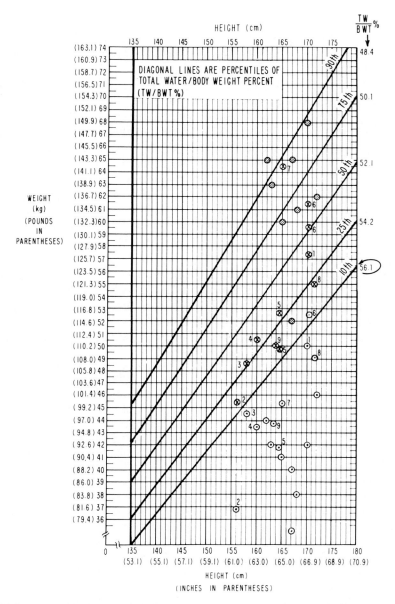

Figure 26-2 The minimum weight necessary for a particular height for restoration of menstrual cycles is indicated by the 10th percentile diagonal line of total water/body weight percent *(56.1)* as it crosses the vertical height line. For example, a 20-year-old woman whose height is 160 cm (63 in) should weigh at least 46.3 kg (102 lb) before menstrual cycles could be expected to resume. Symbols are as follows: ⊙, weights while amenorrheic of patients of one of us (J.W.M.); ⊗, their weights at resumption of regular cycles; ⊘, the weights before occurrence of amenorrhea of subjects; ⊙, their weights while amenorrheic. When two weights are given for a patient, the lower weight is at the first resumed cycle.

1. The patient is requested to keep accurate records of what, where, and when she eats and her emotional response, as well as significant events. Records can be kept on 3×5 cards. These enable the therapist to rely on data rather than memory in evaluating treatment.

2. A collaborative relationship must be established between providers and the patient in which both feel that they have something to gain by treatment. Often patients do not wish a change in weight but may want to feel less depressed, increase their self-esteem, or become more effective in their social relationships.

3. It is important to emphasize simultaneously nutritional rehabilitation and the more general issues that have been mentioned.

The exact method of psychotherapy chosen to supplement nutritional rehabilitation will vary with the therapist's training and with the patient's needs. Some individuals are able to undergo insight-oriented psychotherapy while others may need more supportive and problem-oriented psychotherapy. It is essential to have a firm idea of the lowest acceptable weight for the patient to achieve and not to allow negotiation or manipulation to lead to lower and lower weights in the hope that the situation will improve in the future.

PREVENTION

There is no demonstrated way to prevent anorexia nervosa, but there are a number of plausible possibilities that may be useful. One of the most helpful changes in the last 10 years has been the widespread dissemination of information about the signs and symptoms of anorexia nervosa through the mass media. This has resulted in earlier identification of the disorder by families and affected individuals and has led to earlier treatment.

To change society's emphasis on extreme slimness is difficult in view of the lack of awareness of its origins. There appears to be a dialectic between upper and lower classes regarding a variety of parameters. The early nineteenth-century Dickensian picture of a thin impoverished lower class and a plump well-to-do upper class has now been replaced by a heavier lower class and a slim upper class. This trend can be appreciated in developing countries, where increased socioeconomic status still is associated with increased weight.

Teaching appropriate nutrition and giving facts about anorexia nervosa in grade schools and junior high schools may help prevent some cases. A more practical approach might be to emphasize early identification and treatment. Parents, teachers, and others should be responsive to teenage girls and boys who go on diets that continue beyond reasonable goals and result in preoccupation with food and weight. When extreme slimness becomes manifest and perceptual distortion, amenorrhea, bingeing, and vomiting are present, early intervention is warranted.

The most vulnerable individual usually is an adolescent girl who comes from an upper-middle-class home. The family usually is in crisis and the adolescent has a history of being an ideal child. The diet takes place because of a 5-to-15-pound excess and proceeds to lower and lower limits. The individual affected is intelligent but not gifted or psychologically insightful and often is self-critical and obsessional in style.

The likelihood of developing anorexia nervosa is greatly decreased in individuals who are impulsive, rank below average in intelligence, come from a lower-class background, or are capable of experiencing pleasure freely.

REFERENCES

1. Russell GFM: Modern trends in psychological medicine, vol 2, JH Price, editor, London, 1970, Butterworth & Co (Publishers) Ltd, p 131.
2. American Psychiatric Association: Diagnostic and statistical manual of mental disorders, ed 3, Washington DC, 1980, The Association.
3. Vigersky RA, et al: Anorexia nervosa: behavioral and hypothalamic aspects, Clin Endocrinol Metab **5:**517-535, 1976.
4. Andersen AE: Atypical anorexia nervosa. In Vigersky R, editor: Anorexia nervosa, New York, 1977, Raven Press, pp 11-19.
5. Mecklenburg RS, et al: Hypothalamic dysfunction in patients with anorexia nervosa, Medicine **53:**147-159, 1974.
6. Frisch RE: Food intake, fatness, and reproductive ability. In Vigersky R, editor: Anorexia nervosa, New York, 1977, Raven Press, pp 149-162.
7. Cantwell DP, et al: Anorexia nervosa, Arch Gen Psychiatry **34:**1087-1093, 1977.
8. Russell GFM: Bulimia nervosa: an ominous variant of anorexia nervosa, Psychol Med **9:**429-448, 1979.
9. Casper RC, et al: Bulimia, Arch Gen Psychiatry **37:**1030-1035, 1980.
10. Bruch H: Eating disorders, New York, 1973, Basic Books Inc, pp 87-105.

11. Slade PD, Russell GFM: Awareness of body dimensions in anorexia nervosa: cross-sectional and longitudinal studies, Psychol Med **3**:188-199, 1973.

12. Garfinkel PE, et al: The stability of perceptual disturbances in anorexia nervosa, Psychol Med **9**:703-708, 1979.

13. Metzner RJ: Videotape: Body confrontation in anorexia nervosa. Abstract in Syllabus and scientific proceedings, 133rd Annual Meeting of the American Psychiatric Association, 1980, pp 118-119.

14. Goldblatt PB, et al: Social factors in obesity, JAMA **192**:1039-1044, 1965.

15. Andersen AE: Comprehensive practical treatment of anorexia nervosa and bulimia, Baltimore, 1985, Johns Hopkins University Press.

16. Andersen AE, Margolis S: Eating disorders: obesity and anorexia nervosa. In Harvey AM, et al, editors: The principles and practice of medicine, New York, 1980, Appleton-Century-Crofts, pp 824-834.

17. Frisch RE, McArthur JW: Menstrual cycles: fatness as a determinant of minimum weight for height necessary for their maintenance or onset, Science **185**:949-952, 1974.

CHAPTER 27

Psychiatric Disorders

Alan J. Gelenberg

Nutrition and psychiatry. The juxtaposition of these two words evokes images of cultists and food faddists, richer in dogma than in data. Yet direct links between what we eat and what we perceive, feel, and think are nothing new. Examples abound. Both before and after birth, the developing nervous system requires abundant supplies of protein and calories. Toxins such as heavy metals, which may be included in the diet, can cause damage within the nervous system, particularly in the immature brain. Selective diets also can be used to treat non-nutritional diseases. Elimination diets are prescribed for patients with inborn errors of metabolism: phenylalanine is deleted from the diet of patients with phenylketonuria (PKU), phytols from patients with Refsum's disease, copper from patients with Wilson's disease. For less obvious reasons, children with epilepsy often benefit from a ketogenic diet as an adjunct to anticonvulsant drug therapy.

Too little and too much of various dietary substances can affect behavior in healthy individuals. Dietary deficiencies of specific vitamins and minerals may lead to neuropsychiatric syndromes. Dietary excesses of alcohol, caffeine, and some vitamins also may impair central nervous system functioning.

Another area where diet is relevant to psychiatric practice concerns potential interactions with psychotropic medications. Patients receiving lithium carbonate therapy require a fairly constant sodium intake to maintain a stable serum lithium concentration and to avoid potential toxicity. Patients who take monoamine oxidase inhibitor (MAOI) antidepressants must avoid foods and beverages rich in tyramine and other pressor amines to reduce the risk of a hypertensive crisis. Patients receiving a number of different psychoactive drugs often note an increase in appetite and must curb their intake to avoid weight gain.

The goal of this chapter is to bring these issues to the attention of clinicians. In addition, a final section will present a look to the future, based on research in the present. This will involve the use of dietary precursors of brain neurotransmitters—precursors such as choline, tyrosine, and tryptophan—as substances with potential use in the treatment of nonnutritional neuropsychiatric disorders.

DEFICIENCIES

Deficient diets can result from social disturbances such as war, famine, poverty, or human cruelty. Deficiencies also may reflect psychiatric disturbances, including alcoholism, anorexia nervosa, psychosis, and severe personality disturbances. Unorthodox living patterns might cause the selection of diets that do not meet all of the nutritional requirements for good health. When diet suffers, mental functioning and behavior also may suffer. This section will examine dietary defects that can lead to psychiatric changes, focusing primarily on adults. It is obvious that gross starvation, i.e., protein-energy malnutrition, will lead to disturbances in cognition, sensorium, and psychomotor functioning, but only more selective deficiencies will be considered here. The scientifically unproved "orthomolecular" theories, which claim that certain psychiatric disturbances such as schizophrenia reflect localized cerebral deficiencies in specific nutrients, will be addressed briefly later.

Water-Soluble Vitamins

Vitamins are substances essential for normal metabolic functioning that are not synthesized within the body and hence must be ingested from outside sources. The B vitamin complex and vitamin C are water-soluble, which means the body does not build up large stores in fatty tissues; therefore, regular and constant intake of these substances must be assured for normal functioning.

Thiamine (vitamin B_1). Thiamine plays several important roles in nervous system metabolism. Thiamine deficiency can lead to peripheral neuropathy, beriberi, subacute necrotizing encephalomyelopathy (Leigh's encephalopathy), or the Wernicke-Korsakoff syndrome. The last, not uncommon among alcoholics, is characterized by confusion, ataxia, and ophthalmoplegia in the acute phase (Wernicke's encephalopathy), and by a striking inability to learn new information in the chronic phase (Korsakoff's psychosis). It has been claimed[1] that many American teenagers who are devotees of "junk foods"—high in calories, but lacking in nutritional value—may suffer from thiamine deficiency.

Riboflavin (vitamin B₂). Riboflavin appears important for the development of the fetal brain, but its role in the adult brain is less clear. Isolated riboflavin deficiency in humans is uncommon.

Niacin (vitamin B₃). A deficiency of nicotinic acid—niacin, vitamin B₃—can lead to pellagra, observed in underdeveloped areas of the world, as well as among alcoholics and those who choose eccentric diets. Psychiatric symptoms in pellagra are varied and nonspecific, including apathy and depression, emotional lability and irritability, anxiety, and memory deficits.

Pyridoxine (vitamin B₆). The synthesis of a number of important brain neurotransmitters is dependent on pyridoxine, vitamine B₆. Brain damage and mental retardation can result from B₆ deficiency in infants. Isolated pyridoxine deficiency in adults is unusual. However, patients treated with the antituberculous drug isoniazid can develop B₆ deficiency, leading to excessive somnolence and other neurologic symptoms, as well as to mood changes and even psychosis. It is possible that oral contraceptive medication can lead to B₆ deficiency, and it has been hypothesized that this may cause depression in many women using these contraceptives. There are no naturally occurring human deficiency diseases associated with pantothenic acid or biotin, other B vitamins, but experimental deprivation of both substances has resulted in personality changes and depression.

Cyanocobalamin (vitamin B₁₂). Deficiency of vitamin B₁₂ is well known as the cause of psychiatric symptoms. Nonspecific mental disturbances, such as irritability, memory defects, labile mood, depression, and psychosis, may appear prior to sensory changes or to development of the characteristic megaloblastic anemia.

Therefore, some physicians have suggested that all psychiatric inpatients be screened with serum B₁₂ assays. A similarly wide spectrum of psychiatric symptoms, including psychosis, delirium, and dementia, can occur with deficiencies of folic acid, observed among the elderly or the chronically institutionalized, as well as in patients taking drugs that lower folate levels (e.g., phenytoin, oral contraceptives, or antifolates used as antitumor drugs). As with vitamin B₁₂, serum folate levels are often low among psychiatric inpatients.

Ascorbic acid (vitamin C). Ascorbic acid must be ingested daily, for it is not widely stored in the body. The total body pool has been variously estimated at about 1.5 g. A prolonged deficiency can lead to gingivitis and ultimately to scurvy. Associated mental symptoms may include hypochondriasis and depression.

Fat-Soluble Vitamins

Deficiencies of the fat-soluble vitamins (A, D, E, and K) result from prolonged dietary deprivation or problems of gastrointestinal absorption. Central nervous system symptoms and signs are not prominent in the associated deficiency syndromes.

Mineral Elements

Plasma levels of calcium must be maintained within a fairly narrow range for normal mental and neurologic functioning. Inadequate intake of calcium and vitamin D can result in hypocalcemia, which may be associated with a plethora of mental changes. A deficiency in magnesium can occur with inadequate diet or chronic alcoholism and also can lead to neuropsychiatric disturbances, including irritability and psychosis. It is possible that the minerals calcium, magnesium, and rubidium may be involved in the pathophysiology of periodic psychoses and mood disorders[2]; if so, dietary factors eventually may be found relevant.

Lithium is a monovalent cation that has found an important role in psychiatric chemotherapy. Although lithium is found in small amounts in the environment, it does not have a known physiological function, nor does there appear to be a lithium-deficiency state.

It is conceivable that, as we understand more about normal and abnormal brain function, the role of minerals will assume greater importance than they appear to at present. For more information on trace metals in the body, see the review of Versieck and Cornelis.[3]

EXCESSES

The chronic and regular consumption of large quantities of ethanol constitutes a dietary excess. Alcohol has direct toxic effects on the nervous system, as it does on other body systems. Alcohol abuse can lead secondarily to dietary deficiencies, particularly in certain B vitamins, through a combination of its diminution of appetite and its draining of funds from an individual's food budget. Alcoholism, of course, has many psychosocial ramifications. A full discussion of these aspects of alcohol abuse is beyond the scope of this chapter.

Other dietary excesses also may lead to psychiatric symptoms. Large doses of water-soluble vitamins are usually innocuous, since any amount in excess of metabolic needs can be eliminated by the kidney. However, one group of clinicians[4] has described a neurotoxic syndrome (ataxia and severe sensory dysfunction) that followed daily megadose consumption of pyridoxine (vitamin B_6).

Fat-soluble vitamins, by contrast, do not have this "safety valve," and hypervitaminosis can occur. Although it does not happen often with natural food stuffs, it occasionally is observed in people who take large quantities of vitamin supplements. Vitamin A intoxication can produce psychiatric effects (irritability, anorexia, headache) and symptoms of increased intracranial pressure (drowsiness, obtundation). This is usually a chronic process, but acute vitamin A poisoning has been reported following the ingestion of polar bear liver. Manifestations of vitamin D toxicity are those associated with hypercalcemia; early neuropsychiatric symptoms include weakness, fatigue, lassitude, and headache. It is unclear whether there are any psychiatric sequelae of excessive intake of vitamins K and E.

Even pure water can be drunk to excess. Occasional patients, usually because of delusions, have extreme psychogenic polydipsia and drink themselves into states of severe hyponatremia, leading to convulsions and death.[5]

Excessive intake of various elements—including normal minerals and trace elements—can produce toxicity: this occasionally happens in people who frequent so-called health food

stores. Furthermore, contaminants such as heavy metals have been found in materials sold in these establishments, with resultant toxic effects.

One of the most common dietary excesses associated with psychiatric symptoms involves caffeine. Approximately 100 mg of caffeine is a pharmacologically active dose. The average daily per capita consumption in the United States is about 200 mg, and this figure is even higher in many European countries. It is estimated[6] that 10% of U.S. citizens consume more than 1000 mg of caffeine/day.[6]

The average cup of coffee or tea contains about 100 mg of caffeine, the actual amount depending on the method of preparation.[7] Many soft drinks, such as colas, Dr. Pepper, and Mountain Dew, also contain caffeine, typically 30-60 mg/360 ml (12 oz). A cup of cocoa contains more than 200 mg of theobromine, another xanthine, but one that is less of a central nervous system stimulant than caffeine (though more of a cardiac stimulant). A variety of over-the-counter medications, sold for the relief of headache, allergy, or cold symptoms, contain caffeine, some 15 to 30 mg/tablet or capsule.

It will come as no surprise to learn that caffeine is a stimulant. Many people drink beverages containing caffeine specifically for the "lift" when starting the day or the "pickup" when fatigued. But many individuals experience untoward effects from caffeine ingestion, and not all are aware of the association between the symptoms and their source.

Acute caffeine intake can lead to jitteriness, agitation, and insomnia. Most individuals develop tolerance to these central nervous system–stimulating effects of caffeine and experience them only when caffeine intake exceeds their normal levels. However, chronic caffeine use also has been associated with more generalized and long-lasting symptoms—anxiety, tension, irritability, insomnia, and even depression.[8] Caffeine is not an antidepressant but may turn the psychomotor retardation of depression into agitation.[9] It also can worsen psychosis, counteracting the effects of antipsychotic drugs. Effects in children are largely similar to those observed in adults.[10]

Caffeine has a half-life of approximately 3 hours. When individuals with moderate to high daily caffeine intake discontinue it, withdrawal symptoms typically begin in 18 to 24 hours.

These may include headache, drowsiness and lethargy, irritability, and mild depression.

In addition to counteracting the effects of sedative, antianxiety, and antipsychotic drugs, caffeine and the beverages in which it is contained also can produce pharmacokinetic interactions with psychotropic drugs. For example, coffee and tea form an insoluble precipitate with a number of antipsychotic compounds, thus potentially diminishing the absorption of these agents.[11] In addition, caffeine can affect the renal clearance of lithium, thereby altering serum lithium concentrations.[12]

Physicians should utilize information on caffeine intake in a clinically prudent manner. Questions and information about caffeine intake should form a standard part of the medical history. When symptoms of emotional distress or insomnia are part of a patient's complaints, the level of caffeine intake should be considered as well as the possible effects of caffeine on existing psychiatric and medical disorders, and potential interactions with prescribed drugs.

DIET AND PSYCHOTROPIC DRUGS

Patients taking two types of psychotropic medications need to pay particular attention to their diets to avoid potential toxicity. Those receiving lithium carbonate must maintain a relatively constant sodium intake, whereas patients taking monoamine oxidase inhibitor (MAOI) antidepressants must avoid foods rich in tyramine and other pressor amines. In addition, many patients taking psychoactive drugs must limit calorie intake if they are to avoid weight gain.

Lithium

Lithium carbonate is a mainstay for the long-term maintenance therapy of patients with bipolar affective disorder (i.e., with alternating states of mania and depression). Lithium also is used to treat acute mania, for maintenance therapy in recurrent depressions, and it has been tried experimentally in other psychiatric conditions.

Lithium is not metabolized but instead is eliminated almost entirely by the kidney. Filtered through the glomerulus, lithium is then largely reabsorbed in proximal tubule, with some additional uptake occurring in the loop of Henle. Reabsorption in the proximal tubule occurs by the same mechanisms responsible for the reabsorption of sodium. If a patient taking lithium

suddenly restricts his intake of sodium, the amount of sodium filtered by the glomerulus will drop, the percentage of sodium reabsorbed will rise, and the amount of lithium reabsorbed also will increase. This will result in an increase in the serum lithium concentration. When lithium salts were used as sodium substitutes for patients on salt-restricted diets, deaths resulted that probably were due to lithium toxicity.

Two common clinical examples of the lithium/sodium interaction follow:

A patient has been taking lithium carbonate for some time at a constant dose that results in a stable and therapeutic serum lithium level. On his own, or upon the advice of a physician, the patient elects to restrict his dietary salt intake. Within a few days he has symptoms and signs of lithium toxicity, resulting from a sharp rise in his serum lithium concentration.

Less ominous, but clinically as troublesome, is the case of a patient whose physician cannot find a stable dose of lithium that will achieve a constant serum concentration. On any given dose of lithium, serum concentrations show wide fluctuations, and it is difficult to achieve a desired level. Unknown to the physician, this patient is varying his sodium intake from day to day.

If renal function is normal, a patient's compliance is good, and blood is drawn for serum lithium assays at the same time each day (approximately 12 hr following the last dose of lithium), then sodium intake will be the next most important variable in achieving a stable lithium concentration. (It is also important to attend to possible effects of other drugs, most notably thiazide diuretics, which also can cause sharp upswings in serum lithium concentrations.) This means that patients taking lithium should maintain a relatively constant daily intake of sodium, and therefore that they should be educated about the sodium content of common foods. A visit to a dietitian or use of tables may be particularly helpful for patient education.

Even patients ingesting a low-sodium diet can take lithium safely, provided their sodium intake is consistent and an appropriate dose and blood level are ascertained. A patient on a salt-restricted diet (e.g., 1 g of Na/da) can be stabilized on a given dose of lithium carbonate. Presumably, he will require less lithium each day to achieve a therapeutic level than if he were taking in more sodium. If a patient with unrestricted sodium intake is to decrease his daily intake, lithium serum levels must be monitored carefully and frequently; probably the daily lithium dose will need to be lowered. Patients should be cautioned not to decrease their salt intake without telling the physician who is prescribing lithium. Similarly, they should be instructed to alert the physician if there is a marked increase in salt excretion. For example, in unusually hot weather, when one may be expected to sweat a great deal, or during a bout of diarrhea, it is prudent to monitor serum lithium concentrations more carefully and to adjust both lithium and sodium intake accordingly.

Patients should be informed about common sources of sodium in their diets. Although the salt shaker is familiar and obvious, many people are unaware that processed foods tend to be particularly high in salt. Canned soups, for example, are high in sodium: an average portion may contain more than 1 g.[12] If a bologna sandwich accompanies the soup, another gram of sodium may be ingested.[13] A peanut butter sandwich, however, has less than half as much sodium. "Fast foods" tend to be very high in sodium chloride: Burger King's Whopper contains 1083 mg of sodium; half of a Pizza Hut Pizza Supreme, 1281 mg; an order of fries, up to 590 mg; and a "shake," as much as 685 mg.[14]

The ingestion of sparkling waters is becoming increasingly popular. The amount of sodium can vary considerably, from 0.38 mg/ounce in Perrier Water to 41.4 mg/ounce in Vichy Water.[15] Similarly, the sodium content of vegetable juices is highly variable: Mott's Apple Juice contains 0.34 mg/ounce; V-8 Vegetable Juice, 109 mg/ounce.[16]

In addition to sodium chloride, sodium bicarbonate and monosodium glutamate must be accounted for. Many medications, as well as foods, also contain sodium. The important point is that it is changes or variability in the amount of sodium consumed that can wreak havoc with serum lithium levels.

Another area where attention to diet can help a patient taking lithium is in the management of polyuria.[17] Defined as a daily urine output in excess of 4 liters, polyuria occurs in a substantial percentage (variably estimated as 20% to 70%) of patients receiving long-term lithium therapy. Although not usually serious, the need to urinate frequently and consequently to replenish fluids by frequent drinking can be a constant annoyance in daily life.

Lithium is believed to impair the kidney's ability to concentrate urine by interfering with the effects of antidiuretic hormone (ADH) on the distal tubule. However, the smallest volume of urine a person can produce in 24 hours is determined not only by the maximum urine concentrating capacity of the kidney (frequently diminished by lithium) but also by the quantity of solutes that the kidney is called on to excrete. If the concentration of urine remains constant, the urine volume will vary directly with the solute load. Thus the amount of urine excreted can be decreased by decreasing the amount of solute excreted, which can be done by reducing the daily intake of salt and/or protein.

Therefore, patients with lithium-related polyuria should be told to eat less sodium and protein. Of course, as noted earlier, if sodium intake is to be diminished in a lithium-treated patient, the plasma lithium concentration must be monitored carefully to see whether the lithium dose should be lowered.

An additional dietary interaction with lithium involves caffeine. Like other xanthines, caffeine appears to enhance the renal excretion of lithium. Introduction of caffeine to the diet of a patient with a stable lithium level can, therefore, depress the plasma lithium concentration. Conversely, when caffeine intake has been abruptly discontinued in some lithium-treated patients,* lithium levels have climbed, resulting in such signs of toxicity as increased tremor. In contradistinction to this pharmacokinetic interaction, lithium and caffeine can act pharmacodynamically to increase the likelihood of a fine and rapid "postural" tremor—more common among the elderly and in those with a familial predisposition.

MAO Inhibitors

Three antidepressants available by prescription in the United States—isocarboxazid (Marplan), phenelzine (Nardil), and tranylcypromine (Parnate)—are irreversible inhibitors of the enzyme monoamine oxidase. The drugs are believed to act by inhibiting brain MAO, which results in increased levels of selected neurotransmitters. On the negative side, inhibition of MAO in the gut, liver, and blood vessels compromises

---

*Jefferson JW: Lithium tremor and caffeine intake: two cases of drinking less and shaking more, J Clin Psychiatry **49**:72-73, 1988.

the body's line of defense against ingested pressor amines, normally degraded by this enzyme. Therefore, when a patient taking an MAOI eats or drinks something rich in tyramine or other pressor substances, a hypertensive crisis may ensue.

This potential of MAO inhibitors to raise blood pressure in the presence of certain foods has been called the "cheese effect," because particularly high levels of tyramine are found in ripened cheeses. Cheddar, Emmenthaler, Boursault, Stilton, and Camembert are very rich in tyramine; Limburger, Romano, blue, brick, Brie, Gruyere, mozarella, parmesan, Swiss, and Roquefort are moderately high. Cottage cheese and cream cheese are generally safe. Another dairy product, yogurt, contains barely detectable quantities of tyramine if made by well-known companies. It must be remembered, however, that dairy products left unrefrigerated for an extended period will begin to ferment, and this will increase the content of pressor amines.[18]

In general, meat and fish tend to develop high tyramine levels when they are left unrefrigerated and begin to ferment. Spoiled pickled herring has particularly high levels, and the tyramine concentration in dried salted herring also may be high. Similarly, caviar can be especially dangerous, as can beef and chicken liver if left unrefrigerated. Any dried or pickled fish or unrefrigerated meat may contain moderate tyramine levels, and fermented sausages—bologna, pepperoni, salami, and summer sausage—often contain very high levels.[18]

Fruits and vegetables develop increased tyramine concentrations as they become overripe. In particular, overripe avocados and canned figs should be avoided. Fava and broad bean pods should be avoided because of their dopamine content, but narrow green beans and lima beans are safe. Yeast extracts, such as Marmite, are very high in tyramine, but baked goods are safe.[19]

Among alcoholic beverages, Chianti wine appears to have the highest tyramine content, but one should be cautious about any red wine or sherry. Tyramine content in beer is variable. Patients also have reported reactions to liqueurs such as Chartreuse and Drambuie. In addition, it would be prudent for patients taking MAOIs to restrict their intake of caffeine, which has hypertensive effects, and of chocolate, which

contains the weak pressor agent phenylethylamine.[18]

I always urge my MAOI-treated patients to be particularly cautious when eating out, as opposed to cooking for themselves. One can never be certain as to the freshness of meat and produce, unless one has been personally involved in its storage. When patients do eat out, I encourage them to avoid soups, sauces, gravies, and dressings—in which tyramine and other hidden pressors might lurk.

As part of my teaching to patients taking MAOIs, I emphasize that cheating on their diet is something like playing Russian roulette. The number of chambers loaded (the risk) corresponds to the amount of pressor ingested, which may vary from episode to episode. For example, how much tyramine one ingests is a product both of the concentration of tyramine in that particular food and of the amount of food ingested. Since this may vary from time to time, the likelihood of a hypertensive crisis also is unpredictable, as is the probability that a given rise in blood pressure will result in a serious event, such as a stroke. Thus, I tell patients not to think that, if they cheat once and "get away with it," they can cheat again with impunity.

WEIGHT GAIN

A number of psychiatric syndromes, including endogenous depression and anorexia nervosa, are associated with weight loss. When patients recover from these maladies, weight typically returns to normal. At times, however, the drugs used to treat emotional disorder can promote excessive weight gain, often beyond an individual's normal or premorbid weight.

Several major classes of psychoactive compounds are associated frequently with unwanted weight gain. These are the antipsychotic drugs (also known as neuroleptics or major tranquilizers, including phenothiazines and related compounds), tricyclic MAO inhibitor antidepressants, and lithium carbonate. Among antipsychotic and antidepressant drugs, the lower-potency more sedating agents are increasingly likely to promote unwanted weight increases. Low-potency antipsychotic drugs include chlorpromazine (Thorazine) and thioridazine (Mellaril); by contrast, drugs such as trifluoperazine (Stelazine), fluphenazine (Prolixin), and haloperidol (Haldol) are more potent, less sedating, and probably less likely to add pounds to a patient. The most sedating tricyclic antidepressants are doxepin (Adapin, Sinequan) and amitriptyline (Elavil); less sedating, and probably less likely to promote weight gain, are desipramine (Norpramin, Pertofrane) and protriptyline (Vivactil).

Excessive weight gain associated with antipsychotic and antidepressant compounds probably results from increased appetite. Some patients who take these drugs describe a particular craving for carbohydrates. The mechanism may be related to the drugs' blockage of the histamine H_1 receptor.[20]

Lithium carbonate is another drug that appears to promote weight gain in some patients. The mechanism of this effect is unclear, but some investigators have pointed to the secondary polydipsia often associated with lithium therapy. If increased thirst is quenched by calorie-laden beverages such as soft drinks, the source of weight gain becomes obvious.[21]

Regardless of the mechanism of drug-induced weight gain, the obvious and most direct therapeutic approach is calorie restriction. Patients should be told about the hazards of increased weight and should receive dietary counseling to assist them in maintaining an appropriate body weight.

PSEUDOSCIENCE

Nutrition has come in for more than its share of irrationalism and fads—and so has psychiatry. It should not be surprising, therefore, that nonscientific practitioners of unfounded therapies have made a home for themselves in the treatment of psychiatric syndromes with the use of diets and nutritional therapies.

Megavitamin therapy, which grew into orthomolecular psychiatry, began with a reasonable and rather straightforward hypothesis: that methylated derivatives of normally occurring neurochemicals could lead to hallucinations and, by analogy, to schizophrenia. Therefore, theorists proposed that niacin could serve as a methyl acceptor to spare endogenous epinephrine from methylation into a psychotogenic compound. From this beginning Pauling subsequently hypothesized that schizophrenia was due to cerebral vitamin deficiencies, and from there a motley crew of orthomolecularists has purveyed countless numbers of vitamins, minerals, and who-

knows-what for the treatment of all manner of behavioral and other medical disturbances. The theories and therapies have been well reviewed by Lipton.[22] Suffice it to say that, despite serious attempts to substantiate the efficacy of such treatments, there is no scientific basis for their use.

Another point of contact between diet and psychiatry came with Feingold's hypothesis about hyperactivity.[23] This theory held that hyperactivity (in the current psychiatric nomenclature known as attention deficit disorder) could be alleviated by a diet lacking in artificial food colorings and flavors, as well as by deleting naturally occurring salicylates. Although there is limited evidence that very high concentrations of some additives might cause transient changes in certain behavioral outcomes in selected subjects, the very elaborate diet recommended by Feingold has been shown to be a powerful placebo (demonstrating the importance of psychosocial factors in this syndrome), but the specific diet itself has been found to be of relatively little effect on the behavioral syndrome.[23]

In the never-ending series of unfounded hypotheses is a recent one about refined sugars causing hyperactive behavior in children. This myth appears to have been debunked by a recent scientific study,[24] but some new data have reopened the controversy.[25] Also unproved are frequent patient-generated expectations that a wide range of psychiatric symptoms, including anxiety and depression, are due to hypoglycemia.

Jarvis[26] has explained the tenacity of food faddism as a universal fear of death, coupled with eternal hopes for means to overcome mortality. He emphasizes the victory of symbolism over substance in many faddist preoccupations. As an example, the assumption that honey is superior to sugar, presumably because it is more "natural," has no basis in fact: there is no fundamental nutritional difference between the two sweeteners; and honey can become contaminated with botulism, may be poisonous because of toxic nectar, and is perhaps more cariogenic. Furthermore, points out Jarvis, food faddism is not innocuous. Fatalities have occurred among devotees of Zen macrobiotics and the Temple Beautiful Diet; in children given remedies from Adele Davis, *Let's Have Healthy Children;* from poisonings by laetrile; and through overdoses and misidentification of herbal therapies. Children of overzealous vegetarians have suffered from malnutrition. And last, although not least, the poor are often misled into purchasing "health foods," which typically cost many times more than standard preparations.[26]

With so much to learn about the link between diet and brain function, it is sad that many patients succumb to quackery and charlatanism. In many cases this is the result of lack of effective medical treatments, in others the result of unsympathetic treatment by reputable practitioners. Physicians and health care professionals must accept the responsibility of educating their patients and the broader public about fact and fiction regarding nutrition, lest science cede the territory to witchcraft.

A LOOK TO THE FUTURE

A possible new role for dietary substances in the treatment of neuropsychiatric disorders has emerged from basic science. By adjusting the amount of orally ingested precursors of selected brain neurotransmitters, the brain levels and activity of these neurotransmitters can be altered. The precursors for which this has been shown and which have attracted the greatest interest to date are choline, tryptophan, and tyrosine.[27]

Feeding animals large quantities of choline can lead to increased plasma choline levels, followed sequentially by increased brain uptake of the neurotransmitter acetylcholine. Phosphatidylcholine, contained in lecithin, is the most common sourse of choline in the diet, and lecithin administration has been shown to produce blood and brain changes similar to those found with choline.

Preliminary work in humans suggested that choline and lecithin administration might be useful for increasing brain acetylcholine activity in neuropsychiatric conditions in which such an increase would be therapeutic. Early reports[28] proposed that choline and lecithin could suppress the abnormal involuntary movements of tardive dyskinesia, a syndrome attributed to long-term use of antipsychotic drugs. Some subsequent double-blind studies,[29] however, have come to negative conclusions, and our own more recent study[30] found a definite (though modest) benefit from lecithin as opposed to placebo.

Another possible role for cholinergic agents has been for the treatment of Alzheimer-type dementia, a common form of cognitive deterioration thought to be associated with specific deficits in acetylcholine-containing neuronal systems. Most work with choline and lecithin alone for these conditions has been unimpressive, although there is hope that, together with other agents (e.g., those that diminish the breakdown of acetylcholine [the cholinesterase inhibitors]), lecithin may be useful.[31] Still another tack has been the possible application of lecithin as an adjunctive treatment for mania; but, again, the future of this therapy has yet to be determined.[32]

Tryptophan, an essential amino acid, is the dietary precursor of the neurotransmitter serotonin. Because of theories linking serotonin deficits to the pathophysiology of depression, tryptophan has been employed—both singly and as an adjunct to antidepressant drugs—for the treatment of depressed patients for about 25 years. However, results from controlled studies remain equivocal and contradictory. At present the role of tryptophan in the treatment of depression must remain tentative at best.[33]

Serotonin has also been linked to the induction and maintenance of normal sleep, and for this reason tryptophan has been administered as a hypnotic. Although results are not yet conclusive, a review of current information[34] suggests that tryptophan might act as a mild physiologic sedative. Serotonin also has been implicated in the genesis and alleviation of pain. For this reason, studies[35] are being conducted of tryptophan as a possible analgesic; and, again, preliminary results are encouraging.

The fact that insulin administration, or the elicitation of endogenous insulin by the administration of carbohydrate, can raise the ratio of tryptophan to other large neutral amino acids (with which it competes for uptake in the brain) in plasma has spawned a theory that people who crave carbohydrates may be seeking a surge of brain serotonin activity. Therefore tryptophan might some day be applicable as a treatment for excessive carbohydrate craving. By analogy, carbohydrates can serve as temporary physiologic sedatives, and meals rich in carbohydrate may be more desirable when one seeks to relax or go to sleep whereas meals more heavily skewed toward protein content would be more appropriate when maximum alertness and concentration are desired. Preliminary data do tend to support this hypothesis.[36]

Another neutral amino acid, tyrosine, is the precursor of the catecholamines dopamine, norepinephrine, and epinephrine. Research is proceeding on the possible application of tyrosine as a treatment for Parkinson's syndrome and hyperprolactinemia, in which its effect of inducing an elevation of cerebral dopamine levels might have salutory results. Similarly, a trial of tyrosine as a possible treatment for depression could be conducted based on theories that depression is related (at least in some patients) to inadequate cerebral activity of norepinephrine.[37] Unfortunately, our data do not support the efficacy of tyrosine in treating depression.

The possibility that dietary substances can affect the concentrations and activity of important brain chemicals is interesting from a theoretical perspective, because it suggests that the brain is much less isolated than hitherto believed and much more responsive to the vicissitudes of diet. From a clinical standpoint, if the positive preliminary results described here are confirmed by carefully designed studies in adequate patient samples, a new avenue of treatment may be opened for the treatment of brain diseases.

Several caveats are in order, however.

First, data supporting a role for any of these neurotransmitter precursors in the treatment of nonnutritional brain disorders range from preliminary to purely speculative. Moreover, even though lecithin, tryptophan, and tyrosine are natural food substances, when used to increase brain neurotransmitter levels they are administered in quantities beyond those normally ingested in the diet, so they cannot automatically be assumed to be without hazard. Therefore much additional testing remains to be done before these compounds can be pronounced safe or effective for the treatment of any neuropsychiatric syndrome.

A second caveat has to do with substances available through so-called health food stores. If substances like lecithin, tryptophan, and tyrosine were drugs, they would not be available to practicing physicians and the public until issues of safety, efficacy, and quality control had been resolved to the satisfaction of the U.S. Food and Drug Administration (FDA). However, according to current classifications, these substances are available for purchase without prescription in health food establishments. The quality, quantity, and purity of such materials are not monitored by the FDA.

Practicing physicians are naturally enthusiastic about promising new developments that may bring therapeutic advances. However, there is also a role for a conservative and skeptical spirit, for the dictum *primum non nocere*. It would be prudent for clinicians to watch and wait until this area has matured and more evidence has become available before prescribing or recommending these substances to their patients.

CONCLUSIONS

Psychiatrists, nonpsychiatric physicians, and other clinicians who treat patients with mental disorders are becoming more aware of nutrition. As a factor in general health or pathology in many conditions affecting thought and feelings, diet is being recognized increasingly as a vital fact of everyday life. With that recognition, health professionals are taking better dietary histories from their patients and teaching more about nutrition in the interest of preventive medicine.

REFERENCES

1. Cohn V: Junk food disease, The Washington Post, April 20, 1980.
2. Carmen JS, et al: Calcium and calcium-regulating hormones in the biphasic periodic psychoses, J Oper Psychiatry **11**:5-17, 1980.
3. Versieck J, Cornelis R: Normal levels of trace elements in human blood plasma or serum, Anal Chim Acta **116**:217-254, 1980.
4. Schaumberg H, et al: Sensory neuropathy from pyridoxine abuse, N Engl J Med **309**:445-448, 1983.
5. Rosenbaum JF, et al: Psychosis and water intoxication, J Clin Psychiatry **40**:287-291, 1979.
6. Garfield E: Should we kick the caffeine habit? Curr Contents, Feb 18, 1980, pp 5-9.
7. Ritchie JM: Central nervous system stimulants: the xanthines. In Goodman LS, Gilman A, editors: Pharmacological basis of therapeutics, ed 5, New York, 1975, Macmillan Publishing Co, pp 367-378.
8. Greden JF, et al: Anxiety and depression associated with caffeinism among psychiatric inpatients, Am J Psychiatry **135**:963-966, 1978.
9. Neil JF, et al: Caffeinism complicating hypersomnic depressive episodes, Compr Psychiatry **19**:377-385, 1978.
10. Elkins R, et al: Acute effects of caffeine in normal prepubertal boys. Read at the 133rd Annual Meeting of the American Psychiatric Association, San Francisco, May 4-6, 1980.
11. Kulhanek F, et al: Precipitation of antipsychotic drugs in interaction with coffee or tea (letter), Lancet **2**:1130, 1979.
12. Gelenberg AJ: Caffeine and caffeinism, MGH Newsl Biol Ther Psychiatry **1**:31-32, 1978.
13. Consumer Reports **45**:147, March 1980.
14. Consumer Reports **45**:471, August 1980.
15. Iannaccone ST, et al: Sodium content of bottled sparkling water (letter), JAMA **244**:436-437, 1980.
16. Consumer Reports **44**:509-512, September 1979.

17. Gelenberg AJ: Lithium-induced polyuria: approaches to management, MGH Newsl Biol Ther Psychiatry **6:**7-19, 1983.

18. Monoamine oxidase inhibitors for depression, Med Lett Drugs Ther **22:**58-60, 1980.

19. Folks DG: Monoamine oxidase inhibitors: reappraisal of dietary considerations, J Clin Psychopharmacol **3:**249-252, 1983.

20. Richelson E: Tricyclic antidepressants and neurotransmitter receptors, Psychiatr Ann **9:**16-32, 1979.

21. Vendsborg PB, et al: Lithium treatment and weight gain, Acta Psychiatr Scand **53:**139-147, 1976.

22. Lipton MA, et al: Vitamins, megavitamin therapy, and the nervous system. In Wurtman RJ, Wurtman JJ, editors: Nutrition and the brain. Vol 3. Disorders of eating and nutrients in treatment of brain diseases, New York, 1979, Raven Press, pp 183-264.

23. Lipton MA, et al: Hyperkinesis and food additives. In Wurtman, RJ, Wurtman JJ, editors: Nutrition and the brain. Vol 4. Toxic effects of food constituents on the brain, New York, 1979, Raven Press, pp 1-26.

24. Rapoport JL: Effects of dietary substances in children, J Psychiatr Res **17:**187-192, 1982-1983.

25. Conners DK: Breakfast and sugar effects on cognition in children. Read at the 139th Annual Meeting of the American Psychiatric Association, Washington DC, May 10-16, 1986.

26. Jarvis WT: Food faddism, cultism, and quackery, Annu Rev Nutr **3:**35-52, 1983.

27. Gelenberg AJ: Use of choline, lecithin, and individual amino acids in psychiatric and neurologic disease. In Beers RF Jr, Bassett EG, editors: Nutritional factors: modulating effects on metabolic processes, New York, 1981, Raven Press, pp 239-254.

28. Gelenberg AJ, et al: Choline and lecithin in the treatment of tardive dyskinesia: Preliminary results from a pilot study, Am J Psychiatry **136:**772-776, 1979.

29. Anderson BG, et al: Lecithin treatment of tardive dyskinesia—a progress report, Psychopharmacol Bull **18:**87-88, 1982.

30. Gelenberg AJ, et al: Psychiatric applications: depression and tardive dyskinesia. Read at the 139th Annual Meeting of the American Psychiatric Association, Washington DC, May 10-16, 1986.

31. Thal ALJ, et al: Oral physostigmine and lecithin improve memory in Alzheimer's disease, Ann Neurol **14:**491-496, 1983.

32. Cohen BM, et al: Lecithin diagnosis of mania: double-blind placebo-controlled trials, Am J Psychiatry **139:**1162-1164, 1982.

33. Gelenberg AJ, et al: Neurotransmitter precursors for the treatment of depression, Psychopharmacol Bull **18:**7-18, 1982.

34. Hartmann E: Effects of L-tryptophan on sleepiness and on sleep, J Psychiatr Res **17:**107-114, 1982-1983.

35. Seltzer S, et al: The effects of dietary tryptophan on chronic maxillofacial pain and experimental pain tolerance, J Psychiatr Res **17:**181-186, 1982-1983.

36. Wurtman JJ, Wurtman RJ: Studies on the appetite for carbohydrates in rats and humans, J Psychiatr Res **17:**213-222, 1982-1983.

37. Gelenberg AJ, et al: Tyrosine for the treatment of depression, J Psychiatr Res **17:**175-180, 1982-1983.

CHAPTER 28

Childhood Diseases

George M. Owen
David M. Paige

LOW BIRTH WEIGHT

Survival of low–birth-weight infants has increased markedly over the past 15 years. Nearly three fourths of babies weighing between 650 and 1000 g at birth now survive in newborn intensive care units of major medical centers. This compares with only about 10% in 1970. More important, whereas 70% of infants weighing between 1000 and 1500 g survived in 1970 there is now a better than 95% survival rate. No doubt, disagreement exists as to the relative levels of sophistication of nutritional management and other aspects of neonatal care (respiratory, environmental), but it is true nevertheless that the increased attention to nutritional concerns and feeding techniques has contributed significantly to improved survival of these infants. An understanding of the increasing chemical maturity of the fetus and its associated shift in the composition of fetal weight gains has assisted in estimating nutritional requirements and improving the general prognosis of fetuses. (See Table 28-1.)

In reviewing some of the controversial theories about the feeding of premature infants 25 years ago. Holt and Snyderman[1] stated, "it was long believed, and still is in some quarters, that only breast milk was a suitable food for these infants." The researchers noted the contradictory policies pertaining to levels of caloric intake and types and quantities of protein, fat, and carbohydrate, as well as levels of minerals and vitamins. Today many neonatologists favor the use of human milk to nourish low–birth-weight infants. Human milk contains macrophages, immunoglobulins, enzymes, lactoferrin, and other components or features that protect the newborn from infection. Some of these protective features are lost if the milk is pasteurized or stored, especially if frozen, for any length of time, but the potential advantages of human milk still outweigh any recognized nutritional disadvantages for low–birth-weight infants, at least in the short term.

Nutritional Requirements

Low–birth-weight infants have limited stores of energy and most nutrients. At the same time they are physiologically disadvantaged with respect to maintaining homeostasis. During the

Table 28-1 Estimates of Body Composition of the Reference Fetus

Gestational Age (wk)	Body Weight (g)	Per 100 g of Body Weight				Per 100 g of Fat-Free Weight							
		Water (g)	Protein (g)	Lipid (g)	Other (g)	Water (g)	Protein (g)	Ca (mg)	P (mg)	Mg (mg)	Na (mM)	K (mM)	Cl (mM)
24	690	88.6	8.8	0.1	2.5	88.6	8.8	621	387	17.8	9.9	4.0	7.0
26	880	86.8	9.2	1.5	2.5	88.1	9.4	611	384	17.5	9.7	4.1	7.0
28	1160	84.6	9.6	3.3	2.4	87.5	10.0	610	385	17.4	9.4	4.2	6.9
30	1480	82.6	10.1	4.9	2.4	86.8	10.6	619	392	17.4	9.2	4.3	6.8
32	1830	80.7	10.6	6.3	2.4	86.1	11.3	640	406	17.8	9.1	4.3	6.6
34	2230	79.0	11.0	7.5	2.5	85.4	11.9	675	428	18.3	8.9	4.4	6.4
36	2690	77.3	11.4	8.7	2.6	84.6	12.5	726	460	19.0	8.8	4.5	6.1
38	3160	75.6	11.8	9.9	2.7	83.9	13.1	795	501	20.0	8.8	4.5	5.9
40	3450	74.0	12.0	11.2	2.8	83.3	13.5	882	551	21.1	8.7	4.6	5.7

Modified from Ziegler EE, et al: Growth **40**:329-341, 1976.

early hours of life, provision of water, energy, and electrolytes is essential. Early feeding of low–birth-weight infants is now an established routine in special-care nurseries. Hypoglycemia and jaundice are lessened in infants fed as early as 2 hours after birth compared to those fed later.[2]

Protein and minerals. Advisable intakes of protein and major minerals (Table 28-2) for infants weighing between 1200 and 1800 g are based primarily on the estimated rates of synthesis for new body tissue and gains in weight of low–birth-weight infants equal to those of fetuses (in utero). Dermal, fecal, and urinary losses are also taken into account. Advisable intakes (per kilogram or per 100 kcal) of protein and major minerals for very low–birth-weight infants (less than 1200 g) are 10% to 15% greater than those for larger (1200-1800 g) infants.

Levels recommended (per 100 kcal) are as follows: zinc, 0.55-1.1 mg; copper, 90-120 μg: manganese, 2-8 μg; iodine, 5 μg; vitamin A, 150-250 IU; vitamin D, 60-120 IU; vitamin E, 0.7 IU; vitamin K, 4-15 μg; thiamine, 40-250 μg; riboflavin, 60-400 μg; niacin, 800-5000 μg; vitamin B_6, 35-250 μg; vitamin B_{12}, 0.15 μg; folic acid, 15-60 μg; pantothenic acid, 100 μg; biotin, 1.5 μg; vitamin C, 8-40 mg. Some investigators believe it is preferable to aim for the higher levels in formulas. Others maintain that it is impossible to assure an adequate intake of trace minerals and vitamins in formulas; they argue for supplementation.

Amino acids. Histidine, tyrosine, cystine, and taurine may be essential for the preterm infant. All formulas designed for preterm infants contain ample quantities of histidine and tyrosine provided a suitable energy intake for the formula is achieved. Although hepatic cystathionase and cystinesulfinic acid decarboxylase activities may be lower in the preterm than in the term infant, available evidence indicates that there are some conversions of methionine to cystine and of cystine to taurine. Therefore amounts of cystine and taurine derived from metabolic precursors plus the amounts ingested will adequately meet the low–birth-weight (LBW) infant's needs.[5]

All special formulas for preterm infants are fortified with taurine to ensure a level comparable to that in human milk. In one study,[6] however, the only demonstrated benefit from adding taurine was an improvement in the absorption of fat, especially saturated fatty acids. The LBW infant's requirements for trace minerals and vitamins have been reviewed in detail,[7] and recommendations have been made for levels in formulas.[8,9]

Vitamins. Advisable intakes of vitamin A, vitamin K, thiamine, riboflavin, niacin, vitamin B_6, vitamin B_{12}, vitamin C, pantothenic acid, and biotin for the low–birth-weight infant are those recommended for full-term infants. Although levels of the water-soluble vitamins in human milk can be significantly affected by maternal intake, the relatively limited ingestion of human milk or formula by a low–birth-weight infant mandates the use of a multivitamin supplement enterally, starting by the third or fourth day. Because of rapid skeletal growth, low–birth-weight infants fed human milk or formula should receive between 400 and 800 IU of vitamin D daily. Those fed formula with corn or soy oil as the major source of calories will have relatively high intakes of polyunsaturated fatty acids and should be supplemented with 25 to 30 IU of alpha-tocopherol daily. Because a substantial proportion of low–birth-weight infants have laboratory evidence of mild folic acid deficiency (low serum folate concentration, hypersegmentation of neutrophils), supplementation to ensure a daily intake of between 50 and 60 μg of folic acid may be prudent.

Feeding Low–Birth-Weight Infants

Infants weighing more than 1500 g at birth without evidence of respiratory distress or other disorders can be started on nipple feedings. An

Table 28-2 Advisable Intakes for Low–Birth-Weight Infants

Nutrient	Intake		
	per kg	per 100 kcal	per da
Protein (g)	3.5	2.7*	5.2
Sodium (mM)	3.0	2.3	4.5
Potassium (mM)	2.3	1.8	3.4
Chloride (mM)	2.5	2.0	3.8
Calcium (mg)	185	140	280
Phosphorus (mg)	123	95	185
Magnesium (mg)	8.5	6.5	13

Modified from Ziegler EE, et al: In Suskind RM, editor: Textbook of pediatric nutrition, New York, 1981, Raven Press, pp 29-39.
*Assuming an intake of 130 kcal/kg/day.

initial serving of 10-15 ml of distilled water may be used to monitor the infant's ability to suck and swallow. Feedings should then be given every 3 hours, starting with 10 to 15 ml of 10% glucose solution for two or three feedings and following with feedings of human milk or equal parts of 10% glucose solution and formula, aiming for a total fluid intake of between 65 and 75 ml/kg the third day. Composition of the formula feeding and the volume of intake are progressively changed over 3 to 4 days to achieve intakes of 140 ml and 110 kcal/kg/day. By the end of the first week, the infant should tolerate full-strength formula (between 67 and 80 kcal/dl). It is helpful to monitor urine osmolality and to maintain a level between 300 and 400 mOsm/liter while progressively decresing the proportion of glucose solution and increasing the proportion of formula, and therefore of protein and minerals in the feedings.

Healthy infants weighing between 1200 and 1500 g at birth may not require parenteral fluids, but many will require tube feeding initially. A nasogastric tube can usually be inserted as soon as the infant's temperature and respiratory rate have stabilized, usually within 3 to 6 hours after birth. After an initial feeding of 3-4 ml of distilled water, an additional two feedings of 4 or 5 ml of 5% glucose solution can be given at 3-hour intervals. The stomach should be aspirated before each subsequent feeding to ensure that gastric contents are not accumulating. As with larger infants, it is appropriate to proceed with feedings of human milk or equal parts of 10% glucose solution and formula and progressively change the composition and volumes of formula feeding to achieve intakes of 110 kcal and 140 ml/kg/day from full-strength formula (67-80 kcal/dl) by the end of the first week.

RECENT DEVELOPMENTS

To meet the nutritional needs of low–birth-weight infants, there have been a number of changes in management over the past decade. Among these have been earlier feedings and greater use of continuous (versus bolus) intragastric and transpyloric feeding techniques. Special premature infant formulas are availble at a higher (80 kcal/dl) as well as the usual (67 kcal/dl) caloric density. All special formulas have higher levels of protein, calcium, phosphorus, and sodium per 100 kcal than do routine formulas for term infants. These premature formulas have a portion of carbohydrate as glucose polymers and a portion of fat as medium-chain triglycerides. Absorption of calcium and magnesium is improved in premature infants fed formulas containing medium-chain triglycerides and correlates well with improved fat absorption.[10]

Levels of protein and major minerals in three such premature infant formulas are shown in Table 28-3.

Neither mature human milk (MHM) nor preterm human milk (PTHM) contains sufficient calcium or phosphorus to meet the premature infant's needs.[12,13] Although PTHM has higher concentrations of protein, sodium, and chloride than does MHM,[11] the levels of these nutrients are frequently insufficient for preterm infants.[7,14]

Fortified PTHM has been used increasingly in

Table 28-3 Protein and Major Minerals (per 100 kcal) in Preterm Human Milk and Formulas

	Preterm Human Milk*	Enfamil Premature	Similac Special Care	Preemie SMA
Protein (g)	2.2	3.0	2.7	2.5
Sodium (mM)	2.0	1.7	1.9	1.7
Potassium (mM)	2.2	2.8	3.2	2.3
Chloride (mM)	2.2	2.4	2.3	1.7
Calcium (mg)	37.8	117	177	93
Phosphorus (mg)	18.4	59	89	49
Magnesium (mg)	4.7	10	12	8.6
Osmolality (mOsm/kg H_2O)	300	300†	300†	270

Modified from Lemons JA, et al: Pediatr Res **16**:113-117, 1982.

*Estimates based on an average of samples obtained from women 7 and 14 days after delivery of preterm infants.

†Osmolality at 80 kcal/dl; the figure is 244 mOsm/kg H_2O at 67 kcal/dl dilution.

the 1980s to feed premature infants. Fortification is accomplished by the addition of special formulas for preterm infants,[15] by the use of a special product containing hydrolyzed protein,[16] and by the use of bovine whey protein with various mineral salts.[17] Available evidence[16-20] indicates that infants fed fortified PTHM, just as those fed premature formulas, achieve a growth rate and body composition similar to those of the fetus and tolerate the additional protein without evidence of metabolic aberrations.

Nutrient compositions of two human milk fortifiers marketed in North America are shown in Table 28-4. Additions of the quantities of for-

tifiers indicated in Table 28-3 will yield feedings with very similar nutrient composition.

Overall, clinical experience with premature infant formulas has been favorable: low–birthweight babies show enhanced rates of growth, shortened stays in newborn intensive care units, and a lower incidence of nutritional rickets; metabolic balance studies indicate retention of nitrogen, calcium, and phosphorus in keeping with fetal accretion rates. These medical and economic benefits have been achieved without jeopardizing the health of the infants. Of perhaps even greater importance than the foregoing, however, is the observation that premature infants fed special preterm formula not only are bigger at age 18 months than their counterparts fed routine formula or PTHM but also score higher on developmental evaluation.[21] Further study is needed to determine whether the use of special preterm formula and fortified human milk in early weeks confers long-term advantages.

GROWTH FAILURE

The need for adequate weight gain and body fat for progression of growth and puberty has long been known.[22] The average growth veloc-

Table 28-4 Human Milk Fortifiers of PTHM for Premature Infants

Component	Enfamil Human Milk Fortifier (per 4 packets)*	Similac Natural Care Human Milk Fortifier (per 50 ml)†
Calories (kcal)	14	41
Protein (g)	0.7	1.1
Fat (g)	Trace	2.2
Carbohydrate (g)	2.7	4.3
Calcium (mg)	60	86
Phosphorus (mg)	33	43
Magnesium (mg)	4	5
Copper (μg)	80	102
Zinc (mg)	0.8	0.6
Sodium (mg)	7	21
Potassium (mg)	15.6	57
Chloride (mg)	17.7	37

*Amount added to 100 ml of PTHM to yield 81 kcal/dl of feeding.
†Amount added to 50 ml of PTHM to yield 81 kcal/dl of feeding.

Table 28-5 Average Growth Velocities in Infants, Children, and Adolescents

Age groups (yr)	Height (cm)	Weight (kg)
Infancy		
0-1	25/yr	6.5/yr
1-2	12/yr	2.5/yr
Childhood		
6-12	6/yr	2.5/yr
Adolescence		
Males	1.5-6/6 mo	7/6 mo
Females	1.7-5/6 mo	6/6 mo

From Motil KJ: Clin Nutr **4**:75-84, 1985.

Table 28-6 Nutritional Causes of Short Stature and/or Poor Growth*

	Number of patients	Percentage
Decreased intake	75	73.5
Nonorganic failure to thrive	(20)	(19.6)
Anorexia nervosa	(36)	(35.3)
Fear of obesity	(15)	(14.7)
Other eating disorders	(4)	(3.9)
Chronic inflammatory bowel disease	21	20.6
Hypozincemia	6	5.9

From Lifshitz F: Clin Nutr **4**:40-47, 1985.
*Data are for 102 patients with poor growth and development and/or short stature from nutritional causes. This was defined as a height below the 3rd percentile and a growth rate of less than 4 cm/year with inadequate weight increments or even weight loss. The 102 patients with nutritional causes were derived from a population of 805 patients referred to our center over the past 10 years because of the complaint of short stature; of these, only 272 were found to have a pathologic cause for short stature, including the 102 patients with nutritional causes. Data in parentheses are subtotals for patients with decreased intakes.

ities of infants, children, and adolescents are presented in Table 28-5.[23]

Clearly, undernutrition is the single most important cause of growth retardation throughout the world. The retarded growth is due to a complex of factors involving the lack of food, or of appropriate nourishment, frequently in combination with infection and chronic disease leading to increased catabolic needs and nutrient losses. Poor growth from other nutritional causes usually involves not the classic problems of poverty-related malnutrition as reviewed in Chapter 20 but rather other factors. The nutritional causes and prevalence of short stature and/or poor growth as reported by Lifshitz[24] are noted in Table 28-6.

FAILURE TO THRIVE

A number of patients are often referred for failure to thrive (FTT). They have decreased growth rates and cessation of body weight increments. After evaluation the diagnosis of non-organic failure to thrive (NOFTT) may be established. These cases have varying etiologies, leading to a decreased dietary intake.

Approximately 2% to 3% of pediatric tertiary hospital admissions are due to FTT.[25] Although there is lack of agreement as to the definition of FTT, most health workers would define it as the condition wherein an infant exhibits poor weight gain without an immediate explanation. The term is most often applied to infants less than 2 years of age. It is not a disease state. It is a descriptive term.

Thus "failure to thrive" has frequently been used indiscriminately. The following definition attempts to achieve greater precision[26]:

a rate of gain in length and/or weight less than the value corresponding to 2 standard deviations below the mean during an interval of at least 56 days for infants less than 5 months of age or during an interval of at least 3 months for older infants.

This definition permits careful categorization of children at risk. It also eliminates the misidentification of a large proportion of children who demonstrate normal shifts in growth at some time during the first year.

Careful history-taking and examination may exclude the obvious causes of growth failure (inadequate dietary intake or malabsorption, excessive loss of nutrients). In the absence of overt

clinical problems, a careful protocol should be developed and followed to determine the causes of an infant's failure to grow.

The diagnosis centers on two main lines of investigation. The clinician should explore whether

1. The available calories in the diet are adequate to meet the energy needs of the infant but the infant is not accepting the food provided or is accepting it but regurgitating. The former group may include infants with central nervous system disorders, endocrine disease, congenital defects, or partial intestinal obstruction; the latter, infants whose formula may have been inappropriately prepared (improper dilution) or who may have been exposed to other poor dietary practices that led to inadequate caloric intake.
2. The infant who is receiving a diet adequate to promote satisfactory growth may be failing to achieve expected rates of growth because of inadequate absorption, excessive fecal loss, or calorie requirements that are unusually high.

When appropriate, a period of hospitalization is recommended to classify infants with failure to thrive. A plan of hospital study is outlined in Fig. 28-1.[26]

Over the years since the description of NOFTT in the 1940s, two divergent hypotheses have been developed regarding its etiology. One suggested that lack of weight gain resulted from decreased caloric intake or endocrine factors related to starvation. The other noted lack of weight gain to be due to psychologic factors mediated through decreased intestinal absorption, decreased utilization of calories, or abnormal endocrine function. This latter hypothesis was based on a belief that nutrition was adequate. Most physicians favor a nutritional role for lack of weight gain in NOFTT despite the fact that relatively few data support this. If lack of weight gain is of nutritional origin, the question remains,[27] why did the infants not receive adequate intake?

Only two studies[24,28] have addressed the possibility of abnormal utilization or metabolism. Krieger and Chen[28] determined the metabolic rate in 16 infants with maternal deprivation or NOFTT and concluded that the intake required for accelerated weight gain was similar to that

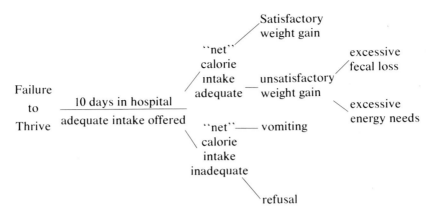

Figure 28-1 Schema for evaluating a hospitalized infant with failure to thrive.

From Fomon SJ: Infant nutrition, Philadelphia, 1974, WB Saunders Co.

in fast-growing normal young infants. Weight gain was linearly related to caloric intake. Neither abnormal metabolism nor malabsorption was demonstrated in NOFTT. Still unexplained, however, is continued lack of weight gain in some hospitalized NOFTT infants on adequate intake.

The only endocrine abnormalities reported in infants with maternal deprivation or NOFTT are elevated cortisol secretion rates and low thyroxine.[29] Although thyroid function and somatomedin are low in severe malnutrition,[30,31] growth hormone is not decreased in infants with maternal deprivation.[32] Confusion about hormonal abnormalities results from grouping NOFTT infants with older children with psychosocial dwarfism in whom decreased growth hormone secretion has been reported.[33] The etiologies of NOFTT and psychosocial dwarfism may be similar, but there are sufficient clinical differences to suggest that the entities not presently be considered a continuum. Endocrine abnormalities are not the primary cause of lack of weight gain in NOFTT.[26]

Mothering

There has been an increasing interest in mother-infant interaction and the reciprocal effect on behavior between the two. Accompanying this interest is a shift in focus concerning the etiology of NOFTT. The emphasis on the underlying cause of NOFTT is now dysfunctional mothering and abnormal mother-infant interaction. Powell[27] further notes that maternal

and social factors in NOFTT are well described but the effects of these factors on the infant are less well defined. No studies have described the mechanism whereby social factors contribute to decreased intake.[34-36] Although Pollitt[37-38] demonstrated a correlation between social factors and decreased caloric intake, he did not show weight gain with increased intake and improved mother-infant interaction.

In the majority of infants decreased intake and dysfunctional interaction may be responsible for the disorder; the question may no longer involve causation but rather treatment aimed at inducing positive social responsiveness. It is necessary to determine whether the infant responds to stimulation or merely receives it. Many infants, especially those with rumination and avoidance of eye contact, are slower in social responsiveness. An infant, once affected by poor environment, may continue to exhibit FFT not only by his contribution to an abnormal interaction but also by not responding to normal types of stimulation.

In most cases an infant with NOFTT is inactive, with little social responsiveness. (1) He or she may not display the usual hunger signals; (2) it may be difficult for the mother to recognize the infant's hunger clues; (3) the mother may simply not take time to feed her infant even when the infant is crying; (4) there may be repeated interruptions of the feeding process; (5) the infant may be a very slow feeder; (6) the mother may not understand the technique or how much caloric intake is needed; (7) she may fail to use feeding times as an opportunity for interaction.

Attentive nursing personnel are often able to identify these problems.[27]

Treatment

The goal of treatment in NOFTT is achieved through a three-part program[27]: treatment of the infant, treatment of the environment, and treatment of the mother-infant interaction.

Infants are generally fed formula alone. This facilitates the calculation of caloric intake. The goal is to have the infant receive 140 kcal/kg/day of the routine formula. It is suggested that caloric intake be based on ideal weight, but such calculations are based on the 50th percentile weight. This is often three to four times the infant's actual weight, resulting in a volume much too large for the infant. If the baby has a milk allergy a soy-based formula or Nutramigen may be fed. Vitamins are given, and if indicated iron. The mother is observed feeding her infant so her feeding techniques can be evaluated and recorded along with her willingness to feed the infant, her recognition of hunger signals, and her nurturing as well as feeding difficulties exhibited by the infant.[27]

Although appetites can vary, most infants have a relatively normal appetite. If 140 kcal/kg/day of formula is not ingested, an increase in caloric density of the formula is required. This is achieved by switching to a commercial preparation with 24 to 27 kcal per ounce. Carbohydrates or lipids, or both, are added to achieve the desired caloric density. In an infant receiving a non–cow's milk formula, ingestion is monitored to assure adequate caloric intake. Vomiting losses are estimated and additional formula is given to compensate for the losses. Infants are monitored daily by weights taken before the first morning feeding, and the appropriate daily weight gain is calculated.[27]

Other treatment of the infant includes identification of the areas of delay. Developmental evaluation is performed immediately after admission, and abnormal behaviors are pinpointed. At the same time, and simultaneously with hospital evaluation of the infant, an environmental evaluation by the social services department should begin. The objective is to identify any family stresses—financial, marital, personal, familial, situational. Support systems are few, and the social services department may aid in decreasing stresses and increasing support systems.[27]

CONSEQUENCES OF FAILURE TO THRIVE

Pollitt[38] has summarized the literature on the consequences of failure to thrive. A group of children who had FTT during infancy were studied approximately 12 years later by Oates et al.[39] and found to be shorter and to weigh less than normal children attending the same schools. The FTT children also scored less well on measures of language, reading, and social maturity and had higher levels of behavioral disturbances. Of interest is the fact that their mothers also had more difficulty with abstract problems and exhibited lower intellectual ability than did the mothers of the control children.

Currently one cannot identify the underlying basis for the cognitive deficits observed in FTT children. They may be the result of a synergism between nutritional insult and emotional deprivation. There are at present no epidemiologic studies on FTT infants and children. Also unknown is the extent to which these patients are those identified simply as "growth retarded" in health and nutritional surveys.

OTHER DISEASES ASSOCIATED WITH GROWTH FAILURE

Long-term nutritional insufficiency in chronic childhood disease states is well recognized. However, unrecognized and untreated conditions also may result in permanent stunting of growth. The diagnostic criteria for growth failure in children are presented in the box.[23]

Chronic Inflammatory Bowel Disease

Chronic inflammatory bowel disease (CIBD) in children may be associated with retardation of linear growth. This occurs in at least 30% of children with the disease, although it has been

---

> **GROWTH FAILURE**
>
> Absolute height more than 2 SD below mean for chronologic age (<5th percentile by National Center for Health Statistics standards)
>
> Linear growth velocity <2 cm/6 mo after 2 yr of age
>
> Bone age more than 2 SD below mean for chronologic age

From Motil KJ: Clin Nutr **4**:75-84, 1985.

reported[40] in up to 85% of patients with Crohn's disease. The growth of these patients may slow down and cease without any other sign or symptom, preceding the gastrointestinal complaints by up to 3 years. Therefore the diagnosis of inflammatory disease of the bowel should always be considered in a child who does not grow adequately even in the absence of gastrointestinal complaints. Lifshitz[24] reports that patients referred to them because of growth abnormalities who were eventually diagnosed as having regional ileitis or ulcerative colitis did not have any gastrointestinal manifestations when first seen.

There are many possible reasons why a child with Crohn's disease may not grow normally. The nutritional causes include impaired absorption of nutrients, decreased nutrient intake, specific nutrient deficiencies, and enhanced protein losses through the gastrointestinal tract.[41] There may also be other causes: growth impairment may be iatrogenic, since steroids often are used in the treatment of these patients; however, growth may improve with steroid therapy, presumably because of suppression of disease activity.

Despite the fact that some children with CIBD have intestinal malabsorption, the majority do not have significant steatorrhea and absorb xylose normally. Thus malabsorption of nutrients does not fully explain poor growth in these patients.[41] A significant problem is anorexia, leading to poor caloric and nutrient intake. Patients may have abdominal pain following meals and prefer to eat frequent small meals or snacks, resulting in a decreased dietary intake and inappropriate caloric balance. Additionally, there may be protein losses through the gastrointestinal tract, leading to hypoalbuminemia. To produce a positive nitrogen balance, up to 1.6 kg/day of protein through intravenous nutrition may be required.[42] These alterations may result in deficiencies of specific vitamins and minerals such as magnesium and zinc, which are essential for normal growth.[43,44] In one study[45] hypozincemia was found in children with poor growth long before any symptoms or other laboratory findings appeared.

Growth retardation in children with CIBD has improved following nutritional rehabilitation. This was done with short-term parenteral nutrition in a hospital setting[46] as well as with long-term home TPN[47]; in both cases height increased and there was marked catch-up growth. We now know that "bowel rest" is not necessary to induce recovery in these patients. Oral feedings of different types may also induce it.[40] Of interest is the fact that with nutritional rehabilitation, not only have the patient's nutritional status and growth improved but a "nutritionally induced remission" of the disease has also been noted.[48] Thus adequate nutrition is needed to control the disease and may allow medications such as sulfasalazine or steroids to exert their therapeutic effect, thereby enabling the patient to assume normal or even catch-up growth. In selected patients resection of a portion of inflamed narrowed intestine may also be necessary for improvement of symptoms. However, surgery is usually not needed for poor growth alone in CIBD patients.[49]

Zinc Deficiency

The zinc deficiency syndrome, first described in Iran and Egypt, has clinical manifestations of dwarfism, hypogonadism, poor hair growth, and roughness of the skin. All these abnormalities are corrected by zinc supplementation.[50] Zinc deficiency has also been found in acrodermatitis enteropathica, a rare autosomal-recessive defect of zinc absorption occurring in infancy. These patients present with severe persistent diarrhea, malnutrition, alopecia, and skin changes of predominantly vesicobullous character localized around the mouth, anus, fingers, and toes, with pustular and eczematoid skin lesions elsewhere.[51] The disorder improves following human milk feeding but is aggravated by cow's milk. The addition of zinc to the diet causes a remission. The mechanism of improved zinc absorption by human milk seems due to the chelation of zinc by some milk components.

The milder manifestations of zinc deficiency associated with growth disorders in childhood are still poorly defined. Ghavani-Maibodi et al.[52] reported favorable results with zinc supplementation in healthy short children. Furthermore, zinc as a supplement to infant formulas has been associated with accelerated weight gain in normal healthy children.[53] However, Lifshitz and Nishi[45] gave oral zinc sulfate to 10 patients with constitutional and familial short stature who had normal serum and urinary zinc levels and found that the supplements over a year had no effect on the growth rate of these patients. Nevertheless, Hambidge et al.[54] described 10 children with a history of poor appetite, decreased taste acuity, short stature, and low hair zinc levels all of whom improved after zinc supplementation. Others[42,55] have not confirmed these observations. At the same time there have been isolated accounts of mineral deficiencies in the etiology of failure to thrive, pica, and various abnormal growth patterns as well as biochemical evidence of insufficient zinc nutrition among preschool low-income children.[56] Thus, although it is possible that zinc deficiency may be found in some patients who do not grow at normal rates,[45,55] in patients with short stature who are growing at normal rates, zinc deficiency is unlikely.

Iron Deficiency

Iron deficiency is the end result of an imbalance between the sum of the patient's iron endowment (including the intake and absorption of this element) and the sum of his iron needs (for growth and replacement of losses) both normal and abnormal. The peak incidence of iron deficiency in childhood is after 6 months of life, with another peak occurring during early adolescence. The daily iron requirements are 0.5 mg in infancy and 2 mg in adolescence; when insufficient iron is ingested or when there are increased losses, iron deficiency may result. The average U.S. diet provides 15-18 mg of iron/day, of which only an average of 10% is absorbed. It is not surprising, therefore, that as many as 10% of normal high school students ingesting various fast food and convenience items have iron-deficiency anemia.

In patients with failure to thrive or poor growth, anemia may be very mild or not present; yet the patient may have iron deficiency, manifesting itself as anorexia and poor growth. Biochemical methods (e.g., serum iron, total iron-binding capacity, ferritin) enable the deficiency to be demonstrated in these patients as well as in the general population with a high degree of reliability.[57] Increased growth and improved appetite may occur after iron replacement.

Iron deficiency interferes with cognitive function and school achievement. Politt[38] specifically reports in his review that infants who are iron-deficient, with or without anemia, obtain lower scores in evaluations of mental development than do iron-replete subjects of the same age. Intramuscular or oral administration of age-appropriate doses of iron for 1-2 weeks to the infants deficient in iron produced significant improvements in the developmental scores as well as increased attention span and cooperativeness.[58-61] Among preschool children, iron deficiency has also been associated with deficits in attention and learning new concepts in problem-solving situations.[62,63] In these cases—as among infants—the deficits in cognition disappeared after controlled and age-appropriate treatment with iron. Iron-deficient schoolchildren also have obtained lower educational achievement test scores than did iron-replete subjects.[64] After iron repletion their achievement scores increased significantly above those of iron-deficient children treated with a placebo.

The biologic reasons for the cognitive deficits observed in the iron-deficient subject are unknown. Iron is an important cofactor in various brain enzymes, and alterations of brain neurochemistry in the presence of iron depletion have been reported. It would appear that some of the iron-dependent enzymes affected by iron deficiency may have systemic consequences, reducing the level of alertness in the organism and thus adversely influencing attention.

Other Mineral Deficiencies

Specific mineral deficiency syndromes have been identified in children with growth failure; they include calcium, phosphorus, magnesium, sodium, potassium, iron, copper, and zinc. It is quite likely that deficiencies of other trace elements necessary for normal growth will be recognized in the future. Trace elements of established importance that have not yet had an impact in clinical practice include manganese, cobalt, molybdenum, selenium, nickel, vanadium, tin, cadmium, silicon, lead, and even arsenic. In some instances considerable information is already available on the biochemistry, physiologic role, and effects of these elemental deficiencies in animals. For example, manganese plays an essential role in mucopolysaccharide synthesis, and its deficiency in young birds causes, among other effects, a variety of skeletal abnormalities with stunted growth.[65] There are data on the effects of selenium deficiency in animals,[66] although only suggestions of possible deficiencies in human infants exist.[16] In the case of other minerals, data are even more limited at present despite the seeming necessity of all these elements to normal growth.

Fear of Obesity

Although malnutrition is a well-recognized cause of poor growth throughout the world, self-imposed malnutrition is becoming a major problem in clinical pediatric practices in developed countries. There has been a proliferation of lay and scientific articles describing poor growth and delayed development among adolescents stemming from various forms of self-imposed restrictions of food intake and fad dieting.[68-70] Pugliese et al.[71] have reported on a group of 14 patients who failed to grow because of malnutrition that was the result of self-imposed restriction of caloric intake arising from a fear of becoming obese. These patients had deteriorating linear growth and failed to attain puberty. The problem was preceded by at least 1-2 years of inadequate weight gain. No organic cause was discovered, but a self-imposed decrease in dietary intake was evident; they ingested only 32% to 91% of the recommended caloric intake for their age, and frequently they skipped meals. Most of their diets were relatively deficient in minerals and vitamin D. Upon investigation, no gross psychiatric disease or anorexia was found. Yet, once the fear of obesity was identified and the patients were given nutritional and psychiatric counseling, they resumed an adequate caloric intake for their age, and recovery occurred (as demonstrated by improved linear growth and sexual development).[71] In one patient, however, there was permanent alteration of height potential because the diagnosis and treatment had been delayed; menarche occurred soon after adequate weight gain was reestablished by appropriate dietary treatment, but the height changed only minimally.[71]

Patients who fear obesity seem to be different from those with other baryphobic syndromes or subclinical anorexia nervosa.[68,70,72] They do not have other features of anorexia (e.g., self-induced vomiting, compulsive exercising, food hoarding, hyperactivity, laxative/diuretic abuse). Nor do they have a distorted body image; they know they are slim and they want to be so!

Pathologic Short Stature

Pathologic short stature accounted for 33% of the short-stature patients referred to the North Shore University Pediatric Endocrine Ambulatory Center. This incidence is high compared to that in the general population[72] but appropriate for a referral center. Pathologic short stature should be suspected in children who do not grow normally (less than 4 cm/yr after age 5) and in those with height below the 3rd percentile. The bone maturation of these patients is usually quite delayed, often even behind that expected for height. The patients with pathologic short stature usually fail to develop normally sexually and the prognosis for ultimate height is dependent on the specific diagnosis. In the North Shore Center the incidence is biased toward nutritional, endocrine, or metabolic disturbances since these are the types of patients referred.[73] Undoubtedly other disturbances known to interfere with growth in children (i.e., renal or cardiac dysfunctions) are preponderant in other respective subspecialty centers.

Metabolic Diseases

Growth failure is usually one of many severe complications arising from a specific underlying primary metabolic disorder. Most of these conditions demonstrate a wide biochemical and clinical spectrum of severity, and the more mildly affected patients often demonstrate only minimum clinical disturbances, one of them being growth failure.

MANAGEMENT OF GROWTH FAILURE

Motil[23] notes that early nutritional intervention is necessary in appropriately managing growth retardation associated with chronic illness. The indications for intervention in nutritionally mediated growth failure are given in the box. Although there is frequently a generalized protein-energy malnutrition, individual nutrient deficiences may also occur, especially in infants and young children, and often there is a complicating progressive growth retardation. Growth failure is multifactorial and can be associated with (1) inadequate dietary intakes, (2) excessive urinary and intestinal losses, (3) abnormal metabolic expenditures, or (4) altered substrate-hormone relationships. Nutritional intervention is indicated in the presence of known chronic

```
┌─────────────────────────────────────────┐
│            WHEN TO INTERVENE              │
│ Height for age <95% of expected          │
│ Weight for height <90% of expected       │
│ Weight for age <90% of expected          │
│ Height velocity <4 cm/yr after 2 yr of age│
│ Weight velocity <15 g/day during first year│
│ Midarm circumference:head circumference  │
│    ratio <0.27                           │
│ Bone age more than 2 yr behind chronologic│
│    age                                    │
│ Anemia                                    │
│ Hypoalbuminemia                           │
└─────────────────────────────────────────┘
```

From Motil KJ: Clin Nutr **4**:75-84, 1985.

illness and failure to demonstrate appropriate linear growth and weight gain during a 6-month to 1-year interval.[23] The prevention of growth retardation can be achieved in chronic disease states by monitoring anthropometric and laboratory indices and when appropriate promptly instituting aggressive enteral or parenteral nutritional rehabilitation. Early aggressive nutritional therapy can reverse the growth arrest associated with chronic diseases of childhood and failure to thrive in infancy.[23]

Reversal of a growth deficiency may be followed by a period of catch-up growth (i.e., supernormal rates of linear and ponderal gains toward the size that would have been attained if the growth lag had not occurred).[75,76] The capacity for catch-up growth after a period of arrest may be limited during early life. For example, infants who are small for gestational age because of maternal alcoholism fail to demonstrate catch-up growth in the postnatal period; by contrast, infants with prenatal growth deficiency that is due to uterine constraint, such as twins, may show postnatal catch-up growth. When the delay is of postnatal onset, there may be dramatic catch-up growth following correction of the deficiency disorder. The accelerated rate of linear growth will continue until the individual's biologic age (bone age) corresponds to his chronologic age. However, total recovery from linear growth arrest may not be accomplished. The extent of recovery will depend on the age of the individual, the etiology, severity, and duration of the growth deficiency, and the type of therapy required to correct the disturbance.[23]

INTELLECTUAL PERFORMANCE AND GROWTH FAILURE

Cognitive and developmental disabilities during the preschool and school-age period have been observed among children born at term with low birth weight. These findings are not, however, uniform in all studies. The developmental risks for infants who have experienced a nutritional insult during the first half of pregnancy are different from those for infants who suffered an insult in the latter half. In both cases, however, the outcomes are probably different from what might have occurred if fetal malnutrition had extended throughout the pregnancy.[37]

A study from Guatemala has indicated that at 3 years of age the cognitive test performance (e.g., discrimination learning, memory, vocabulary) of infants with a ponderal index (weight/$\sqrt[3]{\text{length}} \times 100$) that was adequate for weight and length (denoting symmetrically reduced weight and length throughout the second and third trimesters was both poorer and statistically different from that of control infants. However, in all cognitive tests except one (digit span) the infants with weight reduction in the last trimester only performed as well as the control infants. It is not known whether these differences tended to persist as the children grew older.[37]

Pollitt[37] reports that the significance of small head circumference is controversial. He says some studies of both nutritionally at-risk and well-nourished children have found no relationship between head circumference and cognitive test scores. Conversely, other studies report such a relationship among 4-year-olds designated at birth as large-for-date, small-for-date, or average-sized, particularly in the small-for-date group. The developmental outcome of low birth weight and intrauterine malnutrition is also impacted by the child's social and familial environment.

Social and environmental factors contribute to the final outcome of early nutritional trauma. For example, severe protein and energy deficiency early in life, secondary to a medical condition and independent of social and environmental deprivations, does not leave adverse sequelae in cognitive function. On the basis of the three decades of research, Pollitt[37] concludes that within the low socioeconomic groups there is a small but statistically significant association between growth faltering and below-average performance in tests of mental development.

CONGENITAL DISORDERS
Congenital Heart Disease

Infants and children with congenital heart disease (CHD) are generally underweight and frequently retarded in growth. Those with cyanotic CHD are more likely to manifest retarded growth, especially when congestive failure supervenes.[77] One fourth of all children with CHD have associated (noncardiac) anomalies and 6% are small for gestational age at birth. Though there may be associated anomalies of the gastroenteric tract and kidney, they are no more prevalent in children with CHD than in the general infant population. Some alterations in intestinal function have been found, but there has been no substantive evidence that malabsorption is a common problem in children with CHD.

Many infants with CHD seem unwilling or unable to accept volumes of feeding comparable to those consumed by healthy infants of the same size. Fatigue associated with hypoxia and the dyspnea and tachypnea of congestive heart failure interfere with the infant's ability to suck. Some infants with CHD are hypermetabolic, especially those with labored breathing and/or congestive heart failure and those with significant growth retardation reflecting prenatal and/or postnatal events. Most infants with growth failure attributable to primary malnutrition have high calorie requirements during rehabilitation simply because of the energy cost of catch-up growth.[78]

Nutritional management. The major nutritional problem confronting infants with CHD is achieving an energy intake sufficient to meet expenditures for maintenance and growth without overburdening or taxing the circulatory system. An initial goal is to achieve average calorie intakes of normal infants of the same size. If the infant with CHD demonstrates significant growth retardation, it may be appropriate to base estimates of calorie needs on desired body weight or length. Average energy intakes of healthy infants (in kcal/kg/da) are approximately 120, 110, 105, and 100 during the quarters of the first year, and remain at 100 kcal/kg/day during the second year.[79]

If the younger infant's caloric needs are met by a formula providing approximately 10% of calories as proteins, the infant's protein needs can

be met without imposing an excessive renal solute load. Formulas that include partially demineralized whey may be advantageous in these infants because of the lower levels of minerals per gram of protein in such formulas. Formulas should provide between 35% and 50% of calories from a combination of vegetable oils known to be readily digestible and absorbable. Levels of minerals and vitamins in formulas should be in keeping with those recommended by the National Research Council's Committee on Nutrition.[8]

Sodium intake should be controlled within the range of 6 to 8 mM/day, depending on the use of diuretic agents and the infant's cardiorespiratory status. Great care must be taken to avoid simultaneously restricting sodium and using diuretics, for sodium depletion can occur promptly in infants.

Because an infant with CHD may have difficulty consuming a sufficient volume of formula at regular dilution (67 kcal/dl) to meet caloric requirements, it may be preferable to use a formula that supplies between 90 and 100 kcal/dl. Use of formulas with these higher caloric densities requires careful monitoring of overall water balance and particular attention to extrarenal losses of water. The safety of the infant's diet in these circumstances can be evaluated and monitored by repeated determinations of urinary osmolality, which should be between 300 and 400 mOsm/liter.[80] If these levels are maintained and infants grow satisfactorily, then water balance and nutritional adequacy of the diet have been achieved.

Cystic Fibrosis of the Pancreas

Between 80% and 90% of infants with cystic fibrosis have pancreatic insufficiency; hence the major nutritional problems in these children result from defective digestion and absorption of fat, protein, and carbohydrate. Although there may be some alterations in the intestinal mucosal function, they rarely constitute clinical problems. For example, lactase activity may be decreased somewhat and may need consideration when children with cystic fibrosis have diarrhea that persists during usual management.

Potential consequences of pancreatic insufficiency and maldigestion of fats, proteins, and complex carbohydrates may include retarded growth, hypoalbuminemia and edema, anemia, and vitamin deficiencies (especially of the fat-soluble vitamins A, E, and K). Clinical manifestations of protein and vitamin deficiency are uncommon now; they usually occur in infants with previously unrecognized cystic fibrosis[81] or when supplementary vitamins have not been given as prescribed.[82] Although clinical manifestations of vitamin D deficiency are rare today, many children with cystic fibrosis have low levels of vitamin A (retinol) in blood plasma despite substantial intakes of the vitamin. Many of these children who have received vitamin A supplements have above-normal vitamin levels in the liver. These circumstances reflect impaired production and/or release of retinol-binding protein by the liver.[83] The limited evidence of vitamin D deficiency in children with cystic fibrosis reflects the fact that, with adequate exposure to sunlight, there is no dietary requirement for vitamin D.

Pathologic changes in the spinal cord and deposition of ceroid in smooth muscle, two conditions unique to patients with cystic fibrosis, may indicate vitamin E deficiency that can be prevented by increasing the vitamin E intake.[84]

It has been suggested[85] that intravenous supplementation with fatty acids (soy oil emulsion) may partially correct an error of prostaglandin metabolism in children with cystic fibrosis; however, well-controlled clinical trials have not confirmed this hypothesis.[86]

Children with cystic fibrosis who manifest significant evidence of pancreatic insufficiency should be treated with pancreatic enzyme preparations that contain lipase, amylase, and trypsin. Use of pancreatic enzyme preparations improves the digestion and absorption of fat by 30% to 40%, but effects on nitrogen balance are not clinically significant and effects on starch digestion are difficult to quantitate. Dosage of enzymes is largely empirical, but adjustments are directed at control of overt steatorrhea. It may be necessary temporarily to reduce fat intake in some infants and toddlers until an acceptable dosage of pancreatic enzymes is achieved.

Some attention should be given to the sources of fat in the diet of the child with cystic fibrosis. For example, medium-chain triglycerides are more readily absorbed and have been incorporated in formula products (e.g., Pregestimil) designed for infants and young children with malabsorption disorders. Special diets have been devised for children with cystic fibrosis, including ones based on protein hydrolysates, glucose polymers, and medium-chain triglycerides.[87]

Their potential nutritional advantages are largely offset by the fact that most children refuse to consume them in any quantity for any length of time. Many other children and adolescents have found through experience that only selected foods need be avoided because their ingestion leads to abdominal discomfort and/or steatorrhea.

Infants and children with cystic fibrosis should have calorie and protein intakes 35% greater than those recommended for healthy children of the same age. Fat should probably supply less than 30% of calories: in some cases 15% would be a more realistic figure. Vitamin intakes should be double the usual recommended intakes. With the generous protein allowance, mineral intake (with the possible exception of sodium) from any reasonable selection of foods should be adequate. Sodium depletion, because of sweat losses, was first documented in these children some 30 years ago: since then children with cystic fibrosis generally have been allowed free access to salt or, in the case of infants, the diets consumed have provided sufficient sodium. However, reports[88] have appeared in which several infants with cystic fibrosis became sodium depleted, perhaps reflecting the increase in breast-feeding, delayed introduction of solid foods, and first the reduction and later the elimination of added salt in baby food.

CHRONIC RENAL DISEASE

The average healthy child consumes protein (nitrogen) and major minerals (sodium, potassium, chloride, phosphorus) in excess of metabolic needs. In health the kidney can excrete the excess; but when kidney function is impaired, this is not the case. Attention must then be directed to adjusting intakes to meet needs without imposing excessive loads in children with renal insufficiency. At the same time, as a consequence of altered renal function, and especially the development of uremia, children may not receive sufficient energy intake and may become deficient in essential amino acids and calcium.[89] Deficiencies of major minerals may also develop if tubular disease predominates.

Energy

Partially nephrectomized young rats, a model for renal insufficiency in children, reduce their caloric intake and show retarded growth.[90] In such animals, weight gain in relation to calorie intake may be lower than in healthy animals. Decreased body fat and muscle mass, symptoms of apathy, poor appetite, and in some cases cold intolerance in children with chronic renal disease indicate that they receive a caloric intake well below that required for catch-up growth. These observations suggest that nutrient intake in excess of normal may be required for such children.[91]

Average caloric intakes of children with end-stage renal disease treated by long-term hemodialysis are between 60% and 75% of the RDAs for children of the same height.[92-94] Children whose intakes are less than two thirds of the RDAs grow at an average rate only one third of normal.[92] When these children receive additional calories (carbohydrate and fat) with no additional protein or electrolytes, their caloric intakes increase to an average of 83% of the RDAs. Rate of growth also increases over a period of at least 3 months to an average 90% of normal.[95] If caloric intake of the child with chronic renal disease is less than 50% of the RDAs, growth will cease; if greater than 90%, growth will proceed at an average rate. To achieve normal growth *and* normal body composition, children undergoing chronic hemodialysis may need caloric intakes greater than the RDAs.

Protein

A dietary protein/calorie ratio between 1.5 and 2 g/100 kcal has been suggested for children with uremia who are undergoing chronic hemodialysis. This level of protein, with 40% to 50% as essential amino acids, should meet protein and amino acid needs, including the estimated 2 to 10 g of amino acids lost per dialysis.[96] If protein intake is much greater than 2 g/100 kcal, azotemia is likely to be increased and excess salts will result in expansion of the extracellular fluid volume because of diminished renal tolerance. If protein intake is restricted to 1 g/kg/day, however,[97] it may be difficult to ensure sufficient intake of essential amino acids to meet the child's needs. This reflects the fact that essential amino acids in well-selected diets rarely account for more than 40% of total amino acids. Hence, with a total protein intake of 1 g/kg/day, intake of essential amino acids would be only approximately 0.4 g/kg/day, probably half that required by infants and perhaps three fourths that required by children.

In one report[98] positive nitrogen balance and growth were achieved in a 5-year-old with advanced renal failure by supplementing her diet with essential amino acids for a protein intake of between 0.8 and 1.12 g/kg/day with 60% of total amino acids in the diet being essential. Other investigators[99] have documented improved nitrogen balance in children with chronic renal disease whose diets were supplemented with essential amino acids but have found no significant improvements in growth. Alpha-keto acids have been used to increase protein intake while minimizing nitrogen toxicity in children with chronic renal disease, but it is unclear whether they produced beneficial effects[100] as appears to be the case in adults.[101,102]

Minerals

With the exception of young infants whose only source of nutrition is human milk, most infants and children ingest sodium, potassium, chloride, and phosphorus in excess of need or advisable intake levels.[103] For example, average consumption of sodium among healthy toddlers approximates 7 mM/100 kcal/day[104] whereas the advisable intake is only about 1 mM/100 kcal/day. Children with progressive renal insufficiency lose the ability to excrete excesses, and often their ability to conserve sodium is impaired at very low intakes. The ingestion of sodium, potassium, and chloride in the range of 2-3 mM/100 kcal/day is likely to be tolerated and will meet the needs of these children; but some children with renal tubular disorders will require additional potassium to avoid potassium depletion and hypokalemia.

Intakes of calcium and phosphorus by healthy children average approximately 75 mg/100 kcal/day, amounts that exceed the estimated dietary requirements for calcium and phosphorus by factors of 3 and 6, respectively. In the case of calcium, not more than 40% to 45% is likely to be absorbed from the gut under ordinary circumstances, so control of intake is less important than in the case of phosphorus. However, the reduced glomerular filtration rate increases the resistance to vitamin D and impairs the absorption of calcium from the gastrointestinal tract.[105] Supplementary vitamin D is generally necessary in children with chronic renal insufficiency. Phosphorus is efficiently absorbed; but because phosphorus excretion (renal) is impaired in uremic children, hyperphosphatemia is likely unless net phosphate intake is decreased in proportion to the reduced glomerular filtration.

Children with renal tubular disorders may require supplemental calcium and phosphorus to replace excess renal losses, especially if hypocalcemia or hypophosphatemia and osteomalacia develop.

INFECTION

A synergistic interaction is observed between nutrition and infection. The more depressed the nutritional status of the child, the lower will be the resistance to disease, and therefore the effects of disease will be magnified. *All* infection has some effect on nutritional status, almost always manifested as varying degrees of anorexia, dietary changes, increased metabolic

rate, and a decline in nutrient absorption. The clinical course of intercurrent infections is influenced by their severity and frequency, the nutritional status of the child, and the length of recovery.

Changes in dietary patterns accompanying anorexia often result in weight loss. If anorexia and negative energy-protein balance are prolonged, a decrease in lean body mass may result. Such catabolic phenomena occur somewhat late in the infectious process, and are preceded by changes in which an early host response to infection triggers an increased uptake of plasma amino acids as well as an increase of amino acid metabolism in the liver. Additional losses of amino acids and total nitrogen as well as electrolytes and other minerals also occur via the increased sweating associated with infection. In children with se-

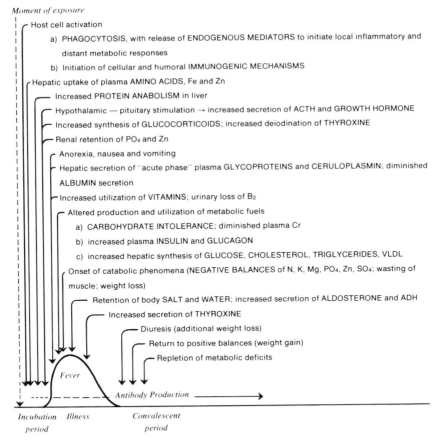

Figure 28-2 Onset times of various metabolic, endocrine, biochemical, and immunologic responses of the patient in relation to the sequential phases of an acute, self-limited, generalized model infectious illness.

From Beisel WR: In McKigney JI, Munro HN, editors: Nutrient requirements in adolescence, Cambridge Mass, 1976, MIT Press.

verely depressed nutritional states, depressed immune response enhances risks of increased morbidity and mortality. The child with protein-energy malnutrition, discussed in detail in Chapter 32, is at greatest risk of developing overwhelming infection from a depressed immune (cellular, humoral, complement) system. The sequence of changes associated with infectious illness in the child is outlined in Fig. 28-2.[106]

THE DEVELOPMENTALLY DISABLED CHILD

Only relatively recently have the special dietary needs of developmentally disabled children been more fully recognized and addressed. Whether the origin of the poor growth patterns of these children is genetic, fetal, maternal, or environmental, the patterns have often been summarily attributed to the metabolic or neurologic deficits, without adequate attention being given to diet.

A child's energy need is not appreciably affected by the nature of a motor dysfunction, which may be ataxic, hypotonic, spastic, or choreoathetotic. If, however, the motor dysfunction is sufficiently severe to cause immobilization, the child's energy requirement is reduced to approximately 75% of that of an average mobile child of similar height. Body length or stature and motor activities, therefore, are more important determinants of energy requirements than is age.[107]

Fluid intake must be monitored in children who will not, or cannot, drink or who are unable to respond adequately to thirst. Constipation is a common problem, and the need for fiber in the diet should be evaluated. Drug intake, insofar as it may interfere with nutrient uptake or modify nutrient metabolism, is of importance in the developmentally disabled child. Anticonvulsants, for example, increase vitamin D requirements and alter folic acid metabolism. Drug-associated fatigue, drowsiness, and torpor, as well as other negative changes linked to drug use, will interfere with appropriate dietary practice.

Mechanical problems frequently bar successful feeding of the developmentally disabled youngster. Difficulty with getting food into the mouth, loss of food from the mouth, poor head and neck control, and difficulty with masticating and salivating, as well as problems with chewing and swallowing, may preclude adequate food intake. Careful attention must be given to the pa-

tient's oral ability, body position, and muscle control; and conscientious menu planning and care-giver instruction must be provided to circumvent, insofar as possible, the impediments to food intake that result in poor growth.

REFERENCES

1. Holt LE, Snyderman SE: The feeding of premature and newborn infants, Pediatr Clin North Am **13**:1103-1115, 1966.
2. Ziegler EE, et al: Body composition of the reference fetus, Growth **40**:329-341, 1976.
3. Wilkinson A, Yu VYH: Immediate effect of feeding on bloodgases and some cardiorespiratory functions in ill newborn infants, Lancet **1**:1083-1085, 1974.
4. Ziegler EE, et al: Nutrition requirements of the premature infant. In: Suskind RM, editor: Textbook of pediatric nutrition, New York, 1981, Raven Press, pp 29-39.
5. Gaull GB, et al: Milk protein; quantity and quality in low–birth-weight infants. III. Effects on sulfur amino acids in plasma and urine, J Pediatr **90**:348-355, 1977.
6. Galeano NF, et al: Taurine supplementation of a premature formula improves fat absorption in preterm infants, Pediatr Res **22**:67-71, 1987.
7. Tsang RC, editor: Vitamin and mineral requirements in preterm infants, New York, 1985, Marcel Dekker Inc.
8. Committee on Nutrition, American Academy of Pediatrics: Nutritional needs of low-birth-weight infants, Pediatrics **60**:519-530, 1977.
9. Committee on Nutrition of the Preterm Infant (ESPGAN): Nutrition and feeding of preterm infants, Acta Paediatr Scand **336**(suppl):1-14, 1987.
10. Tantibhedhyangkul P, Hashim SA: Medium-chain triglyceride feeding in premature infants: effect on calcium and magnesium absorption, Pediatrics **61**:537-545, 1978.
11. Lemons JA, et al: Differences in the composition of preterm and term human milk during early lactation, Pediatr Res **16**:113-117, 1982.
12. Green FR, et al: Bone mineral content and serum 25-hydroxyvitamin D concentration in breast-fed infants with and without supplemental vitamin D, J Pediatr **98**:696-701, 1981.
13. Schanler RJ, et al: Fortified mothers' milk in very low–birth-weight infants: results of macromineral balance studies, J. Pediatr **107**:767-774, 1985.
14. Ziegler EE: Protein requirements of preterm infants. In Fomon SJ, Heird WC, editors: Energy and protein needs during infancy, New York, 1986, Academic Press Inc. pp 69-85.
15. Gross SJ: Bone mineralization in preterm infants fed human milk with and without mineral supplementation, J Pediatr **111**:450-458, 1987.
16. Putet G, et al: Supplementation of pooled human milk with casein hydroysale: energy and nitrogen balance and weight gain composition in very low birth weight infants, Pediatr Res **21**:458-461, 1987.
17. Modanlou HD, et al: Growth, biochemical status and mineral metabolism in very-low–birth-weight infants receiving fortified preterm human milk, J Pediatr Gastroenterol Nutr **5**:762-767, 1986.
18. Schenai JP, et al: Nutritional balance studies in very-low–birth-weight infants: enhanced nutrient retention rates by an experimental formula, Pediatrics **66**:233-238, 1980.

19. Cooper PA, et al: Growth and biochemical response of premature infants fed pooled preterm milk or special formula, J Pediatr Gastroenterol Nutr **3**:749-754, 1984.

20. Hagelberg S, et al: The protein tolerance of very low birth weight infants fed human milk protein enriched mother's milk, Acta Paediatr Scand **71**:597-601, 1982.

21. Lucas A, et al: Multicentre trial on feeding low birth-weight infants: effects of diet on early growth, Arch Dis Child **59**:722-730, 1984.

22. Frisch RE, Revelle R: Height and weight at menarche and a hypothesis of critical body weights and adolescent events, Science **169**:397-399, 1970.

23. Motil KJ: Aggressive nutritional therapy in growth retardation, Clin Nutr **4**:75-84, 1985.

24. Lifshitz F: Nutrition and growth, Clin Nutr **4**:40-47, 1985.

25. English PC: Failure to thrive without organic reason, Pediatr Ann **7**:774-781, 1978.

26. Fomon SJ: Infant nutrition, Philadelphia, 1974, WB Saunders Co, pp 81-83.

27. Powell GF: Nutrition in non organic failure to thrive, Clin Nutr **4**:54-55, 1985.

28. Kreiger I, Chen YC: Caloric requirements for weight gain in infants with growth failure due to maternal deprivation, undernutrition, and congenital heart disease, Pediatrics **44**:647-654, 1969.

29. Kreiger I, Good MH: Adrenocortical and thyroid function in the deprivation syndrome, Am J Dis Child **20**:95-102, 1971.

30. Sterling GA: The thyroid in malnutrition, Arch Dis Child **37**:99-102, 1962.

31. Hintz RI, et al: Plasma somatomedin and growth hormone values in children with protein calorie malnutrition, J Pediatr **92**:152-156, 1978.

32. Kreiger I, Mellinger RC: Pituitary function in the deprivation syndrome, J Pediatr **79**:216-225, 1971.

33. Powell GF, et al: Emotional deprivation and growth retardation stimulating idiopathic hypopituitarism. II, N Engl J Med **276**:1279-1283, 1967.

34. Gaensbauer TH, Sands K: Distorted affective communications in abused/neglected infants and their potential impact on caretakers, J Am Acad Child Psychiatry **18**:236-254, 1979.

35. Vietze PM, et al: Newborn behavioral and interactional characteristics of nonorganic failure-to-thrive infants. In Field TM, et al, editors: High-risk infants and children, New York, 1980, Academic Press Inc, pp 5-23.

36. Gordon AH, Jameson JC: Infant-mother attachment in patients with nonorganic failure to thrive syndrome, J Am Acad Psychiatr **18**:251-259, 1979.

37. Pollitt E: Failure to thrive: socioeconomic dietary intake and mother child interaction data, Fed Proc **34**:1593-1597, 1975.

38. Pollitt E: Nutrition and intellectual performance, Clin Nutr **5**:221-224, 1986.

39. Oates RK, et al: Long-term effects of nonorganic failure to thrive, Pediatrics **75**:36-40, 1985.

40. Rosenthal SR, et al: Growth failure and inflammatory bowel disease: approach to treatment of a complicated adolescent problem, Pediatrics **72**:481-490, 1983.

41. Kirschner BS: Growth retardation in Crohn's disease: the merits of aggressive nutritional therapy, Clin Nutr **2**:26-28, 1983.

42. Layden T, et al: Reversal of growth arrest in adolescents with Crohn's disease after parenteral alimentation, Gastroenterology **70**:1017-1026, 1976.

43. Nishi Y, et al: Zinc status and its relation to growth retardation in children with chronic inflammatory bowel disease, Am J Clin Nutr **33**:2613-2621, 1980.

44. La Sala MA, et al: Magnesium metabolism studies in children with inflammatory disease of the bowel, J Pediatr Res Gastroenterol Nutr. **4**:75-81, 1985.

45. Lifshitz F, Nishi Y: Mineral deficiencies during growth. In de Luca HF, Anast CS, editors: Pediatric diseases related to calcium, New York, 1980, Elsevier/North Holland Inc, pp 305-319.

46. Kelts DG, Grand RJ: Growth failure in intestinal diseases. In Lifshitz F, editor: Clinical disorders in pediatric gastroenterology and nutrition, New York, 1980, Marcel Dekker Inc, pp 305-331.

47. Strobel CT, et al: Home parenteral nutrition in children with Crohn's disease: an effective management alternative, Gastroenterology **77**:272-279, 1979.

48. Morin CL, et al: Continuous elemental enteral alimentation in children with Crohn's disease and growth failure, Gastroenterology **79**:1205-1210, 1980.

49. Homer DR, et al: Growth, course, and prognosis after surgery for Crohn's disease, Pediatrics **59**:717-725, 1977.

50. Prasad AS, et al: Syndrome of iron deficiency anemia, hepatosplenomegaly, hypogonadism, dwarfism, and geophagia, Am J Med **13**:532-546, 1961.

51. Moynahan EJ: Letter: Acrodermatitis enteropathica: a lethal inherited human zinc deficiency disorder, Lancet **2**:339-340, 1974.

52. Ghavani-Maibodi SZ, et al: Effect of oral zinc supplements on growth, hormonal levels, and zinc in healthy short children, Ann Nutr Metab **27**:214-219, 1983.

53. Walravens PA, Hambidge KM: Growth of infants fed a zinc-supplemented formula, Am J Clin Nutr **29**:1114-1121, 1976.

54. Hambidge KM, et al: Low levels of zinc in hair, anorexia, poor growth, and hypogeusia in children, Pediatr Res **6**:868-874, 1972.

55. Solomons NW, Rosenfield RI: Growth retardation and zinc nutrition, Pediatr Res **10**:923-927, 1976.

56. Hambidge KM, et al: Zinc nutrition of preschool children in the Denver Head Start program, Am J Clin Nutr **29**:734-738, 1976.

57. Oski FA: Nutritional anemias of infancy. In Lifshitz F, editor: Pediatric nutrition, New York, 1982, Marcel Dekker Inc, pp 123-138.

58. Lozoff B, et al: The effects of short-term oral iron therapy on developmental deficits in iron-deficient anemic infants, J Pediatr **100**:341-347, 1982.

59. Oski FA, Honig AS: The effects of therapy on developmental scores of iron-deficient infants, J Pediatr **92**:21-25, 1978.

60. Oski FA, et al: Effects of iron therapy on behavior performance in nonanemic, iron-deficient infants, Pediatrics **71**:877-880, 1983.

61. Walter T, et al: Effect of mild iron deficiency on infant mental development scores, J Pediatr **102**:519-521, 1983.

62. Pollitt E, et al: Iron deficiency and cognitive test performance in preschool children, Nutr Behav **1**:137-146, 1983.

63. Pollitt E, et al: Behavioral effects of iron deficiency anemia in children. In Pollitt E, Leibel RL, editors: Iron

deficiency: brain biochemistry and behavior, New York, 1982, Raven Pres, pp 195-208.

64. Pollitt E, et al: Letter: Cognitive effects of iron-deficiency anaemia, Lancet **1**:158, 1985.

65. Leach RM, et al: Studies on the role of manganese in bone formation: effect upon chondroitin sulfate synthesis in chick epiphyseal cartilage, Arch Biochem **133**:22-28, 1969.

66. Rotruck JT, et al: Selenium: biochemical role as a component of glutathione reductase, Science **179**:558, 1979.

67. Collipp PJ, Chen SY: Cardiomyopathy and selenium deficiency in a 2-year-old girl [letter], N Engl J Med **81**:1304-1305, 1981.

68. Button EJ, Whitehouse A: Subclinical anorexia nervosa, Psychol Med **11**:509-516, 1981.

69. Davis R, et al: Diet and retarded growth, Br Med J **1**:539-542, 1978.

70. Smith NJ: Excessive weight loss and food aversion in athletes simulating anorexia nervosa, Pediatrics **66**:139-142, 1980.

71. Pugliese MT, et al: Fear of obesity. A cause of short stature and delayed puberty, N Engl J Med **309**:513-518, 1983.

72. Garner DM, Garfinkel PE: The Eating Attitudes Test: an index of the symptoms of anorexia nervosa, Psychol Med **9**:273-279, 1979.

73. Lacey KA, Parkin JM: Causes of short stature. A community study of children in Newcastle upon Tyne, Lancet **1**:42-45, 1974.

74. Reference deleted in proofs.

75. Prader A, et al: Catch-up growth following illness or starvation, J Pediatr **62**:646-659, 1963.

76. Forbes GB: A note on the mathematics of "catch-up" growth, Pediatr Res **8**:929-931, 1974.

77. Feldt RH, et al: Growth of children with congenital heart disease, Am J Dis Child **117**:573-579, 1969.

78. Krieger I: Growth failure and congenital heart disease, Am J Dis Child **120**:497-502, 1970.

79. Beal VA: Nutritional intake. In McCammon RW, editor: Human growth and development, Springfield Ill, 1970, Charles C Thomas Publishers.

80. Fomon SJ, Ziegler EE: Nutritional management of infants with congenital heart disease, Am Heart J **83**:581-588, 1972.

81. Walters TR, Koch HF: Hemorrhagic diathesis and cystic fibrosis in infancy, Am J Dis Child **124**:641-642, 1972.

82. Keating JP, Feigin RD: Increased intracranial pressure associated with probable vitamin A deficiency in cystic fibrosis, Pediatrics **46**:41-46, 1970.

83. Smith FR, et al: Depressed plasma retinol-binding protein levels in cystic fibrosis, J Lab Clin Med **80**:423-433, 1972.

84. Slater GE, Swaiman KF: Muscular dystrophies of childhood, Pediatr Ann **6**:170-693, 1977.

85. Elliott RB: A therapeutic trial of fatty acid supplementation in cystic fibrosis, Pediatrics **57**:474-479, 1976.

86. Chase HP, Dupont JJ: Abnormal levels of prostaglandins and fatty acids in blood of children with cystic fibrosis, Lancet **2**:236-238, 1978.

87. Allen JD, et al: Nutritional supplementation in treatment of cystic fibrosis of the pancreas, Am J Dis Child **126**:22-26, 1973.

88. Laughlin JJ, et al: Changing feeding trends as a cause of electrolyte depletion in infants with cystic fibrosis, Pediatrics **68**:203-207, 1981.

89. Holliday MA: Management of the child with renal insufficiency. In Lieberman E, editor: Clinical pediatric nephrology, Philadelphia, 1976, J B Lippincott Co, pp 395-423.

90. Chantler C, et al: A rat model for the study of growth failure in uremia, Pediatr Res **8**:109-113, 1974.

91. Spinozzi NS, Grupe WE: Nutritional implications of renal disease. IV. Nutritional aspects of chronic renal insufficiency in childhood, J Am Diet Assoc **70**:493-97, 1977.

92. Simmons JM, et al: Relation of calorie deficiency to growth failure in children on hemodialysis and growth response to calorie supplementation, N Engl J Med **285**:653-656, 1971.

93. Broyer M, et al: Growth in children treated with long-term hemodialysis, J Pediatr **84**:642-649, 1974.

94. Grupe WE: Nutritional considerations in the prognosis and treatment of children with renal disease. In Suskind RM, editor: Textbook of pediatric nutrition, New York, 1978, Raven Press, pp 527-535.

95. Holliday MA: Calorie deficiency in children with uremia: effect upon growth, Pediatrics **50**:590-597, 1972.

96. Holliday MA: Chronic renal disease. In Pediatric nutrition handbook, Evanston Ill, 1979, American Academy of Pediatrics, pp 201-18.

97. Chantler C: Conservative management of renal insufficiency in infants and children, Proc R Soc Med **74**:1047-1079, 1971.

98. Aronson AS, et al: Essential amino acids in the treatment of advanced uremia, Pediatrics **56**:538-543, 1975.

99. Jones RWA, et al: Oral essential amino acid supplements in children with advanced chronic renal failure, Am J Clin Nutr **33**:1696-1702, 1980.

100. Chantler C, et al: Nutritional therapy in children with chronic renal disease. Am J Clin Nutr **33**:1682-1689, 1980.

101. Frohling PT, et al: Conservative treatment with ketoacid and amino acid supplemented low-protein diets in chronic renal failure, Am J Clin Nutr **33**:1667-1672, 1980.

102. Kampf D, et al: Efficacy of an unselected protein diet (25 g) with minor oral supply of essential amino acids and keto analogues compared with a selective protein diet (40 g) in chronic renal failure, Am J Clin Nutr **33**:1673-1677, 1980.

103. Ziegler EE, Fomon SJ: Major minerals. In Fomon SJ, editor: Infant nutrition, Philadelphia, 1974, W B Saunders Co, pp 268-69.

104. Committee on Nutrition, American Academy of Pediatrics: Sodium intake of infants in the United States, Pediatrics **68**:444-445, 1981.

105. DeLuca HF: New developments in the vitamin D endocrine system, J Am Diet Assoc, **80**:231-236, 1982.

106. Beisel WR: The influence of infection or injury on nutritional requirements during adolescence. In McKigney JI, Munro HN, editors: Nutrient requirements in adolescence, Cambridge Mass, 1976, MIT Press, pp 257-263.

107. Howard RB: Nutritional support of the developmentally disabled child. In Suskind RM, editor: Textbook of pediatric nutrition, New York, 1981, Raven Press, pp 577-581.

CHAPTER 29
Diarrheal Diseases

Fima Lifshitz
Hugo da Costa Ribeiro, Jr.

The relationship between nutrition and diarrhea has been apparent since antiquity, when it was recognized that diarrhea could develop in a patient after eating and would improve with fasting. The nutritional management of patients with diarrhea has varied with the medical concepts and fashions of the day. Today it is known that nutrition and diarrhea are interrelated in three ways: (1) nutrition may cause or increase the risk of diarrhea; (2) nutrition may play a role in the manifestation and complications of diarrhea, including protein-energy malnutrition; and (3) nutrition may be important in the management of diarrhea, including dietary objectives, feeding strategies, and water and electrolyte balance. In this chapter we review these factors to provide comprehensive guidelines for the nutritional management of patients with diarrheal disease.

NUTRITION AS A CAUSE OF, OR RISK FACTOR IN, DIARRHEA

Nutrition may cause or increase the risk of diarrhea from common infections induced by food and water ("food poisonings") and food allergies or intolerances. However, nutrition, specifically breast-feeding in infancy, may decrease the causes or risks of diarrheal disease. This is thought to be due to decreased contamination as well as to general and local immune host factors. Breast-feeding may be the most readily available means to reduce the problems of diarrhea and malnutrition. It is also the best way to meet the nutritional, immunologic, and emotional needs of infants, as well as avoid exposure to potentially disease-producing antigens present in other milk formulas.[1-3]

Diarrhea Induced by Food and Water

There is a clear association between the type of food ingested and specific etiologic agents of diarrhea. Infectious diarrhea may be caused by

eating contaminated food—for example, salmonella-induced diarrhea can result from eating contaminated egg products, meat, or poultry salads.[4] Norwalk viruses have been associated with the consumption of raw oysters and bakery products.[5,6] Infection with toxigenic *Escherichia coli* may follow consumption of restaurant food, particularly in foreign countries (as seen in "turista").[7] *Vibrio parahaemolyticus* infection is usually associated with eating shrimp or raw fish,[8] and *Clostridium perfringens* infection may result from eating meat or gravy that has been allowed to cool slowly or remain warm for prolonged periods.[9,10] *Yersinia enterocolitica* has been cultured from ice cream, seafood, canned meats, and slaughterhouse specimens.[11] Finally, *Aeromonas hydrophila* has been shown to produce diarrhea after one consumes contaminated food and water.[12]

Intestinal protozoan infection may be caused by contaminated water or food, particularly salads.[13] Giardiasis, amebiasis, and more recently cryptosporidiasis have been found where sanitary sewerage facilities are absent and water supplies are not properly treated or safeguarded. Symptomatic giardiasis among campers and hikers who drink water from remote mountain streams suggests that wild or domestic animals may also be carriers of this parasite. Cryptosporidiosis has been found to produce diarrhea outbreaks in day care centers and may be the most important protozoan, causing acute diarrhea in up to 7% of cases.[14-17]

Drinking water that contains organic material and is kept without refrigeration may lead to diarrhea from pathogen proliferation. This is of particular importance in the Tropics, where refrigeration may not be available. Thus milk formulas or cow's milk, and even oral rehydration solutions, can be potentially lethal and frequently cause diarrhea and malnutrition in infancy.[1]

447

Food also may be contaminated with toxins or other poisons that induce diarrhea—for example, *Staphylococcus aureus* enterotoxin, has been found in cream-filled pastry and salads. Botulism may occur from eating home-processed foods and should be suspected if a person complains of dizziness, diplopia, descending paralysis, dry mouth, or speech difficulty in addition to diarrhea.[18] Infant botulism, unlike the adult form, may result from ingesting not only the preformed toxin but also the bacterium *Clostridium botulinum*. The spores of this organism germinate in the infant's intestine and produce the toxin in vivo. *C. botulinum* is present in agricultural produce (vegetables and fruits) and may be found in nonessential foods, such as corn syrup and honey. Commercially sterilized low-acid canned foods, including infant formulas, contain no *C. botulinum* or toxin. Scombroid poisoning may follow the eating of tuna or mackerel. In addition to diarrhea, there can be headache, paresthesias, facial flushing, and exanthemas over the upper half of the body. Ciguatera (fish poisoning) may result from eating red snapper or other species; symptoms include paresthesias as well as diarrhea.[19] Cadmium poisoning with diarrhea has followed the intake of food barbecued on a refrigerator tray,[20] and solanine poisoning after the eating of green sprouts or potatoes. Solanine induces diarrhea and vascular collapse, dilated pupils, and hyporeflexia because of cholinesterase inhibition.[21]

Food Intolerances and Allergies

A wide spectrum of symptoms and diseases involving virtually every organ system has been ascribed to practically everything humans eat. Carbohydrates are, by far, the most common dietary component leading to food intolerance. Allergies to particular foods in childhood may produce diarrhea and other reactions ranging from local or systemic anaphylaxis to vague complaints of fatigue and irritability. Not surprisingly, there are wide discrepancies in the reported incidence and prevalence of food allergies, mainly because of their unreproducibility and/or the difficulty of quantifying patient complaints.

Carbohydrate intolerance. Carbohydrate intolerance is characterized by malabsorption that leads to symptoms, particularly diarrhea, and the excretion of acid stools with undigested carbohydrates in the feces following ingestion of dietary sugars. There may also be other complaints such as abdominal pain, failure to thrive, and/or weight loss. It is important to distinguish carbohydrate intolerance from malabsorption of carbohydrates due to oligosaccharidase deficiencies. The latter are laboratory findings that demonstrate diminished intestinal absorption and/or diminished mucosal enzyme concentration. For example, ontogenic lactase deficiency is prevalent among the majority of people throughout the world. Yet they usually do not have clinical problems and may enjoy the nutritional benefits of milk. In contrast, patients with carbohydrate intolerance of any cause will have diarrhea and other pathophysiologic and clinical alterations if they ingest milk.[22,23]

The presence of osmotically active carbohydrate and fermentative products within the lumen is associated with intestinal secretion of fluid and electrolytes until osmotic equilibrium is reached. In addition, there are losses of mucosal cells and intestinal disaccharidases. Organic acids produced by bacterial flora are poorly absorbed by the colon; they, furthermore, increase the osmotic pressure within the lumen and reduce the stool pH. In addition, organic acids interfere with the absorption of water and electrolytes. Increased intestinal motility may develop from the added intraluminal volume, exacerbating the diarrhea. The stools are, therefore, characterized by an acid pH due to organic acids and the presence of unabsorbed carbohydrate. Eliminating the unabsorbed sugar from the diet often breaks the cycle and relieves the diarrhea, regardless of the etiology of the disease.[22,23,30]

The pathogenesis of carbohydrate intolerance may be directly related to the etiology of the primary illness (e.g., gastroenteritis) or to complications of the disease (dehydration and shock). In gastroenteritis, microorganisms usually induce diarrhea by one of a combination of mechanisms leading to epithelial cell injury.[31] The mucosal damage results either from tissue invasion and destruction of the epithelial cells by enteric pathogens or from cell injury by products of bacterial metabolism acting on the foods and host secretions (e.g., deconjugated bile salts, short-chain organic acids, alcohol). The mucosal damage in the small intestine depresses brush-border oligosaccharidases and intestinal transport, leading to carbohydrate malabsorption. The altered epithelial cell membranes contribute to this problem through changed intestinal permeability. In diarrheal disease, other alterations lead to carbohydrate malabsorption even without a decrease in intestinal oligosaccharidases. For example, there may be increased peristalsis, with reduced exposure of the carbohydrates to the action of these enzymes. There may also be interference in the binding of the substrate to the brush border enzymes because of epithelial cell inflammation, anatomic disturbances, or other alterations.

Certain enteric viruses (rotavirus, Norwalk) also induce morphologic and functional changes in the small intestine by penetrating the enterocyte. Rotaviruses seem to be the principal cause of diarrhea and carbohydrate intolerance in infancy. It has been accepted that intestinal lactase is the receptor and uncoating enzyme for these enteric viruses. Before diarrhea occurs, the virus must infect gut epithelium rich in lactase. This concept is consistent with the high prevalence of lactose intolerance in gastroenteritis during infancy whereas in adults, who are usually not sensitive to infection with this virus, lactose intolerance complicating diarrheal disease is infrequent.[32]

Carbohydrate intolerance in diarrhea is frequently specific for lactose, but it may affect other disaccharides such as sucrose, maltose, or even glucose polymers. At times, it may also affect all carbohydrates, including monosaccharides (e.g., fructose).[23] The frequent occurrence of lactose intolerance in diarrheal disease may be due to the fact that lactase is the most superficial enzyme of the brush-border oligosaccharidases; its activity is rate limiting, and its concentrations are considerably lower than those of other brush-border enzymes. In addition, it may be the target enzyme for viral enteritis. Carbohydrate intolerance in diarrheal disease may also be associated with intolerance of other foods. Fat and protein intolerance is thought to be due to a variety of mechanisms (as discussed later). Carbohydrate intolerance may lead to these alterations, or result from them, creating a vicious cycle that induces chronic diarrhea. Therefore recognizing carbohydrate intolerance in infants with diarrhea is of paramount importance for nutritional rehabilitation during the acute stage of the illness as well as after recovery.

Cow's milk protein sensitivity (CMPS). Adverse reactions to milk have been known to occur since Hippocrates recorded that milk could cause vomiting and urticaria.[24] Although there is increasing evidence that cow's milk protein sensitivity results from an immunologically mediated reaction, in clinical practice such evidence is often lacking. CMPS is associated with a range of clinical manifestations, varying from skin eruptions (urticaria, eczema) to respiratory symptoms (wheezing, even asthma) to acute anaphylaxis, which can cause death.

Cow's milk protein sensitivity leading to gastrointestinal manifestations is largely a disease of infancy and is uncommonly diagnosed beyond the age of 3 years. The reported incidence ranges from 0.5% to 7.5% in the general population, and up to 21% in infants referred for "allergic studies." A higher prevalence is recognized as being associated with other atopic conditions and familial allergies,[26] decreased rates of breastfeeding with early introduction of cow's milk in infancy,[27] immunologic abnormalities such as IgA deficiency,[28] and gastroenteritis.[33]

Cow's milk contains three times more protein than human breast milk. The five main proteins that may be highly immunogenic and capable of stimulating a systemic antibody response are bovine serum albumins, bovine serum globulin, bovine casein, alpha-lactoglobulin, and beta-lactoglobulin. The frequency of reactions to these various protein fractions is variable. The most antigenic of them appears to be beta-lactoglobulin, which causes allergic reactions in 66% to 82% of patients. The beta-lactoglobulin protein fraction is not present in breast milk.[34]

The pathogenesis of CMPS continues to be unclear. Therefore the role of the gastrointestinal tract appears to be highly relevant.[35] Under normal circumstances cow's milk protein antigen is not absorbed to any significant extent, because of the gastrointestinal barrier mechanisms (including gastric acidity, proteolytic and lysosomal enzymes, which degrade the antigens, and the normal peristaltic activity). In addition, the host's local secretory IgA immune mechanisms help to neutralize the antigens in the lumen.

Basically, there are two major immunologic pathways thought to be involved in the antigens' role in CMPS: (1) increased permeability of the small intestinal mucosa to the antigen and (2) lack of control of the antigens once they have been absorbed.

CMPS may be primary or secondary. The primary form is caused by an intrinsic disturbance of the local immune system for antigen control. The secondary form is possibly a sequela of intestinal mucosal damage caused by gastroenteritis and leading to excess antigen penetration. However, it should be pointed out that even when there is excess antigen absorption with antibody formation CMPS occurs only in a genetically susceptible host.[34,35]

The clinical pathologic manifestations that occur in CMPS are the consequences of exposure to antigenic proteins leading to their binding to enterocytes, which become the target for killer T cells (a Type I reaginic reaction). CMPS results in structural and functional damage of the small bowel.[34]

In infants with diarrhea it is often difficult to ascertain whether CMPS is the primary event that leads to intestinal mucosal damage, and thus to diarrhea, or a secondary process resulting from intestinal damage from other causes leading to increased permeability to protein antigens and sensitization of a susceptible host. Despite these uncertainties about the relationships among CMPS, carbohydrate intolerance, and diarrheal disease, it is clear that the jejunal mucosa of young infants and of children with diarrhea is sensitive to antigenic proteins (cow's milk, soy, gluten).[29] These observations have important implications for the etiology of the diarrhea as well as the therapy of the patients. They are also pertinent to dietary recommendations in normal infants.

Other intolerances. Dietary fat is frequently indicted as a cause of chronic diarrhea. In situations of high energy needs (e.g., during recovery from diarrhea), low-fat diets may worsen the malnourished state and cause chronic diarrhea by a variety of mechanisms.[36]

Feeding of hyperosmolar formulas or artificial sweeteners, or simply overfeeding normal formula, may also result in loose stools. Overfeeding is frequent in children with diarrheal disease once the anorectic period of the illness is over. When these children are given ad-libitum diets, they often ingest large quantities of formula. Dietary intake in excess of 200 ml/kg/day produces diarrhea and prolongs the disease regardless of the primary etiology. The ingestion of large quantities of fluid per se has also been linked to prolonged diarrhea.[37] Food additives, including flavorings, dyes, and processing material, may cause problems. The abuse of tea, which contains caffeine (75-300 mg/da), may cause diarrhea by stimulation of intestinal secretion via cAMP.[38]

NUTRITION AND THE MANIFESTATIONS AND COMPLICATIONS OF DIARRHEA

Nutrition plays an important role in the immediate as well as the long-term complications of diarrhea. The patient's nutritional intake may determine the presence or absence of these complications as well as the rate of improvement and the eventual outcome of the disease.

The severity and duration of diarrheal disease are related to the quantity and quality of the dietary intake. Specific food intolerances may affect the duration of the illness more directly than the primary agent that triggered the diarrhea illness. For example, diarrhea in acute gastroenteritis may persist as long as lactose is present in the diet. Small molecules of high osmotic pressure (e.g., organic acids) may result from carbohydrate fermentation and contribute to increased fluid losses. The elimination of unabsorbed carbohydrate from the diet brings about prompt recovery.[22,23,30]

Nutritional intake can contribute to specific metabolic problems. The consumption of milk by infants with diarrhea has been associated with hyponatremia, with losses of extracellular sodium and chloride as well as intracellular potassium. Unabsorbed carbohydrates in the intestine potentiate the development of metabolic acidosis. There are several ways that carbohydrate intolerance can lead to this complication. The major source of excess hydrogen ions in children with diarrhea is bacterial carbohydrate fermentation.[39] In addition, the presence of organic acids within the intestinal lumen may stimulate secretion and loss of large quantities of bicarbonate from the serum to neutralize the luminal acid load.

Nutritional Status

Diarrheal diseases are considered the most important inducers of malnutrition because they affect nutrition through a number of mechanisms: (1) reduced food intake, (2) altered digestion and absorption, (3) impaired utilization of nutrients, (4) other metabolic alterations. Each episode of diarrhea has a varying impact on the host economy and nutrition, even when there is no limitation in food availability. Diminished food intake can be substantial during diarrhea, especially among infants and toddlers, because of at least two circumstances: the presence of anorexia and the restriction dictated by medical or popular traditions, beliefs, or taboos. In the latter circumstance the mother, or another person in the family, suppresses food for days or even weeks. However, anorexia appears to be the more important source of diminished food intake. It may be mediated by interleukin-1, a hormone released by macrophages and monocytes after an infection or some other kind of stress. It occurs regardless of the type, severity, or localization of the infection. Most foods are rejected, although breast milk to a lesser extent. The intensity of the anorexia may not correlate with the kind or severity of illness, and a child may become anorectic even with mild diarrhea, lasting for a few hours or for days or weeks. As much as 20% to 70% of food available may be wasted or not eaten during bouts of diarrhea.

Nutritional status is also altered in diarrheal disease through impaired intestinal absorption of nutrients. Even when diarrhea is mild, lactose intolerance is associated with more marked body weight losses.[30] Since 50% of the total caloric requirements in children are derived from dietary carbohydrates, losses of carbohydrates because of diarrhea account for considerable caloric deficits. The presence of unabsorbed carbohydrates in the intestinal lumen also enhances protein and nitrogen losses and decreases nitrogen absorption. This may lead to dilution of bile acid concentrations below the critical micellar level for efficient fat absorption. The association of disaccharidase deficiencies, carbohydrate intolerance, and steatorrhea has long been recognized.

Malabsorption in diarrheal disease leads to increased losses of nutrients and a negative nitrogen balance. Diarrhea results in large losses of nitrogen and other nutrients through the stools. However, urinary losses of nitrogen and other essential nutrients occur with almost any degree of infection. Even during subclinical infections, there may be a negative protein-energy balance, with nitrogen losses of between 0.6 and 1.2 g/kg/day. Patients, especially infants and young children, may lose 10% or more body weight within days. Loss of cells, plasma, amino acids and other nitrogenous substances, vitamins, and hormones may occur when there is intestinal mucosal injury. The dysentery diarrheas often show

a protein-losing enteropathy and exhibit toxic manifestations with weakness and prostration and a high fatality rate.[39a]

In diarrhea, as in other infections, there are anorexia and fever, breakdown of muscle protein, discharge of insulin and glucagon, mobilization of leukocytes, and sequestration of zinc and iron.[39b] Vasoactive intestinal polypeptide (VIP), which inhibits the peristaltic reflex, and other gut hormones (motilin, enteroglucagon, neurotensin) are altered during diarrhea. Prostaglandins are also involved in diarrhea, including mild forms in toddlers.[39c]

Although research on metabolic consequences of diarrhea has been scarce, and this is even more true of endocrine and hormonal interactions, there is reason to believe that they are similar to other infectious diseases.[39b] Metabolic alterations to cope with infection have a grave negative nutritional implication and are costly and slow to correct, particularly when the infection occurs frequently in underprivileged conditions.[1]

Aggravation of Intestinal Malabsorption

Dietary intake may play an important role in the consequences of prolonged diarrhea. Unabsorbed carbohydrates and fermentative products in the small bowel facilitate the colonization and proliferation of enteric bacteria in the upper segments of the intestine. Nonspecific bacterial proliferation of fecal and colonic bacteria is a frequent secondary complication in infants with diarrhea.[31] The disturbed intestinal motility and the presence of free carbohydrates within the lumen may be important factors in enteric bacterial proliferation. This may lead to a further deterioration of intestinal function because the bacteria generate metabolites (deconjugated bile salts, hydroxy fatty acids, alcohol) that are injurious to the proximal portions of the small intestine. Clinically this may aggravate the diarrhea and exacerbate dietary intolerances. A patient with lactose intolerance may become intolerant to other disaccharides, and if the diarrhea persists, monosaccharide intolerance may ensue. Intestinal malabsorption often is intensified in infants who have lactose intolerance for 2-3 weeks before dietary therapy is initiated.[23]

Susceptibility to Other Conditions

Not only do continuing dietary intolerance and nutrient losses impair the infant's ability to recover from the initial illness, they also may increase the susceptibility to other conditions and influence the patient's clinical course. Intestinal or systemic complications may be related to the nutritional intake of patients with diarrhea. The association of pneumatosis intestinalis and necrotizing enterocolitis with feedings was first recognized in infants in whom pneumatosis intestinalis developed during an episode of diarrhea.[40] The infants were being fed milk formula and had lactose intolerance before the appearance of pneumatosis. A similar association of carbohydrate intolerance and necrotizing enterocolitis was subsequently observed in newborn infants. Furthermore, food intolerances such as milk protein hypersensitivity have been associated with necrotizing enterocolitis.[41]

Necrotizing enterocolitis may also result from elemental and hyperosmolar diets. In the majority of patients necrotizing enterocolitis is associated with feedings.[42] It has long been known that intestinal permeability can be altered in gastroenteritis, since there is measurable absorption of egg albumin and milk-protein antibodies frequently present in serum following diarrhea.[33] The increased macromolecular absorption leads to hypersensitivity and allergy to foods in the susceptible host and to toxemia and sepsis when toxins or bacteria cross the intestinal barrier.[35]

The increased intestinal permeability could be related to dietary intolerance. Experimental studies[43] have shown that, under pathophysiologic stress, as in diarrhea, the normal barriers to the intestinal transport of macromolecules may be functionally and structually altered, allowing increased leakage of intact protein across the intestinal epithelium. In diarrheal disease, several alterations (including luminal hyperosmolar gradient, cellular disruption by pathogens, increased levels of deconjugated bile salts, and lactose intolerance) may promote intestinal passage of macromolecules. Thus a child with gastroenteritis and lactose intolerance may become sensitive to food proteins present in the diet.

Indeed, carbohydrate intolerance in diarrheal disease has been associated with food protein hypersensitivity.[33] Lactose intolerance can be associated with milk protein allergy and secretory IgA deficiency. Soy-protein hypersensitivity, apparently acquired during gastroenteritis, also has been associated with monosaccharide intolerance.[44] After rehabilitation the patient may tolerate dietary carbohydrates but still have protein hypersensitivity.

Other conditions can develop as a result of chronic diarrhea and nutritional alterations. Loss of iron from gastrointestinal bleeding may be severe enough to cause anemia. Antibiotic use may impair intestinal synthesis of some vitamins. Deficiencies of folic acid, vitamin B_{12}, and niacin have been reported. Hypoprothrombinemia has also been a complication of these factors. In addition, losses of essential minerals (magnesium, zinc) could lead to deficiencies in these patients and account for other complications.

NUTRITIONAL MANAGEMENT OF DIARRHEA

Nutritional therapy is of great practical value in the patient with diarrhea. Oral rehydration coupled with early restoration of foods and continuity of breast-feeding in infancy are the most basic measures needed to implement an effective treatment of diarrhea.

Fast Versus Feast

"Bowel rest" has long been thought advisable in treating a variety of digestive disorders, particularly diarrheal disease. During the initial treatment for diarrhea, patients were fasted for up to 72 hours "to provide rest" for the gastrointestinal tract. There are no scientific data to support the assumption that dehydrated patients need a period with no oral intake. Moreover, clinicians have long known that breast-feedings should be sustained during diarrhea.

Apart from the undesirable metabolic effects of even a brief fast, withholding oral intake may alter intestinal absorption and disaccharidase activities. Even when total intravenous feedings provide for energy and nitrogen needs, there may be depletion of intestinal digestive enzymes, cell mass, gut growth, bile and pancreatic secretions, release of enteric hormones, and intestinal blood flow. Furthermore, oral feeding plays an important role in the formation of stool bulk, which helps to restore bowel motility.[45] Feedings may be even more critical in a patient with diarrhea, since there are heightened physiologic effects of oral ingestion. For example, intestinal disaccharidases are more sensitive to dietary substrate stimulation during experimental mannitol-induced diarrhea.[46]

Even though feedings may increase stool output and complicate the monitoring of fluid balance in infants with diarrhea, children with acute gastroenteritis who are fed recover faster and with a better body weight than those who are fasted. Oral intake may prevent dehydration in patients with gastroenteritis.[47] Oral feedings also are of value in infants who vomit. Under controlled conditions "bowel rest" was of no benefit compared to oral feedings in altering the course of the illness in patients with chronic diarrhea from inflammatory bowel disease, even when total parenteral nutrition provided all nutrients necessary for nutritional recovery.[48]

Thus fasting may be necessary in patients with diarrhea only when they cannot maintain oral intake because of either anorexia or other complications (e.g., ileus).

Oral Hydration Therapy

Oral hydration is effective regardless of the etiology, nutritional status, or severity of the diarrheal episode or the presence of vomiting. Even the most dehydrated infant with severe deficits of extracellular fluid can be improved with oral hydration and should be continued on breast milk. Parenteral therapy is best reserved for the patient with circulatory failure or CNS damage who cannot take water, salts, and calories by mouth. Also the patient with paralytic ileus or other specific complications may require IV fluids. Oral therapy may fail in the presence of high stool losses (over 10 ml/kg/hr)[49] but is beneficial with lower rates of stool losses.[47] Oral hydration solutions should be employed *to prevent dehydration*. As soon as the patient shows the first symptoms of diarrhea, oral hydration should be started to compensate for the water and electrolyte losses.

There is controversy as to the type of oral hydration to be employed. The discussion regarding solution type is based on the nature and severity of the diarrhea as well as on some practical and theoretical considerations. In a similar manner as intravenous hydration therapy is calculated, the pediatrician should calculate the exact amount of sodium and water that must be replaced by the oral hydration solutions. Deficit replacement by oral fluids, except when the dehydration is hypernatremic, should be rapid (6-8 hr if possible). Replacing deficits in the presence of large stool outputs (secretory diarrhea) requires a relatively higher sodium content of the solutions.[50] The World Health Organization (WHO) currently recommends 90 mEq of sodium/liter for use in oral hydration solutions throughout the world (Table 29-1). Although some authors believe that there should be a single preparation for all circumstances of oral rehydration, this appears to be false.[51] Either 75 or 90 mEq of sodium/liter theoretically is satisfactory as a deficit replacement for infants with severe diarrhea, but a maintenance solution with lower concentrations may be needed when the deficits are not as great or when the losses have been replaced.

In developed countries, where early intervention in diarrhea is usually the case, a lower-content sodium solution should be appropriate. In some experimental studies we have demonstrated that the solution which promotes maximum water transport across the jejunum is the one containing 60 mEq of sodium and 111 mM of glucose (2%). Based on our experimental data[52] a solution containing approximately 60 mEq/liter of sodium and no more than 111 mM/liter of glucose was found to be the most effec-

Table 29-1 Oral Rehydration Solutions and Commercial Products

	Sodium (mEq/liter)	Potassium (mEq/liter)	Chloride (mEq/liter)	Carbohydrate (g/liter)	
WHO recommendations*	90	20	80	Glucose	(20)
Pedialyte	45	20	35	Glucose	(25)
Pedialyte RS	75	20	65	Glucose	(25)
Gatorade	23	3	17	Glucose and sucrose	(59)
LyTren	50	25	45	Glucose and corn syrup	(70)
Hydra-Lyte	84	10	0	Glucose and sucrose	(24)
Cherry Koolaid†	2	0.25	7.5	Sucrose	(109)
Strawberry Jello†	12.5	0.20	0	Sucrose	(152)
Ginger ale	3.5	0.1		Sucrose and corn syrup	(90)

*Sack RB: Am J Clin Nutr **31**:2251-2257, 1978.
†Scanlon JW: Clin Pediatr **9**:508-509, 1970.

tive one. Potassium should be added to deliver about 2 mEq/kg of body weight per day, and a concentration between 15 and 30 mEq/liter of K^+ is suitable. Chloride base should be provided in a ratio of 3:1 or 4:1.

A new preparation of the WHO recommended formula has been released, substituting citrate for bicarbonate to facilitate storage, because the citrate is more stable. An exciting development in the treatment of diarrhea has been the potential to improve oral hydration solutions with substrates, such as glycine, that enhance the absorption of water and sodium from the gut and may thereby reduce the duration of the diarrhea. Also we have demonstrated[53] that alanine is the most effective amino acid in enhancing water absorption across the intestine. However, to date no clinical trials have been done with this amino acid in the oral hydration solution.

Since oral hydration solutions also contain glucose, the possibility of glucose intolerance should be kept in mind.[54] Some 5% to 8% of children with severe diarrhea may have this complication, although fewer than 1% in a clinic setting will have glucose intolerance.[54,55] Such patients do not metabolize these solutions well and excrete stools containing carbohydrates and having an acid pH. Other carbohydrates, such as sucrose, are less effective in the oral rehydration.[56] The stools are larger and correction of deficits is slower. Sucrose intolerance is more common than glucose intolerance in diarrheal disease,[23] yet sucrose (in the form of table sugar) is more readily available and cheaper than glucose and may be an appropriate substitute for the majority of patients.

To maintain water and electrolyte balance and to prevent dehydration, oral therapy should be initiated as soon as there is evidence of disease. When deficits occur, the replacement should be rapid: within 6 to 8 hours if possible, except when dehydration is of the hypernatremic variety. Fever, which often complicates the course of the illness, may increase the risk of hypernatremia, but neither fever nor high environmental temperatures affect the favorable outcome with oral therapy.[47] After dehydration is corrected with oral glucose-electrolyte solution at 125 to 150 ml/kg/day (25-50 kcal/kg), oral feedings should be advanced to formula (Table 29-2), provided stool losses are not severe.

Table 29-2 Principal Components and Cost of Proprietary Milk Formulas

	Carbohydrate (g/100 ml)	Protein (g/100 ml)	Fat (g/100 ml)	Osmolality (mM/liter)	Cost/Liter ($)
Human milk	Lactose (7)	40% casein, 60% whey solids (1.2)	Human milk fat (4)	288	26-52 (from breast-milk bank by prescription)
Cow's milk	Lactose (4.8)	80% casein, 20% whey solids (3.3)	Butterfat (3.7)	276	0.68 (L)
Enfamil 20	Lactose (7)	Nonfat cow's milk (1.5)	80% soy oil, 20% coconut oil (3.7)	286	2.33 (P), 1.70 (L), 4.70 (N)
Similac 20	Lactose (7.2)	Nonfat cow's milk	Coconut oil, soy oil (2.3)	293	1.73 (L), 6.30 (N)
Similac PM 60/40	Lactose (6.9)	Demineralized delactosed whey solids, sodium caseinate (1.6)	Coconut oil, corn oil (3.8)	279	2.33 (P)
SMA	Lactose (7.2)	Demineralized electrodialyzed whey solids, nonfat cow's milk (1.5)	Margarine, coconut, oleic (safflower), soy oils (3.6)	300	2.40 (P), 1.81 (L)
Lonalac	Lactose (4.8)	Casein (3.4)	Coconut oil (3.5)	259	—
Prosobee	Corn syrup solids (6.9)	Soy protein isolate, L-methionine (3.6)	80% soy oil, 20% coconut oil (3.6)	162	2.04 (C)
Nursoy	Sucrose (6.9)	Soy protein isolate, L-methionine (2.1)	Margarine, coconut oil (3.6)	—	1.66

Product	Carbohydrate	Protein	Fat		
Advance	Corn syrup (5.5)	Nonfat milk, soy protein isolate, taurine (2)	Soy oil, corn oil (2.7)	200	1.86
MSUD diet*	Corn syrup solids, modified tapioca starch (8.8)	Free amino acids (1.2)	Corn oil (2.8)	*	—
Product 3200 AB*	Corn syrup solids, modified tapioca starch (8.8)	Casein hydrolysate (2.1)	Corn oil (2.8)	*	—
Product 3200 K*	Corn syrup solids (6.7)	Soy protein isolate (2.1)	Corn oil, coconut oil (3.7)	*	—
Soyalac	Sucrose, corn syrup (6)	Soybean solids, L-methionine (2.1)	Soy oil (4)	275	2.12 (C)
I-Soyalac	Sucrose, tapioca dextrins (6.7)	Soy protein isolate, L-methionine (2.1)	Soy oil (3.8)	617	2.12 (C)
Isomil	Sucrose, corn syrup solids (6.8)	Soy protein isolate, L-methionine (2)	Coconut oil, soy oil (3.6)	242	2.04 (C)
Meat-base formula	Sucrose, modified tapioca starch (6.4)	Beef heart (2.9)	Sesame oil (3.4)	134	4.97 (L)
Lofenolac	84% Corn syrup solids, 16% modified tapioca starch (8.8)	Specially processed casein hydrolysate (2.2)	Corn oil (2.7)	362	4.65 (P)
Nutramigen	72% Sucrose, 28% modified tapioca starch (8.8)	Enzymatically hydrolyzed casein (2.2)	Corn oil (2.6)	481	2.90 (P)
Portagen	73% corn syrup solids, 26% sucrose, 2% other (starch, citrate) (7.8)	Sodium caseinate (2.4)	88% Medium-chain triglyceride oil, 12% corn oil (3.2)	289	2.38 (P)
Pregestimil	85% Corn syrup solids, 15% modified tapioca starch (9.1)	Enzymatically hydrolyzed casein with added L-cystine, L-tyrosine, L-tryptophan (1.9)	60% corn oil, 40% medium-chain triglyceride oil (2.7)	328	3.24 (P)
3232-A†	Modified tapioca starch (2.8)	Enzymatically hydrolyzed casein with added L-cystine, L-tyrosine, L-tryptophan (1.9)	85% Medium-chain triglyceride oil, 15% corn oil (2.7)	*	—
RCF‡	Formula base does not contain carbohydrate (0.1)	4% Soy protein isolate (4 concentrated, 2 standard dilution)	3.5% coconut oil, 3.5% soy oil, (7.0 concentrated, 3.5 standard dilution)	*	1.9 (P)

Note: Probana, Neo-Mull-Soy, and Cho-Free have been withdrawn from the market.

*These products can be obtained as a powder, liquid, nurser, or concentrate.

†To make 20 cal/oz, add 59 g of carbohydrate. Available through Mead-Johnson only (telephone 812-426-6277).

‡This product is made by Ross Laboratories and is the same as Isomil without carbohydrate. It is deficient in iron. An additional 5.3 mg of iron per liter should be supplied from other sources. The osmolality varies depending on quantity and type of carbohydrate used. Dextrose powder has twice the osmolality of table sugar. Polycose glucose polymer is the least osmolar solute of them all. Because this formula base is concentrated, water must be added in proportional amounts to keep the solution isotonic.

Feedings

Human milk. Infants fed human milk have a decreased incidence and severity of diarrhea and carbohydrate intolerance.[57] This is evident even though there is a relatively higher lactose content in human milk (approximately 7%) than in cow's milk (approximately 4%). Human milk contains other ingredients, such as bifidus factor,[58] in concentrations 50 to 100 times higher than in cow's milk. This may account for better tolerance to the lactose in human milk than in cow's milk, both in health and in disease. Moreover, human milk has immunologic advantages that may aid in the treatment of infectious diarrhea and in necrotizing enterocolitis. Other components, such as epidermal growth factor, are thought to stimulate intestinal epithelial tissues. Therefore, breast feedings should be encouraged even during diarrheal disease.

A few infants may be intolerant to human milk during diarrheal disease,[44,59] while those fed breast milk exclusively may also suffer from necrotizing enterocolitis.[60] Therefore, the pediatrician must weigh carefully the use of human milk in infants with severe diarrhea and carbohydrate intolerance.

Cow's milk. Advances in nutritional knowledge have now led to the development of nutritionally and physiologically sound infant formulas for use when breast-feeding is unsuccessful, inappropriate, or stopped early (Table 29-2). Unmodified cow's milk and evaporated milk are not recommended during the first 6 months of life, even in normal infants, since they may cause problems, such as insidious losses of blood in the gastrointestinal tract that lead to iron deficiency. When cow's milk is boiled, or when it is given to older children, this problem does not occur. The renal solute load of boiled cow's milk, which is of little significance to normal infants, may be of concern in patients with diarrheal disease because of the high extrarenal water losses. The lactose and unmodified protein may also be sources of problems in these patients.

Homemade formulas. The use of homemade formulas should be discouraged in areas where proprietary formulas are readily available. Even in hospitals, there may be insufficient dietary backup to prepare adequate homemade diets and to avoid mineral or vitamin deficiencies and other errors. In areas where proprietary formulas are not available, human breast-feedings should be attempted. Reintroduction of breast milk has been useful in the nutritional rehabilitation of infants with acute and chronic diarrhea.

Proprietary formulas. Formulas with special sources or amounts of protein, fat, or carbohydrate have been developed for infants with diarrheal disorders. These special formulas provide all known nutrients required by the infant at levels similar to those of breast milk and of formulas for normal infants, but with specific modifications needed to meet the specific needs of the infant. Most commercially available milk formulas have modified carbohydrates, proteins, and fats to allow for many of the theoretical advantages that should improve tolerance in diarrheal disease. When the carbohydrate is modified, the protein is also modified, as shown in Table 29-2. Lactose-free formulas usually provide a non–cow's milk protein source, or protein hydrolysates, and a different fat content; therefore some of the observed benefits of these formulas may be due to a variety of factors. For example, in an infant with diarrhea, a formula like Nutramigen may effectively treat both lactose intolerance and protein intolerance. However, this formula contains glucose polymers.

Pitfalls of Milk Formulas

A frequent problem in the milk-formula management of infants with diarrhea is the physician's failure to appreciate that different formulas may have the same composition and characteristics though produced by different manufacturers. Frequent formula changes may confuse the clinical course and lead to further problems. Such trials delay the diagnosis while prolonging the diarrhea and leading to further deterioration of intestinal function and clinical status.[61] Therefore formula changes should be made for specific purposes and only after a specific food intolerance has been diagnosed.

The excessive volume and/or rapid advancement of formula intake may also exacerbate diarrhea, leading the physician to conclude that the infant cannot tolerate the particular milk formula. Rather than reducing the amount being fed, the physician introduces further dietary changes, exploring for possible protein, carbohydrate, or fat intolerance. An infant who tolerates one level of formula intake but in whom diarrhea develops at a higher level needs a reduced amount of formula, not a formula change.

Diarrhea may coincide with feedings of full-strength formula after the patient tolerated half-strength. The half-strength approach to nutrition cannot be interpreted rationally, because the volumes taken by the patient may vary considerably. An infant who tolerates dilute formula but has diarrhea at a higher concentration needs a reduced osmotic load and/or volume, not a formula change.

Milk Formula Prescription

A milk formula should be prescribed in accordance with the energy derived (kcal), the volume of intake per kilogram of body weight, and the desired type and concentration of protein, carbohydrate, and fat. An intake of 75 kcal/kg/day is usually sufficient to meet maintenance energy needs and can be established in most cases of severe diarrhea within the first few days of treatment by selecting the appropriate formula. The amount and volume of proprietary milk formula are calculated to provide a proportional amount of water relative to the total energy desired. This usually remains constant (about 1 kcal/1.5 ml of formula), since the provision of nutrients without adequate amounts of fluid will result in dehydration, excessive renal solute load, and inefficient utilization of energy. Furthermore, hyperosmolality of the oral solutions may contribute to diarrhea and other complications such as necrotizing enterocolitis. Therefore a solution of 150 ml of fluid/100 kcal is mandatory, particularly in infants with diarrhea. Increased caloric content should be avoided, even if the patient is underweight, until the diarrhea is controlled.

The amount and frequency of formula feeding may also influence the response. Constant nasogastric administration of a specific milk formula may facilitate the initial stages of nutritional treatment in the very ill malnourished patient, particularly during the anorectic phase of the illness,[62] but feedings by mouth at regular intervals should be given once the patient recovers appetite.

The quantity of formula should be related to the evolution of the disease. Initially, only maintenance energy requirements are attempted. Thereafter, the formula intake may be increased gradually in infants who tolerate oral feedings and who have moderate to milk stool losses (30-50 g/kg/day); the fluid balance is maintained by intravenous fluids and electrolytes. Of equal importance is the character of the stools. Improvement in consistency should allow an advancement in the diet. The number of stools can be misleading, however, and should not be used as a guide in formula changes. It is unrealistic to expect early weight improvement (except that induced by correcting dehydration) as long as diarrheal disease is not improving. In these patients partial peripheral intravenous nutrient supplements can be a useful early adjunct. Very sick infants may benefit from intravenous amino acids or fat when diarrhea is expected to be prolonged and when oral feedings cannot be sustained. However, it is difficult to justify a central venous line and total parenteral hyperalimentation if maintenance energy requirements can be provided as just described. Infection is a major complication and cause of death in patients given central lines. Moreover, an abrupt change to oral feedings may complicate nutritional therapy, which may be precipitated by fever and removal of the catheter.

Formula Selection

Although most patients with diarrhea will respond to cow's milk formula, this may need to be changed in relation to the clinical evolution of the case. Protein and/or carbohydrate intolerance is a primary indication for dietary treatment. As soon as the offending food is identified, it should be eliminated from the diet. This usually results in prompt improvement of diarrhea. Listed in Table 29-2 are the various common milk formulas available in the United States for treatment of specific protein and/or carbohydrate intolerance.

Protein derived from soybean, meat, or chicken has been found useful in treating cow's milk protein hypersensitivity.[22,61] These formulas are often considered to be "hypoallergenic." This is a misconception, since they merely contain a protein source other than cow's milk and may induce further protein intolerance in a susceptible host. Indeed, infants often exhibit multiple food protein sensitivities. Formulas that provide protein hydrolysates instead of whole protein are indicated for patients with severe diarrheal disease resulting from protein intolerance. This type of formula may also avoid multiple food proteins. It is not necessary to use formulas composed entirely of mixtures of free amino acids as the protein source. Sufficient amounts of cytosolic peptidases usually are preserved in the intestinal epithelium to digest, absorb, and tolerate protein hydrolysates. In addition, mixtures of amino acids may be dangerous since they increase the osmolality of the formula and compete for transport mechanisms with other nutrients and with each other.

Infants who have lactose intolerance must be fed a milk formula that contains a disaccharide other than lactose as the carbohydrate source (Table 29-2). Patients who have generalized disaccharide intolerance should be treated with a disaccharide-free formula that contains glucose (dextrose) and/or a combination of glucose polymers. The polymers are very useful in diarrheal disease and can be prepared by an acid enzyme hydrolysis of cornstarch, which yields small amounts of glucose and a variety of glucose polymers. The polymers are attached by a 1,4-glycosidic bond and have a molecular weight of approximately 1000, resulting in a lower osmotic load than would be seen with the equivalent amount of free glucose. They are absorbed directly from the intestine, without the need for special enzyme cleavage during digestion and absorption, since intestinal maltase rapidly hydrolyzes glycose to glucose for absorption. Thus medium-chain glucose polymers offer dietary advantages without the effects (i.e., hyperosmolality) of simple glucose in the formula.

Carbohydrate-free formulas should be reserved for patients who continue to have diarrhea and monosaccharide intolerance. Carbohydrate-free feedings are not without danger: hypoglycemia may ensue as a severe complication during the acute stage or after recovery.[54] Utmost care should be exercised to provide parenteral glucose throughout the time these infants are not fed carbohydrates. Fructose may be added to the formulas of patients with congenital glucose-galactose malabsorption. However, patients with acquired monosaccharide intolerance do not tolerate any carbohydrate, including monosaccharides such as fructose. In fact, the degree of intestinal malabsorption of fructose is more marked, and the intolerance more severe, in those patients since their intestinal permeability is altered by the infectious process that triggers the illness.[23,31] Therefore fructose should be avoided in infectious diarrhea.

Steatorrhea in infants with diarrhea may be due to a failure of micellar solubilization; it can be severe and often prolonged.[63] Consequently medium-chain triglycerides are often desirable in a formula as long as sufficient long-chain fats are used to meet the requirements for essential fatty acids. Most proprietary formulas now provide 1% to 2% of the total energy intake from these sources. Low-fat formulas have no role in the treatment of diarrheal disease, since the fecal energy loss caused by the steatorrhea is transient whereas the limitation of fat intake may lead to chronic persistent diarrhea and malnutrition.[36]

Duration of Treatment

Special formulas should be used only as long as the intolerance lasts. It may subside within a few days or may last for some months after the improvement of diarrhea, with complete disappearance after the child grows older. Therefore, once the diarrhea and body weight improve, these infants should be tested to determine whether they have overcome their intolerance and can be upgraded to one of the conventional milk formulas.[64] An increased number of more complex proteins and carbohydrates may be given soon afterwards. As soon as glucose is tolerated, disaccharides may be introduced; first maltose, then sucrose, and finally lactose. Even patients with severe carbohydrate intolerance following gastroenteritis tolerate lactose within a few weeks of the acute stage of the illness.[61] Prolonged use of vegetable proteins (soy) as the main protein source may result in other nutritional complications (e.g., rickets, carnitine deficiency). Similarly the elimination of dietary carbohydrates for prolonged periods may in itself perpetuate altered absorption of carbohydrates or other nutrients.[46]

Severe Diarrhea

Since intact proteins and lactose in cow's milk can be harmful in diarrheal disease, particularly in infants, formulas that provide protein hydrolysates and are lactose-free have been recommended as the initial treatment for all patients with severe diarrheal disease, unless breast milk is available. The Committee on Nutrition of the American Academy of Pediatrics[65] has recommended a lactose-free diet as the initial feeding for malnourished children with severe diarrhea. These feedings should be instituted, even when there is no proof of lactose intolerance, since malnourished patients are likely to be at a high risk of having this complication. Lactose feedings may lead to more problems than dietary treatment with an alternate carbohydrate source. In infants less than 1 year of age with severe gastroenteritis, initial feeding of lactose-free formula may reduce the duration and severity of the diarrhea.[66] Therefore infants with a short diarrheal course who are not being breast-fed may be given a lactose-free formula. However, those with a prolonged diarrheal course, who usually have a generalized disaccharide intolerance, should be treated with a disaccharide-free formula; once the diarrhea improves, a gradual upgrading to a normal milk formula can be attempted.[61]

There are few data to justify recommending protein hydrolysates as substitutes for cow's milk protein in all infants with severe diarrheal disease. In a large prospective study of patients with severe diarrheal disease[23] the majority improved on a formula with casein as the protein source plus appropriate carbohydrates. Little or no advantage has been demonstrated in using casein hydrolysate formulas for severe diarrhea and malnutrition.[67,68] However, we have reported[61] a declining incidence of acquired monosaccharide intolerance–intractable diarrhea of infancy in the United States, which occurred coincidentally with pediatricians' increased and more rapid use of nutritional rehabilitation of sick infants. It appears that increased feedings of lactose-free protein hydrolysate formulas to patients with diarrhea have been associated with a decline in the number of patient referrals to pediatric gastroenterologists as well as a decrease in the number of patients who have severe chronic diarrhea. This observation is in agreement with the concept of early aggressive nutritional rehabilitation of infants with diarrhea, which we have recommended for a number of years.

Dietary Intake

In older infants and children with diarrheal disease, milk formulas must be supplemented by other foods. The general principles for these dietary supplements should be the same as those applied to formula feedings: a rational approach to introducing specific amounts and types of foods. All too often, simple foods such as broth, gruel, dry toast, apples, bananas, and tea are prescribed, without regard for the energy needs of the patient. In some areas it has been popular to prescribe a "BRATT" diet (based on bananas, rice, applesauce, toast, and tea). The usual portion provides about 1300 calories for an adult—with 317 g of carbohydrate, 15 g of protein, and 3 g of fat. This is hardly a normal intake for human beings, however, and may lead to several detrimental consequences (as described on the preceding pages). Furthermore, the diet is low in energy, nitrogen, and fat but high in carbohydrate and caffeine (75-150 mg/cup of tea), which may perpetuate diarrhea and malnutrition. Nevertheless, it has been advocated on the basis of improvement in stools because of its high pectin content.* The lack of value of such improved stools is beyond the scope of this chapter.

A low-residue diet often is advocated to decrease the frequency and volume of stools, whereas bran is used to increase stool bulk and help restore bowel motility.[45] Dietary fiber also protects the intestine from the strain of defecation, and this may be important in dysenteric diarrhea when small-volume stools are excreted. The use of 25 to 36 g of bran per day may decrease the symptoms of cramping and bowel discomfort[69] although nondigestible bran fiber may cause more flatulence and abdominal distention because of methane production.

Therefore a nutritious well-balanced diet that contains easily digestible material is recommended and should be given in accordance with the needs, likes, and tolerances of the patient once the anorectic phase of the illness improves. If the diarrhea becomes chronic, dietary restriction may have more disadvantages than a normal diet in patients who do not have specific food intolerances. To avoid deficiencies, the diet should provide adequate amounts of all nutrients. The needs are usually increased because of stool losses and higher requirements during diarrhea.

FINAL CONSIDERATIONS

The aforementioned data linking nutritional practices with diarrheal diseases raise several issues. Clearly, preventing the disease through proper food preservation and preparation and thorough improvement of sanitary conditions

---

*Three apples per day yield approximately 2.8 g of pectin, and three bananas about 3.3 g. These quantities are not high compared to those in Kaopectate medication, which contains 130 mg of pectin and 5850 mg of kaolin per ounce.

and refrigeration facilities is of paramount importance. This would automatically result in improved nutritional practices and decreased rates of diarrheal disease and could be achieved by simple measures (e.g., reducing the transmission of pathogens that cause diarrhea and so too reducing the incidence and mortality rate). Since all major diarrhea pathogens are transmitted by the fecal-oral route, measures to reduce transmission must emphasize the traditional triad of improved water supply, improved excretion disposal, and improved domestic and food hygiene. These simple measures may reduce the incidence and mortality rate of diarrhea by 20% to 40%. To strengthen the ability of a child to cope with an infection and to reduce the risk of severe disease and death, breast-feeding, good weaning practices, and certain vaccinations are needed. Recommending that all infants be breast-fed may be at present the most expedient and readily available means of reducing the incidence and severity of diarrheal disease and its complications in childhood but is unlikely to solve the problem in the general population, because of the myriad of etiologies. Unfortunately, the epidemic-like clusters of enteric disease produced by a particular infectious agent will continue to strike the vulnerable patient. Nutritional rehabilitation will continue to be a challenge for all involved in caring for these patients.

The nutritional treatment of patients with diarrhea always will pose a dilemma to the physician: Whereas restricting food may improve diarrhea and reduce stool loss, albeit at the expense of malnutrition and other complications, efforts to meet the patient's nutritional requirements may introduce risks even greater than those of insufficient nutrients. Clinicians therefore should aim at meeting the nutritional needs of the patient safely and effectively during the acute phase of diarrhea in accordance with the patient's clinical course. The recommendations to restrict dietary intake of milk ingredients may be feasible in some areas but impossible where proprietary formulas are not readily available. Moreover, valuable recommendations for a specific patient may at present be impossible to implement on an epidemiologic global scale.

The clinical answer of diet elimination is easy if proprietary formulas are available, but it may be expensive. In Table 29-2 the costs per liter of various formulas are compared. Cost should be considered when prescribing a formula for an individual patient and when making public health recommendations. Furthermore, it should be kept in mind that when changes are made other problems usually are created—for example, cow's milk substitutes, such as soy, also may be highly allergenic. Lactose hydrolysis of cow's milk by commercially available lactase may affect cost, taste, or osmolality; on the other hand, breast-feedings, which are ideal for infants, are not readily available for all.

REFERENCES

1. Mata L: Breast feeding, diarrheal disease, and malnutrition in less developed countries. In Lifshitz F, editor: Clinical disorders in pediatric nutrition, New York, 1982, Marcel Dekker Inc, pp 355-372.
2. Barness LA: Breast milk for all, N Engl J Med **297:**939-941, 1977.
3. Darke SJ: Human milk versus cow's milk, J Hum Nutr **30:**233-238, 1976.
4. Turnbull PCB: Food poisoning with special reference to salmonella. Its epidemiology, pathogenesis, and control. In Lambert HP, editor: Infections of the gastrointestinal tract, Clin Gastroenterol **8:**663-714, 1979.
5. Morse DL, et al: Widespread outbreaks of clam and oyster-associated gastroenteritis—role of Norwalk virus, N Engl J Med **314:**678-681, 1986.
6. Kuritsky JN, et al: Norwalk gastroenteritis: a community outbreak associated with bakery product consumption, Ann Intern Med **100:**519-521, 1984.
7. Gorbach SL, et al: Traveler's diarrhea and toxigenic *Escherichia coli*, N Engl J Med **292:**933-936, 1975.
8. Van Den Brock MJM, et al: Occurrence of *Vibrio parahaemolyticus* in Dutch mussels, Appl Environ Microbiol **37:**438-442, 1979.
9. Gill CO: A review: Intrinsic bacteria in meat, J Appl Bacteriol **47:**367-378, 1979.
10. Barnes EM: The intestinal microflora of poultry and game birds during life and after storage, J Appl Bacteriol **46:**407-419, 1979.
11. Kohl S: *Yersinia enterocolitica* infections in children, Pediatr Clin North Am **26:**433-443, 1979.
12. Agger WA: Diarrhea associated with *Aeromonas hydrophila*, Pediatr Infect Dis **5**(suppl):S106-S108, 1986.
13. Wittner M: Protozoan diarrheas: dientamoebiasis and giardiasis. In Lifshitz F, editor: Clinical disorders in pediatric gastroenterology and nutrition, New York, 1980, Marcel Dekker Inc, pp 315-323.
14. Taylor JP, et al: Cryptosporidiosis outbreak in a day care center, Am J Dis Child **139:**1023-1025, 1985.
15. Jokipu L, et al: Cryptosporidiosis associated with traveling and giardiasis, Gastroenterology **89:**838-847, 1985.
16. Navin TR, Juranck DD: Cryptosporidiosis: clinical epidemiologic and parasitologic review, Rev Infect Dis **3:**313-327, 1984.
17. Mata L: Cryptosporidium and other protozoa in diarrheal disease in less developed countries, Pediatr Infec Dis **5:**5117-5130, 1986.

18. Botulism—United States, 1979-80, Morbid Mortal Weekly Rep **30**(10)121-123, 1981.

19. Bagnis R, et al: Clinical observations on 3,009 cases of ciguatera (fish poisoning) in the South Pacific, Am J Trop Med Hyg **28**:1067-1073, 1979.

20. Samsahl K, Wester PO: Metallic contamination of food during preparation and storage: Development of methods and some preliminary results, Sci Total Environ **8**:165-177, 1977.

21. Oser BL: Natural toxicants in foods, J Am Pharm Assoc **17**:121-123, 1977.

22. Lifshitz F: Carbohydrate malabsorption. In Lifshitz F, editor: Clinical disorders in pediatric gastroenterology and nutrition, New York, 1980, Marcel Dekker Inc, pp 229-247.

23. Lifshitz F, et al: Carbohydrate intolerance in infants with diarrhea, J Pediatr **79**:760-767, 1971.

24. Eastham EJ, Walker WA: Effect of cow's milk on the gastrointestinal tract: a persistent dilemma for the pediatrician, Pediatrics **60**:477-481, 1977.

25. Gerrard JW, et al: Cow's milk allergy: prevalence and manifestations in an unselected series of newborns, Acta Paediatr Scand (suppl) **234**:1-21, 1973.

26. Jakobssen I, Lindberg T: A prospective study of cow's milk protein intolerance in Swedish infants, Acta Paediatr Scand **68**:853-859, 1979.

27. Stintzing G, Zetterstrom R: Cow's milk allergy; incidence and pathogenic role of early exposure to cow's milk formula, Acta Paediatr Scand **68**:383-387, 1979.

28. Kolulkko A: IgA deficiency and infantile atopy, Lancet **2**:668-669, 1973.

29. Falchuk ZM, Strober W: Gluten sensitive enteropathy systems of antigliadin antibody in vitro, Gut **15**:947-952, 1974.

30. Kumar V, et al: Carbohydrate intolerance associated with acute gastroenteritis, Clin Pediatr **16**:1123-1127, 1977.

31. Lifshitz F: Enteric flora in childhood disease—diarrhea, Am J Clin Nutr **30**:1811-1818, 1977.

32. Holmes IH, et al: Is lactase the receptor and uncoating enzyme for infantile enterits (rota) viruses? Lancet **1**:1387-1388, 1976.

33. Iyngkaran N, Abdin Z: Intolerance to food proteins. In Lifshitz F, editor: Clinical disorders in pediatric nutrition, New York, 1982, Marcel Dekker Inc, pp 449-483.

34. Walker-Smith JA: Cow's milk protein intolerance in infancy. In Chandra RK, editor: Food intolerances, New York, 1984, Elsevier Science Publishing Co Inc, pp 119-136.

35. Walker WA: Role of the mucosal barrier in toxin/microbial attachment to the gastrointestinal tract, Ciba Found Symp **112**:34-56, 1985.

36. Cohen SA, Chronic nonspecific diarrhea. Dietary relationship, Pediatrics **64**:402-407, 1979.

37. Greene LG, Tazz KG: Excessive fluid intake as a cause of chronic diarrhea, J Pediatr **102**:836-840, 1983.

38. Krause MV, Mahan LK: Nutritional care for patients with intestinal disease. In Food, nutrition, and diet therapy, Philadelphia, 1979, WB Saunders Co, pp 484-503.

39. Lugo-de Rivera C, et al: Studies on the mechanism of sugar malabsorption in infantile infectious diarrhea, Am J Clin Nutr **25**:1248-1253, 1972.

39a. Dupont HL, et al: Immunity in shigellosis. II. Protection induced by oral live vaccine or primary infection, J Infect Dis **125**:12-16, 1972.

39b. Beisel WR: Metabolic effects of infection, Progr Food Nutr Sci **8**:43-75, 1983.

39c. Dodge JA, et al: Toddler diarrhea and prostaglandins, Arch Dis Child **56**:705-707, 1981.

40. Coello-Ramirez P, et al: Pneumatosis intestinalis, Am J Dis Child **120**:3-9, 1970.

41. DePerger E, Walker-Smith J: Cow's milk intolerance as necrotizing enterocolitis, Helvet Paediatr Acta **32**:507-515, 1977.

42. Lifshitz F: Necrotizing enterocolitis and feedings. In Lifshitz F, editor: Clinical disorders in pediatric nutrition, New York, 1982, Marcel Dekker Inc, pp 513-530.

43. Teichberg S: Penetration of epithelial barriers by macromolecules: the intestinal mucosa. In Lifshitz F, editor: Clinical disorders in pediatric gastroenterology and nutrition, New York, 1980, Marcel Dekker Inc, pp 185-202.

44. Goel K, et al: Monosaccharide intolerance and soy protein hypersensitivity in an infant with diarrhea, J Pediatr **93**:617-619, 1978.

45. Painter NS: The high fiber diet in the treatment of diverticular disease of the colon, Postgrad Med J **50**:629-635, 1974.

46. Pergolizzi R, et al: Interaction between dietary carbohydrates and intestinal disaccharidase in experimental diarrhea, Am J Clin Nutr **30**:482-489, 1977.

47. Hirschhorn N: The treatment of acute diarrhea in children: a historical and physiological perspective, Am J Clin Nutr **33**:637-663, 1980.

48. Dickinson RJ, et al: Controlled trial of intravenous hyperalimentation and total bowel rest as an adjunct to the routine therapy of acute colitis, Gastroenterology **70**:1199-1204, 1980.

49. Palmer DL, et al: Comparison of sucrose and glucose in the oral electrolyte therapy of cholera and other severe diarrheas, N Engl J Med **297**:1107-1110, 1977.

50. Finberg L: Water and electrolyte alterations in diarrheal disease and malnutrition. In Lifshitz F, editor: Clinical disorders in pediatric nutrition, New York, 1982, Marcel Dekker Inc, pp 427-437.

51. Nichols BL, Soriano HA: A critique of oral therapy of dehydration due to diarrheal syndromes, Am J Clin Nutr **30**:1457-1472, 1977.

52. Lifshitz F, Wapnir RA: Oral hydration solutions: experimental optimization of water and sodium absorption, J Pediatr **106**:383-389, 1985.

53. Wapnir RA, et al: Oral hydration solutions (OHS): effectiveness of alanine in a model of osmotic diarrhea, Pediatr Res **20**:252A, 1986.

54. Lifshitz F, et al: Monosaccharide intolerance and hypoglycemia in infants with diarrhea. I. Clinical course of 23 infants, J Pediatr **77**:595-603, 1970.

55. Hirschhorn N, et al: Ad-libitum oral glucose-electrolyte therapy for acute diarrhea in Apache children, J Pediatr **83**:562-571, 1973.

56. Malin DR, et al: Comparison of sucrose with glucose in oral therapy of infant diarrhea, Lancet **2**:277-279, 1978.

57. Okuni M, et al: Studies on reducing sugars in stools of acute infantile diarrhea, with special reference to differences between breast fed and artificially fed babies, Tohoku J Exp Med **107**:395-402, 1972.

58. Gyorgy P: Hitherto unrecognized biochemical difference between human milk and cow's milk, Pediatrics **11**:98-108, 1953.

59. King F: Intolerance to lactose in mother's milk, Lancet **2**:335, 1972.

60. Moriarty RR, et al: Necrotizing enterocolitis and human milk, J Pediatr **94**:295-296, 1979.

61. Lifshitz F: Nutrition for special needs in infancy. In Lifshitz F, editor: Nutrition for special needs in infancy, New York, 1985, Marcel Dekker Inc, pp 1-10.

62. Green HL, et al: Protracted diarrhea and malnutrition in infancy: changes in intestinal morphology and disaccharidase activities during treatment with total intravenous nutrition or oral elemental diets, J Pediatr **87**:695-704, 1975.

63. Jonas A, et al: Disturbed fat absorption following infectious gastroenteritis in children, J Pediatr **95**:366-372, 1979.

64. Lifshitz F, et al: Response of infants to carbohydrate loads after recovery from diarrhea, J Pediatr **79**:612-617, 1971.

65. Barness LA, editor: Pediatric nutrition handbook, Evanston Ill, 1979, American Academy of Pediatrics.

66. Dagan R, et al: Lactose-free formula for infantile diarrhea, [letter], Lancet **1**:207, 1980.

67. MacLean WC, et al: Nutritional management of chronic diarrhea and malnutrition: primary reliance on oral feeding, J Pediatr **97**:316-322, 1980.

68. Graham GG, et al: Lactose-free medium-chain triglyceride formulas in severe malnutrition, Am J Dis Child **126**:330-335, 1973.

69. Brodribb AJM, Humphreys DM: Diverticular disease: three studies. Part I—Relation to other disorders and fiber intake; Part II—Treatment with bran; Part III—Metabolic effect of bran in patients with diverticular disease, Br Med J **1**:424-430, 1976.

CHAPTER 30
Diseases of Aging

Howard N. Jacobson

A characteristic of our time is the increasing prevalence of older persons in society. Indeed the elderly constitute its fastest-growing segment. At present, more than 1 in 10 Americans are 65 years of age or older* (nearly 60% of these are women), and the proportion over 65 will remain high for the rest of the twentieth century.[1] In this chapter the elderly segment of the population is arbitrarily defined as those over 65 years of age (with due regard to the heterogeneity of the group). Today's growing challenge in health and nutritional care, therefore, is to confront the diseases and handicaps of elderly persons and the aging process itself with an eye toward enabling more individuals to face the inevitable, not just in the "usual" manner but "successfully."[2]

Aging is often accompanied by the emergence of various disease states, some of which are so common as to be considered more disorders than diseases (e.g., osteoporosis, cataracts, gastric atrophy). The effects of various disease states and aging disorders on the nutritional status of the older person can be devastating. Elderly people often suffer an array of disabilities, and a complete workup and diagnosis may take several hours (but seldom will be reimbursable).[4]

Prolonged hospitalization is not uncommon with older persons, and their nutritional status in all likelihood declines during such confinements, just as it has been shown to do with younger patients.[5] Added to the problem of physical disability and disease in aging are the problems of social isolation and depression, following the loss of a spouse and friends in death, and rejection by the younger generation. The lack of social integration and of the opportunity to play a useful role in society often leads to anorexia and decreased food intake. Compounding these prob-

lems, the loss of teeth, ill-fitting dentures, and a declining and altered sense of taste or smell have frequently been cited as factors promoting decreased intakes of food. Older people often report tasting substances as bitter or sour, which makes eating an unpleasant experience.[3] Thus both physical and mental factors arise in old age that can have an important impact on the dietary intake and nutritional status of the older person.

The reported dietary intakes, derived from the National Institutes of Health Lipid Research Clinic population studies in elderly men and women contrasted with younger individuals, are presented in Table 30-1.[6]

Additionally in the elderly, medication and ethanol intake and their effects on appetite and the absorption and metabolism of nutrients are a problem. In one study[7] the nutritional status of hospitalized elderly patients with chronic obstructive pulmonary disease was found to be as bad as that of patients with cancer. This may have been due in part to the large number of drugs these patients were given (in another survey the average number taken daily was seven), with the consequential effect of depressed appetite and altered metabolism of essential nutrients.[8]

Despite the foregoing litany of problems, there is also an increasing amount of information pertaining to the way many persons overcome the challenges of growing old, and thus it is additionally important that we in the health care professions distinguish clearly between "usual" and "successful" aging.*

COMMON HEALTH PROBLEMS OF THE ELDERLY

Only 5% of persons over the age of 65 are in nursing homes or other institutions. Indeed, most

---

*Of added note is the recent finding (Bidlack) that in 1986 there were some 37,000 persons over 100!

*Rowe JW, Kahn RL: Human ageing: usual and successful, Science **237**:143-149, 1987.

Table 30-1 Dietary Intake in the United States

	Men (yr)			Women (yr)		
	20-24	50-54	70+	20-24	50-54	70+
Calories/day	3335	2541	1933	2101	1688	1548
Calories/kg/day	45.7	31.7	26.2	35.7	26.7	25.8
Protein (% of cal)	13.7	15.8	15.0	15.1	16.5	15.9
Carbohydrate (% of cal)	43.5	39.7	43.0	43.1	41.2	44.9
Starch (% of cal)	17.1	18.3	19.5	17.2	17.3	18.2
Sucrose	10.7	7.7	6.1	10.1	7.5	7.4
Saturated fat (% of cal)	14.9	15.1	13.4	15.0	14.0	13.5
Monounsaturated fat (% of cal)	15.3	15.5	14.6	15.1	14.6	14.0
Polyunsaturated fat (% of cal)	6.0	6.5	6.7	6.9	7.0	6.4
Cholesterol (mg/da)	481	468	372	355	314	285
Alcohol* (% of cal)	10.3	10.2	10.3	8.3	13.0	12.1

Based on Lipid Research Clinic population studies data book. Vol II. The prevalence study—nutrient intake (NIH Publ 82-2014), Bethesda Md, 1982, National Institutes of Health.
*Intake among drinkers only.

of the noninstitutionalized elderly describe themselves as in fair to good health.[2] The relative importance of nutrition in the clinical management of elderly patients may be judged from the incidence of nutrition-related complaints. In a study of 374 residents of a retirement center who were described as financially secure, educated, and having received good medical care all of their lives,[9] the frequencies of disorders commonly seen were as follows: Cardiovascular complaints accounted for 13% of physician visits; another 13% were accounted for by muscle, tendon, joint, and bone disorders. This figure was thought to understate the prevalence of these problems, inasmuch as it referred only to patients with significant impairments. Most patients have some osteoarthritis, and most are noted to accept it as a fact of long life. About 11% of office visits were for skin problems, about 9% were for urinary tract diseases, about 15% were prompted by the need for an annual checkup or screening session, 5% were for problems with vision and hearing, 5% for respiratory problems, 10% for gastrointestinal disturbances, and the remainder (classified as miscellaneous) were for overt emotional problems (mostly depressive) and, finally, chronic alcoholism (which had about the same prevalence as might be found in any adult population of comparable background and affluence). Thus almost half of these complaints might have had a nutritional component.

The diseases resulting from malnutrition as well as the disorders influenced by nutrition are listed in Table 30-2.[10]

Table 30-2 Diseases and Nutritional Disorders in the Elderly

Resulting from Malnutrition	Influenced by Nutrition
Iron-deficiency anemia	Cardiovascular diseases
Macrocytic anemias	Diabetes
Folic acid deficiency	Hypertension
Vitamin B_{12} deficiency	Osteoporosis
Specific nutrient deficiency	
Avitaminoses	
Protein deficiency	
Underweight (caloric deficiency)	
Overweight (caloric excess)	

From Lamy PP: Clin Nutr **2**:9-14, 1983.

DIGESTION, ABSORPTION, AND METABOLISM IN AGING

The efficiency of digestion and absorption of nutrients by the aged gut is an area in need of study. Fecal fat levels have been shown to be high among elderly persons,[11,12] but the pathophysiology behind this phenomenon is unclear. Decreased secretion of pancreatic enzymes, inefficient intraluminal mixing of fat with bile and pancreatic enzymes, and bacterial overgrowth may be partial explanations. However, the effect of declining blood flow to the small intestine must also be considered. The effect of poor blood circulation on the ability of the intestinal epithelial cells to synthesize brush border enzymes or passively or actively to absorb nutrients is unclear. It was demonstrated[13,14] that the aged gut has a reduced mucosal surface area and the time taken for cells to travel from the crypt to the villous tip is prolonged. However, correlations with gut function in terms of absorption were not made.

Gastric atrophy is a relatively common problem among the elderly, occurring in about 30% of those over the age of 60.[15] Investigations in people ranging from 15 to 65 years of age [16] have demonstrated a yearly increase in the frequency of atrophic gastritis of 1.25%. The effect of relative hypochlorhydria on absorption of certain nutrients (e.g., iron, folate) is mainly speculative. Since a higher intraluminal pH in the small intestine is known to inhibit the absorption of folic acid, possibly hypochlorhydria in the elderly leads to a more basic pH in the proximal duodenum and impairment in the folate absorption.[17] It is notable that low serum levels of folate are common among the elderly, occurring in about 20% of apparently healthy aged persons living in a United Kingdom community.[18] Among poor black old people in Florida,[19] 60% were found to have low red blood cell folate levels. The impact of changes in the aging gut on nutritional status of the elderly must be understood before more rational recommended dietary allowances can be established for this age group.

In addition to lack of knowledge of gut function in aging, there is an equal ignorance of nutritional metabolism in aging. One investigation [20] has shown that the aged kidney is less responsive to parathyroid hormone in terms of stimulating 1,25-dihydroxyvitamin D synthesis. This may be a factor (among many) leading to the development of osteoporosis in the elderly. There is very little known about how aging affects the metabolism of other vitamins. Absorption of vitamin A appears to increase in rats as the animals get older.[21] However, nothing is known about the aged liver's ability to handle an increased load of this vitamin. If the aging liver has reduced uptake and storage capacity for vitamin A, it is possible that toxicity with vitamin A might be a problem in the elderly, especially in those 30%-40% of elderly Americans who take vitamin supplements routinely.[22] In the case of vitamin C, it is not clear whether supplementation with ascorbate is of clinical use in the elderly—even among people with lower than normal white blood cell levels. In one study[23]

supplementation with 80 mg of ascorbate/day over and above that contained in the diet was needed in old people to attain white cell ascorbate levels equivalent to those of younger people. This result implies a problem in getting vitamin C across the white cell membrane. However, no clinical benefits have been demonstrated for the vitamin C–supplemented elderly. It is possible that subclinical deficiency of vitamin C over long periods may be detrimental; further work is needed to document such effects before recommending a rise in the dietary requirement for vitamin C in the older age group.

Changes in metabolism of macronutrients with aging are also a fruitful area of study. Preliminary work[24] has suggested that old people may need higher protein intakes to maintain nitrogen balance. Certainly they require a more carefully selected nutrient-dense diet because of their decreased energy expenditure.

SKELETAL DISORDERS AND LOSS OF MOBILITY

Most elderly patients have some degree of osteoarthritis, and most accept it, even if it is symptomatic, as a part of growing old. In women osteoporosis frequently presents with pain from compression and overt fracture of the dorsal and lumbar vertebrae. A disproportionately large percentage of femoral neck damage is due to minor falls with a twisting motion. Sit-down injuries, such as pelvic fractures, with poorly localized pain, are frequently encountered. By the ages of 70 to 80 years, men catch up with women in the frequency of osteoporosis. More often than in women, in men the fracture site is the femur, not the vertebrae[9]; and if the spine is involved, carcinoma of the prostate must be considered before a diagnosis of osteoporosis is made with certainty. In both men and women with osteoporosis, the diagnosis of Paget's disease must be entertained. Experience has shown that, by themselves, most skeletal problems are likely to be accepted but when combined with vision and hearing deficits that impede activities on which elderly persons thrive, such as reading, watching television, or writing, they bring out sensitivities to physical symptoms that otherwise might have been ignored.[9] Loss of mobility also seriously restricts the opportunities for the elderly to do comparison shopping and limits their food selection, which further impacts on their diets.

Some loss of bone is now being seen as an inevitable part of human aging: by the fifth decade, bone loss is a general phenomenon, that progresses faster in women than in men.[25] Indeed, it has been suggested[26] that the amount of bone found in old age is related to the amount present in early adult life and not to the level of subsequent calcium intake. Nevertheless, reports abound[27] that calcium supplements have led to increased calcium retention, with some relief of symptoms.

It has long been known that inactivity, immobilization, and weightlessness all are accompanied by loss of bone mass; however, only recently has the converse situation—increased activity, exercise, and weight-bearing—been recognized as promoting the accumulation of bone mass. Thus, in the last several years it has been shown[28] that (1) exercise is beneficial in elderly postmenopausal women and (2) women who have been active throughout their lives develop less osteoporosis than do similarly aged sedentary ones. The synergistic effects of exercise and calcium supplementation have been convincingly demonstrated in clinical trials utilizing densitometry as a more sensitive means to measure change.[29] All these findings lead to the conclusion that the most effective long-term approach begins with efforts to acquire as much bone mass as possible before menopause and to maintain it thereafter.[30] Measures to be used include regular weight-bearing exercises and a varied diet that contains 1-1.5 g of calcium/day.[28]

MUSCLE MASS

Both muscular strength and the total mass of muscle decline with age. Usually muscle mass is replaced by fat tissue, and thus the percent of total body weight attributable to lean body mass diminishes relative to that represented by fat. On average, in men the lean body mass decreases regularly from about 60 kg at age 25 to less than 50 by the age of 65 to 70; in women it is preserved in the range of 40 kg from the ages of 25 to 55, with a diminution to 35 kg in the age range 65 to 70.[31]

It has long been held that an adequate intake of all nutrients, with an emphasis on protein, and physical activity are essential ingredients of any program designed to maintain the mass of lean body tissue. More recently it has been shown

that exercise training reduces body fat and increases lean body mass. Thus, on average, an active exercise program of 4 months' duration might be expected to decrease total body weight by approximately 1%, decrease body fat stores by 4% to 10%, and increase lean body mass by around 1%.[32]

CARDIOVASCULAR DISEASES

The chief causes of death in the United States are those associated with cardiovascular disease, and arteriosclerotic heart disease is the most frequent cardiac problem encountered among elderly persons. Coronary heart disease underlies about half the cases of congestive heart failure. Atrial fibrillation and other arrhythmias may often be due to difficulties in controlling digitalis or diuretic dosage or too little potassium replacement.[9] The dietary management of these patients continues to be nonspecific; and for patients seeking relief from dyspnea, edema, orthopnea, weakness, or angina, a careful regimen of rest, drug therapy, and diet control may prove effective. The diet should be designed to maintain normal weight. Any anemia or other oxygen-restricting condition(s) should be treated vigorously. Patients' activities, including scheduled bed rest, carefully planned walks, and sedentary periods following meals and prior to exercise, should be scheduled in accordance with their cardiac capacities.

In a careful study performed in the Netherlands[33] on some 40 people in the tenth decade of life, total caloric and total protein intakes were found to be in line with general recommendations—specifically, for men 75 years old and older, about 2000 kcal/day and, for women, 1600 kcal/day. The protein intakes in these elderly people averaged 68 g/day for men and 56 g/day for women, which were in line with Dutch recommendations but would be considerably more than the present-day RDAs for adults in the United States. The total fat intake was higher for both sexes, at the cost of carbohydrates, whereas the intake of polyunsaturated fats was far below that recommended and of cholesterol relatively above, especially for men. A selectional bias in this study existed insofar as the diet of these elderly people was determined by the central kitchens in the two homes in which they lived, although it generally followed the dietary pattern of the population at large.

The findings about cholesterol in this study were surprising. Despite the high fat intake and the relatively high dietary cholesterol levels in both men and women, the mean values of total cholesterol were much lower than those reported in most middle-aged Western population groups. One key question that remained unanswered was whether this low total cholesterol level constituted an aging trend or had been present for decades. Furthermore, the study revealed no relation between plasma cholesterol and cholesterol intake. As compared to total cholesterol in this group, the HDL fraction was normal and the ratio of total to HDL cholesterol was comparable to that found in healthy American population groups below the age of 30.

DIABETES

The incidence of abnormal glucose tolerance gradually increases with age in both men and women. Indeed, if the standard for young adults were used, 50% to 80% of the elderly would be diagnosed as diabetic.[34,35] Whether these abnormalities represent diabetes or a new standard needs to be applied to the elderly has been a controversy for many years. A comprehensive review of the subject is found in Chapter 39.

ALCOHOL

Chronic alcoholism is a problem among elderly persons. The combination of alcohol abuse with severe social and personal difficulties can be disastrous. More amenable to management is the situation in which counseling for the families of the elderly can point out that there are no medical contraindications to the moderate use of alcohol. A frequent cause of depression among old people living in families is when the family members, as part of a general pattern of deprecating the elderly, forbid even a dinner highball, often while they themselves are freely partaking of one.

DISEASE EFFECTS ON DRUG-FOOD MANAGEMENT

Several disease states aggravate drug-food interactions and make patient management more difficult. Examples are presented in Table 30-3.[10]

Table 30-3 Diseases that Heighten the Risk of Drug-Food Interactions

	Management Risk
Cardiovascular	Electrolyte disturbance; decreased K^+ and Mg^{+2}, increased Ca^{+2}
Depression	Anticholinergic (antidepressant) drugs can cause dry mouth, sour or metallic taste, constipation, nausea and vomiting; possible reduced food intake and electrolyte disturbance can follow
Gastrointestinal	Heavy use of antacids and laxatives can change nutritional status
Infectious	Possible high sodium and potassium intake (via antibiotics)
	Disturbance of natural flora by antibiotics
	Nausea, vomiting, diarrhea (from treatment) can lead to electrolyte disturbances
Respiratory	High-carbohydrate low-protein diet can change theophylline kinetics
Rheumatoid	High aspirin dose can deplete iron stores
	Phenylbutazone can induce sodium retention

From Lamy PP: Clin Nutr **2**:9-14, 1983.

DRUGS AND DRUG-FOOD INTERACTIONS

Data by Lamy[10] indicate that yearly per capita usage of prescription drugs by persons over 70 years of age has risen to 17.9 and that not only the number but also the size of the prescriptions has increased. This finding is attributed to the higher incidence of chronic diseases. Thus the elderly are being given more drugs than any other segment of the U.S. population, and these drugs can have more deleterious effects on people who may be less fit to bear them. Lamy's findings[10] also indicate that multiple chronic conditions accompanied by polymedications can be especially harmful in old people because of the interacting effects of primary aging (normal attritional and physiologic changes), secondary aging (accumulation of trauma, injury, and pathophysiologic changes over time), and "sociogenic" aging (effects of losses, which often lead to depression and adversely influence drug action). Perhaps more important, changes in body composition, kidney and liver function, and immune status make predicting drug action in the elderly a difficult process.

Older patients respond to drug therapy in a more individualized fashion than do younger ones, and there is greater variability of responses.[37] Therefore any factor that can reduce this variation should be pursued by physicians who prescribe. One factor, among many, that can influence drug effectiveness is food. Food changes drug action, sometimes in an unanticipated manner. It is thus important to become familiar with the effects of foods on drug action.[10]

Clearly drug-food interaction is of great importance in the elderly,[36] and one particularly important aspect is the effectiveness/risk ratio of the drug. This is altered in older patients, especially when the drug is taken at or near mealtimes. The drug risk increases and its effectiveness decreases. Since drugs are among the most cost-effective modalities of disease management in long-term care, this situation calls attention to the need for more effort (on the part of physicians) to make drug action as efficient and effective as possible.[37] It also means that more stress needs to be placed on the importance of having a good supportive dietary substrate when treating the elderly.

Drug actions influence the nutritional status of the elderly both directly and indirectly. For example, there are many drugs that have anticholinergic side effects. They reduce salivary flow, which is already reduced with advancing age, leading to difficulties with mastication, so the person eats less. Furthermore, decreased salivary flow leads to problems with dentures; thus, again, the person eats less, and a vicious cycle occurs.[38]

With the increasing recognition of drug-food interactions, it is essential to know about a patient's total drug intake. Patients should be asked to give the clinician an inventory of their medicine cabinets as often as every 6 months, since drug intake by the elderly can be voluminous. An examination of the patient's history and the inventory may often reveal explanations of, or contributions to, the patient's complaints. Of particular importance is the intake of such drugs as salicylates, antacids, corticosteroids, antibiotics, laxatives, anorexic agents, and anticonvulsant drugs. (See also Chapter 3.)

Diuretics

Many diuretics increase the urinary excretion of potassium. Patients on diuretics must consume ample dietary potassium, which can be provided through a wide variety of fruits and vegetables. Careful attention needs to be paid to the vehicle for potassium, since one of the side effects of the diuretics themselves may be anorexia, gastrointestinal disturbances, and difficulties with taste.

Cardiovascular Drugs

Cardiovascular drugs characteristically lead to gastrointestinal symptoms, including anorexia, nausea, vomiting, and diarrhea. Great care must be taken to separate these side effects from symptoms of toxicity, which also include anorexia, nausea, vomiting, and diarrhea.

Analgesics

Aspirin is probably the drug used with the greatest frequency in elderly patients, and its most common side effect is gastric irritation. More importantly, high levels of salicylate intake can increase the urinary loss of ascorbic acid, potassium, and amino acids.[39,40]

Laxatives

Frequent use of laxatives has serious nutritional implications, either through nonabsorption of food, which passes unchanged through the GI tract, or through solubility factors, which modify their availability for absorption. The identification of the laxative should lead to the appropriate management. In the case of mineral oil, the fat-soluble vitamins (A, D, E, K) and carotene become dissolved in the mineral oil and hence unavailable for absorption. Other cathartic agents may lead to increased intestinal loss of calcium and potassium.[39]

Other Drugs

A partial list of possible drug interferences with food and the mechanism of activity in the elderly is presented in Table 30-4.[41]

Vitamin and Mineral Supplementation

Several studies have estimated that about 50% of the elderly population in the United States may be using nutrient supplements and that many individuals may consume doses well in excess

Table 30-4 Drug Interferences with Foods

Drug(s)	Mechanism of Interference	Effect
Antihistamines		
Cyproheptadine	Appetite stimulation	Weight gain
Antihypertensives		
Ganglionic blockers	Impaired or enhanced gastrointestinal motility	Generalized malabsorption
Antiinfectives		
Aminoglycosides	Enzyme inactivation	Decreased carbohydrate absorption
Chloramphenicol	Impaired nutrient metabolism and utilization	Inhibition of protein binding
Griseofulvin	Appetite suppression	Growth retardation, weight loss
Isoniazid	Altered nutrient excretion	Pyridoxine deficiency
Lincomycin	Appetite suppression	
Neomycin	Interference with bile acid activity	Decreased absorption of vitamin B_{12}, carotene, iron, sugar, and triglycerides
	Enzyme inactivation	Decreased carbohydrate absorption
Tetracycline	Impaired nutrient metabolism and utilization	Decreased bone growth
Trimethoprim (prolonged)	Impaired nutrient metabolism and utilization	Folate deficiency, accumulation of phenylalanine
Antineoplastics		
Aminopterin	Damage to intestinal mucosa	Decreased absorption of vitamin B_{12}, carotene, cholesterol, lactose, D-xylose; megaloblastic anemia; steatorrhea
Bleomycin	Damage to intestinal mucosa	Same as Aminopterin
Cisplatin	Damage to intestinal mucosa	Same as Aminopterin
Methotrexate	Damage to intestinal mucosa	Same as Aminopterin
	Impaired nutrient absorption	Decreased folic acid synthesis
Antirheumatoids		
Colchicine	Damage to intestinal mucosa	Same as Aminopterin
Penicillamine	Appetite suppression	Growth retardation, weight loss
	Altered nutrient excretion	Sodium depletion in adrenally suppressed patients
Central nervous system stimulants/ depressants		
Amphetamines	Appetite suppression	Growth retardation, weight loss
Benzodiazepines	Appetite stimulation	Weight gain
Levodopa	Competition for uptake at blood-brain barrier	Decreased phenylalanine and tyrosine absorption
Phenobarbital	Impaired nutrient metabolism and utilization	Vitamin D deficiency
Phenothiazines	Appetite stimulation	Weight gain
Phenytoin	Impaired nutrient metabolism and utilization	Osteomalacia
Primidone	Impaired nutrient metabolism and utilization	Folate deficiency, neurologic complications (possibly peripheral neuropathy, psychological effects ranging from irritability to paranoid psychosis)
Tricyclic antidepressants	Appetite stimulation	Weight gain

Based on data from Hartz SC, Blumberg J: Clin Nutr **5:**130-136, 1986.

Continued.

Table 30-4 Drug Interferences with Foods—cont'd

Drug(s)	Mechanism of Interference	Effect
Gastrointestinal stimulants/depressants		
Aluminum hydroxide gel	Complexation of nutrient by drug	Decreased phosphate absorption
Antacids	Altered gastrointestinal pH	Thiamine deficiency
Anticholinergics	Impaired or enhanced gastrointestinal motility	Generalized malabsorption
Cathartics	Impaired or enhanced gastrointestinal motility	Calcium and potassium loss
Cholestyramine	Interference with bile acid activity	Vitamin A, D, E, and K deficiencies
Clofibrate	Enzyme inactivation	Decreased carbohydrate absorption
	Appetite suppression	Growth retardation, weight loss
	Interference with bile acid activity	Decreased absorption of vitamin B_{12}, carotene, iron, sugar, triglycerides
Immunosuppressants		
Cytotoxic	Appetite suppression	Growth retardation, weight loss
Steroids	Altered nutrient excretion	Sodium depletion in adrenally suppressed patients

of the recommended dietary allowances. Without question, supplementation can reduce the dangers of inadequate nutrient intake in elderly persons. However, there is also a risk (albeit slight) that toxicity from unsupervised high consumption may develop. If high intakes occur elsewhere in the diet or the individual is especially susceptible to the adverse effects of a particular nutrient, such supplementation may induce an allergic response; but the problem of overdosage is not great, because most all-purpose nutrient supplements have a built-in margin of safety. Exceptions are single-entity preparations of vitamins A and D, selenium, and iodine. These have smaller margins of safety.[41]

It is important to note that the lack of documented toxicity in healthy individuals from single or multiple megadose supplements does not imply that such use is beneficial or without drawbacks. Adverse nutrient-nutrient and drug-nutrient interactions must be considered whenever supplements are prescribed. Additionally, the expense of purchasing these over-the-counter items may deflect funds that could otherwise be spent on diverse and high-quality foodstuffs.

The prevalence of frequent (four or more times/wk) and chronic nutrient supplementation among Boston elderly is presented in Table 30-5.[41] Three-day median dietary intakes were comparable between users and nonusers of supplements. Supplement users equaled or exceeded their estimated 3-day median dietary intake for all vitamins and minerals (except for calcium, phosphorus, and magnesium) through the use of supplements alone. Thus the proportions of elderly subjects whose dietary intake alone was considered inadequate were similar between users and nonusers of nutrient supplements. The ingestion of nutrient supplements did, however, markedly decrease the prevalence of total nutrient intakes that fell below two thirds of the RDAs.[41]

ADDITIONAL CONSIDERATIONS IN NUTRITION MANAGEMENT
Income

Nutritional deficits may reflect a preponderance of socioeconomic factors rather than intrinsic disease. Undernutrition in the elderly is often a result of insufficient funds. For the elderly, especially those living on fixed incomes, the only part of the budget that can be adjusted is the amount spent on food.[42] Rent must be paid, utilities must be paid, and medical expenses must be paid. Thus, fewer and fewer dollars can be spent for food. Too often, elderly persons are faced with the reality of poor nutrition resulting from poverty.[43]

Table 30-5 Frequent and Chronic Nutrient Supplement Use Among Boston Elderly

	Men		Women	
	% Frequent users	Mean duration (yr)	% Frequent users	Mean duration (yr)
Vitamin A	23	6.0	29	9.8
Thiamin	24	8.1	32	9.5
Riboflavin	24	8.1	32	9.5
Niacin	24	8.0	32	9.5
Vitamin B_6	22	7.5	33	9.4
Vitamin B_{12}	23	7.7	33	9.3
Vitamin C	29	9.0	37	9.5
Vitamin D	23	6.2	28	9.5
Vitamin E	24	7.4	36	8.7
Folic acid	18	8.2	20	9.4
Iron	15	8.7	20	9.9
Calcium	11	10.2	16	8.0
Phosphorus	10	10.7	10	7.4
Magnesium	10	9.0	14	9.6
Zinc	15	7.2	17	8.8

From Hartz SC, Blumberg J: Clin Nutr **5**:130-136, 1986.
Nutrient may be taken as a single supplement or as part of a combination product.

Lack of transportation is another factor that contributes to undernutrition in the elderly. As neighborhoods change and supermarkets relocate, areas in which the elderly often live are transformed and it becomes more difficult to shop. Loss of familiar local food stores further dislocates established shopping patterns. The dietary habits of older persons, already precarious, are further eroded.[42]

Immobility

Physical inactivity, with resulting or accompanying depression, may also lead to impaired nutritional status. The decreased activity results in a moderation of the usual range of environmental stimuli. There are fewer inducements to move about, and this contributes to increasingly sedentary habits, with a consequent loss of muscle tone that adds to the continuing downward spiral. The result is easier fatigability and depression. The lethargy that follows can reduce the levels of all vital funtions, further accentuated by insufficient sensory stimulation.[44]

Anorexia

A decrease in or loss of appetite is a common problem, often magnified by drugs, disease, and depression and also aggravated by the fact that elderly persons usually have dry mouth from di-minishing salivary gland activity. Adding to the problem is reduced secretion of hydrochloric acid in the stomach, which may lead to gastritis and bacterial overgrowth in the small intestine and eventually to megaloblastic anemia because of vitamin B_{12} deficiency.[42] Impaired digestion may also result, from a weakening of the smooth muscle of the stomach and intestine.[43]

Chewing and Digestion

An inability to chew food without experiencing pain may lead to inadequate food intake. There are many reasons for chewing problems — infected or decayed teeth, dysfunction of the temporomandibular articulation, ill-fitting dentures. (Frequently old dentures no longer fit the bony ridges for which they were made.) As a result of these problems the actual work of chewing may exceed the physical stamina of the individual. The most common cause for loss of dentures is well known in long-term care institutions: at mealtime the denture is removed, placed on the tray (usually wrapped in a napkin), and discarded with the leftovers at the end of the meal.

Intrinsic diseases of the gastrointestinal tract also may be the cause of dietary deficiencies. Presbyesophagus and reflux esophagitis prevent adequate passage of food into the stomach. Celiac disease can be a problem, but it does not occur frequently. Diverticulosis, by far the most common cause of intrinisic malabsorption, may be a result of diarrhea, unpredictable food intolerances, or the impact of unacceptable dietary restrictions (often self-imposed).[42]

Mental Hygiene

Depression, agitation, petulance, and aggression in an elderly patient may signal a shift in the mental health of that person. Loneliness, too, may be a confounding factor. When an elderly individual visits his physician, his complaint must be taken seriously. Old people do not complain unnecessarily. They almost always have a good reason for going to the trouble of visiting their physician: loneliness is a good reason in itself.[42]

During an office visit, patients should be encouraged to talk about their families, hobbies, whatever interests them; and physicians should remember that medical practice is a "hands on" art. The human touch is reassuring. Hospital staff might be instructed to take a pulse, even though it is not needed. Getting to know the patients not only helps in learning about their diets but also makes it easier to spot personality changes or recognize the first signs of senile dementia.[42]

Federal Programs

The multifaceted and complex nature of the nutrition and health problems of elderly persons has resulted in the passage of federal legislation addressing these issues. The federal agency charged with coordinating and integrating programs directed at the elderly is the Administration on Aging. It also serves to coordinate federal, state, and local programs as well as functions as a center for information. The Nutrition Program for the Elderly was authorized as part of the comprehensive Older Americans Act of 1965.[45] Title III of this legislation as amended through 1981 directs agencies to provide congregate nutrition services as well as home-delivered meals (Meals on Wheels). The daily energy and nutrient intakes furnished by these programs are listed in Table 30-6.[46]

Dependent Noninstitutionalized Elderly

Various authors[46] have shown that participants in congregate meals programs have a signifi-

Table 30-6 Daily Energy and Nutrient Intakes Provided by Congregate Meals

	Percentage of Total Intake	
	Men	Women
Energy	41 ± 3.2*	48 ± 1.9
Protein	54 ± 3.4	59 ± 2.0
Fat	41 ± 3.0	49 ± 2.4
Calcium	48 ± 3.5†	61 ± 2.8
Phosphorus	47 ± 3.4†	56 ± 1.9
Iron	46 ± 3.0	52 ± 2.1
Vitamin A	49 ± 5.0	59 ± 3.4
Thiamin	39 ± 3.2	42 ± 2.2
Riboflavin	50 ± 3.2	56 ± 2.3
Niacin	53 ± 3.6	54 ± 2.2
Ascorbic acid	36 ± 4.6	44 ± 3.9

From Harrill I, et al: Aging **311**:36-41, 1980.
*Mean ± standard error (SEM).
†Significantly different from women (P <0.05).

cantly higher intake of energy and nutrients than do socioeconomically comparable nonparticipants. In each of these programs educational efforts and materials are geared to this population and provide guidance in making appropriate food choices.

The educational component of the congregate meals programs has been successful in improving the nutritional knowledge of many participants.[47] Home-delivered meals are provided, along with educational materials that recommend additional intake based on the typical contribution of the meals delivered and written to be understood by persons with minimum independence and income. The educational materials usually recommend that the recipient eat "at least" certain other foods in addition to the delivered meal.[47]

The homebound elderly account for nearly 10% of old people living in their own homes in the United States and are the largest single group at risk of nutritional problems, which are frequently accentuated by limitations of transportation and by isolation.[48] The many and varied nutrition-related concerns of the homebound elderly have received increasing recognition. For example, a pilot program in Philadelphia aimed at maximizing such persons' self-care abilities and enhancing their community supports has been favorably received and is considered a useful approach. Programs of this kind will be in greater demand as public-supported activities of social and health services for the frail elderly continue to be expanded.[49]

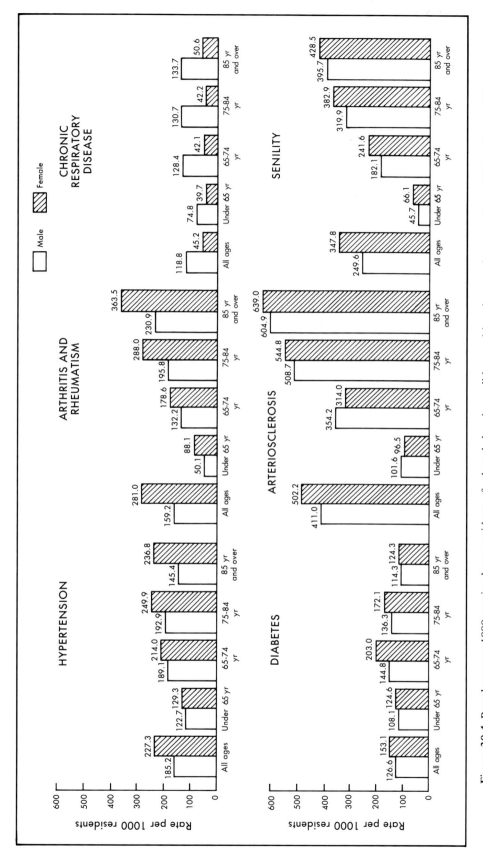

Figure 30-1 Prevalence per 1000 nursing home residents of selected chronic conditions and impairments, by age and sex, United States, 1977.

From National Center for Health Statistics: (DHHS Publ 81-1712), Vital Health Stat [13], pp 4-10, 1981.

INSTITUTIONAL CARE OF THE ELDERLY

Nutritional care in nursing homes is an important area of concern. The number of elderly patients in institutional care has steadily increased. Nursing home surveys have found that vitamin A, riboflavin, thiamine, and iron intakes are low among residents.[50] Calcium intakes have also been reported to be low.[51] Infrequent servings of green and yellow vegetables, the low ascorbic values of some foods, and infrequent availability of citrus fruits have been implicated in the low vitamin A and vitamin C values found.[52]

Refusal of food or limited daily consumption suggests that these people have special needs that require the attention of a dietitian. The nature and scope of the medical complications of elderly persons in institutionalized care are extensive (Fig. 30-1),[53] and the dietitian's services are important for ensuring the nutritional well-being of all elderly populations in nursing homes. Dietary assessment and monitoring should be key elements in the overall care of the institutionalized elderly.

CONTINUING NUTRITIONAL CARE OF THE DISCHARGED PATIENT

A frequent cause for hospital readmission of patients with chronic diseases is inadequate discharge planning and follow-up, which result in exacerbation of their disease after discharge. In an attempt to reduce readmissions for this reason, many hospitals have developed continuing care services.[54] These services are designed essentially to assist patients, especially older ones, in following their medical regimens after discharge. The care plan is devised by a team headed by the nursing staff and with a dietitian as a member. The physician assumes primary responsibility and besides supervising the patient's medical management, is responsible for defining the goals and objectives to be achieved. Social workers are involved as appropriate, and occupational therapists and physical therapists also participate.

Early in their hospital stay, patients are assessed from the standpoint of their health-care needs, activities of daily living, and understanding of their own medical condition. In determining the continuing care requirements of these patients, it is important to consider several alternative plans (1) discharge to home with family support, (2) a coordinated home-care program through agencies like the visiting nurse association or other community services, and (3) a specific level of extended care. The discharge plan should include a discussion of these possibilities with the patient and an agreement on the best possible way to meet the patient's individual home-care needs; and to facilitate communication among the team members, it is becoming increasingly accepted that all members of all disciplines involved in the continuing care of the discharged patient use the patient's progress notes in the medical record to assist in communications and recording of information pertinent to the patient's progress.[42]

REFERENCES

1. Weiner MB, et al: Working with the aged, Englewood Cliffs NJ, 1978, Prentice-Hall Inc.
2. Bidlack WR: Nutritional requirements and nutritional status of the elderly. In Dobernz AR, et al, editors: Food and agricultural research opportunities to improve human nutrition, Newark Delaware, 1986, University of Delaware Press, p A31.
3. Shank RE: Nutrition and aging. In Ostfeld AM, et al, editors: Epidemiology of aging, DHEW Publ (NIH) 75-711, p 199, 1975.
4. Supplement to On health and medicine, Employment outlook: the graying of America, The New York Times, Nov. 3, 1985.
5. Weinsier RL, et al: Hospital malnutrition: a prospective evaluation of general medical patients during the course of hospitalization, Am J Clin Nutr 32:418-426, 1979.
6. Lipid Research Clinic population studies data book. Vol II. The prevalence study—nutrient intake (NIH Publ 82-2014), Bethesda Md, 1982, National Institutes of Health.
7. Bushman L, et al: Malnutrition among patients in an acute-care veterans facility, J Am Diet Assoc 77:4462-465, 1980.
8. Hynak MR, et al: Nutritional assessment among patients with chronic obstructive pulmonary disease [abstract], Clin Res 28:596A, 1980.
9. Eckstein D: Common complaints of the elderly, Hosp Pract, April 1976, pp 67-74.
10. Lamy PP: Nutrition, drugs, and the elderly, Clin Nutr 2:9-14, 1983.
11. Werner I, Hambroens L: The digestive capacity of elderly people. In Carlson LA, editor, Nutrition in old age, Uppsala, 1972 Almqvist & Wiksell, pp 55-60.
12. Pelz KS, et al: Intestinal absorption studies in the aged, Geriatrics 23:149-153, 1968.
13. Lesher S, Sacher GA: Effects of age on cell proliferation in mouse duodenal crypts [abstract], Exp Gerontol 3:211, 1968.
14. Warren PM, et al: Age changes in small-intestinal mucosa, [letter], Lancet 2:849-850, 1978.
15. Cornet A, et al: La muqueuse gastrique des sujets agés, Arch Mal Appar Digest 53:365-376, 1964.

16. Siurala M, et al: Pernicious anemia and atrophic gastritis, Acta Med Scand **166:**213-223, 1960.

17. Russell Rm, et al: Influence of intraluminal pH on folate absorption: Studies in control subjects and in patients with pancreatic insufficiency, J Lab Clin Med **93:**428-436, 1979.

18. Webster SGP, Leeming JT: Erythrocyte folate levels in young and old, J Am Geriatr Soc **27:**451-454, 1979.

19. Bailey LB, et al: Folacin and iron status and hematological findings in predominately black elderly persons from urban low-income households, Am J Clin Nutr **32:**2346-2353, 1979.

20. Slovik DM, et al: Deficient production of 1,25-dihydroxy-vitamin D in elderly osteoporotic patients, N Engl J Med **305:**372-374, 1981.

21. Hollander D, Morgan D: Aging: its influence on vitamin A intestinal absorption in vivo by the rat, Exp Gerontol **14:**301-305, 1979.

22. Yearick ES, et al: Nutritional status of the elderly: dietary and biochemical findings, J Gerontol **35:**663-671, 1980.

23. Andrews J, et al: Vitamin C supplementation in the elderly: a 17 month trial in an old persons' home, Br Med J **2:**416-418, 1969.

24. Young VR: Impact of aging on protein metabolism. In Armbrecht HJ, et al, editors: Nutritional intervention in the aging process, New York, 1985, Springer-Verlag, Inc, p 27.

25. Garn SM: Bone loss and aging. In Garn SM, editor: The physiology and pathology of human aging, New York, 1975, Academic Press Inc.

26. Committee on Dietary Allowances, Food and Nutrition Board, National Research Council: Recommended dietary allowances, ed 9, Washington DC, 1980, National Academy of Sciences.

27. Albanese AA: Bone loss: Causes, detection, and therapy, New York, 1977, Alan R Liss.

28. Dairy Council Digest: Diet, exercise, and health, vol 56, May-June, 1985.

29. Anderson JJB, Tylavsky FA: Diet and osteopenia in elderly caucasian women. In Christiansen C, et al, editors: Osteoporosis. Proceedings of the Copenhagen International Symposium on Osteoporosis, June 3-8, 1984, Glostrup Hospital, Denmark.

30. Avioli LV: Calcium supplementation and osteoporosis. In Armbrecht HJ, et al, editors: Nutritional intervention in the aging process, New York, 1985, Springer-Verlag New York Inc, p 183.

31. Munro HN, Young VR: Protein metabolism in the elderly, Postgrad Med **63:**143-148, 1978.

32. Shepard JW Jr: Interrelationship of exercise and nutrition in the elderly. In Nutritional intervention in the aging process, *op cit,* reference 30, p 315.

33. Danner SA: Methuselah's secret—cardiovascular health in the tenth decade. A study of the Dutch Heart Foundation, Amsterdam, 1977, Drukkerij Cliteur BV.

34. Bierman EL: Obesity, carbohydrate, and lipid interactions in the elderly. In Winick M, editor: Nutrition and aging, New York, 1976, John Wiley & Sons Inc.

35. Hodkinson HM: Biochemical diagnosis of the elderly, New York, 1977, John Wiley & Sons Inc.

36. Roe DA: Drug-induced nutritional deficiencies, Westport Conn, 1976, AVI Publishing Co Inc.

37. Lamy PP: Prescribing for the elderly, Littleton Mass, 1980, PSG Publishing Co Inc.

38. Lamy PP: Nutrition, drugs and the elderly. Occasional report series, Chapel Hill NC, 1982, Institute of Nutrition, University of North Carolina, p 6.

39. March DC: Handbook: Interactions of selected drugs with nutritional status in man, Chicago, 1976, The American Dietetic Association.

40. Hethcox JM, Stanaszek WF: Interactions of drugs and diet, Hosp Pharm **9/10:**373-383, 1974.

41. Hartz SC, Blumberg J: Use of vitamin and mineral supplements by the elderly, Clin Nutr **5:**130-136, 1986.

42. Eckstein D, Hesla T: Nutritional care of the elderly, Clin Nutr **2:**19-25, 1983.

43. Assessing nutritional status of the elderly: state of the art. Ross roundtable on medical issues, Columbus Ohio, 1982, Ross Laboratories.

44. Mooltin SE: Nutrition in the elderly. In Mooltin SE, editor: The geriatric imperatives, New York, 1981, Appleton-Century-Crofts.

45. Older Americans Act of 1965, as amended through Dec 29, 1981, Washington DC, 1982, Government Printing Office.

46. Harrill I, et al: The nutritional status of congregate meal recipients, Aging **311:**36-41, 1980.

47. Folds CC: Practical aspects of nutritional management of the elderly, Clin Nutr **2:**15-18, 1983.

48. Exton-Smith, AN: Eating habits of the elderly. In Turner M, editor: Nutrition and lifestyles, London, 1980, Applied Sciences Publishers, p 179.

49. Glanz K, Scharf M: A nutrition training program for social workers serving the homebound elderly, Gerontologist **25:**455-459, 1985.

50. Brown PT, et al: Dietary status of elderly people, J Am Diet Assoc **71:**41-45, 1977.

51. Himniks B, Cate HD: Nutrient content of foods served vs foods eaten in nursing homes, J Am Diet Assoc **59:**126-129, 1971.

52. Leighton MM, Harrill J: Nutrient content of food served in nursing homes, J Am Diet Assoc **53:**465-468, 1968.

53. National Center for Health Statistics: Characteristics of nursing home residents, health status, and care received: National Nursing Home Survey, United States, May-December, 1977 (DHHS Publ 81-1712), Vital Health Stat [13], pp 4-13, 1981.

54. Goodhue PJ, et al: Continuing nutritional care for the discharged patient, Dietetic Currents, Ross Timesaver **3**(1):1-4, 1977.

CHAPTER 31
Enteral and Parenteral Nutrition

Cleon W. Goodwin
Douglas W. Wilmore

OVERVIEW

Determination of energy requirements and the method of nutrient administration depends upon the patient's nutritional status, expected length of illness, available gastrointestinal tract, and metabolic response to the disease process. Techniques for review of dietary adequacy and for assessment of body fat, lean body mass, and visceral protein, as well as immune competence are described elsewhere in this manual and indicate the necessary intensity of nutritional support. In unstable patients, correction of tissue hypoxia, electrolyte imbalance, and hypovolemia takes precedence over institution of vigorous nutritional support. Once such patients are stabilized, nutrients should be administered by the safest and most effective route.

Choice of Caloric Goals

Three levels of nutritional support are practicable in the hospital setting: hypocaloric feeding, maintenance diets, and supranormal energy balance–weight gain diets (Table 31-1).

The hypocaloric, nitrogen-containing diet provides 400 to 1800 kcal/day, which is generally 1000-2000 kcal/day less than the metabolic expenditure of the hospitalized patient. Such diets minimize the weight loss, erosion of lean body mass, and ketosis induced by starvation. This level of nutritional support is quite acceptable for postoperative feeding of patients undergoing elective surgery, in whom immediate recovery and return to customary oral feeding is expected soon thereafter, and is provided by peripheral infusions of 5% or 10% dextrose solutions with or without amino acids in volumes usually well tolerated by postoperative patients.

The maintenance diet achieves energy and nitrogen balance. The patient is given nutrients to satisfy his caloric requirements as determined by the response to a particular illness plus an additional allowance of energy to provide for treatment and physical activity (usually 25% of the resting energy expenditure). Except in children, in whom growth also is desired, the goals of this program are to preserve body mass and to maintain body weight. For seriously ill patients, maintenance diets provide the optimal balance between energy administration and incidence of complications.

Supranormal dietary intake aims for positive balance of both energy and nitrogen. To meet this goal, the patient must be provided sufficient calories to meet his resting energy expenditure, plus 25% of resting expenditure for physical activity, plus an additional 1000 kcal/day. Such a

Table 31-1 Methods for Administering Varying Levels of Caloric Support

Route	Hypocaloric, Nitrogen-Containing	Maintenance or Positive Energy and Nitrogen Balance
Enteral	Ad-lib food intake from hospital trays Low-volume or dilute tube feedings	High-calorie high-protein diet with between-meal supplements Defined-formula diet, either orally or by tube feeding
Parenteral	Peripheral vein infusions containing amino acids	Hypertonic glucose and amino acids infused into central vein Fat-containing peripheral vein infusions in non-stressed patients

regimen results in a weight gain of approximately 0.5-1 kg/week. This level of support may be difficult to administer and potentially hazardous to patients who are severely catabolic. Hyperglycemia is common and energy support in excess of energy requirements occasionally results in lipogenesis with increased CO_2 production and respiratory failure.[1,2] As critically ill patients stabilize and begin to respond to treatment, metabolic needs decrease, and diets that previously met only maintenance requirements now provide positive balances of nitrogen and energy. At this time, such supranormal diets may be tolerated safely and, if continued at the same level, allow the patient to restore fat and lean body mass.

Steps for Planning Long-Term Metabolic Support

Although many complicated formulas have been utilized to calculate metabolic require-

ments, a systematic approach utilizing a few simple nomograms is convenient for predicting the needs of patients suffering a wide variety of illnesses.[3]

1. Determine the body surface area from the patient's weight and height (Fig. 31-1).
2. Find the basal metabolic rate based on the patients age, sex (Table 31-2), and surface area (Fig. 31-2).
3. Ascertain the effect of the specific disease on the basal metabolic rate to determine the patient's resting metabolic expenditure (Fig. 31-3). Alternatively, the resting metabolic expenditure can be measured by indirect calorimetry.
4. Increase the resting metabolic expenditure by 25% to allow for activity or treatment requirements. (This may not be necessary for patients heavily sedated or paralyzed and on a ventilator.)
5. Decide on the degree of caloric support

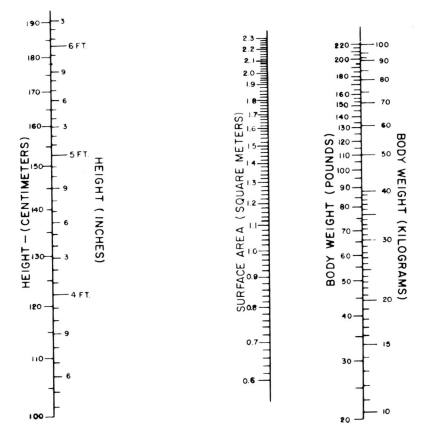

Figure 31-1 Surface area computation. To determine body surface area from the height *(left-hand scale)* and weight *(right-hand scale),* connect these readings with a straightedge and note the result on the middle scale.

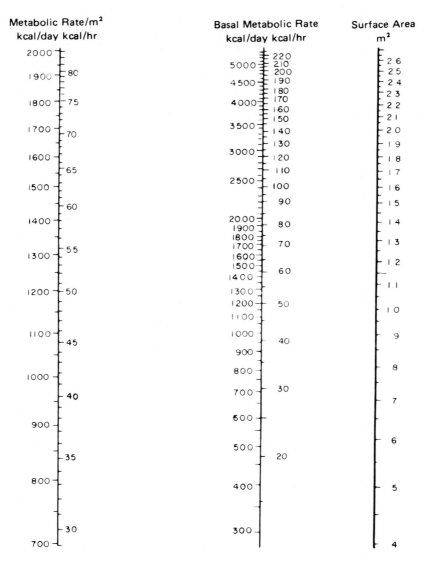

Figure 31-2 To predict daily basal metabolic requirements, determine the surface area *(right-hand scale)* and with a straightedge note the BMR by aligning with the metabolic rate *(left-hand scale)*.

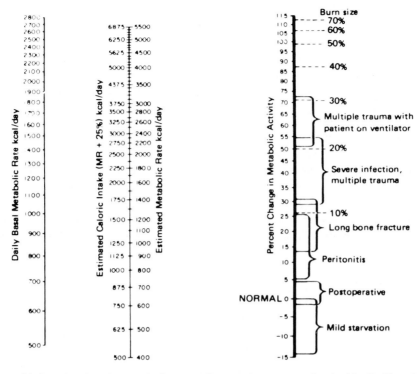

Figure 31-3 Estimating the metabolic expenditure and energy needs of critically ill patients.

Table 31-2 Standard Metabolic Rates (kcal/m²/hr)

Age (yr)	Men	Women	Age (yr)	Men	Women
1	53.0	53.0	17	40.8	36.3
2	52.4	52.4	18	40.0	35.9
3	51.3	51.2	19	39.2	35.5
4	50.3	49.8	20	38.6	35.3
5	49.3	48.4	25	37.5	35.2
6	48.3	47.0	30	36.8	35.1
7	47.3	45.4	35	36.5	35.0
8	46.3	43.8	40	36.3	34.9
9	45.2	42.8	45	36.2	34.5
10	44.0	42.5	50	35.8	33.9
11	43.0	42.0	55	35.4	33.3
12	42.5	41.3	60	34.9	32.7
13	42.3	40.3	65	34.4	32.2
14	42.1	39.2	70	33.8	31.7
15	41.8	37.9	75 and over	33.2	31.3
16	41.4	36.9			

From Wilmore DW: The metabolic management of the critically ill, New York, 1977, Plenum Press Inc, pp 171-233.

(i.e., maintenance versus positive balance) and the proportion of dietary fat and carbohydrate calories.

6. Determine the nitrogen requirements by choosing an appropriate nitrogen/calorie ratio, usually 1:150 for seriously ill patients (Fig. 31-4).
7. Add maintenance vitamins, minerals, and essential fatty acids.
8. Decide on the safest delivery system that will furnish the required nutrients.

General Concepts of Nutrient Utilization

Although individual requirements for calories, nitrogen, vitamins, and trace elements and their respective deficiency syndromes are discussed elsewhere in this manual, the understanding of certain additional general principles will aid in planning nutritional support. Carbohydrate (and, to a lesser degree, glycerol) has a specific protein-sparing effect when administered alone. Sugars maintain hepatic glycogen stores, which protect hepatocytes from hypoxia and toxins, and this effect may apply to other organs as well. In the absence of amino acids, exogenously administered fat does not appear to spare protein except for that related to its glycerol content.[4,5] When fat and amino acids are administered together, variable degrees of protein sparing occur depending on the patient's underlying metabolic

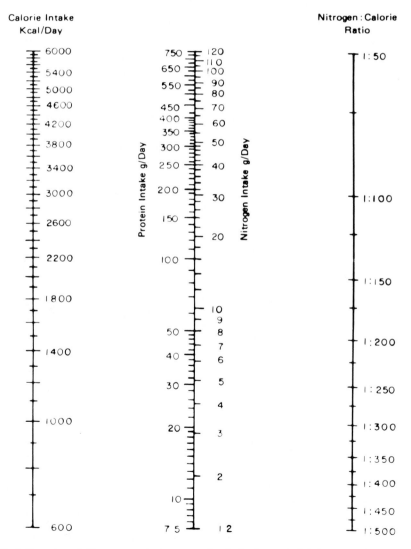

Figure 31-4 Quantity of dietary protein in terms of caloric demand *(left-hand scale)* and nitrogen requirements *(right-hand scale)*.

state and level of nitrogen intake. In general, as patients become increasingly hypermetabolic, they are less able to utilize fat as a nonprotein calorie source to conserve nitrogen, and in severely stressed patients, fat does not initiate nitrogen retention until resting metabolic expenditures are met by the provision of energy in the form of carbohydrate.[6] For depleted chronically ill patients with minimal hypermetabolic response, exogenous fat comprising up to 83% of nonprotein calories is as effective as carbohydrate in maintaining nitrogen balance.[7,8] In addition, fat intake is necessary to provide essential fatty acids and is an effective calorie source for restoring body fat mass once the catabolic phase of injury has abated. Endogenous protein is a poor energy store and under a wide variety of stresses provides 15% to 20% of caloric requirements.[9] Because of this obligatory loss as an energy source, exogenous protein must be supplied for the synthesis of enzymes and new structural protein.

ENTERAL FEEDING

The method of feeding depends on the status of the gastrointestinal tract and the quantity of calories required. Since enteral feeding promotes more efficient utilization of nutrients and better preservation of intestinal integrity than does parenteral administration, the gut is the preferred route when it is functioning and accessible.[10] Enteral alimentation is generally safer and more economical than parenteral alimentation and, when tolerated, is the preferred route of nutrient administration for patients requiring intensive nutritional support.[11] With currently available products the large caloric requirements of severely hypermetabolic patients can be met completely by enteral support.[12]

Oral Feeding

When feasible, spontaneous oral consumption of a regular diet is the safest and most effective method for nutrient administration. Although most hospital diets contain up to 60-80 g of protein and approximately 2200 kcal/day, a high-calorie high-protein diet can be devised by adding supplements to the prepared food to provide 100-120 g of protein and 3000 kcal/day. The attending physician should ensure that the patient is not oversedated and should treat severe depression, both of which depress the appetite. The dietitian can increase patient cooperation and

food consumption by catering to food preferences and selecting high-calorie food items. If necessary, dietary composition, calories, and food texture can be altered further to meet certain requirements (e.g. a mechanically soft diet, lactose restriction, a low-sodium diet).

However, critically ill patients who can eat rarely consume more than they were accustomed to eating before becoming ill. Since such patients usually have increased energy needs, spontaneous eating provides only a portion of required calories. Anorexia and food boredom, which often accompany a prolonged illness, further depress spontaneous intake. Oral intake can be supplemented by interval liquid nutrient feedings, which are available as high-calorie high-protein milk shakes fortified with carbohydrate and protein modular supplements or as commercially available formulas meeting specific requirements. The latter are particularly useful in cases of lactose intolerance, a common occurrence with critically ill patients. These liquid supplements are given around the clock by the nursing staff and should replace all low-calorie fruit juices or soft drinks.

Fat must be an integral component of both hospital tray food and interval supplements. Diets containing less than 25% of calories as fat generally are unpalatable and will not elicit long-term patient cooperation. Although long-chain fatty acids require bile salts and micelle formation for absorption, medium-chain triglycerides (MCTs) are easily hydrolyzed without bile salts or pancreatic enzymes and are useful caloric sources in patients with fat malabsorption. MCTs are absorbed directly into the portal circulation and apparently stimulate insulin secretion, which may promote nitrogen conservation. However, unlike long-chain triglycerides, MCTs are not stored in fat depots and hence are ineffective in restoring body triglyceride mass.

Tube Feeding

For patients who cannot or will not eat, but who have a functioning gastrointestinal tract, tube feeding provides an effective and increasingly utilized alternative to parenteral alimentation. With the advent of pliable small-caliber feeding tubes and defined-formula diets, the indications for tube feeding overlap those of parenteral feeding and include patients whose diseases are expected to persist for a long time, are best treated with slow enteral infusion of an unpalatable formula, or are expected to preclude, temporarily or permanently, oral intake:

High-Risk Conditions Requiring Intensive Nutritional Support

Gross underweight, below 80% for height standard

Recent loss of more than 10% of usual body weight, including obese individuals

Nutritional intake of only low-calorie intravenous solutions (5%-10% dextrose) for over 10 da

Sustained nutrient losses
  Short-bowel syndrome
  Malabsorption syndromes
  Enterocutaneous fistulas
  Draining wounds and abscesses

Hypermetabolic processes
  Massive burns and multiple trauma
  Massive infection (e.g., peritonitis)
  Sustained febrile syndromes

Chronic alcoholism

Use of drugs that promote catabolism or poor nutrition
  Corticosteroids
  Antineoplastic agents
  Immunosuppressants

Infants, especially if premature, and children under age 2 yr

Nasoenteric tube. Nasogastric tubes are the most common means of intubating the gastrointestinal tract, both for drainage and for alimentation. These tubes can be left in place for continuous feeding or can be inserted intermittently by the patient for periodic feeding. Large rubber or polyethylene tubes are uncomfortable and elicit poor patient cooperation. New small-caliber (5-8 French) tubes of silicone elastomer are well tolerated and can be left in place with little patient discomfort. Mercury weights on the tips aid in passage through the stomach into the duodenum and jejunum.[13] Nasoduodenal and nasojejunal tubes are particularly useful for instituting early postoperative feeding and for aiding nonsurgical closure of high enteric fistulas.[14] If the fistula is proximal to the jejunum, continuous jejunostomy feeding decreases stomal drainage, decreases intestinal secretions, provokes less nausea and vomiting, and lessens the risk of aspiration more effectively than does gastric feeding. Fluoroscopy or gastroscopy are effective methods for guiding the tube past the pylorus into the small bowel.

Cervical esophagostomy. With cervical esophagostomy, the feeding tube is inserted through a stoma placed in the piriform recess.[15] The surgical procedure is minor and usually is performed with local anesthesia. Cervical esophagostomy is less complex and more convenient than a gastrostomy. For long-term feeding a cervical esophagostomy tube is tolerated better than a nasogastric tube.

Gastrostomy. Although the newer silicon feeding tubes have decreased the use of gastrostomy, this method remains one of the best for prolonged or permanent feeding, especially in patients who have undergone major abdominal surgery. It has also been used effectively in catabolic patients with large burns, inhalation injury, repeated pulmonary aspiration, and severe fungal pharyngitis. Since large-bore tubes usually are employed, inexpensive blenderized diets can be utilized. If the tube is removed inadvertently, it is easily replaced without the need for a sophisticated guidance system or abdominal surgery. Gastrostomies gradually close spontaneously after the tube is removed. The surgical procedure can be done with local anesthesia in critically ill patients. In a modification of the gastrostomy technique,[16] small-bore catheters have been introduced percutaneously through the abdominal wall into the stomach under endoscopic control. Although this avoids the formal laparotomy incision, the technique offers only selective advantages over the older open procedures.

Percutaneous catheter jejunostomy. With percutaneous catheter jejunostomy, one end of a small-bore catheter is inserted directly into the jejunal lumen through a serosal tunnel while the opposite end is passed through the abdominal wall, where it is secured.[14,17] Although this type of feeding tube usually is a part of other major abdominal surgical procedures, a needle catheter jejunostomy may be placed as a primary step, even in high-risk patients. The indications for such a tube are essentially those of the transnasal jejunostomy, and the technique is especially useful for early postoperative fluid and nutrient infusion.[18] The narrow caliber of the catheter precludes the use of other than low-viscosity nutrient solutions.

Instituting Tube Feeding

Following insertion of the feeding tube, its location is confirmed by aspiration of luminal contents or by listening for the sound of injected air. If small bowel feeding is planned, the location of the tip usually must be confirmed by abdominal roentgenograms. The tube should be secured in place to prevent displacement and subsequent injection of the feeding solution into the upper esophagus, trachea, or abdominal cavity.

Although many patients can tolerate intermittent bolus tube feedings, continuous infusion through a small caliber enteral tube represents the safest and most reliable method of administering nutrients to critically ill patients and to patients with repeated pulmonary aspiration, fistulas, malabsorption, and short bowel syndrome. Constant infusion is tolerated better and results in small residuals, and the use of an infusion pump ensures uniform flow. Initially, tube feedings are administered in dilute concentrations at a low infusion rate. Most patients will initially tolerate 20 to 30 ml/hour, and these rates can be increased incrementally every 12 hours up to 200 ml/hour. Once the desired infusion rate has been attained and is tolerated well, the concentration of the feedings is increased slowly to full strength. During this time the patient must be assessed continuously for gastrointestinal stasis, residual feeding volume, and abdominal distension or discomfort.

Meticulous care of the tube is critical.[19] The tube should be aspirated every 6 hours. Following routine aspiration and the administration of medications, the tube is irrigated with saline. The patient should be fed in a semireclining position to prevent aspiration, which is less likely to occur if the tube has been advanced into the small bowel. Infusion sets should be changed daily.

Complications of Tube Feedings

Diarrhea is the most common complication of tube feeding and is most apt to occur following the rapid administration of hyperosmolar solutions directly into the small bowel. This unwanted effect can be minimized by beginning enteral feedings slowly with dilute solutions to allow the bowel to adapt to the osmolar load. The osmolarity of the feedings can be reduced by substituting glucose polymers for the simple sugars and by including fat as a major source of nonprotein calories. Enteral feedings with high fiber content have been shown[20] to be effective in minimizing diarrhea in hypermetabolic patients requiring increased enteral feedings to

meet caloric requirements. Bacterial overgrowth in the feeding solution can cause explosive diarrhea and is particularly likely to occur after prolonged storage of home-prepared blenderized diets. The commercial formulas are packed sterilely and can be left open for up to 12 hours if chilled. Feeding schedules and solution preparations should be so arranged that these formulas do not remain in administration sets for any longer than this time. Lactose intolerance presents with flatulence and diarrhea and can develop in patients who normally have tolerated milk products. Avoidance of lactose is made convenient by the availability of many commercial lactose-free defined-formula diets. Diarrhea in patients with fat malabsorption can be reduced by using medium-chain triglycerides as the source of fat. Minor degrees of diarrhea can be treated with opiates or kaolin-pectin, which can be added directly to the tube feedings. Pseudomembranous colitis presents with intractable diarrhea and may follow an epidemic pattern in closed critical care units. This diarrhea is associated with the use of multiple antibiotics and possibly sustained use of antacids to prevent stress ulceration.[21] Overgrowth of the gastrointestinal tract with *Clostridium difficile* is the suspected cause of the diarrhea, which is treated by the oral administration of vancomycin.

The risk of pulmonary aspiration is highest when the tip of a large-caliber feeding tube lies within the stomach. The nasogastric tube apparently acts as a "wick" around which gastric contents pass up the esophagus to be inhaled. That this is not the sole mechanism, however, is reflected by the not infrequent episodes of aspiration associated with tube gastrostomies, especially if the feedings are administered by the bolus technique. The most effective maneuvers for avoiding this complication are continuous feeding of the patient in the upright position and utilization of a small-bore feeding tube that has been placed into the small bowel.

If retention of more than 100 ml of tube feedings occurs, the rate of administration should be reduced or temporarily terminated for 2 hours. Predisposing factors (e.g., hypokalemia, ileus, obstruction, anticholinergic drugs) should be eliminated and feedings slowly reinstituted. When large residuals occur with intragastric feedings, the same volume of fluid frequently can be administered into the small bowel after a period of adaptation. Less frequent complications associated with tube feeding include esophagitis, parotitis, and otitis media. Their frequency is reduced by using small-caliber feeding tubes.

The metabolic complications of tube feedings are similar to those associated with parenteral alimentation. Hypokalemia and hyperglycemic and hyperosmolar dehydration are the most frequent and potentially most serious disorders accompanying enteral alimentation, especially if diarrhea is present.

Food Supplements and Liquid Formula Diets

The selection of a product for enteral feeding depends on the expected mode of administration and the patient's underlying nutritional difficulty. The avenue and rate of administration, osmolarity, and content of the feedings must be considered. Patients with dysphagia have no special content requirements and require only liquefied food. Patients with malabsorption or a shortened gastrointestinal tract, however, require slow and continuous administration of a chemically defined diet. Palatability determines whether a formula is consumed orally or by tube feeding.

Blenderized food from regular family fare can be used conveniently by patients with no digestive or absorptive disorders and is an effective and cheap dietary form for patients who have a permanent tube gastrostomy or who insert large nasogastric tubes themselves for intermittent feedings. Feeding tubes of large caliber are required because of the large size of the food particles. Blenderized diets are available as commercial formulas (Compleat-B Vitaneed, Formula 2), which have the advantage of being packaged sterilely. Homemade blenderized diets are susceptible to bacterial overgrowth and should be used soon after preparation. All these feedings contain whole beef and/or vegetables as well as a moderate amount of indigestible residue. Because commercially available blenderized diets now cost approximately the same as homemade preparations, the latter currently are seldom used.

Defined-formula diets, including chemically defined and elemental diets, are made by combining known amounts of individual nutrients in a fixed polymeric formula (Table 31-3). All are commercially manufactured and are offered as nutritionally complete liquid formula diets. All suffer the drawback, however, of a fixed composition that may not meet the individual patient's specific needs. Protein content varies from intact protein in hydrolysates and amino acids. Carbohydrate content likewise varies (with most products containing sucrose, corn syrup, and/or maltodextrins) and provides 40% to 90% of the calories. Very few commercial defined-formula diets contain glucose, which must be utilized in high concentrations to achieve adequate caloric density. Hyperosmolarity is avoided by utilizing starches, dextrins, and glucose polymers, which have a high caloric density but are less osmotically active. These polysaccharides do not require amylase for digestion but are hydrolyzed in the intestinal mucosa and absorbed directly. Since glucose oligosaccharides have very little taste, they can be used in high concentrations and are especially suitable in patients with dumping symptoms. Although lactose is used as a carbohydrate source in some preparations, most formulas contain no lactose and are available for use in lactase-deficient patients.

Fat provides 10% to 50% of the nonprotein calories of the commercial formulas. Most contain purified long-chain mono- and diglycerides and mixed triglycerides in the form of corn, soy, or safflower oil. When tolerated, fat is a very effective caloric source, since it is calorically dense (8.1 kcal/g) and osmotically inactive. Fats improve palatability, and fat-free elemental diets are so distasteful that most require tube administration. Medium-chain triglycerides are an effective source of lipid for patients with fat malabsorption.

Although most general-purpose defined-formula diets (not including Amin-Aid or Hepatic Aid) contain vitamins in fixed amounts, none contain vitamin K, which must be supplemented separately. All contain trace elements, but supplements may be needed as indicated by regular serum determinations in some patients with malabsorption or with high volume fistulous drainage. Most formulas contain electrolytes in fixed amounts.

Several special purpose formulas can meet the nutritional requirements of patients with specific diseases. Amin-Aid is offered for use in patients with renal insufficiency. It contains carbohydrate, small amounts of fat, and the eight essential amino acids plus histidine. When reconsti-

Table 31-3 Approximate Composition of Defined-Formula Diets and Modular Supplements

Diet or Supplement	Caloric Density (kcal/ml)	Carbohydrate (g/liter)	Carbohydrate Source	Fat (g/liter)	Fat Source	Protein (g/liter)	Protein Source	N/kcal Ratio	Osmolality (mOsm/kg)	Na (mEq/liter)	K (mEq/liter)
Whole Food Base											
Compleat B	1	120	Vegetables fruit, maltodextrins, lactose, sucrose	40	Corn oil, milk	40	Beef, nonfat milk	1:156	390	52	33
Formula 2	1	123	Vegetables, fruit, lactose, sucrose, starch	40	Corn oil, egg yolk	38	Beef, nonfat milk, egg yolk	1:164	475	26	45
Vitaneed	1	130	Vegetables, fruit, maltodextrins, corn syrup solids	40	Soy oil, monoglycerides, diglycerides	35	Beef, calcium caseinate	1:179	400	24	32
Milk Base											
Nutri-1000	1	101	Corn syrup solids, sucrose, lactose	55	Corn oil, monoglycerides, diglycerides	40	Skim milk, sodium caseinate	1:156	500	23	39
Meritene Liquid	1	115	Corn syrup solids, sucrose, lactose	33	Corn oil, monoglycerides, diglycerides	60	Skim milk, sodium caseinate	1:104	600	40	43
Carnation Instant (powder)*	1	135	Corn syrup solids, sucrose, lactose	31	Milk fat	58	Milk, soy protein, sodium caseinate	1:107	600	40	70
Lactose-Free, Intact Protein											
Ensure	1.1	143	Corn syrup solids, sucrose	37	Corn oil	37	Soy protein, sodium and calcium caseinate	1:186	450	32	38
Ensure Plus	1.5	197	Corn syrup solids, sucrose	53	Corn oil	55	Soy protein, sodium and calcium caseinate	1:171	600	32	34
Sustacal Liquid	1	138	Corn syrup solids, sucrose	23	Soy oil	60	Soy protein, sodium and calcium caseinate	1:104	625	40	53

Continued.

Note: Composition varies with individual lot and with flavoring. Osmolality is approximately one-quarter larger than osmolarity.
*Reconstituted as recommended by manufacturer to give the stated caloric density.

Table 31-3 Approximate Composition of Defined-Formula Diets and Modular Supplements—cont'd

Diet or Supplement	Caloric Density (kcal/ml)	Carbohydrate (g/liter)	Carbohydrate Source	Fat (g/liter)	Fat Source	Protein (g/liter)	Protein Source	N/kcal Ratio	Osmolality (mOsm/kg)	Na (mEq/liter)	K (mEq/liter)
Enrich	1.1	162	Soy polysaccharide, sucrose, hydrolyzed corn starch	37	Corn oil	40	Soy protein, sodium and calcium caseinate	1:156	480	37	40
Isocal	1	130	Glucose, oligosaccharides, corn syrup solids	44	Soy oil, MCTs	34	Soy protein, sodium and calcium caseinate	1:183	350	23	33
Osmolite	1	144	Corn syrup solids	38	Corn oil, soy oil, MCTs	40	Soy protein, sodium and calcium caseinate	1:186	300	25	23
Nutri-1000 LF	1	101	Corn syrup solids, sucrose	55	Corn oil, soy oil, monoglycerides, diglycerides	38	Soy protein, sodium and calcium caseinate	1:164	380	31	38
Magnacal	2	250	Corn syrup solids, sucrose, maltodextrins	80	Soy oil, monoglycerides, diglycerides	70	Sodium and calcium caseinate	1:179	520	43	32
Precision Isotonic	1	144	Glucose oligosaccharides, sucrose	30	Soy oil, monoglycerides, diglycerides	29	Egg albumin solids, sodium caseinate	1:208	300	33	25
Precision HN	1	217	Maltodextrins, sucrose	1.3	Soy oil, MCTs monoglycerides, diglycerides	44	Egg albumin solids	1:149	560	43	23
Chemically Defined											
Flexical	1	154	Sucrose, dextrins	34	Soy oil, MCTs, monoglycerides, diglycerides	23	Casein hydrolysate, amino acids	1:272	550	15	32
Nutramigen (powder)*	0.67	86	Sucrose, tapioca starch	26	Corn oil	22	Casein hydrolysate	1:284	440	14	17

Vital	1	185	Glucose oligo- and polysaccharides, sucrose, hydrolyzed corn starch	10	Sunflower oil, MCTs	42	Whey solids, soy and meat protein hydrolysates, amino acids	1:149	460	17	30
Elemental											
Vivonex	1	226	Glucose oligosaccharides	1.4	Safflower oil	20	Amino acids	1:313	550	37	30
Vivonex HN	1	211	Glucose oligosaccharides	0.9	Safflower oil	43	Amino acids	1:149	810	34	18
Vipep	1	170	Corn syrup solids, sucrose, corn starch	25	Corn oil, MCTs	25	Amino acids, oligopeptides, polypeptides	1:250	520	33	22
Special Formula											
Amin-Aid	2	324	Maltodextrins, sucrose	70	Partially hydrogenated soy oil	19	Essential amino acids	1:643	900	<3	<3
Hepatic Aid	1.6	287	Maltodextrins, sucrose	36	Soy oil, lecithin, monoglycerides, diglycerides	43	Amino acids	1:240	900	0	0
Lofenalac	0.67	86	Corn syrup	27	Corn oil	22	Casein hydrolysate	1:284	920	14	17
Modular Supplements											
MCT Oil	8	0	—	933	MCTs	0	—	—	20	0	0
Microlipid	4.5	0	—	500	Safflower oil	0	—	—	32	0	0
Polycose Liquid	2	500	Glucose oligosaccharides	0	—	0	—	—	850	27	6
Sumacal Plus	2.5	625	Glucose syrup solids, maltodextrins	0	—	0	—	0	860	12	11
Controlyte (powder)*	2.1	298	Corn starch hydrolysates	100	Vegetable oil	0.2	—	—	590	2.5	0.5
EMF (liquid)	2 (protein)	0	—	0	—	500	—	—	690	106	10
Citrotein (powder)*	0.7	129	Sucrose, maltodextrins	2	Vegetable oil, monoglycerides, diglycerides	43	Egg solids	1:102	500	32	20

tuted as recommended by the manufacturer, its caloric density is 2 kcal/ml. Amin-Aid contains no indigestible bulk, no electrolytes, and no vitamins and, even with flavorings, is quite unpalatable. Hepatic Aid, used in patients with liver disease, contains high concentrations of branched-chain amino acids and decreased amounts of aromatic amino acids. This amino acid composition potentially corrects the opposite configuration frequently seen in such patients. Like Amin-Aid, it contains no vitamins, minerals, or trace elements. Other products deficient in a single specific nutrient are used to treat inborn errors of metabolism (e.g., Lofenalac for phenylketonuria).

Except for the blenderized food-based formulas and Enrich, all the diets in Table 31-3 contain little or no residue. Since they are finely dispersed, the defined-formula diets can be administered through small-caliber tubes and are well tolerated over prolonged periods. Enrich, which has a high fiber content, frequently plugs small feeding tubes, and care must be taken to continually irrigate such tubes to maintain patency. Specific nutrient deficits in these diets can be rectified by adding appropriate modular supplements. Carbohydrate, fat, and protein modules are available in powder and liquid form and can be added in amounts producing the desired caloric density, nitrogen/calorie ratio, and osmolarity.

PARENTERAL FEEDING

The parenteral route of nutrient administration is utilized when the gastrointestinal tract is not accessible or is not functioning or is partially functioning but not capable of absorbing sufficient nutrients to meet the patient's metabolic requirements. This method may be the sole means of alimentation or may supplement inadequate enteral feedings. Intravenous feeding as the sole means of nutrition can provide total metabolic support of the critically ill patient.[22] Although parenteral feeding is normally carried out in a carefully supervised hospital environment, complete home programs are feasible for some patients requiring permanent total parenteral nutrition (TPN).

Components of Parenteral Solutions

Carbohydrate. Glucose is the carbohydrate most commonly used as a calorie source in par-

enteral solutions. It is readily available, inexpensive, and well tolerated in high concentrations after a period of adaptation. Complete oxidation of glucose yields 4.1 kcal/g. Fructose (and sorbitol, which is metabolized to fructose) occasionally is used as an alternative to glucose, but its use predisposes the patient to lactic acidosis, hypophosphatemia, hyperuricemia, and liver dysfunction. Recently, parenteral solutions containing 3% glycerol have been used as a source of nonprotein calories. Glycerol-containing solution may cause hemolysis and renal failure and should be used with extreme caution in patients with liver and kidney disease.

Lipid. Lipids for parenteral administration are now available in the United States as 10% or 20% emulsions of either soybean or safflower oil (Table 31-4). These emulsions consist of the triglycerides of long-chain saturated and unsaturated fatty acids. Since the triglycerides exert little osmotic activity, glycerol is added in a 2.5% concentration to provide sufficient osmolarity to the solutions. The emulsions provide 1.1 or 2 kcal/ml. Although the recommended maximum dose for adults is 2.5 g/kg/day, up to 4 g/kg/day may be tolerated by patients for prolonged periods in quantities exceeding 50% of caloric requirements. High proportions of lipid emulsions may cause elevations in serum triglycerides and phospholipids, whose long-term significance is unknown. In patients requiring prolonged parenteral nutritional support, these lipid emulsions effectively prevent the occurrence of essential fatty acid deficiencies if the fatty acid component supplies at least 4% of the caloric requirements.[23] The major essential fatty acid in both commercial preparations is linoleic, and 500 ml of 10% lipid emulsion infused two or three times weekly meets most patients' requirements. Studies[24,25] have shown that medium-chain triglyceride (MCT) emulsions are more effective than their long-chain counterparts in maintaining lean body mass. The MCTs demonstrate more rapid elimination kinetics, increased ketone production, and greater lack of fatty deposition in the tissues than the long-chain triglyceride emulsions do.

The lipid emulsion usually is refrigerated until used and may be infused into the venous catheter system or by a separate peripheral vein. Because the emulsion will block most infusion filters, it must be infused beyond the filter. If administered

Table 31-4 Composition of Intravenous Fat Emulsions (10%)

	Intralipid	Liposyn
Lipid content		
Triglyceride	10% soybean oil	10% safflower oil
Phospholipid	1.2% (egg)	1.2% (egg)
Glycerol	2.5%	2.5%
Fatty acid composition (%)		
Linoleic (18:2)*	55	77
Oleic (18:1)	26	13
Palmitic (16:0)	9	7
Other	10	3
Osmolarity (mOsm/liter)	280	300
Caloric content (kcal/ml)	1.1	1.1

*18 carbons, 2 double bonds.

in combination with aqueous solutions, the less dense lipid emulsions must be elevated above the other bottles. When parenteral lipid furnishes a major portion of daily caloric requirements, it is convenient to infuse the emulsions for 20 hours each day (e.g., 8 AM to 4 AM) to allow a sufficient interval for lipid clearance so that routine laboratory blood tests are not contaminated.

A number of adverse reactions may accompany the use of the fat emulsions. All are rare and disappear with reduction or cessation of the infusate. Pyrogenic reactions occur in less than 1% of patients. A coagulopathy manifested by thrombocytopenia rarely causes clinically important bleeding problems. Hyperlipidemia may occur when doses exceed 3 g/kg/day. Pulmonary diffusion capacity may fall with rapid administration of the emulsion to patients with preexisting pulmonary insufficiency.[26] The fat overload syndrome associated with use of the older parenteral fat emulsions (Lipomul) is rarely seen with the newer emulsions. With prolonged administration, fat pigment deposition and microgranuloma formation in the liver not infrequently occur but are not associated predictably with liver dysfunction. The long-term consequences of these histologic changes is not known. Liver dysfunction, which is rare, may cause moderate elevation of bilirubin, alkaline phosphatase, and enzymes. The emulsions contain high concentrations of phosphate and must be used with caution in patients with renal failure. Parenteral lipid influsions should not be used in patients with (1) abnormalities of lipid transport and metabolism, (2) diabetes mellitus, (3) liver disease, (4) coagulopathy with thrombocytopenia, and (5) severe pulmonary disease.

Nitrogen. Although protein hydrolysates formerly were used as a source of nitrogen, they have been replaced by crystalline amino acid solutions. A variety of these solutions is now available, each with its unique spectrum of amino acid composition and concentration (Table 31-5). Infants and children require a higher fraction of total amino acids as essential ones (0.4 versus 0.2 for adults), and all commercial preparations are formulated to meet the higher requirements of children (including histidine). Nephramine does not contain arginine, which may have to be added separately to obtain optimal nitrogen balance in uremic patients.[27] Certain amino acids (e.g., aspartate, glutamate) are absent from most commercial preparations, and abnormal plasma patterns of uncertain physiologic significance may result. Trophamine contains glutamic acid, as well as taurine and tyrosine (from N-acetyl-L-tyrosine), a formulation that is proposed to produce a unique tophic effect on growing tissues. Studies[28] have shown that glutamine may have a major importance in the maintenance of the integrity of the small bowel. Following administration of a glutamine-enriched parenteral diet, the small intestine demonstrates a net uptake of glutamine associated with an increase in small bowel mucosal weight, DNA content, and villous height. This increase in mucosal mass may improve small bowel function, facilitate enteral nutrition, and maintain an effective barrier against escape of luminal bacteria from the gut. FreAmine I contains the basic amino acids as hydrochloride salts, and although its use not infrequently causes metabolic acidosis, especially in children, it occasionally is

Table 31-5 Amino Acid Content of Parenteral Solutions

Amino Acids (g/100 ml)	Aminosyn* 10%	FreAmine II 8.5%	Nephramine 5.4%	Travasol* 8.5%	Veinamine 8%
Essential					
L-Isoleucine	0.720	0.590	0.560	0.406	0.493
L-Leucine	0.940	0.770	0.880	0.526	0.347
L-Lysine (free base)	0.720	0.620	0.640	0.394	0.534
L-Methionine	0.400	0.450†	0.880	0.492	0.427
L-Phenylalanine	0.440	0.480	0.880	0.526	0.400
L-Threonine	0.520	0.340	0.400	0.356	0.160
L-Tryptophan	0.160	0.130	0.200	0.152	0.080
L-Valine	0.800	0.560	0.640	0.390	0.253
TOTAL (g/100 ml)	4.700	3.940	5.901	3.242	2.694
Nonessential					
L-Alanine	1.280	0.600	—	1.760	—
Aminoacetic acid (glycine)	1.280	1.700	—	1.760	3.387
L-Arginine	0.980	0.310	—	0.880	0.749
Aspartic acid	—	—	—	—	0.400
L-Cysteine/HCl/H$_2$O	—	0.020	<0.020	—	—
Glutamic acid	—	—	—	—	—
L-Histidine‡	0.300	0.240	0.250	0.372	0.237
L-Proline	0.860	0.950	—	0.356	0.107
L-Serine	0.420	0.500	—	—	—
L-Tyrosine	0.044	—	—	0.034	—
TOTAL (g/100 ml)	5.164	4.320	0.270	5.162	5.306
Percentage of total that is EAA	47	48	100†	39	34
Total nitrogen (g/liter)	15.7	13.0	8.5	13.2	12.6
Osmolarity (mOsm/liter)	1000	810	440	860	950

*Available as less concentrated solutions with amino acid concentrations in proportion, with or without added electrolytes.

†As DL-methionine.

‡Histidine is an essential amino acid in infants.

beneficial in patients with metabolic alkalosis.[29] FreAmine II employs acetate as the corresponding amino acid salt and has added phosphate (20 mEq/liter), which must be considered in the daily determinations of phosphate requirements. Amino acid solutions are normally low in electrolytes, but several commercial formulations are available with fixed quantities of added electrolytes. Trace elements are present in varying amounts only as contaminants and their concentration varies with each lot of any single brand.

Albumin provides a usable but prohibitively expensive source of nitrogen. It is rapidly degraded after administration, and its amino acid components are added to the body nitrogen pool. If given in sufficient amounts, exogenous albumin can achieve positive nitrogen balance.[30] Administration of red blood cells provides little nutritional protein. Plasma, like purified albumin, is an impractical source of nitrogen. The use of plasma to replace trace elements is expensive and unnecessarily exposes the patient to the risk of hepatitis and acquired immune deficiency syndrome. Trace element solutions based on the individual patient's specific needs are formulated easily in the hospital pharmacy.

Vitamins. Parenteral vitamins can be supplied by several commercial preparations whose composition is based on various empirical standards. Most do not contain a full spectrum of vitamins, and familiarity with the concentrations in each formulation is essential. Overdosage of vitamins A and D and omission of folate, biotin, and vitamins K and B$_{12}$ cause the most frequent vitamin derangements in hospitalized patients. One preparation (MVI-12) contains all the vitamins except K in doses that meet the Nutritional Advisory Group/American Medical Association guidelines for maintenance requirements (Table 31-6).[31] In stressed patients, requirements for some vitamins may be increased, especially those for vitamin C, which may be supplemented (up to 500 mg/da). Vitamin K is administered orally or parenterally

Table 31-6 Intravenous Multivitamins for Daily Maintenance

Vitamin	Units	Infants or Children under 11 Years	Older Children and Adults
A	IU	2300	3300
D	IU	400	200
E	IU	7.0	10
K	mg	0.2	—
Ascorbic acid	mg	80	100
Thiamine	mg	1.2	3
Riboflavin	mg	1.4	3.6
Niacin	mg	17	40
Pyridoxine	mg	1	4
Pantothenic acid	mg	5	15
Folic acid	μg	140	400
B_{12}	μg	1	5
Biotin	μg	20	60

From Shils ME: Bull Parenter Drug Assoc **30**:226-233, 1976.

once each week. Measurement of plasma vitamin concentrations as a guide to replacement may be misleading, since low concentrations of the carrier protein may mask a normal active level. Parenteral vitamins should be administered slowly and in higher doses because of high urinary loss.

PERIPHERAL INFUSIONS

Alimentation by peripheral infusion is used most effectively as a weight maintenance diet for nonhypermetabolic patients (basal energy expenditure less than 1800 kcal/da), as a preliminary mode before central infusion, and as a supplement to tube feeding. In addition, hypocaloric peripheral infusions minimize protein breakdown in stable postoperative patients who are expected to return to an adequate oral diet within 10 days. Parenteral nutrition by peripheral vein avoids the hazards of catheters placed in central veins. The limnits to peripheral nutrition are the high tonicity and volume of infusate required to meet caloric demands. Prolonged infusions into low flow peripheral veins are possible with solutions of less than 500 mOsm/liter (10% dextrose in water has a tonicity of 530 mOsm/liter). The use of solutions with greater tonicity is associated with the rapid onset of phlebitis and thrombosis.

Peripheral Vein Nutrition

The availability of fat emulsions has permitted peripheral total parenteral nutrition in some pa-

tients. However, most ill patients will utilize no more than 50% to 60% of total caloric intake as fat, and the remaining nutritional intake must be supplied as carbohydrate and nitrogen. Since most adult patients cannot safely tolerate more than 3 liters of fluid per day, peripheral feedings can supply, at best, 2200 kcal/day (e.g., 150 g of lipid, 150 g of dextrose, 80 g of amino acids in 3 liters of solution). Such formulations are markedly hypertonic (900 mOsm/liter), and the peripheral infusion sites usually must be changed every 48 hours to minimize phlebitis. Until usable peripheral veins are exhausted, such techniques frequently will meet the energy requirements of resting starved patients. Peripheral feedings will not meet the requirements of critically ill hypermetabolic patients or of debilitated patients who require long-term hypercaloric support to meet existing metabolic requirements and to restore body weight. Even in burn patients whose high evaporative water loss allows the administration of large fluid volumes (5-6 liters/da), peripheral vein nutrition ordinarily will not meet resting energy requirements.[32]

Protein-Sparing Therapy

Peripheral intravenous feeding with isotonic amino acids alone has been proposed as a nutritional regimen that uniquely conserves body protein.[33,34] In those studies, amino acid solutions administered at a rate of 1 to 2 g/kg/day blunted nitrogen loss and in some patients temporarily induced positive nitrogen balance. Equicaloric amounts of glucose were not as effective in improving nitrogen balance. Insulin concentrations were decreased, and fatty acid and ketone levels were increased in patients receiving the glucose-free isotonic amino acid solutions. These conditions allowed lipid mobilized from fat stores to serve as an energy source. Since glucose stimulates insulin production and its subsequent antilipolytic effects, it was proposed that glucose increased protein catabolism.

Protein sparing is not unique with infusions of amino acid alone, and the effect of amino acids is not related to the degree of endogenous fat mobilization.[35,36] The addition of either glucose or fat to the infusion regimen does not increase negative nitrogen balance, and at fixed amino acid infusion rates, increasing glucose intake increases nitrogen retention and protein synthesis.[32,37,38] In general, this technique does not totally reverse negative nitrogen balance, and most of the administered amino acid is catabolyzed and excreted as urea.[39] The increased nitrogenous breakdown products may be hazardous to patients with renal or hepatic failure. The maximum improvement in nitrogen balance seems to occur predominately in depleted patients, and isotonic amino acid solutions do not meet the energy and amino acid requirements of hypermetabolic patients.

COMBINED ENTERAL AND PARENTERAL FEEDING

Parenteral infusion, usually by peripheral vein, can be used to supplement the enteral intake of patients with inadequate gastrointestinal function or with limited body stores in the face of increased metabolic demands. Such patients include those with partial small bowel obstruction, malabsorption, intractable diarrhea, depressed appetite following trauma, renal or liver dysfunction, marked hypermetabolism, and those receiving chemotherapy. Every attempt should be made to utilize the enteral route, including continual infusion of defined formula diets. If such round-the-clock feeding does not meet the patient's nutritional needs adequately, parenteral administration of the remaining required nutrients is initiated. Parenteral infusions may be continuous, or intermittent with the use of a heparin lock. Although carbohydrate and nitrogen requirements are met by the enteral portion of the diet, parenterally administered lipid

emulsions may effectively supplement caloric intake. Vitamins and trace elements usually are included in the enteral feedings.

CENTRAL INFUSIONS

Total parenteral nutrition (TPN) by prolonged and continuous central vein infusion is the only means to meet complete nutritional requirements when enteral feeding is not feasible. Although central infusions can be used to supplement enteral diets, peripheral infusion is safer in this context because it avoids the hazards of a central venous catheter. The term intravenous hyperalimentation often is used as a synonym for central TPN, but it implies that caloric support is administered in excess of the patient's energy requirements. However, the therapeutic goal of TPN in most situations is maintenance of body mass rather than its gain, and the term TPN provides a more applicable general description of this form of nutritional support.

Indications

Current nutrition texts list many specific diseases for which TPN has been found to be useful.[40] In many cases, some of these indications are relative, and with the recent availability of nonreactive small-caliber feeding tubes and defined formula diets, enteral feedings often can be substituted for TPN. General indications can be separated into categories for childhood and adult age groups. In infants, TPN is effective in three groups of patients. (1) "Surgical neonates" in whom gastrointestinal tract dysfunction prevents enteral feeding for 10 to 14 days require TPN beginning as soon following delivery as is feasible. Infants in this category include those with omphalocele, gastroschisis, bowel atresia, and short bowel syndrome following resection for midgut volvulus. (2) TPN can reverse the severe malnutrition of infants and small children with chronic diarrhea and malabsorption syndromes. During TPN, a complete workup of the underlying disease should be carried out. (3) Low–birth-weight infants with initial poor feeding behavior may benefit from TPN until a mature suckling response develops.

Most of the indications for TPN in adults are included in the following categories: (1) TPN should be administered to patients with surgically correctable diseases that have caused a weight loss exceeding 10% of the ideal or usual body weight.[41] Examples are chronic bowel obstruction and peptic ulcer. Following surgical correction, TPN should be continued if the patient is not expected to be able to eat within 7 to 10 days postoperatively. (2) TPN is efficacious for patients with chronic gastrointestinal diseases that produce excessive weight loss or in whom enteral intake activates the disease process. These diseases include regional enteritis, radiation enteritis, enteric fistulas, and chronic pancreatitis. (3) TPN is indicated in patients with greatly increased metabolic demands that cannot be satisfied by enteral feedings, and in whom resolution of the disease process is a distant prospect. These diseases include burns, multiple trauma, and peritonitis. A somewhat controversial indication involves patients with diseases in which anabolism may increase healing or beneficially modify the pathologic process. In these diseases, which include renal failure, hepatic insufficiency, and cancer, correction of abnormal laboratory values and restoration of normal body composition have been achieved with TPN, but the data so far are inconsistent and insufficient to confirm improved survival.[42,43]

Calculation of TPN Feedings

The daily patient diet utilizing TPN can be constructed easily by following a logical sequence of calculations.

1. Determine the patient's daily fluid requirements.
2. Determine the patient's energy expenditure (by direct measurements or from nomograms that reflect the effect of specific diseases) and the goal of nutritional support (hypocaloric versus maintenance versus weight gain).
3. Decide on the composition of the nonprotein calorie source. In addition to glucose, up to 50% of the caloric requirement can be administered as fat to patients whose energy expenditures do not exceed 25% of their normal rates.
4. Decide on the optimum nitrogen/calorie ratio, approximately 1:150 for most critically ill patients, although may be lower in hypocaloric feeding. Nitrogen is administered as crystalline amino acids.
5. Distribute glucose and amino acids evenly in the fluid to be administered (excluding the volume to be given as a fat emulsion).

Table 31-7 Daily Maintenance Requirements

	Infants (per kg)	Adults (per kg)
Calories (kcal)	90-125	30-40
Protein (g)	2-3.5	1-1.5
Water (ml)	100-200	30-40
Electrolytes*		
Sodium (mEq)	2-4	1-2
Potassium (mEq)	2-3	0.7-2
Magnesium (mEq)	0.3-0.5	0.3-0.4
Calcium (mEq)	0.3-0.5	0.2-0.3
Phosphorus (mM)	0.5-0.8	0.3-0.5

*Extremely variable; adjust to maintain normal serum concentrations.

6. Add vitamins, electrolytes, and essential fatty acids as indicated by known daily requirements and timely laboratory determinations.

Relative requirements of infants and small children are proportionately larger than those of adults (Table 31-7). As always, these calculations are guidelines only, to be modified by continual clinical and laboratory assessment.

Solution Preparation

Two approaches to the preparation of parenteral solutions commonly are employed in most hospitals: basic unit formulation and individual formulation. The basic unit contains prescribed quantities of calories, nitrogen, and electrolytes per unit volume and is usually available in several standard compositions (low sodium, high potassium, etc.). The individual formulation, although more expensive, allows the use of solutions that meet the individual patient's specific requirements (Table 31-8). Although standard basic units meet the needs of the majority of patients, individual formulations can meet unusual needs of particular patients, and most hospital pharmacy departments use both methods.

Solutions should be prepared in a special section of the hospital pharmacy department by a pharmacist who is a member of a multidisciplinary team with primary responsibility for advanced hospital nutrition support techniques. Most methods utilize partially filled evacuated bottles of components that are added in the desired quantities with closed transfer sets. The

Table 31-8 Typical Composition of 1 Liter of TPN Solution for Central Vein Infusion in Adults

Volume	1000	ml
Energy	1000	kcal
Dextrose	250	g
Amino acids	42.5	g
Nitrogen	6.25	g
Electrolytes		
Sodium (chloride, acetate, lactate, bicarbonate)	40-50	mEq
Potassium (chloride, acetate, lactate, acid phosphate)	30-40	mEq
Magnesium (sulfate)	6-10	mEq
Phosphate (potassium acid salt)	12-18	mM
Calcium (gluconate)	4-8	mEq
Trace elements*		
Vitamins† (additions to 1 unit daily)		
Vitamin A	3300	USP units
Vitamin D	200	USP units
Vitamin E	10	IU
Vitamin C‡	100	mg
Thiamine	3	mg
Riboflavin	3.6	mg
Niacinamide	40	mg
Pantothenic acid	15	mg
Pyridoxine	4	mg
Folic acid	400	μg
Biotin	60	μg
B_{12}	5	μg

Note: Commercial kits containing 500 ml of 50% dextrose and 500 ml of 8.5% crystalline amino acids commonly are utilized to approximate TPN solution.

* Trace elements are present in commercial amino acid solutions in variable amounts and should be supplemented as dictated by serum concentrations.

† Vitamin K (5 mg) is administered orally or by intramuscular injection once weekly.

‡ Vitamin C may be required in higher levels in critically ill patients.

additions are carried out under laminar flow hoods, which reduce the incidence of solution contamination. The glucose and amino acid portions should not be combined until shortly before use. If these two ingredients are allowed to remain mixed for prolonged periods, they combine to form glucosamines (Maillard reaction), which discolor the solutions and bind zinc and copper following infusion.[44] The risk of solution contamination rises after storage for 12 hours at room temperature, and the daily fluid requirement should be packaged so that no single bottle

is hung for more than that length of time. The prepared solutions may be stored safely at 4° C for up to 48 hours before use. Because ventricular fibrillation can occur with infusion of cold fluid directly into the heart, refrigerated solutions must be rewarmed before infusion through a central venous cannula.

Solution Administration

Although solutions can be administered by gravity flow, calibrated pumps ensure accurate flow rates and provide a variety of alarms to signal an empty container or potential air embolism. However, tape with incremental delivery times should be placed on the fluid containers to serve as a monitor of infusion pump accuracy. The pumps are not without hazard, since they will continue to force fluid through a cannula that has extravasated into the pleural space or subcutaneous tissue until sufficient back pressure has developed.

Hypertonic nutritional solution administration should be instituted at a relatively slow infusion rate (1 liter/24 hr). Gradually, the rate of infusion is increased to the maximal levels of fluid tolerance, usually around 3 liters/day. The speed with which the infusion rate can be increased is determined by the patient's tolerance and renal threshold to glucose. With each increment, small doses of insulin may be administered subcutaneously or added to the infusion to facilitate normoglycemia. Later, as the patient's endogenous insulin production increases, the exogenous insulin may be decreased or eliminated.

Central Venous Catheter Insertion

The most important technical advance in TPN was the realization that a catheter placed in a high flow central vein allowed rapid dilution of the infused hypertonic nutrient solutions. Although the catheter can be introduced safely through the internal jugular and external jugular veins, the percutaneous infraclavicular subclavian vein is the most popular approach for long-term parenteral nutrition.[45] In this location the catheter is most reliably secured and least obtrusive to the patient. Following central vein cannulation, the tip of the catheter is placed in the superior vena cava at its junction with the right atrium.[46] Although the inferior vena cava approached through the femoral vein may be used as a temporary expedient in patients with difficult to cannulate superior vena cava tributaries, the long-term use of this route is associated with a higher incidence of thrombosis and infection.[47] Furthermore, the central venous cannula should not be threaded through a peripheral vein into the superior vena cava. The peripheral vein commonly develops thrombophlebitis, and movement of the joints over which the catheter traverses produces a back and forth motion of the catheter tip, which eventually can puncture the wall of the superior vena cava.

Many papers describe the technique of central venous cannulation, and the details of insertion will not be described here. Subclavian vein catheterization (or any comparable method) is not a technique that should be read about and then performed. Rather, after a thorough review of the pertinent regional anatomy, this procedure should be learned under the guidance of an experienced physician (more than 1000 insertions) who daily uses this technique. However, there are a few points that should be emphasized, since they often help avoid a number of complications.

Catheter insertion is a sterile surgical procedure, and the operator should wear a gown, gloves, and a mask. As in any preoperative preparation, the skin at the insertion site is shaved, defatted, and disinfected. If tolerated, the patient should be placed in the Trendelenburg position to dilate the subclavian vein maximally for easier insertion and to decrease the risk of air embolism. If the patient is being treated with positive-pressure ventilation, the patient should be disconnected briefly from the respirator, if possible, to decrease the risk of puncturing the pleura. Although many original descriptions of catheter placement emphasized the lateral approach directed toward the sternal notch, a higher rate of success and few complications may be obtained by insertion at the medial one third of the clavicular border and aiming one finger breadth cephalad of the sternal notch.[48] A 2-inch needle mounted on a 3 ml syringe should be used. A longer needle can be passed inadvertently across the midline, producing serious injury, and the small syringe more effectively detects the "flashback" of blood upon entering the subclavian vein than does a large syringe, which may obscure entry into the vein by causing it to collapse. No attempt should be made to withdraw a nonfunctioning catheter while the needle remains inserted into the patient. Rather, if the catheter cannot be advanced easily, both needle and catheter should be withdrawn as a single unit. Failure to follow this dictum may lead to severance and subsequent embolism of the catheter. After the catheter has been inserted and the needle withdrawn, the infusion bottle should be lowered beneath the level of the patient to verify by the free return of blood that the catheter is in the vein. If no blood return occurs, the entire catheter assembly should be removed and replaced with a new apparatus. Following successful placement, the catheter should be sutured in the skin and covered with a small dressing. A chest roentgenogram will confirm catheter tip location and detect potential mechanical complications. The use of an introducer system facilitates safe subclavian vein catheterization of infants and children.[49] In stable patients without infection, a well-functioning catheter can last from weeks to months.[50]

Catheter Maintenance

For patients requiring long-term TPN, the central venous catheter is best cared for by members of the nutrition support team especially trained for this responsibility. The catheter site is inspected and cleansed every 48 hours (or three times weekly). The old tape and dressings are removed by personnel wearing masks, gloves, and gowns, and the insertion site is defatted and disinfected. An antibiotic ointment and sterile dressings are reapplied. If gross contamination of the dressings is expected (as from an adjacent draining wound), an adherent plastic surgical drape may be placed over the dressing.

Monitoring the Patient Receiving TPN

Frequent monitoring of patients is necessary because of the potentially high incidence of dangerous complications associated with TPN. In addition, a systematic monitoring protocol facilitates assessment of the efficacy of nutritional support. It should be pointed out that many of the monitoring requirements for TPN also apply to those for continuous enteral feeding with defined formula diets. Although Table 31-9 lists the recommended frequencies of specific tests, the frequency should be altered according to the patient's immediate condition and response to therapy. The patient's nutrient and fluid needs must be reviewed daily and correlated with laboratory data. Overzealous reliance on blood analysis can lead to introgenic anemia from excessive blood sampling and to neglect of clinical assessment.

The most important variable to be evaluated following institution of TPN is the patient's response to the hypertonic glucose infusion. Testing the urine for glucose every 4 to 6 hours usually provides an adequate estimate of the patient's glucose tolerance and need for insulin. However, concomitant plasma determinations may be required initially to determine the threshold for glucose "spillage." Urine chemistry determinations provide a convenient means for monitoring other nutritional variables. Nitrogen excretion reflects nutritional status. Administration of sufficient potassium to produce urinary losses of approximately 40 mEq/day generally reflects adequate potassium intake, although acutely tramatized patients (e.g., burns) may lose up to 600 mEq/day unrelated to intake. Patients receiving fat emulsions as a major caloric source should have more frequent determinations of serum lipids than are recommended in Table 31-9.

Complications of TPN

Mechanical. Mechanical complications related to catheter malposition usually are not hazardous to the patient initially. Instead of turning down into the superior vena cava, the cannula inserted through the subclavian vein may course into the internal jugular vein or, rarely, into the opposite subclavian vein. Before infusion of hy-

Table 31-9 Variables to be Monitored During Parenteral Alimentation

	Frequency of Monitoring	
	First Week	Thereafter
Energy balance		
Weight	Daily	Daily
Indirect calorimetry	As needed	As needed
Fluid balance		
Volume of infusate	Daily	Daily
Oral intake (if any)	Daily	Daily
Urinary output	Daily	Daily
Other losses	Daily	Daily
Metabolic variables		
Blood measurements		
Plasma electrolytes (Na^+, K^+, Cl^-)	Daily	3 × weekly
BUN	3 × weekly	2 × weekly
Creatinine	Daily	3 × weekly
Osmolarity	Daily	3 × weekly
Total calcium and inorganic phosphate	3 × weekly	2 × weekly
Glucose	Daily	3 × weekly
Liver profile	3 × weekly	2 × weekly
Total protein and fractions	2 × weekly	Weekly
Acid-base status	As indicated	As indicated
Hemoglobin	Weekly	Weekly
Ammonia	As indicated	As indicated
Prothrombin time	Weekly	Weekly
Magnesium	2 × weekly	Weekly
Triglyceride	Weekly	Weekly
Urine measurements		
Glucose	4-6 × daily	2 × daily
Specific gravity or osmolarity	2-4 × daily	Daily
Urea (for balance studies)	As indicated	As indicated
Prevention and detection of infection		
Clinical observations (activity, temperature, symptoms)	Daily	Daily
WBC count and differential	As indicated	As indicated
Cultures	As indicated	As indicated

pertonic fluids, the misplaced catheter should be repositioned into the superior vena cava, where maximum flow and dilution of infusate occur. Pneumothorax is the most common and potentially dangerous mechanical complication. Others are as follows:

Pneumothorax
Hemothorax
Arterial or venous laceration
Air embolism
Cardiac perforation and tamponade
Hydromediastinum
Subclavian vein or superior vena cava thrombosis
Catheter embolism
Pulmonary embolism
Thoracic duct laceration
Cardiac arrhythmias
Subcutaneous emphysema
Nerve injury (brachial plexus, phrenic, vagus)
Improper location

As with most of the mechanical complications, the incidence of pneumothorax is related to physician experience with catheter placement.[51,52] The incidence of pneumothorax following subclavian catheterization by members of an experienced nutrition support team is commonly less than 1% or 2%. Excessive bleeding can occur in patients with severe thrombocytopenia (platelet count less than 25,000/ml,) and if central venous catheterization is imperative, platelet transfusions should be administered. Most potential complications can be prevented or detected early by adhering to the checks of a strict insertion protocol and by obtaining a post-insertion roentgenogram.

Infectious. The most serious late complication of TPN is catheter sepsis, which is defined as a febrile episode unexplained by another identifiable septic focus and is relieved by removal of the catheter. Others are as follows:

Endocarditis
Septic thrombophlebitis
Septic embolism
Septicemia arising from contaminated catheter or
contaminated parenteral solution

Although patients receiving TPN often have diseases and are being given medications that predispose them to infection, the adherence to a strict protocol of catheter care can reduce the incidence of catheter sepsis to under 5%. The central venous cannula should not be used for hemodynamic monitoring, the infusion of blood products, blood sampling, or the administration of medications or other parenterals. The parenteral solutions are excellent culture media and should be freshly prepared or refrigerated until used. In-line filters may reduce the incidence of catheter-related infection. The 0.45 μm filter will remove air bubbles, particulate contaminants, and most bacteria except *Pseudomonas*. A 0.22 μm filter will remove *Pseudomonas*, but its use requires an infusion pump for fluid delivery. If the central venous catheter must be used for both TPN and hemo-access in certain critically ill patients, the increased risk of infection requires more frequent replacement of the cannula. If such patients have invasive infection and frequent bacteremias, the catheters may require replacement every 48 or 72 hours.[53] If the catheter must be removed because of suspected catheter sepsis, it should be replaced in a new anatomic location rather than over a guidewire through the same insertion site.

If a patient receiving TPN becomes unexpectedly febrile or displays other signs of sepsis, such as hypothermia or sudden glucose intolerance, catheter sepsis must be suspected and investigated in a systematic fashion. A thorough history and physical examination is carried out to detect other potential sources of infection. If a source unrelated to the catheter is found, it is treated and the TPN infusion continued. If the TPN apparatus is suspected and the patient otherwise is stable, the infusate and tubing are replaced and cultured. Blood is obtained from a peripheral site and through the catheter for bacterial and fungal cultures. If the patient has multiple positive blood cultures and no source is discernible, the catheter should be removed. Even in the absence of positive blood cultures, if fever persists for 4 to 12 hours or if the patient's condition deteriorates, the catheter should be removed. A peripheral infusion containing 5% to 10% dextrose is administered to prevent hypoglycemia. Additional blood cultures should be obtained after the catheter is removed, and appropriate antibiotics are administered as indicated by blood culture results and/or the patient's condition.

Metabolic. Numerous metabolic complications have been associated with the administration of specific nutrients. The major ones with their causes and remedies appear on p. 498.

Metabolic Complication	Possible Causes	Remedies
Glucose		
Hyperglycemia, glycosuria, hyperosmolar dehydration	Excessive rate of infusion of glucose; inadequate endogenous insulin; sepsis; glucocorticoids; hypokalemia	Reduce glucose infusion rate; administer insulin; utilize fat emulsion as a portion of calories; replace potassium; correct fluid deficit
Ketoacidosis	Inadequate endogenous insulin response; insufficient exogenous insulin therapy	Give insulin; reduce glucose administration
Postinfusion (rebound) hypoglycemia	Persistence of increased insulin secretion rates by islet cells following abrupt cessation of hypertonic glucose infusions	Administer 5%-10% glucose before infusions discontinued
Fat		
Pyrogenic reaction	Fat emulsion	Exclude other causes of fever
Altered coagulation	Hyperlipemia	Restudy after fat has cleared from bloodstream
Hyperlipemia	Rapid infusion, decreased clearance	Decrease rate of infusion; reassess after lipid has cleared from bloodstream
Impaired liver function	Possibly fat emulsion, but more likely underlying disease process	Exclude other causes of hepatic dysfunction
Essential fatty acid deficiency	Absent or inadequate administration of essential fatty acid, especially linoleic; vitamin E deficiency	Enteral or topical safflower oil; parenteral lipid emulsions
Amino acid		
Hyperchloremic acidosis	Excessive chloride content of some crystalline amino acid solutions	Administer Na^+ and K^+ as acetate or lactate salts
Hyperammonemia	Deficiencies of specific amino acids in TPN solutions, especially arginine; primary liver disease	Reduce total amino acid intake; administer specific amino acid (arginine)
Prerenal azotemia	Excessive amino acid infusion with inadequate nonprotein calories	Reduce amino acid intake; increase glucose calories
Amino acid imbalance	Optimal amino acid mixtures not yet determined for specific disease processes	Utilize low concentrations (2%-3%) of amino acids; experimental amino acid solutions

Hyperglycemia is the most common metabolic complication and is accentuated by sepsis, hypovolemia, hypokalemia, and certain drugs. Pronounced hyperglycemia leads to glycosuria and an osmotic diuresis, resulting in dehydration and hyperosmolarity. Hyperglycemia following the institution of TPN is treated with exogenous insulin and/or a reduction in the rate of glucose administration. Often, hyperglycemia can be avoided by slowly increasing the daily glucose dose to the desired caloric levels, allowing the pancreas to adapt gradually to new endogenous insulin requirements. If this regimen is unsuccessful, insulin is administered in dosages usually determined by the degree of glycosuria. For most patients, urine glucose of 3+ is treated with 5 units of regular insulin and 4+ with 10 units. If the patient has a high renal threshold for glucose, which can be determined by simultaneously obtained blood glucose concentrations, or if the patient has diabetes mellitus with a known insulin requirement, proportionally higher doses of insulin will be needed.

Except in patients with diabetes mellitus, ketonemia and ketonuria do not often accompany hyperglycemia. When ketosis occurs, it can be prevented by the use of hypertonic glucose and rarely will occasion the need for additional insulin. Initially the insulin should be administered subcutaneously, since sharp fluctuations of plasma glucose reflect the very short activity half-life of insulin given intravenously as a bolus. Alternatively, the insulin can be infused continuously with a syringe pump. Once the daily dose of insulin stabilizes, it can be placed in the TPN solutions in evenly divided amounts. Although this approach suffers from the theoretical disadvantage of insulin adherence to the container, the amount lost tends to be constant and is easily replaced as guided by routine chemistry determinations. Fasting blood glucose should be maintained between 150 and 200 mg/dl if hypoglycemia can be avoided. Once the patient's endogenous hormonal response has adapted to the added glucose load and any acute process has resolved, the need for exogenous insulin may be eliminated or at least reduced.

If the severely stressed patient receiving TPN becomes hyperglycemic with glycosuria and dehydration, it is virtually impossible to treat his hyperglycemia without first correcting the deficit of free water and intravascular volume. This means using 5% dextrose solutions and correcting any electrolyte imbalances. The azotemia often associated with hyperglycemic hyperosmolar dehydration readily responds to fluid replacement. Glucose-free solutions should not be used in most cases, since sudden and unexpected hypoglycemia may occur. When the patient's fluid and electrolyte abnormalities have returned to normal and body weight is restored, TPN can be resumed slowly, with additional insulin if necessary.

When lipids are omitted from the diet for periods exceeding 1-2 weeks, unsaturated fatty acid deficits occur and cause a characteristic syndrome. This essential fatty acid deficiency presents with dermatitis, hemolytic anemia, thrombocytopenia, impaired wound healing, loss of hair, and early death. The deficiency can be prevented with parenterally administered lipid emulsions or enterally administered safflower oil, as mentioned on page 498. Medium-chain triglycerides (MCTs) lack essential fatty acids, which must be supplemented separately. In addition, MCTs may cause ketoacidosis and must be utilized with caution, especially in patients with liver disease or portacaval shunts.

The hyperammonemia associated with protein hydrolysates and the metabolic acidosis with the hydrochloride salts of amino acids are now rarely encountered. Occasionally, these complications, as well as azotemia, occur in infants and small children receiving large volumes of amino acid solutions deficient in histidine and arginine. The disorders can be treated by ensuring that adequate nonprotein calories are administered with amino acids (which should include histidine and arginine) or by decreasing the rate of administration of the amino acid solutions.

Most major electrolyte (Na^+, K^+, Cl^-) abnormalities can be avoided by careful monitoring and by a familiarity with typical maintenance requirements (Table 31-7). Vitamin overdosages (especially with A and D) and deficiencies are avoided by the daily administration of recommended allowances and by clinical and laboratory assessment.

Daily calcium requirements vary, but the amount given must prevent bone demineralization while avoiding soft tissue calcification. Increased protein intake and immobilization accentuate calcium loss in the urine. Hypercalcemia may be caused by excessive vitamin D, phosphate deficiency, inactivity, and overzealous calcium administration. Phosphate deficiency usually arises from inadequate administration. Sudden infusion of a large glucose load (as with the inappropriate institution of TPN) may elicit a profound drop in serum phosphate; conversely, hyperphosphatemia may occur when glucose administration is reduced.[54] Adequate phosphate intake is essential for nitrogen retention, with approximately 85 mg of phosphate required for each gram of nitrogen incorporated.[55] Severe hypophosphatemia (less than 1 mg/dl) causes reduced erythrocyte concentrations of 2,3-diphosphoglycerate and increased oxygen affinity for hemoglobin, hemolytic anemia, altered phagocytosis, hyperventilation, seizures, and coma.[56] Magnesium, for which there is a well-established requirement, is frequently overlooked when planning TPN. The administration of amphotericin, carbenicillin, cisplatin, and other drugs accentuates urinary magnesium losses, which must be replaced. Since magnesium is an intracellular cation, serum determinations may not reflect acute losses. Balance studies calculated from urine and drainage collections will provide a more accurate quantification of daily magnesium requirements.

Hepatic dysfunction may occur during TPN administration.[57] Affected patients become jaundiced without pruritus or prominent hepatomegaly. Although the serum bilirubin may be markedly elevated (exceeding 10 mg/dl), alkaline phosphatase usually exhibits only a mild and transient rise. Liver histology reflects fatty infiltration and intrahepatic cholestasis. The hepatic steatosis secondary to TPN may be treated by lowering the glucose concentration and/or increasing the amino acid concentration of the infusion or by administering glucose-free amino acid solutions.

HOME TPN

Patients utilizing home TPN usually have undergone a massive bowel resection or had severe malabsorption following radiation or inflammatory bowel disease[58] and are clinically stable; but whereas some will eventually experience intestinal adaptation to normal eating, others will be dependent on home TPN for the remainder of their lives. For these persons the cuffed silicone catheter[59,60] provides safe home delivery of parenteral nutrients for as long as 5 years. The catheter is introduced through a subcutaneous tunnel and inserted into the cephalic, subclavian, or jugular vein. Fibrous tissue grows around it and into the Dacron cuff, thus fixing it to place and retarding bacterial spread along its course.[61] When this catheter only has been used for TPN, catheter-related sepsis has occurred in less than 5% of patients and the patients have become very adept at cleaning it aseptically.

TPN solutions can be prepared sterilely at home by using vacuum-sealed containers in kits. Many patients use intermittent infusions while asleep, so that during the daylight hours they will be free of the administration system. The intermittent infusion must be tapered over the last 1 to 2 hours to avoid rebound hypoglycemia. Patency of the catheter is maintained by a heparin lock. Alternatively, with an appropriate harness and portable battery-driven or gas-pressure pumps, TPN solutions can be infused continuously. The daily administration rate and volume of the nutritional solutions should be regulated to maintain body weight. Infusion protocols must include all nutrients, along with trace elements, lest deficiencies occur during prolonged home TPN.

ASSESSMENT OF THE HOSPITALIZED PATIENT RECEIVING NUTRITIONAL SUPPORT

Measurements of body weight not only yield accurate information about the patient's nutritional status prior to hospitalization but, when performed daily, also allow continuous monitoring of the efficacy of intensive nutritional support once treatment is instituted. Rapid changes in weight almost always arise from alterations in body water balance, and only after the patient has reached a clinically stable period during his illness do body weight determinations accurately reflect his nutritional balance. An increase in weight exceeding 0.4 kg/day indicates water accumulation, and even smaller increments during the first several weeks of refeeding the depleted patient often represent only an increase in body water. Gradual accumulation of edema may mask a continued erosion of lean body mass. However, when fluid balance calculated from intake and output records is compared with changes in daily weight, an accurate estimate of body mass can be deduced in most situations.

Nitrogen balance studies reflect alterations in body protein stores. Nitrogen balance is the algebraic sum of the daily intake and of nitrogen loss. A positive value implies net gain in body protein; a negative value denotes erosion of body protein mass. Nitrogen intake is calculated easily from the known nitrogen content of food items and the amount administered. Nitrogen loss is more difficult to quantify and must include that lost from urine, feces, skin, exudates, and drainage. Eighty percent of nitrogenous wastes appear in the urine as urea. Thus a rough calculation of nitrogen loss can be obtained by measuring the 24-hour urinary excretion of urea and adding 2 to 4 g to account for other unmeasured losses. However, large quantities of nitrogen may be lost from nonurinary sources, such as from recently burned skin, from which losses may contribute up to 25% of total nitrogen deficit.[62] In such cases, all body effluents must be collected and nitrogen content determined. Currently available instrumentation using automated micro-Kjeldahl or chemiluminescence techniques permits determination of all nitrogen-containing compounds, including urea, uric acid, ammonia, amino acids, and intact protein.

Calorie counts are carried out by the dietitian and dietary technicians working with the nutrition support team. By careful supervision of food tray distribution and retrieval and by monitoring fluid balance records, an accurate measurement of calories, nitrogen, and other essential nutrients can be made. When combined with daily weight determinations and nitrogen balance studies, the overall effectiveness of nutritional support in

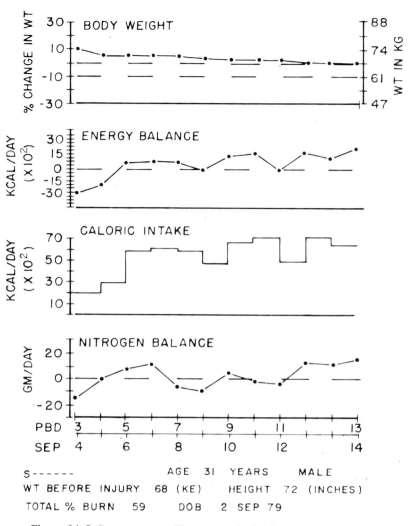

Figure 31-5 Computer surveillance record of daily nutritional support.

preserving or restoring body mass can be assessed on a continuous basis (Fig. 31-5).

Anthropometric measurements are most helpful for assessing the nutritional state of patients with long-standing illnesses. In this role, these techniques yield an accurate indication of the degree of depletion before nutritional therapy is instituted and are effective monitors of patient response during a long period of dietary support. A variety of standardized tests can estimate proportions of body fat and protein and are discussed in Chapters 9 and 10. Anthropometric measurements are usually less applicable to critically ill or injured patients, who develop sepsis or cardiopulmonary insufficiency or who require multiple surgical procedures.

A number of laboratory tests are utilized to assess plasma proteins, which reflect in part the capability of the liver to synthesize protein. The plasma concentrations of transport proteins, including albumin, transferrin, prealbumin, and retinol binding protein, may correlate with the degree of nutritional sufficiency, but are also affected by disease state. Although less well studied, the production of acute phase proteins, including α_2-macroglobulin and α_1-antitrypsin, may reflect the ability to synthesize hepatic protein and, by inference, structural protein for enzymes and muscle. A variety of immunologic defects accompany malnutrition, and the patient's response to alimentation can be assessed by serial measurements of immunologic function. Specific tests are described in Chapters 2 and 32.

Computer monitoring of nutritional support provides a means for accurate record keeping and for quality control and evaluation of techniques and diets. The data files store information about the carbohydrate, protein, fat, vitamin, mineral, and other nutrient contents of all table foods, defined formula diets, food supplements, and parenteral solutions. All pertinent laboratory data, including both blood and uring determinations, are entered and stored daily. When accurate intake and output records are provided, precise balance measurements are calculated automatically. Body weight and anthropometric measurements are correlated with the balance studies. The computer surveillance program also monitors all important complications of the various alimentation techniques, and these complications should be reviewed periodically.

REFERENCES

1. Kinney JM, et al: Use of the ventilatory equivalent to separate hypermetabolism from increased dead space ventilation in the injured or septic patient, J Trauma 20:111-119, 1980.
2. Robin AP, et al: Influence of parenteral carbohydrate on fat oxidation in surgical patients, Surgery 95:608-618, 1984.
3. Wilmore DW: The metabolic management of the critically ill, New York, 1977, Plenum Press Inc, pp 171-233.
4. Brennan MF, et al: Glycerol: Major contributor to the short term protein sparing effect of fat emulsions in normal man, Ann Surg 182:386-504, 1975.
5. Brennan MF, Moore FD: An intravenous fat emulsion as a nitrogen sparer: Comparison with glucose, J Surg Res 14:501-504, 1973.
6. Long JM, et al: Effect of carbohydrate and fat intake on nitrogen excretion during total intravenous feeding, Ann Surg 185:417-422, 1977.
7. Jeejeebhoy KN, et al: Metabolic studies in total parenteral nutrition with lipid in man, J Clin Invest 57:126-136, 1976.
8. Elwyn DH, et al: Some metabolic effects of fat infusions in depleted patients, 29:125-132, 1980.
9. Duke JH Jr, et al: Contribution of protein to caloric expenditure following injury, Surgery 68:168-174, 1970.
10. Johnson LR, et al: Structural and hormonal alterations in the gastrointestinal tract of parenterally fed rats, Gastroenterology 68:1177-1183, 1975.
11. Heymsfield SB, et al: Enteral hyperalimentation: An alternative to central venous hyperalimentation, Ann Intern Med 90:63-71, 1979.
12. Larkin JM, Moylan JA: Complete enteral support of thermally injured patients, Am J Surg 131:722-724, 1976.
13. Dobbie RP, Hoffmeister JA: Continuous pump-tube enteric hyperalimentation, Surg Gynecol Obstet 143:273-274, 1976.
14. Page CP, et al: Continual catheter administration of an elemental diet, Surg Gynecol Obstet 142:184-188, 1976.
15. Graham WP, Royster HP: Simplified cervical esophagostomy for long term extraoral feeding, Surg Gynecol Obstet 125:127-128, 1967.
16. Ruge J, Vazques RM: An analysis of the advantages of Stamm and percutaneous endoscopic gastrostomy, Surg Gynecol Obstet 162:13-16, 1986.
17. Delany HM, et al: Jejunostomy by a needle catheter technique, Surgery 73:786-790, 1973.
18. Hoover HC Jr, et al: Nutritional benefits of immediate postoperative jejunal feeding of an elemental diet, Am J Surg 139:153-159, 1980.
19. Orr G, et al: Alternatives to total parenteral nutrition in the critically ill patient, Crit Care Med 8:29-33, 1980.
20. Williamson J, et al: The GI tolerance of a fiber supplemented tube feeding formula in burn patients, Proc Am Burn Assoc 17:29, 1985.
21. Grube BJ, et al: Clostridium difficile diarrhea in critically ill burned patients, Arch Surg 122:655-661, 1987.
22. Dudrick SJ, et al: Can intravenous feeding as the sole means of nutrition support growth in the child and restore weight loss in an adult? An affirmative answer, Ann Surg 169:974-984, 1969.
23. Caldwell MD, et al: Essential fatty acid deficiency in an infant receiving prolonged parenteral alimentation, J Pediatr 81:894-898, 1972.
24. Johnson RC, Cotter R: Metabolism of medium-chain triglyceride lipid emulsion, Nutr Int 2:150-158, 1986.
25. Cotter R, et al: A metabolic comparison of pure long-chain triglyceride lipid emulsion (LCT) and various medium-chain triglyceride (MCT)-LCT combination emulsions in dogs, Am J Clin Nutr 45:927-939, 1987.
26. Wilmore DW, et al: Clinical evaluation of a 10% intravenous fat emulsion for parenteral nutrition in thermally injured patients, Ann Surg 178:503-515, 1973.
27. Bergstrom J, et al: Intravenous nutrition with amino acid solutions in patients with chronic uremia, Acta Med Scand 191:359-367, 1972.
28. Hwang TL, et al: Preservation of small bowel mucosa using glutamine-enriched parenteral nutrition, Surg Forum 37:56-58, 1986.
29. Heird WC, et al: Metabolic acidosis resulting from intravenous alimentation mixtures containing synthetic amino acids, N Engl J Med 287:943-948, 1972.
30. Allen JG, et al: Similar growth rates of litter mate puppies maintained on oral protein with those on the same quantity of protein as daily intravenous plasma for 99 days as only protein source, Ann Surg 144:349-355, 1958.
31. Shils ME: Parenteral multivitamins: time for changes, Bull Parenter Drug Assoc 30:226-233, 1976.
32. McDougal WS, et al: Effect of intravenous near isosmotic nutrient infusions on nitrogen balance in critically ill injured patients, Surg Gynecol Obstet 145:408-414, 1977.
33. Blackburn GL, et al: Protein sparing therapy during periods of starvation with sepsis or trauma, Ann Surg 177:588-594, 1973.
34. Blackburn GL, et al: Peripheral intravenous feeding with isotonic amino acid solutions, Am J Surg 125:447-454, 1973.
35. Greenberg GR, et al: Protein-sparing therapy in postoperative patients, N Engl J Med 294:1411-1416, 1976.

36. Felig P: Intravenous nutrition: fact and fancy, N Engl J Med **294**:1455-1456, 1976.

37. Sim AJ, et al: Glucose promotes wholebody protein synthesis from infused amino acids in fasting man, Lancet **1**:68-71, 1979.

38. Elwyn DH, et al: Protein and energy sparing of glucose added in hypocaloric amounts to peripheral infusions of amino acids, Metabolism **27**:325-331, 1978.

39. Wolfe BM, et al: Substrate interaction in intravenous feeding, Ann Surg **186**:518-540, 1977.

40. Duke JH Jr, Dudrick SJ: Parenteral feeding. In American College of Surgeons, editors: Manual of surgical nutrition, Philadelphia, 1975, WB Saunders Co, pp 285-317.

41. Askanazi J, et al: Affect of immediate postoperative nutritional support on length of hospitalization, Ann Surg **203**:236-239, 1986.

42. Wilmore DW, Dudrick SJ: Treatment of acute renal failure with intravenous essential L-amino acids, Arch Surg **99**:669-673, 1969.

43. Meguid MM, et al: Nutritional support in cancer, Lancet **2**:230-231, 1983.

44. Stegink LD, Pitkin RM: Placental transfer of glucose–amino acid complexes present in parenteral solutions, Am J Clin Nutr **30**:1087-1093, 1977.

45. Dudrick SJ, Wilmore DW: Long-term parenteral feeding, Hosp Pract **3**:65-78, 1968.

46. Sasaki TM, et al: The relationship of central venous and pulmonary artery catheter position to acute right-sided endocarditis in severe thermal injury, J Trauma **19**:740-743, 1979.

47. Warden GD, et al: Central venous thrombosis: a hazard of medical progress, J Trauma **13**:620-626, 1973.

48. Borja AR, Hinshaw JR: A safe way to perform infraclavicular subclavian vein catheterization, Surg Gynecol Obstet **130**:673-676, 1970.

49. Filston HC, Grant JP: A safer system for percutaneous subclavian venous catheterization in newborn infants, J Pediatr Surg **14**:564-570, 1979.

50. Wilmore DW, Dudrick SJ: Safe long-term venous catheterization, Arch Surg **98**:256-258, 1969.

51. Herbst CA: Indications, management, and complications of percutaneous subclavian catheters, Arch Surg **113**:1421-1425, 1978.

52. Bernard TW, Stahl WM: Subclavian vein catheterizations: a prospective study, Ann Surg **173**:184-190, 1971.

53. Pruitt BA Jr, et al: Diagnosis and treatment of cannula-related intravenous sepsis in burn patients, Ann Surg **191**:546-554, 1980.

54. Sheldon GF, Grzyb S: Phosphate depletion and repletion: Relation to parenteral nutrition and oxygen transport, Ann Surg **182**:683-689, 1975.

55. Rudman D, et al: Elemental balances during intravenous hyperalimentation of underweight adult subjects, J Clin Invest **55**:94-104, 1975.

56. Knochel JP: The pathophysiology and clinical characteristics of severe hypophosphatemia, Arch Intern Med **137**:203-220, 1977.

57. Sheldon GF, et al: Hepatic dysfunction during hyperalimentation, Arch Surg **113**:504-508, 1978.

58. Jeejeebhoy KN, et al: Total parenteral nutrition at home: studies in patients surviving 4 months to 5 years, Gastroenterology **71**:943-953, 1976.

59. Riella MC, Scribner BH: Five years' experience with a right atrial catheter for prolonged parenteral nutrition at home, Surg Gynecol Obstet **143**:205-208, 1976.

60. Howard L, et al: A review of the current national status of home parenteral and enteral nutrition from the provider and consumer perspective, J Parenter Enter Nutr **10**:416-424, 1986.

61. Heimbach DM, Ivey TD: Technique for placement of a permanent home hyperalimentation catheter, Surg Gynecol Obstet **143**:634-636, 1976.

62. Soroff HS, et al: An estimation of the nitrogen requirements for equilibrium in burned patients, Surg Gynecol Obstet **112**:159-172, 1961.

CHAPTER 32

Parenteral Nutrition in Infancy and Childhood

Alan M. Lake

It is estimated that more than one third of children admitted to the hospital today have significant nutritional compromise.[4] Nutritional therapy must frequently be adapted to a restricted enteric functional capacity. In Fig. 32-1, taken from Heird and Winters,[5] the range of nutritional options is matched to the spectrum of enteric compromise.

As enteric function and appetite begin to decline, the first option is introduction of high-caloric oral supplements (Chapter 13). As appetite declines with reduced enteric function, tube feeding can be initiated. Decreasing enteric function will further require intravenous nutrition supplements, often by peripheral vein. Only as enteric function essentially ceases does total parenteral nutrition become necessary.

It is worth emphasizing that the "total" aspect of TPN applies only at the one end of this spectrum. Further, the patient's position on this spectrum is rarely fixed and nutritional adjustments must be made in response to the alterations in enteric function.

INDICATIONS FOR INITIATION OF TPN

The criteria for initiation of parenteral nutrition fall into three broad categories: (1) sustaining nutritional adequacy, (2) meeting extraordinary metabolic demands, and/or (3) serving as primary medical therapy. Common clinical situations included in these categories are as follows:

Sustaining nutritional adequacy
    Low–birth-weight neonates
    Necrotizing enterocolitis
    Intractable diarrhea
    Postoperative bowel resection
    Cancer
    Intestinal pseudoobstruction
    Anorexia nervosa

Meeting extraordinary metabolic demands
    Sepsis, trauma, or burns
    Renal or hepatic failure
    Cardiopulmonary disease
    Malnutrition
    Cystic fibrosis
Primary nutritional therapy
    Inflammatory bowel disease
    Enteric fistula
    Chylothorax or chylous ascites
    Pancreatitis

The disease states included in the broad category of sustaining nutritional adequacy are bound by a common mandate for prospective nutritional therapy, often mandating TPN. The duration of need may vary from a few days to years. The indications for TPN are greater in children than in adults with similar disease because of the demands of growth.

The diseases with extraordinary metabolic demands may be acute or chronic. Together they share a continuing, if not unique, demand for extraordinary caloric delivery. It is dangerous to group these conditions because the pathophysiology of each disease must be considered to a far greater degree than in routine TPN use. For example, the fluid and protein requirements of a burn patient have little resemblance to that of a patient in hepatic failure.

The diseases in our third category share the need for relatively strict bowel rest. The duration of exclusive TPN may be brief, as in pancreatitis, or prolonged, as in Crohn's disease with enterocutaneous fistula. At this time, exclusive TPN is a cornerstone of medical management of these patients.[6]

Although a list of absolute contraindications to TPN is not useful, surely the presence of intact enteric function and appetite is a relative contraindication. An even greater dilemma is the

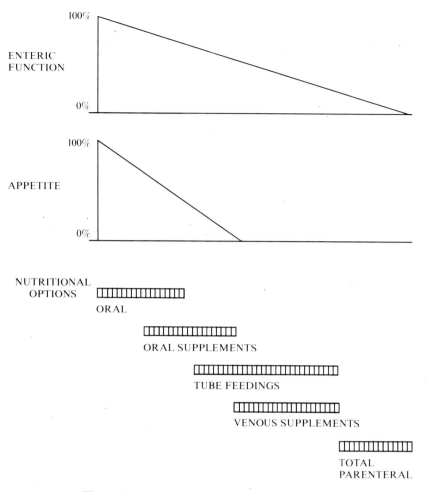

Figure 32-1 Spectrum of nutritional need.

From Heird WC, Winters RW: J Pediatr **86**:2-16, 1975.

justification of initiating TPN in patients with irreversible disease. Does it ease the burden, prolong the inevitable, or provide, via complications, a modus exitus?

PATIENT ASSESSMENT FOR TPN

The application of TPN should be individualized to today's status and tomorrow's need. The profile of patient need includes

Nutritional assessment
Enteric function
Fluid limits
Caloric requirements
Venous access
Specific metabolic limitations
Immunologic limitations
Psychosocial status

The nutritional assessment of the patient is the first task, and its techniques and applications are outlined in Chapter 9. In this phase one seeks to determine "where we have been" in a nutritional sense. Dietary assessment is a critical component of this phase as well and is discussed in Chapter 11.

Objective assessment of residual enteric function is the next step. This phase entails combining clinical status: appetite, caloric intake, stool frequency, etc., with biochemical parameters of absorptive ability: fecal losses, serum proteins or lipids, immune function, as well as other clinical parameters. Approximates are all that is sought, for one can spend weeks trying to quantify an enteric capacity that may change daily. The enteric function that persists must literally be nourished, with a commitment to maximally sustaining enteric nutrient delivery.

The next step is to determine the limits of the patient's fluid tolerance. Obvious limitations in fluid delivery are present in premature infants, children with chronic renal or cardiopulmonary disease, and patients with increased intracranial pressure. Of note, in 1981, we reviewed our patient population on TPN in the Johns Hopkins Children's Center and found that fluid limitations were the rate-limiting factor in TPN delivery in nearly 70%.

The caloric requirements of the child must next be determined. Because the RDA for calories is based on median intake of normal children, there are adjustments required to correct for both disease and prior malnutrition. In the child, the demands of growth must not be ignored even in the face of acute disease.

The compensation for increased metabolic demand is reviewed below. It is not uncommon to seek intakes in excess of 175 kcal/kg/day, though such are rarely required.

Venous access is a significant issue in children, especially when intravenous medications are also required. Peripheral venous nutrition is ideally suited to supplementation of enteric feedings and rarely sustains long-term TPN in infancy. The new generation of long-term, double lumen venous catheters has greatly facilitated long-term TPN and ushered in the era of practical home parenteral nutrition. Line care remains a major concern in childhood TPN and usually demands a specific nursing team.

Specific metabolic limitations may be imposed by inborn errors or acquired organ dysfunction. These issues are addressed in the sections on systemic diseases and specific disease states. Examples of alterations in energy demands are as follows:

1. Growth catch-up:

   Ideal caloric intake $\times \dfrac{\text{Ideal weight for height}}{\text{Actual height}}$
2. Moderate infection, fractures: 10% to 25% increase
3. Severe infection, multiple trauma: 30% to 50% increase
4. Mechanical ventilation: 50% to 75%
5. Burns: Up to 100% based on burn size

Since acquired organ failure may develop in the course of the basic disease, prospective monitoring of organ function is a critical component of TPN.

The patient's immune status may be a function of infection (Chapter 23), age (Chapter 30), or severity of malnutrition (Chapter 34). Although cellular immune function is usually improved while the patient is receiving TPN, the septic complications of TPN are all too apparent. Immune deficiency is not a contraindication to TPN.

The psychologic implications of TPN must not be underestimated. One must acknowledge and address not only the patient's response to TPN but that of his family and community. In the infant, the initiation of TPN all too often implies a "fragility" to his or her life. The adolescent, on the other hand, often misinterprets the initiation of TPN as an emphasis on disability rather than a hope for habilitation. Healthy adaptation requires a shared sense of limitations, realistic goals, and anticipated problems. Emphasis on health must exceed acknowledgement of handicaps. The capacities of the family to support the patient financially, emotionally, and physically must be maximized.

INITIATION OF TPN

The decisions on specific therapy are best made by a single person with the support of a team of dietitians, social workers, and nurses.

The technique for delivery, peripheral versus central line, will be determined by the total caloric demand and anticipated duration of such need. As a guideline, in children, peripheral lines can easily deliver up to 80 kcal/kg/day and are thus appropriate when enteric feedings will be progressively increased within 2 weeks. The new double-lumen long-term central vein lines are most appropriate if chronic blood sampling or drug delivery is anticipated in the face of sustained enteric compromise.

Total caloric demand is a function of both age and associated disease. Thus the premature infant's requirement begins at 90 kcal/kg/day and increases up to 180 kcal/kg/day in the face of chronic bronchopulmonary dysplasia. In early childhood, intakes of 60-90 kcal/kg/day are desired, whereas in adolescence requirements range from 40-60 kcal/kg/day. Increased caloric demands are anticipated in many diseases. After major surgery, a 20% to 30% increase in caloric demand is assumed, with increases of 50% common in sepsis and up to 100% in burns or in long-term malnutrition. In the absence of specific data on a child's disease, it is usually safe to assume a 30% increase in caloric need with a commitment to frequent reassessment of response.

Volume restrictions, as noted, are often rate limiting. With limitations exceeding 150 ml/kg/day, parenteral nutrition is generally successful. If, on the other hand, volume limits are lower than 80 ml/kg/day, enteric nutrient delivery is usually mandated. Fluid limits are reviewed regularly to compensate for fecal or renal output, fever, nasogastric or chest tube drainage, or increased renal solute load.

COMPOSITION OF TPN SOLUTION

To custom-design the TPN solution requires close cooperation of the physician and pharmacist. The use of "standard hyperal" solutions is to be discouraged. This approach forces the responsible physician to precisely think about and review what is being ordered. Requirements for carbohydrate, protein, lipid, vitamins, electrolytes, minerals, and trace elements will vary with age, basic disease, enteric capacity, and preexisting nutritional deficiency. The ordering system utilized at Johns Hopkins will be reviewed shortly.

Carbohydrate. Carbohydrate is now generally supplied in TPN as dextrose, though experience with other carbohydrate sources is increasing. Intravenous fructose or sorbitol is now rarely used since dramatic increases in lactic acid have been reported. Alcohol, at concentrations up to 1%, offers the advantages of minimum osmolality and volume while providing energy at 7 kcal/g. Disadvantages result from incomplete metabolism, especially in the newborn, in whom lethargy and apnea are noted. Studies on galactose and maltose, while encouraging to date, are quite preliminary.

The infusion of glucose is adjusted to minimize the risk of hyperglycemia while progressing to provide at least 40% to 45% of total calories. In infancy, the TPN infusion is generally begun at 8-10 mg/kg/min and increased to 12-15 mg/kg/min. In the absence of alternative carbohydrate sources, insulin may be required in young infants with hyperglycemia at inadequate caloric levels.

Under routine conditions, the protein sparing effect of glucose is well documented. However, in burn or septic situations, hypertonic glucose is often ineffective while complicating treatment by increasing carbon dioxide production, oxygen consumption, and norepinephrine excretion.[8]

Protein. Protein was initially provided in TPN as casein or fibrin hydrolysate. Residual short peptide chains, however, remained antigenic and were not fully metabolized. As a result crystalline amino acids have become the major protein source in commercial TPN products. In 1985 commercial sources for individual amino acids became available. At present, in the absence of great experience, the temptation to design one's own TPN protein is to be discouraged.

The commercial amino acid preparations were originally standardized to casein and/or adult plasma amino acid levels after oral or intravenous administration. For the neonate, new products standardized to breast milk amino acid composition are now in production. As noted in Chapter 31, infants and children require a higher percentage of total amino acids as essential amino acids (40%) than adults (20%). In the newborn, cysteine and taurine supplements are encouraged.

Protein infusions at 2.5 to 4 g/kg/day are used, with 8% to 12% of total calories as protein. In severely catabolic patients, infusions up to 15% of total calories may be utilized. When intakes exceed 5-6 g/kg/day, hyperammonemia, plasma amino acid elevations, acidosis, and lethargy are noted.[9] With the use of 8% to 15% of protein calories, the ratio of nonprotein to protein calories ranges from 288:1 to 142:1, well within advised limits. The amino acid compositions of standard commercial preparations are noted in Table 31-5.

Essential amino acid formulations are now available for use in children with aminoacidopathy, hyperammonemia, or renal failure. Some of these children have demonstrated normal growth on 5% protein calories; however, close monitoring is required.

Solutions high in branched-chain and low in aromatic amino acids have been used in patients with hepatic failure (Chapter 13) and demonstrated to normalize plasma amino acid levels. Similarly, after burns or other severe metabolic stress, increased oxidation of and hence demand for branched-chain amino acids is documented. The long-term effectiveness of branched-chain amino acid enrichment and its influence on growth in children are not documented.

Lipid. The delivery of lipids in TPN is reviewed extensively in Chapter 31 and summarized in Table 31-4. Both 10% and 20% lipid emulsions in glycerol (2.5%) are commercially available. Early studies[10] documented the capacity for these emulsions to meet essential fatty acid requirements with infusions at 1 g/kg/day. Thus, when 6% of total calories are delivered as lipid, essential fatty acid deficiency can be prevented; and when 10% are so delivered, such deficiency can be reversed.

Lipid infusions can be progressively advanced to a level of 40% of total calories with monitoring of serum triglycerides. The higher level of lipid infusion is often mandated by severe metabolic stress, marked fluid restriction, or the desire to maximize peripheral vein caloric delivery.

Maximum fatty acid oxidation at the mitochondrial level requires L-carnitine, a material only recently available for use in TPN solutions and known to be low in neonates.[11] The significance of low plasma levels of carnitine versus low tissue levels and the potential benefits of carnitine supplementation have yet to be determined.

To optimize triglyceride clearance by endothelial lipoprotein lipase, lipid emulsion infusions in excess of 2 g/kg/day are generally delivered over 16-20 hours. Elevated serum lipid emulsion concentrations have been associated with decreased arterial oxygenation, deposition of lipid in macrophages, and displacement of bilirubin from albumin.[10]

Vitamins. Vitamin supplements available for TPN use are summarized in Table 31-6, and RDAs for age are noted in Appendix I. Excessive supplementation may lead to specific toxicity or toxicity from the propylene glycol used as a stabilizer in many commercial products. The vitamin deficiency states are summarized in Chapter 35. Commercial vitamin supplements do not contain iodine or iron, and increased biotin requirements are common with prolonged TPN.

Electrolytes. Electrolyte requirements are generally equivalent to standard intravenous delivery. The parenteral needs for calcium, phosphorus, and magnesium are less than oral needs; however, compatibility and precipitation problems often mandate oral supplements, especially in the neonate.

Table 32-1 Daily Trace Element Supplements ($\mu g/kg$)

	Weight of Child		
	<3 kg	3-12 kg	>12 kg
Zinc	300	100	3 (mg)
Copper	20	20	1.2 (mg)
Manganese	6	6	0.5 (mg)
Chromium	0.17	0.17	12

Trace minerals. These are defined as minerals comprising less than 5 g per adult or 0.01% of total body weight. Early TPN solutions lacked trace minerals and deficiency states were frequent (Chapter 36). Guidelines for trace mineral delivery have been issued by the AMA[12] and are summarized in Table 32-1 as recommended daily supplements as a function of weight. Molybdenum requirements are poorly defined, though isolated case reports of deficiency in chronic TPN exist. Routine selenium supplements have not been advised since significant selenium is found "contaminating" most commercial amino acid preparations. Trace element requirements are increased in a number of chronic inflammatory diseases, so close monitoring and awareness of deficiency symptoms are critical.

ORDER FORMS

The Johns Hopkins Hospital order sheet for pediatric venous alimentation is reproduced for comparison to ordering systems available to the reader (Fig. 32-2). All such systems should share the capacity for individual therapy in a structured system to avoid chaos, confusion, and error in the pharmacy.

In this model, the physician first notes the fluid limitation in ml/kg/day followed by the total caloric intake (kcal/kg/da) desired for the next 24-hour period. For routine care, this system proposes that 10% of total calories be provided as protein (equivalent to 2.5 g/kg at 100 kcal/kg/da). This percentage is easily increased for metabolic stress or decreased for cases of renal or hepatic dysfunction. With lipid emulsion providing up to 40% of total calories, dextrose provides from 50% to 90%.

Standard electrolyte, mineral, vitamin, and trace element supplements are provided. The

THE JOHNS HOPKINS HOSPITAL
Department of Pediatrics
PEDIATRIC ALIMENTATION SOLUTION
ORDER SHEET

Page No. | Patient Name & History Number

1. This order sheet is to be used for hyperalimentation orders only.
2. All orders must be written by 10 AM daily.
3. Routine start time is between 12 N and 4 PM daily.
4. New orders received after 5 PM will automatically start at 10 AM the next day.
5. Changes in existing solutions will be made as Pharmacy is able.
6. New orders must be written for any change in the existing solution.
7. ALL ORDERS ARE FOR A 24 HOUR SUPPLY. Pharmacy will automatically supply sufficient quantities for administration.

DATE: | TIME: | PATIENTS WEIGHT: | Kg. | CENTRAL LINE: | Yes | No

Summary of routine IV/Oral Fluids per day: (DO NOT USE FOR PAS CALCULATIONS)
IV: _____ ml/kg, _____ ml/day, _____ Kcal/day; PO _____ ml/kg, _____ ml/day, _____ Kcal/day.

GUIDELINES:
MAXIMUM ALLOWABLE SOLUTIONS
Caloric density of Total Alimentation Fluids [Kcal/ml] × Fluid requirement [ml/kg/day] = Tot Kcal/day

CENTRAL ADMINISTRATION:
—No Fat: 1.5 Kcal/ml
—With 20% Fat: 1.5 Kcal/ml
—With 10% Fat: 1.2 Kcal/ml

PERIPHERAL ADMINISTRATION:
—No Fat: 0.4 Kcal/ml
—With 20% Fat: 0.6 Kcal/ml
—With 10% Fat: 0.5 Kcal/ml

CALORIC CONTENT SUGGESTED:
10% Kcal as Amino Acids
90% Kcal Non-Protein
  as 50-90% Dextrose
  40- 0% Fat
TOTAL CONTENT = 100%

TOTAL ALIMENTATION FLUIDS:
Should be > 50 ml/kg/day to provide adequate Kcal.

INFUSE 1/3-1/2 Total Kcal on day 1, 2/3 on day 2, 100% desired on day 3; or as tolerated.

ADDITIVE CONTENT:
—Na: 3-4 mEq/kg/day
—K: 2-3 mEq/kg/day
—Mg, Ca, P: Added as standard concentrations based on age, weight, and caloric content.
THESE IONS MUST BE MONITORED FREQUENTLY; CONTACT PHARMACY SHOULD ABNORMALITIES NEED CORRECTION.
—[Na] = [Cl] routinely

HYPERALIMENTATION CAN BE A VALUABLE ADJUNCT TO THERAPY IF CAREFULLY PLANNED AND MONITORED. PLEASE DIRECT ANY QUESTIONS ABOUT FORMULATION, MONITORING OR MODIFICATIONS TO STANDARD ADDITIVES TO THE PHARMACY PRIOR TO INITIATION.

PLEASE PREPARE THE FOLLOWING PEDIATRIC ALIMENTATION SOLUTION:

A TOTAL ALIMENTATION FLUID REQUIREMENT: PER 24 HOURS:
_____ ml/kg/day × _____ kg. = | ml

B CALORIC CONTENT:
Total/day = _____ Kcal/kg × _____ kg. = | Kcal

AMINO ACIDS:*
Total Kcal _____ × _____ % ÷ 4 (Kcal/Gm) = AA | Gm

DEXTROSE:
Total Kcal _____ × _____ % ÷ 3.7 (Kcal/Gm) = Dex | Gm

FAT EMULSION:
Total Kcal _____ × _____ % ÷ 11 (Kcal/Gm) = Fat | Gm

C ADDITIVE CONTENT:
Na = | Na | mEq
K = | K | mEq
Check desired: | Mg | mEq
_____ Standard Mg° | Ca | mg
_____ Standard Ca° | P | mg
_____ Standard P°
_____ Standard Vitamins°
_____ Standard Trace Elements°
_____ Max [Cl] or _____ Max [Acetate]

D FLUID CONTENT:
TOTAL ALIMENTATION FLUIDS (as A. above) = | ml

1. 10% Fat Emulsion: _____ Gm × 10 ml/Gm.
   or
   20% Fat Emulsion: _____ Gm × 5 ml/Gm. = Fat | ml
2. PAS Solution: (Total Vol. – Fat Vol.) = PAS | ml
3. RATE: PAS @ _____ ml/hr for 24 hr
   Fat Emulsion @ _____ ml/hr for _____ hr.

E MODIFICATIONS:
*Requires Pharmacy consult for the use of Essential A.A.
°Requires Pharmacy consult for modifications.

PHYSICIAN SIGNATURE

Pharmacy JHHX25-0268 | Copy 1: CHART | Copy 2: PHARMACY

Figure 32-2 Pediatric alimentation solution order sheet.

Courtesy The Johns Hopkins Hospital, Baltimore, Md.

physician is also reminded that lipid emulsion is either 80% or 90% water, a factor that must be considered in total fluid intake. Consultation with the Nutrition Support Service and Pharmacy is required for modification of amino acid content. All orders must be prepared daily, and monitoring protocols must be recorded on the patient's chart.

MONITORING THE TPN PATIENT

The monitoring system presented in Table 31-9 is quite applicable to the child. Such surveillance is required not only to detect metabolic derangements but also to confirm clinical response. In children daily weights and weekly anthropometrics should be performed even with relatively short-term TPN.

None of the presently available amino acid preparations will produce a "normal" plasma amino acid profile. Indeed, the assumption that TPN sustains normal organ function is just that—an assumption. Alterations in organ uptake of amino acids, lipids, minerals, and glucose should be anticipated. The liver and the skeletal system are two very sensitive organ systems in long-term TPN. The influence on brain growth, intestinal regeneration, and immune competency is under active investigation.

The metabolic and microbiologic complications of TPN are listed on pp. 497 and 498. They are relatively independent of the duration of treatment but relatively dependent on the underlying disease.

TRANSITION TO ENTERIC NUTRITION

A plan for transition to enteric nutrition must be developed as soon as TPN is begun. This is generally a gradual process with increasing enteric workload demanded. A major consideration in this transition is the avoidance of severe enteric mucosal atrophy. The fasted patient, on TPN alone, will have up to a 50% reduction in mucosal mass within the first week. Since enteric compromise is often the indication for TPN, such atrophy only impedes the rate of recovery.

The initiation of enteric nutrition will be controlled by degree of residual enteric function, as reviewed prior to the initiation of TPN. A safe starting point is a challenge of 20 kcal/kg/day to the intestine. This may be too liberal with extreme "short-gut syndrome" or too conservative with modest intestinal inflammation. This

may be delivered either orally or by tube, by continuous infusion or bolus, in dilute or concentrated form.

In most children on TPN, the degree of enteric compromise is initially so great that continuous infusion techniques are used to maximize substrate-enzyme integration and minimize the role of gastric emptying and colonic stimulation. The products available for tube feeding or oral liquid nutrition are summarized in Table 31-3, including composition, distribution of nutrient, electrolyte content, and modular supplements.

Regrettably, the ideal product probably does not exist. The first issue is composition. Protein is optimally absorbed from the lumen in the form of dipeptides and oligopeptides. But it is rarely protein that limits enteric tolerance. Lipid can be delivered as medium chain triglyceride to minimize bile micelle requirements and lymphatic function, but only at the sacrifice of osmolality and with the realization that essential fatty acids are long chain triglycerides.

Carbohydrate composition is thus usually the primary factor in enteric tolerance. Of the brush border enzymes, glucose-D-amylase and maltase are the most resistant to injury and thus maximize the tolerance of glucose polymers and starch. Sucrase activity is often spared and is substrate-inducible. Lactase is the most sensitive, and recovery is often genetically restricted. As a result lactose-containing products are rarely utilized early in enteric alimentation. The availability of noninvasive carbohydrate breath testing offers great promise in documentation of residual enzyme activity and clinical tolerance.[13]

Other significant factors in the choice of enteric formula include palatability, osmolality, cost, and availability. Degree of residue may also be critical with chronic intestinal inflammation or obstruction. Additional comments on the choice of formulations are found in Chapters 12 and 29.

Enteric feedings are advanced as tolerated with stepwise increases in enteric workload. Increases may be made either by increasing volume or concentration but not both simultaneously. Increments of 5-10 kcal/kg are usually attempted on a daily basis. Despite the temptation, transition to bolus oral feeding is rarely justified until total volume and caloric needs have been met by continuous infusion.

The transition to bolus feeding may be initiated by gradual increases in oral offerings while slowing the rate of infusion, or by gradually shortening the interval of infusion (e.g., giving 4 hr worth of feeding over 3 hr, then 2 hr, then 1 hr). This latter technique is especially valuable in young infants with sensitive gastric emptying. Parenteral nutrition is continued until enteric delivery is assured.

HOME NUTRITIONAL SERVICES

With both parenteral and enteral nutrition, financial and personal costs can be reduced markedly by outpatient management.[14] This is now technically possible with the availability of long-term venous catheters, less expensive pumping devices, and home health care delivery services. Patient and family education, home monitoring, and reassessment are best supervised by a multidisciplinary nutritional support service.[15]

REFERENCES

1. Helfrick FW, Abelson NM: Intravenous feeding of a complete diet in a child, J Pediatr **25**:400-402, 1944.
2. Dudrick SJ, et al: Long-term total parenteral nutrition with growth, development, and positive nitrogen balance, Surgery **64**:134-138, 1968.
3. Wilmore DW, Dudrick SJ: Growth and development of an infant receiving all nutrients exclusively by vein, JAMA **203**:140-143, 1968.
4. Merritt RJ, Suskind RM: Nutritional survey of hospitalized pediatric patients, Am J Clin Nutr **32**:1320-1325, 1979.
5. Heird WC, Winters RW: Total parenteral nutrition: the state of the art, J Pediatr **86**:2-16, 1975.
6. Rosenberg IH: Profiles in nutritional management: the G.I. patient, Chicago, 1981, Medical Directions Inc.
7. Kerner JA, editor: Manual of pediatric parenteral nutrition, New York, 1983 John Wiley & Sons Inc.
8. Hassett J, et al: Multiple systems organ failure: mechanisms and therapy, Surg Ann **14**:27-72, 1982.
9. Committee on Nutrition, American Academy of Pediatrics: Commentary on parenteral nutrition, Pediatrics **71**:547-552, 1983.
10. Committee on Nutrition, American Academy of Pediatrics: Use of intravenous fat emulsions in pediatric patients, Pediatrics **68**:738-740, 1981.
11. Mitchel ME: Carnitine metabolism in human subjects. I. Normal metabolism, Am J Clin Nutr **31**:293-296, 1978.
12. American Medical Association: Guidelines for essential trace element preparations for parenteral use, JAMA **241**:2051-2054, 1979.
13. Newcomer AD, et al: Prospective comparison of indirect methods for detecting lactose deficiency, N Engl J Med **293**:1232-1236, 1975.
14. Wateska LP, et al: Cost of a home parenteral nutrition program, JAMA **244**:2303-2305, 1980.
15. Shils ME: A program for total parenteral nutrition at home, Am J Clin Nutr **28**:1429-1435, 1975.

CHAPTER 33

Home Parenteral Nutrition

Marvin E. Ament

It has been more than a decade and a half since the publication of the first case report[1] of a patient with short-bowel syndrome who was sent home receiving parenteral nutrition. In the early years this case was rapidly followed by the experiences of Jeejeebhoy et al.,[2] Broviac and Scribner,[3] Grundfest and Steiger,[4] and Byrne et al.[5] with the at-home management of adults and children who required parenteral support. Subsequent to the safe establishment of this technique in university medical centers during the 1970s, the use of home parenteral nutrition spread rapidly in the 1980s to community hospitals. It is now estimated[6] that 3000 patients are currently receiving home total parenteral nutrition. The number of patients receiving home parenteral nutrition has been slowly and steadily increasing each year as physicians have become more comfortable with the idea of managing at home patients who, in past times, were kept in the hospital strictly because of their need for parenteral support. As experiences with relatively healthy patients who required home total parenteral nutrition (HTPN) accumulated, physicians began to broaden their concept of the types of sick patients who could be sent home and placed on a total parenteral nutrition (TPN) program to include patients who were formerly believed to be manageable only in the hospital. Examples of such patients are those with graft-versus-host disease after bone marrow transplantation and patients with acquired immunodeficiency syndrome who have intractable diarrhea. During the past 15 years our techniques for managing patients at home have been developed and refined and our knowledge of the special nutritional needs of such patients has evolved.

INDICATIONS

There are six main categories or conditions of adult patients who might qualify and benefit from home parenteral nutrition[7-12]:

Short-bowel syndrome
  Secondary to superior mesenteric artery thrombosis
  Secondary to mesenteric vein thrombosis
  Midgut volvulus with infarction
    Congenital
    Secondary to adhesions from previous abdominal surgery
  Secondary to intestinal fistulas
Crohn's disease
  Diffuse disease with diarrhea and abdominal pain refractory to medical management
  Short-bowel syndrome
  Fistula formation immediately following resection and reanastomosis
  To estabalish weight gain and accelerate growth in adolescents with delayed bone age and failed medical treatment
Motility disorder of the intestinal tract
  Chronic intestinal pseudoobstruction syndrome
    Primary from myopathic or neuropathic involvement of GI tract
    Secondary to scleroderma
  Secondary to radiation injury of the intestine
  Following surgery for peptic ulcer disease when stomach fails to empty
  Postoperative intestinal fistulas
Small intestinal mucosal injury
  Unclassified sprue
  Hypogammaglobulinemia sprue
  Eosinophilic gastroenteritis
Other indications
  Graft-versus-host disease
  AIDS
  Intestinal lymphangiectasia with intractable diarrhea
  Gastrointestinal bleeding secondary to hereditary hemorrhagic telangiectasia

There are a number of causes of short-bowel syndrome in the adult patient besides Crohn's disease. The most common are those arising secondary to thromboses of the superior mesenteric artery and mesenteric vein. Occasional cases of short-bowel syndrome develop secondary to midgut volvulus, with strangulation and infarction from previous abdominal surgery. Least common are those that require intestinal resections to correct obstruction after the development of intestinal fistulas from multiple intestinal surgical procedures.

Patients with Crohn's disease most frequently requiring HTPN commonly have short-bowel syndrome and/or diffuse disease that is refractory to all medical therapy and thought to be nonoperable.[13-15] Patients in both categories are usually younger. Those with medically refractory diffuse Crohn's disease may enter a prolonged remission after 90 to 180 days of HTPN. Remission for 1 or more years occurs in approximately 33% of such patients.[16] This treatment may be considered heroic by some, but it is possibly the only way to manage such patients effectively. It may also be used as a form of treatment for fistulas that develop immediately after resection and anastomosis of a diseased bowel. HTPN is used as a means to bring about weight gain, accelerated growth, and sexual development in adolescents with delayed bone age who have failed to mature secondary to inadequate nutrient intake.

The third major category of patients requiring HTPN comprises those with intestinal motility disorders. Included are chronic intestinal pseudoobstruction syndrome caused by primary myopathic or neuropathic involvement of the gastrointestinal tract or motility problems due to scleroderma.[17-19] These disorders may appear at any time, and patients often require either total or partial support to maintain their nutritional status effectively.

Patients can also have motility disorders secondary to radiation injury of the intestine, causing fibrosis that impedes motility and leads to obstructive symptoms. Patients who have undergone a Billroth procedure for treatment of severe peptic ulcer disease may experience gastroparesis, which may require repeat operations to correct the defect. They may subsequently have major problems with the formation of inoperable fistulas. Intestinal or pancreatic fistulas that develop in patients after abdominal procedures may heal successfully if the bowel is kept at rest for up to 6 months. Most fistula, however, close within a month.

The fifth category includes persons in whom a severe small intestinal mucosal injury develops. This represents a relatively minor group of patients. They are usually nonresponsive to a gluten-free diet, and a generalized malabsorption syndrome that cannot be managed by diet develops. There are occasional patients in whom a severe allergy to all types of food protein develops, and they can be effectively managed only by elemental diets or by the use of HTPN. This last group of patients presents some rare situations and has broadened our scope of HTPN use. Patients with graft-versus-host disease after bone marrow transplantation as well as those with AIDS or intractable diarrhea may make up a sizable group of individuals receiving home support.[20,21]

CONTRAINDICATIONS

There are four groups of patients for whom home total parenteral nutrition is contraindicated: (1) senile, (2) psychotic, (3) depressed and unable or unwilling to master the necessary techniques for home care, and (4) without family members who can assist in performing the techniques. Physicians must carefully assess patients before the initiation of a home program so the inappropriate ones will not be referred. Senile patients pose a major problem, since they cannot safely master the techniques for home care and may not have familial resources to assist them. Psychotic patients are dangerous to themselves because they may bring about their own death by some misadventure with technique.

There are some patients who are unable or unwilling to master the techniques of home care and do not have family members to assist them. These patients are often difficult to place. There are very few extended-care facilities that can care for patients who require home parenteral nutrition, because such patients need a higher level of nursing skill and their medical management requires additional time. In most instances reimbursement for this is not available. During the more than a decade of our home parenteral nutrition program, we have only rarely found extended-care facilities that wanted to care for these patients and who did so without major

Table 33-1 Standard HTPN Formulations for Adult Patients at UCLA

	Amino acids (%)	Dextrose (%)	Na (mEq/liter)	K (mEq/liter)	Ca (mg/dl)	Mg (mEq/liter)	Cl (mEq/liter)	P (mg/dl)	Acet (mEq/liter)	Cu (mg/liter)	Zn (mg/liter)	Se (μg/dl)	Cr (μg/dl)
HP25	4.25	25	35	30	10	10	35	30	64	1	2	40	10
AH10	3.5	10	35	30	10	10	35	30	55	1	2	40	10
AH15	3.5	15	35	30	10	10	35	30	55	1	2	40	10
AH20	3.5	20	35	30	10	10	35	30	55	1	2	40	10
AH25	3.5	25	35	30	10	10	35	30	55	1	2	40	10

Se and Cr are not added to 1-liter bags of AH10 through AH25.

problems. More often than not, septic conditions developed in patients placed in these institutions. If a decision is made to place a patient in an extended-care facility, physicians and nurses responsible for the care and/or training of the patient must certify that such an institution is capable of providing the care. Finally, patients who have widespread metastic disease may be better off left in the hospital than brought home, because of the amount of care they may require besides HTPN.

SOLUTIONS FOR HOME TOTAL PARENTERAL NUTRITION

In most instances the decision for a patient to receive HTPN is made while the patient is hospitalized. Formulation of the solution has been determined during the hospitalization. The major step in this instance is to ensure that the solution is the simplest one possible and to minimize the additives that the patient may be required to inject into the TPN solution.[22] Such additives can increase both the cost and the risk of contamination.

Patients who are malnourished will be provided appropriate calories and amino acids to normalize weight and total-body protein. Once this point is reached, the nutrient contents of solutions need to be readjusted to prevent obesity. This is especially important in the long-term HTPN patient.

Depending on the diagnosis necessitating HTPN, function of the intestinal tract may gradually improve digestion and absorption to the point that the volume or dextrose concentration of TPN can be reduced.

Table 33-1 shows the content of the standard solutions available to our patients. Typically only vitamins need to be added just before the 2- or 3-liter bag of solution is suspended.

Lipid emulsion is provided to most patients in a dose believed to prevent essential fatty acid deficiency.[23-25] An amount equal to 4% of the day's calories is necessary for normal nutritional support, which figure is then multiplied by 7 days to arrive at the weekly requirement. This is given once a week as a 10% or 20% fat emulsion. Some patients who are more dependent on HTPN for their nutritional needs than most may be provided lipid emulsions on a daily or every-other-daily basis. This, in part, is determined by their ability to tolerate dextrose loads and various volumes of TPN solutions. Certain elderly persons will tolerate infusion of HTPN better if the volume of solution is restricted and the concentration of nutrients raised. It is in these patients that more lipid emulsion is likely to be used.

Essential Trace Metals

The trace metals are a subgroup of the trace elements that occur in the human body. Trace elements can be defined as those that constitute less than 0.01% of the human body—i.e., less than 7 g in a 70 kg man. Fifteen trace metals have been shown[26] to be of biologic importance in mammalian systems. However, not all these elements are minerals and not all have been confirmed as essential nutrients in humans. Nutritional deficiency syndromes in humans have been recognized for iron, zinc, copper, selenium, molybdenum, and possibly chromium. Trace elements have diverse biochemical and physiologic functions. Most trace metals express their biologic roles as part of metalloenzymes (i.e., enzymes with stoichiometric amounts of one or more trace minerals firmly bound to the protein and required for maximal enzymatic activity).

Trace elements can also participate in metabolism as soluble ionic cofactors. Examples are zinc and manganese or specialized nonprotein organic molecules such as chromium. A common feature of many trace minerals is that there is inefficient absorption from dietary sources. Substantial differences exist between the amounts that must be taken in (the RDAs) and the amounts that must be absorbed daily to replace normal losses.

Clinical deficiencies of trace metals can develop when one or more mechanisms occur often simultaneously. With TPN, issues of gastrointestinal absorption are moot, although some patients who are on a mixed nutrient intake for enteral and parenteral nutrition may receive sufficient trace metals from both sources to avoid a deficiency state. There are four possible mechanisms by which a low circulating concentration of trace metal nutrients can develop: deficient intake, enhanced loss, redistribution from the vascular space to the tissues, and deficient maintenance of the circulating binding protein.

Trace metal deficiency syndromes rarely occur in patients who receive short-term TPN. In addition, most hospitals currently give two to four trace metals as part of their routine TPN solutions as a means of avoiding these syndromes. Complex surgical conditions or chronic medical disorders for which TPN is prescribed may bring about nutrient depletion if the patient is not given sufficient replacement for excess loss of trace metals. Patients with massive catabolic loss (e.g., those with infection and/or inflammation) may become depleted of macronutrients, micronutrients, and trace metals. In infants and children receiving TPN, sufficient amounts of trace minerals must be available to replace deficits to permit growth. An early sign of nutrient deficiency in a child being given seemingly adequate parenteral intake may be failure to grow at the normal rate.

Iron

Iron deficiency may be difficult to assess by laboratory means in patients undergoing TPN.[27] Anemia can be caused by a number of nutritional factors other than iron deficiency in diseases for which TPN is employed. Many of the diseases themselves can cause bone marrow hypoplasia. In this situation anemia is not necessarily a specific sign of iron deficiency. Because transfer and saturation depend on the concentration of protein as well as the quantity of circulating iron, protein deficiency will artifactually raise the percentage of saturation even in the face of iron deficiency. Serum ferritin has been related to the amount of iron in deposits. However, tumors and inflammatory conditions produce elevations of ferritin. When it is absolutely necessary to know iron status, bone marrow aspiration may be required. Alternatively, the use of iron absorption tests with radiolabeled iron and whole body counting serve to indicate iron deficiency when the patient has a sufficient segment of small intestine to absorb the iron.[28] Total body iron stores are normally regulated by the intestine. There is no efficient mechanism for excretion of excess iron. Bypassing the gut with parenteral iron creates substantial risk of iron overload and the production of cirrhosis. In long-term multiyear HTPN, achieving a net mean daily intake of iron in a narrow range of approximately 1 mg is optional. This can be done by periodically having the patient add small amounts of iron dextran to the TPN solution to provide the necessary requirement of iron. The patient may also periodically receive an infusion of iron dextran given in saline over 4 to 6 hours that will fill the body's iron stores.

Zinc

The biochemical functions of zinc fall into three categories: metalloenzyme formation, RNA conformation, and membrane stabilization. At least 70 metalloenzymes of zinc have been identified.[29] Zinc nutriture in humans is important because it participates in cell growth and proliferation, sexual maturation and reproduction, dark adaptation and night vision, gustatory acuity, wound healing, and hemostasis. By far the most commonly used index of zinc nutriture is the circulating zinc concentration. Blood plasma and serum (a relatively accessible fluid) are analyzed by atomic absorption spectrophotometry to provide an accurate and precise method of quantifying zinc in biologic materials. Zinc levels depend on the availability of the circulating binding protein, specifically albumin. Hypoalbuminemia per se can account for low zinc level. Despite these pitfalls, circulating zinc concentration does have a reasonable role to play in the assessment of patients undergoing TPN when care is taken to avoid the technical errors and when serial determinations beginning prior to the implementation of TPN are utilized.

Patients receiving TPN who have low zinc levels will show depression of alkaline phosphatase, a zinc metalloenzyme.[30] This may even be a guideline to the diagnosis and treatment of zinc deficiency. The clinical manifestations of zinc deficiency are protean and can include the following[31]: growth retardation, hypogonadism, hypospermia, alopecia, skin lesions, diarrhea, mental depression/apathy, glucose intolerance, night blindness, impaired taste sensation/perception, impaired wound healing, impaired leukocyte chemotaxis, impaired T-lymphocyte function, and cutaneous anergy. These manifestations of zinc deficiency are no longer common in patients receiving long-term parenteral nutrition since zinc supplementation is almost universally given. The zinc needs of patients vary depending on the age and maturity of the patient. Adults typically receive 2 mg of zinc per liter,[31] newborn infants 400 mg/kg/day. A minimum of 3 mg of zinc per day is required in adults to maintain zinc nutriture. In our patients the average amount of zinc varies from 4 to 6 mg/day because they generally receive 2-3 liters of TPN solution per day. Infants and children are given proportionally more based on weight.

Since this has been done, we have not seen a clinically apparent case of zinc deficiency syndrome in over a decade; and with monitoring of serum zinc levels we have seen no measurable zinc deficiency in our patients.

Copper

The adult human body contains about 82-200 mg of copper. The main site of copper storage, distribution, and regulation is the liver. Copper is transported in the circulation and delivered to tissues by the protein ceruloplasmin.[32] It is excreted with the bile into the fecal stream and thus eliminated from the body via the intestinal tract. Copper expresses its biochemical function as a component of copper metalloenzymes. It may also play a role in bone mineralization and as an antioxidant. The common feature of cuproenzymes is their utilization of molecular oxygen or derivative species to effect an oxidation reaction. The best method of assessing copper status is to determine the serum copper concentration and the serum ceruloplasmin level. Some 94% of circulating copper is in the form of ceruloplasmin.[33] Whatever influences the levels of ceruloplasmin will determine the serum or plasma total copper levels as well. Again, external contamination during the obtaining, handling, or processing of blood samples must be avoided. Copper determinations are less sensitive to hemolysis than are zinc determinations. Corticosteroid therapy tends to lower copper levels; but a number of conditions increase circulating copper/ceruloplasmin concentration: acute and chronic infections, pregnancy, oral contraceptive agents, and smoking. Hair copper is a poor index of copper nutriture.

The most common clinical signs in acquired human copper deficiencies are anemia and neutropenia.[34] The anemia is a microcytic hypochromic type, in which the patient presents with depigmented hair, skin pallor, hypotonia, hypothermia, and growth retardation. Bone disease can predispose to fractures.[32,35] Swelling and deformity of bones from subperiosteal bleeding have been documented.[32] Copper is provided to adults at a dosage of 1 mg/liter of parenteral nutrition solutions, which should meet the needs of most patients, except those who have excessive losses in biliary drainage. Clinical copper deficiency has not been seen in our patients for more than a decade.

Manganese

Manganese is a component of two metalloenzymes, superoxide dismutase and pyruvate carboxylase.[36] It functions as an antioxidant as well as in energy metabolism and is important in the formation of connective tissue. No clearcut definitive incidence of clinical manganese deficiency in humans has been reported, and it is unknown to what extent whole body nutriture is reflected by circulating or whole blood manganese levels.

Selenium

Selenium is involved in protection of the cell from oxidant stress. Its antioxidant functions mimic to some extent those of vitamin E in preventing the extension of lipid peroxidation in the membranes of cells and their intracellular organelles.[37] Selenium is a constituent of the selenoenzyme glutathione peroxidase. Plasma or serum selenium concentration is one practical means by which selenium status is assessed,[38] although erythrocyte glutathione peroxidase activity also is used to accomplish this. Without question, patients undergoing TPN for prolonged intervals have a gradual decline in their selenium levels. Normal plasma selenium is in the range of 5-15 μg/dl. TPN-induced selenium deficiency has been recognized in association with ascites, muscle pain, intense pallor of fingernails and nailbeds, and cardiac arrhythmias followed by cardiac dilation. Congestive heart failure is another rare manifestation of selenium deficiency,[39] and deficiency of this metal has been associated with macrocytosis without the development of anemia as well as with decreased hair color and skin pigmentation. All these findings—cardiomyopathy, peripheral muscle myositis, macrocytosis, decreased skin and hair coloration—have been reversed by the administration of selenium.[40,41] Furthermore, T-lymphocyte function has been shown to be compromised in selenium-deficient patients. TPN solutions should therefore be supplemented with 40-60 μg of selenium per liter.

We have recognized biochemical selenium deficiency in virtually all of our long-term HTPN patients who absorb less than 25% of their nutrition enterally. Adults have had both macrocytosis and lightening of hair color, which were reversed with selenium treatment. Cardiomyopathy was not recognized in our patients. Clinically apparent selenium deficiency was seen in three children who took virtually nothing by mouth, and in whom lightening of hair and skin color and macrocytosis without anemia developed. Cell volumes in all were above 115 fl (femtoliters). There was no evidence of increased hemolysis. Liver dysfunction, with transaminase elevation, has also been described. In every case the symptoms were reversed with supplementation of selenium to cancel the deficit.

Chromium

Chromium is not a component of any metalloproteins. Its main biologic action appears to be the potentiation of the action of insulin. It is thought to participate in the hormonal transmission of insulin at the level of the receptor cell. Deficiency of chromium may lead to impaired glucose tolerance.[42,43] Whenever plasma, serum, and red cells are collected for chromium determinations, great care is necessary to avoid contaminating the specimens. Containers must be trace metal–free, and the needles and syringes with which they are drawn likewise must be free of the trace metal. Overestimation of chromium in tissues has occurred as a result of contamination. Normal levels of chromium are less than 0.1 μg per liter, or 1 μg/dl. In two patients who had been receiving long-term HTPN for 5 and 34 months, a peripheral sensory and motor neuropathy developed, including the classic picture of diabetic neuropathy. They showed reversal of both the neuropathy and the glucose intolerance when supplementation was used to correct the deficiency. After the initial administration of 3100 and 9000 μg of Cr, respectively, they were able to maintain glucose control without insulin and to reduce their caloric intake by 200 and 1000 kcal. However, none of the glucose-intolerant children requiring insulin whom we have treated showed improvement with chromium supplementation.

Molybdenum

Molybdenum is important in the oxidative metabolism of purines and sulfur-containing compounds into forms that can be excreted by the kidney.[44] It is a constituent of three metalloenzymes in mammals: xanthine oxidase, sulfate oxidase, and aldehyde oxidase. Analytic determinations of molybdenum in organic fluids and tissue matrices are difficult and not widely available. Neutron activation analysis represents the method of choice for determining it, and in recent years the consensus has developed that normal circulating molybdenum levels are less than 1 μg/liter. Obstructive hepatocellular disease produces an elevation in serum molybdenum concentrations, and this makes it difficult to assess molybdenum nutriture in certain patients undergoing HTPN. Molybdenum deficiency has been described in a 24-year-old man with short-bowel syndrome secondary to Crohn's disease while receiving prolonged parenteral nutrition. A syndrome of intermittent headache, night blindness, central scotomas, nausea, vomiting, tachycardia, and tachypnea developed progressing to edema, disorientation, and coma. The syndrome was precipitated by crystalline amino acid solutions and was associated with a tenfold rise in plasma methionine concentration.

Vitamins

We have evaluated all fat-soluble and water-soluble vitamin levels in patients who receive parenteral nutrition on a 5-7 day/week basis and found that the currently available preparations containing fat- and water-soluble vitamins provide them in sufficient quantities to maintain normal to slightly elevated blood levels. Our data indicate that the vitamin A levels in patients being given multiple vitamin infusions are up to 25% higher than normal. None of our patients could be said to be biochemically vitamin deficient. (Vitamin E levels, however, were at the lower range of normal.) After more than a decade of our HTPN program, we have not recognized any vitamin deficiencies in patients as long as they took their vitamins at the level prescribed. We have seen two patients from other programs who were incorrectly prescribed vitamins and in whom obvious biotin deficiency developed. This should not occur, because all the preparations currently available contain this essential vitamin. It is critical for patients who receive premixed solutions to add the vitamins just before infusion; this will minimize the loss caused by allowing the vitamins to stand in a parenteral nutrition solution.

CENTRAL VENOUS CATHETERS

Venous access for the administration of parenteral nutrition solutions is achieved through the placement of silicone catheters.[45-46] Although the typical location for such catheters is the right atrium, at times this site is not available. Access through the central venous circulation can be made by placing the catheter in the axillary, external jugular, or internal jugular or the femoral and saphenous veins. Patients who have received parenteral support for a number of years may have had catheters placed in a variety of sites. Some persons, particularly young women and men who are especially concerned about their physical appearance and sexual attractiveness, may prefer that the catheter be placed in the femoral-saphenous vein area and threaded up the inferior vena cava to just below the level of the diaphragm. There is no evidence that catheters placed in these areas are any more prone to infection or thrombosis than catheters placed in the veins draining the upper half of the body.

Patients and/or their families are taught the technique for catheter care and the administration of parenteral nutrition solutions. Most patients participating in such programs need dressing changes on either a daily or an every-other-daily basis. Both have been found effective in preventing the development of localized skin infections.[47-50] There are some persons who will be sensitive to certain cleaning agents and bacteriostatic or bactericidal ointments; they may use simple cleaning measures (sterile water and bacteriostatic soaps) but not antiseptic ointments or antibacterial ointments, because of their sensitivity to them.

PATIENT MANAGEMENT

Goals of managing an adult patient on a home parenteral nutrition program are to provide the amount of nutrients necessary for either weight maintenance or weight gain until optimum weight is reached and to provide those nutrients in a safe manner that is free of complications. Most patients on home parenteral nutrition regimens receive their solutions overnight during 8-to-14-hour periods. Factors that must be considered include the capability of the patient to manage the parenteral nutrition infusions without help, the life-style of the patient, and the time of day or night that is most convenient for the patient or family members to manage the care.

Some elderly patients do not like to be awakened during the night by the need to reset their infusion pumps, and/or they may dislike having to arise to void several times during the night. Some may prefer to receive their infusion during the daytime hours so they do not have to get up at night, which interferes with their sleep. Others may be fearful of complications that might occur during the night and worry about their inability to contact appropriate nursing and medical staff during these hours. All these fears must be considered in the establishment of an appropriate time to receive parenteral support. Most adults, however, who work during the day and homemakers who wish to care for their families will elect to receive TPN at night.

After it has been determined when the patient is to receive parenteral nutrition, the physician in charge must set up a schedule for gradually providing the solution at a more rapid rate of infusion over progressively fewer hours. Gradual reduction allows adaptation of the patient's pancreas to provide insulin for the progressively increasing rate of delivery of dextrose to the systemic circulation.[51] A rate of infusion exceeding 350 ml/hour cannot be tolerated in most persons. Adults receiving 2 liters of a 25% dextrose solution generally can tolerate an infusion rate of 250 ml/hour for 8 hours without difficulty. This may be given with the addition of a lipid emulsion if necessary.

Some patients will require the administration of additional fluids to compensate for losses from ostomies. These fluids may be simultaneously administered or given rapidly at the completion of the TPN infusion.

To avoid reactive hypoglycemia at the termination of a TPN infusion, most patients need to have a gradual reduction in the rate of infusion. Hypoglycemia may still develop in occasional patients with a slower rate of tapering, and these patients may be better managed by reduction of the concentration of dextrose they receive and reliance on a greater proportion of calories from a lipid infusion.

At the completion of the infusion, all catheters should be flushed with a heparin solution to prevent clots from forming. Most catheters can be filled with a solution of heparin containing 100 units per milliliter. Commonly used mixtures are 250-300 units or 2.5 to 3 ml of heparin solution per lumen.

The catheters must be flushed with heparin after use and carefully secured to the body to prevent dislodgment (of the catheter or the catheter cap). This can be done by placing adhesive tape between the cap and the catheter itself. Patients with central venous catheters can shower, bathe, swim, and participate in athletic activities if they wish, provided the catheter is properly secured. After participation in any of these activities, however, the catheter may have to be resecured and the insertion site cleaned and dried.

PEDIATRIC HOME PARENTERAL NUTRITION

In the pediatric population the major indications for parenteral nutrition at home are as follows[52-57]: (1) short-bowel syndrome that cannot be managed by either oral or continuous drip infusion of elemental formulas; (2) Crohn's disease refractory to drug therapy, short-bowel syndrome secondary to resection, and postoperative enterocutaneous fistula; (3) generalized motility disorders of the intestinal tract; (4) intractable diarrhea that occurs during infancy (neonatal/postnatal) and beyond infancy; (5) malignant tumors with intestinal or gastric obstruction or radiation damage to the intestinal tract; (6) graft-versus-host disease after bone marrow transplantation; and (7) miscellaneous disorders.

The decision to place an infant or child on a home parenteral nutrition program starts when the attending physician realizes or recognizes that the patient cannot be successfully nourished by mouth or by drip infusion of elemental formulas. Sometimes this is recognized immediately after the resection of a considerable length of intestine, and at other times it may not be recognized or apparent until after feeding has failed. In virtually all the conditions listed the physician's recognition of the patient's inability to use the digestive tract, in whole or in part, is the deciding factor.

Once it is determined that a pediatric patient needs home total parenteral nutrition, a conference should be held with the family member or members who will be providing the care. The purpose of the meeting should be to present the concept of HTPN to the parents and the patient, if the latter is old enough to understand. Each member of the nutritional support service who will aid in training the parent/patient and/or providing part of the care should be present. Typically this will include the training nurse, the social worker, the pharmacist, and the nutritionist. Their roles in the establishment of the HTPN program should be presented and time should be left for the parents or caregivers to ask questions.

The most frequently asked questions are (1)

How long will my child require such care? (2) How many hours per day will it require? (3) How dangerous is it? (4) Can my child take a bath or shower with the catheter in place? (5) What do we do if there's a fire in our house or apartment when the patient is receiving HTPN? (6) What do we do if the power fails? (7) How expensive is it? (8) Who will pay for it? (9) Who will do the HTPN care if I am sick and cannot do it? (10) What if I need to be away from my child for a week and there is no one available to help do the HTPN? (11) How is it mixed?

These are some of the questions typically asked. Suggested responses can be based on information contained in the ensuing discussions.

Pediatric Infusion Devices

Central venous catheters made of silicone are the most commonly chosen infusion devices because of their flexibility, decreased thrombogenicity, and supposedly decreased risk of contamination. The most commonly used are the Broviac and the Hickman catheters. The differences between them relate to their length and internal diameter and to whether the external part is a single lumen, with or without a protective sheath. The Hickman catheter has the greater internal diameter and thicker walls, and it does not have a protective sheath.

Both the Hickman and the Broviac catheters have a Leur-Lok fitting on the end, which allows them to be easily capped off or connected to an injection cap when not being used. Each has a Dacron cuff on the external portion that adheres to the subcutaneous tissue on the chest and lower abdominal wall and prevents dislodgment.

The infant-size Broviac is the smallest of all catheters. It is satisfactory for placement in patients less than 1 year old. The standard Broviac is better for use after the first year of life. The Hickman catheter is best for patients who may require blood products in addition to HTPN and who often require drawing of blood samples. It cannot be used in infants.

Placement of the catheter depends, in part, on the sites available, the presence or absence of ostomies, and in some instances the cosmetic appearance. Teenagers especially may object to catheter placement in the jugular or subclavian veins because the exit site on the chest is easily seen and may impose limitations as to the type of clothing that can be worn.

Catheter exit sites adjacent to ileostomies, colostomies, or jejunostomies have a theoretically greater risk of becoming infected from cross-contamination. However, meticulous attention to hand washing should reduce the risk. There are at least eight sites that can be used for catheter placement: two external jugular, two internal jugular, two subclavian, and two femoral.

Another type of infusion device recently used in a limited way for HTPN is the Port-A-Cath. This is an implantable drug-and-solution-delivery system that is placed completely under the skin. It allows drugs and fluids to be administered directly into the circulatory system. Its advantages are that it is completely under the skin (not readily visible) and does not require frequent care and special dressings, as with the Broviac and Hickman catheters. A Port-A-Cath does not interfere with bathing and swimming, as does a Hickman or Broviac catheter. The Port-A-Cath does require the placement of a needle through the skin and into the diaphragm. Some 2000 punctures with a 22-gauge Huberpoint needle are said to be the number that can be tolerated by the diaphragm without leaking. Some patients who would not like the minor discomfort caused by the need to prick the skin to access the Port-A-Cath on a daily basis may be poor candidates for this system.

Experience with the Port-A-Cath for long-term HTPN daily or five times per week is limited, in both children and adults. Complications have occurred that are similar to those with the Hickman or Broviac catheters, except for the tunnel and catheter insertion site infections typical of the Broviac and Hickman.

Formulating Parenteral Nutrition Solutions

Parenteral nutrition solutions for use at home may be no different from those used in the hospital. Only the addition of certain trace metals (selenium, chromium), which are typically used only in patients receiving HTPN for more than 30 days, makes them unique.

The number of calories to be provided parenterally depends on the patient's age, ideal or usual body weight, and estimated or measured absorptive capacity of the intestine. Even in patients who have only a duodenum anastomosed to the colon, 5% of the needs should be calculated or absorbed enterally to allow for oral or tube feeding from the beginning. In infants readjustments of calories provided must be done frequently because of their rapid growth. In the first 3 months of life readjustment should be done every week; in the second 3 months, every 2 weeks; during the last half of the first year, monthly; and in the second year and thereafter, every 3 months.

The fluid volume necessary to provide water depends on the patient's weight and whether there are reasons to restrict or provide extra fluid. If the patient has excess losses from an ostomy, we prefer to give this fluid as a separate replacement solution. If fluids must be restricted, it may be necessary to increase the concentrations of other nutrients.

Energy calories are usually provided in the form of dextrose. However, a minimum of 4% of calories should be provided as lipid emulsion to prevent essential fatty acid deficiency. The final concentration of dextrose used depends on the variables just mentioned and may range from 10% to 35%. The proportion of calories provided by lipid emulsions should not exceed 25% on a long-term basis. The physician must carefully determine whether the emulsion is being cleared from the circulation and is not progressively increasing. Failure to follow triglyceride levels may result in a serious complication, the lipid overload syndrome.

The amino acid concentration used depends on the patient's age and needs for growth. Amino acid preparations specifically designed for infants are probably preferable for use during infancy. Beyond infancy standard balanced amino acid preparations are adequate.

Electrolytes, Calcium, Magnesium, Phosphate

Electrolytes, calcium, magnesium, and phosphate are added to the solution according to the recognized requirements of infants and children based on weight in kilograms. Additional electrolytes, as needed because of losses from ostomy or diarrhea, should be provided in a separate solution and given intravenously by "IV piggyback," either during or after the infusion of TPN solutions.

Vitamins

Specific infant formulas of intravenous vitamins should be given to all infants who weigh less than 10 kg.

Infants >3 kg and children less than 11 years of age
  Absorbic acid—80 mg
  Vitamin A—0.7 mg (2300 USP units)
  Ergocalciferol (D_2)—10 μg (400 USP)
  Thiamine (B_1)—1.2 mg
  Riboflavin (B_2)—1.4 mg
  Pyridoxine (B_6)—1.0 mg
  Niacinamide—17.0 mg
  Dexpanthenol—5.0 mg
  Vitamin E—7.0 mg (7 USP)
  Biotin—20 μg
  Folic acid—140 μg
  Cyanocobalamin (B_{12})—1 μg
  Phytonadione (K_1)—200 μg
Pediatric patients 11 years of age or older
  Ascorbic acid—100 mg
  Vitamin A—1 mg (3300 USP)
  Ergocalciferol (D_2)—5 μg (200 USP)
  Pyridoxine (B_6)—4 mg
  Riboflavin (B_2)—3.6 mg
  Thiamine (B_1)—3.0 mg
  Niacinamide—40 mg
  Dexpathenol—15 mg
  Vitamin E—10 mg (10 USP)
  Biotin—60 μg
  Folic acid—400 μg
  Cyanocobalamin (B_{12})—5 μg

For infants who weigh more than 10 kg, a multivitamin formulation for adults will provide the necessary levels of vitamins, except for vitamin K, which may need to be supplemented periodically. Ten milliliters is the customary quantity. To minimize the degradation of certain fat-soluble vitamins, they should be added to the solution just before it is administered.

Trace Metals

Four trace metals are routinely added to the parenteral nutrition solution: zinc, copper, chromium, and selenium. The dose schedule used is as shown*:

	Amount (μg/kg/da)
Zinc	100
Copper	20
Chromium	0.14-0.2
Manganese	2-10
Selenium	1.4

Patients with large ostomy output and/or voluminous diarrhea may require additional supplementation, especially of zinc and selenium. Measurement of zinc and selenium in ostomy effluent

*Term infants >3 kg same as for children to 18 years.

and diarrhea fluid may be useful in helping to determine the daily requirements for certain patients whose zinc and selenium status indicates deficiency in spite of standard supplementation.

Patients receiving long-term HTPN have been found to be deficient in a number of other trace been metals, but the role of these elements in biologic processes is unknown and therefore the patients do not receive supplements. These trace elements include nickel, rubidium, cobalt, and manganese.

Other Additives

A variety of other additives may be added to the TPN solutions without altering the solution and may be helpful in the overall management of the patient. The two most common are insulin and histamine$_2$ blockers.

Infusion Pumps

All parenteral nutrition solutions should be administered with a volumetric infusion pump to ensure the patient's safety. Infusion pumps with cassettes are the safest and most accurate and should be used for all children less than 10 years of age. Children older than 10 years may be infused with pumps that do not involve cassettes; these pumps, however, have a 6% to 10% error rate and usually deliver extra solution.

Cyclic Parenteral Nutrition

Since the goal for patients receiving HTPN is to assume as normal a life as possible, it seems only appropriate that they be disconnected from the infusion system as often as possible. To accomplish this, a period of physiologic readjustment needs to take place. In most patients the TPN solutions are infused at home over an 8-to-12-hour period depending on the volume to be infused and the body's ability to handle the glucose load.

Typically the number of hours of infusion is decreased by 1 or 2 per day as determined by the patient's response to the progressively increasing infusion rate and calculated by the following formula:

$$\text{Rate per hour} = \frac{\text{Volume to be infused (ml)}}{\text{Hours of infusion}}$$

At the completion of the infusion period the rate is reduced by 50%; after another 15 minutes it is reduced by another 50%. Fifteen minutes after the second reduction the pump is turned off; and after a period during which the catheter is aseptically cleaned, flushed with 300 units of heparin, and capped, the patient is disconnected from the infusion system.

The blood sugar value should be determined just before the infusion rate is reduced and at the end of the second 15-minute infusion cycle. If the blood glucose value decreases to less than 60 mg/dl and/or if symptoms develop, a longer period of stepping down the rate or a reduction in the concentration of dextrose in the TPN solution may be necessary. This should always be done in the hospital. Patients in whom hypoglycemia develops must remain in the hospital. The problem must be resolved before discharge. Seldom do problems develop long after discharge. Symptoms of hypoglycemia become apparent either to the parent or to the patient and may consist of irritability when the TPN solutions are tapered and discontinued, difficulty in arousing from sleep, and (rarely) diaphoresis.

In certain cases when TPN is not required on a nightly basis, or as the bowel adapts, nights can be chosen when parenteral nutrition is not given. Most families logically choose at first to have the weekend nights free of TPN infusion. It is possible for a patient to go without an infusion for 2 nights.

The specific hour at which the infusion is started may vary from day to day without any risk to the patient, as long as the solutions are given at the established rate. It is quite possible for the rate to vary by ±10% per day without serious consequences.

Teaching Family Members

Parents of children who receive HTPN must go through a program of rigorous training to ensure their capability of flawlessly administering the solutions in an aseptic manner and that they understand what to do if emergency situations occur or there is a malfunction of the equipment or catheter. They must be closely supervised and should practice daily under direct supervision until their technique is flawless. They must then perform in the hospital independent of direct nursing supervision. The duration of training and supervision may vary from as little as 10 to more than 40 hours. Typically, our parents manage the entire care for a week or more alone before the patient is discharged.

DISCHARGE PLANNING

It is the job of the medical social worker to help make the arrangements for home care, determining who is responsible for payment and helping to direct the family to appropriate state agencies or private insurance companies. This person also determines whether the family has adequate space at home for the storage of supplies and an adequate refrigerator to hold enough solution for 2 to 4 weeks. If the family does not have an adequate refrigerator, the social worker may help find the means to pay for a new one. If the family needs transportation to attend the clinic, this may be arranged; and if necessary, visits to the home by the Visiting Nurses Association may be coordinated with the patient's early days at home. Finally, there may be the occasional infant who requires care in a foster home because its parents are not capable of executing the procedures or are not committed to providing this kind of care, and these plans must be devised.

LONG-TERM OUTPATIENT CARE

After discharge an infant or child who receives HTPN is seen within 1 week. Visits after this time are dependent on the patient's age, nutritional status at the first visit, and whether problems have developed that were not anticipated. Infants are seen on a prearranged schedule. After infancy follow-up visits should be no less than one in 3 to 6 months. At each visit the infant or child is weighed and its height measured. Occipital frontal circumference is measured until the infant is 2 years of age. For infants and children these data are plotted on nomograms (e.g., the Iowa growth grids) for age and sex to determine the adequacy of growth and weight gain.

Parents are questioned about any problems with the use of the infusion pump or clearing of the catheter when it is flushed with heparin. The catheter insertion site is checked for tenderness, fluctuation, or discharge of purulent or serosanguineous material.

The physical examination is completed after a check for signs of vitamin deficiency and other indicators of malnutrition. The abdomen is palpated for assessment of liver size, because hepatomegaly is not atypical in patients receiving HTPN who are overfed.

The contents of nutritional support solutions are reviewed and adjustments made, depending on the patient's needs.

Blood samples are taken for a CBC and evaluation of electrolytes and calcium and magnesium levels. Liver function tests are done as indicated or every 3 months. Trace metal determinations are done every 6 to 12 months.

Bone age testing is performed every 6 to 12 months to ascertain whether the patient is maturing at a rate comparable with chronologic age.

Feeding by mouth should be encouraged as much as possible to promote oral gratification and facilitate the transition to full enteral nutrition when possible.

Child development specialists should see these patients at regular intervals to track their progress and to help with the counseling of parents. School-age children may require routine consultation with child psychiatrists to deal with problems they encounter at home and school because of their unique situation.

SUPPORTING PERSONNEL
Medical Social Worker

Home parenteral nutrition programs training two or more patients per month find that it is important either to have a medical social worker (MSW) assigned exclusively to work with such patients, if the program warrants, or to delegate a MSW in the hospital to become involved in the program. After discharge, this person acts as a liaison between the patient and the other members of the home parenteral support team, providing progress reports on the transition from hospital to home.

Nurse

Nurses are key to the success of a home parenteral support program. They are responsible for all patient teaching, and they have other functions (e.g., providing a medical link between the patient and the physician responsible). They are the first line of defense, and the ones the patient learns to call first if problems develop. The HTPN nurse, when listening to a patient's problem, can determine whether there is immediate need for medical intervention or whether the complaint is minor and can wait to be assessed in the clinic. The nurse's role is also supportive in a psychologic sense.

Pharmacist

The pharmacist's role in home parenteral support programs is to help the physician determine the optimum solution and nutrients to be given a patient and to provide these in a form that is easy to administer and requires the fewest additives.[29]

In some programs the pharmacist provides training and helps teach formulation to the patient and/or advises the physician on formulations. The pharmacist's role after discharge is to expedite any changes in the solutions proposed by the physician and to help monitor the patient with the physician and nursing staff. The pharmacist helps ensure that the patient maintains the correct stock of solution additives and supplies and that they are received.[9]

Visiting Nurse

After discharge from the hospital patients are usually seen on the first and/or second day by a visiting nurse. It is that person's job to determine whether the patient's transition to the home has been successful. The visiting nurse can provide additional nursing services to patients who in the physician's opinion need it. By the time most of our patients are discharged, they are confident in their abilities and require no more than a token visit.

FOLLOW-UP VISITS

Patients usually return within a week after discharge. Depending on their condition at that time the following are performed and an appointment may be made for a visit in a week or later as needed:

Weight
  Triceps skinfold thickness, middle arm circumference, mid–arm muscle circumference (optional)
Nutrients infused
  Days per week
  Hours per day
  Tapering technique used
Review
  Social, financial, family situations
  Problems
    Delivery of solutions and supplies
    Reaching staff
    Pump, catheter, or solution
Laboratory tests
  Electrolytes, calcium, magnesium, phosphorus, CBC
  Liver function
  Trace metals (once or twice yearly)
Readjust fluid and nutritional needs as indicated

Gradually reduce parenteral nutritional fluid while increasing enteral intake
Reduce number of nights of HTPN as indicated by patient's weight gain and/or stability or by increased enteral or oral intake

The frequency of visits is determined by the patient's medical or surgical condition, how often adjustments in the solutions need to be made, and the psychologic status of the patient. In most instances patients who are followed for 6 or more months are seen on a bimonthly or quarterly basis. After the second year they are often seen on a twice-a-yearly basis. At each visit the physician or pharmacist should review with the patient the nutrients infused and the rate and number of hours of infusion. Patients may try to change their own infusion schedule and volume if they are independent; this needs to be discouraged. The physician recalculates the nutritional support to determine if it is what has been prescribed. For patients receiving enteral and parenteral nutrition these data are also collected. After a physical examination decisions are made as to whether a change in the solutions or volumes being administered is indicated.

All members of the parenteral support service should talk with the patient, if possible, when such a service is provided. Otherwise, it is the responsibility of the physician who cares for the patient to function in multiple roles as needed.

HOME VENDOR SELECTION

The choice of whether to use a private vendor or a hospital-based HTPN support service depends on what is available in the community. In some institutions the entire home support program is offered by the medical center; in others private vendors are used. At the University of California–Los Angeles we provide premixed solutions and all supplies, as is done by HTPN vendors. At discharge the patients are given a list of the supplies and solutions they will need and the amount of these to be ordered on a bimonthly basis. Patients are taught how to take stock of their supplies and solutions and are given specific instructions as to when to reorder either supplies or solutions. A phone number is given for them to call so they have direct contact with a knowledgeable person in the pharmacy who works strictly on the program. The frequency with which solutions and supplies are delivered is based in part on the storage capacity of the family's home and the refrigeration facilities. Patients who live close to the Medical Center may on their own choose to come and obtain solutions more frequently. Those who live some distance away may have them delivered. Patients have the choice of obtaining solutions that are premixed or learning to mix their own. In our program all except one or two patients have chosen premixed solutions. Both are effective ways of delivering parenteral nutrition. Careful analysis has not been made of the complication rates between using solutions manufactured by major national home care support services and using those by smaller local companies. Nor are data available comparing the quality of support in hospital-based programs versus that in home support services, or even whether the two are comparable.

DURATION OF HTPN

Nearly one third of the adult patients in our experience at UCLA have received home total parenteral nutrition for less than 6 months, but one fourth (25%) have participated in such a program for more than half a decade and 2% for more than a decade.

Although many patients admitted to a HTPN program will receive it for a limited time, those who usually require it for a year are unlikely ever to discontinue it. This is because patients with short-bowel syndrome who are going to adapt fully to enteral nutrition usually do so within a year. An occasional patient with a very short and small bowel (>12 cm but <25 cm with the ileocecal valve, or >25 cm without the valve) may ultimately adapt, but this may take up to 5 years.

MORBIDITY

During 1985 and 1986, 25% of our patients at UCLA receiving home parenteral nutrition had to be readmitted for problems related to home total parenteral nutrition. Most were admitted only once, but some were admitted multiple times. Catheter occlusion and fever secondary to catheter sepsis were the two most common reasons for admission. No patients were admitted because of electrolyte imbalance. This was because abnormalities found in blood chemistry determinations at follow-up visits were corrected on an outpatient basis. Our experience is comparable to what has been reported by others in the home parenteral nutrition (HPN) registry.[25]

All our patients use premixed solutions, and thus there have been no complications secondary to incorrect compounding of solutions. Over a year's time three episodes of contamination of solutions premixed by a commercial vendor did occur. All three patients had candidemia. Surprisingly, the HPN registry shows no real difference in risk of complications and readmissions between premixed and self-mixed solutions.[25] However, reporting by members of the registry may not be complete.

Infections

When patients were admitted because of suspected catheter sepsis, three sets of blood cultures were obtained from the peripheral veins and the central venous catheter. Antibiotics were then started. Antibiotics used most frequently were vancomycin hydrochloride and gentamicin, because of their antistaphylococcal and gram-negative coverage. In cases identified as caused by staphylococci, vancomycin was the drug of choice. Once the patient had been afebrile for a minimum of 24 hours, he or she was taught how to administer the intravenous antibiotics and was sent home to complete a month's course of antibiotics. Patients were instructed to take and record their temperature four times a day and to notify the physician if it exceeded 37.8° C.

Our overall sepsis rate is one episode for every 4.5 years of HTPN and is comparable to results compiled by the HPN registry.[25] Some patients have received HTPN up to 12 years without any infection, which demonstrates the safety of this technique.

Although most infections have been secondary to staphylococci, a variety of other bacterial organisms and fungi (e.g., *Candida*) have been recognized to cause sepsis. When *Candida* is found, the catheter is almost always removed and amphotericin administration is begun and continued for a full course. A new catheter is placed once the blood cultures fail to grow fungi.

Subcutaneous tunnel infections accounted for 20% of all our cases and were difficult to eradicate. They commonly led to catheter removal because of the difficulty of removing the nidus from the Dacron cuff.

Whenever several veins have already been used, patients may be treated with multiple courses of antibiotics in an effort to maintain the catheter. During the past 12 years only 4 of 700

Table 33-2 Causes of Death at UCLA Among Patients Receiving HTPN (1985)

Non–TPN related	28
Metastatic carcinoma	11
Gastric	2
Hepatic	1
Esophageal	1
Colonic	2
Ovarian	2
Unspecified	3
Leukemia	2
Graft-versus-host disease	1
AIDS	5
Hemorrhage from fistulas	1
End-stage liver disease	3
End-stage pulmonary disease	1
Intractable bleeding from fistulas	2
Following liver transplantation	2
TPN related	2
Fat-overload syndrome	1
Sepsis	1

Table 33-3 Current Status of 116 HTPN Patients at UCLA with Nonmalignant Disease (1986-87)

Working full time at occupation	18
Full-time homemaker	12
Retired	14
Attending preschool	7
Attending elementary school	7
Attending high school	3
Attending college	1
Out of school	2
Not working because of illness	52

Table 33-4 Discontinuation of HTPN in 22 Patients at UCLA (1986)

Crohn's disease	10
Short-bowel syndrome	4
Enterocutaneous fistulas	3
Intractable disease	2
Colitis	1
Motility disorders	3
Pseudoobstruction	2
Scleroderma	1
Pancreatitis	3
Short-bowel syndrome	1
Mesenteric artery thrombosis	1
Postoperative enterocutaneous fistulas	3
Hyperemesis gravidarum	1
Bone-marrow transplantation	1

patients required thoracotomy for placement of a central venous line when no other access routes were available.

MORTALITY

In our experience at UCLA 28 of 30 deaths were due to the patients' primary disease (Table 33-2). Only two could be directly related to the use of HTPN. In one patient with Crohn's disease a sepsislike condition with hypertriglyceridemia developed after a 2-week period during which 500 ml of 20% lipid emulsion was administered on a daily basis. No organism was ever isolated from the blood, but the patient had a disseminated intravascular coagulation–like condition and died of pulmonary and renal failure.[32-34] Another patient died of sepsis that was secondary to catheter contamination with a gram-negative organism. There was a delay in diagnosis, which may have prevented successful eradication of the organism.

Among the patients who died of complications from metastatic disease, we could not predict with any accuracy when this was likely to occur. The duration and survival varied from 2 weeks to 14 months. Some patients with metastatic disease confined to the gastrointestinal tract survived for prolonged periods, even up to 6 months. Those with metastatic ovarian carcinoma generally survived 18 months. Most patients with cancer lived far longer than had been estimated by their oncologists, which made it difficult to anticipate the degree of care that would be required by the patient. Of the patients with AIDS, most survived between 1 and 6 months. Those with graft-versus-host disease (GVHD) had lingering illnesses that persisted up to 6 months after discharge.

WORK, SCHOOL, AND SOCIAL STATUS

Most patients less than 40 years of age who did not have a malignant disease were able to work full or part time, be full time homemakers, or attend school (Table 33-3). All children of school age attended the appropriate school for their age.

All patients with active malignant disease or GVHD and adult patients with primary and secondary pseudoobstruction and pancreatitis were too incapacitated by their disease and its complications to work. Many of these patients were febrile, had large volumes of diarrhea, and were beset with other complicating factors that made it difficult to do anything but care for their own needs.

No divorces occurred in any family with a member participating in an HTPN program. Only one of our unmarried patients who was less than age 40 married, and only one became pregnant, while receiving HTPN.

DISCONTINUATION OF HTPN

Parenteral nutrition was successfully discontinued in 22 patients at our center (Table 33-4). Those with short-bowel syndrome successfully adapted after 6 to 12 months of TPN. Each had between 75 and 100 cm of small intestine and no ileocecal valve. Enterocutaneous fistulas secondary to operative procedures closed in 6 to 12 weeks in each instance. Two patients with intractable Crohn's disease went into clinical remission and were able to resume eating normally. In two of the three patients with pancreatitis the pain and diarrhea were resolved. One continues to have intractable pain and, because of failure to comply with techniques, was removed from the program. For unexplained reasons, two patients with primary pseudoobstruction syndrome and one with scleroderma had sufficient improvement in their bowel function to try to support themselves entirely by the enteral route.

REFERENCES

1. Shila ME, et al: Long-term parenteral nutrition through an external arteriovenous shunt, N Engl J Med **283**:341-344, 1970.
2. Jeejeebhoy KN, et al: Total parenteral nutrition at home for 23 months without complication and with good rehabilitation, Gastroenterology **65**:811-820, 1973.
3. Broviac JN, Scribner BH: Prolonged parenteral nutrition in the home, Surg Gynecol Obstet **139**:24-28, 1974.
4. Grundfest S, Steiger E: Home parenteral nutrition, JAMA **244**:1701-1703, 1980.
5. Byrne WJ, et al: Home parenteral nutrition, J Pediatr Surg **12**:359-366, 1977.
6. Howard L, Hichalek AV: Home parenteral nutrition, Annu Rev Nutr **4**:69-99, 1984.
7. Byrne WJ, et al: Home parenteral nutrition, Surg Gynecol Obstet **149**:593-597, 1979.
8. Steiger E, et al: Total parenteral nutrition and fluid/electrolyte therapy in the home, Cleve Clin Q **52**:317-327, 1985.
9. Cannon RA, et al: Home parenteral nutrition in infants, J Pediatr **96**:1098-1104, 1980.
10. Vargas JH, et al: Long-term home parenteral nutrition in

pediatrics—Ten years experience in 102 patients, J Pediatr Gastroenterol Nutr **6**:24-33, 1987.
11. Ostro MJ, et al: Total parenteral nutrition and complete bowel rest in the management of Crohn's disease, J Parenter Enter Nutr **9**:280-287, 1985.
12. Lake AM, et al: Influence of preoperative parenteral alimentation on postoperative growth in adolescent Crohn's disease, J Pediatr Gastroenterol Nutr **4**:182-187, 1985.
13. Fleming CR: Home parenteral nutrition as primary therapy in patients with extensive Crohn's disease of the small bowel and malnutrition, Gastroenterology **73**:1077-1081, 1977.
14. Jarnum S, Ladefoged K: Long-term parenteral nutrition, Scand J Gastroenterol **16**:903-911, 1981.
15. Matsueda K, et al: A long-term follow-up of home hyperalimentation for short bowel syndrome and its therapeutic application in inflammatory bowel disease. In Shohei BV, et al, editors: Parenteral and enteral hyperalimentation, New York, 1984, Elsevier Science Publishing Co Inc.
16. Strobel CT, et al: Home parenteral nutrition in children with Crohn's disease: An effective management alternative, Gastroenterology **77**:272-278, 1979.
17. Schuffler MD, Deitch EA: Chronic idiopathic intestinal pseudo-obstruction, Ann Surg **192**:752-761, 1980.
18. Anuras S, et al: A familial visceral myopathy with dilatation of the entire gastrointestinal tract, Gastroenterology **90**:385-390, 1986.
19. Vargas HJ, et al: Chronic intestinal pseudo-obstruction syndrome in pediatrics: Results of a North American survey, Gastroenterology. (In press, 1987.)
20. Durack DT: The acquired immune deficiency syndrome, Adv Intern Med **30**:29-52, 1984.
21. Riella MC, Scribner BH: Five years experience with a right atrial catheter for prolonged parenteral nutrition at home, Surg Gynecol Obstet **143**:206-208, 1976.
22. Louie N, Niemiec PW: Parenteral nutrition solutions. In Rombeau JL, Caldwell MD, editors: Parenteral nutrition, vol 2, Philadelphia, 1986, WB Saunders Co, pp 272-305.
23. Cox KK, et al: Hyperalimentation during pregnancy: a case report, J Parenter Enter Nutr **5**:246-249, 1981.
24. Pitkin RM: Nutritional support in obstetrics and gynecology, Clin Obstet Gynecol **19**:489-513, 1976.
25. Howard L, et al: A review of the current national status of home parenteral and enteral nutrition from the provider and consumer perspective, J Parenter Enter Nutr **10**:416-422, 1986.
26. Mertz W: The essential trace elements, Science **18**:1332-1338, 1981.
27. Sayers MH, et al: Supplementation of total parenteral nutrition solution with ferrous citrate, J Parenter Enter Nutr **7**:117-121, 1983.
28. Valber LS, et al: Cobalt test for the detection of iron deficiency anemia, Annu Intern Med **77**:181-187, 1972.
29. Mills CF: Biochemical roles of trace elements, Prog Clin Biol Res **77**:179-188, 1981.
30. Kararskis EJ, Schuna A: Serum alkaline phosphatase after treatment of zinc deficiency in humans, J Clin Nutr **33**:2609-2612, 1980.
31. McClain CJ: Trace metal abnormalities in adults during hyperalimentation, J Parenter Enter Nutr **5**:424-429, 1981.
32. Delves HT: The microdetermination of copper in plasma protein fraction, Clin Chim Acta **71**:495-500, 1976.

33. Fleming CR: Essential fatty acid, copper, zinc and tocopheral deficiencies in total parenteral nutrition, Acta Chir Scan (Suppl) **466:**20-21, 1976.

34. Tasman-Jones C, et al: Zinc and copper deficiency, with particular reference to parenteral nutrition, Surg Ann **10:**23-52, 1978.

35. Blumenthal I, et al: Fracture of the femur, fish odour, and copper deficiency in a preterm infant, Arch Dis Child **55:**229-231, 1980.

36. Versieck J, et al: Determination of manganese in whole blood and serum, Clin Chem **26:**531-532, 1980.

37. Rotruck JT, et al: Selenium: biochemical role as a component of glutathione peroxidase, Science **179:**588-590, 1973.

38. Hahn HK, et al: Determination of serum selenium by means of solvent extraction combined with activation analyses, J Lab Clin Med **80:**718-722, 1972.

39. Johnson RA, et al: An occidental case of cardiomyopathy and selenium deficiency, N Engl J Med **304:**1210-1212, 1981.

40. Kien C, Ganther HE: Manifestations of chronic selenium deficiency in a child receiving total parenteral nutrition, Am J Clin Nutr **37:**319-328, 1983.

41. King WW, et al: Reversal of selenium deficiency with oral selenium [letter], N Engl J Med **304:**21-22, 1981.

42. Freund H, et al: Chromium deficiency during total parenteral nutrition, JAMA **241:**496-498, 1979.

43. Jeejeebhoy KN, et al: Chromium deficiency, glucose intolerance and neuropathy reserved by chromium supplementation in a patient receiving long-term total parenteral nutrition, Am J Clin Nutr **30:**531-538, 1977.

44. Abumrad NN, et al: Amino acid intolerance during prolonged total parenteral nutrition reversed by molybdate therapy, Am J Clin Nutr **34:**2551-2559, 1981.

45. Grundfest S, Steiger E: Experience with the Broviac catheter for prolonged parenteral nutrition, J Parenter Enter Nutr **3:**45-47, 1979.

46. Pollack PF, et al: 100 patient years experience with the Broviac silastic catheter for central venous nutrition, J Parenter Enter Nutr **5:**32-36, 1981.

47. Hickman RO, et al: A modified right atrial catheter for access to the venous system in marrow transplant recipients, Surg Gynecol Obstet **145:**871-875, 1979.

48. Sanders JE, et al: Experience with double lumen right atrial catheters, J Parenter Enter Nutr **6:**95-99, 1982.

49. Forlan L: Parenteral nutrition in the critically ill child, Crit Care Q **3:**7, 1981.

50. Jarrard MM, et al: Daily dressing change effects on skin flora beneath subclavian catheter dressing during total parenteral nutrition, J Parenter Enter Nutr **4:**391-392, 1980.

51. Byrne WJ, et al: Adaptation to increasing loads of total parenteral nutrition: metabolic endocrine, and insulin receptor responses, Gastroenterology **80:**947-956, 1981.

52. Fleming CR, et al: Home parenteral nutrition as primary therapy in patients with extensive Crohn's disease of the small bowel and malnutrition, Gastroenterology **73:**1079-1081, 1977.

53. Jeejeebhoy KN, et al: Total parenteral nutrition at home: studies in patients surviving 4 months to 5 years, Gastroenterology **71:**943-953, 1976.

54. Riella MC, Scribner BH: Five years' experience with a right atrial catheter for prolonged parenteral nutrition at home, Surg Gynecol Obstet **143:**295-300, 1976.

55. Byrne WJ, et al: Home parenteral nutrition, Surg Gynecol Obstet **149:**593-597, 1979.

56. Byrne WJ, et al: Home parenteral nutrition, J Pediatr Surg **12:**359-366, 1977.

57. Cannon RA, et al: Home parenteral nutrition in infants, J Pediatr **96:**1098-1104, 1980.

VI

NUTRITIONAL DEFICIENCIES AND ABNORMALITIES

CHAPTER 34
Protein-Energy Malnutrition

Fernando E. Viteri
Benjamin Torún

Protein-energy malnutrition (PEM) encompasses a wide spectrum of general nutritional conditions that range clinically from almost unrecognizable symptoms to the florid pictures of starvation and kwashiorkor.

PEM can be primary or secondary (i.e., the result of a *deficit of available food* or the consequence of some *alteration that impairs* intake, absorption, or utilization, or that increases energy and/or protein needs or losses). This chapter focuses on primary PEM, a prevalent nutritional deficiency condition among populations in most developing countries. PEM generally is associated with poverty, limited availability of food, unsanitary environments, high rates of infection, and marked socioeconomic inequalities. Clearly it can assume epidemic proportions as a consequence of natural, political, or sociodemographic calamities. Famine then becomes a "social scandal" worthy of dramatic remedial efforts. Unfortunately, the fundamental issue in resolving the causes of chronic socioeconomic disadvantage and marginalization of large population groups remains relegated.

The clinician can diagnose PEM among population groups by being aware of characteristic social settings (even in the absence of specific clinical signs), functional consequences and patterns of morbidity and mortality. Affected population groups are generally deprived. Food intake is monotonous and food often is scarce. Physiologic performance is suboptimal (i.e., poor growth, high prevalence of small babies at term, substandard mental performance, lower relative physical activity levels in tasks that demand energy). A few cases of severe, clinically evident PEM are seen, the endemic rate of infections (mostly gastrointestinal and respiratory) is elevated, and infant and preschool mortality rates are high.

At the individual level, the diagnosis of mild or even moderate PEM is often difficult without adequate information about the setting and conditions of the family and the community as a whole. Even then, in the isolated patient, PEM is often an exclusion diagnosis arrived at after chronic infection, malignancy, eating disorders, other secondary causes, and primary nonnutritional alterations in physiologic performance have been discarded.

Another problem in diagnosing PEM is the duration of the process as well as its sequelae. Acute and severe PEM is often superimposed on chronic mild to moderate PEM. Frequently sequelae related to the inadequate environment and previous PEM (stunted poorly developed individuals) lead to the diagnosis of PEM when it is no longer present. At the population level these sequelae can be functionally significant. Thus large-scale prevention, early detection, and prompt and effective correction of protein and energy deficits are imperative.

ETIOLOGY

Primary PEM results from prolonged deprivation of essential amino acids and total nitrogen and/or of energy substrates. The limiting nutritional factor(s) at the onset of the process leading to PEM can be protein-nitrogen (essential amino acids and nonessential nitrogen) and/or total energy. Each of these deficiencies may occur singly (i.e., in the presence of adequate or even excessive amounts of the other nutrients) or be combined. Often they are added to one or more pathologic and/or socioeconomic deprivation states. However, as the severity and duration of a specific deficiency advance, the other factors also become deficient. For example, in pure energy deficiency, protein nutriture can be spared initially; but in more advanced energy deficiency, protein is utilized for energy. Similarly, as protein-nitrogen becomes less available, the efficiency of energy utilization declines. In practice, then, except for very acute situations, the vast majority of cases with moderate to severe PEM present with a combined protein-nitrogen and energy deficiency either part of which still may predominate.[1]

In the absence of complicating factors, which could alter the absorption, transport, and utilization of protein-nitrogen and energy, the cause of these deficits at the cell level is inadequate intake. Inadequate intake is defined as intake not sufficient to meet the individual's needs. The levels of essential amino acids, total nitrogen, and energy have been defined (Chapters 1 and 2) in terms of both minimum requirements and recommended intakes.

Conditioning Factors

From the standpoint of the deficiency or adequacy of protein and energy intakes in relation to the etiology of PEM, several conditioning factors must be considered: First, the staple foods and preparation techniques typical of individual cultures, together with other cultural determinants of total food intake, must be known so energy and protein intakes can be evaluated at the population level. Second, although total food intake may be adequate for the population as a whole, it may be inadequate for certain groups that require more protein or energy per kilogram of body weight. This consideration takes into account the importance of food intake patterns at different ages, intrafamilial food distribution, protein and energy density of foods, differences in food preparation techniques, and food bulk and satiety.

Finally, protein sources must be known to enable one to judge whether they provide adequate amounts of the essential amino acids in balanced proportion (protein quality) as well as adequate amounts of total nitrogen. Protein quality is especially important when protein needs are higher per kilogram of body weight (early childhood). In this age group animal protein is normally fed (breast milk, other milk preparations) to satisfy protein needs. Other animal or selected vegetable sources of protein, which are often mixed to complement their essential amino acid contents, can serve as substitutes for milk (e.g., corn and beans, providing 50% of protein

from each source; formulated vegetable protein mixes).

The causes of inadequate food intakes that lead to PEM now can be analyzed from the standpoints of the individual, the family unit, and the population as a whole.

Causes of PEM in Infants and Children

The persons most often afflicted with PEM are children under 5 years of age.[2] They appear to be the most vulnerable group because both the proportion of the population afflicted and the incidence of severe PEM are higher in this group than in any other age group. This situation is determined by host, environmental, and agent factors.[3]

Host factors. The host factors that can be implicated in PEM are as follows:
1. A child under the age of 5 years has high protein and energy requirements on a body weight basis, particularly if he/she was small at birth (premature, small for date, or both).
2. A child under 5 years of age has a limited capacity to ingest large amounts of food at a single sitting.
3. A 5-year-old or younger child has no access, or only limited access, to food at will.
4. Once the child is malnourished, his/her condition is complicated further by lowered defenses against infectious agents, resulting in more frequent illness, anorexia, irritability, listlessness, and deterioration of appearance and affective interaction with caregivers as time elapses.

Environmental factors. The environmental factors implicated in PEM include the following:
1. A woman malnourished prior to and/or during pregnancy and lactation is more likely to produce an underweight baby.[4] Lactation in these cases often is inadequate, and affective interaction is impaired.
2. Poverty almost always is an underlying cause of PEM. Living quarters are overcrowded, the environment is often dirty and lacks the most basic hygienic conditions (particularly in slums and camps), and often the parents do not care for the child. Thus the child is weaned at an early age and is exposed to infection due to lack of proper attention. Substitute food preparations under these circumstances are added sources of infection and of improper nutrition. Infection and undernutri-

tion act synergistically to aggravate both conditions.[5]

3. Cultural considerations in poverty-stricken populations are essential in the analysis of environmental factors in PEM. On the one hand, in more "primitive" cultures, where breast-feeding is still universal and lasts for the greater part of the first 12-24 months of the child's life, PEM begins during the third and fourth month of life and is progressive, because often among these marginally nourished mothers breast milk production is smaller than among well-nourished women in the industrialized world.[6] Under these circumstances, frequently associated with high infection rates, breast milk alone cannot provide enough energy and protein beyond 3-4 months of age. Although complementary foods are essential, often they are introduced late and inappropriately. Thus, weaning becomes a critical nutritional period. On the other hand, socioeconomic demands and improper practices of assimilation, particularly in urban settings, have resulted in a marked decline in breast-feeding. Improper feeding practices (nonhygienic preparation of overdiluted formula or substitution of milk for unsanitary sugar water or starch gruels) result in early-age severe PEM. The whole weaning process encompasses a very delicate period for the child under these circumstances; but, even after weaning, in the face of scarcity, the small child receives the smallest and most inadequate proportion of the family pot. Moreover, cultural practices often dictate a restricted food intake when the child is sick; such children may be given only "medicinal" or "safe" beverages that have essentially no nutritional virtues and that even may be toxic.

Agent factors. The primary agents in these cases are the scarcity and/or poor quality of the diet ingested by the child.

1. Insufficient intake occurs in the child principally as a result of one of three causes: (a) the child is offered little food and is still unable to get more by him/herself (e.g., restricted intake during illnesses or prolonged exclusive breast-feeding); (b) the child is offered ample food but of an improper quality for his/her needs, resulting from low protein and/or low energy densities or from improper preparation for the gastrointestinal and general functional capacity at his/her age (e.g., diluted formula, cereal-based and root-based gruel or porridge, unmodified cow's milk given to newborns and premature babies, and improperly prepared complementary foods fed to infants); and (c) the child is given food to satiety only a few times per day or when he/she is anorectic, resulting in diminished total intake in either case. The anorexia of infection in children that are repeatedly ill is particularly damaging.

2. Children frequently ingest a poor-quality diet because they often are given overdiluted milk formulas and/or foods that are bulky, starchy, and poor in protein content, a result of a low protein concentration (low protein density) and/or an imbalanced amino acid composition. In this case the proportion of protein utilized for synthetic purposes is, at best, that of its most limiting amino acid (see Chapter 1). In terms of energy, food preparations that are rich in starches and undigestible fiber, bulky, and very poor in fat content (low energy density) usually cannot provide the required energy. Moreover, imbalanced diets produce anorexia. Protein-poor but carbohydrate-rich foods are particularly likely to induce acute severe protein deficiency[7] through mechanisms to be discussed under "Pathophysiology" (p. 538).

Causes of PEM in Older Children and Adults

In addition to children under the age of 5 years (and especially under 3 yr), the elderly, pregnant and lactating women, and adolescents are also vulnerable groups for some of the same reasons already discussed but also for the following specific factors more prevalent for their different ages and physiologic conditions.

The elderly. Elderly persons often are unable to care for themselves properly, and with advancing age their energy requirements fall as a consequence of inactivity and of slight reductions in maintenance requirements. Their protein needs, however, do not seem to diminish at the same rate. Therefore the food consumed must be more carefully balanced in terms of protein density and quality. In addition, a more sedentary life, the frequent existence of other nutritional deficiencies, and alterations in behavior frequently lead to anorexia and neglect in eating habits.

Pregnant and lactating women. Pregnant and lactating women require both more energy and more protein than nonpregnant nonlactating women of reproductive age do. At the same time, pregnant women often suffer nausea in the early periods of pregnancy and their gastric capacity is somewhat reduced as pregnancy advances. In primitive cultures pregnant and lactating women remain active and probably do not reduce their energy output as much as those women in developed societies do. Adequate energy and protein intakes appear to be essential during pregnancy and lactation to ensure satisfactory reproductive performance.[8]

Adolescents. In primitive societies adolescents participate in the labor-intensive chores of adults and at the same time undergo rapid growth often complicated by teenage pregnancy. Therefore adolescents' protein and energy needs are high. In developed societies the abundance of diet fads can predispose teenagers to some degree of PEM.

Older children and adults. Older children and adults in developing countries, although nutritionally less likely to be afflicted with PEM, also often suffer moderate, and predominantly mild, energy deficits. These deficiencies can result in lower physical activity both at school or work and outside, with consequences more evident in the spheres of productivity, social and family interactions, and community development activities.

Family and Community Etiologic Factors

Since describing PEM from the family or community standpoint is not the primary purpose of this chapter, the factors conducive to primary PEM at family and community levels will be analyzed only briefly. In general, PEM affects the family as a unit even though different members may present with varying degrees of severity. Often families and communities have no clear concept of the limits of normal for individuals of different ages and sex. This makes it difficult or impossible for them to detect the early stages of PEM. For example, the families may recognize malnutrition earlier in boys than in girls; a nutritionally deteriorated child after an episode of diarrhea may be considered "normal" for that situation. Where poverty and ignorance are prevalent, malnourished mothers with severely malnourished children are a common

sight; however, obese mothers with severely malnourished children also are seen. Mothers of the latter type may relate the beginning of PEM to an infection that was followed by repeated bouts of diarrhea, anorexia, and progressive PEM. In these cases older or younger siblings often appear healthy or only mildly malnourished. An analysis of the situation may disclose that the mother progressively had withdrawn foods from the sick child while the child was being given medicines and multivitamin preparations prescribed by physicians or other health workers, employees at drug stores, traditional healers, or relatives. The point is that, just as the woman appears ignorant of her own and her family's dietary practices, there is also ignorance and a general impression of impotence in trying to bring health back to severely malnourished children once a vicious cycle of PEM and other diseases is established. (See "Pathophysiology" [p. 538] for a discussion of the role of infection as a precipitating cause in severe PEM.)

Families of malnourished children are often disorganized, usually with uneducated parents. Alcoholism and other social diseases are evident among many malnourished families. In general, the presence of a malnourished child clearly indicates a lack of well-being in the family as a whole; the family must be investigated and must become the center of rehabilitative measures. The same general thinking applies to the community in which malnourished families exist. Malnutrition implies social disease and requires prompt attention.

Many schemes have been drawn to explain the factors that, at a macro-level (community-national-regional), are conducive to PEM.[9] All indicate multiple interactions among poverty, population growth, food production and general food policies, food preservation and distribution, health status, education, and migration. Improper planning and execution of cash-crop agroindustrial complexes can have a negative nutritional effect on populations who previously derived subsistence from their own small plots of land.[10] The schemes all seem to indicate that malnutrition is the ultimate result and, at the same time, often a perpetuating factor in very complex and diverse social-political-economic conditions originating far back in the development of cultures and nations or as a result of recently developed pressures. Consequently, abolishing malnutrition requires diverse and often bold actions. Malnutrition in urban Pakistan, northwestern Argentina, tropical Africa, India, and even rural and urban Guatemala is the result of different yet often comparable etiologic factors. Therefore it is essential to understand the details in each region to design effective strategies for controlling and preventing PEM.

EPIDEMIOLOGY

Based on the etiologic considerations just discussed, most of the epidemiologic characteristics of PEM can be described in terms of global magnitude, general trends in populations undergoing rapid urbanization, and effective food distribution.[11]

Global Magnitude

The global magnitude of PEM is difficult to estimate with precision. However, rough estimates of the affected populations in different regions and countries can be obtained by evaluating the proportion of individuals who chronically consume food in amounts that provide less than 1.2 times their basal energy expenditures. This estimate is based on a series of assumptions that make it somewhat imprecise. Two main variables are the precision by which chronic food intake is measured and the value of individual basal energy expenditures used as cutoff points. The variance from these factors can easily add up to 30%. Yet despite these limitations, the figure of 1.2 times basal energy expenditure is useful as a relative standard that, in theory, is the minimum intake necessary to live a very sedentary life.[12] Therefore it reflects the lower limit below which energy deficiency undoubtedly will occur. There are various terms for this level, one of which is physiologic energy need (PEN). Food intake at the population level, however, must be enough to allow the population to fulfill its function properly, in accordance with its life-style and optimum developmental rate. Many persons can fulfill their PENs but still be limited in functional performance by their food intakes. The number of malnourished people can be much higher according to this criterion (the recommended energy allowance or REA) than that computed on the basis of the PENs. Therefore, in spite of inaccuracies, the estimate based on PEN may still be conservative, particularly when it is realized that developing societies often de-

pend on energy-intensive life-styles and thus on relatively high REAs.[13]

Population Trends

With this understanding in mind, the proposed next step links income and poverty to food (energy) intake and projects the estimated population that, on the basis of income or poverty level, cannot acquire enough food to fulfill its physiologic energy needs. The inaccuracy of these projections extends beyond the simple fulfillment or nonfulfillment of PENs. However, it links the estimate of destitute populations, or of marginal populations in "extreme poverty" or "extreme underdevelopment," to the nutritional component. Obviously, populations in these categories not only are undernourished but, in general, are desperate from the standpoints of life fulfillment and of health as defined by the World Health Organization (WHO).

The Food and Agricultural Organization (FAO)[14] and the World Bank have provided estimates of the global magnitude of PEM. These estimates indicate a total number of PEM victims at between 450 million and 1 billion persons. Almost all of these people are in developing countries; 56% are in developing countries classified as "most seriously affected" in terms of the world economic crisis.

The population distribution by regions as of 1972-74, according to the Fourth World Food Survey,[14] is presented to serve as a baseline for comparison with figures pertaining to the next 10 years:

Region	Number below PEN (millions)	Percentage of Population
Far East	297	29
Africa	83	28
Latin America	46	15
Near East	20	16

The prevalence of PEM for the years 1979-81 as compared to 1969-71 is reported in the Fifth World Food Survey.[15] During that decade the estimated number of undernourished individuals increased by 10-20 million, primarily in Africa and the Far East, even though in both regions the proportions of malnourished individuals remained stable or actually declined (4%-6% in the Far East). All nations belonging to the least developed group suffered an increase of PEM both in absolute numbers and as a percentage of the population (accounting for nearly 80 million malnourished persons). Low-income developing countries showed little change in the percentage of their population affected, but the few middle- to high-income developing countries reduced both their PEM rates and the actual numbers of people affected.

Food Distribution

Estimates of food availability, translated into energy and protein supplies, can be summarized for the years 1969-71 from the 1974 UN World Food Congress[16] as follows:

The energy supply (kcal/person/da) and the protein supply (g/person/da) data available from 33 developed countries showed that the lowest energy intake was in Japan: 2510 kcal/person/day (107% of the estimated requirements). The overall mean energy intake, based on country means, was 3136 kcal/person/day (SD 280). The percentage of estimated supplies to fulfill requirements ranged from 99 to 136. In terms of protein, the range was from 74 g/person/day in Albania to 109 g/person/day in New Zealand.

By contrast, data available from 95 developing countries showed a wide range of values in both energy and protein supply. Only 37 (39%) of these countries averaged energy supplies above 100% of estimated requirements. Of these countries, 13% had dietary energy supplies below 2000 kcal/person/day, which is lower than 86% of estimated requirements (range, 72%-85%). In terms of protein, the range is from 33 to 106 g/person/day; however, only 9 of 93 developing countries with available data had 74 g of protein supply/person/day, the lowest level found among the developed countries.

Global projections of future food supply indicate that the current differences between countries with different degrees of development will increase. Projected food demands showed increases of 26% for developed countries and 70% for developing countries between 1970 and 1985. Given these conditions, even at a calculated high rate of increase in food availability, the global per capita supply would be stationary at best. The situation becomes more serious for developing than for developed societies because the former have a near threefold increase in demand rate and the distribution of food and resources is known to be unequal between more affluent groups and those with scarce-assets.

As indicated previously, in the face of food scarcity, young children (infants and preschoolers), the elderly, pregnant and lactating women, and adolescents are more vulnerable to PEM.

PEM INDICATORS IN CHILDREN

Growth retardation, weight and height in relation to age, type of infant feeding, and mortality rates are a few indices of the relative magnitude and severity of PEM.[17]

Growth Retardation

A manifestation of PEM in children is growth retardation. If PEM occurs for a prolonged time in relation to the child's age and occurs early in life, when linear growth rate is higher, stunting is one result. The recovery or catch-up in linear growth is a slow process and can occur only in situations that ensure optimum conditions in terms of health, nutrition, and general stimulation. However, acute severe PEM at any age causes weight loss, and mild to moderate PEM at least reduces weight gain. Under adequate conditions catch-up in weight can be dramatic and complete. PEM, therefore, affects both components of growth—linear and body mass increments—but these components are affected differently and in such a way that the attained stature at a given age determines the maximum body mass (weight) a child can achieve. Weight, then, generally should be interpreted in terms of height (as weight-for-height).

Weight and Height

When only a child's weight is available and it is below normal, it can mean, in terms of PEM, that the child either *is* or *was* malnourished. If the height is also below normal, the process has been chronic, but one still cannot determine whether the process exists in the present or existed in the past. If weight and height are compared and weight is found to be adequate for height, this being subnormal, the child previously has been stunted by PEM but currently has adequate body mass for height. If the body weight is below normal for the child's subnormal height, the child *is* and *has been* malnourished.

Most estimates of PEM prevalence are based only on weight determinations. On this basis, children with weight deficits greater than 40% for their age and/or with edema are considered to be suffering from severe PEM. Those with deficits between 10% and 40% may be moderately malnourished, but the risk exists of calling them malnourished when they are only stunted from previous PEM and now have adequate weight for height. With these limitations on the estimates, roughly 75% of preschool children in developing countries show some degree of PEM. In any case, they have been malnourished, which emphasizes the poor overall community situation. Roughly 3% of the children in Asia, Africa, and Latin America present with severe PEM (range, 0.05% to 20% according to 25 different surveys from 1963 to 1973) and 20% present with moderate forms (range, 3.5% to 46.4% according to the same surveys).[2]

Another survey based on anthropometric measurements obtained from 33 developing countries[18] showed that up to 78% of children below 5 years of age were stunted because of chronic PEM (peaking in the fourth year of life, with a median of 39% of children affected). Similarly, up to 26.9% of children were found to have low weight for height (wasting), also because of PEM (peaking in the second year of life, with a median of 9.6% of children affected). Wasting was more prevalent in East Asia and Africa, indicating the greater severity of PEM in those countries, since generally wasting increases almost exponentially whereas stunting increases but linearly. The major demand presented by these findings is for prompt intervention to restore the lost body weight.

Infant Feeding and Age

In populations at risk, PEM is generally seen at a later age among children who have been breast-fed than among those who have been bottle-fed. In these PEM cases energy deficiency is predominant and is aggravated by frequent bouts of infectious diarrhea. Severe marasmus is the predominant form of PEM in early infancy and kwashiorkor occurs later in the weaning period or in preschoolers.[19]

Mortality Rates

Mortality patterns also reflect malnutrition in childhood. Four characteristics are particularly useful: the total mortality in children under 5 years of age; the ratio of infant mortality to that of 1-to-4-year-old children and, within the infant group, the ratio of neonatal to postneonatal mortality; the mortality rate associated with low birth weight and "immaturity"; and the mortality rate due to diarrheal disease. Inter-American research on mortality in childhood has illustrated the usefulness of two of these characteristics[20]: mortality in children less than 5 years of age and the ratio of mortality in infants versus that in 1-4 year old children.

Mortality in children less than 5 years of age. Total mortality in children under 5 years of age was 48 and 50/1000 in rural Bolivia and rural El Salvador, respectively; in Sherbrooke, Quebec, Canada, and suburban California it was only 4.1/1000. Santiago, Chile, and San Juan, Argentina, each had a total mortality of 13/1000.

Infant/1-4 year old child mortality ratio. The ratio of infant mortality to that of the 1-to-4-year-old children was lowest in the rural areas of El Salvador and Bolivia (4.6 and 5.7/1000, respectively) and highest in the cities of San Juan and Santiago (33.8 and 30.5/1000). Sherbrooke and suburban California each showed a ratio close to 23/1000. These data suggest that late chronic PEM exists predominantly in areas with low infant/child mortality ratios, which areas also have high mortality rates in both age groups. In San Juan and Santiago, infant mortality was almost three times higher than in Sherbrooke and suburban California; the 1-4 year old group mortality rate was nearly twice as high in San Juan and Santiago as in Sherbrooke and suburban California, showing that early urban malnutrition is a predominant problem in Santiago and San Juan.

Neonatal/postneonatal mortality ratios further clarify this problem: in Sherbrooke and suburban California the neonatal mortality was nearly three times higher than the postneonatal mortality. In Santiago and San Juan this ratio was near 1 and in rural El Salvador and rural Bolivia it was 0.7 and 0.4.

The statistics illustrate a well-known fact: as child health and medical care improve, mortality in children under 5 years is concentrated in the neonatal group. The statistics also show that poor child health and nutrition shift the highest mortality rate to the postneonatal period because the less favorable circumstances extend the elevated death rate beyond the first year of life. Conversely, mortality in the 1-4 year old group is the first to be reduced as nutrition and other preventive health measures directed to the child improve.

PATHOPHYSIOLOGY

Four basic concepts define the pathophysiology of PEM[1,21-25]:

1. PEM is a dynamic condition to which the subject adapts and survives.
2. Severe deficiencies or the superimposition of stressful situations can cause decompensation, which is translated into severe disease.
3. PEM induces harmonic changes in (a) intracellular energy and amino acid metabolism, (b) intracellular electrolyte concentrations, (c) changes in enzyme activities (organ-specific as well as general), (d) hormone levels and end-organ action, and (e) body composition with all its functional consequences.
4. Adaptation to deficiencies in protein and/or energy imply functional repercussions and alter host-environment interactions.

Energy Equilibrium

In the compensated reduced–energy intake state energy equilibrium is achieved by reducing expenditure. Depending on the severity of the deficit, diverse mechanisms come into play: mild deficits can result in only a diminution of physical activity and/or a slightly increased energy reserve (adipose tissue) mobilization; as deficits become more severe, the impact on these mechanisms increases, protein synthesis declines, and utilization of body protein (primarily muscle) for energy begins. This process, together with utilization of visceral protein, is greatly accentuated in severe energy deficits (starvation). In these cases a prompt initial reduction in basal metabolic rate is followed by a progressive reduction that parallels the diminution in body protein (lean body and active tissue masses).

Energy Reserve Mobilization

Mobilization of energy reserves is accomplished by neurohormonal mechanisms, including decreased insulin activity due to diminished stimulation from food intake, increased epinephrine and norepinephrine production, decreased intracellular potassium, and elevated free fatty acid levels as a result of increased growth hormone, glucagon, glucocorticoid, and catecholamine levels. These hormonal changes also favor the mobilization of amino acids from muscle and their visceral utilization for gluconeogenesis; moreover, amino acid nitrogen is spared

by more efficient recycling, by the promotion of specific transamination reactions, and by a reduction in urea cycle enzyme activities. As the need for oxygen declines, the hypothalamic-pituitary-thyroidal axis diminishes thyroxine and triiodothyronine levels: peripheral T_4 metabolism decreases and reverse T_3 increases. In elderly persons thermoregulation is impaired by undernutrition.[26] This general adaptation mechanism can be upset by infection, which induces hormonal alterations that lead to diminished utilization of fat and increased dependence on carbohydrate metabolism and amino acid catabolism for energy purposes.[27]

Theories as to the mechanism by which infection and nutritional status interact[28,29] have centered on the production and metabolic effects of cytokinins and prostaglandins, with special reference to interleukin 1. This acute-phase protein is diminished in PEM, and this may block the normal reaction to infection in these patients. Impaired thymic hormone production has also been reported.[30] Carbohydrate intake produces increased insulin activity and a consequent decrease in the hormonal mechanisms that lead to lipolysis and amino acid transport from muscle to viscera. Insulin promotes lipogenesis and amino acid deposition in muscle, thus upsetting the internal adaptive shift of protein synthesis from muscle to viscera. This, in turn, causes acute amino acid depletion at the visceral level and decompensation (manifested by decreased synthesis of albumin, apolipoprotein, and other transport proteins and by a reversal of the enzymatic systems that increased the efficiency of amino acid utilization at the visceral level).

Protein metabolism in malnourished and infected children has been studied in depth.[31]

Kwashiorkor and Marasmus

Characteristics. The differences between kwashiorkor (decompensated PEM) and marasmus are primarily the presence of edema and of fatty liver. Edema results from sodium retention and excessive extracellular fluid accumulation with absolute intracellular fluid deficit (paralleling the reduction in body cell mass) but elevated cell water per gram of cell solids; intravascular spaces are preserved or even decreased (hypovolemia). Relative increases in extracellular fluid volume in the absence of clinical edema occur in marasmus and in moderate PEM. The roles of hypoalbuminemia, increased aldosterone and renin activities, altered renal and cardiac functions, and defects in the cell sodium pump as explanations for increased sodium retention are still debatable.*

Potassium and magnesium deficits and mild levels of acidosis also are present in both kwashiorkor and marasmus and have two origins[33,34]: (1) a decreased intracellular capacity to retain potassium associated with protein deficiencies and an accumulation of free acids (metabolites, amino acids) and (2) excessive losses of potassium, magnesium, bicarbonate, and other electrolytes as consequences of diarrhea and altered renal functions.

Fatty liver results primarily from a decrease in beta-lipoprotein synthesis and, thus, decreased fat mobilization from the liver. It has also been proposed that liver fat synthesis increases.

The decline of albumin and other protein synthesis is associated with an overall reduction in the catabolism of proteins. Thus, total protein turnover is markedly depressed in malnutrition. During recovery, protein synthesis increases while protein catabolism lags behind, increasing later as protein repletion proceeds. In fact, with accelerated rates of growth, parallel increases in protein turnover occur, which also depend more on the levels of protein intake than on the levels of energy intake.[35]

Causes. Many of the clinical manifestations and fatal consequences of severe decompensated malnutrition result from infection and/or forced carbohydrate feeding without adequate protein intake. However, many functional manifestations of malnutrition, whether mild, moderate, or severe, result either from alterations of functional capacity (conditioned, in part, by the changes in body and organ composition already referred to) or from the progressive adaptation of enzyme systems and organ function to a persistently reduced stimulus (e.g., chronic meager food intake or, specifically, extremely reduced fat intake; lack of physical activity; reduced tissue O_2 needs because of progressive loss of active tissue mass) upon which a chronic force of infection is superimposed. Thus hemoglobin pro-

duction and red cell production are reduced to assure the necessary levels of O_2 transport as demanded by the lower oxygen requirements of the diminished active tissue mass in malnourished children. Yet, both red cell production and hemoglobin production respond to hypoxia even in the presence of severe PEM; pancreatic lipase production is reduced but can be stimulated to high levels by administering fat; antibody production may be substantial in the presence of infection despite severe PEM; the pituitary/thyroid system may be less active but responds well to hypothalamic thyrotropin-releasing factor; cardiac function is reduced but may respond to moderately increased circulatory demands, although the low cardiac reserve and a reduced oncotic pressure easily result in "wet lungs" and dependent edema. In other words, with the proper stimulation many functions "adaptatively" depressed in PEM can respond to additional demands, even in the presence of severe protein and energy deficiencies, albeit with certain limitations.[1,36]

An important alteration in severe PEM is the inadequate response to bacterial infection,[24,37] an alteration particularly critical in the gastrointestinal and respiratory tracts, which have their own ecologies as open systems. Bacterial overgrowth takes place in both systems, increasing the incidences of diarrhea and of both upper and lower respiratory infections. In the intestine the mucosal cells are shorter and have slower turnover rates (as is the case for all mucosal and rapid-turnover cell systems), the production of local antibodies is reduced, bacterial overgrowth raises the free (unconjugated) bile acid levels in the upper intestine, and the micellarization capacity for fat is reduced. This last process is essential for long-chain fatty acid absorption. In addition, because free bile acids are toxic to the gut cells, severe PEM reduces the rates at which facilitated and active transport mechanisms absorb carbohydrates.[38] The gastric and enteric barriers to bacterial penetration are faulty and thus the gastrointestinal tract becomes an important source of bacteremia, urinary tract infections, and septicemia, with fatal consequences. In the respiratory system "wet lungs" clearly promote bacterial overgrowth. Cell-mediated immunity in general is impaired. Leukocyte migration, phagocytic capacities, and T-cell production and function are reduced, leading to defective tissue

---

* An interesting unifying theory for the development of edema[32] considers an increased rate of production of free radicals and a diminished capacity to reduce membrane peroxidative damage.

defense mechanisms, including delayed hypersensitivity reactions.[39]

HISTOPATHOLOGY

Acute infections (respiratory, gastrointestinal, urinary, septicemic) and superimposed specific nutrient deficiencies often are evident macroscopically and upon histopathologic examination.

General pathology reveals tissue atrophy without any specificity except for fatty infiltration of the liver, edema, and skin changes evident in severe protein deficiency.[40] More atrophy occurs in tissues with greater turnover (intestinal mucosa, red bone marrow, pancreatic acini, testicular epithelium). Periportal fat appears first and advances centripetally as severity increases. The skin changes consist of dermal atrophy, ecchymoses, ulcerations, and hyperkeratotic desquamation, seen primarily in areas subjected to irritation and not necessarily restricted to exposed areas, as in the case of pellagra. Intestinal villi are flattened, and the enterocytes lose their columnar appearance. Gastric, colonic, and rectal mucosal atrophy is evident. Special staining techniques and electron microscopy reveal many other minute alterations, not all of which result specifically from primary protein-energy malnutrition but do reflect generalized atrophy and the effects of infection as they affect specific cell types.

With nutritional recovery, these states revert to normal, although some residual lesions may persist (e.g., at the diaphyseal-epiphyseal junctions). There is some disagreement about the completeness of pancreatic and intestinal recoveries.

CLINICAL SYNDROMES
Mild PEM

As mentioned under "Etiology," mild PEM cannot be diagnosed clinically with certainty. In children apathy, some retardation in growth, and decreased physical activity plus a history of inadequate food intake and frequent infections can lead to a tentative diagnosis of mild PEM. The whole socioeconomic structure of the community and the family, as well as the presence of other specific nutritional deficiencies such as vitamin A and iron, may also suggest the diagnosis. In older children and adults PEM is often difficult to diagnose.[28]

Moderate PEM

Moderate PEM accentuates the symptoms of mild PEM: greater deficiencies in height and weight with certain losses in lean body mass, flaccidity, apathy, repeated infections, and signs of other associated deficiencies. In women inadequate weight gain during pregnancy, the delivery of small-for-date babies, and poor lactation performance all suggest the diagnosis of moderate PEM.

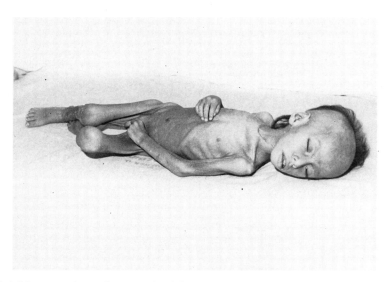

Figure 34-1 Marasmus in a 16-month-old child. Note the lack of skin changes and edema. The principal feature is emaciation.

Severe PEM

Severe PEM[41] is the end result of a continuum that, when compensated by the efficient operation of adaptive mechanisms, is primarily manifested as tissue wasting that produces the clinical picture of marasmus in a small child and emaciation in older children and adults (e.g., as seen in World War II concentration camp victims). The marasmic child is very lean, hypotonic, hungry and "monkey-faced" with a disproportionately big abdomen and head and very thin limbs, very evident rib cage, and sunken cheeks and eyes. Severely marasmic children may suck their thumbs and other fingers or may be too apathetic even to do that; they may be interested in their environment and cry actively, or may be depressed to the point of coma. Normally, severely marasmic children are constipated or may pass small mucous stools, but these children also can suffer diarrhea and dehydration. Generalized infection and septic death are not uncommon. Hair is thin, dry, and fragile, like that of a doll, and falls out easily (Fig. 34-1).

The uncompensated state (kwashiorkor)[42] results from acute severe protein deficiency. This deficiency can exist alone (in cassava-eating populations or where children are force-fed starch or other carbohydrate-rich, protein-deficient foods) or as a consequence of infection. Kwashiorkor is characterized by edema, soft hepato-

megaly (the fatty liver possibly extending down to the iliac crest), extreme apathy and irritability, and hair discoloration (reddish blond) with bands of dark and light hair reflecting the past nutritional history (flag sign), mucosal and cutaneous lesions that range from thinness, dryness, scaliness, and depigmentation through hyperkeratotic large-scale skin desquamation of pigmented mosaic-like lesions to deep ulcerations. Petechiae and ecchymoses are not infrequent with infection (Figs. 34-2 and 34-3). In both kwashiorkor and severe marasmus, patients can present with acute corneal ulceration as a result of infection superimposed on severe vitamin A deficiency. These signs may result from (1) malnutrition per se or (2) sequestration of vitamin A in the liver, as occurs also with fat, because of the marked deficiency of transport apoproteins (retinol-binding protein and beta-lipoproteins).

Laboratory Findings

Hematologic, clinical, and nutritional chemistry findings can be summarized as follows[40-42]:

1. In the erythron, low hemoglobin concentration and low hematocrit are the rule, although the values may be within normal ranges. A diagnosis of anemia from protein deficiency usually is false since hematopoietic-factor deficiencies responsible for anemia interact with hemodilution as a result of the PEM. Iron and folate deficiencies, singly or together, are not

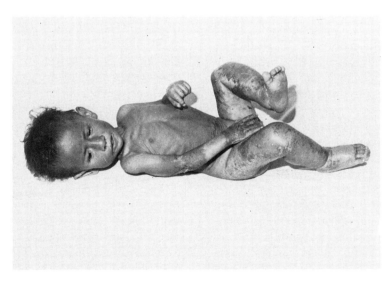

Figure 34-2 Kwashiorkor/marasmus in an 18-month-old child. Note the skin lesions, edema, and loss of fat around the rib cage.

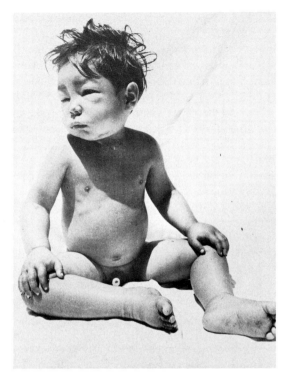

Figure 34-3 Acute kwashiorkor ("sugar-baby" type) in a 32-month-old child. Note the mild skin changes, generalized edema, and preservation of subcutaneous fat.

uncommon, particularly when these substances are not provided in adequate amounts during nutritional recovery, which is accompanied by rapid expansion of the erythron.[1]

2. White cell and platelet changes compatible with folate deficiency are not uncommon and lymphopenia (especially of T-cells) is the rule in severe PEM accompanied by thymic atrophy. In children with severe PEM the leukocytic response to infection may be curtailed, but changes from septicemia and intravascular coagulation are noted as clearly as in well-nourished children with massive infections.

3. When protein intake is low and no renal impairment is present, the blood urea level is low. When PEM is decompensated, levels of serum albumin and transport proteins (transferrin, apolipoproteins, retinol-binding protein, transcortin) are low. In contrast, gammaglobulins may be elevated, particularly if infections are or have been present. Plasma amino acids are low, the branched-chain amino acids and tryosine being more affected. Some nonessential amino acids may be present in higher concentrations. Serum enzymes (cholinesterase, alkaline phosphatase, amylase, lipase) are diminished.

4. When protein intake is low and muscle mass reduced, urinary excretion of urea and creatinine, respectively, is low. Timed creatinine excretion relative to that of a normal child of the same height can help estimate the degree of muscle mass deficit; this estimate gives results similar to those determined by total-body potassium. Urinary hydroxyproline and 3-methylhistidine are also reduced, indicating low protein turnover (collagen and muscle, respectively); unfortunately, infection can alter these nutritional indicators.

5. Serum levels of the fat-soluble vitamins A and E as well as prothrombin time (responsive to vitamin K administration) are compatible with deficiencies of these nutrients. However, often they improve as protein nutrition improves and, because of transport proteins synthesis, they are mobilized from accumulated fat in the liver. Biochemical indicators of water-soluble vitamin and mineral (trace element) deficiencies frequently are reported in different parts of the world, where such deficiencies tend to be more prevalent even among otherwise well-nourished populations.

PEM CLASSIFICATIONS

For different reasons several classifications of malnourished children have been proposed. A Mexican group[43] suggested classifying them on the basis of body weight for age, by which *children with a clinical diagnosis of malnutrition* would be ranked on the basis of their risk of death.[42] Malnourished children were clasified as grades 1, 2, or 3 if their weight-for-age deficits were 10%-25%, 25%-40%, or greater than 40%. Children with edema also were classified as grade 3.

This system has been used clinically and in survey work to identify nutritional deficiencies at the family and community levels. It has been misused, however, when, on the basis of body weight for age alone, *children with no evidence of clinical malnutrition* were classified as presently malnourished (see "Etiology").

As discussed, weight and height for age must

Table 34-1 Protein-Energy Malnutrition

Condition	Body Weight (% of Standard)*	Edema	Deficit in Weight for Height
Underweight	80-60	0	Minimal
Nutritional dwarfing	<60	0	Minimal
Marasmus	<60	0	Severe
Kwashiorkor	80-60	+	Severe
Marasmic kwashiorkor	<60	+	Severe

From a report to the Wellcome Trust, 1968. FAO/WHO Expert Committee on Nutrition: Eighth report, WHO Tech Rep Ser 477, 1971.

*Standard taken as the 50th percentile of the Harvard values.[45]

+ Weight for height = (weight of patient)/(weight of normal subject of same height) × 100.

be known so the history of malnutrition and its type (marasmus, kwashiorkor, and marasmic kwashiorkor) can be precisely determined as well as the completeness of recovery monitored. The Joint FAO/WHO Expert Committee on Nutrition[44] proposed the classification shown in Table 34-1.

These classifications are useful, but they obscure the fact that PEM is a continuum on which a progressive energy deficit results primarily in loss of fat and (only when late and very severe) in a substantial loss of protein whereas protein deficiency results primarily in loss of muscle protein in the presence or absence of body fat deficit.

To simplify, the following generalizations can be made: the greater the weight-for-age deficit in a malnourished population of children, the higher is the risk of death; the greater the deficit in height, the more chronic and earlier-appearing is the problem of malnutrition; and the larger weight-for-height deficit, the more severe present malnutrition is. Height and weight must be considered before attempting to evaluate the immediate correction of present malnutrition (by weight-for-height changes) and the long-term correction of chronic malnutrition (by height-for-age and weight-for-age changes).

PROGNOSTIC FACTORS

Infection, dehydration and electrolyte imbalances, hypothermia, obnubilation, extreme emaciation and flaccidity, jaundice, petechiae, and eye lesions from vitamin A deficiency are poor clinical prognostic signs. Septicemia, anuria, heart failure, hypovolemic shock, and markedly impaired liver function are actually emergency situations demanding heroic measures. Bio-

chemically albumin levels below 1 g/dl and elevation of serum ferritin levels, coupled with diminished red-cell glutathion reductase activity, indicate an extremely poor prognosis.

TREATMENT

The treatment of a severely malnourished child is divided into three phases: emergency, initiation of cure, and nutritional consolidation.[46-48]

Emergency Phase

The emergency phase deals with complications that normally hospitalize a child with PEM: infection, water and electrolyte disturbances, hypoglycemia and hypothermia, cardiac, renal, and respiratory failures, and other associated nutritional deficiencies.

Infection. Suspected infection and septicemia in any severely malnourished child can lead to septic death. Careful clinical examination and auxiliary laboratory analyses, and their interpretation, must be accompanied by the awareness that normal responses to infection, such as leukocytosis and fever, often are depressed. The presence of petechiae, hypothermia and hypoglycemia, diarrhea, shock, or general hypotonia usually indicate severe infection. At the slightest suspicion of infection, start aggressive treatment; investigate the identity of the infective organism, but do not delay treatment with broad-spectrum antibiotics while waiting to institute more specific therapy. Treat septicemia and intravascular coagulation syndromes aggressively, regardless of the nutritional condition of the patient.

Water/electrolyte disturbances. Water and electrolyte disturbances have two origins: (1) the nutritional status per se and (2) the associated alterations as a result of infection and diarrhea. The first of these alterations, intracellular potassium deficits and whole-body sodium excess associated with hyposmolality, are corrected during nutritional recovery. Then the superimposed dehydration accompanied by aggravation of the potassium deficit (which would reduce total-body K^+ to below 30-35 mEq/kg and could be reflected in hypokalemia) and the magnesium deficiency are treated with oral rehydration plus, if necessary, intravenous fluids. Various solutions have been proposed and shown to be successful in treating this complication. Generally the primary aim of rehydration is to maintain renal function. No more than 5 (and no less than 3) mEq of Na^+/kg/day, together with 4% to 5% dextrose and approximately 1 mEq of magnesium/kg/day, can be safely administered by mouth or intravenously to provide between 120 and 140 ml of water/kg/day. If renal function is adequate, 4-8 mEq of potassium can be administered without surpassing 40 mEq KCl/liter of solution. If impending shock and anuria are detected, rapidly administer 30-40 ml/kg of Hartman's solution or (in its absence) saline solution, giving 20 ml/kg in the first half hour. If hypoalbuminemia is extremely severe (less than 1 g/dl), plasma can be added in repeated 20 ml doses.

Cardiac, renal, and respiratory failures. If a child is severely anemic (hemoglobin concentration <5 g/dl) and/or shows signs of impending cardiorespiratory decompensation, administer small transfusions of packed red cells or whole blood, taking care not to bring the hemoglobin concentration above 8-10 g/dl.

In the process of oral rehydration, essentially the same fluids can be fed as were administered by vein, but potassium content can be raised to provide up to 8-10 mEq/kg/day. Do not raise sodium intake (or sodium administered parenterally) above 5 mEq/kg/day, since a child's body contains a large amount of sodium and greater concentrations of this cation may be fatal.

Careful rehydration and evaluation of other causes of cardiac failure can prevent this complication. Administer diuretics only if necessary and only after careful evaluation. Rapid digitalization can proceed (always with extreme care) if hypokalemia is not present.

Liver failure in connection with malnourishment is extremely rare but, when it exists, a careful progression in protein intake should be used, together with all other measures routinely used in liver failure in nonmalnourished populations.

Other nutritional deficiencies. Keep in mind other acute specific nutritional deficiencies, particularly severe vitamin A deficiency, which can develop rapidly into keratomalacia. For this reason it is advisable to administer routinely 50,000 units of a water-dispersable preparation of vitamin A to a malnourished patient upon admission. Hypocalcemia, hypomagnesemia, and zinc, copper, and chromium deficiencies have been described; keep these deficiencies in mind if muscle twitching, tetany, convulsions, hyperglycemia and glycosuria, cutaneous ulcers, or leukopenia are present. Diet therapy should include all the aforementioned trace minerals and vitamins and essential fatty acids in amounts sufficient to achieve the four- to fivefold rate of normal tissue growth induced by adequate nutritional repletion; otherwise, secondary vitamin and mineral deficiencies are easily precipitated (Ca^{+2}, vitamin D, folate, Fe^{+2}, Mg^{+2}, Cu^{+2}).

Initiation of Cure

Start diet therapy as soon as possible, keeping in mind the following three general principles:

1. The malnourished child has reached this stage through prolonged adaptation. Therefore, metabolic systems cannot handle sudden energy and protein loads.
2. Anorexia is a very common sign of uncompensated and complicated malnutrition. Patience in feeding these children, together with corrections of complications, will result in progressively larger intakes and smooth recovery.
3. Severely malnourished children with diarrhea of infectious origin can present with decreased lactose tolerance. Therefore, carefully evaluate milk tolerance initially. Also, avoid osmolar loads in these children. Use calcium caseinate (half-milk/half-casein), low-lactose milk, and/or other animal or vegetable protein mixtures of high protein quality to start diet therapy. Actual intolerance to physiologic milk intake and to progressively administered whole or fat-rich milk preparations is rare and its prevalence has been exaggerated; however, genetically determined lactose intolerance may be important in certain populations.

Simple schemes for progressively increasing protein and energy intakes are effective in treating severely malnourished children. A common program starts with 1 g of protein/kg/day, 50-75 kcal/kg/day, 20%-30% of which is provided by fat (preferably rich in polyunsaturated fatty acids), with supplementary vitamins and minerals. Depending on the child's tolerance and appetite, greater concentrations of nutrients can be administered at 2- to 4-day intervals, as follows:

Protein (g/kg)	Energy (kcal/kg)
2	100-150
3	150-200
4	200-300

Nutritional Consolidation

The consolidation of cure in terms of nutrition can start as soon as edema disappears and the child begins to gain weight rapidly. One should rapidly and progressively introduce other foods, taking into account local eating habits, to lead to a varied and healthy diet.

Throughout recovery, the child must be stimulated both mentally and physically to promote physical activity and emotional well-being.

Ideally, severely malnourished children without complications should be treated at home, and both food assistance and nutritional/health education should be provided for the family. The child with complications that merit hospitalization should be kept in the hospital only as long as necessary, and efforts should be made to ensure his/her complete nutritional rehabilitation as well as that of the family. Longer hospitalization increases the chance of further infection and is unhealthy from the standpoint of physical, mental, and emotional recovery and development. Since many of these children suffer from poor general care, health personnel can take advantage of this contact to promote immunizations and other necessary health and hygienic measures in addition to caring for the immediate problem; however, nutritional recovery must precede immunizations in children with severe PEM.

Children with PEM often have intestinal parasites. Unless there are clinical reasons to suspect massive loads or clinical signs of protozoal disease (amebiasis, giardiasis), delay treatment until the child is well into nutritional recovery. However, if there are clinical signs of malaria it should be treated immediately.

SEQUELAE

It has been suggested[49] that children who have suffered from severe or moderate PEM are not normal even when they have recovered fully. These children have been deprived not only of nutrition but also of opportunities for development, and they may have missed the critical period for acquisition of different concepts, abilities, and reactions that lead to a harmonic maturation, both physically and mentally. Physically these children usually show retarded development, primarily in height, bone age, and sexual maturation.[50,51] Weight for height can be restored easily, but this still leaves a child who is dwarfed and underweight for age. Malnourished children may grow and tend to mature at their biologic age rather than at their chronologic age; in other words, if a 5-year-old child has the stature and bone maturation of a 3-year-old child, his rate of growth and maturation will be more like that of a 3-year-old. Mentally, severely malnourished children appear to have residual problems in terms of creativity and social interaction; however, the roles of malnutrition and poor environment are not easily dissociated. Adolescent children who were previously malnourished often exhibit altered neural function.[52]

Persistent altered insulin secretion, increased glucose intolerance, and chronic pancreatic insufficiency have been suggested as long-term sequelae of severe PEM, but the validity of many of these observations has been questioned.

REFERENCES

1. Viteri FE: Primary protein-energy malnutrition: clinical, biochemical, and metabolic changes. In Suskind RM, editor: Textbook of pediatric nutrition, New York, 1981, Raven Press, pp 189-215.
2. DeMaeyer EM: Protein-energy malnutrition. .In Beaton GH, Bengoa JM, editors: Nutrition in preventive medicine, Geneva, 1976, World Health Organization, pp 23-54.
3. Scrimshaw NS, Behar M: Protein malnutrition in young children, Science **133**:2039-2047, 1961.
4. Raman L: Influence of maternal nutritional factors affecting birthweight, Am J Clin Nutr **34**:775-783, 1981.
5. Mata LJ: Malnutrition-infection interactions in the tropics, Am J Trop Med Hyg **24**:564-574, 1975.
6. Aebi H, Whitehead R, editors: Maternal nutrition during pregnancy and lactation, Nestle Foundation publications series, Bern, 1980, Hans Huber Publishers.
7. Waterlow JC: Fatty liver disease in infants in the British West Indies, Medical Research Council Special Report Series 263, London, 1948, Her Majesty's Stationery Office.
8. Committee on Dietary Allowances, Food and Nutrition Board, National Research Council: Recommended dietary allowances, ed 9, Washington DC, 1980, National Academy of Sciences, p 185.

9. Joy JL, Payne PR: Nutrition and national development planning, Food Nutr (FAO) **1**:2-10, 1975.

10. Victora CG, et al: Child malnutrition and land ownership in Southern Brazil, Ecol Food Nutr **18**:265-275, 1986.

11. Scrimshaw NS, Behar M: Worldwide occurrence of protein malnutrition, Fed Proc **18**:82-88, 1959.

12. Reutlinger S, Selowsky M: Malnutrition and poverty—magnitude and policy options, (World Bank occasional paper 23), Baltimore, 1976, Johns Hopkins University.

13. United National University/World Hunger Program: The uses of energy and protein requirement estimates: Report of a workshop, Food Nutr Bull **3**:45-53, 1981.

14. Food and Agriculture Organization of the United Nations: Fourth World Food Survey, Food Nutr (FAO) **10**:128, 1977.

15. Food and Agricultural Organization of the United Nations: Fifth World Food Survey, Rome, 1985, FAO.

16. United Nations World Conference: Assessment of the world food situation, present and future, Rome, Nov 5-16, 1974.

17. Waterlow JC: Classification and definition of protein-energy malnutrition, WHO Monog Ser **62**:530-555, 1976.

18. Keller W, Fillmore CM: Prevalence of protein-energy malnutrition, World Health Stat Q **36**:129-167, 1983.

19. McCance RA, Widdowson EM, editors: Calorie deficiencies and protein deficiencies, London, 1968, J & A Churchill Ltd, p 386.

20. Puffer RRR, Serrano CV: Patterns of mortality on childhood, Washington DC, 1973, American Health Organization, p 470.

21. Alleyne GAO, et al: Protein-energy malnutrition, London, 1977, Edward Arnold Publishers Ltd, p 244.

22. Waterlow JC, Alleyne GAO: Protein malnutrition in children: advances in knowledge in the last ten years, Adv Protein Chem **25**:117-241, 1971.

23. Gardner LI, Amacher P, editors: Endocrine aspects of malnutrition, Santa Ynez, Calif, 1973, Kroc Foundation, p 520.

24. Young VR, et al: Mechanisms of adaptation to protein malnutrition. In Blaxter K, Waterlow JC, editors: Nutritional adaptation in man, London, 1985, John Libbey & Co Ltd, pp 189-217.

25. Waterlow JC: Metabolic adaptation to low intakes of energy and protein, Annu Rev Nutr **6**:495-526, 1986.

26. Fellows IW, et al: The effect of undernutrition on thermoregulation in the elderly, Clin Sci **69**:525-532, 1985.

27. Neufeld HA, et al: The effect of bacterial infections on ketone concentrations in rat liver and blood and on free fatty acid concentrations in rat blood, Metabolism **25**:877-884, 1976.

28. Clowes GHA, et al: Muscle proteolysis induced by a circulating peptide in septic and traumatized patients, N Engl J Med **308**:545-552, 1983.

29. Baracos V, et al: Stimulation of muscle protein degradation and prostaglandin E2 released by leukocyte pyrogen (interleukin-1): a mechanism for the increased degradation of muscle proteins during fever, N Engl J Med **308**:553-558, 1983.

30. Martinez-Cairo Cueto S, et al: Activity of serum thymic factor in undernourished newborn infants, Arch Invest Med (Mex) **16**:199-207, 1985.

31. Tomkins AM, et al: The combined effects of infection and malnutrition on protein metabolism in children, Clin Sci **65**:313-324, 1983.

32. Golden MHN: The consequences of protein deficiency in man and its relationship to the features of kwashiorkor. In Blaxter K, Waterlow JC, editors: Nutritional adaptation in man, London, 1985, John Libbey & Co Ltd, pp 169-188.

33. Nichols BL, et al: Clinical significance of muscle potassium depletion in protein-calorie malnutrition, J Pediatr **80**:319-330, 1972.

34. Montgomery RD: Magnesium metabolism in infantile protein malnutrition, Lancet **2**:74-75, 1960.

35. Waterlow JC, et al: Protein turnover in mammalian tissues and in the whole body, Oxford, 1978, North Holland Publishing Co, p 804.

36. Viteri FE, et al: El problema de la desnutrición proteínico-calorica en el istmo centroamericano, Rev Col Med (Guatemala) **21**:137-245, 1970.

37. Suskind RM, editor: Malnutrition and the immune response, New York, 1977, Raven Press, p 468.

38. Viteri FE, Schneider RE: Gastrointestinal alterations in protein-calorie malnutrition, Med Clin North Am **58**:1487-1505, 1974.

39. Chandra RK: Immunology of nutritional disorders, London, 1980, Edward Arnold (Publishers) Ltd, p 110.

40. Viteri FE, Torún B: Protein-calorie malnutrition. In Goodhart RS, Shils ME, editors: Modern nutrition in health and disease, ed 6, Philadelphia, 1980, Lea & Febiger, pp 697-720.

41. Viteri FE, et al: Clinical aspects of protein malnutrition. In Munro HN, Allison JB, editors: Mammalian protein metabolism, vol 2, New York, 1964, Academic Press Inc, pp 523-568.

42. Trowell HC, et al: Kwashiorkor, London, 1954, Edward Arnold & Co, p 308.

43. Gomez F, et al: Mortality in second and third degree malnutrition, J Trop Pediatr **2**:77-83, 1956.

44. FAO/WHO Expert Committee on Nutrition: Eighth report, WHO Tech Rep Ser 477, 1971.

45. Nelson WE: Textbook of pediatrics, ed 8, Philadelphia, 1964, WB Saunders Co, pp 48-53.

46. Torún B, Viteri FE: Tratamiento de niños hospitalizados con desnutrición proteínico-energética severa, Rev Col Med (Guatemala) **27**:42-62, 1976.

47. Picou DM: Evaluation and treatment of the malnourished child. In Suskind RM, editor: Textbook of pediatric nutrition, New York, 1981, Raven Press, pp 217-228.

48. Wharton BA: Difficulties in the initial treatment of kwashiorkor. In McCance RA, Widdowson EM, editors: Calorie deficiencies and protein deficiencies, London, 1968, J & A Churchill Ltd, pp 147-158.

49. Bengoa JM: Significance of malnutrition and priorities for its prevention. In Berg A, et al, editors: Nutrition, national development, and planning, Cambridge Mass, 1971, MIT Press, pp 103-128.

50. Alvear J, et al: Physical growth and bone age of survivors of protein energy malnutrition, Arch Dis Child **61**:257-262, 1986.

51. Galler JR, et al: A follow-up study of the effects of early malnutrition on subsequent development. 1. Physical growth and sexual maturation during adolescence, Pediatr Res **19**:518-523, 1985.

52. Galler JR, et al: A follow-up study of the effects of early malnutrition on subsequent development. 2. Fine motor skills in adolescence, Pediatr Res **19**:524-527, 1985.

CHAPTER 35
Vitamin Deficiencies

Fernando E. Viteri

Vitamin deficiencies should be considered part of a greater problem of general undernutrition and malnutrition. The rule is for several deficiencies to be present simultaneously. In developed or industrialized countries, some vitamin deficiencies are the consequence of small pockets of malnourished populations, but most often are the result of concomitant diseases, such as alcoholism, chronic liver disease, and malabsorption syndromes, and of food faddism. Vitamin B_{12} deficiency, however, poses a different problem, since it is most often due to genetically determined specific vitmin B_{12} malabsorption. In developing countries, most deficiencies of public health importance are the consequence of inadequate intake complicated by infection and/or malabsorptive diseases. It is evident, then, that in the development of vitamin deficiencies, several factors related to the host, to the environment, and to the agent play important and different roles.

Fat-soluble vitamins (retinol, ergo- and cholecalciferols, tocopherol, and phyllo- and menaquinone as specific compounds for vitamins A, D_2, D_3, E, and K_1 and K_2, respectively) are all soluble in lipids and organic solvents and often constitute a family of compounds with similar biologic activity. Fat solubility determines their sources, their systems of intestinal absorption and transport within the body, their storage characteristics, and their metabolism and actions. Deficiency of these vitamins arises when fat intake is very small and/or when there is any kind of fat malabsorption. This group of vitamins, in contrast to the water-soluble vitamins, can become toxic when ingested in large quantities for long periods of time. Although their functions are not as well defined as those of most B vitamins, the syndromes caused by their deficiencies in humans are well defined, and recent advances have greatly clarified their diverse modes of action.

Water-soluble vitamins (thiamine, riboflavin, niacin, pyridoxine, folic acid, cyanocobalamin, ascorbic acid, pantothenic acid, biotin, choline, inositol, carnitine, certain bioflavonoids, and other still controversial factors) are ubiquitous in natural foods, and their deficiencies generally result from poor dietary habits, including food preparations that either remove or destroy the vitamins. Interestingly, the opposite case (when food preparation improves vitamin nutrition), as with alkali treatment of corn by native American cultures, which prevents niacin deficiency, is also true among the water-soluble vitamins. With few exceptions, water-soluble vitamins are less prone than lipid-soluble vitamins to becoming deficient because of malabsorption but they are more susceptible to alterations in utilization as a consequence of alcohol intake and other drug uses. In general, the basic metabolic role of each of the water-soluble vitamins is well defined and the clinical consequences of their naturally occurring deficiencies constitute well-recognized syndromes. However, natural deficiency situations in the human have been described for the first seven water-soluble vitamins listed, although not for the rest of them, some of which are still dubiously categorized as vitamins.

FAT-SOLUBLE VITAMINS
Vitamin A and Carotenes

Vitamin A is a generic term for the biologically active compounds retinol (vitamin A_1), dehydroretinol (vitamin A_2), retinal (vitamin A_1 aldehyde), retinoic acid, and the esters of retinol and dehydroretinol. Different forms of vitamin A are more biologically active in different systems: retinal is the active compound in the rods and cones of the retina. Retinol (vitamin A_1) appears to be the most active compound in reproductive function, while retinoic acid appears to be the most active form in all other vitamin A functions. Retinoic acid is not interconvertible with retinol or retinal and cannot be stored, in contrast to the previous forms.

The carotenes are provitamin A compounds that are converted to vitamin A by an enzyme-catalyzed oxidative split of the molecule between the 15 and 15′ carbons. There are over 400 carotenoids, among which nearly 60 have provitamin A activity, the most important being α-, β-, and γ-carotenes and cryptoxanthin. The discovery[1] that fish and other lower animals can produce beta-carotenes through reductive metabolism of xanthophylls has completed the vitamin A synthetic chain in the animal kingdom.

The old nomenclature for quantification of vitamin A was in international units, which are equivalent to 0.3 μg of retinol or 0.6 μg of β-carotene. However, studies have been contributing to a better definition of the vitamin A activity of many carotenoid compounds present in foods. Older methods of carotene determinations overestimated provitamin A activity by up to 10 times its true value in food.

Because of the presence of different compounds, vitamin A activity in foods is expressed as retinol equivalents. Preformed vitamin A is found primarily in liver oils, in animal fats, including those found in milk, butter, cheese, and egg yolk, and in liver. Some fatty fish are excellent sources of preformed vitamin A. Vegetables are also a source of carotenoids, particularly green and yellow vegetables, in which carotene is present in association with chlorophyll. Some seed and palm oils are also rich in carotene. White lard, vegetable oils, white corn and other cereals, beef, and most legumes, jams, and other carbohydrate sources are very poor in vitamin A activity. The vitamin A losses that occur during ordinary cooking are small, particularly if cooking takes place in neutral or alkaline solutions protected from light and from metals that can catalyze oxidation.[2]

Carotenoids diminish photolysis of nutrients in food and similarly protect the skin by quenching excited photosensitizing compounds.[3] Carotenes also undergo photodegradation, which can lead to significant losses of these provitamins.

Absorption and metabolism. Preformed vitamin A (retinol) and carotenes are absorbed as fat micelles in conjunction with bile acids. These molecules are first hydrolyzed from their esters by the action of pancreatic and proximal intestine brush-border mucosal hydrolases.[4]

About 90% of ingested retinol and 60% of ingested carotenes enter the intestinal mucosa. Control of vitamin A absorption is poor; absorption of carotenes decreases as ingested amounts increase. Retinol absorption is mediated by a specific cellular retinol-binding protein, Type II (CRBP-II), which is present in the epithelial cell layer of the small intestinal villi.[5] All-*trans* retinol is then reesterified by a specific microsomal enzyme, acyl-CoA–retinol–acyltransferase. This enzyme is inhibited by retinoic acid and other retinoids, and its activity is increased in fasting and by the ingestion of retinol and fat. Reesterified retinol enters the lymphatics as chylomicrons, and then the general circulation, being captured by the liver parenchymal cells as chylomicron remnants, through intracellular hydrolysis and binding by retinol-binding protein (RBP) and transfer to parasinusoidal stellate cells, where it is again reesterified and stored if vitamin A nutrition is satisfactory. Normally these cells contain 80%-90% of liver retinol. In vitamin A deficiency the accumulated retinyls (fatty acid esters of retinol) are hydrolyzed and transferred back to the parenchymal cells until there are no more esters. By then these cells have accumulated apo-RBP, because of a block in its secretion into the plasma. Any newly arrived retinol is bound to the available apo-RBP and secreted as holo-RBP into the plasma, where it binds to prealbumin (thyroxin-binding prealbumin [transthyretin, TTR]). Liver retinyl-ester hydrolases are elevated in vitamin A and E deficiencies and are supressed by vitamin E. Holo-RBP plasma levels are homeostatically regulated when liver retinol concentration is between 20 and 300 μg/g of liver. A fall in serum retinol occurs when liver reserves are lower, and a rise occurs when they are higher. Both responses tend to be linear. Biliary excretion of vitamin A metabolites is very low and stable when liver vitamin A concentration is below 30 μg/g, and it rises rapidly up to eightfold as this increases, reaching a new plateau at liver vitamin A concentrations of nearly 140 μg/g. Plasma holo-retinol does not continue to rise with increasing levels of vitamin A intake (as in vitamin A intoxication). In these cases plasma vitamin A is transported as lipoprotein-bound retinyl esters.[6,7] Extensive recycling of retinol between liver, plasma, and tissues normally occurs.[8] Almost half the circulating holoretinol originates in the liver. The other half is derived from other tissues, where holoretinol delivers the retinol moiety to cells that trap it into cellular retinol-binding proteins (CRBPs). A total of six of these specific CRBPs have been identified; along with CRBP-II and RBP, they are present in essentially all tissue cells, except ileal mucosa, muscle, and seminiferous germ cells. Cellular retinoic acid–binding protein (CRABP) exists in high concentrations in the eye, pituitary, ovary, testicular germ cells, prostate, and uterus but is absent from adult muscle and liver cells, from jejunal and ileal mucosal cells, and from Sertolli cells (in the testes). This explains why retinal is ineffective in restoring fertility to vitamin A–deficient animals.[6,9] CRBP and CRABP deliver retinol and retinoic acid, respectively, to the nucleus and maintain an intracellular vitamin A pool.[10] Retinal and interphotoreceptor (interstitial) retinol-binding proteins (CRALBP and IRBP) are the other cellular vitamin A–binding proteins. They have very special functions in vitamin A metabolism in the retina.

Evidence from several studies[18-20] has indicated that both retinol and retinoic acid are involved in allowing normal genomic expression (e.g., epithelial differentiation, fibronectin mRNA transcription in hepatocytes, and preservation of sites selected by RNA polymerase in testicular chromatin). Similarly, they are involved in the secretion of insulin by the beta islet cells.[21] (Retinoic acid also increases the binding sites for 1,25-dihydroxyvitamin D_3 in osteosarcoma cells, which may explain the well-known overlapping effect of vitamins A and D in bone tissue metabolism.[22]) Vitamin A appears to be essential for the operation of normal infection-defense mechanisms: In animals different aspects of the immune response are altered in vitamin A deficiency. These include reduced leukocytic, lysozymal, phagocytic, and bactericidal activities; reduced secretion of biliary immunoglobulin A[23]; and a diminution in the lymphocyte transportation capacity and number of T lymphocytes. However, infections often impede the absorption of vitamin A, and the circulating levels of retinol and RBP fall with fever and common infections. Of particular importance is measles, in which, even in mild cases, there is a viral corneal infection that with vitamin A deficiency may accelerate corneal liquefaction and ulceration. In analogous fashion vitamin A deficiency in animals facilitates upper respiratory infections and bacteriuria.[24] Natural and synthetic carotenoids with and without provitamin A activity are the object of increasing attention as chemopreventive agents for certain types of cancer and as quenchers of singlet oxygen, reducing free-radical oxidative damage.[25]

Vitamin A deficiency. Vitamin A deficiency is recognized when liver deposits of vitamin A are below 20 µg/g and circulating retinol levels are below 100 µg/liter.[26] To assess liver reserves of vitamin A, which are not reflected by plasma retinol (except when clearly deficient), a retinol dose response (RDR) test has been devised. It is based on the plasma increase of vitamin A after a standard dose of retinol over the fasting levels. Low liver reserves are detected by the relatively greater RDR (normal between 14% and 20%), because of its rapid entry into the circulation as holo-RBP.[7,28] Chronic vitamin A deficiency in animals is associated with impaired growth, anorexia, and increased rate of infections and morbidity and other sequelae that have been also documented in depletion studies in humans. Deficient humans suffer from night blindness (the earliest-appearing sign), follicular hyperkeratosis, alterations in taste and smell, loss of equilibrium, and increased cerebrospinal fluid pressure. In animals, congenital malformations and sterility are most often produced in vitamin A deficiency, and severe vitamin A deficiency also produces anemia secondary to altered iron metabolism. There is also evidence suggesting that iron metabolism is similarly altered in vitamin A deficiency in humans. Iron appears to be sequestered in the depot cells and poorly transported and utilized for hemoglobin synthesis, as happens in chronic infection. Finally, xerophthalmia, which denotes an advanced degree of vitamin A depletion, is the most devastating and dreaded manifestation of deficiency if not adequately controlled. (See Chapter 21.)

Public health significance. Estimates based on a series of prevalence studies of vitamin A deficiency suggest that there are 250,000 cases of blindness due to xerophthalmia every year in four major Asian countries. Some 8 million to 9 million people suffer from xerophthalmia not involving the cornea. Millions of children and adults have serum vitamin A levels below 100 µg/liter, which places them at risk of severe deficiency and xerophthalmia, particularly in the presence of protein-energy deficiency and infections.[28] Sun exposure has been noted to induce photodegradation of carotenes in humans.

Through this process exposure to the sun can thus possibly increase vitamin A requirements and the incidence of vitamin A deficiency in populations at risk as well as decrease chemoprotective effects of carotenes.[29] Prevalence, expressed as percent of preschool children between 6 months and 6 years of age, is useful in determining the public health significance of xerophthalmia and vitamin A deficiency: night blindness, $>1\%$; Bitot's spots, $>0.5\%$; corneal xerosis/ulceration and keratomalacia, $>0.1\%$; corneal scars, $>0.05\%$; plasma vitamin A less than 100 μg/liter, $<5\%$.

Retinoic acid exists in the body as a consequence of its intake and absorption (and its production from β-carotene in the intestine and retinol in most other cells). Its absorption and transport resemble those of free fatty acids, plasma albumin being the main carrier. It is not stored in the liver or in any other tissue.[11,12]

A large proportion of carotenes are converted to vitamin A at the intestinal cell level through the activity of two enzymes: 15,15'-dioxygenase, which splits the β-carotene molecule, yielding two retinal molecules (10% of which are converted to retinoic acid), and retinaldehyde reductase, which acts to yield two retinol molecules. Bile acids or lecithin, NADH or NADPH, and oxygen are required in the process. Unsplit dietary β-carotene leaves the intestinal cells as chylomicrons, enters the lymphatic channels, and then follows the general unspecific lipoprotein transport system to reach most cells (the brain in only trace amounts) and be deposited in adipose tissue and other lipid-rich or secretory cells (e.g., the mammary glands). Tissue and liver conversion of carotenes to vitamin A−active compounds is very slow, which explains the lack of toxicity of excess carotene intakes and hypercarotenemia.[6,7]

Vitamin A metabolism occurs by oxidation to retinoic acid in most tissues, and within the liver retinol as well as retinoic acid form glucuronides, which are excreted in the bile. Retinoic acid can also undergo decarboxylation and further catabolism to a series of poorly identified compounds, including CO_2. Vitamin A glucuronides are partially reabsorbed in the gut, although the majority are hydrolyzed by β-glucuronidases from bacteria and then excreted in the feces as a mixture of vitamin A compounds and catabolites.[13] The turnover of retinol in children averages about 2.5 mg/week or about 370 μg/day. In the adult it is between 500 and 600 μg/day. Once retinol and retinal are converted to retinoic acid, the reaction is irreversible and turnover is rapid.[14]

Functions of vitamin A. Vitamin A has generalized functions throughout the body and a specialized function in the retina as an important component of the visual system. This topic is considered more fully in Chapter 21.

Outside the visual cycle, vitamin A, through the compound retinol-phosphate-mannose, provides mannose in the synthesis of glycoproteins, which are essential for the mucus secretion of epithelial cells.[15] Vitamin A also appears to be involved in the synthesis of glycogen, acetate, lactate, and glycerol, probably in connection with an ill-defined role it has in steroid metabolism. Vitamin A deficiency increases the synthesis of coenzyme Q and squalene in the liver but reduces the synthesis of cholesterol, a precursor for steroid hormones necessary in gluconeogenesis.[16] Vitamins A and E both appear important in the stabilization of membranes and therefore in keeping the cell lysosomes inactive.[17] Retinoic acid is involved in the synthesis of muscle and serum proteins.

Studies by Sommer et al.[30-32] and by others[33] have given a new dimension to moderate vitamin A deficiency. Indonesian and Indian children presenting with even mild xerophthalmia had greater incidence and severity of diarrhea (in Indonesia) and respiratory infections (in both sites). Risk of death in such children was increased fourfold relative to similar children without xerophthalmia. This applied to all children, including those otherwise apparently well nourished. Moreover, periodic administration of therapeutic oral vitamin A doses to Indonesian children not only corrected the xerophthalmia but reduced morbidity and mortality in relation to control populations. These studies are being expanded and replicated in other parts of the world to determine the worldwide significance of their findings.

The seriousness of this nutrition problem has inspired special efforts to control and prevent vitamin A deficiency and xerophthalmia. Among the important public health measures dedicated to this aim are (1) strategies for periodic dosing of vitamin A, such as capsules or oil preparations containing 200,000 IU given about every 6 months, (2) vitamin A fortification of different vehicles, such as sugar, monosodium glutamate, and skim milk, (3) educational programs urging greater consumption of green and yellow vegetables, and (4) promotion of horticulture for carotene-rich foods.[34,35]

An important consideration is that the detection of xerophthalmia must lead to active treatment of the affected individual not only to relieve the syndrome but also to increase his/her liver reserves. WHO[24] proposes the following treatment schedule:

Immediately on diagnosis: 110 mg of retinyl palmitate or 66 mg of retinyl acetate (200,000 IU) orally, or 55 mg retinyl palmitate (100,000 IU) by injection

The following day: 110 mg of retinyl palmitate or 66 mg of retinyl acetate (200,000 IU) orally

Prior to discharge (or if clinical deterioration occurs 2 to 4 wk later): 110 mg of retinyl palmitate or 66 mg of retinyl acetate (200,000 IU) orally

Vitamin A requirements are dealt with in other chapters of this manual but can be summarized as follows: The requirement for an adult man to prevent xerophthalmia is 600 μg/day or a retinol equivalent of 1200 μg/day β-carotene. Twice that amount ensures vitamin A levels in serum above 300 μg/liter, which are the desirable levels.

There is an ongoing controversy concerning the recommended dietary intakes, RDIs (versus allowances, RDAs) of vitamin A equivalents. New RDIs propose figures in general lower than the 1980 RDAs: about 9% lower for infants, 10%-30% lower for children, 30% lower for adult men, 25% lower for adult women. More important, recommended intakes during pregnancy are lower because of demonstrated teratogenic effects of vitamin A doses in early pregnancy.[26,34]

Hypervitaminosis A. Hypervitaminosis A can occur acutely after a massive dose, but most often chronic hypervitaminosis A is seen when individuals habitually take doses in excess of 20 times the RDAs. The symptoms are transient hydrocephalus and vomiting or generalized malaise, listlessness, lethargy, abdominal discomfort and constipation, joint and bone pains, severe headache, insomnia, emotional lability, and an array of ill-defined symptoms. On physical examination, exophthalmos may be present together with edema, dry and rough skin, and

mouth fissures. Exostoses, hair loss, and brittle nails are not uncommon.[37] With excess carotene intake the only symptom is yellow-colored skin, especially of the palms and soles, that disappears upon discontinuation of the excess intake. The differential diagnosis includes jaundice of diverse etiologies.

Vitamin D

The antirachitic factor contained in cod liver oil was given the name of vitamin D. Subsequent identification of its chemical structure and different properties led to the realization that ergocalciferol, or vitamin D_2, was the product of ultraviolet irradiation of ergosterol. Similarly, vitamin D_3, or cholecalciferol, is the product of ultraviolet irradiation of 7-dehydrocholesterol. This process, which takes place almost fully in the epidermis, is less effective in persons with pigmented skin and the elderly. Prolonged skin exposure to sunlight partially destroys provitamin D_3 levels. Some 10%-20% of the skin's provitamin D_3 is finally converted to cholecalciferol, and its plasma levels increase 12 to 24 hours after sun exposure.[38] This compound is broken down to the active metabolite 1,25-dihydroxyvitamin D_3, which is considered a hormone because it is produced almost exclusively in the kidney and has as target organs predominantly the bone and the intestine (although many endocrine, secretory, reproductive, and hematolymphopoietic tissues are also responsive to 1,25-$(OH)_2D_3$). Under normal conditions 1,25-$(OH)_2D_3$ can also be produced by the placental decidua and by some of the target cells for the active metabolite (i.e., bone cells). In pathologic states associated with hypercalcemia, extrarenal 1,25-$(OH)_2D_3$ can be produced by abnormal cells. Such is the case for lymphomatous cells, sarcoid lymph nodes, alveolar macrophages, and possibly also cellular elements of other granulomatous reactions.[39,40] Thus vitamin D is a nutrient and a prohormone. It is needed as a nutrient only when exposure to sunlight is insufficient to produce enough vitamin D_3 internally from irradiation of dermal 7-dehydrocholesterol. All functions and metabolic transformations mentioned as D_3 derivates occur as well for vitamin D_2.[41] Animal fats, in particular fish liver oils, are rich in vitamin D. The amount present in animal fat, organs, tissues, and milk depends on the vitamin D status of the animal producing them. Similarly, a breast-fed infant can have rickets if the vitamin D status of the mother is inadequate and thus breast milk is poor in the vitamin.

Absorption and metabolism of vitamin D. The daily recommended intake is 400 units (10 μg)/day. Ingested vitamin D is absorbed together with dietary fats and is subjected to the same limitations indicated for vitamin A and fats in general. Bile must be available for vitamin D absorption, which takes place in the lower small intestine (jejunum or ileum).

The vitamin is then transported, as chylomicrons, through the lymphatic and vascular systems, where approximately 50% of it is bound to an alpha-1 globulin with specific vitamin D affinity known as vitamin D–binding protein (DBP). The rest is bound to other lipoproteins and to albumin. Vitamin D is rapidly captured by the liver, where it undergoes hydroxylation in position 25 (25-OH-D_3). This reaction is poorly regulated, and thus essentially all liver vitamin D_3 is hydroxylated. A proportion of this metabolite again reaches the plasma, bound to DBP, and constitutes the predominant form of vitamin D in the blood; this explains why circulating levels of 25-OH-D_3 reflect liver vitamin D content. However, 1,25-(OH)$_2$$D_3$ diminishes the activity of the 25-hydroxylase and thus promotes further hydroxylation of 25-OH-D_3 (to 1,25-(OH)$_2$$D_3$), the most active form of vitamin D, by the enzyme 25-hydroxyvitamin D_3–1α-hydroxylase. This enzyme is located mostly in the mitochondria of the proximal renal tubule and is activated (with elevation of 1,25-(OH)$_2$$D_3$ levels) by parathyroid hormone, low serum inorganic phosphate, ionized calcium and thyroid hormones, and increased circulating calcitonin, glucocorticoids, insulin, and growth hormone. Opposite serum concentrations of these factors and higher levels of 1,25-(OH)$_2$$D_3$ diminish the enzyme's activity. Pregnancy also elevates the enzyme's activity, along with its blood levels, possibly through increased circulating Ca^{+2} and P^{+5} and greater placental production. The dihydroxy form of vitamin D_3 is also the fastest-acting metabolite (responses obtained within 3 hr). It is 10 times more active than vitamin D_3 and 2-5 times more active than 25-OH-D_3 in terms of promoting calcium absorption by the intestine.

Other hydroxylated compounds (e.g., 24,25-dihydroxyvitamin D_3) also have vitamin D action but less than that of 1,25-(OH)$_2$$D_3$. These are metabolites or catabolites of the active vitamin D, which is inactivated in several tissues by side chain oxidation to calcitroic acid, by 24-hydroxylation, and by formation of a 24-oxo–23,26-lactone derivative and other polar metabolites (monoglucuronides in bile). There is a small degree of enterohepatic circulation, but most of the hydroxylated vitamin is excreted through the bile. Only about 3% of an intravenous dose may appear in the urine.[40-47]

Mechanisms of action. The prevailing concept, based on a number of articles, is that the active vitamin D metabolite has a series of functions besides the classic role of regulating Ca^{+2} and P^{+5} metabolism. All these functions are related to the presence of cellular vitamin D–binding proteins (CDBPs), which selectively bind 1,25-(OH)$_2$$D_3$ in the cytoplasm and transfer it, in a phosphorylated state, to the nuclei of a great variety of cells: enterocytes, osteoblasts, distal renal tubular cells (possibly also islet), cells of the parotid gland, muscle, brain, skin, and reproductive organs (testes, ovaries, placenta, uterus, mammary glands), and monocytes, macrophages, thymoblasts, and T- and B-lymphocytes upon activation. The CDBPs apparently protect 1,25-(OH)$_2$$D_3$ from degradation by 24-hydroxylation; they then transfer the vitamin to the nucleus, where it controls DNA transcription and processing of mRNA (enhancing the activity of DNA-dependent RNA polymerase II) and thereby affects the production of specific proteins (e.g., Ca-binding protein in the enterocyte and distal tubular cell, gamma-carboxyglutamic acid [GLA] protein in bone interacting with vitamin K, lymphokines, osteoblast-derived resorption proteins, skeletal growth factor, 24-hydroxylase [P-450], alkaline phosphatase, and interleukins 1 and 2). In addition, the vitamin influences peptide hormone secretion, collagen production, and cell differentiation. The end results of all this activity[39-51] are increased Ca^{+2} and P^{+5} intestinal absorption (the latter by a newly defined sodium-dependent saturable component); Ca^{+2} extrusion through the basolateral membrane of the enterocyte; renal tubular reabsorption of Ca^{+2}, P^{+5}, Na$^+$, and HCO$_3$$^-$; increased calcium entry into muscle cells and neurons (producing adequate muscle tone and improved cell excitation); bone remodeling and cartilage ossification (preventing osteoporosis in the elderly), by modulation of osteoblast activity (while bone cell number is modulated by parathyroid hormone); maintenance of normal serum Ca^{+2} levels (in concert with parathyroid hormone and calcitonin); redirection of monocyte differentiation and maturation, fusion of macrophages, and production of osteoclasts; increased interleukin 1 and decreased interleukin 2 production (which increase inflammatory responses and Ca^{+2} reabsorption and arrest lymphocyte proliferation, respectively); and increased insulin production through enhanced beta cell activity.

Vitamin D deficiency. The clinical result of chronic vitamin D deficiency in the growing child is rickets.[52] Rickets is characterized by disorganization of calcification at the endochondral surfaces of long bones, which become swollen by excessive noncalcified osteoid tissue. Reduced periosteal calcification and abnormal osteoid deposition beneath the periosteal surface also occur. This, plus active bone decalcification resulting from compensatory secondary hyperfunctional parathyroid glands aimed at maintaining normal serum calcium levels in the face of poor calcium absorption, produces soft bones that become deformed by weight bearing and normal muscle pulls. Characteristically, osteoblast alkaline phosphatase secretion is increased and the blood levels of this isozyme are elevated. In mild cases, calcium and phosphorus concentrations in the blood may be within normal limits, although in severe cases they are lower than normal. The levels of 25-OH-D$_3$ are usually below 5 mg/liter. Mild cases may show only biochemical alterations and slight radiographic signs of rickets. Clinically the infant appears well nourished, often obese. His or her skin reflects an absence of exposure to the sun, and the child is hypotonic, sometimes assuming unnatural postures. Anemia and both a higher incidence and greater severity of infections are the rule (because of impaired immune mechanisms).[47] The abdomen is distended, and diarrhea is not infrequent. Bony deformities are most characteristic; enlarged and painless diaphyseal-epiphyseal junctions (particularly the costochondral [rachitic rosary], distal radial and femoral, and proximal tibial) are easily detectable upon inspection and palpation. The shafts of long bones and the flat bones of the skull are also deformed, with flattening of the sides where the head most often rests on the pillow (craniotabes) and bossing of frontal and parietal bones; closing of the anterior fontanelle is delayed. The softening of the rib cage results in protrusion of the sternal area at inspiration while the lateral costal region is sucked into the chest from diaphragmatic pull (Harrison's groove), accentuating the sternal prominence (pigeon chest). This situation can seriously impair cardiorespiratory function, particularly in the presence of infection, which is favored by weakened coughing and pseudocroup from cartilaginous softening of air passages. There is also retardation in motor development (sitting and standing occur later than normal) and dental eruption. In older children who already stand, bowing of the tibia and other bone deformities occur. These remain as residual evidence of earlier rickets.

Renal and liver disease in adults and children can lead to functional vitamin D deficiency.[53] Severe chronic liver disease impairs the 5-hydroxylation of vitamin D$_3$ and chronic renal disease with azotemia is associated with impaired synthesis of 1,25-(OH)$_2$D$_3$. The administration of this active metabolite is successful in treating calcium malabsorption and secondary hyperparathyroidism in both diseases. Also, in the case of chronic liver disease, the administration of 25-OH-D$_3$ is effective, since 1-hydroxylation can proceed in the kidney. In chronic renal failure the administration of the synthetic 1α-hydroxyvitamin D$_3$ is also effective, since 25-hydroxylation can occur in the liver. In general, 1α-OH-D$_3$ is easier to synthesize than the other vitamin D coenzymes and can be used therapeutically except in liver disease.[54]

Osteomalacia is the clinical manifestation of vitamin D deficiency in adults. It affects primarily women of childbearing age who become calcium deficient after repeated pregnancies.[52] As with rickets in childhood, inadequate exposure to direct sunlight is the primary cause of this disease. Women complain of persistent skeletal pain, muscle weakness, and skeletal deformities. The main item in the differential diagnosis is osteoporosis, which occurs usually in older women beyond reproductive age. It has none of the biochemical features of osteomalacia (which are similar to those of rickets) and does not respond to vitamin D administration. Also compression and other bone fractures are common, with normal healing in osteoporosis, although in osteomalacia bone fractures are relatively uncommon and, when they occur, healing is delayed.[41]

Thanks to health education and to vitamin D fortification of milk, the presence of rickets in temperate climates has been essentially eradicated. The disease may still occur in developing countries among the urban poor, when children are locked in at home while both parents work, and in certain cultures that maintain children indoors or cover them from sunlight when they come outdoors.

Rickets and vitamin D deficiency have been documented among immigrants from the Indian subcontinent to industrialized cities in the United Kingdom as well as among the urban poor in many cities of the developing world. The consumption of calcium-deficient diets accelerates the body turnover of vitamin D and increases the relative values of circulating $1,25\text{-}(OH)_2D_3$. These diminish 5-hydroxylase activity and thus aggravate marginal vitamin D deficiencies caused in part by less effective skin production of vitamin D_3 in the face of lowered exposure to the sun. This mechanism may also be operating in elderly persons, in whom evidence is disclosing a high prevalence of vitamin D deficiency and even osteomalacia complicating osteoporosis and bone fractures. There is enough evidence also as to the benefits of better calcium and vitamin D nutrition in the elderly.[55-58]

Vitamin D is rapidly catabolized to inactive metabolites in subjects receiving anticonvulsant drugs chronically. These patients require vitamin D supplementation.[59]

Other therapeutic applications of vitamin D metabolites. Vitamin D metabolites and derivatives are essential therapeutic agents in various congenital diseases of vitamin D metabolism.[60] In vitamin D–resistant rickets (or familial hypophosphatemia) there is a blunted response of $1,25\text{-}(OH)_2D_3$ to the lower blood P^{+5} levels, and successful treatment is achieved with physiologic or larger doses of this compound together with increased phosphate intake. Rickets patients suffer from impaired 25-hydroxylation of vitamin D_3. Again, the administration of physiologic doses of $1,25\text{-}(OH)_2D_3$ (0.05 μg/kg/da) is successful treatment.

Two types of hereditary hypocalcemic vitamin D–resistant rickets are now known: Type I is due to a genetic error in the kidney's 1-hydroxylase level. Type II, more rare, is due to impaired CDBP production or DNA binding of the vitamin D–CDBP complex. Responses are attained with high doses of 1,25.[46] The administration of $25\text{-}OH\text{-}D_3$, $1\alpha\text{-}OH\text{-}D_3$, and dihydrotachysterol can be effective in controlling idiopathic or acquired hypoparathyroidism by (1) favoring calcium intestinal absorption and renal tubular reabsorption and (2) supplying active vitamin D metabolites, which are low in hypoparathyroidism.

Vitamin D toxicity. Vitamin D toxicity is due to high circulating levels of $25\text{-}OH\text{-}D_3$, which increase calcium transport and give rise to hypercalcemia and calcium deposition in soft tissue, including the kidney (nephrocalcinosis). These effects can be due to the ingestion of a massive dose or to the chronic intake of as little as five times the recommended allowance, for example, 2000 units of vitamin D (50 μg) per day. Serum calcium is usually above 120 mg/ liter. The individual, usually a child, is anorexic, presents with nausea and vomiting and alternating diarrhea and constipation, most often is irritable and depressed, and may complain of tingling sensations around the mouth and of generalized aches and pains. If the process is chronic, malnutrition and wasting can develop and may progress to death, which can also be the outcome of acute intoxication. Treatment consists of cessation of vitamin D intake, a low-calcium diet, systemic steroids, hydration, and intravenous administration of calcium chelating agents. The availability of synthetic calcitonin, which can be administered parenterally, has added an important new resource to the management of hypercalcemia. It should be used in acute intoxications, with careful monitoring of serum calcium.[61]

A certain proportion of hypertensive patients will show relatively low ionized serum calcium, elevated levels of circulating $1,25\text{-}(OH)_2D_3$ and sodium, and diminished renin activity and salt sensitiveness. These patients usually respond to calcium administration with a lowering of blood pressure and circulating vitamin D. Experimental evidence has demonstrated that $1,25\text{-}(OH)_2D_3$ directly affects vascular tone, which indicates that it is responsible for the blood pressure elevation in these cases. Obese subjects and blacks generally have increased muscularity, bone mass, and circulating levels of vitamin D and parathyroid hormone, together with relatively low levels of serum and urinary calcium. They are salt-sensitive also, in terms of blood pressure. Thus vitamin D and the calcium-regulating system may be crucial in unifying a specific subgroup of calcium-responding hypertensives.[40,62-64]

Some children receiving the recommended periodic prophylactic doses of vitamin D (600,000 units every 3-5 mo) have hypervitaminosis D and hypercalcemia. In view of the possible long-term undesirable effects of hypervitaminosis D, these doses should be lowered.[65]

Vitamin E

Alpha-tocopherol is most often referred to as vitamin E; but there are a total of eight tocopherols with vitamin E activity: the tocols and the tocotrienols (each with four forms, α-, β-, γ-, and δ-, depending on the number and position of methyl groups on the ring molecule). Compared to α-tocopherol activity, β- and γ-tocols and α-tocotrienol have, respectively, 37%, 7%, and 22% activity. The others have even less.[66] Vitamin E was isolated from the nonsaponifiable fraction of wheat germ oil. Alpha-tocopherol is generally present in various vegetable oils in proportion to the linoleic acid content of the triglycerides; an exception is corn oil, which contains primarily γ-tocopherol. Some of the normal vitamin E content of oils is lost in processing.

Vitamin E is found in all cell membranes, and evidence exists that its main function is to prevent oxidation of polyunsaturated fatty acids; a more general action, however, as an effective terminator of free-radical chain reactions, has also been established.[67] Deficiency of the vitamin is accelerated by ingesting large amounts of polyunsaturated fatty acids as well as by conditions that increase free-radical formation.[68] Cell damage occurs from free-radical molecular interactions, including cross-linking and decreased fluidity of membranes, from structure-function activities of membranes (redox disturbances, receptor-enzyme interactivations), and from the formation of diffusable biologically toxic products that spread the damage, including the deposition of lipofuscin (or ceroid) pigments.[69] Evidence that peroxidation of lipids in tissues can alter DNA[70] has been published, providing further links between free-radical damage and cancer.

Nutritional requirements, therefore, vary with the total amount of polyunsaturated bonds derived from fatty acid intake.[71] It has been suggested that a ratio of 0.6 mg of α-tocopherol per gram of polyunsaturated fatty acid be present in the diet. This is particularly important among persons who eat large amounts of fish oils, which have elevated peroxidative potential and low vitamin E contents. Vitamin C, selenium, and sulfur amino acid intakes spare vitamin E requirements by virtue of their antioxidant roles. The main dietary sources of vitamin E are vegetable oils; animal products generally are rather poor. Various tocopheryls (fatty acid esters of tocopherol) and free tocopherols are absorbed in the intestine in the free form and are digested and absorbed as lipids, although some (e.g., α-tocopherol acetate) are partially absorbed unchanged. In plasma the vitamin is transported as low-density and very low-density lipoproteins and becomes incorporated in the lipid components of cell membranes. The capacity of the cells to incorporate vitamin E is determined by their lipid composition and cannot be exceeded by increased availability of tocopherols at the cell level.[72] Vitamin deposits occur in both peripheral and visceral body fat, in the approximate proportion of 1 mg of tocopherol per gram of lipid.[73] The vitamin is metabolized to inactive oxidation products (quinones, etc.) that are excreted in the urine.

Vitamin E deficiency. Given the wide distribution and nonspecific action of vitamin E as a protector of cell membranes against free radicals, the signs of its deficiency appear in many cells and tissues. In animals these signs are observed in the reproductive, muscular, nervous, vascular, and hematopoietic systems.[74] Males typically show degenerative changes in the seminiferous tubules; females, fetal reabsorption after implantation. Paralysis and creatinuria, indicative of muscular lesions, may be severe. Skeletal muscle as well as the myocardium becomes ischemic, with deposition of calcium and lipofuscin; one of these fatty pigments, ceroid, may also appear in visceral smooth muscle. Nutritional encephalomalacia, another nervous system sign of vitamin E deficiency evident in chickens, may be accompanied by pigmentary deposition in and degeneration of the anterior horns of the spinal cord, the vestibular nuclei, and the pyramidal tracts. Increased capillary permeability with hemorrhages (exudative diathesis) is common in vitamin E–deficient chickens. Alterations in red cell production, hemolysis in vivo, and increased sensitivity to hemolysis in the presence of peroxide in vitro are observed early. All these defects are magnified when polyunsaturated fatty acids are added to the vitamin E–deficient diet.

There are few clear signs of vitamin E deficiency in humans. In premature infants[75,76] deficiency may be associated with the development of bronchopulmonary dysplasia, hemolytic anemia, edema, skin lesions, and morphologic changes in the erythroid series; but these respond quickly to vitamin E administration, although they may be aggravated or precipitated by the administration of polyunsaturated fatty acid–rich formula and/or iron compounds. A study also has shown that immature children supplemented with vitamin E have a lower incidence of retrolental fibroplasia. Occasional reports[77,78] of adults and older children with muscular alterations and creatinuria, encephalomalacia, and hemolytic anemia that responded to vitamin E administration suggest that possibly severe vitamin deficiency in humans under special circumstances (e.g., associated folic acid deficiency) can produce lesions similar to those observed in deficient animals. An exception to this appears to be the lack of effect on the reproductive organs and function even in moderately vitamin E–deficient humans. Administration of vitamin E in complicated pregnancies has consistently met with failure.[79]

There is doubt regarding the levels of circulating α-tocopherol that will induce signs of vitamin E deficiency. When the plasma tocopherol is below 5 mg/liter, peroxide hemolysis tests become positive; and when it is equal to or below 2 mg, most likely in vivo hemolysis occurs.[71]

Because of the pivotal role that vitamin E plays in protecting cells from free-radical damage, the known cellular effects of these radicals and of conditions accelerating their production have been explored relative to the consequences of vitamin E deficiency, sufficiency, and excess. In some studies the interaction between the vitamin and other nutrients that are also protective against free-radicals (β-carotene, ascorbic acid, Se, Cu, Mn, Zn, Fe, sulfur amino acids) has been explored. Free radicals are constantly being produced in oxidative processes in all cellular compartments and organelles. Exposure to ionizing or photoexcitatory radiation, high oxygen tensions, or conditions that accelerate oxidative processes (x rays, sunlight, physical exercise, hyperthyroidism, hyperthermia) can increase free-radical production and damage. Such damage results from the numerous processes that affect health: exposure to ozone, smoke, or other pollutants, leading to lung cancer and emphysema; cataract formation; phototoxicity; platelet and lipoprotein aggregations that accelerate the development of atherosclerosis; sequelae of reoxygenation following ischemia. Many epidemiologic and experimental studies have shown predicted associations between high levels of free-radical formation and damage and the prevalence of pathologic conditions. Also implicated has been "inadequate nutritional protection" (i.e., insufficient intake of the protective nutrients, including vitamin E). However, at the same time, few studies have been able to even suggest a beneficial effect from higher-than-recommended intakes of these nutrients in terms of decelerating the aging process or reducing free-radical damage beyond that accomplished with the recommended levels.[68,69,80-83]

The only well-known pharmacologic action of vitamin E is as an inhibitor of vitamin K; therefore care must be exercised not to give added oral doses of vitamin E to patients being anticoagulated.[84] Chronic administration of pharmacologic doses has not generally been associated with any toxic effect, although in very low–birth-weight babies increased incidence of sepsis and necrotizing enterocolitis has been associated with prolonged pharmacologic vitamin E serum levels.[85,86]

Vitamin K

Vitamin K activities are shared by several related compounds, which include naphthoquinones. Vitamin K_1, or phylloquinone, which is the original form in the vegetable kingdom, is slightly soluble in water and easily soluble in organic solvents. Vitamin K_2, a product of bacterial metabolism, consists of a family of menaquinones with isoprenol units on the side chain numbering 4 to 13. The original vitamin K_2, isolated from putrid fish, is menaquinone-7. Synthetic vitamin K (menadione) has no isoprenol side chains, and only about 1% of it is converted to biologically active menaquinone.

The most important dietary sources of vitamin K are green leafy vegetables, beef liver, and foods in which bacterial putrefaction has taken place. About 50% of the vitamin K in the human liver is considered to result from endogenous biosynthesis by the gastrointestinal bacterial flora.[87] The requirement for this vitamin is 0.15-0.4 μg/kg of body weight/day for adults. The mean requirement for infants is 5 μg/day. The total body pool of vitamin K in adult men is only 70-100 μg, with a rapid turnover of approximately 30 hours.[88,89]

All vitamin K compounds are absorbed in micellar form with other dietary fats. They enter the lymph ducts as chylomicrons and are released at the liver, whence they go into the general circulation associated with β-lipoproteins. Normally 40%-70% of ingested vitamin K is absorbed. It is widely distributed among the body cells and becomes associated with mitochondrial and microsomal membranes. Catabolism of the vitamin occurs primarily via the bile and feces, which contain about 60% of a parenteral dose, whereas other metabolites, amounting to about 30% of the dose, appear in the urine. Nearly 30% of the excreted vitamin K_1 remains as phylloquinones. Vitamin K is normally synthesized by colonic and lower small intestinal flora in both animals and humans, and some of it is absorbed in the lower jejunum and ileum. Colonic absorption is minimal. The importance of this source of vitamin K in humans is demonstrated by the fact that patients receiving antibiotics that reduce intestinal bacterial flora often suffer from vitamin K deficiency.[90]

Functions of vitamin K. Vitamin K's role as a cofactor in the liver synthesis of prothrombin (Factor II) and other coagulation factors (VII, IX, and X) is well documented.[87] After these proteins have been synthesized at the ribosomal level, the vitamin induces carboxylation of glutamate residues to form gamma-carboxyglutamates by a reaction that takes place in the 10 glutamate residues on the N-terminal side of the prothrombin molecule. This carboxylase system is bound to the microsomal membranes and requires CO_2, oxygen, a peptide substrate, and vitamin K hydroquinone (which can be substituted by vitamin K plus NADH). The active incorporation of CO_2 does not involve biotin, ATP, or bicarbonate.[91] Peptides containing GLA have a calcium-binding ability and are present not

only in the four clotting factors just mentioned (II, VII, IX, X) but also in three circulating proteins (C, S, and Z)* as well as in muscle, kidney, placenta, skin, lung, and bone, and in both eukaryotic and prokaryotic ribosomal proteins. Since reduced vitamin K appears to be an essential cofactor in the formation of gamma-carboxyglutamate residues, its function may be more general than just in clotting reactions (i.e., also in calcium binding). Osteocalcin, a vitamin D-regulated bone protein that apparently interacts with hydroxyapatite in the process of calcification of bone, has been found to contain GLA residues. A similar protein is present in the bone-hydroxyapatite matrix and in normal urine, but its precise role is not yet known.[92]

Vitamin K deficiency. The diagnosis of vitamin K deficiency is usually established by measurement of prothrombin time. However, both prothrombin and des-GLA-prothrombin can now be measured directly in plasma, and their ratio detects vitamin K deficiency states before these affect prothrombin times.[93] In fact, two defective prothrombins, which do not bind calcium because they lack γ-carboxyglutamyl residues, have been identified in the liver of warfarin-treated rats and are postulated to be precursors of normal prothrombin produced when vitamin K-dependent carboxylase is blocked by the antagonist.[94]

Primary vitamin K deficiency is essentially unknown in otherwise healthy human adults. In contrast, newborn breast-fed infants who still lack intestinal bacteria sometimes have long prothrombin times because of vitamin K deficiency.[95] This usually is true in the first week of life and is due to the poor placental transfer of vitamin K, the sterility of the gut, and the fact that human milk is a poor source of this vitamin.

The most common vitamin K deficiencies are those secondary to impaired fat absorption or severe liver disease. Among the first type of disorders, biliary obstruction or fistula, pancreatic insufficiency, celiac disease, tropical and nontropical sprue, pellagra, regional enteritis, ulcerative colitis, and blind loop syndromes all can

---

*These are found in bovine and human plasma. They contain GLA and are of differing sizes and electrophoretic mobilities. Their precise function is not yet known. They are not clotting factors, but serve to point up the ubiquitousness of GLA proteins and the many vitamin K functions yet to be defined.

cause vitamin K deficiency. Gut sterilization also produces vitamin K deficiency.

Vitamin K is important because its antagonists (e.g., dicumarol, warfarin) inhibit, by still ill-defined mechanisms, the carboxylation of glutamate residues in the precursors of coagulation factors. Vitamin K has some therapeutic value when overdoses of antagonists occur and in the treatment of hemorrhagic disease of the newborn. Oral or parenteral vitamin K_1 must be given in these cases. The routine use of vitamin K, and particularly of some of its water-soluble analogues, in newborns has been discontinued because they may contribute to neonatal hyperbilirubinemia and kernicterus[95]; however, vitamin K deficiency has also been identified in increasing numbers of breast-fed neonates, and this measure thus is being advised again.[96-98] When fat malabsorption is the cause of the deficiency, the intramuscular route is essential.

Vitamin K deficiency is more frequently recognized among elderly debilitated patients and in persons with osteoporosis whether or not they have major bone fractures.[99,100] There is need for concern as to vitamin K nutrition in these cases and wherever bone formation may be desirable.

WATER-SOLUBLE VITAMINS
Thiamine (Vitamin B_1)

The discovery by Funk (1912) of thiamine, an active amine present in rice polishings, gave rise to the name *vitamin* for the series of essential nonmineral nutrients required in very small amounts.

Intestinal absorption of thiamine into the portal system occurs by both active transport and passive diffusion. Absorption is reduced in the presence of diarrhea, alcoholism, and folate deficiency.[101,102] A total of about 30 mg of thiamine is present in normal adults, over 75% of it as the pyrophosphate. This pool can be depleted in about 2 weeks or even faster if there is no intake and a high-carbohydrate diet is established. Thiamine metabolites, numbering over 20 different compounds, appear in the urine.[101]

The best sources of thiamine are yeast, whole grain cereals, legumes, and meat. Some fruits and vegetables also contain good amounts of this vitamin. Enriched wheat flour is an important source. Diets that provide 0.25 mg/1000 kcal protect against thiamine deficiency, and an intake of 0.5 mg of thiamine/1000 kcal from the diet is recommended. In any case, intake should be more than 1 mg per day.

Thermolabile and thermostable antithiamine factors have been identified in certain foods and bacteria. Thermolabile thiaminases exist in the viscera of fresh fish, shellfish, and certain bacteria. The thermostable variety is found in plants associated with caffeic and tannic acids and in animal tissues associated with hemoglobin, myoglobin, and hemin.[103] About 25% of the thiamine in foods is lost in normal cooking.

Biologic activity. Thiamine pyrophosphate is a coenzyme involved in the oxidative decarboxylation of α-keto acids to aldehydes. This reaction is particularly important in the generation of acetyl-CoA from pyruvate and of succinyl-CoA from α-ketoglutarate. The reaction proceeds in three steps: thiamine is involved in the first (active aldehyde formation); lipoic acid in the second; and coenzyme A in the third.[104] Another important function of thiamine is as a coenzyme in the process of transketolation in the phosphogluconate pathway, which generates glyceraldehyde-3-phosphate and sedoheptulose-7-phosphate from two pentoses. This pathway is also important in the generation of reduced nicotinamide adenine dinucleotide phosphate (NADPH). Thiamine also is a cofactor in other decarboxylation and transketolation reactions in bacteria.

Thus thiamine is an important coenzyme in carbohydrate metabolism and in the normal operation of the energy-yielding tricarboxylic acid cycle, which explains why its deficiency can be accelerated by high carbohydrate intakes and retarded by substituting fat for carbohydrate as an energy source.

Thiamine deficiency. Classically thiamine deficiency is known as beriberi, which has two essential forms[105]: chronic polyneuropathy (dry beriberi) and acute or subacute high-output cardiac failure (wet beriberi). Under natural conditions these forms characteristically occur in outbreaks in a community or among groups of individuals consuming similar diets, usually based on polished rice. When thiamine deficiency is seen in a small infant, its characteristic features identify it as infantile beriberi. Thiamine deficiency occurs also in alcoholics,[106] in persons with chronic vomiting and/or diarrhea, particularly if they are maintained with carbohydrate-rich fluids, in hyperemesis gravidarum, and in an occasional person who lives in social isolation and consumes a peculiar diet (e.g., the elderly, the young drug addict). Thiamine deficiency of this type also presents with the clinical picture of polyneuropathy, heart failure (which may be not only high output but also associated with toxic cardiomyopathy), and acute and chronic encephalopathy, known as the Wernicke-Korsakoff syndrome. This syndrome appears to have some genetic predisposition associated with a reduced affinity for thiamine-containing cofactor among variants of apotransketolase.[107] Furthermore, the apotransketolase is unstable in the acid pH resulting from pyruvic and lactic acid accumulations in the brain with thiamine deficiency.[108]

Often a single clinical form of thiamine deficiency will be present or at least markedly predominant over the others. Only rarely are all the syndromes present together. Polyneuropathy is present primarily in persons subsisting chronically on diets slightly low in thiamine. When the depletion is more acute or is complicated by cardiomyopathy, wet beriberi develops. Apparently this form of the disease also occurs most often in individuals engaged in physically demanding tasks, wherein because of inadequate pyruvic acid metabolism both pyruvate and lactate accumulate at the muscle level, thus producing intense vasodilation. Severe lactic acidosis accelerates cardiac failure, giving rise to yet a third form of the disease, a fulminating syndrome called Shoshin beriberi. Encephalopathy can be the first manifestation in sedentary people, especially in alcoholics.

Specific diagnosis of thiamine deficiency can be obtained by laboratory determinations of erythrocyte transketolase activity in the absence and presence of thiamine pyrophosphate. Concomitant findings are elevated pyruvate and lactate levels, although in chronic dry beriberi the blood pyruvate can be within normal limits. Diminished urinary excretion of thiamine metabolites and a dietary history of low-thiamine high-carbohydrate intakes also favor the diagnosis. Proof of diagnosis is the rapid improvement observed with thiamine administration, although this may not be the case in the polyneuropathy

and encephalopathy syndromes (particularly in Korsakoff's psychosis).*

All severe forms of thiamine deficiency have common clinical features as early manifestations: anorexia, malaise, weakness, decreased attention span, calf tenderness upon weight bearing and the application of pressure to the gastrocnemius, burning and numbness of the extremities with associated altered tendon reflexes, and in general a lower work efficiency. Often some degree of dependent edema appears, together with a full pulse and tachycardia, particularly upon mild exercise. If polyneuropathy progresses, there is marked muscle weakness and aggravation of the symmetric paresthesia, persistence of touch sensations (which are distorted), and painful nerve tracts and burning sensations, together with anesthesia over the anterior tibial surface. Walking is impaired and the patient may become bedridden. Foot and wrist drop are common. Usually by this stage the patient is cachectic and prone to fatal infections. In prisoners of war, Wernicke's and Korsakoff's encephalopathies were described together with this syndrome.

Beriberi heart disease can progress more rapidly if the patient leads a physically active life, exercises (moderately or vigorously), or suffers from febrile episodes. The most notable features of wet beriberi are edema, which involves not only the legs but also the trunk and the face, and capillary dilation, which is evident as reddened face and extremities. Palpitation and shortness of breath are the usual features, together with pain upon movement of the legs and increased calf tenderness with weight bearing or pressure. Pulse pressure is high, because of both an increase in systolic and a decrease in diastolic. Auscultation over large arteries may disclose a "pistol shot" sound. As cardiac failure becomes more severe, characteristic features include bounding venous pulse in dilated neck veins, cold extremities, and cyanosis because of skin vasodilation brought on by lactic acidosis. Low

---

*This condition includes an acute component that responds rapidly to thiamine administration and a chronic one that does not respond satisfactorily or responds but slowly. The first component is supposed to represent only biochemical and physiologic abnormalities caused by thiamine deficiency, the second to imply anatomic brain damage.[106]

voltages and other alterations suggestive of myocardial ischemia may appear on the electrocardiogram. Oliguria is common. When toxic cardiomyopathy is superimposed by alcoholism or excessive lactic acid accumulation, low output failure results and the patient becomes acutely ill with severe dyspnea and a sudden increase in edema; death may follow shortly.

The infantile form of beriberi can also be acute, with a predominant symptomatology of acute cardiac failure, cyanosis, dyspnea, and death within a few days. This is often preceded by convulsions and coma and partial or complete aphonia. The chronic form of infantile beriberi is manifested primarily by gastrointestinal alterations (severe constipation and vomiting that occurs repeatedly throughout the day). The child appears agitated, sleeps poorly, and may have signs of mild cardiac failure that can progress suddenly to death. Infantile beriberi is more common between 2 and 5 months of age and is caused by thiamine deficiency in the mother, with consequent low milk thiamine content.

The manifestations of nonoriental beriberi polyneuropathy are no different from those of oriental beriberi but usually are associated with other nutritional deficiencies (pellagra, vitamin B_6 deficiency, folate deficiency) and with damage produced by toxic factors, including alcohol. Differential diagnoses include polyneuropathies from other metabolic diseases, different poisonings, iatrogenic diseases (large doses of isoniazid), infections (including leprosy), and various neoplastic and genetic disorders.[109]

The encephalopathy can be acute, characterized by ophthalmoplegia, nystagmus, ataxia, disorientation, coma, and death. Chronic encephalopathy is characterized by psychosis, severe learning and memory disturbances, and often confabulation. Memory lapses are fundamentally of recent events and the patient often covers these lapses with confabulation. The encephalic lesions are symmetric areas of myelin degeneration with small hemorrhages; in severe cases complete necrosis occurs in various parts of the brainstem, diencephalon, cerebellum, mamillary bodies, thalamus, and periaqueductal grey matter. These lesions, in different stages of development, are common to the acute and chronic manifestations of encephalopathy from thiamine deficiency.[106,110]

The treatment of wet beriberi is essentially bed rest and 25 mg of intramuscular thiamine hydrochloride twice daily for 2-3 days. Oral doses of 10 mg 3-4 times a day should also be given from the beginning. The response to treatment is prompt, clear improvement being noticeable in a few hours. Occasionally diuretics and digitalis may be needed, but these are ineffective without thiamine administration. The same vitamin and dietary treatment should be applied to the polyneuropathy, but recovery is slow. The fact that other vitamin and mineral deficiencies are often present must be kept in mind. The best treatment for infantile beriberi, if the child is being breast-fed, is 10 mg of thiamine intramuscularly to the baby and 20-30 mg a day of thiamine by mouth to the mother. For encephalopathy, treatment is essentially the same although the intravenous route can also be used.[110,111] Thiamine is essentially devoid of toxic effects, even when large doses are administered parenterally.

Riboflavin

Riboflavin, or vitamin B_2, is the prosthetic group of the "active yellow respiratory enzymes" of Warburg and Christian. In pure form it is composed of an alloxazine ring with dimethyl ribitil; it is moderately soluble in water. Its two active coenzyme forms (flavin mononucleotide, or FMN, and flavin adenine dinucleotide, FAD) are highly soluble in water. The three compounds are destroyed by alkaline solutions, particularly in the presence of light and heat. The most important sources of riboflavin are yeast, meat extracts, wheat bran and whole grains, legumes, egg yolk, and most animal tissues. Riboflavin and FMN are readily absorbed from the upper intestine (FAD less well) and from then on they are transported bound mostly to albumin or free in the plasma and are distributed throughout the body tissues.[112]

Biochemical function. The riboflavin-containing mono- and dinucleotides are part of the electron transport chain, being the prosthetic group in a series of oxidation-reduction enzyme systems, including glutamate reductase, amino-acid oxidases, xanthine oxidase, and succinic-acid dehydrogenase and involves beta oxidation of fatty acids, purine catabolism, and oxidative phosphorylation.[113]

Metabolism. Riboflavin is easily absorbed

from the intestine. FMN and FAD must first be dephosphorylated at the brush border of the upper intestine. Intracellularly (in the gut as well as in the liver) riboflavin is phosphorylated to FMN. It is then distributed throughout the body and is excreted primarily in the urine as a free vitamin. It also appears in feces, together with metabolites produced primarily from bacterial action. A significant fraction of FAD is tightly bound to flavoproteins that have enzymatic functions and is released only when proteolysis takes place.[114,115] In riboflavin deficiency, very small amounts of the vitamin appear in the urine, probably from these sources. This characteristic also may explain the relative paucity of signs and symptoms in riboflavin deficiency despite the central biochemical role this vitamin plays.

Tissue content of riboflavin may be chronically depleted when daily intake is less than 1.2 mg in adults. Riboflavin is retained when there is positive nitrogen balance and its excretion is increased, as indicated before, when there is proteolysis with nitrogen loss.[71,116] Thus there is some discussion as to whether requirements for this vitamin should be related to energy intake, body size, or protein or total nitrogen requirements. In any case, the allowances are set now at 0.6 mg/1000 kcal regardless of age. However, a minimum intake of 1.2 mg is recommended in adults. Slight increases of riboflavin intake are recommended during pregnancy and lactation, the total recommended allowance being increased by 0.3 and 0.5 mg/day, respectively under those conditions.

Riboflavin deficiency. Riboflavin deficiency is established by measuring the glutathione reductase activity in red cells in the absence and in the presence of FAD.[117] Also, erythrocyte flavin nucleotides, particularly FMN, and urinary riboflavin excretion before and after a load are depressed when this vitamin is deficient. Surprisingly, riboflavin deficiency in humans produces a few characteristic signs and symptoms, some of which are still not clearly specific for vitamin B_2 deficiency. In a study of riboflavin using volunteer subjects, extensive corneal vascularization was seen that was similar to what has been observed in rats, but other studies failed to indicate that riboflavin deficiency produced any changes in the general capillary bed. Riboflavin deficiency exhibits no neurologic abnormalities or behavioral changes.

A syndrome of angular stomatitis, glossitis, and seborrheic dermatitis around the nose and scrotum, together with corneal vascularization has been generally accepted as the clinical picture of riboflavin deficiency, but it is not reproducible in every case and is not aggravated by increasing levels of carbohydrate intake or energy expenditure. In animals cessation of growth is apparent, along with eczematous skin alterations around the eyelids, nose, and mouth, conjunctivitis, corneal opacities, and pericorneal arched vascularization. Irreversible damage to reproductive organs has also been substantiated.[118] Riboflavin deficiency during recovery from protein-energy malnutrition in children has been associated with abnormal red cell precursors and with anemia that responds to riboflavin administration.[119]

In riboflavin deficiency substantial increases in lipid peroxides have been documented. This is associated with deactivation of many FMN- and FAD-requiring enzymes that are involved in oxidation-reduction processes and in free-radical formation and inactivation.[120] Among newborns undergoing phototherapy, riboflavin is photodegraded and deficiency can be induced.[121] This vitamin is essentially free of toxicity in humans. When deficiency exists, and is not due to chronic diarrhea or severe malabsorptive syndromes of various sources, oral intake of 10-15 mg of riboflavin/day for 1 week should cure it. Parenteral preparations can be used when absorptive defects are severe.

Nicotinic Acid and Nicotinamide

Pyridine-3-carboxylic acid and its amide, respectively labelled nicotinic acid and nicotinamide, or niacin and niacinamide, are the active compounds also known as pellagra-preventive factors (PP). Niacin is also accepted as a generic term for pyridine-3-carboxylic acid and its biologically active derivatives. In the body, nicotinic acid is easily converted to nicotinamide, which is the physiologically active form of the vitamin. This conversion takes place through the formation of desamido-nicotinamide adenine dinucleotide and the activity of glycohydrolases on niacinamide in cells of the intestine and other tissues. Nicotinamide combined with two ribose molecules and either two or three phosphoric acid residues forms the dinucleotide (NAD) and the trinucleotide (NADP), respectively. Important antagonists are 3-acetylpyridine and pyridine-β-sulfonic acid.

Nicotinic acid is soluble in water and alcohol and is very heat stable. Niacinamide has similar characteristics but is even more soluble in water and alcohol.

Biochemical function. NAD and NADP both exist in the oxidized and reduced (NADH, NADPH) states, executing essential functions in the intracellular respiratory electron-transport system as hydrogen and electron acceptors and donors. NADH mainly transfers electrons and hydrogen further along the electron-transport chain for the release of energy whereas NADPH donates electrons and hydrogen primarily for synthetic purposes, especially in the production of fatty acids. NAD is also a coenzyme for the enzymatic joining of DNA strands.[122]

Although NAD and NADP can be coenzymes for electron and hydrogen transfer in multiple reactions, they perform this function with different efficiencies and specificities. NAD is the preferred coenzyme for the conversion of lactic to pyruvic acid, α-ketoglutaric acid to succinic acid, and both β-hydroxybutyric acid and alcohol to acetaldehyde. NADP is essential in the formation of phosphogluconate from glucose-6-phosphate and is preferred in the conversion of citric acid to α-ketoglutaric acid.[112]

Niacin metabolism. Niacin is present in small amounts in most foods and in larger amounts in viscera, meats, fish, whole grain cereals, and legumes. Coffee (particularly when roasted) and tea are also good sources; and, because it can be transformed into niacin by the body, tryptophan likewise is a good source. Thus it can be said that the lower the intakes of niacin and tryptophan the more efficient will be the conversion of tryptophan to niacin and vice versa. Approximately 60 mg of tryptophan can replace 1 mg of nicotinic acid in the diet. Consequently the term niacin equivalent is used to refer to all niacin-active compounds, including one sixtieth of the dietary tryptophan.[112,123] This proportion appears not to apply in the case of pregnant women and women taking oral contraceptive steroids, who apparently can metabolize tryptophan to niacin with three times "normal" efficiency because estrogens stimulate tryptophan oxygenase.[124,125]

In many cereals, particularly corn, niacin appears to be bound to peptides and complex carbohydrates. Alkaline treatment or roasting releases this bound niacin and explains why corn-eating cultures throughout Latin America, which treat whole corn with lime or ashes prior to the preparation of different foods, do not suffer from niacin deficiency or pellagra. In contrast, pellagra reached epidemic proportions in the southern United States and Europe when corn was eaten after removal of the germ and without prior alkaline treatment.[126] There is evidence that zein, the predominant nongerm protein in corn, and sorghum protein have an imbalanced amino acid composition, with excess leucine (which, together with a relatively low amount of tryptophan, can accelerate niacin deficiency). Alkaline treatment hydrolyzes some of the proteins and releases leucine into wash water, leaving a residual protein that is better balanced in terms of tryptophan and leucine.[127]

Both niacin and niacinamide are rapidly absorbed from the stomach and upper intestine by simple diffusion. They enter the circulatory system and reach all the cells, where NAD and NADP are then synthesized. Catabolism of niacin and niacinamide results in a series of compounds that are excreted in the urine, the main compounds being N′-methyl nicotinamide and its oxidation products (N′-methyl pyridone carboxamides) and nicotinuric acid.[128]

As is the case with thiamine, requirements and recommended intakes of niacin are related to energy intake. Various studies suggest that 4.4 mg of niacin equivalents/1000 kcal protect all persons from pellagra. The recommended intake is 6.6 mg of niacin equivalents/1000 kcal.

Niacin deficiency. In severe forms niacin deficiency produces the classic syndrome of pellagra, the disease of the 4 Ds: dermatitis, diarrhea, dementia, and death. Mild and early cases may lack any of the three initial components of the syndrome, and certainly the last. Pellagra is still a problem in parts of Africa and India, where epidemics are usually associated with sun exposure, periods of epidemic diarrhea, and consumption of maize and millet during periods of food scarcity. Pellagra is classically a multiple deficiency syndrome. With many of the manifestations due to multiple vitamin, protein, and mineral deficiencies, although the niacin deficit predominates. In the southern United States, where pellagra reached epidemic proportions early in the twentieth century, it has been eradicated by flour fortification with niacinamide and an improved diet. In most countries, however, occasional cases of pellagra are evident among alcoholics and food faddists, and are associated with severe malnutrition, malabsorption syndromes, carcinoid and other tumors, thyrotoxicosis, diabetes, chronic administration of isoniazid and 3-mercaptopurine, and the genetically determined Hartnup disease.[128,129]

The patient with a mild case of pellagra appears generally malnourished, apathetic, anorexic, and depressed and presents with general aches and pains. Some degree of symmetric dermatitis on exposed surfaces may be present, although it may be absent if the subject has not been exposed to sun. Dermatitis around the natural orifices (stomatitis, proctitis, vulvovaginitis, erythrematous scrotal macerations) is, however, almost universal. In severe deficiency with sun exposure the dermatitis may be prominent, resembling a symmetric severe burn, with scaly flakes and secondary infections. Typically the hands and forearms up to the elbow and the skin around the neck and upper thorax are affected (Casal's necklace). Diarrhea is common, and the entire gastrointestinal mucosal membrane is inflamed and atrophied. Marked pancreatic dysfunction is present.[130] Buccal angular fissures are common with inflammation, as is secondary infection with pain and frequent small hemorrhages. Vaginitis and amenorrhea also are common. Diarrhea induces malabsorption of most nutrients, aggravating the chronic general malnutrition. In mild cases the neurologic manifestations consist of depression and irritability, anxiety, general weakness, and mild tremor. In severe cases delirium and dementia occur. Bilateral peripheral neuropathy affecting both motor and sensory nerves is often present, leading to spasticity, ataxia, loss of position and vibratory senses, paresthesia, persistance of touch sensations, and dysesthesias. As deficiency becomes severe and chronic, different degrees of spinal cord involvement have been described, up to the syndrome of combined cord degeneration. This, however, may be due to severe concomitant vitamin B_{12} deficiency. Seizures and coma can precede death.

Laboratory analyses do not necessarily help in the diagnosis of pellagra. However, low plasma tryptophan levels, low excretion of N-methylnicotinamide and its pyridone, and in particular the ratio of the pyridone to N-methylnicotinamide urinary excretion are useful tests. The last test may be necessary for early diagnosis of deficiency since the pyridone decreases even in subclinical deficiency. Normally this ratio is higher than one, and a ratio lower than one is indicative of blatant niacin deficiency.[131]

Therapy involves the administration of 300-500 mg of nicotinamide daily plus a well-balanced diet with supplementary vitamins and minerals. Initially the diet should be soft. Dramatic results of this therapeutic regimen are very rewarding.

A biochemical form of diabetes has been described with the chronic intake of large doses of nicotinic acid. Massive doses of niacin (but not the amide) have been used pharmacologically to produce peripheral vasodilation and to reduce serum cholesterol levels.[132] It is known that these massive doses reduce serum cholesterol levels (lowering VLDL and LDL while increasing HDL), inhibit lipolysis, and enhance carbohydrate utilization by muscle. In carefully conducted studies[133] the chronic intake of nicotinic acid in hyperlipemic individuals accomplished a slight reduction in the incidence of myocardial events, although the overall and general mortality remained unchanged.

Vitamin B_6 (pyridoxine, pyridoxal, and pyridoxamine)

Vitamin B_6 is present in nature in three forms: in the vegetable kingdom as pyridoxine and in the animal kingdom mostly as pyridoxal and pyridoxamine. Pyridoxine is soluble in water and stable in acid solutions. It is rapidly destroyed by alkaline treatment in the presence of heat and light. It is widely distributed in essentially all foods. The best sources are animal viscera, egg yolk, soy and many beans, peanuts, bananas, and avocados.[112,134-136]

Vitamin B_6 is rapidly absorbed from the small intestine and distributed throughout the body. Red cells play an important role in the transport and metabolism of pyridoxine and pyridoxal and their active phosphates. Hemoglobin and albumin bind these components in blood. The active form is pyridoxal-5-phosphate (PLP), produced in all tissues by the action of ATP-pyridoxal kinase and by flavin-dependent oxidase acting on pyridoxine and pyridoxamine phosphates. Brain, liver, and kidney are most active in producing

PLP. This coenzyme is "stored" in muscle as part of the glycogen-phosphorylase enzyme in that tissue, constituting the major component of the body's pyridoxine pool. The stored PLP is, however, not available to the rest of the organism if B_6 intake is low. PLP leaves the muscle reservoir when muscle glycogen is broken down, typically during exercise, or when muscle-protein wastage takes place (i.e., during starvation[137,138]). Vitamin B_6 is extensively metabolized to several end products that appear in the urine. The major metabolite is 4-pyridoxic acid, which accounts for about one third of daily vitamin B_6 catabolism.[139]

The recommended daily allowance is 2 mg of vitamin B_6 for adult men and women. This is increased to 2.5 mg/day during pregnancy and lactation. In formula-fed infants the recommended allowance has been 0.4 mg/day. Human milk provides between 0.1 and 0.25 mg/liter, which appears ample for normal nutritional status of infants. The production of vitamin B_6 deficiency by means of vitamin B_6–free diet requires 2 months or more and can be accelerated by increasing nitrogen intake. However, eating more does not affect the rate of vitamin B_6 deficiency[140] although several conditions can accelerate its development. Experimentally the administration of B_6 antagonists, such as 4-deoxypyridoxine, and the intake of steroid hormones, including those in oral contraceptives, can lead to biochemical indications of vitamin B_6 deficiency; the same effect is seen during pregnancy and in individuals taking isoniazid (for the treatment of tuberculosis), penicillamine, semicarbazide, hydralazine, and cycloserine. Many of these drugs react with PLP, forming complexes that are then excreted. Several of them are carboxyl "trapping."[141,142]

Biologic activity. The active vitamin is pyridoxal phosphate (PLP), but occasionally pyridoxamine phosphate is found and performs the same functions. The active form of vitamin B_6 is a coenzyme to a large number of enzymes involved in the synthesis and catabolism of amino acids: aminotransferases or transaminases, hydrolases, carboxylases, decarboxylases, desulfhydrases, racemases, dehydrases, and synthases.* The major enzyme group, how-

ever, is aminotransferases or transaminases. Most of the transamination reactions lead to utilization of the amino acid carbon skeleton in energy-yielding reactions while the nitrogen moiety is excreted in urea. PLP-dependent decarboxylases play important roles in the synthesis of amino acid–derived metabolites with biologic activities, such as dopamine, serotonin, γ-aminobutyric acid, taurine, and nicotinic acid (from tryptophan). Other important reactions in which vitamin B_6 is required are the synthesis of δ-aminolevulinic acid, a precursor of heme; the conversion of cysteine to pyruvic acid; and the conversion of oxalate to glycine. A large proportion of vitamin B_6 is found in muscle, bound to phosphorylase, the enzyme that catalyzes the first step in the breakdown of glycogen. Apparently its role is to stabilize the structure of this enzyme.

Vitamin B_6 deficiency. Deficiency of vitamin B_6 caused by dietary inadequacies under natural conditions is extremely rare. It can occur, however, with chronic severe diarrhea or alcoholism and among socially abandoned indigent individuals or food faddists. In adults the natural syndrome produces an ill-defined clinical picture in which irritability, nervousness, insomnia, difficulty in walking, and weakness are the predominant signs and symptoms. In infants, widespread B_6 deficiency occurred when a feeding formula was prepared without vitamin B_6. The children presented a picture of inadequate growth, nervousness, irritability, and seizures, and they had abnormal electroencephalographic patterns.[143] Oxaluria may occur in vitamin B_6 deficiency induced by the chronic intake of isoniazide or 4-deoxypyridoxine, by large intakes of leucine, and by chronic uremia and liver disease.[135,144] Adults and children respond dramatically, within 24 hours, to the administration of pyridoxine.

Experimentally induced deficiencies have replicated the same clinical pictures and have produced hypertrophy of the filiform lingual pillae, nasolabial seborrhea, angular stomatitis, and intertrigo under the breast and in moist skin areas. Occasionally, with the use of pyridoxine antagonists, hyperpigmented pellagra-like dermatitis has also been observed. Typical peripheral neuropathy has also been produced by the use of antagonists. In addition, increased susceptibility to infections and impairment of antibody syn-

---

*References 112, 134, 135.

thesis have been described.[145-147] Biochemically, tryptophan metabolites prior to the synthesis of niacin are excreted in the urine in large amounts whereas niacin metabolites are not. Plasma and blood levels of vitamin B_6 fall drastically, and aminotransferase activity, both in plasma and in red cells, is lowered. The in vitro addition of PLP to red cells significantly increases the transaminase activity. Measurements of these parameters are the preferred biochemical tests for detecting vitamin B_6 deficiency.[148,149]

Genetic conditions affecting vitamin B_6 metabolism. There is a series of clinical conditions that markedly improve or disappear upon the administration of large doses of vitamin B_6. They are vitamin B_6–responding syndromes and are not to be confused with pyridoxine deficiency syndromes. Prominent among them is sideroblastic anemia (or PLP-responsive anemia), characterized by a blood picture identical to that of iron deficiency except that there are sideroblasts (iron-loaded red cell precursors) in the bone marrow and ferritin levels are extremely elevated. This condition is caused by an abnormal δ-aminolevulinic acid synthetase that blocks the production of heme. It responds to the administration of over 2 g of PLP daily. A second syndrome, which occurs among children who have been recognized to require large doses of vitamin B_6 starting at birth, includes convulsions and brain damage, and the children die unless properly treated. They may have abnormal glutamic acid decarboxylase that does not bind PLP and therefore reduces γ-aminobutyric acid synthesis.[143,150] In addition, various congenital disorders associated with mental retardation, deformities, thrombotic problems, osteoporosis, and visual defects have been associated with congenital anomalies in the structure and function of apoenzymes that bind with PLP. Some of these disorders, and the levels of urinary metabolites indicative of them, respond to large doses of vitamin B_6. They include xanthurenic aciduria, homocystinuria, cystathioninuria, homocysteinemia, homocystinemia, and hypermethioninemia.[151] It is interesting that both children with homocystinuria and rabbits injected with homocysteine suffer from premature arteriosclerosis.[143,152]

Subclinical vitamin B_6 deficiency has been described among chronic users of anovulatory steroids and pregnant women in the developing world. During pregnancy the response to incubation with PLP or serum diamine oxidase (placentally produced) appears to be a sensitive test for pyridoxine deficiency.[153]

Vitamin B_6 toxicity is essentially unknown, but excess pyridoxine can reduce the clinical effects of levodopa in the treatment of Parkinson's disease.[154]

Folic Acid

Folic acid (folacin, pteroylglutamic acid [PGA]) is the simplest of the compounds involved in promoting one-carbon transfers that are generically known as folates. It is present in nearly all natural food, but the richest sources are yeast, liver and other organ tissues, and fresh green vegetables. Protracted cooking or food processing can destroy up to 95% of the food content of folacin. Food folates are naturally in the polyglutamate form, but the monoglutamate is liberated by the activity of conjugases present in vegetables as well as in mammalian tissues, one of which is the brush border of the intestinal cell.

The folic acid requirement in infants and children is 5 μg/kg/day, and tissue reserves are maintained in adults with 100-200 μg of folacin/day. Since only about a fourth to a half of dietary folacin is nutritionally available, 400 μg is the recommended intake. During pregnancy these amounts should be doubled, and during lactation they are increased to 500 μg/day.[155,156] A series of studies and newly available data have suggested that these amounts are unnecessarily high except during pregnancy. Suggested recommended intakes are otherwise nearly half the 1980 RDAs.[157]

Metabolic functions. Typically, folate coenzymes participate as one-carbon donors in purine and thymidine biosynthesis and in hystidine-glutamate, serine-glycine, and homocysteine-methionine interconversions. Of special importance is the methylation of homocysteine to methionine, which through cyclic methionine demethylation serves in a large number of methylation reactions. It is of primary importance in explaining the folate–vitamin B_{12} metabolic interrelations, since it requires vitamin B_{12} as a cofactor and is inhibited by tetrahydrofolate (THF).[158] Methionine synthesis from 5-methyl-THF, with regeneration of the THF, is the only pathway whereby this folate metabolite is used, since it is produced exclusively by the reduction of 5,10-methylene-THF (catalyzed by methylene-THF reductase, with NADPH and FADH$_2$ as coenzymes). Both these reactions are irreversible, and the latter is exquisitely regulated by adenosylmethionine feedback. In vitamin B$_{12}$ deficiency 5-methyl-THF not only is underutilized but even is produced in excess from 5,10-methylene-THF. As a consequence this latter metabolite is depleted, which leads to depressed synthesis of thymidylate and thereby serves as a rate-limiting step in nucleic acid synthesis. The excess 5-methyl-THF is excreted. It is this general mechanism that explains the occurrence of folate deficiency when vitamin B$_{12}$ is deficient and is known as the "methyl-folate trap." The interrelationships also explain folate sparing of methionine when vitamin B$_{12}$ is deficient.[159-161]

Evidence has been accumulating over the past few years that polyglutamates rather than the folyl-monoglutamates are the preferred coenzyme form and that the polyglutamate side chain regulates one-carbon metabolism. Intracellular folyl-polyglutamates also are the storage form of the vitamin, having increased affinity for folyl-polyglutamate synthase but not serving as a substrate for the enzyme. Through this mechanism a form of end product inhibition is established, which explains the new steady intracellular folyl-polyglutamate levels that are attained when folate availability to the cell changes. 5-Methyl-THF is a poor substrate for the polyglutamate synthase; as a consequence, when that is the markedly predominant form of folate metabolites (i.e., when the methyl folate trap is operating), intracellular folate levels decline.[162] Insulin and adrenal steroids increase the synthesis of folyl-polyglutamates, and cyclic-AMP decreases it.[163]

Extensive reviews of the participation of folate in one-carbon metabolism are available in the literature.[164,165] The interrelationships of folate and vitamin B$_{12}$ metabolic reactions are described further under "Vitamin B$_{12}$"; for now it is enough to note that vitamin B$_{12}$ and folate deficiencies produce similar defects in DNA synthesis, resulting in abnormal nuclear chromatin and asynchronism between nuclear and cytoplasmic maturation (generally known as megaloblastic changes) in all actively DNA-generating cells. These changes reflect impaired DNA polymerization and arrest cell maturation.

The discovery that exposure to nitrous oxide produced megaloblastic anemia that could be ameliorated by administering large doses of formyl-THF opened a productive channel of research in the mechanisms of megaloblastosis. It has been proved, for instance, that nitrous oxide oxidizes vitamin B$_{12}$ (in the coenzyme-I form of the vitamin) and inhibits B$_{12}$-dependent enzyme functions. Vitamin B$_{12}$ deficiency can thus be produced in experimental animals; and this includes an almost total inhibition of methionine synthase activity, the accumulation of 5-methyl THF, and the consequent development of folate deficiency.[159,165-167]

There are several techniques for measuring folate content in blood and tissues. Normal human serum folacin activity is between 7 and 20 ng/ml. Normal folate concentrations in red cells average about 160 ng/ml, reflecting the general intracellular accumulation of polyglutamates. In vitamin B$_{12}$ deficiency the accumulation of 5-methyl-THF in bone marrow cells and transformed lymphocytes is impaired.

Folate metabolism. Folates are actively absorbed as monoglutamates throughout the small intestine but primarily in its proximal third. Cell transport and conjugase activity may, however, be inhibited by acid pH and by certain factors present in beans, yeast, and other foods that reduce folate absorption.[169] Anticonvulsants and alcohol also impair intestinal absorption of folacin. After absorption, folates are transported in the plasma either free or bound to low- or high-affinity binders. The latter-type binders are present in leukocytes, from which they are released to the serum and may play a role in diminishing folate availability. In serum the most abundant folate compound is 5-methyl-THF, which is transferred to body cells by active transport and then converted to THF prior to the synthesis of intracellular polyglutamate (the storage form of folates). The total body folate pool is 5-10 mg, half of which is liver folates. The excretion routes for folate are urine and bile. About 100 μg/day is excreted in bile and normally reabsorbed. Alcohol interferes with this enterohepatic cycle and apparently with redelivery of 5-methyl-THF from storage.[158]

Folate deficiency. Folate malabsorption and vitamin B$_{12}$ deficiency secondary to its malabsorption are the most common causes of nutritional folate deficiency. Besides occasional persons who ingest a bizarre folate-deficient diet, alcoholics suffer from folate deficiency, not only because of impaired folate absorption and poor diet but also because of metabolic blocks in 5-methyl-THF release, decreased methionine synthesis, and impaired formate oxidation. This reaction is dependent on formyl-THF dehydrogenase.[170] During pregnancy women become more susceptible to folate deficiency because of increased requirements and higher urinary losses of 5-methyl-THF.[171] Persons receiving anticonvulsant therapy also are more susceptible because of impaired absorption and metabolism of folates. Oral contraceptives and folacin antagonists can precipitate severe deficiencies when given to persons who already have increased requirements for folate because of preexisting rapid cell turnover, as in hemolytic anemias and with certain tumors. For example, in chronic myelogenous leukemia high-affinity binders are often present in the cells and are secreted, making folate less available.

The syndrome of folate deficiency was experimentally self-induced by Herbert,[172] who observed that in 3 weeks serum folate decreased below 3 ng/ml, in 7-10 weeks white cell hypersegmentation was evident, in 12-16 weeks urinary excretion of formiminoglutamic acid was elevated (demonstrating a block in the reactions leading from histidine to glutamic acid), in 17 weeks red cell folate concentration was markedly decreased, and in 18-20 weeks megaloblastic anemia with macroovalocytosis appeared.

Early in the induction of folate deficiency, apathy, irritability, depression, and forgetfulness are also evident. Megaloblastic changes occur rapidly in tissues with highest rates of cell replication (e.g., bone marrow, reproductive organs, GI tract, genital mucosa), which appear thin, inflamed, and often secondarily infected.

Dramatic therapeutic results are obtained when folate-deficient patients are administered 100 μg of folacin/day, orally or parenterally in cases of suspected malabsorption. This dose will not produce a response when vitamin B_{12} deficiency is present. Doses as high as 1 mg of folacin/day are indicated when folate requirements are increased, as in pregnancy and hemolytic anemias and with tumors or hypermetabolic states. However, doses larger than 1 mg/day are not indicated. Typically reticulocytosis and correction of all manifestations of megaloblastic bone marrow changes occur within a week of the initiation of therapy, by which time all symptoms are also markedly improved.

The prevention of folate deficiency could be accomplished by the routine inclusion of fresh fruit and a vegetable in the daily diet of the world population. However, in populations with malabsorption (e.g., tropical enteropathy, sprue) and particularly during pregnancy, folacin administration either as a supplement or through food fortification programs appears highly desirable and is both inexpensive and effective.[173]

The administration of folate in doses larger than 100 μg/day to vitamin B_{12}–deficient subjects may precipitate neurologic symptoms characteristic of severe combined posterolateral cord degeneration. Therefore caution must be exercised in the prescription of folate supplements when the possibility of vitamin B_{12} deficiency exists.[165]

The only toxic effect of folate reported in the literature[174] has been convulsions after parenteral administration of massive doses of folacin in persons receiving anticonvulsant drugs because of epilepsy. Large doses of folacin, however, may also reverse anticonvulsant-drug effects.

Vitamin B_{12}

Vitamin B_{12}, whose structure was elucidated in 1964, is the product of bacterial synthesis concentrated by the animal kingdom within the natural food chain. Vegetables, greens, fruits and legumes are devoid of vitamin B_{12} unless they are contaminated by bacteria. (Thus, contaminated vegetables may be an adequate source of vitamin B_{12} in vegans, as may fecal contamination of the environment among humans living in poor hygienic conditions.) Shellfish accumulate vitamin B_{12} from plankton and bacteria-rich seaweeds, and bacteria in the rumen and the intestinal tract of animals synthesize vitamin B_{12}; thus the best sources of this vitamin are organ meats (particularly liver), clams, and oysters. These sources provide more than 10 μg of vitamin B_{12}/100 g. All other animal foods provide vitamin B_{12} in smaller quantities. Some seaweeds can provide vitamin B_{12} to strict vegetarians. Losses of vitamin B_{12} during cooking are accelerated by an alkaline medium and by prolonged exposure to high temperatures.[175]

Metabolic functions. Both vitamin B_{12} and folate coenzymes are required in the synthesis of DNA. The key role of vitamin B_{12} in this metabolic process is as a B_{12}-containing enzyme that carries the methyl group from 5-methyl-THF to homocysteine, to produce methionine. In the process tetrahydrofolic acid (THF) is regenerated and becomes available for the synthesis of 5,10-methylene-THF, required in the synthesis of thymidine from deoxyuridine. Since this is the only way by which methyl groups can be removed from THF, when vitamin B_{12} is deficient transmethylation is blocked and 5-methyl-THF cannot be used. This causes a "methylfolate trap" (i.e., 5-methyl-THF levels dramatically increase in liver and plasma and large urinary excretion of this compound occurs). Thus folate deficiency, particularly of 5,10-methylene-THF, occurs, making the final biochemical damage from both deficiencies the same: impaired thymidine synthesis. Methyl–vitamin B_{12} is the active coenzyme in this reaction.[159,176]

The interrelations between vitamin B_{12} and folate are, however, more complex than suggested by the "methyl trap." Evidence has accumulated to establish the critical role of vitamin B_{12} in methionine and formate metabolism as bases for additional explanations of the pathology associated with vitamin B_{12} deficiency: cobalamins appear indispensable for the provision of formate in folyl-polyglutamate synthesis, probably through (1) the generation of formate from the reconversion of methylthioribose to methionine and (2) the oxidation of methionine's methyl group in the process of synthesizing polyamines. Formate either provides single carbon units or is oxidized by CO_2. In both cases folate coenzymes are required. Formate utilization in synthetic pathways, however, is impaired by vitamin B_{12} deficiency. In vitamin B_{12} deficiency or inactivation with nitrous oxide, an "escape" from the methyl-folate trap has been documented as due to the induction of betaine-methyl transferase and the consequent elevation of methionine levels. It is important to remember also that formate can originate from oxidation of methyl groups to methanol, glycine, serine, sarcosine, glycolate, and glyoxylate.[177,178]

5'-Deoxyadenosyl vitamin B_{12} becomes the B_{12} coenzyme to methylmalonyl-CoA mutase in the reversible reaction between L-methylmalonyl-CoA and succinyl-CoA. Thus vitamin B_{12} is involved in energy liberation from both carbohydrate and fat metabolisms. Furthermore, inadequate myelinization may take place with impaired propionic acid utilization in the synthesis of odd-chain fatty acids because of the inadequate interconversion between methylmalonyl-CoA and succinyl-CoA.[179]

The role of nervous tissue methyl group deficit as a contributor to the neurologic damage characteristic of vitamin B_{12} deficiency is still not well defined. Inhibition of the synthesis of adenosylmethionine by the administration of cycloleucine reproduces the lesions and symptoms of vitamin B_{12} deficiency, and methionine administration ameliorates any neuropathy of induced cobalamin deficiency. However, the nervous system takes up methionine at the expense of liver uptake of the amino acid and converts it effectively into adenosylmethionine, maintaining the levels for prolonged periods in vitamin B_{12} deficiency states.* B_{12} also may affect fat metabolism, through the synthesis of methionine and its subsequent methyl transfers to choline and betaine, which are lipotropic substances. In addition, there is evidence that B_{12} helps maintain the levels of reduced glutathione in the liver and red cells, and it also appears essential in the production of intracellular folyl polyglutamates from THFA. Detailed accounts of the many metabolic roles of vitamin B_{12} are available in the literature.[159,175,183,184]

Vitamin B_{12} metabolism. Vitamin B_{12} is normally absorbed in the terminal ileum when it is delivered to these intestinal cells in a complex dimer with gastric intrinsic factor, and in the presence of calcium and a pH above 6. (Intrinsic factor is a glycoprotein secreted by normal gastric parietal cells.) For this to occur, the natural vitamin B_{12} in foods, which is normally attached to polypeptides, must first be hydrolyzed in the stomach and upper intestine, where it binds with intrinsic factor. At the ileal cell the vitamin B_{12} is freed from the polypeptide complex, with the participation of bile acids, and is transported into venous blood, where it attaches to vitamin B_{12}– binding proteins. This mechanism handles less than 3 μg of vitamin B_{12} at a single time but regenerates its power in a few hours. Besides, about 1% of free vitamin B_{12} is absorbed by diffusion throughout the length of the small intestine. This fact can be used for the oral ad-

---

*References 175, 177, 180, 181, 182.

ministration of large doses of vitamin B_{12} in the treatment of its deficiency, although the gastrointestinal route is less reliable than the intramuscular route. Approximately 5 μg of vitamin B_{12} per day is excreted in the feces even in vitamin B_{12}–deficient subjects. It is the product of colonic bacteria and includes some isomers with no biologic activity.[185-187]

There are three classes of vitamin B_{12}–binding proteins in serum that are involved in vitamin B_{12} transport: transcobalamins I, II, and III. Only transcobalamin II is involved in the delivery of vitamin B_{12} to the body cells, including the bone marrow and nervous tissue. It is a β-globulin synthesized in the liver, and it normally holds 10% to 20% of the circulating vitamin B_{12}; its turnover is intermediate between those of the other two transcobalamins, which are glycoproteins mostly synthesized by white cells and which appear to have different functions: transcobalamin III–bound vitamin B_{12} has a rapid turnover (minutes) whereas the transcobalamin I–bound vitamin has a long turnover (days). Both these glycoproteins are abnormally elevated whenever the body neutrophil pool is increased, as in leukemia and other myeloproliferative disorders. All cells have receptor sites for transcobalamin II, and liver cells have receptor sites for transcobalamin III also. These transport proteins thus play a role in the delivery of vitamin B_{12} to the liver, where it is normally stored.[188,189]

Vitamin B_{12} averages about 4 mg (1 μg/g of liver), and its whole-body turnover is between 0.1% and 0.2% of the body pool per day. Vitamin B_{12} is secreted through the bile, reaching the small intestine and being reabsorbed almost in its entirety. This explains why it takes many years to produce deficiency, except in the absence of ileal function and/or intrinsic factor, or in the presence of pancreatic disease, when both bicarbonate and various proteolytic enzymes are defectively produced, thereby impairing the liberation of vitamin B_{12} from its peptide linkages and preventing induction of a favorable pH for ileal absorption.[190] Under these conditions, in persons beginning with normal liver reserves, vitamin B_{12} deficiency may still take more than 3 years to develop.

Average daily intakes of vitamin B_{12} are about 5 μg/day, of which some 25% is absorbed. The recommended dietary allowances are 3 μg/day for adults, 0.15 μg/100 kcal for infants and children, and 4 μg/day for pregnant and lactating women, to allow a margin of safety for increased requirements from elevated metabolic activity and fetal demands as well as for daily output during lactation. A smaller recommended intake has been suggested[155,191] for adults while keeping these values unchanged for infants, children, and pregnant women.

Vitamin B_{12} deficiency. Vitamin B_{12} deficiency can occur from inadequate intake, as among vegans living in very hygienic conditions, and among some food faddists and populations whose intake of the vitamin is derived from overprocessed milk (e.g., Mexican young adults). It can also occur as a consequence of poor absorption due to hereditary autoimmune gastric lesions (which cause inadequate production of intrinsic factor), gastric atrophy, or total gastrectomy. Malabsorption resulting from small intestinal disease requires impairment of distal ileal function. Absorption may also be blocked by abnormal binders and drugs, such as para-aminosalicylic acid, ethanol, and possibly oral contraceptives. Inadequate intestinal conditions for vitamin B_{12} absorption may be found in pancreatic insufficiency and in other specific genetically determined diseases.[189]

A curious form of B_{12} deficiency is produced by infection with the tapeworm *Diphyllobothrium latum* or by blind loops populated with vitamin B_{12}–avid bacteria. The vitamin also can be destroyed by excessive doses of ascorbic acid, or deficiency may occur from alterations in transport because of faulty transcobalamins, congenital enzymatic deficiencies, biologically inactive analogues (e.g., N_2O inhalation), or inadequate binding with increased renal excretion.* The classic vitamin B_{12} deficiency is the Addison-Biermer pernicious anemia,† characterized by the presence of megaloblasts (which reflect alterations in the synthesis of DNA produced by either folate or vitamin B_{12} deficiency). This alteration occurs in replicating cells throughout the body and denotes failure of DNA chain elongation, although the capacity to begin the synthesis of this molecule is still preserved. Apparently thymidylate concentrations are not adequate for elongation by DNA polymerases. In

*References 166, 167, 189.
†References 159, 165, 192.

addition, the deoxythymidine triphosphate pool is depleted whereas the deoxyuridyl triphosphate pool is enlarged so the latter nucleotide is misincorporated into DNA. Frequent breaks occur in single- and double-stranded DNA. The classic picture is of pancytopenia (anemia, leukopenia, thrombocytopenia), ineffective erythropoiesis with intra–bone-marrow hemolysis, increased serum bilirubin, and increased urinary excretion of methylmalonic acid. Serum and red cell vitamin B_{12} levels are decreased (to levels below 100 pg/ml). The oxyuridine suppression test has been devised for definitive diagnosis of B_{12} or folate deficiencies. It detects relative responses of DNA synthesis to the addition of either of these vitamins and is particularly useful in disclosing past vitamin B_{12} deficiencies by incubation of lymphocytes, which in resting phases reflect the B_{12} nutrition at the time of their production. In both folate and vitamin B_{12} deficiency the urinary excretion of glycinamide ribonucleotide (GAR) and 5-amino-4-imidazole carboxamide ribonucleotide (AICAR) may be elevated. Studies[193] suggest that the urinary excretion of more than 5 μg/day of methylmalonic acid is diagnostic of vitamin B_{12} deficiency (highly sensitive and specific).

The person with classic megaloblastic anemia appears pale, with a yellowish tint, has glossitis and thin irritated mucosae, complains of weakness and tiredness, may present with either diarrhea or constipation (more common in folate and B_{12} deficiencies, respectively), may be irritable and forgetful (more profound in folate deficiency), and often manifests combined degeneration of the posterolateral columns of the spinal cord (in the case of B_{12} deficiency), which is due to nervous system damage both centrally (in the posterior and lateral columns) and peripherally (in the myelinated nerves). The lesion begins insidiously and includes paresthesias and numbness of the hands and feet, usually a diminution of vibrational and positional senses, ataxia, moodiness, poor memory, confusion, and depression. The condition ultimately can evolve into delusions, hallucinations, and an overt psychosis. The peripheral nerve disease is in most cases bilateral and symmetric. Characteristically, indigent people who consume overall poor diets develop anemia and neurologic symptoms more or less in a balanced form whereas individuals whose diet is very good but who have

specific B_{12} deficiency may suffer almost exclusively from the neurologic syndrome. This is also the case for vitamin B_{12}–deficient vegetarians.

Therapy with parenteral B_{12} (100 μg or more) will produce a dramatic remission in deficiency patients. When the cause of deficiency is impaired absorption, monthly injections of 100 μg of the vitamin prevent further recurrences. Vitamin B_{12} is nontoxic even in huge doses.

Vitamin C

Vitamin C is a simple carbohydrate ($C_6H_8O_6$) with the name L-ascorbic acid. It is very soluble in water, stable in acid media, and destroyed by alkali and oxygen, particularly in the presence of catalysts, such as ionic copper. Its oxidized form, dehydro-L-ascorbic acid can correct vitamin C deficiency, since it is reversibly reduced to L-ascorbic acid. In certain species ascorbate sulfate also shows vitamin C activity; however, in some populations and under experimental conditions,[194-196] high intakes and elevated serum levels of dehydro-L-ascorbic acid have been associated with higher rates of diabetes mellitus. In the process of oxidation, L-ascorbic acid is first converted to dehydro-L-ascorbic acid. Further oxidation gives origin to diketogulonic and oxalic acids, CO_2, L-xylose, and other derivatives that have irreversibly lost all vitamin C activity. At lower intakes of L-ascorbic acid, oxalic acid is the predominant urinary metabolite; at higher intakes, urinary excretion of ascorbic acid increases proportionally.[196-197]

Ascorbic acid is widely distributed, primarily in the vegetable kindgom, where it is easily synthesized and is present in large amounts of fresh and growing plants. Dormant plant foods, such as cereal grains, seeds, and nuts, are relatively poor sources of vitamin C. Vegetable sources of vitamin C have been divided into three convenient categories—excellent, good, and fair—which on a 100 mg basis provide, respectively, 100 or more, 50 to 100, and 30 to 50 mg. In the first category are the berry family, black currants, guava, sweet peppers, broccoli, and brussels sprouts. The second category includes cabbage, cauliflower, mustard greens, beet greens, spinach, water cress, and most of the juicy citrus fruits. In the third category are asparagus, lima beans, potatoes, turnips, and a few fruits, such as tomatoes, melons, grapefruit, and lime. Even though some of these foods contain little vitamin

C, the fact that they are eaten in large quantities, as is the case with potatoes, makes them an important source of this vitamin.

Most animal flesh contains vitamin C, but in small quantities. Only a few animals are unable to convert L-gulonolactone to L-ascorbic acid; these species require the vitamin in their diet. They include humans, monkeys, guinea pigs, Indian fruit-eating bats, and the red-vented bulbul, as well as some other birds. There is discussion as to whether the inability to produce ascorbic acid by humans is total and universal. Suggestions have been made that certain individuals and persons with certain physiologic conditions (i.e., pregnancy and lactation) can produce small amounts of ascorbic acid.

At present, recommended dietary allowances are 60 mg/day for adults, 100 mg for pregnant and lactating women and premature infants (to prevent transient tyrosinemia), and 45 mg for children.[155]

Interpretation of available data on vitamin C nutrition suggests that the recommended dietary intakes can be lower than the 1980 RDAs and still maintain an adequate ascorbic acid pool and prevent deficiency. Arguments also exist[199-203] as to the need for higher intakes to optimize certain endocrine and reproductive functions, facilitate iron absorption from diets with low iron bioavailability, and increase the protective role of the vitamin as an inhibitor of nitrosamine formation in the gastrointestinal tract. Persons continually exposed to increased oxidative risks (free-radical damage), such as smokers, require higher levels of ascorbic acid intake.[67-69,204]

Biochemical function. Vitamin C is a powerful reducing agent, and its biologic function is linked to this important property in both plants and animals. Ascorbic acid and dehydroascorbic acid are involved in setting the oxidation-reduction potential in the cell, which appears to be importantly linked to the oxidation and reduction of the tripeptide glutathion. Vitamin C's role as a water-soluble antioxidant is important in protecting other antioxidants, even though they may be lipid-soluble, such as vitamin A, essential fatty acids, and vitamin E. It also is involved in maintaining the folacin coenzymes dehydro- and tetrahydrofolic acids in a reduced form, and possibly iron in the ferrous state during its absorption. Ascorbic acid is important as an electron donor for transfer across membranes to reduce

prosthetic metal ions of enzymes involved in many hydroxylation reactions, among which are those that explain several of the clinical signs and symptoms of scurvy as they become less active: production of C-terminal amidated peptides in the pituitary and epinephrine in the adrenal medulla, the production of hydroxyproline from proline in collagen, the oxidation of tyrosine by parahydroxyphenylpyruvic-acid oxidase, the hydroxylation of tryptophan to 5-OH-tryptophan and then to serotonin, II-beta-hydroxylation and steroid secretion by the adrenals and ovaries, and the metabolism of 3,4-dihydroxyphenylethylamine to norepinephrine. (These last two compounds are important neurotransmitters.) Some studies* further indicate that ascorbic acid can inactivate lipase in the presence of ATP and magnesium chloride. Even though the adrenals are rich in vitamin C, and upon secretion of corticosteroids large amounts of vitamin C are lost from them, the specific biochemical link of vitamin C with steroid production and/or secretion has not been clearly identified. Importantly, many features of scurvy are still unexplained by these defects.[197]

Ascorbic acid metabolism. Ascorbic acid is readily and rapidly absorbed in the upper small intestine and very little fecal loss occurs normally. The processes of facilitated diffusion at the brush border and active transport at the basolateral membrane, similar to those operating in the absorption of simple hexoses, are involved in the absorption of ascorbic acid by the intestinal cell as well as the renal tubular cell. In the intestine, dehydroascorbate is reduced to ascorbic acid in humans and species that do not synthesize vitamin C.[207] Studies with small doses of ^{14}C-L-ascorbic acid have shown most of its excretion to occur through the urine as ascorbic acid or several metabolites, with only minute amounts appearing in feces, sweat, and expired CO_2. The dynamics of kidney reabsorption show clear threshold and maximum reabsorptive capacities; total reabsorption takes place when the concentration in plasma is less than 15 mg/liter. Consequently, large loads of ascorbic acid in the intestine and the kidney tubule result in poor absorption and tubular reabsorption, respectively, and in significant fecal and renal losses.[208]

---

*References 201, 205, 206.

After absorption ascorbic acid is taken up by all cells of the body, reaching different concentrations in different tissues. The glandular tissues (adrenals, pancreas, salivary glands, testes, spleen) generally concentrate ascorbic acid, although large accumulations also occur in the eye (lens and aqueous humor), brain, pituitary, and liver. The average body pool is 1.5 g in persons receiving around 75 mg of ascorbic acid per day, and 3% of it is catabolized daily. If the diet provides 30 mg of ascorbic acid/day, the total body pool is around 1 g. In a classic study[209] of experimental vitamin C deficiency, after about 60 days on a vitamin C–free diet the subjects' mean fell to 300 mg and the daily catabolic rate was below 9 mg. At this level, deficiency signs began to appear.

Serum, plasma, white cell, or buffy coat ascorbic acid levels are used for evaluating vitamin C status. It is generally agreed that vitamin C deficiency can be diagnosed only when its levels are below 2 mg/liter of serum or below $2 \mu g/10^8$ white cells. Vitamin C levels in human connective tissue are markedly depressed when blood levels reach these limits.[210] Plasma ascorbate reflects intake whereas white cell ascorbate reflects cellular levels.[211] Plasma levels are lower among elderly men than among elderly women on the same intakes.[212]

Vitamin C deficiency, or scurvy. Vitamin C deficiency was well described in medical writings of ancient cultures because it affected primarily sailors and soldiers and thus greatly influenced the development of history. It also occurred in mild epidemic forms, the last having been in the late 1800s among infants fed boiled and pasteurized milk. At present, scurvy is seen only in indigent persons or in children and the elderly who are fed unusual diets. Occasionally it follows discontinuation of megadoses of vitamin C because of induced continued high rate of ascorbic acid catabolism.[109,213]

The first manifestations of scurvy appear after about 60 days of no ascorbic acid intake, and consist of small recurrent ecchymoses and petechiae that progressively coalesce to form larger ecchymoses later. Typically, many of these petechiae are perifollicular, surrounding a hyperkeratotic follicle containing a plug or a corkscrew-like hair. which may also be broken. Follicular hyperkeratosis also becomes apparent on the back of the arms, buttocks, thighs, and calves. About this time the gums also become swollen, hemorrhagic, and finally necrotic; this change occurs only when teeth are present, begins at the molar areas, and is retarded by good hygiene. Secondary periodontal infection can take place.

Under natural circumstances, scurvy in adults develops in 120-150 days of a vitamin C–poor diet. By this time, white-cell vitamin C levels are essentially zero. Plasma vitamin C reaches very low levels much earlier, in about 4 weeks. Other early manifestations of scurvy are weakness; anorexia; aching bones, joints, and muscles; and mental depression, listlessness, apathy, and hysteria. Hemorrhages are also evident in old scars, which in extreme cases may actually reopen, as has been described also for old healed bone fractures (because of bone resorption in the presence of impaired formation of bone trabeculae). Loosening of teeth and dental fillings, dryness of the mouth and eyes, loss of hair, and skin dryness with pruritus can also develop (Sjögren's syndrome). Vasomotor instability, engorgement of capillary beds, oliguria, dependent edema, and hemorrhages from small blood vessel ruptures are common. Sudden cardiovascular death may be seen in full-blown scurvy. When hemorrhages occur in nerve sheaths, peripheral neuropathy can develop; when they occur in the subperiosteal region, tender bone swellings, particularly in the upper humerus and distal femur and around the diaphyseal-epiphyseal cartilage and costochondral junctions, are characteristic, primarily in infants. In infantile scurvy the child typically assumes a froglike position, with pseudoparalysis, is extremely apprehensive of being handled because of periosteal pain, is irritable and anorexic, and may have petechiae. Hemorrhagic manifestations are common, including epistaxis, bloody diarrhea, hematuria, bleeding gums around erupting teeth, and retrobulbar bleeding.

Subperiosteal separation and hemorrhages with absence of calcification in the diaphyseal-epiphyseal junction constitute the "corner sign of Park," which is an almost pathognomonic radiologic sign of infantile scurvy. Thickened diaphyseal lines with subepiphyseal atrophy, linear transverse fractures, and radiolucent ossification centers are also typical. In extreme cases the sternum, together with the cartilaginous ribs, suffers posterior subluxation and the anterior bony extremes of the ribs form a sharp angle with the cartilage.

Anemia is a common feature in scurvy, possibly because of hemorrhages, alterations of folate metabolism, and impaired iron absorption.

The prevention and treatment of scurvy have become classic nutritional feats. The preventive value of lemon juice, of fresh vegetables, of fruits, and of foods in general, and even a decoction of pine needles and bark, have been known since the sixteenth century, but it was only in the late eighteenth century that specific measures were taken by the British navy to prevent scurvy. A prompt and sustained improvement in scorbutic signs has been obtained with doses of vitamin C ranging from 5 to 60 mg/day, so a therapeutic scheme of 100 mg of ascorbic acid three times a day by mouth or, if necessary, parenterally, is more than ample. Once the diagnosis is established, therapy should be instituted promptly because of the danger of sudden death.

Toxicity. Vitamin C is essentially free of acute toxic effects, but the following alterations have been described as a consequence of the sustained intake of masssive doses (in the gram range) of this vitamin: diarrhea of the osmotic type, caused by poor absorption; impaired absorption of vitamin B_{12}; increased urinary oxalic acid excretion, possibly increased formation of calcium oxalate stones, and precipitation of uric acid; reversal of anticoagulant effects of heparin in vitro and dicumarol in vivo; possible chronic iron overload; reduction of copper-containing reagents used in the detection of glycosuria, giving false-positive or false-negative reactions in tests for glycosuria based on glucose oxidase; increased serum cholesterol; and enzyme induction of catabolic reactions, so that upon withdrawal of C megadoses, blood concentrations become abnormally low and there is a conditioned deficiency, with relative lack of responsiveness to normal doses of the vitamin.[213]

Pauling et al.[214] have advocated the ingestion of massive vitamin C doses as a prevention for infection and treatment of colds. The overwhelming evidence, however,[197,215] is that this "orthomolecular medicine" is totally ineffective or its benefits may be so slight as not to be justified. Inadequate evidence exists also at present to attribute a preventive role to ascorbic acid in the development and progression of cancer and atherosclerosis.[197] By contrast, some rather convincing evidence[216] has begun to accumulate on the preventive role of vitamin C intake in the development of bone demineralization and osteoporosis.

REFERENCES

1. Goodwin TW: Metabolism, nutrition and functions of carotenoids, Annu Rev Nutr **6**:273-279, 1986.
2. Olson JA: The metabolism of vitamin A, Pharmacol Rev **19**:559-596, 1967.
3. Mathews-Roth MM: Photoprotection by carotenoids, Fed Proc **46**:1890-1893, 1987.
4. Goodman DS, et al: The intestinal absorption and metabolism of vitamin A and β-carotene in man, J Clin Invest **45**:1615-1623, 1966.
5. Ong DE: A novel retinol-binding protein from rat: purification and partial characterization, J Biol Chem **259**:1476-1482, 1984.
6. Pitt GAJ, editor: Biological roles of retinol and other retinoids. Society/Host Colloquim, Biochem Soc Trans **14**:923-945, 1986.
7. Olson JA: Serum levels of vitamin A and carotenoids as reflectors of nutritional status, J Natl Cancer Inst **73**:1439-1444, 1984.
8. Green MH, et al: A multicompartmental model of vitamin A kinetics in rats with marginal liver vitamin A stores, J Lipid Res **26**:806-818, 1985.
9. Ong DE, Page DL: Quantitation of cellular retinol binding protein in human organs, Am J Clin Nutr **44**:425-430, 1986.
10. Ong DE: Vitamin A binding proteins, Nutr Rev **43**:225-232, 1985.
11. Fidge NW, et al: Pathways of absorption of retinal and retinoic acid in the rat, J Lipid Res **9**:103-109, 1968.
12. Mandani KA: Retinoic acid: a general overview, Nutr Res **6**:107-123, 1986.
13. DeLuca HF, Roberts AB: Pathways of retinoic acid and retinol metabolism, Am J Clin Nutr **22**:945-952, 1969.
14. Smith JE, et al: The plasma transport and metabolism of retinoic acid in the rat, Biochem J **132**:821-827, 1973.
15. DeLuca LM, et al: Biosynthesis of phosphoryl and glycosyl phosphoryl derivatives of vitamin A in biological membranes, Fed Proc **38**:2535-2539, 1979.
16. Wiss O, Gloor U: Vitamin A and lipid metabolism, Vitam Horm **18**:485-498, 1960.
17. Roels OA, et al: The effect of vitamin A deficiency and dietary alpha-tocopherol on the stability of rat-liver lysosomes, Biochem J **97**:353-359, 1965.
18. Chytil F, Ong EE: Intracellular vitamin A binding proteins, Annu Rev Nutr **7**:321-335, 1987.
19. Kim HY, Wolf G: Vitamin A deficiency alters genomic expression for fibronectin in liver hepatocytes, J Biol Chem **262**:365-371, 1987.
20. Porter SB, et al: Vitamin A status affects chromatin structure, Int J Vitam Nutr Res **56**:11-20, 1986.

21. Chertow BS, et al: Effects of vitamin A depletion and repletion on rat insulin secretion in vivo and in vitro from isolated cells, J Clin Invest **79:**163-169, 1987.

22. Petkovich, et al: Retinoic acid stimulates 1,25-dehydroxyvitamin D$_3$ binding in rat osteosarcoma cells, J Biol Chem **259:**8274-8280, 1984.

23. Puengtomwatanakul S, Sirisinha S: Impaired biliary secretion of immunoglobulin A in vitamin A-deficient rats, Proc Soc Exp Biol Med **182:**437-442, 1986.

24. World Health Organization: Control of vitamin A deficiency and xerophthalmia. Report of a Joint WHO/UN-ICEF/ISAID Helen Keller International/IVACG Meeting, WHO Tech Rep Ser 672, 1982.

25. Olson JA: Carotenoids, vitamin A, and cancer, J Nutr **116:**1127-1130, 1986.

26. Olson JA: Recommended dietary intakes (RDI) of vitamin A in humans, Am J Clin Nutr **45:**704-716, 1987.

27. Amedee-Manesme O, et al: Relation of the relative dose response to liver concentrations of vitamin A in generally well nourished surgical patients, Am J Clin Nutr **39:**898-902, 1984.

28. Sommer A, et al: Increased risk of xerophthalmia following diarrhea and respiratory disease, Am J Clin Nutr **45:**977-980, 1987.

29. Roe DA: Photodegradation of carotenoids in human subjects, Fed Proc **46:**1886-1889, 1987.

30. Sommer A, et al: Increased mortality in children with mild vitamin A deficiency, Lancet **2:**585-588, 1983.

31. Sommer A, et al: Increased risk of respiratory disease and diarrhea in children with preceding mild vitamin A deficiency, Am J Clin Nutr **40:**1080-1095, 1984.

32. Sommer A, et al: Impact of vitamin A supplementation on childhood mortality, Lancet **1:**1168-1173, 1986.

33. Milton RC: Mild vitamin A deficiency and childhood morbidity—an Indian experience, Am J Clin Nutr **46:**827-829, 1987.

34. Arroyave G, et al: Evaluation of sugar fortification with vitamin A at the national level, Sci Publ 384, Washington DC, 1979, Pan American Health Organization.

35. Solon FS, et al: Planning, implementation and evaluation of a fortification program, J Am Diet Assoc **74:**112-118, 1979.

36. Lammer EJ, et al: Retinoic acid embryopathy, N Engl J Med **313:**837-841, 1985.

37. Muenter MD, et al: Chronic vitamin A intoxication in adults. Hepatic, neurologic and dermatologic complications, Am J Med **50:**129-136, 1971.

38. Holick MF: Photosynthesis of vitamin D in the skin: effect of environmental and life-style variables, Fed Proc **46:**1876-1882, 1987.

39. Editorial: The vitamin D endocrine system and the hematolymphopoietic tissue, Ann Intern Med **100:**144-146, 1984.

40. Bell NH: Vitamin D endocrine system, J Clin Invest **76:**1-6, 1985.

41. DeLuca HF: Vitamin D. In Goodhart RS, Shils ME, editors: Modern nutrition in health and disease, ed 6, Philadelphia, 1980, Lea & Febiger, pp 160-170.

42. Kuman R: The metabolism and mechanism of action of 1,25-dihydroxyvitamin D$_3$, Kidney Int **30:**793-803, 1986.

43. DeLuca HF: The metabolism, physiology, and function of vitamin D. In Kumar R, editor: Vitamin D: basic and clinical aspects, Hingham Mass, 1984, Martin Nijhoff Publishers, pp 1-68.

44. Avioli LV, et al: Metabolism of vitamin D$_3$–3H in vitamin D–resistant rickets and familial hypophosphatemia, J Clin Invest **46:**1907-1915, 1967.

45. DeLuca HF: Vitamin D: the vitamin and the hormone, Fed Proc **33:**2211-2219, 1974.

46. Pike JW: Intracellular receptors mediate the biologic action of 1,25-dihydroxyvitamin D$_3$, Nutr Rev **43:**161-168, 1985.

47. Haussler MR: Vitamin D receptors: nature and function, Annu Rev Nutr **6:**527-562, 1986.

48. Wongsurawat N, Armbrecht HJ: Insulin modulates the stimulation of renal 1,25-dihydroxyvitamin D$_3$ production by parathyroid hormone, Acta Endocrinol **109:**243-248, 1985.

49. Matsumoto T, et al: Role of insulin in the increase in serum 1,25-dihydroxyvitamin D concentrations in response to phosphorus deprivation in streptozotocin-induced diabetic rats, Endocrinology **118:**1440-1444, 1986.

50. Cade C, Norman AW: Vitamin D$_3$ improves impaired glucose tolerance and insulin secretion in the vitamin D-deficient rat in vivo, Endocrinology **119:**84-90, 1986.

51. DeLuca HF: The role of vitamin D and its relationship to parathyroid hormone and calcitonin, Recent Prog Horm Res **27:**479-516, 1971.

52. Davidson S, et al: Rickets and osteomalacia. In Human nutrition and dietetics, New York, 1979, Churchill-Livingstone Inc, pp 276-282.

53. Avioli LV, editor: Vitamin D metabolites: their clinical importance, Arch Intern Med (special issue) **138:**835-888, 1978.

54. Holick MF, et al: 1α-Hydroxy derivative of vitamin D$_3$. A highly potent analog of 1α,25-dihydroxyvitamin D$_3$, Science **180:**190-191, 1973.

55. Sitrin MB, Rosenberg IH: Vitamin D. In Warren KN, Mahmoud AAF, editors: Tropical and geographical medicine, New York, 1984, McGraw-Hill International Book Co.

56. Clements MR, et al: A new mechanism for induced vitamin D deficiency in calcium deprivation, Nature **325:**62-65, 1987.

57. McKenna MJ, et al: Hypovitaminosis D and elevated serum alkaline phosphatases in elderly Irish people, Am J Clin Nutr **41:**101-109, 1985.

58. Chapuy MC, et al: Calcium and vitamin D supplements: effects on calcium metabolism in elderly people, Am J Clin Nutr **46:**324-328, 1987.

59. Hahn TJ, et al: Serum 25-hydroxycalciferol levels and bone mass in children on chronic anticonvulsant therapy, N Engl J Med **292:**550-554, 1975.

60. Haussler MR, McCain TA: Basic and clinical concepts related to vitamin D metabolism and action, N Engl J Med **297:**974-983, 1041-1050, 1977.

61. Milhaud GE: In Talmage RV, Berlanger LF, editors: Parathyroid hormone and thyrocalcitonin (calcitonin), New York, 1968, Excerpta Medica Foundation.

62. Resnick LM: Calcium and vitamin D metabolism in the pathophysiology of human hypertension. In Levander OA, editor: AIN Symposium Proceedings, Nutrition '87, Bethesda, 1987, American Institute of Nutrition, pp 110-114.

63. Bell NH, et al: Evidence for alteration of the vitamin D–endocrine system in blacks, J Clin Invest **76**:470-473, 1985.

64. Merke J, et al: 1,25-$(OH)_2$-D_3 receptors and actions in endothelial and smooth muscle cells of arterial vessels, Abstract 908, Eleventh Scientific Meeting of the International Society of Hypertension, Heidelberg, 1984.

65. Markestad T, et al: Intermittent high-dose vitamin D prophylaxis during infancy: effect on vitamin D metabolites, calcium and phosphorus, Am J Clin Nutr **46**:652-658, 1987.

66. Horwitt MK: Vitamin E. In Goodhart RS, Shils ME, editors: Modern nutrition in health and disease, Philadelphia, 1980, Lea & Febiger, pp 181-191.

67. McCay PB: Vitamin E: interactions with free radicals and ascorbate, Annu Rev Nutr **5**:323-340, 1985.

68. Machlin LJ, Bendich A: Free radical tissue damage: protective role of antioxidant nutrients, FASEB J **1**:441-445, 1987.

69. Slater TR: Free radical-mediated tissue damage. In Levander OA, editor: AIN Symposium Proceedings, Nutrition '87, Bethesda, 1987, American Institute of Nutrition, pp 46-50.

70. Summerfield FW, Tappel AL: Effects of dietary polyunsaturated fats and vitamin A on aging and peroxidative damage to DNA, Arch Biochem Biophys **233**:408-416, 1984.

71. Horwitt MK: Interpretations of requirements for thiamin, riboflavin, niacin-triptophan, and vitamin E plus comments on balance studies and vitamin B_6, Am J Clin Res **44**:973-985, 1986.

72. Burton GW, et al: Is vitamin E the only lipid-soluble, chain-braking antioxidant in human blood plasma and the erythrocyte membranes? Arch Biochem Biophys **221**:281-290, 1983.

73. Harris PL, Embree ND: Quantitative consideration of the effect of polyunsaturated fatty acid content on the diet upon the requirement for vitamin E, Am J Clin Nutr **13**:285-292, 1963.

74. Mason KE, Horwitt MK: Effects of deficiency in man. In Sebrell WH, Harris RS, editors: The vitamins, vol 5, New York, 1972, Academic Pres Inc, pp 293-309.

75. Oski FA, Barness LA: Vitamin E deficiency: a previously unrecognized cause of hemolytic anemia in the premature infant, J Pediatr **70**:211-220, 1967.

76. Hassan H, et al: Syndrome in premature infants associated with low plasma vitamin E levels and high polyunsaturated fatty acid diet, Am J Clin Nutr **19**:147-157, 1966.

77. Johnson L, et al: The premature infant, vitamin E deficiency and retrolental fibroplasia, Am J Clin Nutr **27**:1158-1173, 1974.

78. Binder HJ, et al: Tocopherol deficiency in man, N Engl J Med **273**:1289-1297, 1965.

79. Horwitt MK, et al: Erythrocyte survival time and reticulocyte levels after tocopherol depletion in man, Am J Clin Nutr **12**:99-106, 1963.

80. Machlin LJ: Protective role of vitamins against free radical tissue damage. In Levander OA, editor: AIN Symposium Proceedings, Nutrition '87, Bethesda, 1987, American Institute of Nutrition, pp 51-54.

81. Halliwell B: Oxidants and human disease: some new concepts, FASEB J **1**:358-364, 1987.

82. Gay KF, et al: Plasma levels of antioxidant vitamins in relation to ischemic heart disease and cancer, Am J Clin Nutr **45**:1368-1377, 1987.

83. Gohil K, et al: Vitamin E deficiency and vitamin C supplements: exercise and mitochondrial oxidation, J Appl Physiol **60**:1986-1991, 1986.

84. Corrigan JJ, Marcus FI: Coagulopathy associated with vitamin E ingestion, JAMA **230**:1300-1303, 1974.

85. Farrrell PM, Bieri JG: Megavitamin E supplementation in man, Am J Clin Nutr **28**:1381-1386, 1975.

86. Johnson L, et al: Relationship of prolonged pharmacologic serum levels of vitamin E to incidence of sepsis and necrotizing enterocolitis in infants with birth weight 1,500 grams or less, Pediatrics **75**:619-638, 1985.

87. Suttis JW, Olson RE: Vitamin K. In Olson RE, et al, editors: Present knowledge of nutrition, Washington DC, 1984, The Nutrition Foundation Inc, pp 241-259.

88. Bjornsson TD, et al: Disposition and turnover of vitamin K_1 in man. In Suttie JW, editor: Vitamin K metabolism and vitamin K–dependent proteins, Baltimore, 1980, University Park Press, pp 328-332.

89. Olson JA: Recommended dietary intakes (RDI) of vitamin K in humans, Am J Clin Nutr **45**:687-692, 1987.

90. Ansell JE, et al: The spectrum of vitamin K deficiency, JAMA **238**:40-42, 1977.

91. Olson RE, Suttie JW: Vitamin K and carboxyglutamate biosynthesis, Vitam Horm **35**:59-108, 1977.

92. Lian JB, Prien EL Jr: γ-Carboxyglutamic acid in the calcium binding matrix of certain kidney stones, Fed Proc **35**:1763, 1976.

93. Blanchard KA, et al: Immuno assay of human prothrombin species which correlate with functional coagulation activities, J Lab Clin Med **101**:242-255, 1983.

94. Graves CB: Immunochemical isolation and electrophoretic characterization of precursor prothrombines in H-35 rat hepatoma cells, Biochemistry **19**:266-272, 1980.

95. Oski FA, Naiman JL: Hematologic problems in the newborn, ed 2, Philadelphia, 1972, WB Saunders Co.

96. Owen CA: Vitamin K, pharmacology and toxicology. In Sebrell WH Jr, Harris RS, editors: The vitamins, vol 3, New York, 1971, Academic Press Inc, pp 492-509.

97. Chaow WT, et al: Intracranial hemorrhage and vitamin K deficiency in early infancy, J Pediatr **105**:880-884, 1984.

98. Committee on Nutrition: American Academy of Pediatrics, Nutrition needs of low birth weight infants, Pediatrics **75**:976-986, 1985.

99. Hart JP, et al: Electrochemical detection of depressed circulating levels of vitamin K_1 in osteoporosis, J Clin Endocrinol Metab **60**:1268-1269, 1985.

100. Dodds RA, et al: Effects on fracture healing of an antagonist of the vitamin K cycle, Calcif Tissue Int **36**:233-238, 1984.

101. Neal RA, Sauberlich HE: Thiamin. In Goodhart RS, Shils ME, editors: Modern nutrition in health and disease, ed 6, Philadelphia, 1980, Lea & Febiger, pp 191-197.

102. Thomson AD, et al: Folate-induced malabsorption of thiamin, Gastroenterology **60**:756, 1971.

103. Tanphaichitr V, Wood B: Thiamin. In Olson RE, et al, editors: Present knowledge in nutrition, Washington DC, 1984, The Nutrition Foundation Inc, pp 273-284.

104. Sauberlich HE: Biochemical alterations in thiamin deficiency–their interpretation, Am J Clin Nutr **20**:528-546, 1967.

105. Davidson S, et al: Beriberi and the Wernicke-Korsakoff syndrome. In Human nutrition and dietetics, ed 7, New York, 1979, Churchill-Livingstone Inc, pp 283-288.

106. Thomson AD, et al: Possible role of toxins in nutritional deficiency, Am J Clin Nutr 45:1351-1360, 1987.

107. Blass JP, Gibson GE: Abnormality of A thiamine-requiring enzyme in Wernicke-Korsakoff syndrome, N Engl J Med 297:1367-1370, 1977.

108. Jeyasingham MD, et al: Reduced stability of rat brain transquetolase after conversion to the apo form, J Neurochem 47:278-281, 1986.

109. Sandstead HH: Clinical manifestations of certain classical deficiency diseases. In Goodhart RS, Shils ME, editors, Modern nutrition in health and disease, ed 6, Philadelphia, 1980, Lea & Febiger, pp 685-696.

110. Victor M, Adams RD: Etiology of the alcoholic neurologic diseases, Am J Clin Nutr 91:379-397, 1961.

111. Whitfield CL, et al: Detoxification of 1,024 alcoholic patients without psychoactive drugs, JAMA 239:1409-1410, 1978.

112. Sebrell WH, Harris RS, editors: The vitamins. Chemistry, physiology, pathology, methods, New York, 1972, Academic Press Inc, p 961.

113. Rivlin RS, editor: Riboflavin, New York, 1975, Plenum Press Inc.

114. Slater EC, editor: Flavins and flavoproteins, New York, 1966, American Elsevier Publishing Co Inc.

115. Rivlin RS: Riboflavin. In Olson RE, et al, editors: Present knowledge in nutrition, Washington DC, 1984, The Nutrition Foundation Inc, pp 285-302.

116. Horwitt MK: Nutritional requirements of man with special reference to riboflavin, Am J Clin Nutr 18:458-466, 1966.

117. Sauberlich HE, et al: Application of the erythrocyte glutathione reductase assay in evaluating riboflavin nutritional status in a high school population, Am J Clin Nutr 25:746-762, 1972.

118. Horwitt MK: Riboflavin. In Goodhart RS, Shils ME, editors: Modern nutrition in health and disease, ed 6, Philadelphia, 1980, Lea & Febiger, pp 197-203.

119. Foy H, Kondi A: Comparison between erythroid aplasia in marasmus and experimentally induced erythroid aplasia in baboons by riboflavin deficiency, Vitam Horm 26:653-684, 1968.

120. Yagi K, et al: Flavins and flavoproteins. In Massey V, Williams CH Jr, editors: Seventh International Symposium, New York, 1982, Elsevier Science Publishing Co Inc, pp 402-409.

121. Sisson TRC: Photodegradation of riboflavin in neonates, Fed Proc 46:1883-1885, 1987.

122. Zimmerman SB, et al: Enzymatic joining of DNA strands: a novel reaction of diphosphopyridine nucleotide, Proc Natl Acad Sci USA 57:1841-1848, 1967.

123. Horwitt MK, et al: Tryptophan-niacin relationships in man, J Nutr 60(suppl 1):1-43, 1956.

124. Rose DP, Braidman IP: Excretion of tryptophan metabolites as affected by pregnancy, contraceptive steroids and steroid hormones, Am J Clin Nutr 24:673-683, 1971.

125. Horwitt MK, et al: Niacin tryptophan relationships for evaluating niacin equivalents, Am J Clin Nutr 34:423-427, 1981.

126. Darby WJ, et al: In Present knowledge in nutrition, ed 4, New York, 1976, The Nutrition Foundation Inc, pp 162-174.

127. Gopalan C, Jaya Rao KS: Pellagra and amino acid imbalance, Vitam Horm 33:914-919, 1975.

128. Narasinga Rao BS, Gopalan C: Niacin. In Olson RE, et al, editors: Present knowledge in nutrition, Washington DC, 1984, The Nutrition Foundation Inc, pp 318-331.

129. Sandstead HH: Clinical manifestations of certain classical deficiency diseases. In Goodhart RS, Shils ME, editors: Modern nutrition in health and disease, ed 6, Philadelphia, 1980, Lea & Febiger, pp 685-696.

130. Singh M: Effect of niacin and niacin-tryptophan deficiency on pancreatic acinar cell function in rats in vitro, Am J Clin Nutr 44:512-518, 1986.

131. Sauberlich HE, et al: Laboratory tests for the assessment of nutritional status, Cleveland, 1974, CRC Press Inc.

132. Miller ON, et al: Investigation of the mechanism of action of nicotinic acid on serum lipid levels in man, Am J Clin Nutr 8:480-490, 1960.

133. Coronary Drug Project Research Group: Clofibrate and niacin in coronary heart disease, JAMA 321:360-381, 1975.

134. Gregory JF, Kirk JR: Vitamin B_6 in foods: assessment of stability and bioavailability. In Human vitamin B_6 requirements, Washington DC, 1978, National Academy of Sciences, pp 72-77.

135. Ink SL, Henderson LM: Vitamin B_6 metabolism, Annu Rev Nutr 4:455-470, 1984.

136. Tryfiates GB, editor: Vitamin B_6 metabolism and role in growth, Westport Conn, 1960, Nutrition Press.

137. Black AL, et al: The behavior of muscle phosphorylase as a reservoire for vitamin B_6 in the rat, J Nutr 109:670-677, 1978.

138. Mancra MM, et al: Vitamin B_6 metabolism as affected by exercise in trained and untrained women fed diets differing in carbohydrates and vitamin B_6 content, Am J Clin Nutr 46:995-1004, 1987.

139. Reynolds RD, Leklem JE, editors: Vitamin B_6: its role in health and disease, Curr Top Nutr Dis 13:526, 1985.

140. Sauberlich HE, et al: Human vitamin B_6 nutriture, J Sci Ind Res 29(suppl 8):S28-S37, 1970.

141. Cornish HH: The role of vitamin B_6 in the toxicity of hydrazines, Ann NY Acad Sci 166:136-145, 1969.

142. Gershoff SN: Vitamin B_6. In Present knowledge in nutrition, ed 4, New York, 1976, The Nutrition Foundation Inc, pp 140-161.

143. Snyderman SE, et al: Pyridoxine deficiency in the human infant, Am J Clin Nutr 1:200-207, 1953.

144. McCoy EE, et al: The excretion of oxalic acid following deoxypyridoxine and tryptophan administration in mongoloid and nonmongoloid subjects, J Pediatr 65:208-214, 1965.

145. Merrill AH Jr, Henderson JM: Diseases associated with defects in vitamin B_6 metabolism or utilization, Annu Rev Nutr 7:137-157, 1987.

146. Hodges RE, et al: Factors affecting human antibody response, Am J Clin Nutr 11:187-199, 1962.

147. Ha C, et al: The effect of vitamin B_6 deficiency on host susceptibility to Maloney sarcoma virus-induced tumor growth in mice, J Nutr 114:938-945, 1984.

148. Sauberlich HE, et al: Laboratory tests for the assessment of nutritional status, Cleveland, 1974, CRC Press Inc, p 136.

149. LeKlem JE, Reynolds RD: Vitamin B_6 methodology

and nutritional assessment, New York, 1981, Plenum Press Inc.

150. Scriver CR, Whelan DT: Glutamic acid decarboxylase (GAD) in mammalian tissue outside the central nervous system, and its possible relevance to hereditary vitamin B_6 dependency with seizures, Ann NY Acad Sci **166**:83-96, 1969.

151. Mudd SH: Pyridoxine-responsive genetic disease, Fed Proc **30**:970-976, 1971.

152. Gyorgy P: Developments leading to the metabolic role of vitamin B_6, Am J Clin Nutr **24**:1250-1256, 1971.

153. Hunt IF, et al: Zinc, vitamin B_6, and other nutrients in pregnant women attending prenatal clinics in Mexico, Am J Clin Nutr **46**:563-568, 1987.

154. Cotzias GC: Metabolic modification of some neurologic disorders, JAMA **210**:1255-1262, 1969.

155. Committee on Dietary Allowances, Food and Nutrition Board, National Research Council: Recommended dietary allowances, ed 9, Washington DC, 1980, National Academy of Sciences.

156. Krumdieck CL: Folic acid. In Present knowledge in nutrition, New York, 1976, The Nutrition Foundation Inc, pp 175-190.

157. Herbert V: Recommended dietary intakes (RDI) of folates in humans, Am J Clin Nutr **45**:661-670, 1987.

158. Herbert V, et al: Folic acid and vitamin B_{12}. In Goodhart RS, Shils ME, editors: Modern nutrition in health and disease, ed 6, Philadelphia, 1980, Lea & Febiger, pp 229-259.

159. Shane B: Vitmin B_{12}–folate interrrelationships, Annu Rev Nutr **5**:115-141, 1985.

160. Fujii K, et al: Accumulation of 5-methyl-tetrahydrofolate in cobalamin-deficient L1210 mouse leukemia cells, J Biol Chem **257**:2144-2146, 1982.

161. Stokstad ELP, et al: Role of methylenetetrahydrofolate reductase in regulation of folic acid metabolism and its relation to the methyl trap hypothesis. In Blair AJ, editor: Chemistry and biology of pteridines, Hawthorne NY, 1983, Walter DeGruyter Inc, pp 241-245.

162. Kisliuk RL: Pteroylpolyglutamates, Mol Cell Biochem **39**:331-345, 1981.

163. Galivan J: Hormonal alteration of methotraxate polyglutamate fermation in cultured hepatoma cells, Arch Biochem Biophys **230**:355-362, 1983.

164. Butterworth DE Jr, et al: A study of folate absorption and metabolism in man utilizing carbon-14–labeled polyglutamates synthesized by the solid phase method, J Clin Invest **48**:1131-1142, 1969.

165. Chanarin I: The megaloblastic anemias, ed 2, St. Louis, 1979, Blackwell-Mosby Book Distributors.

166. O'Sullivan H, et al: Human bone marrow biochemical function and megaloblastic hematopoiesis after nitrous oxide anesthesia, Anesthesiology **55**:645-649, 1981.

167. Amos RJ, et al: Prevention of nitrous oxide-induced megaloblastic changes in bone marrow using folinic acid, Br J Anesthesiol **56**:103-107, 1984.

168. Deacon R, et al: Impaired deoxyuridine utilization in the B_{12} inactivated rat and its correction by folate analogues, Biochem Biophys Res Commun **93**:516-520, 1980.

169. Tamura T, Stokstad ELR: The availability of food folate in man, Br J Hematol **25**:513-532, 1973.

170. Eells JT, et al: Methanol poisoning and formate oxidation in nitrous oxide treated rats, J Pharmacol Exp Ther **217**:57-61, 1981.

171. Pritchard JA, Macdonald PC: Williams obstetrics, ed 15, New York, 1976, Appleton-Century-Crofts.

172. Herbert V: Experimental nutritional folate deficiency in man, Trans Assoc Am Phys **75**:307-320, 1962.

173. Colman N, et al: Prevention of folate deficiency by food fortification. IV. Identification target groups in addition to pregnant women in an adult rural population, Am J Clin Nutr **28**:471-476, 1975.

174. Ch'ien LT, et al: Harmful effect of megadoses of vitamins: electroencephalogram abnormalities and seizures induced by intravenous folate in drug-treated epileptics, Am J Clin Nutr **28**:51-58, 1975.

175. Herbert V: Vitamin B_{12}. In Olson RE, et al, editors: Present knowledge in nutrition, Washington DC, 1984, The Nutrition Foundation Inc, pp 347-364.

176. Deacon R, et al: The effect of folate analogues on thymidine utilization by human and rat marrow cells and the effect on the deoxyuridine suppression test, Postgrad Med J **57**:611-617, 1981.

177. Chanarin I, et al: Cobalamin-folate interrelations: a critical review, Blood **66**:479-489, 1985.

178. Chanarin I, et al: Vitamin B_{12} regulates folate metabolism by the supply of formate, Lancet **2**:505-508, 1980.

179. Frenkel EP: Abnormal fatty acid metabolism in peripheral nerves of patients with pernicious anemia, J Clin Invest **52**:1237-1245, 1973.

180. Scott JM, et al: Pathogenesis of subacute combined degeneration: a result of methyl group deficiency, Lancet **2**:334-337, 1981.

181. Van der Westhuyzen J, Metz J: Tissue S-adenosylmethionine levels in fruit bats *(Rosettus aegyptiacus)* with nitrous oxide-induced neuropathy, Br J Nutr **50**:325-330, 1983.

182. Small DH, Carnegie PR: A new understanding of the role of vitamin B_{12} in methylation of proteins in the nervous system, Proc Nutr Soc Aust **5**:178-184, 1980.

183. Beck WS: Metabolic features of cobalamin deficiency in man. In Babior BM, editor: Cobalamin biochemistry and pathophysiology, New York, 1975, John Wiley & Sons Inc, pp 403-450.

184. Shin YL, et al: The relationships between vitamin B_{12} and folic acid and the effect of methionine on folate metabolism, Mol Cell Biochem **9**:97-108, 1975.

185. Herbert V: Detection of malabsorption of vitamin B_{12} due to gastric or intestinal dysfunction, Semin Nucl Med **2**:220-234, 1972.

186. Kanazawa S, et al: Enhancing effect of human bile on the uptake of free vitamin B_{12} and intrinsic factor-B_{12} by receptors on the small bowel epithelial cells, Blood **60**:30a, 1982.

187. Herbert V: Vitamin B_{12}, Am J Clin Nutr **34**:971-972, 1981.

188. Allen RH: Human vitamin B_{12} transport proteins, Prog Hematol **9**:57-84, 1975.

189. Cooper BA, Rosenblatt DS: Inherited defects of vitamin B_{12} metabolism, Annu Rev Nutr **7**:291-320, 1987.

190. Heyssel RM, et al: Vitamin B_{12} turnover in man. The assimilation of vitamin B_{12} from natural foodstuff by man and estimates of minimal dietary requirements, Am J Clin Nutr **18**:176-184, 1966.

191. Herbert V: Recommended dietary intakes (RDI) of vitamin B_{12} in humans, Am J Clin Nutr **45:**671-678, 1987.

192. Herbert V: Biology of disease: megaloblastic anemias, Lab Invest **5:**3-19, 1985.

193. Matchar DB, et al: Isotope dilution assay for urinary methylmalonic acid in the diagnosis of vitamin B_{12} deficiency, Ann Intern Med **108:**707-710, 1987.

194. Hodges RW: Ascorbic acid. In Goodhart RS, Shils ME, editors: Modern nutrition in health and disease, ed 6, Philadelphia, 1980, Lea & Febiger, pp 259-273.

195. Mooradian AD, Morley JE: Micronutrient status in diabetes mellitus, Am J Clin Nutr **45:**877-895, 1987.

196. Jaffe GM: Vitamin C. In Machlin LJ, editor: Handbook of vitamins: nutritional, biochemical and clinical aspects, New York, 1984, Marcel Dekker Inc, pp 199-244.

197. Levine M: New concepts in the biology and biochemistry of ascorbic acid, N Engl J Med **314:**892-902, 1986.

198. Olson JA, Hodges RE: Recommended dietary intakes (RDI) of vitamin C in humans, Am J Clin Nutr **45:**693-703, 1987.

199. Burns JJ: Biosynthesis of L-ascorbic acid: basic defect in scurvy, Am J Med **26:**740-748, 1959.

200. England S, Seifter S: The biochemical functions of ascorbic acid, Annu Rev Nutr **6:**365-406, 1986.

201. Levine M, Morita K: Ascorbic acid in endocrine systems, Vitam Horm **42:**1-64, 1985.

202. Kyrtopoulos SA: Ascorbic acid and the formation of N-nitroso compounds: possible role of ascorbic acid in cancer prevention, Am J Clin Nutr **45:**1344-1350, 1987.

203. Oshima H, Bartsch H: Quantitative estimation of endogenous nitrosation in humans by monitoring N-nitrosoproline excreted in the urine, Cancer Res **41:**3658-3662, 1981.

204. Kallner AB, et al: On the requirements of ascorbic acid in man: steady-state turnover and body pool in smokers, Am J Clin Nutr **34:**1347-1355, 1981.

205. Matsuo M, et al: Novel C-terminally amidated opioid peptide in human phaeochromocytoma tumor, Nature **305:**721-723, 1983.

206. Russel J, et al: Electron transfer across posterior pituitary neurosecretory vesicles, J Biol Chem **260:**226-231, 1985.

207. Rose R: Transport and metabolism of ascorbic acid in mammalian tissues, Fed Proc **45:**36-37, 1986.

208. Baker EM, et al: Metabolism of ^{14}C- and ^{3}H-labeled L-ascorbic acid in human scurvy, Am J Clin Nutr **24:**444-454, 1971.

209. Hodges RW, et al: Clinical manifestations of ascorbic acid deficiency in man, Am J Clin Nutr **24:**432-443, 1971.

210. Sauberlich HE: Vitamin C status: methods and findings, Ann NY Acad Sci **258:**438-450, 1975.

211. Jacob RA, et al: Biochemical indices of human vitamin C status, Am J Clin Nutr **46:**818-826, 1987.

212. VanderJagt DJ, et al: Ascorbic acid intake and plasma levels in healthy elderly people, Am J Clin Nutr **46:**290-294, 1987.

213. Hodges RW: Ascorbic acid. In Present knowledge in nutrition, ed 4, New York, 1976, The Nutrition Foundation Inc, pp 119-130.

214. Pauling L: The significance of the evidence about ascorbic acid and the common cold, Proc Natl Acad Sci USA **68:**2678-2681, 1971.

215. Dykes MHM, Meier P: Ascorbic acid and the common cold. Evaluation of its efficacy and toxicity, JAMA **231:**1073-1079, 1975.

216. Freudenheim JL, et al: Relationships between usual nutrient intake and bone-mineral content of women 35-65 years of age: longitudinal and cross-sectional analysis, Am J Clin Nutr **44:**863-876, 1986.

CHAPTER 36
Mineral Deficiencies

Noel W. Solomons

The minerals can be divided into two classes: the major minerals, those occurring in the adult in quantities greater than 7 g; and the trace minerals, those occurring in quantities less than 7 g.[1] The extracellular fluid concentration of many minerals is regulated homeostatically, thus complicating the diagnosis of mineral deficiency or excess. This is especially true for sodium and potassium, whose concentrations can be regulated effectively by the kidneys. Similarly, the circulating concentration of calcium is maintained strictly through an interplay of various regulatory hormones, including parathyroid hormone, calcitonin, and vitamin D. Magnesium, iron, zinc, and copper levels are maintained within certain limits by a type of homeostatic control, except with total-body mineral depletion or overload. Thus, in the diagnosis of total-body mineral nutriture, it is often necessary to go beyond the determination of circulating levels.

The hospital-based clinician should become aware of the pervasive association of total parenteral nutrition (TPN) and depletion of both major and trace minerals. In fact, certain mineral deficiency syndromes have been recognized only in the context of TPN. Theoretically, in parenteral nutrition, mineral deficiencies could be induced by several mechanisms (Fig. 36-1): (1) insufficient intake of the mineral caused by improper formulation of the nutrient solutions; (2) excessive loss of nutrient as a result of some component of the intravenous diet or metabolic adjustment; (3) decline in the serum binding capacity; or (4) redistribution of the mineral from the circulation to the peripheral tissue. Any of these mechanisms is possible during TPN, but undoubtedly, the failure to provide a given nutrient in sufficient quantities to maintain mineral balance is the most frequent. Patients requiring TPN are often in states of extreme catabolism or anabolism, greatly increasing the demand for a given nutrient. Clinicians attending such patients must remain alert to the possible development of mineral deficiencies.

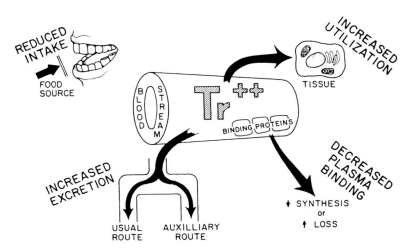

Figure 36-1 Mechanisms for the development of decreased circulating levels of minerals in total parenteral nutrition. Tr^{++}, Trace mineral ion.

THE MAJOR MINERALS

Six minerals—sulfur, sodium, potassium, calcium, phosphorus, and magnesium—occur in the body in amounts greater than 7 g. Sulfur is important as a component of sulfur-containing amino acids, or as a constituent of such trace moieties as biotin and taurine. The electrolytes—sodium and potassium—are discussed in detail in Chapter 2. The focus here is on calcium, phosphorus, and magnesium.

Calcium

The total calcium content of fat-free body tissue averages 20.7 to 24.8 g/kg, with 99% of it found in the crystalline structure of bone. Thus, not only does calcium provide the strength and plastic rigidity of the skeleton and teeth, but bone calcium plays an active role in acid/base and phosphorus homeostasis. Bone is constantly being reabsorbed and redeposited, at maximum rates during early childhood and more slowly in adult life. The catabolic component of bone turnover becomes predominant in the later years.

Calcium is present in bone as (1) the crystallized bone mineral, resembling hydroxyapatite $(Ca_{10}(PO_4)_6(OH)_2)$, that is predominant in adults and (2) an amorphous pool of hydrated calcium phosphate that is predominant at early ages and in young bones. The latter is the precursor to the crystalline phase, which becomes deposited on the bone matrix and which consists of collagen fibers and a mucopolysaccharide gel. The process of bone turnover and remodeling normally recycles from 0.25 to 1 g of calcium/day by the continuous transformation of resting undifferentiated bone cells to osteoblasts and osteoclasts as a response to the level of secretion of parathyroid hormone (PTH). This hormone induces greater transformation to osteoclasts, activated by the vitamin-hormone $1,25\text{-}(OH)_2D_3$ in response to low ionized calcium plasma levels. Calcitonin, or thyrocalcitonin, on the other hand, inhibits osteoclastic activity. As a result of parathyroid hormone secretion, serum calcium levels increase, and bone calcium is released. At the same time, calcium absorption from the intestine is increased, and the production of $1,25\text{-}(OH)_2D_3$ at the kidney level increases, so renal tubular calcium reabsorption is more effective. Thus, calcium homeostasis is maintained by regulation of its absorption, bone formation or bone destruction, and urinary excretion. In general, un-der normal conditions, calcium absorption and its regulation are more important than renal excretion in maintaining calcium balance.

In addition to being present in bone, calcium is present in membrane structures and cellular cement substances and is an activator of several enzymes, particularly those involved in neuromuscular function. Rasmussen[2] has reviewed the role of calcium movement and intracellular concentrations involving calmodulin and membrane phospholipids as a messenger for enzyme regulation. Calcium is involved in various phases of blood coagulation and as an activator of other terminally carboxylated proteins, such as osteocalcin.[3]

A safe intake of calcium is still debatable. Nevertheless, the Committee on Dietary Allowances of the National Research Council[4] in 1980 established an intake allowance of 800 mg/day for adults, with an additional 400 mg/day recommended for women during pregnancy and lactation. Calcium intake of 60 mg/kg of body weight is recommended for infants below 1 year of age, and 800 mg/day is recommended for children between 1 and 10 years of age. During periods of rapid growth a standard of 1.2 g/day has been set. Although the current RDA for adults is 800 mg, it is estimated that 1000 mg of daily calcium intake is needed to maintain balance in adult women before menopause and 1400 mg thereafter.[5]

Factors that influence absorption of calcium are of primary importance. The leading sources of calcium in Western diets are milk and dairy products. The biologic availability of the calcium in these items is high. It is known that the milk sugar, lactose, promotes the absorption of milk calcium by enhancing its passive diffusion in the lower small intestine. The tortilla prepared from lime-soaked corn, as used in southern Mexico and Central America, and the Ethiopian grain teff are also rich sources of absorbable dietary calcium. Calcium solubilized from fish bones is also a rich source of calcium in some diets. Certain amino acids and short-chain fatty acids enhance calcium absorption whereas phytic acid (inositol phosphate), cellulose, alcohol, anticonvulsants, antacids, and tetracycline depress calcium uptake. Oxalate of green leafy vegetables is a major inhibitor of calcium bioavailability. Thus, much of the calcium in leaves is not available for absorption. The amount of calcium in a meal conditions the fractional absorption of the mineral: the higher the load, the lower the proportion absorbed by the intestine. In pregnancy, adaptive changes in the intestine increase the efficiency of calcium absorption. Senile changes in the gut reduce the absorptive caapacity for calcium. Vitamin D status is an important factor in calcium uptake in humans; this vitamin governs the active transport of calcium in the upper intestine.

Epidemiologic and experimental studies have provided preliminary evidence that higher calcium intakes, both within the range of recommended allowances and beyond that range, can exert a "protective" effect against certain specific diseases in susceptible persons. Hypertensive syndromes and colonic neoplasms are two such potential "calcium-responsive" entities. McCarron et al.[6] showed an inverse correlation between dietary calcium and blood pressure in data from the second National Health and Nutrition Examination Survey (HANES II). Villar et al.[7] reviewed the data regarding calcium intake and toxemia of pregnancy. Prospective experimental studies in both normotensive and hypertensive subjects have revealed beneficial blood-pressure–lowering effects of calcium supplementation of about 1 g daily.[7]

Garland and Garland[8] present geographic evidence of an inverse correlation, both within populations and among nations, between higher sun exposure and higher calcium intakes and lower rates of colonic carcinoma. A direct effect of oral calcium supplementation, reducing the tendency of colonic mucosa to proliferate, also has been shown in persons with familial colonic cancer.[9]

Although there are norms for the full complement of total-body calcium at any given age and sex, the definition of a "calcium deficiency" syndrome, per se, has been elusive. Osteoporosis, which involves the loss of both bone mineral and bone matrix, with relatively normal maintenance of mineral density in the remaining bone, is considered to be tantamount to a whole-body calcium deficit. Hypocalcemia results from a failure of homeostatic regulation of circulating calcium, but is not equivalent to a "deficiency" and can occur when bone calcium is at peak levels. Accepting the difficulty of a precise definition, we note that calcium deficiency occurs when a combination of factors negatively and

---

CALCIUM DEFICIENCY

Predisposing Conditions

Deficiency or malutilization of vitamin D
Very-low–birth-weight prematurity
TPN-induced hypercalciuria
Long-term extracoporeal dialysis
Postmenopausal bone loss
Short bowel syndrome
Jejunoileal bypass

Tests of Calcium Nutriture

Cortical thickness assessment by standard roentgenograms
Bone density assessment by photon beam
Whole-body neutron activation analysis
Quantitative histology of bone biopsies

---

chronically affects calcium balance. Conditions predisposing to calcium depletion are shown in the box. TPN-induced hypercalciuria has been documented.[10,11] Urinary losses of calcium in excess of intake from intravenous solutions lead to reduced bone mass and skeletal pain. Theoretically loss of sufficient absorption surface will reduce the capacity of an individual to remain in calcium balance, and calcium malabsorption in short bowel syndrome has been documented.[12] Certain diseases also induce secondary hyperparathyroidism and/or intestinal malabsorption of calcium (pronounced in diarrhea with steatorrhea).

Very low–birth-weight infants (those weighing around 1000 g) lack 80% of the normal full-term complement of skeletal calcium.[13] In the growing child both calcium deficiency and hypophosphatemia can induce muscle weakness, bone pain, and impaired mineralization of bone. Hypocalcemia also can induce tetany in the infant. In the adult, deficiency can induce bone atrophy or osteoporosis, which is more common in postmenopausal women. It is possible that osteoporosis can be diagnosed early if, as has been suggested, spontaneous periodontal disease is an early sign of bone atrophy. It is believed now that high intakes of calcium and lower intakes of protein, together with estrogen/progestogen administration, may prevent the development of, and even possibly improve the conditions conducive to, osteoporosis in women.[14] However, the degree of excess risk of endometrial cancer has not been assessed fully.

The assessment of total-body calcium nutriture is not clear-cut. Circulating calcium levels are controlled homeostatically. Hypocalcemia and tetany should be considered not as signs of calcium deficiency, but rather as the result of abnormal redistribution. Calcium nutriture is reflected in skeletal mineral mass. Calcium nutriture assessment techniques are listed in the box. Osteopenia can be caused by deficiency of nutrients other than calcium, namely ascorbic acid and copper in children and vitamin D in any age group. Calcium deficiency is clinically manifested as bone loss, osseous fractures and pseudofractures, bone pain, and rarefaction of bone by x ray.

The management of calcium depletion depends on the cause. Very premature infants require vitamin D supplementation complemented by massive levels of dietary calcium and phosphorus. TPN-induced hypercalciuria has been reversed by stopping vitamin D therapy or discontinuing intravenous feeding.[10,11]

Phosphorus

The phosphorus content of fat-free body tissue averages 11 to 14 g, resulting in a total-body amount of about 700 g in a 70 kg man. As with calcium, most of the phosphorus resides in the skeleton. The additional physiologic role of phosphorus is as a constituent of membranes (as phospholipid) and as part of intracellular phosphate esters, including the vital high-energy phosphorus compounds essential for the storage and release of energy in carbohydrate, lipid, and protein metabolism. In plasma and urine, phosphates are important in the maintenance of acid/base equilibrium.

PTH is also important in the homeostatic regulation of circulating levels of phosphorus. By mobilizing osteoclasts, this hormone releases bone phosphorus. Its effect on the kidney is to decrease tubular reabsorption of filtered phosphorus levels, often decreased in hyperparathyroid states. Overall, renal mechanisms are more important than intestinal ones in regulating body phosphorus reserves. Normally, two thirds of the dietary phosphorus intake appears in the urine, with peak excretion early in the morning (it appears to be controlled by cortisol excretion). Normally, also, about 90% of the phosphate load passing through the renal tubule is reabsorbed, with maximum tubular reabsorption capacity as high as 8 mg/minute. Typically, renal excretion

of phosphorus is increased by PTH, estrogen, thyroid hormones, steroid therapy, and elevations in serum calcium. Vitamin D deficiency also results in decreased tubular phosphate reabsorption, both through decreased direct vitamin D action and through secondary hyperparathyroidism consequent to lower calcium levels.

The RDA for phosphorus (milligrams) in adults is equivalent to the corresponding allowance for calcium.[14] Net intestinal absorption of dietary phosphate is 70%, although the phosphorus in the plant constituent, phytic acid (inositol hexaphosphate) is poorly absorbed. This poor phytate-phosphorus absorption is observed when unrefined cereal diets are fed in metabolic balance studies. The leavening and baking of flour into bread, however, reduce the amount of intact phytate, liberating its phosphorus for absorption. Excess calcium, or aluminum hydroxide, markedly impairs phosphorus absorption, as does iron.

In infants fed human milk, up to 85% of the phosphorus is absorbed. Human milk is relatively low in phosphorus, and the ratio of calcium to phosphorus in this vital food is much higher than that in cow's milk. In early life, parathyroid responses to low calcium levels are still inadequate, which may explain the development of hypocalcemic tetany in infants fed cow's milk.

An important issue with phosphorus nutrition is the feeding of very low–birth-weight premature infants (weighing less than 1500 g). The problem has been to provide, by an oral or enteral route, the amounts of calcium and phosphorus that would allow the same mineral accretion and skeletal development as would have occurred during normal intrauterine development. Two recent publications[15,16] have shown that suitably soluble formulas with the amounts of calcium and phosphorus needed to achieve in utero rates of bone growth can be provided. In both studies, net retention of phosphorus was related to the amounts administered, and retention was over 95% of that absorbed. Hypophosphatemia and hypercalciuria were seen in one of the studies.[15]

Conditions predisposing to phosphate deficiency, the clinical manifestations of phosphate depletion, and techniques for evaluating phosphorus status are given in the box. In adults, TPN is an unlikely situation in which to observe hypophosphatemia. In very low–birth-weight infants, a positive balance of phosphorus (and calcium) to provide for skeletal accretion at rates equivalent to those in utero can be achieved.[17]

The clinical manifestations of phosphorus depletion are shown in the box. The assessment of phosphate nutriture by laboratory means is complicated, since circulating concentrations also are regulated homeostatically; moreover, hormone-directed redistribution of circulating concentrations—in the absence of total-body depletion, as in parathyroid disease—is not uncommon. A major problem is that, although circulating phosphate levels do fall in true deficiency, they also decline as a result of internal redistribution in a host of metabolic disorders such as carbohydrate loading, alkalosis, sepsis, and volume expansion. In theory, measurement of intracellular concentrations of organic phosphates could serve as indices of phosphorus nutriture. Nutritional repletion in phosphate deficiency states can be accomplished with intravenous phosphate in TPN or oral solutions of inorganic phosphates.

Magnesium

Half the total adult magnesium complement of 25 to 27 g is found in bone; the rest is a soluble ionic form, both intracellular and extracellular, participating as a cofactor in countless enzymatic reactions of energy metabolism. For men 350 mg of daily dietary magnesium intake is recommended.[4] The conditions that predispose to human magnesium deficiency are shown in the box. Once again, faulty formulation of TPN

PHOSPHATE DEFICIENCY

Predisposing Conditions

Alcoholism
Chronic liver disease
Protein-energy malnutrition
Vomiting and diarrhea
Malabsorption syndrome
Ingestion of phosphate-binding antacids
Metabolic acidoses, including ketoacidosis
Diuretics
Hyperparathyroidism
Renal tubular defects

Clinical Manifestations

Acute brain syndrome
Convulsions
Cranial nerve palsies
Peripheral neuropathy
Ascending paralysis
Myopathy and rhabdomyolysis
Glucose intolerance
Decreased tissue oxygenation
Hemolysis
White cell defects
Thrombocytopenia and platelet dysfunction
Hypoparathyroidism
Osteomalacia
Pseudofractures
Hypercalciuria

Tests of Phosphate Nutriture

Circulating phosphate concentration
Erythrocyte 2,3-diphosphoglycerate (?)
Erythrocyte adenosine triphosphate (ATP) (?)

MAGNESIUM DEFICIENCY

Predisposing Conditions

Improper formulation/administration of TPN
  solutions
Chronic alcoholism
Malabsorption syndrome
Kwashiorkor
Diabetes
Acute diarrhea
Cancer
Cisplatin chemotherapy
Diuretics
Renal tubular defects

Clinical Manifestations

Central nervous system
  Apathy
  Depression
  Memory impairment
  Delirium
  Convulsions
  Coma
Neuromuscular
  Myopathy
  Muscle twitching
  Paresthesias
  Tetany (positive Chvostek's sign)

Tests of Magnesium Nutriture

Magnesium balance
Circulating magnesium concentration
Erythrocyte magnesium content
Leukocyte magnesium content
Magnesium load test
Exchangeable magnesium turnover (^{28}Mg)
Muscle analysis (biopsy)

regimens can lead to mineral deficiency. An important cause of magnesium depletion is thiazide diuretics.[18,19] Use of potassium/magnesium–sparing diuretics, however, can act to prevent excessive renal loss of magnesium.[19] In a survey of hospitalized patients hypomagnesemia was found in a surprisingly high number.[20] With erythrocyte magnesium as the index of magnesium status, magnesium deficiency was also diagnosed in over 20% of a sample of unselected elderly persons whose median age was over 80 years.[21] In both series hypertension and the use of diuretics were associated with a higher probability to manifest deficiency.

The manifestations of magnesium deficiency are somewhat protean (see box) because of concomitant redistribution of calcium and the influence on intracellular potassium. An important concern in hypomagnesemia is ectopic ventricular cardiac arrhythmias and other conduction abnormalities.[18,22] Two important mineral/mineral interactions are associated with magnesium depletion. First, hypocalcemia may not reverse itself until a concomitant magnesium deficiency is repleted. Second, magnesium depletion may also impair the restoration of a concurrent intracellular potassium deficiency. Both these factors can be important in explaining the cardiac arrhythmias associated with magnesium depletion.

The laboratory tests for assessing magnesium status are listed in the box. Our understanding of the clinical consequences of deficiency comes from work with experimental volunteers by Shils,[23] who noted that circulating magnesium levels are tightly regulated homeostatically and their decline is seen only with extreme states of depletion. In the study of elderly persons by Touitou et al.,[21] red cell magnesium was depressed more than twice as often as circulating concentrations. White cell magnesium content determination is another possible way to overcome the confounding factors of homeostatic regulation in serum. The magnesium load test has been proposed[24,25] for detecting less severe degrees of deficiency. Intense physical exercise has been shown[26] to exert an immediate and dramatic, but transient, effect on magnesium metabolism. A shift of magnesium from the plasma into the red cells caused a 7% decrease in the Mg concentration of the former; urinary magnesium excretion was also increased. Both abnormalities reversed themselves rapidly after the cessation of strenuous activity.

Magnesium depletion can be managed by the intravenous or oral administration of magnesium salts. Oral doses should be given in moderation since large doses have a laxative effect. Concomitant hypocalcemia cannot be reversed until the magnesium status has been corrected. Magnesium toxicity is not uncommon. Many antacids and laxative preparations have magnesium salts as the active ingredient.

TRACE ELEMENTS

The trace elements of nutritional importance in humans are iron, zinc, copper, selenium, chromium, manganese, iodine, fluorine, molybdenum, vanadium, nickel, silicon, tin, lithium, and cobalt. The last is of nutritional importance only as a component of vitamin B_{12}. Iodine and fluorine are not, strictly speaking, minerals. The nutritional issues related to iodine are presented in Chapter 17. Further reference to trace minerals is made in Chapter 22, in connection with diseases of the skin. This section amplifies on the subject of trace mineral deficiency. Since iron nutrition is covered in Chapter 37, it will not be treated here.

Zinc

The human body contains 2 to 3 g of zinc in adulthood. Muscle, bone, skin, and liver combined account for most of the body reserves. Zinc from the first three compartments, however, is mobilized with difficulty for nutritional purposes. The physiologic functions subtended by zinc include cell growth and replication; fertility, reproduction, and sexual maturation; immune defenses; dark adaptation; and taste and appetite.[27] At a biochemical level the primary role of this mineral is to be a component of zinc metalloenzymes. Many enzymes of the nucleus involved in genetic information transfer, protein synthesis, and cellular replication are metalloenzymes of zinc.[28] Zinc as an ionic species may also play a role in membrane stabilization of cells and subcellular organelles. Furthermore, it appears to regulate serum thymic factor (thymulin),[29] an important messenger in immunologic regulation, and to play a role in glucose homeostasis as well.

The RDA for zinc in adults is 15 mg,[4] although surveys have shown that few Americans ingest the requisite amount. Since only 2.5 to 4 mg of zinc need be absorbed daily, however, there is a margin of safety. The determining factor is

ZINC DEFICIENCY

Predisposing Conditions

Prematurity
Bizarre food selection pattern
Anorexia nervosa
Diets high in fiber and phytic acid
Geophagia
Improper formulation/administration of
  TPN solutions
Protein-energy malnutrition
Down's syndrome
Cystic fibrosis
Pancreatic insufficiency
Acute pancreatitis
Acrodermatitis enteropathica
Celiac sprue
Short bowel syndrome
Chronic diarrhea
Intestinal parasitism
Crohn's disease
Ulcerative colitis
Pancreatic-cutaneous fistulas
Acquired immunodeficiency syndrome
  (AIDS)
Alcoholism
Alcoholic cirrhosis
Viral hepatitis
Sickle cell anemia
Thalassemia
Thiazide diuretics
Nephrotic syndrome
Treatment with systemic chelating agents
  such as D-penicillamine
Extracorporeal dialysis with zinc-deficient
  dialysate

Exfoliative dermatoses
Psoriasis
Thermal burns and scalds
Neoplasia
Pregnancy
Lactation

Clinical Manifestations

Growth retardation
Delayed sexual maturation
Hypospermia and hypogonadism
Alopecia
Skin lesions
Diarrhea
Glucose intolerance
Mental depression/apathy
Impaired wound healing
Impaired dark adaptation (night
  blindness)
Impaired taste acuity (hypogeusia)
Impaired phagocytic chemotaxis
Impaired T-lymphocytic function
Cutaneous anergy

Tests of Zinc Nutriture

Plasma or serum zinc concentration
Erythrocyte zinc content
Leukocyte zinc content
Platelet zinc content
Hair zinc concentration
Salivary zinc concentration
Zinc metalloenzyme activity
  Alkaline phosphatase (serum)
  Carbonic anhydrase (red cell)

whether the bioavailability of zinc from a zinc-poor diet is sufficient to maintain zinc balance. Dietary fiber and phytic acid—components of unrefined foods—can impair zinc absorption and actually produce a net negative zinc balance. Premature infants and pregnant and lactating women are at especially high risk for zinc depletion. Dermatologic (Chapter 22), gastrointestinal, hematologic, renal, neoplastic, and iatrogenic conditions can predispose to zinc depletion (box). Zinc deficiency also has been the presenting manifestation of acquired immunodeficiency syndrome (AIDS).[30] Short bowel syndrome, Crohn's disease, and jejunoileal bypass produce frank zinc malabsorption.[31] Alcoholic and viral liver disease, burns, nephrotic syndrome, and various hemolytic anemias may aggravate a major loss of zinc in the urine and lead to excess daily absorption. As with iron, how-ever, there seems to be a compensatory uptake and retention of zinc in the presence of total-body depletion.[32]

Increasing concern about marginal or deficient zinc states during pregnancy have been voiced; teratogenesis and adverse pregnancy outcomes have been associated, by some investigators,[33] with inadequate gestational zinc nutriture. Zinc deficiency is also thought to be a cofactor in the development of fetal alcohol syndrome.

Total parenteral nutrition, unless properly managed, places the patient at risk of zinc depletion. The intrinsic zinc of intravenous nutrient solutions is variable.[34] Circulating levels of zinc declined in the majority of patients receiving unsupplemented TPN observed serially.[35,36] Florid signs of zinc deficiency syndrome have been described in patients undergoing TPN. Most of the published cases of TPN-related zinc depletion occurred in individuals after abdominal surgery or with inflammatory bowel diseases. For the stable adult, 2.5 to 4 mg delivered intravenously daily generally will maintain balance.[37] In catabolic states (fever, stress, surgery) an additional 2 mg should be given. However, when fluid loss from either the small or the large bowel is involved, an additional 12 and 17 mg of zinc, respectively, is required per liter of fluid lost.[38] Nitrogen balance and insulin secretions tend to improve when patients receive adequate zinc.[38]

The clinical manifestations of zinc deficiency are shown in the box. Stunted growth and hypogonadism in children and adolescents in the Middle East were the first documented.[39] The acute manifestations are seen more commonly in the hospital setting. Even in the absence of a genetic predisposition, skin lesions identical to those of acrodermatitis enteropathica may occur in acute zinc deficiency states.[40,41] Night blindness, reduced taste sensitivity, and delayed wound healing are functional consequences; but only in the presence of zinc deficiency are any of these manifestations likely to respond to administration of the element. Each disorder has a number of other nutritional and nonnutritional etiologies.

The long list of predisposing factors appears to warrant constant surveillance for zinc deficiency in patients, and even in selected susceptible populations. Potentially useful tests for the assessment of zinc nutriture (box) include, by far the most common, the index of circulating zinc (i.e., plasma or serum concentration). As an indicator of total-body zinc status, however, circulating zinc has severe limitations. Because plasma and serum zinc are homeostatically regulated, factors such as hemolysis of red blood cells, chronic venous occlusion, and prolonged fasting artifactually increase zinc levels whereas corticosteroids, estrogens, and oral contraceptives as well as infectious or inflammatory conditions and recent meals may decrease levels. The concentration and binding affinities of serum albumin can influence zinc levels in either direction, independent of body stores. Detailed and prolonged isotopic turnover studies with radioactive zinc would be, in theory, the most accurate indicator of true body zinc, but such an approach is both invasive and impractical for routine application.[42] The box contains other commonly used laboratory indices for assessing zinc status. In diagnostic decision-making a combination of tests often provides the best picture of zinc nutriture.[27] For patients receiving TPN, urinary excretion of zinc is a promising guide to zinc status.[43]

Despite the array of analytic technology, a supplemental trial of zinc is often the best final arbiter of whether a zinc deficiency state existed at the time of initial reference. Since body-fluid and tissue concentrations of zinc may increase with supplementation, whether the status was low or adequate, functional indices (based on the physiologic defects of zinc deficiency) have been explored.[44] In vivo indices of dark adaptation, taste and olfactory acuity, sperm production, nitrogen retention, insulin production, rates of experimental wound healing, and intestinal zinc uptake—if initially deficient or defective—may be used as a measure of the response to the unique supplementation of zinc. In vitro tests of leukocyte chemotaxis, lymphocyte mitogen response, platelet aggregation, and red cell zinc uptake may also serve as functional indices of zinc status during a therapeutic challenge.

When zinc deficiency is suspected on a clinical or laboratory basis, supplementation is indicated. If it occurs in the context of TPN, infusions should be adjusted according to the guidelines just enumerated. Various preparations are available for oral supplementation. Despite claims by manufacturers, no conclusive evidence of the superiority of various salts and organic complexes over zinc sulfate exists. Zinc sulfate dosage in the range of 660 mg/day (150 mg of Zn^{+2}) has been associated with dyspepsia, epigastric burning, nausea, and occasionally gastric erosion. Taken over a long time (i.e., several years[45]) or in enormous doses for a shorter time,[46] $ZnSO_4$ can induce a competitive interaction with copper, leading to copper deficiency. To avoid this complication, it has been recommended[47] that chronic, routine zinc supplementation be limited to 40 mg of the mineral per day.

Copper

Copper reserves of the adult constitute between 80 and 150 mg. The safe and adequate daily dietary intakes (SADDIs) for adults are estimated[4] to be 2 to 3 mg. Surveys[48] have shown that the average daily copper intake in the United States is on the order of 1.2 to 1.3 mg. Foods such as shellfish and legumes are rich in copper. Milk, both human and bovine, is extraordinarily poor in copper; hence copper deficiency is a problem in the very low–birth-weight premature infant. Soluble forms of copper are absorbed at the level of the stomach,[49] but since most of the copper in the diet is in complex organic compounds in a protein-bound form it is not liberated for intestinal absorption until the meal has reached the jejunum.

The liver, which contains from 8% to 15% of total-body copper, is the central terminal for the uptake of dietary copper, for its mobilization as a nutritionally relevant metal, and for the excretory regulation of copper reserves of the whole organism.[50] The physiologic functions related to copper are numerous. They include erythropoiesis and leukopoiesis, skeletal mineralization and connective tissue formation, melanin synthesis, oxidative phosphorylation, thermal regulation, myelin formation, catecholamine metabolism, antioxidant protection, cholesterol metabolism, immune function, glucose homeostasis, and myocardial function.[50] At a biochemical and cellular level, copper—like zinc—has its primary nutritional and metabolic role as a component of a host of copper metalloenzymes.[27,50]

Conditions predisposing to human copper depletion are listed in the box. Copper deficiency in humans was first described in Peruvian toddlers recovering from severe protein-energy malnutrition on milk-based diets reconstituted with water from a plastic pipe system that had replaced copper tubing.[51] Not uncharacteristic of trace mineral deficiencies, copper depletion during TPN is a major concern.[52,53] The first case of copper deficiency in an adult was seen in the context of TPN. Generally, TPN solutions have nearly undetectable amounts of copper,[34] and a predictable decline in plasma and serum copper will occur with prolonged administration of unsupplemented TPN formulas. The aminoaciduria that occurs with TPN also promotes renal loss of copper.

The clinical signs of copper deficiency listed in the box include the most common and earliest manifestation, a reduction in circulating neutrophils. A hypochromic microcytic anemia, morphologically similar to iron deficiency anemia but unresponsive to iron supplementation, is also common. In children, bone changes reminiscent

---

COPPER DEFICIENCY

Predisposing Conditions

Prematurity
Protein-energy malnutrition
Chronic diarrhea
Short bowel syndrome
Jejunoileal bypass
Celiac disease
Tropical sprue
Improper formulation/administration of TPN solutions
Treatment with systemic chelating agents such as D-penicillamine
Excessive zinc supplementation
Chronic oral alkali therapy
Primary hyperparathyroidism
Nephrotic syndrome
Pregnancy

Clinical Manifestations

Hypochromic microcytic anemia
Neutropenia
Depigmentation of hair and skin
Arterial aneurysms
Defective elastin formation with arterial aneurysms
Central nervous system abnormalities
Hypotonia
Hypothermia
Skeletal demineralization
Subperiosteal hemorrhages
Epiphyseal separation

Tests of Copper Nutriture

Hemoglobin or hematocrit
Reticulocyte count
Leukocyte count and differential
Plasma or serum copper concentration
Serum ceruloplasmin
Leukocyte copper content
Erythrocyte copper content
Copper metalloenzyme activity
  Superoxide dismutase (erythrocyte)
  Amine oxidase (serum)
  Cytochrome C oxidase (leukocyte)

---

of scurvy are seen. The other manifestations have been reported only in premature infants with copper deficiency and are similar to the signs of the congenital X-linked disease of copper metabolism, known as Menkes' steely hair syndrome. Menkes' disease is fatal within the first 2 years of life. (See Chapter 22.)

The diagnosis of copper deficiency should be suspected when anemia and neutropenia (with or without osteopenia in young children) occur in the setting of one of the predisposing conditions listed in the box. As with zinc, interpretative problems limit the utility of circulating copper levels as an index of total-body nutriture. Copper levels probably are regulated homeostatically to some extent. More important, however, is that 94% of copper in the circulation is firmly bound to ceruloplasmin.[54] False elevations of copper levels, not indicative of changes in nutriture, can be produced by infection and inflammation, smoking, oral contraceptive use, and pregnancy. In Wilson's disease (hepatolenticular degeneration) the failure to release ceruloplasmin from the liver produces constant hypocupremia, without any reduction in total-body copper reserves (which, in fact, are increased). It has been demonstrated[55] that premature infants, although susceptible to true copper deficiency, have an inherent maturation delay in ceruloplasmin release. This prevents the attainment of normal circulating copper levels until the child has reached the postconceptional age equivalent to full term. Hair shafts bind environmental copper and represent a poor index of nutriture. As determination of copper metalloenzymes becomes more widespread, a greater reliance on these indicators should be assumed.

Copper deficiency during TPN requires appropriate supplementation. The American Medical Association[37] recommends 0.5 to 1.5 mg of intravenous copper daily for stable adults receiving TPN. Shike et al.,[56] however, found in metabolic studies on TPN patients that balance was achieved at a delivery of about 0.4 mg daily. They caution against higher rates of delivery, especially if biliary excretory function is at all compromised. Oral copper can be given as copper sulfate, but the doses must be small because copper is a powerful emetic in doses as low as 10 mg. In some cases a cause such as excessive zinc or parenteral chelating agent can be adjusted or eliminated to relieve copper imbalance.

Chromium

The total-body content of chromium is estimated to be 6 to 10 mg. The recommended safe limit for daily chromium intake by adults is 0.05 to 0.2 mg.[4] Estimates of daily dietary chromium intakes in Western societies have come from Canada and the United States. Gibson et al.[57] found that postmenopausal women in Ontario consumed a median level of 77 µg of the element daily (range 21-274 µg). Only 22% had intakes below the 50 µg lower limit of the SADDIs.

Adult subjects in Maryland[58] consumed an average 28 µg of chromium, or only 50% of the SADDI level. More than 90% of all diets had below 50 µg of chromium. Under certain circumstances "contamination" of the diet with inorganic chromium from stainless steel cooking utensils can contribute to chromium intakes from meals. The utilization of this latter chemical species, however, is in doubt since there has been speculation as to the possibility that dietary chromium exists in two forms: a highly absorbable organic form (preformed glucose tolerance factor) and a poorly absorbable inorganic (salt) form. The chemical form of chromium in human milk is not precisely known, but the concentration varies from 0.2 to 0.3 ng/ml and daily intakes by the end of the first month for breast-fed infants would be around 0.19 µg per day.[59]

The primary role of chromium in human metabolism appears to be its participation as a glucose tolerance factor in insulin metabolism. A role in the binding of insulin to receptors has been postulated. Chromium is transported in the circulation on transferrin. In conditions of total-body iron overload (e.g., hemochromatosis) the competition between iron and chromium for binding sites can lead to chromium depletion.[60]

The most common situation in which human chromium deficiency can appear is TPN. The clinical manifestations seen in the two confirmed reports of a chromium-responsive deficiency syndrome presenting during intravenous alimentation[61,62] were glucose intolerance, peripheral neuropathy, and metabolic encephalopathy. Chromium depletion has also been seen in severe infantile protein-energy malnutrition and has been suspected to occur in pregnancy, in insulin-dependent diabetics, and with increasing age. The increased beta-cell sensitivity and the enhanced peripheral utilization of glucose seen in glucose-intolerant elderly patients studied with

---

CHROMIUM DEFICIENCY

Tests of Chromium Nutriture
Plasma chromium concentration
Serum chromium concentration
Erythrocyte chromium content
Whole-blood chromium content
Hair chromium content
24-Hour urinary chromium excretion
Urinary chromium/creatinine ratio

a hyperglycemic insulin clamp technique, when they were supplemented for 12 weeks with 200 µg of chromium as $CrCl_3$,[63] suggest that the glucose intolerance of senescence may be in part a consequence of chromium depletion or its redistribution. However, 10 weeks of supplementation with 5 µg of chromium as brewer's yeast, 200 µg of chromium as $CrCl_3$, or a placebo to 23 healthy elderly persons failed to effect any change in glucose tolerance.[64] A possible role for marginal chromium intake (chronic) as an etiologic factor in cardiovascular disease has been discussed.[65,66]

The clinical assessment of chromium status is particularly difficult, mainly because of problems with quantitative analysis of chromium in body fluids and tissues. The prevailing analytic technique during the past decade has been atomic absorption spectrophotometry. As a result of problems with contamination during collection and processing of materials and with background correction during the spectrophotometry, the majority of reported values for chromium in blood, urine, and hair are much greater than those obtained by more meticulous collection methods to avoid contamination (e.g., neutron activation analysis).[67] With resolution of the analytic problems involving the quantification of chromium in biologic materials, it is now possible to think of several approaches to the assessment of chromium nutriture in humans. Potential indices of chromium nutriture are listed in the box. Several "functional" tests of chromium nutriture, also involving measurement of chromium, have been proposed. These include the response of circulating chromium and urinary chromium to an oral glucose load. As noted, the change in glucose tolerance and serum lipids with chromium supplementation may also represent functional measures of initial chromium status.

Since TPN presents a risk of chromium depletion, it has been recommended[37] that 10 to 15 µg of chromium be administered daily in TPN infusions. Brewer's yeast is rich in biologically available glucose tolerance–factor chromium and has been used as a source of the mineral when oral supplementation was deemed appropriate. More recently, however, doubt has been cast on the role of chromium per se in whatever moieties in yeast might act in vivo and in vitro to improve the action of insulin. Thus it is impossible to be sure with present evidence that

chromium is a component of mammalian glucose tolerance factor.

Selenium

The total amount of selenium in the body is estimated to be 6 to 10 mg. The specific limits of daily selenium intake (the SADDIs) are 0.05 to 0.2 mg. Levander et al.,[68] in metabolic studies, have shown that 60 µg of daily oral intake of selenium from a conventional diet is sufficient to maintain balance in residents of California. In countries with hyposeleniferous soil (e.g., New Zealand, Finland) adults remain in apparent good health on intakes of about half this amount of selenium. In usual foods selenium is found in organic form (selenoamino acids such as selenomethionine); but in livestock feeding, inorganic salts such as sodium selenite are used. Organic selenium in the diet has a high efficiency of absorption, approaching 90%.[69] Foods like haddock, tuna, and oysters contain appreciable amounts of selenium.

The primary role of selenium in mammalian metabolism is as a component of the metalloenzyme glutathione peroxidase, which acts to re-

---

SELENIUM DEFICIENCY

Predisposing Conditions

Improper formulation/administration of TPN
　solutions
Cystic fibrosis
Thermal burns
Alcoholism
Alcoholic cirrhosis
Cancer
Semisynthetic diets for disease such as
　phenylketonuria or maple syrup urine
　disease

Clinical Manifestations

Myalgias and myositis
Cardiomyopathy
Hemolytic anemias
Decreased leukocyte bactericidal activity
Depressed cellular immunity

Tests of Selenium Nutriture

Plasma or serum selenium concentration
Whole blood selenium concentration
Erythrocyte selenium concentration
Erythrocyte glutathione peroxidase activity
Platelet glutathione peroxidase activity
Serum creatine kinase activity
Serum creatinine phosphokinase activity

duce inorganic and organic peroxides and thus aborts oxidative damage to cells. A list of the conditions predisposing to selenium depletion and the clinical manifestations of selenium deficiency are shown in the box. Again, TPN is the major context for the occurrence of these signs.[70] An epidemiologic association between seleniferous soils and a lowered rate of neoplasia is being studied. Willett et al.[71] found an interaction between midlife plasma selenium levels and subsequent development of malignancy. Keshan disease, a seasonal acute cardiomyopathy endemic to certain hyposeleniferous regions of China, is prevented by prophylactic use of oral selenium.

As with other trace elements, assessment of human selenium status by laboratory methods is inexact. The platelet glutathione peroxide activity is a promising index and has been shown[72] to respond to dietary selenium supplementation in apparently healthy Finnish men with a chronically low selenium intake. In overt myositis or cardiomyopathy of selenium deficiency, concentration of the muscle-related enzymes creatine kinase and creatinine phosphokinase, respectively, can be followed in serum as a guide to the response to selenium therapy.

Several fatalities from selenium deficiency cardiomyopathy have been reported in TPN patients.[73-75] For prophylactic or therapeutic use in intravenous nutrition, selenious acid can be used. Levander[76] recommends a dose of 50 to 60 μg of selenium daily for maintenance therapy during TPN. For oral supplementation, selenized *Torula* yeast preparations are available commercially.

Manganese

A safe and adequate daily dietary intake of 2.5 to 5.0 mg has been established for manganese in adults. Postmenopausal women in Ontario consumed upwards of 5 mg daily,[57] largely attributable to the high consumption of tea, which is an abundant source of this metal. Manganese is a component of two mammalian enzymes (pyruvate carboxylase and superoxide dismutase) as well as a soluble cofactor in certain biochemical reactions. Deficiency in humans has not been described extensively. One case of accidental manganese depletion was reported[77] in a man undergoing nutritional experimentation with a formula diet. He experienced weight loss, dermatitis, nausea, hypocholesterolemia, and changes in the color and growth of hair and beard. These signs and symptoms responded to manganese supplementation. In theory, a pregnant woman might be more susceptible to marginal manganese intakes, since in utero teratogenic effects involving the connective tissue structures of the inner ear have been observed in experimental animal models of manganese restriction.

Despite the absence of a clear deficiency syndrome, it is recommended[37] that 0.15 to 0.8 mg of manganese be included in TPN regimens. However, a high content of contaminant manganese in intravenous solution constituents may make additives superfluous.[78]

Molybdenum

Molybdenum is involved as a component of two mammalian enzymes, sulfite oxidase (which functions in the degradation of sulfur from amino acids) and xanthine oxidase (which functions in the degradation of purine nucleotides to uric acid).[79] In the liver, molybdenum is incorporated into an organic cofactor that is inserted posttranslationally into these enzymes.[80] A lethal inborn error of metabolism caused by absence of hepatic molybdenum cofactor has been described. The syndrome combines dislocation of the ocular lens with metabolic abnormalities of purines and sulfur. A case suggestive of molybdenum deficiency was reported in a 20-year-old patient with short bowel syndrome after 18 months of TPN.[81] The clinical manifestations in the case were headache, irritability, night blindness, lethargy, coma, abnormal metabolism of sulfur-containing amino acids, and abnormal degradation of nucleic acids. The syndrome responded to a total dose of 150-250 μg of molybdenum administered as ammonium molybdate.

Nickel, Vanadium, Tin, and Lithium

Although confirmed in laboratory animals, no clinical syndrome of human deficiencies of nickel, vanadium, tin, and lithium have been observed.[82,83] Surveys suggest that the usual concentrations of nickel in U.S. diets are in a range that would prevent nickel deficiency in laboratory animals, but human consumption of vanadium may be marginal compared to the requirements in animal species. Tin intake depends on the contamination from food containers. Data on spontaneous lithium consumption are scarce at present.

REFERENCES

1. Mertz W: The essential trace elements, Science **213:**1332-1338, 1981.

Calcium

2. Rasmussen H: The calcium messenger system, N Engl J Med **314:**1094-1101.
3. Hauschka PV: Osteocalcin: The vitamin K–dependent Ca^{2+}-binding protein of bone matrix, Haemostasis **16:**258-272, 1986.
4. Committee on Dietary Allowances, Food and Nutrition Board, National Research Council: Recommended dietary allowances, ed 9, Washington DC, 1980, National Academy of Sciences.
5. Allen LH: Calcium and age-related bone loss, Clin Nutr **5:**147-152, 1986.
6. McCarron D, et al: Blood pressure and nutrient intake in the United States, Science **224:**1392-1398, 1984.
7. Villar J, et al: Calcium and blood pressure, Clin Nutr **5:**153-160, 1986.
8. Garland CF, Garland FC: Calcium and colon cancer, Clin Nutr **5:**161-166, 1986.
9. Lipkin M, Newmark H: Effect of added dietary calcium on colonic epithelial-cell proliferation in subjects at risk for familial colonic cancer, N Engl J Med **313:**1381-1384, 1985.
10. Shike M, et al: Metabolic bone disease in patients receiving long-term parenteral nutrition, Ann Intern Med **92:**343-350, 1980.
11. Klein GL, et al: Bone disease associated with total parenteral nutrition, Lancet **2:**1041-1044, 1980.
12. Ladefoged K, et al: Calcium, phosphorus, magnesium, zinc, and nitrogen balance in patients with severe short bowel syndrome, Am J Clin Nutr **33:**2137-2144, 1980.
13. Chesney RW, et al: Rickets of prematurity: supranormal levels of serum 1,25-dihydroxyvitamin D, Am J Dis Child **135:**34-37, 1981.
14. Christensen C, et al: Prevention of early postmenopausal bone loss: controlled 2-year study in 315 normal females, Eur J Clin Invest **10:**273-279, 1980.

Phosphorus

15. Towe JC, et al: Achievement of in utero retention of calcium and phosphorus accompanied by high calcium excretion in very low birth weight infants fed a fortified formula, J Pediatr **110:**581-585, 1987.
16. Giles MM, et al: Sequential calcium and phosphorus balance studies in preterm infants, J Pediatr **110:**591-598, 1987.
17. Vileisis RA: Effect of phosphorus intake in total parenteral nutrition infusates in premature neonates, J Pediatr **110:**586-590, 1987.

Magnesium

18. Dyckner T, Wester PO: Potassium/magnesium depletion in patients with cardiovascular disease, Am J Med **82** (suppl 3A):11-17, 1987.
19. Ryan MP: Diuretics and potassium/magnesium depletion. Directions for treatment, Am J Med **82** (suppl 3A):38-47, 1987.
20. Whang R: Magnesium deficiency: pathogenesis and prevalence and clinical implications, Am J Med **82** (suppl 3A):24-29, 1987.
21. Touitou Y, et al: Prevalence of magnesium and potassium deficiencies in the elderly, Clin Chem **35:**518-523, 1987.

22. Hollifield JW: Magnesium depletion, diuretics and arrhythmias, Am J Med **82** (suppl 3A):30-37, 1987.
23. Shils ME: Experimental human magnesium depletion, Medicine (Baltimore) **48:**61-85, 1969.
24. Caddell JL, et al: Parenteral magnesium load evaluation of malnourished Thai children, J Pediatr **83:**129-135, 1973.
25. Caddell JL, et al: Parenteral magnesium test in postpartum Thai women, Am J Clin Nutr **26:**612-615, 1973.
26. Deuster PA, et al: Magnesium homeostasis during high-intensity anaerobic exercise in men, J Appl Physiol **62:**545-550, 1987.

Zinc

27. Solomons NW: Zinc and copper. In Shils ME, editor: Modern nutrition in health and disease, ed 7, Philadelphia, 1987, Lea & Febiger.
28. Valee BL, Falchuk KH: Zinc and gene expression, Philos Trans R Soc Lond (Biol) **B294:**185-197, 1981.
29. Dardenne M, et al: A zinc-dependent epitope on the molecule of thymulin, a thymic hormone, Proc Natl Acad Sci USA **82:**7035-7038, 1985.
30. Tong TK, et al: Childhood acquired immune deficiency syndrome manifesting as acrodermatitis enteropathica, J Pediatr **108:**426-428, 1986.
31. McClain CJ: Zinc metabolism in malabsorption syndromes, J Am Coll Nutr **4:**49-64, 1985.
32. Cousins RJ: Toward a molecular understanding of zinc metabolism, Clin Physiol Biochem **4:**20-30, 1986.
33. Solomons NW, et al: Zinc needs during pregnancy, Clin Nutr **5:**63-71, 1986.
34. Solomons NW: Trace minerals. In Rombeau JL, Caldwell MD, editors: Parenteral nutrition. Vol 2. Clinical nutrition, Philadelphia, 1986, WB Saunders Co, pp 169-197.
35. Solomons NW, et al: Plasma trace metals during total parenteral alimentation, Gastroenterology **70:**1022-1025, 1976.
36. Fleming CR, et al: A prospective study of serum copper and zinc levels in patients receiving total parenteral nutrition, Am J Clin Nutr **29:**70-77, 1976.
37. American Medical Association: Guidelines for essential trace element preparations for parenteral use, JAMA **241:**2052-2054, 1979.
38. Wolman SL, et al: Zinc in total parenteral nutrition. Requirements and metabolic effects, Gastroenterology **76:**458-467, 1979.
39. Prasad AS, et al: Zinc metabolism in normals and patients with the syndrome of iron deficiency anemia, hypogonadism and dwarfism, J Lab Clin Med **61:**537-549, 1963.
40. Takagi Y, et al: Clinical studies on zinc metabolism during total parenteral nutrition as related to zinc deficiency, J Parenter Enter Nutr **10:**195-202, 1986.
41. Winston E, et al: Zinc deficiency during parenteral hyperalimentation, Ill Med J **168:**161-163, 1968.
42. Aamodt RL, et al: Effects of oral zinc loading on zinc metabolism in humans. I. Experimental studies, Metabolism **31:**326-334, 1982.
43. Main AN, et al: Clinical experience of zinc supplementation during intravenous nutrition in Crohn's disease: value of serum and urine zinc measurement, Gut **23:**984-991, 1982.
44. Solomons NW: Assessment of nutritional status: functional indicators of pediatric nutriture, Pediatr Clin North Am **32:**319-334, 1985.

45. Hoogenraad TU, et al: Copper responsive anemia, induced by oral zinc therapy in a patient with acrodermatitis enteropathica, Sci Total Environ **42**:37-43, 1985.

46. Patterson WP, et al: Zinc-induced copper deficiency: megamineral sideroblastic anemia, Ann Intern Med **103**:385-386, 1985.

47. Sandstead HH: Zinc interference with copper metabolism [editorial], JAMA **240**:2188-2189, 1978.

Copper

48. Klevay LM, et al: Evidence of dietary copper and zinc deficiency, JAMA **241**:1916-1918, 1979.

49. Van Berge Henegouwen GP, et al: Biliary secretion of copper in healthy man: quantitation by an intestinal perfusion technique, Gastroenterology **72**:1228-1231, 1977.

50. Solomons NW: Biochemical, metabolic, and clinical role of copper in human nutrition, J Am Coll Nutr **4**:83-105, 1985.

51. Cordano A, et al: Copper deficiency in infancy, Pediatrics **34**:324-326, 1964.

52. Joffe G, et al: A patient with copper deficiency anemia while on prolonged intravenous feeding, Clin Pediatr **20**:226-228, 1981.

53. Levy J, et al: Epiphyseal separation simulating pyoarthritis, secondary to copper deficiency in an infant receiving total parenteral nutrition, Br J Radiol **57**:636-638, 1984.

54. Delves HT: The microdetermination of copper in plasma protein fraction, Clin Chim Acta **71**:495-500, 1976.

55. Hillman LS, et al: Effect of oral copper supplementation on serum copper and ceruloplasmin concentrations in premature infants, J Pediatr **98**:311-313, 1981.

56. Shike M, et al: Copper metabolism and requirements in total parenteral nutrition, Gastroenterology **81**:290-297, 1981.

Chromium

57. Gibson RS, et al: Dietary chromium and manganese intakes of a selected sample of Canadian elderly women, Hum Nutr Appl Nutr **39**:43-52, 1985.

58. Anderson RA, Kozlovsky AS: Chromium intake, absorption and excretion of subjects consuming self-selected diets, Am J Clin Nutr **41**:1177-1183, 1985.

59. Casey CE, et al: Studies in human lactation: zinc, copper, manganese and chromium in human milk in the first month of lactation, Am J Clin Nutr **41**:1193-1200, 1985.

60. Sargent T III, et al: Reduced chromium retention in patients with hemochromatosis, a possible basis of hemochromatotic diabetes, Metabolism **28**:70-79, 1979.

61. Jeejeebhoy KN, et al: Chromium deficiency, glucose intolerance, and neuropathy reversed by chromium supplementation, in a patient receiving long-term total parenteral nutrition, Am J Clin Nutr **30**:531-538, 1977.

62. Freund H, et al: Chromium deficiency during total parenteral nutrition, JAMA **241**:496-498, 1979.

63. Potter JF, et al: Glucose metabolism in glucose-intolerant older people during chromium supplementation, Metabolism **34**:199-204, 1985.

64. Offenbacher EG, et al: The effects of inorganic chromium and brewer's yeast on glucose tolerance, plasma lipids, and plasma chromium in elderly subjects, Am J Clin Nutr **42**:454-461, 1985.

65. Newman HA, et al: Serum chromium and angiographically determined coronary artery disease, Clin Chem **24**:541-544, 1978.

66. Simonoff M: Chromium deficiency and cardiovascular risk, Cardiovasc Res **18**:591-596, 1984.

67. Shapcott D, Hubert J: Chromium in nutrition and metabolism, New York, 1979, Elsevier/North-Holland Inc, pp 1-14.

68. Levander OA, et al: Selenium balance in young men during selenium depletion and repletion, Am J Clin Nutr **34**:2662-2669, 1981.

69. Barbezat GO, et al: Selenium. In Solomons NW, Rosenberg IH, editors: Absorption and malabsorption of mineral nutrients, New York, 1984, Alan R Liss Inc, pp 232-258.

70. Triplett WC: Clinical aspects of zinc, copper, manganese, chromium and selenium, Nutr Int **1**:60-67, 1985.

71. Willett WC, et al: Prediagnostic serum selenium and risk of cancer, Lancet **2**:130-134, 1983.

72. Levander OA, et al: Bioavailability of selenium to Finnish men as assessed by platelet glutathione peroxidase activity and other blood parameters, Am J Clin Nutr **37**:887-897, 1983.

73. Johnson RA, et al: An Occidental case of cardiomyopathy and selenium deficiency, N Engl J Med **304**:1210-1212, 1981.

74. Fleming CR, et al: Selenium deficiency and fatal cardiomyopathy in a patient on home parenteral nutrition, Gastroenteroloogy **83**:689-693, 1982.

75. Quercia RA, et al: Selenium deficiency and fatal cardiomyopathy in a patient receiving long-term home parenteral nutrition, Clin Pharm **3**:531-535, 1984.

76. Levander OA: The importance of selenium in total parenteral nutrition, Bull NY Acad Med **60**:144-155, 1984.

Manganese

77. Doisy RA Jr: Effects of deficiency in manganese upon plasma levels of clotting proteins in man. In Hoekstra WG, et al, editors: Trace elements in animals, ed 2, Baltimore, 1974, University Park Press, pp 749-751.

78. Kuttel T, et al: Micronutrient adequacy in home parenteral nutrition patients, Am J Clin Nutr **39**:679, 1984.

Molybdenum

79. Rajagopalan KV: Chemistry and biology of the molybdenum cofactor, Biochem Soc Trans **13**:401-403, 1985.

80. Beemer FA, et al: Absence of hepatic molybdenum cofactor. An inborn error of metabolism associated with lens dislocation, Ophthalmic Paediatr Genet **5**:191-195, 1985.

81. Abumrad NN, et al: Amino acid intolerance during prolonged total parenteral nutrition reversed by molybdate therapy, Am J Clin Nutr **34**:2551-2559, 1981.

Other Trace Metals

82. Nielsen FH: Possible future implications of nickel, arsenic, silicon, vanadium, and other ultratrace elements in human nutrition. In Prasad AS, editor: Clinical, biochemical and nutritional aspects of trace elements, New York, 1982, Alan R Liss Inc, pp 379-404.

83. Solomons NW: The other trace minerals: manganese, molybdenum, vanadium, nickel, silicon, and arsenic. In Solomons NW, Rosenberg IH, editors: Absorption and malabsorption of mineral nutrients, New York, 1984, Alan R Liss Inc, pp 269-295.

CHAPTER 37
Anemias

Victor Herbert

Nutritional anemias are conditions in which the hemoglobin content of the blood is lower than normal owing to a deficit in a specific nutrient.[1] There are three simple nutritional anemias: those resulting from deficiencies of iron, folate, and/ or vitamin B_{12}.[23] The two vitamins are closely interrelated biochemically in DNA synthesis, and iron is indirectly involved.[4] Partly for this reason, and partly because a patient may have more than one of these deficiencies, all three nutrients must be considered whenever a patient presents with deficiency of any one of them.[5]

In treating nutritional anemia, if one aims high-dose therapy at the wrong deficiency the real deficiency may be masked, with disastrous results. For example, folate therapy may obscure vitamin B_{12} deficiency by improving the blood picture but may allow neurologic damage involving all myelinated neurons to progress unchecked. The result is a multisystem disease that sometimes presents as "megaloblastic madness."[5] At the same time, "shotgun" therapy aimed at all three, on the assumption that at least one is bound to be present, runs many of the same risks as therapy aimed improperly at only one or two—with the added risk of iron overload and possible intractable heart failure.

Despite their sometimes confounding interrelationship, the nutritional anemias are usually completely curable when properly diagnosed.[1] Specific diagnostic tests, coupled with sound clinical judgment, ensure early and accurate diagnosis.[4,6-8] Proper follow-up can verify that the specific therapy has corrected the anemia, thereby confirming the diagnosis. Often the root cause of the nutrient deficiency can be identified and corrected to provide an ultimate cure. Even when the root cause cannot be corrected, continuing therapy can usually sustain a normal nutritional status and thereby avert the consequences of deficiency.

CRITERIA FOR NUTRITIONAL ANEMIA

A simple nutritional anemia must meet two criteria: (1) by itself, deficiency or lack of the nutrient must produce the anemia; and (2) providing only the nutrient must correct the anemia.

By these criteria, some anemias that may appear nutritional really are more complex. For example, leucopenia and thrombopenia associated with copper deficiency are not produced by a diet lacking only copper, and children with Menkes' disease copper deficiency do not become anemic.[9] A copper-corrected anemia associated with multiple nutrient deficiencies occurs in infants fed a copper-deficient milk diet that is also protein- and iron-deficient. This anemia, which occurs in generalized malnutrition, can also occur after intestinal bypass surgery or parenteral alimentation.[9] It is therefore not generally counted among the simple nutritional anemias.

The anemia of protein-energy malnutrition is also not included among the true nutritional anemias because it is physiologic rather than pathologic. The fall in red cell mass results from lower oxygen requirements of the reduced body mass; less tissue means less tissue hypoxia to trigger red cell formation.[11] In a pathologic anemia, the total red cell mass is below the norm required for adequate oxygenation of the given total body mass.[11]

A hemolytic anemia is seen in premature infants who receive large amounts of oxidant agents (e.g., iron), usually together with substantial amounts of PUFA (polyunsaturated fatty acids) and inadequate vitamin E to metabolize the PUFA. This hemolytic anemia is corrected by oral administration of 50 to 200 mg of alpha-tocopherol, but it responds as well to a reduction in the formula content of iron and PUFA.[12] In addition, it fails to meet the criteria of a true nutritional anemia because it is due to factors other than simply a lack of vitamin E; it is more a nutrient-responsive anemia than a nutrient-deficiency anemia. Occasional sideroblastic (sideroachrestic) anemias also are nutrient-responsive to 50-200 mg of pyridoxine daily or to pyridoxal-5-phosphate.[9,13]

The distinction between nutrient-responsive and nutrient-deficiency anemias is illustrated by the interrelationship between the folate and vitamin B_{12} deficiencies. Anemia resulting from either responds to therapy with the other, although not primarily caused by lack of the other. Failure to make this crucial distinction in the past has led to improper treatment of patients with anemia from vitamin B_{12} deficiency (i.e., they were given folate). Since this anemia responds to folate, these patients showed hematologic improvement but suffered progressive neurologic damage because folate did not correct the vitamin B_{12} deficiency.[14] Only vitamin B_{12} can arrest and (up to a point) reverse the neurologic damage.

ETIOLOGY AND CLASSIFICATION

Etiologically, all the nutritional anemias fall into one of six categories: inadequate ingestion, absorption, or utilization of a particular nutrient and increased requirement, excretion, or destruction of the nutrient.[15] Besides correcting the deficiency, the aim must be to determine the cause and, where possible, correct it.

Iron Deficiency

In the United States, iron deficiency anemia, resulting mainly from inadequate intake for rate of growth or rate of blood loss, is found in up to 25% of infants, 6% of children, 3% of menstruating women, and 10% of pregnant women.[10] Iron depletion of insufficient degree to cause anemia may exist in as many as half of all infants and menstruating women and in 90% of pregnant women.[9,16]

The peak incidence of iron deficiency in childhood is between 6 months and 2 years of age, with another peak during early adolescence. In the case of very young children, the two specific causes generally cited are absent or low iron stores at birth and a diet consisting mainly of cow's milk, which is low in absorbable iron and at times may irritate the intestine. The peak in early adolescence stems mainly from increased body requirements because of the growth spurt;

Table 37-1 Estimated Dietary Iron Requirements (mg/da*)

Normal men and nonmenstruating women	5-10
Menstruating women	7-20
Pregnant women	20-48†
Adolescents	10-20
Children	4-10
Infants	1.5 mg/kg‡

From: Herbert V: Hosp Pract **125**:65-89, 1980.
*Assuming 10% absorption.
†More than can be derived from the diet; mandates iron supplementation in the latter half of pregnancy.
‡To a maximum of 15 mg.

at the same time, intake may be relatively deficient. The daily oral iron requirement ranges from 5 mg in infancy to 20 mg in adolescence (Table 37-1). In the United States the average adult diet provides only 15 to 18 mg of iron per day, of which an average of only 10% (1.5-1.8 mg) is absorbed.[16] It is not surprising therefore that up to 10% of female high school students in some low-income areas have iron deficiency anemia.

It is also not surprising that women in the childbearing years, whose daily absorbed iron requirement may be 2 mg because of menstrual blood loss, have a high incidence of iron depletion. Women taking oral contraceptives have less menstrual blood loss and, therefore, a lower incidence of iron depletion. Pregnancy aggravates the situation because the fetus takes from the mother the iron that it requires, regardless of her status. The iron lost during lactation, however, is offset by the associated amenorrhea. The total iron "cost" of a normal pregnancy has been put at 440 to 1050 mg.[9,16,17]

Only 0.2% of adult men in the United States have iron deficiency anemia.[10] The daily dietary requirement for men is about 10 mg, and the average diet provides nearly double this amount.[17] Therefore iron deficiency in men and nonmenstruating women should be considered secondary to blood loss, usually from the gastrointestinal tract, until proved otherwise.

Certain other conditions are frequently associated with iron-deficiency anemia. The most common is alcoholism. About 50% of alcoholics, estimated to number 2 to 10 million in the United States, have iron depletion if not anemia. Iron deficiency also is associated with hookworm infestation. Although largely of historical interest in the United States, hookworm is still a major cause of iron deficiency whenever people walk barefoot, particularly in poor and underdeveloped nations, where up to 90% of the population may have iron deficiency from this parasitic infestation.[9]

Folate Deficiency

Folate deficiency may arise from as many as 50 subcategories of the six basic etiologies of nutrient deficiency, but most cases result from inadequate ingestion, inadequate absorption, or increased requirement.[5,15,16,18]

Inadequate folate ingestion is the most common cause despite the fact that this nutrient is found in nearly all raw foods. Folate is readily destroyed by cooking, especially when the foods are small particles with large surface areas exposed to cooking temperatures, e.g., beans and rice. The folic acid content of the average diet varies widely, depending on its raw food content, how the food is prepared, and factors in the food that inhibit or enhance folate absorption. These factors, plus the increased metabolic requirements of pregnancy, mean that folate deficiency and megaloblastic anemia can develop in about one third of all pregnant women. Therefore a pregnant woman whose daily diet does not include either fresh or fresh-frozen uncooked fruit or fruit juice or a fresh, raw, or lightly cooked vegetable, or anyone whose food is all cooked more than 15 minutes, must be presumed folate deficient until proved otherwise. Folate deficiency is also seen in some 90% of hard-liquor alcoholics, most beer and wine alcoholics, and perhaps half of narcotic addicts. The main reason is low intake of nutritious food.[18,19]

Inadequate folate absorption is possible even with adequate intake, when the ingested form (predominantly the polyglutamates) cannot be split into absorbable form (mainly monoglutamate). Inadequate folate absorption results from inhibition of the intestinal conjugase enzyme, which removes the extra glutamate residues so that absorption may occur. Inhibition may be caused by acidic foods, such as orange juice, which lower the intestinal pH, or by a heat-stable heat-activated conjugase inhibitor found in beans and other legumes. In addition, absorbability not only of polyglutamates but also of monoglutamates varies among food sources so foods of

equally high folate content may differ widely in quantity of absorbable folate.[18]

Increased utilization of folate, a third cause of deficiency, appears to be the main factor in a newly recognized iatrogenic syndrome, hyperalimentation-associated megaloblastic anemia. This type of anemia develops too rapidly to be caused entirely by inadequate intake; the alcohol in the infusion fluid may increase folate losses in the bile.[19]

Folate deficiency, as well as vitamin B_{12} deficiency resulting in megaloblastic anemia, is seen in tropical sprue. This disease is endemic in the Caribbean and in Southeast Asia. A person born in an endemic area who acquires the disease may have remissions and exacerbations throughout life, regardless of where he or she may subsequently live. Reinfection from close association with conationals may be a factor, so a person born in Puerto Rico or another endemic area who develops megaloblastic anemia in the continental United States should be considered to have tropical sprue until diagnosed otherwise.

Vitamin B_{12} Deficiency

Of the three nutritional anemias, the one caused by vitamin B_{12} deficiency is the least common in the United States, since this nutrient is found in all foods of animal origin, including meat, poultry, fish, eggs, and dairy products. Vitamin B_{12} is not destroyed by usual cooking.[15,16] Intestinal reabsorption of the vitamin from bile contributes significantly in meeting the body's requirements.[5] The comparatively large enterohepatic circulation of the vitamin explains why deficiency occurs slowly (20-30 yr) in those whose dietary intake is minimal but occurs comparatively rapidly (3-6 yr) in those whose absorption (and therefore reabsorption) is cut off.

Strict vegetarians are the only notable group in the United States whose vitamin B_{12} intake is essentially nil, but this is not a sizable group. Of 37,000 Seventh Day Adventists, only 2% were pure vegetarians (29% were lactoovovegetarians, 25% ate meat rarely, 29% ate meat one to four times per wk, 15% ate meat five or more times per wk).* Strict vegetarianism itself does

*Johnston PK, et al, editors: Proceedings. First International Congress of Vegetarian Nutrition, Am J Clin Nutr (suppl), September 1988.

not always entail B_{12} deficiency. In southern India, the vitamin B_{12} requirements of many strict vegetarians are partly met by contamination of food and water by fecal and other animal matter and by microorganisms in the nodules of legumes. In the United States, some cereals and soy are "spiked" with B_{12}.

In the United States vitamin B_{12}–deficiency anemia usually means inadequate absorption. Vitamin B_{12} normally is liberated from the food by digestion. It combines with intrinsic factor secreted by the gastric parietal cells and with nonintrinsic factor–vitamin B_{12}–binding glycoproteins called R-binders or cobalophilins, which are mainly salivary in origin. The bound complexes then pass down the intestine, where the nonintrinsic factor binder is destroyed at alkaline pH by pancreas enzymes, and the freed vitamin B_{12} combines with intrinsic factor. When the intrinsic factor–vitamin B_{12} complex reaches the ileum, in the presence of calcium, it attaches to enterocytes and is transported through the ileal epithelial cell into the circulation. Despite the complexity of the absorptive process, malfunctions stem from only three major factors, involving as many sites: (1) a structural or functional gastric defect, leading to insufficient intrinsic factor secretion; (2) an ileal defect, leading to inadequate absorption even in the presence of adequate intrinsic factor; or (3) pancreatic disease, in which optimum conditions for the absorption of the vitamin are not met despite the presence of other requisite factors.[20,21]

Malabsorption in the stomach usually means pernicious anemia (i.e. insufficient secretion of intrinsic factor from unknown causes) usually associated with gastric atrophy. This disease is commonly age-dependent and is seen with increasing frequency after age 50 years. Both the tendency to gastric atrophy and the age at which it becomes manifest are genetically determined. There is also an autoimmune component in pernicious anemia, and two different types of intrinsic factor antibody have been described in the disease. One, a blocking antibody, reacts only with intrinsic factor apoglycoprotein and prevents the initial binding of vitamin B_{12}. The other, a binding antibody, combines with intrinsic factor at a site distal to the vitamin B_{12}–binding site and binds to either apoglycoprotein or the intrinsic factor–vitamin B_{12} complex.

Any stomach condition (e.g., severe chronic gastritis) that reduces acid and pepsin secretion may inhibit vitamin B_{12} absorption. The resulting disease is distinguishable from classic pernicious anemia by the fact that the Schilling test is normal when the patient is fed crystalline radioactive vitamin B_{12}, but subnormal when the radioactive vitamin B_{12} is in eggs or meat, and by the fact that the aspirated gastric juice contains appreciable intrinsic factor.[5,8] In gastrectomy, intrinsic factor secretion usually is reduced in proportion to the parietal cell mass that is removed. Total gastrectomy means a complete loss of intrinsic factor, of course, with eventual severe vitamin B_{12} deficiency unless vitamin replacement therapy is instituted by injection.

Ileal or small bowel conditions that lead to vitamin B_{12} malabsorption usually involve either stasis of luminal content, with consequent overgrowth of bacteria, known as the "blind loop syndrome," or an effective reduction in the ileal absorptive surface, such as occurs in regional enteritis. Vitamin B_{12} malabsorption in intestinal bacterial overgrowth may be caused in part by direct interference of the bacterial toxins and in part because the bacteria themselves take up the vitamin, making it unavailable to the host.

Any procedure that shortens the ileum, such as some operations for intractable obesity, can appreciably reduce vitamin B_{12} absorption by reducing the available absorptive surface. Again, such malabsorption is to be expected, and the usual practice is to provide replacement therapy. Almost any type of bowel surgery may be followed by the stagnant bowel syndrome, which should be considered in any patient with vitamin B_{12} deficiency and previous abdominal surgery.

The intestinal absorptive surface may also be reduced by deficiency of either vitamin B_{12} itself or folate. The megaloblastosis (resulting from impaired DNA synthesis) affects all of the dividing cells of the body, including those of the intestinal lumen. The result is an effective atrophy of the absorptive cells, so that the induced malabsorption "feeds upon itself." This type of malabsorption can be remedied by administering vitamin B_{12} (or folate, as the case may be); but once a vitamin B_{12} or folate deficiency has developed, the deficiency may become self-perpetuating, producing a secondary deficiency of the other vitamin caused by reduced absorption. This vicious cycle also can lead to diagnostic difficulties. The diagnosis of vitamin B_{12}

malabsorption is usually based on the patient's failure to absorb radiolabeled vitamin B_{12}, whether given alone or with intrinsic factor. In some 40% of cases, the malabsorption is secondary to vitamin B_{12} or folic acid deficiency, not the result of primary intestinal malabsorption. Thus, after vitamin therapy, the test with added intrinsic factor reverts to normal.[20]

Vitamin B_{12} deficiency is also common in tropical sprue, as just noted. In about one third of cases, it is associated with a secondary gastric lesion resulting in reduced or absent intrinsic factor secretion. The defect can usually be remedied with broad-spectrum antibiotic therapy, which corrects the absorption defect, presumably by killing the unknown causative organism.

The vitamin B_{12} malabsorption arising from pancreatic disease may result in part from inadequate secretion of bicarbonate. Absorption of the vitamin occurs only in an alkaline milieu, and the pancreas must provide sufficient bicarbonate to neutralize the gastric acid that pours into the small bowel. Pancreatic trypsin also is essential to vitamin B_{12} absorption. This enzyme must destroy the nonintrinsic factor–vitamin B_{12} binders, releasing their vitamin B_{12} so it can bind to intrinsic factor.[21]

Several drugs, including neomycin, colchicine, paraaminosalicylic acid, slow-release potassium chloride, metformin, and ethanol, have been associated with malabsorption of vitamin B_{12}. In short-term drug therapy, malabsorption is usually not of clinical significance, but long-term therapy with either paraaminosalicylic acid or an oral antidiabetic drug may result in anemia. The mechanism of malabsorption in these drug-induced deficiencies is not always clear. It is clear, however, that they are not usually rectified by supplying intrinsic factor, so the presumption is that either ileal uptake or transport is impaired.[5,20]

With the widespread use of vitamin C, a few patients taking megadoses have been found to have unexpectedly low serum vitamin B_{12} concentrations. Thus, some persons ingesting large doses of vitamin C for long periods may risk a vitamin B_{12} deficiency. Recently, it has been found that mixing vitamin B_{12} with vitamin C or certain other vitamins and minerals converts a variable amount of the vitamin B_{12} to analogues.[22] Some of these analogues may have anti–vitamin B_{12} action.

PATHOLOGY

Each nutritional anemia produces a specific pathologic picture that provides a ready distinction between iron deficiency anemia and anemia caused by one or both of the vitamin deficiencies. However, as noted at the outset, the picture can be quite confounding if, as often happens, iron deficiency coexists with a deficiency of one or both of the other nutrients. If folate and/or vitamin B_{12} deficiency is also present, the clinical and laboratory picture can be clarified only by the proper sequence of tests plus appropriate therapy.[4,15,16]

Iron Deficiency

The iron of the body is found almost exclusively bound to protein—either in transferrin (a transport form) or ferritin (a storage form)—or in heme (hemoglobin, myoglobin, or heme enzymes). Hemoglobin alone accounts for some two thirds (2.5 g) of the total-body iron, whereas about 1 g in men and 0.3 g in women is in reserves, partly as ferritin but mainly as hemosiderin, a more stable, less available, form of storage iron. Only about 3% is found in myoglobin, some 0.5% in heme enzymes, and about 0.1% in transferrin. The total-body iron content is about 50 mg/kg of body weight in men and 35 mg/kg in women. Iron tends to remain relatively fixed; otherwise, iron deficiency or iron overload (hemosiderosis) results. Iron is not excreted in the usual sense, being tenaciously conserved and lost only when cells are lost. A practical consequence of this tenacious conservation is that iron requirements are relatively modest.[9,17,23]

Central to iron metabolism is its role in hemoglobin synthesis. The iron contained in the red cells is salvaged at the end of the 120-day life-span of these cells by the reticuloendothelial system and is either stored for a time or delivered to transferrin.

The biosynthesis of hemoglobin requires that its three components (iron, comprising 0.33% of its weight, protoporphyrin, and globin) be provided in optimum amounts. Normally the main source of the iron for hemoglobin synthesis is that carried by the plasma in transferrin. If the transferrin is less than 15% saturated with iron, red cell production is reduced, and the cells that are produced are at first microcytic and then also hypochromic. Such cells in the peripheral blood smear are hallmarks of inadequate hemoglobin synthesis. Iron deficiency therefore is not the only condition so characterized; others include the anemia of chronic disorders, thalassemia major and minor, hemoglobin C or E disease, and the sideroblastic anemias.[23-27]

Combined Iron and Vitamin Deficiency

If iron deficiency is accompanied by vitamin B_{12} deficiency, large oval red cells (macroovalocytes) may be present in a blood smear, as well as neutrophils with hypersegmented nuclei, since the characteristic feature of both vitamin B_{12} and folate deficiencies is a bone marrow megaloblastosis resulting from slowed DNA synthesis in which the progeny of megaloblasts are macroovalocytes. Another feature of megaloblastic hematopoiesis is megaloblastic myelopoiesis, as evidenced by the presence in the bone marrow of many giant metamyelocytes, whose progeny in the blood are neutrophils with hypersegmented nuclei. Normally, cells capable of reproducing are in a resting state and usually contain one unit of DNA. When they reproduce, they double their DNA, divide, and return to the resting state. Hence, at any given moment, 100 normal nucleated cells contain, say, 101 units of DNA, since all but one of the cells are most likely to be in the resting state. However, in vitamin B_{12} or folate deficiency, very few cells are in the resting state. Instead, many are slowly trying to double their DNA, with frequent arrest of the process in the synthesis phase, since vitamin B_{12} and folate are essential to the process. The result is a larger cell containing more than one unit of DNA (i.e., a megaloblastic cell). Microscopically such cells have more than the normal amount of DNA despite their defective DNA synthesis. Since their ability to synthesize RNA is relatively unimpaired, the cytoplasm is larger than the nucleus and more mature in appearance. This nuclear-cytoplasmic synchrony or dissociation results in the finely particulate nuclear chromatin (or "young nucleus") typical of erythroid megaloblasts at every cytoplasmic maturation stage and differentiates them from normoblasts, which have coarsely clumped ("old") nuclear chromatin as the cytoplasm matures and starts making hemoglobin.[5,15]

If the deficiency-induced megaloblastic anemia is overlaid with iron deficiency, as is the case in about one-third of the vitamin B_{12}–deficiency anemias and in about one-half of the

cases resulting from folate deficiency, the blood cell picture is mixed. When the vitamin deficiency is dominant, the pathologic picture may be one of iron overload, because the slowed DNA synthesis and anemia mean that iron requirements are greatly reduced. Thus iron that would be insufficient to sustain a normal red cell mass may be excessive for the reduced red cell mass of the anemia. Some patients, however, may have intermediate megaloblastosis in the bone marrow, with the macroovalocytic progeny mixed with hypochromic microcytes in the blood, a "dimorphic" anemia. A key morphologic feature that may be used to recognize the presence of vitamin B_{12} or folate deficiency, even in the face of dominant iron deficiency, is myeloid megaloblastosis in the bone marrow. The latter is characterized by the production of hypersegmented polymorphonuclear leukocytes (or "hypersegmented polys") that, unlike macroovalocytes, are not masked in the peripheral blood by concomitant iron deficiency. The hypersegmented polymorphonuclear leukocytes are commonly defined by a rule of fives: if more than 5% neutrophils have five or more lobes, hypersegmentation is present. A more elaborate method involves calculating the lobe average per 100 polymorphonuclear leukocytes, with hypersegmentation diagnosed if the average is 3.5 or higher, since the normal lobe average is 3.2 ± 0.15.[5,6]

Vitamin Deficiency

Since the vitamin deficiency–induced megaloblastic anemias result from inadequate erythropoiesis, the hemolytic component and the seeming iron overload also provide important diagnostic clues. The increased "fetal" death rate of erythroid cells may be evidenced by the presence of up to 25% reticulocytes among bone marrow erythrocyte precursors, as contrasted with 1% or less in the blood. Blood chemistry findings include increased serum lactate dehydrogenase from cells destroyed in the bone marrow and modestly elevated serum bilirubin from cells destroyed in the blood.[5]

The ineffective use of available iron that is characteristic of both folate- and vitamin B_{12}–deficiency anemia results in an increased saturation of the iron-binding capacity and an increase in iron stores, which produce a picture that mimics iron overload. Therefore, if a patient with megaloblastic anemia has normal rather than elevated serum iron and bone marrow hemosiderin, often with an elevated total iron-binding capacity as well, coincident iron deficiency should be suspected. Both serum and bone marrow iron should be reevaluated after 1 month of vitamin therapy to determine whether iron deficiency has been unmasked. The vitamin therapy may have drawn the stored iron into hemoglobin synthesis, and the hemoglobin may have risen toward normal but then leveled off at still anemic values.[4]

Just as megaloblastic atrophy of the intestinal epithelial surface area reduces the absorptive surface for folate and vitamin B_{12}, gastric atrophy associated with deficiency of iron, vitamin B_{12}, or folate may reduce the production of intrinsic factor necessary for vitamin B_{12} absorption, thus creating another of the vicious cycles that may tend to be self-perpetuating.

A primary defect found only in vitamin B_{12} deficiency, and not in folate deficiency, is an inability to synthesize myelin. The result is the insidious development of a demyelinating neuropathy, usually commencing in the peripheral nerves, progressing to the posterior and lateral columns of the spinal cord, and ultimately reaching the cerebrum. Folate has no helpful effect on this neuropathy, and incorrect therapy can lead to irreversible damage.[14] The damage stems from the inability to synthesize myelin, but inadequate myelin synthesis causes the deterioration of the axon and eventually of the nerve head. Short of the point of nervehead deterioration, the process is reversible. Work in Dublin has shown that vitamin B_{12}–deficiency nerve damage in monkeys can be prevented by methionine and that the "folate trap"[29] is involved.[14,30]

DIAGNOSIS
Iron Deficiency

The tests that may be used to determine iron deficiency with or without resultant anemia depend on the stage or severity of the deficiency. In general, four distinct stages have been described* (Fig. 37-1).

Initially, there is simply negative balance with depletion of iron stores. If these are not replenished, iron-deficient erythropoiesis (iron deficiency without anemia) ensues. Anemia ultimately will develop.

At the next stage there is a fall in bone marrow storage iron (and in the plasma ferritin, with which it is in equilibrium) and a rise in unsaturated iron-binding capacity. Simultaneously, the ability to absorb iron begins to rise. The serum iron content, reflecting parenchymal iron and the hemoglobin level, remains within normal range, and transferrin remains approximately one third saturated with iron.

At the third stage, as iron-deficient red cell synthesis

*References 5, 17, 23, 24.

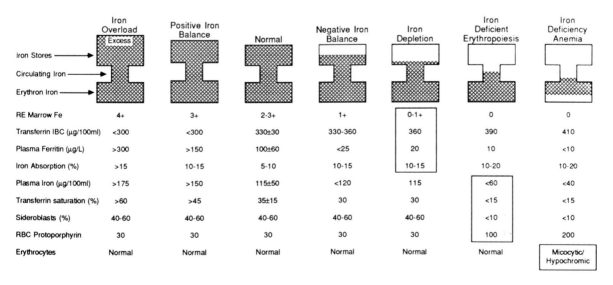

	Iron Overload	Positive Iron Balance	Normal	Negative Iron Balance	Iron Depletion	Iron Deficient Erythropoiesis	Iron Deficiency Anemia
Iron Stores	Excess						
Circulating Iron							
Erythron Iron							
RE Marrow Fe	4+	3+	2-3+	1+	0-1+	0	0
Transferrin IBC (μg/100ml)	<300	<300	330±30	330-360	360	390	410
Plasma Ferritin (μg/L)	>300	>150	100±60	<25	20	10	<10
Iron Absorption (%)	>15	10-15	5-10	10-15	10-15	10-20	10-20
Plasma Iron (μg/100ml)	>175	>150	115±50	<120	115	<60	<40
Transferrin saturation (%)	>60	>45	35±15	30	30	<15	<15
Sideroblasts (%)	40-60	40-60	40-60	40-60	40-60	<10	<10
RBC Protoporphyrin	30	30	30	30	30	100	200
Erythrocytes	Normal	Normal	Normal	Normal	Normal	Normal	Micocytic/ Hypochromic

Figure 37-1 Sequential stages of iron status. The boxes enclose the abnormalities whose appearance indicates the onset of that particular stage of negative balance.

sets in, the serum iron level falls, and the percentage of transferrin saturated with iron drops below one sixth. At the same time the free erythrocyte protoporphyrin triples, indicating a lack of sufficient iron to convert it to hemoglobin; the loss of iron is also manifested by a drop in sideroblasts to below 10%.

Finally, when frank anemia has developed, the red cells take on the characteristic hypochromic-microcytic appearance.

Thus anemia is the final manifestation of iron deficiency. It is also the easiest of the four stages of such deficiency to diagnose definitively, and an additional definitive test—response to iron therapy—is available. In the absence of anemia, the lack of bone marrow iron suggests iron-deficient erythropoiesis. However, diagnosing iron depletion requires that two of the laboratory tests be abnormal if bone marrow iron is present. If the transferrin saturation is less than 15%, the free erythrocyte protoporphyrin greater than 100 μg/100 ml, and the serum ferritin less than 12 ng/ml, the patient is clearly iron deficient even in the absence of anemia. Yet each of these tests in isolation may indicate a condition other than iron deficiency. Free erythrocyte protoporphyrin, for example, is greatly elevated in the early stages of lead poisoning. For this reason, lead poisoning should always be considered in the differential diagnosis of patients with the findings of anemia, especially children from an urban environment and adults who may have been removing old paint. Serum ferritin also may be elevated in acute and chronic inflammatory diseases and in liver disease, even in the presence of an underlying iron deficiency.[9,23]

The most direct test for anemia is the hemoglobin, and most physicians use it in screening; the hematocrit and the red cell count are less commonly used alternatives. If any one of the three indicates anemia, it is imperative to determine the underlying cause. The next step, therefore, should be a look at the peripheral blood smear, followed by determination of the mean corpuscular volume (MCV). Low MCV at face value means inadequate hemoglobin synthesis; and, statistically, most such cases represent iron deficiency, with a minority caused by thalassemia, lead poisoning, sideroblastic anemia, or chronic inflammatory disease. The average MCV in normal adults is 90 femtoliters (fl), with 80 fl the lower limit of normal; in adolescents, the average is 88 fl, with a lower limit of 78 fl;

in infants, it averages 77 fl, rising in children to 86 fl, just before adolescence.[25-27]

A low MCV mandates determination of iron and iron-binding capacity, free erythrocyte protoporphyrin levels, or serum ferritin levels. Since anemia is known to be present, one need not do all three tests; any one will do because response to iron therapy constitutes a second (and the best) test. If there is a possibility of lead poisoning, the free erythrocyte protoporphyrin test is perhaps the most accurate of the three. If it is elevated, one should immediately assay blood lead or delta-aminolevulinic acid dehydrase to rule out possible plumbism.[23-27] Hair lead is a poor test: it is elevated later, and, when elevated, may be so from hair dyes or adventitious lead.

The blood smear should be examined at this point. If the cells are small and undercolored, the diagnosis in a majority of patients is iron-deficiency anemia. The remainder will prove to have thalassemia or one of the other conditions that may result in microcytic or hypochromic anemia. In combined iron deficiency and deficiency of vitamin B_{12} and/or folate, red cells may be normochromic and normocytic; or they may be dimorphic (some small and uncolored because of iron deficiency, others macroovalocytic because of vitamin deficiency).

Even if all the tests point to iron deficiency anemia, the definitive diagnostic test remains therapeutic trial. Oral iron therapy should be used for at least 6 months to assure replenishment of body stores, even though laboratory indicators revert to normal in less than half this time.[2,9] The reticulocyte count, for instance, rises within 3 to 10 days, but if the anemia is mild, the rise may be small and difficult to detect. Also, serum ferritin does not immediately reflect the size of the iron stores. It can be used to detect the occasional case of iron overload, however, provided the test is done at two dilutions to avoid the "high dose hook effect."

Thus, it is obvious that a low MCV and anemia in and of themselves are not sufficient for a diagnosis of iron deficiency anemia. Treatment based on these two measurements alone carries the risk of using iron to treat a condition in which iron excess is already present. Medicinal iron should never be used as a "tonic," and patients should be cautioned against self-medication with iron on the basis of advertising claims. Iron taken by a person who already has excessive iron stores

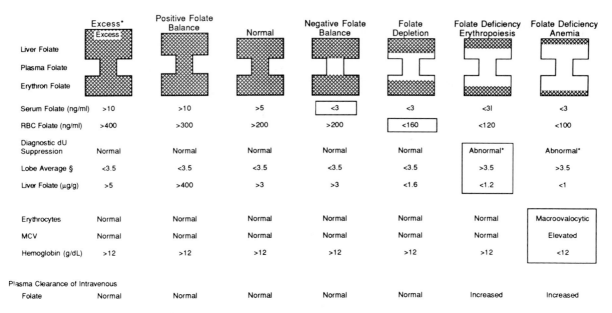

	Excess*	Positive Folate Balance	Normal	Negative Folate Balance	Folate Depletion	Folate Deficiency Erythropoiesis	Folate Deficiency Anemia
Liver Folate							
Plasma Folate							
Erythron Folate							
Serum Folate (ng/ml)	>10	>10	>5	<3	<3	<3l	<3
RBC Folate (ng/ml)	>400	>300	>200	>200	<160	<120	<100
Diagnostic dU Suppression	Normal	Normal	Normal	Normal	Normal	Abnormal*	Abnormal*
Lobe Average §	<3.5	<3.5	<3.5	<3.5	<3.5	>3.5	>3.5
Liver Folate (µg/g)	>5	>400	>3	>3	<1.6	<1.2	<1
Erythrocytes	Normal	Normal	Normal	Normal	Normal	Normal	Macroovalocytic
MCV	Normal	Normal	Normal	Normal	Normal	Normal	Elevated
Hemoglobin (g/dL)	>12	>12	>12	>12	>12	>12	<12
Plasma Clearance of Intravenous Folate	Normal	Normal	Normal	Normal	Normal	Increased	Increased

* Dietary excess of folate reduces zinc absorption.

Figure 37-2 Sequential stages of folate status. The boxes enclose the abnormalities whose appearance indicates the onset of that particular stage of negative balance.

Stage:	Excess*	Positive B12 Balance	Normal	Negative B12 Balance	B12 Depletion	B12-Deficient Erythropoiesis	B12-Deficiency Anemia
Liver B12							
HoloTC II							
RBC+WBC B12							
HoloTC II (pg/ml)	>50	>40	>30	<20	<20	<12	<12
TC II % sat.	>5%	>5%	>5%	<5%	<2%	<1%	<1%
Halohap (pg/ml)	>500	>300	>150	>150	<150	<100	<100
dU Suppression	Normal	Normal	Normal	Normal	Normal	Abnormal	Abnormal
Hypersegmentation	No	No	No	No	No	Yes	Yes
TBBC† % sat.	>50%	>40	>15%	>15%	>15%	<15%	<10%
Hap % sat.	>50%	>40	>20%	>20%	>20%	<20%	<10%
RBC Folate (ng/ml)	>160	>160	>160	>160	>160	<140	<100
Erythrocytes	Normal	Normal	Normal	Normal	Normal	Normal	Macroovalocytic
MCV	Normal	Normal	Normal	Normal	Normal	Normal	Elevated
Hemoglobin	Normal	Normal	Normal	Normal	Normal	Normal	Low
TC II	Normal	Normal	Normal	Normal	Normal	Elevated	Elevated
Methylmalonate ↑≠	No	No	No	No	No	?	Yes
Myelin Damage	No*	No	No	No	No	?	Frequent

* Cyanocobalamin excesses (injected or intranasal) produce transient rise in B12 analogues on B12 delivery protein (TC II); the significance of such rises is unknown (Herbert et al, 1987). Cyanocobalamin acts as an anti-B12 in a rare congenital defect in B12 metabolism.
≠ In serum and urine.
† TBBC= Total B12 binding capacity.

Figure 37-3 Sequential stages of vitamin B12 status. Biochemical and hematologic sequence of events as negative vitamin B12 balance progresses. The boxes enclose the abnormalities whose appearance indicates the onset of that particular stage of negative balance.

only hastens the development of iron overload and possibly such serious complications as intractable heart disease. The public should be warned that over-the-counter iron should follow, and not precede, diagnosis of iron deficiency.

Always determine iron status (Fig. 37-1) before treating. Feeling tired and rundown occurs in many conditions, including iron overload.[5,24]

Vitamin Deficiency

Fig. 37-2 presents the biochemical and hematologic sequence of events in developing folate deficiency and Fig. 37-3 does the same for developing vitamin B_{12} deficiency. The box lists the diagnostic tests used in the differential diagnosis of vitamin B_{12} deficiency from folate deficiency.[5,8] A diagnostic "pearl" is that early vitamin B_{12}–deficiency nerve damage may be recognized by loss of ability to perceive vibrations of a 256 vps tuning fork and loss of ability to perceive whether the index toes are moved up or down. These losses may precede by up to 6 months loss of the ability to perceive vibrations of a 128 vps tuning fork or the direction of great toe passive movement.

If examination of the peripheral blood shows the macroovalocytes and hypersegmented neutrophils indicative of megaloblastic anemia, the cause in 95% of cases will be vitamin B_{12} or folate deficiency, or both. However, a high proportion of these patients proves to have iron deficiency as well, so all of them should be tested for it also at the outset and again after a month of vitamin therapy. In an unknown but large percentage of these patients, it will be impossible to diagnose the coexisting iron deficiency straightaway. Rather, there is a seeming iron overload or seemingly normal iron status because of the ineffective erythropoiesis. Only after the vitamin deficiency has been adequately treated will iron utilization become effective so that one can diagnose iron deficiency. The rule to remember is that if the patient with megaloblastic anemia has laboratory results indicating normal iron instead of iron overload he probably does not have enough iron in his body to get hemoglobin levels back to normal with vitamin therapy, so his iron status must be reevaluated after 1 or 2 months of vitamin therapy. At that time the laboratory tests will probably show iron deficiency requiring iron therapy.

As indicated by examination of the peripheral

DIAGNOSTIC TESTS TO DIFFERENTIATE VITAMIN B_{12} DEFICIENCY FROM FOLATE DEFICIENCY

Before Therapy Only

Serum vitamin B_{12} (radioassay): normal 200-900 pg/ml

Serum folate: normal 7-16 ng/ml

Erythrocyte folate: normal >150 ng/ml

Methylmalonate in urine or serum: increase usually means vitamin B_{12} deficiency

Formiminoglutamate and urocanate in urine after oral histidine load: increased in vitamin B_{12} deficiency, folate deficiency, liver disease

Deoxyuridine suppression test (in vitro therapeutic trial) on bone marrow: cells abnormal, corrected by missing vitamin

Before or After Therapy

Gastric analysis: acid, pepsin, quality, quantity, intrinsic factor content

Tests of radioactive vitamin B_{12} absorption after physiologic dose of radioactive vitamin B_{12} orally (Schilling test, etc.)

Circulating antibody to human intrinsic factor (normally absent)

Deoxyuridine suppression test on lymphocytes (may remain abnormal up to 2 mo after start of therapy)

Lymphocyte folate (may be low as long as lymphocyte deoxyuridine suppression test remains abnormal)

Adapted from Herbert V: *Hosp Pract* **125**:65-89, 1980.

---

blood smear, about one quarter of the patients with an elevated MCV have macrocytic (not macroovalocytic), round (rather than oval) red cells caused by hyperthyroidism, hypoplastic anemia, hemolytic anemia, sideroblastic anemia, neoplasia, liver disease, or some other condition often associated with reticulocytosis. If both the MCV and the peripheral blood smear indicate megaloblastic anemia, the next steps are to draw blood for serum vitamin B_{12} and folate levels and red cell folate and to examine a bone marrow aspirate to confirm megaloblastosis.

It is desirable to make three routine laboratory measurements (serum vitamin B_{12} and folate, plus red cell folate) rather than just two in evaluating megaloblastic anemia. The purpose is to attempt to separate four clinical situations, and only by use of the three tests can this be done, as indicated in Fig. 37-3.

Table 37-2 Need for Serum Vitamin B_{12} and Folate Plus Red Cell Folate in Differential Diagnosis

Clinical Situation	Serum Vitamin B_{12}	Serum Folate	Red Cell Folate
Normal	Normal	Normal or low	Normal
Vitamin B_{12} deficiency	Low	Normal or high	Low
Folic acid deficiency	Normal	Low	Low
Deficiency of both	Low	Low	Low

As suggested by Table 37-2, a low serum folate level is diagnostic only for negative folate balance and not for folate deficiency. Thus, the folate level may be low in many people whose tissue folate content and metabolism are normal but who simply have had poor appetite for several weeks. This explains the fact that two thirds of patients in acute-care hospitals have low serum folate levels. Their red cell and tissue folate levels are usually normal, and their serum folate levels will return to normal without folic acid treatment as they regain appetite.

Simultaneous radioassays for serum vitamin B_{12} and folate make these two determinations operatively just one laboratory procedure, with results available the same day.[31] Separately measuring red cell folate (by measuring whole blood folate and using the appropriate formula to calculate red cell folate)[32] is the second procedure to be done on the same original blood specimen.

Many persons, including commercial suppliers, frequently erroneously refer to the vitamin radioassays as "radioimmunoassays." Vitamin radioassay is competitive inhibition radioassay.[5,8] Radioimmunoassay is a subgroup of competitive inhibition radioassay, in which the binding agent is antibody. Antigen-antibody reaction makes a radioassay a radioimmunoassay; it is not a radioimmunoassay when no immunologic reaction is involved.[5]

The Deoxyuridine (dU) Suppression Test

The peripheral blood and bone marrow aspirate are being used increasingly to provide direct biochemical evidence of megaloblastosis by demonstrating impaired DNA synthesis in the deoxyuridine suppression test, which compares the incorporation of tritiated thymidine into the DNA of cultured lymphocytes (or bone marrow cells) preincubated in the presence and in the absence of nonradioactive deoxyuridine.[4,8,33,34] If folate coenzyme function (indicating normal folate and vitamin B_{12} activity) is normal, thymidylate synthetase converts the nonradioactive deoxyuridine to thymidine. This means that a reduced proportion of the thymidine pool is radioactive and there is a consequent "suppression" of the amount of radioactivity that is incorporated into the DNA. Vitamin B_{12} activity is assayed indirectly since it is an essential component in one of the reactions that converts the circulating form of folate into one that is involved in thymidine synthesis.[4] If either folate or vitamin B_{12} is deficient, there is less suppression of radioactive thymidine incorporation into DNA by the deoxyuridine.

Thus, if the deoxyuridine "suppression" is normalized by adding folate in methylfolate form to the culture, the diagnosis is folate deficiency; if vitamin B_{12} in hydroxocobalamin form normalizes the suppression, this vitamin is deficient; if both are required, there is combined deficiency.[4,8,33] The peripheral blood dU suppression test is of particular value in diagnosing folate or vitamin B_{12} deficiency concealed by iron deficiency,[4] in diagnosing vitamin B_{12} or folate deficiency even after a month of vitamin therapy,[33] and in diagnosing deficiency of vitamin B_{12} or folic acid despite falsely normal serum levels of vitamin.[5,8,15,33,39]

In its original form, this procedure required 50 ml of peripheral blood, from which the lymphocytes were then separated. Now a very small volume of blood (0.1 ml) suffices for each test tube in the test, and there is no need to separate the lymphocytes.[35] This means that the test can now be done as a routine laboratory procedure, even in pediatric patients. The dU suppression test on bone marrow measures current status with respect to vitamin B_{12} and folate; on lymphocytes, the test measures long-term or chronic status.[33] Vitamin therapy normalizes the deficient bone marrow vitamin status in less than 24 hours, but it may take more than 2 months to normalize the lymphocyte vitamin status.

Since the test, in effect, is a therapeutic trial in a test tube, it can obviate the need for a clinical therapeutic trial to distinguish folate deficiency from vitamin B_{12} deficiency. Essentially, the clinical therapeutic trial involves eliminating sources of folate and vitamin B_{12} from the diet for a period of 10 days, then starting therapy with either 1 μg of vitamin B_{12} daily or 100 μg of folic acid daily, depending on which is considered more likely to be deficient, and reevaluating the situation 5 to 12 days later, with reticulocyte counts every 2-3 days.

Such a trial, it should be noted, requires a minimum of 10 days' hospitalization: the deoxyuridine procedure does not require hospitalization and provides results in 1 day when done on bone marrow cells and in 4 days when done on peripheral blood lymphocytes.[35]

Other Tests

Other aids that may be useful in differentiating folate and vitamin B_{12} deficiency include the admission reticulocyte count, which commonly is below 1% in vitamin B_{12} deficiency but 1.5% to 8% in folate deficiency; and formiminoglutamic aciduria, which is seen not only in folate deficiency but in primary vitamin B_{12} deficiency, as well as in liver disease. Tests that may aid in differentiating the two anemias from those arising from other factors, but not from each other, include reduced haptoglobin, hyperbilirubinemia, increased stercobilin, elevated serum lactate dehydrogenase, loss of gastric acid, abnormal liver function, and intestinal malabsorption.[5,8,15,25-27]

Also, in vitamin B_{12} deficiency the serum level of the vitamin directly reflects the tissue level, whereas the serum folate is so sensitive that it becomes low after only 3 weeks of a poor diet. However, the red cell folate reflects tissue levels. Results must be interpreted in light of the possible interrelationships between the two vitamins. Thus, a vitamin B_{12} serum level of less than 100 pg/ml is essentially diagnostic of a deficiency of that vitamin, but a diagnosis of folate deficiency would require both a serum folate level of less than 3 ng/ml and a red cell folate level of less than 150 ng/ml. The reasons are as follows: vitamin B_{12} is required to keep folate in

the cells, so a low red cell folate level may be seen with vitamin B_{12} deficiency alone; also, the serum folate level may fall before the tissue level. When the serum levels of both vitamins are low, as is often the case, the primary deficiency may still be of only one, with the resulting megaloblastosis causing malabsorption or a decreased secretion of intrinsic factor, or both, with a consequent secondary deficiency.

These intricate interrelationships are often seen in the megaloblastic anemia of pregnancy, in which case the levels of both vitamins may be low but treatment with folate alone results in a gradual rise of vitamin B_{12} levels.[36] Also, the red cell folate level may be normal, despite an actual deficiency, because of a lag in replacing normal- with low-folate red cells as the pregnancy progresses, because of either the presence of high-folate cells (reticulocytes or transfused cells) or an iron deficiency anemia.[5,36]

RADIO-B_{12} ABSORPTION TESTS

If pernicious anemia is suspected, either an absence of intrinsic factor on in vitro assay, a typical Schilling test result (failure to absorb radioactive vitamin B_{12} when fed alone, corrected by feeding it with intrinsic factor) or the presence of circulating antibody to intrinsic factor in the serum will confirm the diagnosis.[5,8,36] Again, however, it must be borne in mind that primary intestinal malabsorption of either vitamin B_{12} or folate may result in a secondary loss of intrinsic factor, which returns to normal after therapy with the appropriate vitamin.[20] If the gastric juice aspirated 45 minutes after histamine stimulation has a pH higher than 5, is viscous, and has a volume under 25 ml, pernicious anemia is suggested. Such gastric juice is usually deficient in intrinsic factor.

When there is apparent vitamin B_{12} malabsorption of any kind, including pernicious anemia, the simplest means of sorting out possible causes is the Schilling test.[20] The patient is given a small oral dose of radioactive vitamin B_{12} (0.5-2 μg), followed immediately by a 1000 μg parenteral dose of nonradioactive vitamin. The nonradioactive vitamin B_{12} binds to most available receptor sites in the liver and other body tissues, and thus any of the radioactive dose that is absorbed enters the bloodstream but is soon passed out into the urine, in the absence of binding sites. The amount of radioactivity in the patient's 24-

hour urine collection provides an index of the degree of malabsorption.

If this first stage of the test demonstrates malabsorption, it is repeated, but this time the patient is given a dose of intrinsic factor concentrate in addition to the vitamin B_{12}. If absorption becomes normal, the patient lacks sufficient intrinsic factor of his own. If the added intrinsic factor fails to correct the malabsorption, the defect lies in either the ileum or the pancreas. If the pancreas is at fault, absorption could be normal in a third-stage test, in which pancreatic enzymes or bicarbonate are given with the vitamin. If not, ileal malfunction is diagnosed by exclusion. Both stages of the Schilling test may be executed simultaneously, with two different radioisotopes of vitamin B_{12}.[20,21]

There is at least one major pitfall in the Schilling test. Almost half the patients with pernicious anemia show subnormal second-stage test results (intrinsic factor fails to normalize vitamin B_{12} absorption). Such patients have intestinal malabsorption arising from the slowed DNA synthesis characteristic of vitamin B_{12} deficiency, with consequent atrophy of the absorptive cells in the gut.[20] If the results of the second-stage Schilling test are equivocal, but the presumptive diagnosis remains pernicious anemia, the patient should be given parenteral vitamin B_{12} for about 2 months and the second-stage Schilling test then should be repeated. If the test results become normal, it will be apparent that the patient's only disease is pernicious anemia, for the parenteral vitamin B_{12} will have corrected the malabsorption resulting from megaloblastic changes in the intestine. If the first-stage Schilling test (vitamin B_{12} alone) is repeated at this point, it will still show malabsorption.

As observed previously, folate deficiency may also "feed on itself." Patients with tropical sprue, for example, with malabsorption of folate and of vitamin B_{12}, may develop megaloblastic changes in both stomach and intestinal cells. The gastric changes may lead to a secondary intrinsic factor insufficiency that is correctable with adequate folate therapy.

Caveats

A caveat regarding serum vitamin B_{12} assay is that the physician should rely on clinical judgment when it conflicts with the laboratory report. In megaloblastic anemia resulting from vitamin B_{12} deficiency, the serum vitamin B_{12} level may be normal if the patient has a liver disorder or a myeloproliferative disorder that releases into the plasma binding proteins that hold vitamin B_{12} (and sometimes folic acid) in the serum without delivering these vitamins to deprived tissues.[8,15,16] In addition, the serum contains not only "true vitamin B_{12}" (metabolically active for humans) but also analogues of vitamin B_{12}, which may be inactive for humans or even may act as anti–vitamin B_{12} molecules.* With occasional exceptions,[38] "true" vitamin B_{12} is measured by microbiologic assay or by radioassay with either pure intrinsic factor or intrinsic factor concentrate "spiked" with nonradioactive analogue to "tie up" its nonintrinsic factor vitamin B_{12} binders. The latter are capable of binding analogues of vitamin B_{12}, leaving available only the intrinsic factor portion, which can only bind true cobalamins.[37] Radioassays using serum not adequately pretreated to destroy endogenous vitamin B_{12} binders and endogenous antibody to intrinsic factor may give erroneously high results in patients with pernicious anemia, and erroneously low results in patients with increased endogenous vitamin B_{12} binders.

A caveat regarding the Schilling test is that vitamin B_{12} in food is not crystalline B_{12} and as people age they lose the ability to split vitamin B_{12} from food (and therefore the ability to absorb this vitamin from food) before they lose the ability to absorb crystalline B_{12}.[5] Thus for elderly persons the Schilling test is better done with an omelet containing radioactive vitamin B_{12} than with crystalline B_{12}.[5]

If the patient has been properly evaluated, specific therapy should present few problems.

Iron Deficiency

In the case of iron deficiency, therapy, for at least 6 months, should begin with the most inexpensive iron preparation, ferrous sulfate (300 mg four times/da, after meals and at bedtime).[2,4,23] About 8% of patients on iron therapy have side effects, ranging from nausea and vomiting to diarrhea and severe stomach cramps. It is sometimes suggested that other iron salts may be less toxic than ferrous sulfate, but this is not usually the case. They are less toxic not by dint

---

*References 8, 24, 37, 38.

of being different salts but simply because they contain less ionic iron per dose. Ionic iron is responsible for both iron absorption and iron toxicity.[2,9,23] Therefore, if toxicity is seen with ferrous sulfate, the simplest remedy is to reduce the dose. Usually, it is best to eliminate the bedtime dose. In addition, one might give the remaining doses with, rather than between, meals. Giving the dose with meals reduces the amount of free ionic iron, which reduces toxicity and iron absorption; the repletion of iron stores takes somewhat longer, but this will also occur if an ostensibly less toxic (less free ionic) form of iron is used.

In an occasional patient with chronic blood loss from the gastrointestinal or genital tract, for example, oral iron may prove inadequate. Too little can be absorbed to compensate for the loss, and parenteral iron may be advisable. In contrast to the overall safety, efficacy, and low cost of oral iron, parenteral iron is expensive and may be hazardous. Intramuscular preparations may cause pain at the injection site, skin discoloration, and local inflammation. Systemic toxicity may occur in up to 0.8% of patients treated with parenteral iron. The risk may be slightly higher with intravenous than with intramuscular administration. Specific manifestations may include headache, muscle and joint pain, hemolysis (caused by unbound iron), faintness, nausea and vomiting, dyspnea, hypotension, dizziness, and circulatory collapse. Anaphylaxis may occur with any type of parenteral iron, and one should always have a syringe of epinephrine close at hand. Since unbound iron in the parenteral preparation is the main cause of side effects, it is good practice (when possible) to give iron from a batch that recently has been used safely.[2,9,23]

Whatever the type of therapy used, every effort should be made to find and correct the cause of the iron deficiency, since in adults it is almost invariably blood loss. Failing this, replacement must be continued indefinitely. If the underlying cause is corrected, replacement therapy should be continued only until iron balance has been restored, which takes about 6 months.[2]

Vitamin B$_{12}$ Deficiency

Therapy for the anemia of vitamin B$_{12}$ deficiency is usually divided into two stages: primary and maintenance.[3] The normal practice in primary therapy is to administer a minimum of 1 μg/day vitamin B$_{12}$ parenterally for a period of 10 days, adding a minimum of 50-100 μg folate if that is also deficient. Unless hematopoiesis is suppressed by infection, alcohol, or some other factor, reticulocytosis starts to appear in about 3 days and should peak in about 7 days. The hemoglobin gradually rises and should be approximately normal in about 1 month. The low platelet count in most patients and the low white blood cell count in about 10% of them spike to above normal in the first week and then settle back to normal.

In patients with megaloblastic anemia so severe as to cause dyspnea, congestive failure, and occasionally angina (the hematocrit in such cases is usually below 15%), immediate therapy is advisable. The rapid administration of packed red cells, with simultaneous withdrawal of a slightly lesser volume of blood to reduce the danger of circulatory overload, brings rapid and dramatic relief of symptoms. With the use of a 50 ml syringe and a three-way stopcock, red cells may be infused at the rate of one unit every 5 minutes, alternately injecting 50 ml of packed cells, withdrawing 50 ml of whole blood, and monitoring venous pressure. The net effect of simultaneous administration and withdrawal is that packed cells with a hematocrit of about 80 are exchanged for whole blood with a hematocrit of less than 15, and venous pressure falls slightly rather than rises toward congestive failure levels.

Immediate therapy with vitamin B$_{12}$, folate, or both is also advisable in the patient with severe megaloblastic anemia and bleeding (with a platelet count below 50,000/mm^3) or infection and leukopenia (with a white cell count of less than 2000/mm^3). It is also advisable in patients with severe infection, coma, serious disorientation, marked neurologic damage, severe liver disease, uremia, or other markedly debilitating illness. If therapy must be undertaken before an etiologic diagnosis can be made, blood should be drawn immediately for subsequent vitamin assays, and therapy should begin with at least 30 μg of vitamin B$_{12}$ (cyanocobalamin) and 1 mg of folic acid intramuscularly, followed by 1 mg of folic acid by mouth each day for a week. After a week of therapy, which should take the patient from a critical state to one of relative well-being, all vitamin therapy should be stopped until the vitamin assays on the blood drawn prior to the therapy are reported. Other appropriate tests then should be done to define the patient's nutritional status etiologically.

The patient found to lack intrinsic factor or to have a noncorrectable structural or functional lesion of the ileum resulting in vitamin B_{12} malabsorption requires lifelong maintenance therapy. The usual practice is to administer a minimum of 30 μg of vitamin B_{12} parenterally once a month. The most commonly used form of the vitamin in the United States is cyanocobalamin, but in Europe hydroxocobalamin appears to be preferred. There is little evidence that one is better than the other in the monthly oral doses given. Cyanocobalamin tends to be less expensive. Oral preparations of vitamin B_{12} plus intrinsic factor should not be used for long-term therapy. The vitamin B_{12} in such preparations is not absorbed by patients with structural or functional disorders of the small bowel, and absorption of the vitamin B_{12} is unreliable in patients with pernicious anemia. Patients with pernicious anemia are likely to become refractory to such preparations, since they develop a local intestinal antibody to such exogenous intrinsic factor.[3]

Folate Deficiency

Therapy for folate deficiency per se may be started with 1 mg/day of pteroylglutamic acid (folacin) parenterally for 10 days, after which oral therapy in the same dosage may be substituted. This regimen is sufficient to maintain body folate stores, even with a suboptimum absorption rate, since the daily need for folate is only about 50 μg.[3,17,18]

Summary

The three simple nutritional anemias may be so intertwined biochemically and pathologically in a patient that the initial clinical and laboratory picture may allow only partial diagnosis. Newer and more specific tests have made diagnosis less uncertain, but it still must be pursued in reasoned sequence to yield valid results. All patients diagnosed as just iron-deficient should be reevaluated for vitamin B_{12} or folate deficiency after a month of iron therapy, and those diagnosed as vitamin-deficient should be reevaluated for iron deficiency. Similarly, specific agents are available for all three nutritional anemias; but in virtually all instances therapy must be administered as part of the ongoing diagnostic process, for the cure of one deficiency may unmask another. In the worst of circumstances, therapy for folate deficiency may mask a B_{12} deficiency and allow resulting damage to proceed unchecked.

REFERENCES

1. WHO Scientific Group on Nutritional Anemias: Nutritional anemias, WHO Tech Rep Ser [405], 1968.
2. Herbert V: Drugs effective in iron-deficiency anemia and other hypochromic anemias. In Goodman LS, Gilman A, editors: The pharmacological basis of therapeutics, ed 5, New York, 1975, Macmillan Publishing Co, pp 1309-1323.
3. Herbert V: Drugs effective in megaloblastic anemias. In Goodman LS, Gilman A, editors: The pharmacological basis of therapeutics, ed 5, New York, 1975, Macmillan Publishing Co, pp 1324-1349.
4. Das KC, et al: Unmasking covert folate deficiency in iron-deficient subjects with neutrophil hypersegmentation: dU suppression tests on lymphocytes and bone marrow, Br J Haematol **39**:357-375, 1978.
5. Herbert V: Nutrition science as a continually unfolding story: the folate and vitamin B_{12} paradigm, 1987 Herman award lecture, Am J Clin Nutr **46**:387-402, 1987.
6. Herbert V: The megaloblastic anemias, New York, 1959, Grune & Stratton Inc.
7. Herbert V: Nutritional anemias of childhood—folate, B_{12}: the megaloblastic anemias. In Suskind RM, editor: Textbook of pediatric nutrition, New York, 1981, Raven Press, pp 133-144.
8. Herbert V: B_{12} and folate deficiency. In Rothfeld B, editor: Nuclear medicine in vitro, ed 2, Philadelphia, 1983, JB Lippincott Co, pp 337-384.
9. Hillman RS, Finch CA: Drugs effective in iron deficiency and other hypochromic anemias. In Gilman AG, et al, editors: The pharmacological basis of therapeutics, ed 7, New York, 1985, Macmillan Publishing Co, pp 1308-1322.
10. Cook JD, et al: Estimates of iron sufficiency in the US population, Blood **68**:726-731, 1986.
11. Herbert V: Blood in hypothyroidism. In Werner SC, Ingbar SH, editors: The thyroid, ed 5, Philadelphia, 1986, JB Lippincott Co, pp 1162-1168.
12. Oski FA: Vitamin E in infant nutrition. In Suskind RM, editor: Textbook of pediatric nutrition, New York, 1981, Raven Press, pp 145-152.
13. Hines JD, Cowan DH: Anemia in alcoholism. In Dimitrov NV, Nodine JH, editors: Drugs and hematologic reactions, New York, 1974, Grune & Stratton Inc, p 141.
14. Scott JM, Weir DG: The methyl folate trap: a physiological response in man to prevent methyl group deficiency in kwashiorkor (methionine deficiency) and an explanation for folic-acid–induced exacerbation of subacute combined degeneration in pernicious anemia, Lancet **2**:337-340, 1981.
15. Herbert V, Colman N: Folic acid and vitamin B_{12}. In Shils ME, Young VE, editors: Modern nutrition in health and disease, ed 7, Philadelphia, 1988, Lea & Febiger, pp 388-416.
16. Herbert V: Hematology and the anemias. In Schneider HA, et al, editors: Nutritional support of medical practice, ed 3, New York, 1988, Harper & Row Publishers.
17. Herbert V: Recommended dietary intakes of folate, vitamin B_{12}, and iron in humans, Am J Clin Nutr **45**:661-668, 1987.
18. Food and Nutrition Board, National Research Council: Folic acid: biochemistry and physiology in relation to the human nutrition requirement, Washington DC, 1977, National Academy of Sciences.

19. Colman N, Herbert V: Dietary assessments with special emphasis on prevention of folate deficiency. In Botez HI, Reynolds EH, editors: Folic acid in neurology, psychiatry, and internal medicine, New York, 1979, Raven Press, pp 63-74.

20. Herbert V: Detection of malabsorption of vitamin B_{12} due to gastric or intestinal dysfunction, Semin Nucl Med **2:**200-234, 1972.

21. Herzlich B, Herbert V: The role of the pancreas in cobalamin (vitamin B_{12}) absorption, Am J Gastroenterol **79:**489-493, 1984.

22. Herbert V, et al: Multivitamin/mineral food supplements containing vitamin B_{12} may also contain analogues of vitamin B_{12}, N Engl J Med **307:**255-256, 1982.

23. Bothwell TH, et al, editors: Iron metabolism in man, St. Louis, 1979, Blackwell-Mosby Book Distributors.

24. Herbert V: Staging nutrient status from too little to too much by appropriate laboratory tests. In Livingston GE, et al, editors: Nutritional status assessment of the individual, 1988. (In press.)

25. Williams WJ, et al, editors: Hematology, ed 3, New York, 1983, McGraw-Hill International Book Co.

26. Wintrobe MM, et al, editors: Clinical hematology, Philadelphia, 1981, Lea & Febiger.

27. Nathan DG, Oski FA, editors: Hematology of infancy and childhood, ed 2, Philadelphia, 1981, WB Saunders Co.

28. Lindenbaum J, Nath B: Megaloblastic anemia and neutrophil hypersegmentation, Br J Haematol **44:**511-513, 1980.

29. Das KC, Herbert V: Vitamin B_{12}–folate interrelations, Clin Haematol **5:**697-715, 1976.

30. Scott JM, et al: Pathogenesis of subacute combined degeneration: a result of methyl group deficiency, Lancet **2:**334-337, 1981.

31. Jacob E, et al: Evaluation of simultaneous radioassay for two vitamins: folate and vitamin B_{12}, Clin Res **25:**537A, 1977; Am J Clin Nutr **30:**616, 1977.

32. Longo DL, Herbert V: Radioassay for serum and red cell folate, J Lab Clin Med **87:**138-151, 1976.

33. Das KC, Herbert V: The lymphocyte as a marker of past nutritional status: persistence of abnormal lymphocyte deoxyuridine (dU) suppression test and chromosomes in patients with past deficiency of folate and vitamin B_{12}, Br J Haematol **38:**219-233, 1978.

34. Colman N, Herbert V: Abnormal lymphocyte deoxyuridine suppression test: A reliable indicator of decreased lymphocyte folate levels, Am J Hematol **8:**169-174, 1980.

35. Das KC, et al: Simplifying lymphocyte culture and the deoxyuridine suppression test by using whole blood (0.1 ml) instead of separated lymphocytes, Clin Chem **26:**72-77, 1980.

36. Chanarin I: The megaloblastic anemias, St. Louis, 1979, Blackwell-Mosby Book Distributors.

37. Kolhouse JF, et al: Cobalamin analogues are present in human plasma and can mask cobalamin deficiency because current radioisotope dilution assays are not specific for true cobalamin, N Engl J Med **299:**785-793, 1978.

38. Herbert V, Colman N: Evidence humans may use some analogues of B_{12} as cobalamins (B_{12}): pure intrinsic factor (IF) radioassay may "diagnose" clinical B_{12} deficiency when it does not exist, Clin Res **29:**571A, 1981.

39. Herbert V: The nutritional anemias, Hosp Pract **125:**65-89, 1980.

CHAPTER 38
Inborn Errors of Metabolism

David Valle
Grant A. Mitchell

The phrase "inborn error of metabolism" was used first in 1908 by Sir Archibald Garrod to signify a disorder that resulted from an inherited abnormality of a specific enzyme.[1] Garrod's thinking was far ahead of his time. For example, in an era when little was known about biochemical pathways, genes, or inheritance patterns, he predicted that alkaptonuria was caused by a genetically determined deficiency of an enzyme that catalyzed the degradation of homogentisic acid. Fifty years later, Garrod's hypothesis was confirmed when a deficiency of homogentisic acid oxidase was demonstrated in the liver of patients with alkaptonuria.[2]

Since Garrod's time, our knowledge of intermediary metabolism and genetics has increased greatly. We now know that genes are the basic units of genetic function and contain the information necessary for the synthesis of specific ribonucleic acid (RNA) molecules, which in turn direct the synthesis of specific polypeptides. Also, in some cases, the RNA molecule itself may be the final gene product, as with the ribosomal RNAs. A mutation in a gene leads to an alteration in the polypeptide product. A modern definition of inborn errors of metabolism would include genetically determined biochemical disorders that result in specific inherited abnormalities in the structure and/or function of protein molecules. Although most studies of inborn errors have focused on enzymatic deficiencies, defects of all types of proteins, including structural proteins, transport proteins, and regulatory proteins, are included in this definition.[3]

The extent to which our knowledge has increased since Garrod's time is demonstrated by an examination of the seventh edition (1986) of McKusick's *Mendelian Inheritance in Man*,[4] which lists almost 4000 definitely or probably inherited disorders. Although this is an impressive number, the genes defined by these disorders represent only a small fraction of the estimated 30,000 to 50,000 genes required for the normal development and function of the human body.

GENETIC PRINCIPLES

Each diploid cell in the body has a chromosome complement of 46, which consists of 22 pairs of nonsex chromosomes, or *autosomes,* and one pair of sex chromosomes (XX in females and XY in males). In general, each cell has a pair of functional genes for each polypeptide it synthesizes, one of maternal and one of paternal origin. Each gene may have several alternate forms, or *alleles,* any one of which can be found at the specific site or chromosomal locus for that gene. The allele that occurs most frequently in the general population and that directs the synthesis of a polypeptide with normal function is called the *wild-type allele*. Additional alleles arise from mutations of the wild-type gene or its ancestor.

Many alleles for a particular gene may be present in the general population, but this has been studied extensively for only a few genes. For example, more than 100 alleles exist for both β-globin and glucose-6-phosphate dehydrogenase.[4] The occurrence of each of these different alleles varies; most are quite rare (<0.01) whereas a few occur frequently (>0.01). Assuming these genes are representative, the potential for variability at any given locus is great. These variant alleles include some that have little effect on the function of the polypeptide and are therefore "harmless"; others cause moderate or severe reduction in the amount and/or function of the encoded polypeptide and are therefore "harmful." Since each cell has a pair of alleles for any given autosomal gene, the members of the pair may be identical or different. If identical, the cell or individual is referred to as *homozygous* for the specified gene; if different, *heterozygous*

609

for the gene. In females (XX) this holds true for genes with loci on the X chromosome whereas in males (XY) all the genes on the X chromosome are present only as a single copy, and the cell or individual is referred to as *hemizygous* for the specified X-linked gene.

Most inborn errors involving enzymes are inherited as either autosomal or X-linked recessive traits. *Recessive* indicates that the clinical picture or phenotype is abnormal only when both alleles for a given gene present in the cells of an individual are defective. The clinically normal parents of an individual affected with an autosomal recessive disorder are heterozygous (or carriers) for the particular disorder, with one normal allele and one defective allele. This contrasts with autosomal dominant inheritance, in which the phenotype is abnormal when one member of the pair is defective (i.e., the heterozygote is symptomatic). It should be emphasized that the terms "dominant" and "recessive" refer to the clinical phenotype.

The dominance or recessiveness of a particular trait depends not only on the degree to which the mutation disrupts the function of the gene product, but also on the capability of the relevant metabolic and homeostatic systems to tolerate a partial reduction in the function of the polypeptide encoded by the mutant gene. If the functional level of the gene product in normal persons is substantially more than required to meet normal metabolic requirements, a 50% reduction in function will not result in a clinical abnormality. Since many enzymes are present in excess, a heterozygous individual with approximately 50% of normal activity will have sufficient function of the gene product to meet normal demands and will be clinically normal. For some recessive disorders, the heterozygous person normally without symptoms may develop them if the metabolic demands are greatly increased. For example, females heterozygous for the X-linked deficiency of the urea cycle enzyme, ornithine transcarbamylase, may develop headache, nausea, and even coma and death if large quantities of protein are ingested.[5]

As more and more genes are being cloned and characterized, the exact nature of the deleterious mutations is being determined for an increasing number of disorders. Again, studies of the β-globin locus led the way,[6] but information is now available for several enzyme deficiencies, including phenylketonuria,[7,8] the Lesch-

Nyhan syndrome,[9] Tay-Sachs disease,[10,11] citrullinemia,[12] and ornithine transcarbamylase deficiency.[13] At each well-characterized locus several different mutations have been described, confirming and extending the expectations for mutational heterogeneity and partly explaining the variation between patients affected by the "same" inborn error of metabolism.

INDIVIDUAL VARIABILITY

Despite the organizational benefit of grouping all patients with a particular inborn error, it is important to realize that heterogeneity, not homogeneity, is the rule. Appreciation of the tremendous variability among individuals is essential for proper "tailoring" of nutritional therapy to each patient. This variability occurs at three levels: (1) genetic differences among the mutant alleles causing reduced function of a particular polypeptide (variability at the particular locus); (2) differences in the genetic makeup of all the loci other than that responsible for the inborn error (variability within the genome); and (3) different habits, customs, and experiences (environmental variability).

Examples of the influence of each type of variability on the prognosis and nutritional management of persons with inborn errors of metabolism are readily apparent. The extent of variability in the number and types of mutant alleles, all of which lead to reduced function of a particular polypeptide, has already been described. Such differences among mutants probably account for differences in the amount of residual activity or function of the mutant polypeptide. Thus a patient with classic maple syrup urine disease (MSUD) may have less than 2% of normal branched-chain keto-acid decarboxylase activity and require severe limitation in intake of branched-chain amino acids. In contrast, other patients with MSUD have 10%-15% residual enzyme activity and can tolerate nearly normal intake of branched-chain amino acids.[14] Similarly, qualitative differences among the mutant alleles explain why some mutant polypeptides can be stabilized or made more active by supraphysiologic concentrations of vitamin cofactors. For example, some patients with homocystinuria caused by cystathionine-β-synthase deficiency respond to pharmacologic doses of pyridoxine (vitamin B_6) whereas others show no response and require treatment with a methionine-restricted diet.[15]

Variability elsewhere in the genome is also a potent source of difference among individuals with a particular inborn error of metabolism. Although all humans share much genetic information, no two are exactly alike except for identical twins. Individuals are heterozygous at approximately 20% of the loci in the genome because several alleles that have no major deleterious effect are present relatively often at certain loci.[16] Subtle differences in homeostatic and physiologic capabilities caused by these highly variable genes may be accentuated by the unusual stress of an inborn error. Thus variability in genes affecting diverse processes, such as the transepithelial transport and blood-brain barrier permeability of amino acids, maturation of the central nervous system, and enzymes involved in alternative metabolic pathways, may influence the outcome and treatment of a patient with an inherited disorder in amino acid metabolism. Such differences may account for the occasional untreated patient with classic phenylketonuria who has only mild intellectual deficits.[17]

Environmental differences provide a third level of variability among individuals. This broad category includes in utero variables, differences in infant and adult feeding patterns, and exposure to drugs and other chemicals. The sum of an individual's experiences with these environmental variables is unique and may greatly influence the effects and treatment of a given inborn error. For example, the significance of glucose-6-phosphate deficiency depends on exposure to hemolysis-provoking agents such as fava beans and certain drugs. Alternatively, nutritional therapy with a severely restricted diet may be accepted readily by one patient and his family and not by another, depending on the family's dietary customs and disciplinary habits.

PATHOPHYSIOLOGY OF INBORN ERRORS OF METABOLISM

A rational approach to nutritional therapy for inborn errors of metabolism requires an understanding of the pathophysiologic mechanisms involved (Fig. 38-1). Although in most instances the specific mechanisms are not understood completely, four general mechanisms are possible: (1) accumulation of a toxic precursor (excess *A* in Fig. 38-1), (2) alternate pathway overproduction (excess *Y* in Fig. 38-1), (3) product deficit (deficient *C* in Fig. 38-1), or (4) some combination of these. The strategy of nutritional therapy depends on which of these mechanisms is thought to be important. For example, the goal in galactosemia is to reduce the accumulations of a toxic precursor (galactose-1-phosphate) and the product of an alternative pathway (galactitol).[18] In biotinidase deficiency the goal of therapy is to supply a deficient product (biotin).[19] In Type I glycogen storage disease the goal is to supply the deficient product (glucose) and to decrease accumulated products (lactate, cholesterol, triglycerides) of overactive alternate pathways.[20]

In some inborn errors experimental nutritional therapy has been attempted before the pathologic mechanisms were known. A favorable response not only suggested that the therapeutic approach was valid but also provided insight into the pathophysiology of the disease. In infants with argininosuccinic-acid lyase deficiency, the good response to therapy with pharmacologic doses of arginine* was an indication that ammonia and not argininosuccinate might be the major toxic metabolite in this disorder.[21]

---

*Arginine reduces the concentration of ammonia while increasing the accumulation of argininosuccinate.

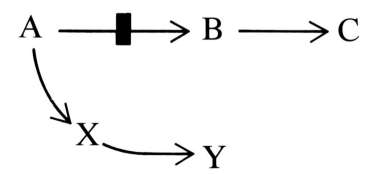

Figure 38-1 Schematic metabolic pathway with an inborn error affecting the enzyme catalyzing the conversion of Substance *A* to Substance *B*.

REQUISITES FOR NUTRITIONAL THERAPY OF INBORN ERRORS

In most instances, nutritional therapy for inborn errors of metabolism is directed at correcting imbalances of substrates or products by (1) reducing an accumulated precursor either by dietary restriction or by stimulation of an alternative metabolic pathway or (2) providing a deficient product. Not all inborn errors are amenable to such approaches. For example, restriction of dietary glycine in nonketotic hyperglycinemia has no effect on the biochemical or clinical features of this devastating disorder, presumably because glycine is a nonessential amino acid that is synthesized readily in the body. Thus, for disorders in which precursor toxicity is the major pathogenic factor, a requisite for dietary therapy is that the diet be the sole or most significant source of the metabolite. Disorders of essential amino acids, certain sugars (galactose and fructose), and a few other substances meet this criterion. Conversely, if the disorder stems from product deficit, a requisite for therapy is that some biologically usable form of the product can be supplied in the diet. For example, it is possible to treat Type I glycogen storage disease with dietary glucose but impossible to treat albinism with melanin.

The vitamin-responsive inborn errors represent a special subgroup in which nutritional therapy is directed at the mutant protein. Requisites for this type of therapy obviously include (1) a mutant polypeptide that is stabilized or activated by supraphysiologic concentrations of its vitamin cofactor and (2) a sufficient margin between therapeutic and toxic levels of the vitamin cofactor. Other inborn errors directly involve vitamin metabolism. For example, late-onset multiple-carboxylase deficiency has been shown to result from a deficiency of the bioavailable form of biotin, a cofactor for all carboxylase enzymes.[19] This results from inactivity of biotinidase, an enzyme that regenerates biotin from its inactive protein-bound form (biocytin). Phar-

Table 38-1 Inborn Errors of Metabolism Responsive to Nutritional Therapy

Disorder	Therapy
Transepithelial transport	
Gastrointestinal	
Chloride diarrhea	Salt supplementation
Hypomagnesemia	Magnesium supplementation
Lactose intolerance	Lactose restriction
Sucrose-isomaltose intolerance	Sucrose restriction
Glucose-galactose malabsorption	Glucose-galactose restriction
β-Sitosterolemia	Plant sterol restriction
Hartnup's disease	Nicotinamide
Methionine malabsorption	Methionine restriction
Folic acid transport defect	Folic acid parenterally
Pernicious anemia	Vitamin B_{12} parenterally
Renal	
Hypophosphatemia	Vitamin D phosphorus
Vitamin D–dependent rickets	Vitamin D_2 or D_3
Cystinuria	Fluid, alkali
Dibasic aminoaciduria	Protein restriction, citrulline
Glutamate-asparate transport defect	Glutamine
Plasma transport	
Abetalipoproteinemia	Vitamins A, D, E, K; medium-chain triglycerides
Hypobetalipoproteinemia	Vitamins A, D, E, K; medium-chain triglycerides
Transcobalamin II deficiency	Vitamin B_{12} parenterally

Data from Holtzman NA, et al: In Goodhart RS, Shils ME, editors: Modern nutrition in health and disease, Philadelphia, 1980, Lea & Febiger, pp 1193-1219; McKusick VA: Mendelian inheritance in man, ed 7, Baltimore, 1986, Johns Hopkins University Press; Rosenberg LE: In Bondy PK, Rosenberg LE, editors: Metabolic control and disease, Philadelphia, 1980, WB Saunders Co, pp 73-102; and Scriver CR, Rosenberg LE: Amino acid metabolism and its disorders, Philadelphia, 1973, WB Saunders Co. (This list is not necessarily complete.)

Table 38-1 Inborn Errors of Metabolism Responsive to Nutritional Therapy—cont'd

Disorder	Therapy
Intermediary metabolism	
Carbohydrate	
Hereditary fructose intolerance	Fructose avoidance
Fructose-1, 6-diphosphatase deficiency	Frequent glucose feedings
Galactokinase deficiency	Galactose avoidance
Galactosemia	Galactose avoidance
Galactose-epimerase deficiency	Galactose avoidance
Glucose-6-phosphate dehydrogenase deficiency	Avoidance of fava beans
Glycogen storage disease	
Type IA glucose-6-phosphatase deficiency	Frequent glucose feeding, starch
Type IB glucose-6-phosphatase receptor defect	Frequent glucose feeding
Type III amylo-1, 6-glucosidase deficiency	Frequent glucose feeding, high protein
Type VI phosphorylase deficiency	Frequent glucose feeding
Type VIII phosphorylase kinase deficiency	High protein
Pyruvate carboxylase deficiency	Biotin
Pyruvate dehydrogenase deficiency	Lipoic acid, high fat, thiamine
Amino acid	
β-Alaninemia	Pyridoxine
Alkaptonuria	Ascorbic acid
Cystathioninuria	Pyridoxine
Glutaric acidemia I	Protein restriction
Glutaric acidemia II	Protein and fat restriction, riboflavin, carnitine
Gyrate atrophy of choroid and retina	Arginine restriction, pyridoxine
Histidinemia	Histidine restriction
Homocystinuria	
Cystathionine-β-synthase deficiency	Pyridoxine and methionine restriction, betaine
5,10-methylene tetrahydrofolate reductase deficiency	Betaine, methionine supplement
Hypervalinemia	Valine restriction
Isovaleric acidemia	Leucine and/or protein restriction
β-Ketothiolase deficiency	Isoleucine restriction
Maple syrup urine disease	See text
Methylmalonic acidemias	
Methylmalonyl-CoA mutase deficiency	Protein restriction, carnitine
Methylmalonyl-CoA racemase deficiency	Protein restriction
Impaired synthesis of 5'-deoxyadenosylcobalamin	Hydroxocobalmin
Multiple-carboxylase deficiency	Biotin, low protein (see text)
Phenylketonuria	See text
Propionic acidemia	Protein restriction, carnitine
Pyroglutaric acidemia	Protein restriction
Tyrosinemia	Phenylalanine and tyrosine restriction
Urea cycle disorders	See text
Lipid	
Adrenoleukodystrophy	See text
Familial hypercholesterolemia	Cholesterol restriction
Refsum's disease	See text
Systemic carnitine deficiency	See text
Lipoprotein disorders	
Long-chain acyl-CoA dehydrogenase deficiency	Fat restriction, riboflavin, carnitine
Medium-chain acyl-CoA dehydrogenase deficiency	Fat restriction, riboflavin, carnitine
Other	
Ehlers-Danlos syndrome VI (lysyl hydroxylase deficiency)	Ascorbate
Periodic paralysis	
Hypokalemic	Carbohydrate restriction, potassium
Normokalemic	Salt
Hyperkalemic	Carbohydrate supplementation
Porphyria, acute, intermittent	Carbohydrate supplementation
Pyridoxine-dependent seizures	Pyridoxine
Xanthinuria	Purine restriction

macologic, and possibly even physiologic, doses of biotin replace the product deficit and quickly induce a clinical cure in this condition, which, if untreated, will lead to exfoliative dermatitis, acidosis, and neurologic disturbances.

The inborn errors for which nutritional therapy is indicated are summarized in Table 38-1.[22] Only selected examples will be discussed in detail in the ensuing sections.

DISORDERS OF AMINO ACID METABOLISM

Amino acids are organic compounds with molecular weights in the range of 75 to 350 daltons. Characteristically, their structure includes a free carboxylic group, an unsubstituted amino group often on the α-carbon, and a variable side chain. Two important amino acids, proline and hydroxyproline, have a substituted instead of a free amino group and often are referred to as *imino acids*. Amino acids can be divided into two major groups depending on whether they are constituents of proteins. There are 20 amino acids that normally are utilized for protein synthesis (Table 38-2). These protein amino acids often

Table 38-2 Amino Acids

Protein Amino Acids	Nonprotein Amino Acids (partial listing)
Acidics	
Aspartic acid	Ornithine
Glutamic acid	Citrulline
Neutrals	Argininosuccinic acid
Threonine*	γ-Aminobutyric acid
Serine	Taurine
Asparagine	
Glutamine	
Proline	
Glycine	
Alanine	
Valine*	
Cysteine	
Methionine*	
Isoleucine*	
Leucine*	
Tyrosine	
Phenylalanine*	
Tryptophan*	
Basics	
Histidine†	
Lysine*	
Arginine	

*Essential in humans.
†Essential in human infants.

are subdivided further on the basis of their charge at physiologic pH into acidics, neutrals, and basics. This chemical characteristic is of physiologic significance in that specific transepithelial and transcellular transport systems exist for each of the three groups.[23] In addition to the protein amino acids, more than 150 known nonprotein amino acids exist, some of which play important roles in metabolism (Table 38-2).

An important metabolic characteristic of each of the protein amino acids is whether it can be synthesized by the human organism. The 12 protein amino acids that can be synthesized in humans at a rate sufficient for growth are referred to as nonessential (i.e., not required or "essential" in the diet). The eight protein amino acids that cannot be synthesized in adequate amounts are referred to as *essential* amino acids (i.e., must be supplied in the diet). Histidine is essential during the rapid growth of infancy and possibly nonessential when growth requirements diminish.

The classification of amino acids as essential or nonessential assumes a complete complement of amino acid–metabolizing enzymes. In a patient with an inborn error involving an enzyme in the synthetic pathway of an amino acid, that normally nonessential amino acid becomes essential. In this manner, cysteine is an essential amino acid in patients with inborn errors in the pathway by which methionine normally is converted to cysteine (homocystinuria caused by cystathionine-β-synthase deficiency), and tyrosine is essential in patients deficient in phenylalanine hydroxylase activity (phenylketonuria).

Dietary Requirements for Protein and Essential Amino Acids

Normal growth requires an adequate intake of essential amino acids, an additional nitrogen source, calories, vitamins, and minerals. Normally these requirements are fulfilled by a well-balanced diet. Nutritional therapy for inborn errors of metabolism often involves highly artificial and restrictive diets, and scrupulous attention must be paid to these requirements and to the patient's growth. Estimated daily dietary protein requirements are presented in Chapter 1. These estimates provide guidelines under normal circumstances. Additional stresses, such as recovery from a catabolic state, pregnancy and lactation, the biologic value of the ingested protein, and genetic factors, all influence the actual requirement. Each patient must be monitored closely with growth measurements and plasma amino acid determinations.

The protein requirement is a function of the need for essential amino acids and nitrogen. The requirements for essential amino acids have been measured by several methods.[24] The values presented in Table 38-3 were obtained in studies of healthy subjects with intact metabolic pathways. At the lower limit of adequate intake, most of the available amino acid is utilized for protein synthesis, obligatory losses, and synthesis of other small molecules and not by the catabolic pathways (Fig. 38-2), although some catabolism is likely. To that extent, these estimates will be high in a patient with an inborn error blocking the catabolic pathway. Thus, when estimating the requirement for the particular amino acid in such a patient, it is prudent to start at the lower limit of the recommended range and utilize

growth and plasma amino acid concentration to adjust the intake to the actual requirement for each patient.

Distribution of Amino Acids

Plasma concentrations of amino acids customarily are used to assess total body pools of free amino acids. To interpret these values, it should be remembered that the plasma concentration of an amino acid varies with the time of day and is influenced by hormonal factors such as insulin and glucagon as well as by the interval after ingestion of a meal containing amino acids.[23] Optimally, therefore, measurements should be made in standardized fashion (8 AM plasma samples following an overnight fast for children and older individuals and just before feeding for infants). Furthermore, the plasma compartment contains only a small fraction of the total body pool of free amino acids, most of which is found

Table 38-3 Estimated Requirements for Essential Amino Acids

Amino Acid	Infancy (mg/kg)	Childhood (g/da)	Adult (g/da)
Leucine	76-226	1.0-1.5	0.17-1.1
Isoleucine	17-126	1.0	0.25-0.45
Valine	65-115	0.6-0.9	0.23-0.8
Phenylalanine*	47-94	0.4-0.8	0.12-0.6
Threonine	45-87	0.8-1.0	0.1-1.5
Tryptophan	13-40	0.06-0.1	0.05-0.25
Histidine	16-34	Nonessential	Nonessential
Methionine†	20-85	—	0.75-0.35
Lysine	90-200	1.2-1.6	0.05-1.2

Data from Irwin MI, Hegsted DM: J Nutr **101:**539-566, 1971; and Scriver CR, Rosenberg LE: Amino acid metabolism and its disorders, Philadelphia, 1973, WB Saunders Co.

*The requirement for phenylalanine assumes tyrosine intake.

†The requirement for methionine assumes adequate cystine intake. Increase by approximately a factor of 2 if cystine intake is negligible.

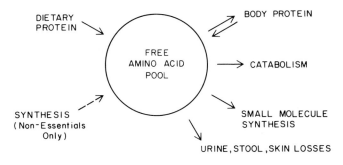

Figure 38-2 Origins and fates of free amino acids in humans.

in the intracellular fluid of muscle and liver.[23] Thus a small permanent change in plasma concentration may reflect a quantitatively large change in the total body pool.

Metabolic Fates of Amino Acids

A general scheme for the metabolic fates of amino acids is shown in Fig. 38-2.

The requirement for protein synthesis is for a net increase in total body protein (protein accretion). In the reference male infant protein accretion is about 3.5 g/day from birth to 4 months and decreases to 3.1 g/day between 4 and 12 months.[23] Protein synthesis also occurs in adults; however, the amino acid need is met by the breakdown of endogenous protein. The normal adult turns over about 400 g of protein/day without protein accretion. There are no known inborn errors in the protein synthetic pathways of humans. These might well be lethal.

Amino acids also play an important role as synthetic precursors of other small molecules, such as nonessential amino acids, nonprotein amino acids, neurotransmitters, hormones, and polyamines.[23] There are several examples of inborn errors affecting this fate of amino acids. For example, defects in the synthesis of glutathione, melanin, and thyroid hormone have been described. In general, such defects are not accompanied by increased concentration of the precursor amino acid, since the total flux in these pathways is generally small and the catabolic pathways remain intact.

A third major fate of amino acids involves obligatory losses in urine, stool, and through the skin. The amount of nitrogen normally lost daily by these routes is 165 mg/kg.[23] A 3 kg infant loses approximately 375 mg, a 10 kg child 925 mg, and a 70 kg adult 4000 mg of nitrogen/day in this manner. Since nitrogen accounts for 16% of protein weight, these losses represent an equivalent of 2.3, 5.8, and 25 g of protein/day. These losses can be increased in special circumstances, such as renal transport defects and exfoliative dermatitis.

Catabolic pathways are available for all amino acids. The carbon skeleton ultimately is oxidized in the tricarboxylic acid cycle or utilized for the synthesis of glucose and/or ketone bodies. In this regard, most amino acids are glucogenic, except for isoleucine, lysine, phenylalanine, and tyrosine (which are both glucogenic and ketogenic) and leucine (which is only ketogenic).

Selected Inborn Errors of Amino Acid Metabolism

More than 50 distinct inborn errors of amino acid metabolism now are known. The phenotypes of these disorders range from benign (many individuals with histidinemia are without symptoms) to insidious intellectual impairment (as in phenylketonuria) to severe and rapidly lethal disorders (e.g., some of the organic acidemias or the urea cycle disorders). Many of these diseases respond to nutritional therapy (Table 38-1). Three examples are discussed.

Phenylketonuria (PKU). Phenylketonuria, a defect in phenylalanine metabolism, is a common inborn error of amino acid metabolism with a frequency of approximately 1:15,000 live births in the United States. It first was described in 1934, and deficiency of hepatic phenylalanine hydroxylase was reported in 1953[25] (Fig. 38-3). The phenotype of untreated individuals has been well documented. Severe mental retardation (mean IQ, 40 ± 3) is the rule, although a few patients are in the mildly retarded or dull normal range.[17] Developmental delay is apparent in the first months of life. However, before the advent of neonatal screening, the diagnosis often was not made until after 6 to 8 months of age. Fair pigmentation, an eczematoid dermatitis, and seizures are present in more than 50% of untreated cases.[17]

The enzymatic lesion responsible for classic PKU is a reduction in phenylalanine hydroxylase activity to values less than 1% of normal (Fig. 38-3). In PKU patients ingesting a normal diet, this enzyme deficiency results in 25- to 40-fold increases in plasma phenylalanine (normal, 55 ± 10 μM) and, after the first few weeks of life, excretion of phenylpyruvic acid and its metabolites. Tyrosine, an essential amino acid in PKU patients, is present in normal concentrations (54 ± 21 μM). The hyperphenylalaninemia can be detected reliably within 2 to 3 days of institution of protein feedings. Almost all patients with classic PKU now are detected by neonatal screening using the blood spot test developed by Guthrie and Susi.[26]

In addition to this "classic" PKU phenotype, many infants detected by neonatal screening have only moderate elevations of plasma phenylalanine. These hyperphenylalaninemic individuals have plasma values ranging from 200 to 1200 μM. Hepatic phenylalanine hydroxylase activity has been measured in a few such infants

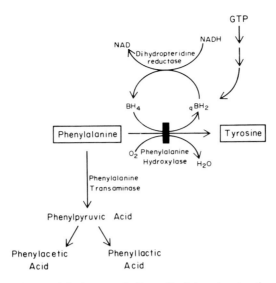

Figure 38-3 Pathways of phenylalanine metabolism. *Dark bar* denotes the site of the enzymatic deficiency in classic phenylketonuria; *BH_4*, tetrahydrobiopterin; *GTP,* guanosine triphosphate; *qBH_2*, quinonoid dihydrobiopterin.

and found to be higher that in patients with classic PKU, although still greatly reduced.[27] Intellectual function is generally normal in these patients without treatment. Additional inborn errors detected by neonatal screening for hyperphenylalaninemia include defects in the synthesis (biopterin synthetic defects) and recycling (dihydropteridine reductase deficiency) of the phenylalanine hydroxylase cofactor, tetrahydrobiopterin.[28] Patients with these disorders have neurologic impairment even if their phenylalanine levels are controlled. They can be distinguished from patients with classic PKU by their heightened response to exogenous tetrahydrobiopterin (plasma phenylalanine falls within hours of administration) and/or by analysis of urinary pterins using high-performance liquid chromatography.[29,30]

The pathophysiologic mechanisms in PKU are not well understood. A toxic effect of the accumulated precursor, phenylalanine, is thought to be a major mechanism.[17] This is partly because untreated patients have normal plasma tyrosine concentrations and because those whose plasma phenylalanine is reduced by a phenylalanine-restricted diet have a good outcome.

The rationale in nutritional therapy for PKU is similar to that for other disorders of essential amino acid catabolism: dietary intake is restricted to an amount just sufficient to meet the requirements for growth, small-molecule synthesis, and obligatory losses.[31] In addition, adequate amounts of tyrosine must be supplied.

Therapy is monitored by following growth parameters, intellectual development, and plasma amino acid concentrations. Plasma phenylalanine concentration is maintained between 100 and 500 μM.[32] Overzealous restriction will lead to phenylalanine deficiency, growth failure, and dermatitis.[17,32] Maintenance of plasma concentrations two to four times above normal provides a buffer against phenylalanine deficiency and does not appear to be harmful. Transient catabolic episodes associated with intercurrent infections produce increases in plasma phenylalanine concentration to values as high as 1200 μM. The typical course of an infant with classic PKU is shown in Fig. 38-4.

The mainstay of nutritional therapy for PKU in the United States is Lofenalac (Mead-Johnson), a complete infant formula when mixed at the recommended dilution (0.67 calorie/ml) except for the reduced content of phenylalanine (at the standard dilution, Lofenalac contains 3.74 mg of phenylalanine per ounce).[33] An intake of Lofenalac sufficient to provide 120 calories/kg of body weight/day supplies approximately 20 mg of phenylalanine/kg/day. Plasma phenylalanine concentrations fall rapidly as phenylalanine is used for growth and is lost through urine, stool, and skin. Although hospitalization is not mandatory, the physician can use inpatient time to determine the normal formula intake for the patient, follow daily weight changes, and counsel the family.

When plasma phenylalanine values fall to less

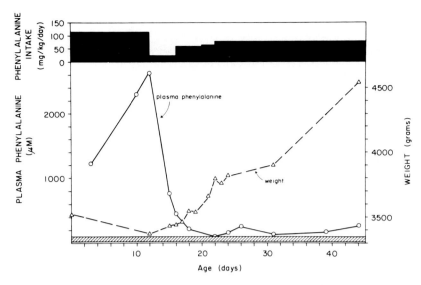

Figure 38-4 Early management of an infant with classic phenylketonuria. The *crosshatched area* indicates the normal range for plasma phenylalanine concentrations. Values at ages 3 and 10 days represent the initial neonatal screening and a repeat measurement for verification. This patient was admitted to hospital at 12 days of age, and a phenylalanine-restricted diet was instituted. On day 16, natural protein in the form of whole cow's milk was added to the formula to bring the infant's intake up to that required for growth; she was discharged on day 24.

than 500 μM, additional phenylalanine must be added to the diet to meet the requirements. In the neonatal period, this can be supplied by adding whole cow's milk (172 mg of phenylalanine/dl)[34] or another protein source (evaporated milk, standard infant formula). An electric blender with a volume scale (in milliliters) and an additional graduated volume measure (in milliliters) are extremely useful in preparing the formula. As the patient grows older, the rate of protein accretion decreases and phenylalanine intake must be reduced accordingly, as indicated by the plasma values. Measured amounts of solid foods can be started at the usual time using an exchange system.[32,35] High-protein foods such as meat are avoided. As the amount of solid foods is increased, the natural protein source in the formulas is decreased. Eventually, the formula can be changed to a preparation that contains no phenylalanine (Phenyl-Free, Mead-Johnson). As long as the patient ingests a phenylalanine-restricted diet, the special formula will be the major dietary protein source.

The outcome of PKU patients treated with a phenylalanine-restricted diet from the first 2 to 3 weeks of age is remarkably good when compared with untreated PKU patients. In a study of 132 children treated before 65 days of age

and well-controlled throughout therapy, the mean IQ was 98 at 6 years of age.[36]

The optimum duration for a phenylalanine-restricted diet in PKU patients is uncertain.[17,37] Our ignorance of the actual pathophysiologic mechanisms and the influence of genetic variability makes this question particularly difficult to answer. Good biochemical control is progressively more difficult to maintain after the child enters school and becomes more independent. In the past, many clinics discontinued diet therapy at approximately 6 years of age. Although some patients appear to tolerate this without problems, there are reports suggesting that slowly progressive intellectual deterioration occurs in some PKU patients following diet discontinuation.[37] Additional knowledge is needed in this area. The most recent report from the Collaborative Study for the Treatment of Children with PKU showed that in this group of patients, all of whom were on a phenylalanine-restricted diet for the first 6 years of life, IQ measured at 8 and/or 10 years of age was inversely related to age at cessation of dietary control.[37] Thus the current practice in most clinics is to recommend a phenylalanine-restricted diet for life.

An additional facet of PKU of great interest is the deleterious effect of high maternal phe-

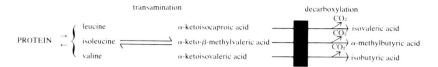

Figure 38-5 The metabolic block in maple syrup urine disease.

nylalanine concentration on the developing fetus. Mental retardation has been found in 90%, and congenital heart disease in 12%, of the offspring of women with plasma phenylalanine concentrations greater than 1200 μM.[38] Theoretically, treatment of the prospective mother with a phenylalanine-restricted diet and adequate tyrosine should allow normal fetal development.[39] Currently, a large prospective study of this entity of "maternal PKU" is underway and should yield information on optimum treatment, maternal plasma phenylalanine levels, and the nuances of maintaining acceptable control under rapidly changing nutritional requirements of pregnancy. This information will be vital for the best treatment of the many intellectually normal PKU women now reaching reproductive age.

Maple syrup urine disease (MSUD). MSUD, a rare (approximately 1:150,000 live births) autosomal recessively inherited disorder, was described by Menkes.[14,40] His interest was piqued by a lethargic neonate, several of whose siblings had died of a similar illness and whose mother reported that her sick infants all had had an unusual body odor. Typically infants with MSUD exhibit lethargy, anorexia, vomiting, and ketosis in the first few weeks of life. Metabolic acidosis may be present but is often lacking. Their urine and sweat have a sweetish syruplike odor. The symptoms may wane if protein intake is decreased. Without treatment, metabolic acidosis and central nervous system depression result in death. Some patients have milder symptoms and exhibit a more prolonged or intermittent course.[14]

The biochemical phenotype of MSUD results from deficient activity of the branched-chain keto-acid decarboxylase (Fig. 38-5). This thiamine-dependent enzyme catalyzes a decarboxylation reaction common to the catabolic pathway for the keto acids of all three branched-chain amino acids (leucine, isoleucine, valine). Because the transamination reactions are freely reversible, both the keto acids and the correspond-

ing amino acids accumulate in MSUD patients. The keto acids are excreted in urine, resulting in positive tests for ferric chloride or 2,4-dinitrophenylhydrazine and in the sweet odor. Special techniques are required for their measurement in plasma, where the concentrations during decompensations may reach 2 mM.[23] Plasma amino acids are strikingly abnormal during an acute episode, with tenfold-to-fortyfold increases in leucine and threefold-to-fivefold increases in isoleucine and valine. Alloisoleucine, a metabolite whose plasma concentration is negligible in normal persons, is present in appreciable amounts (up to 200 μM). Alloisoleucine accumulates because the keto acid of isoleucine has two asymmetric carbon atoms and when this keto acid accumulates in untreated MSUD, it undergoes keto-enol tautomerism and subsequent reversal of the transamination reaction to form L-alloisoleucine.

The pathophysiology of MSUD is not well understood, but clinical symptoms correlate with accumulation of the precursor keto and amino acids. Leucine accumulation is particularly striking and correlates best with the clinical abnormalities. Product deficiency does not seem to be a factor.

The rationale for nutritional therapy in MSUD is similar to that in PKU. Leucine, isoleucine, and valine are all essential amino acids. Their dietary intake is restricted to an amount just sufficient to maintain normal growth. Plasma amino acid concentrations and growth parameters must be monitored carefully. Plasma concentrations of the three amino acids should be maintained between normal and three times normal values. Lethargy and exfoliative dermatitis may result from deficiency of the branched-chain amino acids.

Management of the acute problems of an MSUD patient, either in infancy at the time of diagnosis or during childhood episodes resulting from dietary indiscretion or intercurrent illness, requires intensive nutritional and medical attention. Fluid and electrolyte imbalances must be corrected, and adequate amounts of calories and protein must be supplied to prevent ongoing catabolism of endogenous proteins. This is accomplished best by feeding the patient a formula devoid of branched-chain amino acids but otherwise complete (e.g., MSUD Diet Powder, Mead-Johnson). Peritoneal or hemodialysis may be necessary in the severely acidotic or comatose patient. Thiamine should be given (100 mg/da) to determine if the patient is one of the few thiamine-responsive cases.[23] As the plasma concentrations of the branched-chain amino acids fall in response to this management, care must be taken to avoid deficiency and resultant excessive protein catabolism. Valine and/or isoleucine usually become normal or subnormal several days before leucine does, and they should be added at the lower limit of the estimated requirement for age when their plasma concentrations decrease below the normal mean values. Subsequent dietary changes should be based on frequent measurements of plasma amino acids.

Chronic nutritional management of MSUD patients involves preparation of a formula suitable for the individual's particular needs. MSUD Diet Powder or a similar preparation, mixed at the recommended dilution, will supply all necessary nutrients except for the branched-chain amino acids. These are supplied by adding to the formula a measured amount of natural protein

(cow's milk contains 350 mg of leucine, 228 mg of isoleucine, and 245 mg of valine/dl).[35] Because the leucine content of many proteins is higher than either the isoleucine or the valine content, it may be necessary to add one or both of these amino acids separately. This can be accomplished by supplying the parents with capsules or a solution of the appropriate amino acids to be added to the formula. As the child grows older, measured amounts of low-protein solid foods can be added by an exchange system.[35,41] As solids are added, natural protein can be subtracted from the formula to maintain the appropriate intake of branched-chain amino acids.

As with the inborn errors of metabolism, management of MSUD patients requires close cooperation among physician, metabolic specialist, nutritionist, and the biochemical laboratory specialist. Rapid and accurate plasma amino acid determinations are necessary, particularly during acute episodes. Little information is available on the long-term outcome of nutritional management, but experience suggests that an excellent outcome can be achieved if irreversible damage does not occur in the neonatal period.[42]

Urea Cycle Disorders

The Krebs-Henseleit urea cycle provides a mechanism for converting ammonia (primarily derived from amino acid catabolism) to the readily excretable compound, urea (Fig. 38-6).

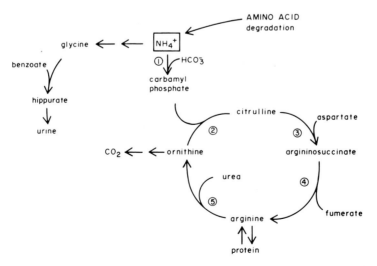

Figure 38-6 The urea cycle and the alternate pathway of waste nitrogen excretion in the formation of hippurate. The enzymes indicated by the numbers are as follows: *1,* carbamyl-phosphate synthase I; *2,* ornithine transcarbamylase; *3,* argininosuccinic-acid synthase; *4,* argininosuccinic-acid lyase; *5,* arginase.

Five enzymes are required for normal urea cycle function, and genetic defects of each have been described.[21] Although each disorder is relatively rare, as a group they may occur with a frequency of approximately 1:25,000 live births. All are inherited as autosomal recessive traits except for deficiency of ornithine transcarbamylase, which is X linked. The typical clinical presentation of patients with severe deficiencies of enzymes *1* to *4* in Fig. 38-6 is similar. Lethargy, anorexia, vomiting, respiratory alkalosis, and coma usually occur within the first few days or weeks of life. If treatment is not instituted, apnea and death ensue. Brusilow and Valle[43] briefly describe an integrated approach to infants with this phenotype. Deficiency of arginase (enzyme *5* in Fig. 38-6) usually is not associated with hyperammonemia and is beyond the scope of this discussion. Severity varies, and milder phenotypes with intermittent vomiting, nausea, and headache in older children have been described.[21,44] Argininosuccinic-acid lyase deficiency has the additional clinical feature of sparse, brittle, and microscopically abnormal hair (trichorrhexis nodosa).

The common biochemical abnormalities in each of these four inborn errors are marked hyperammonemia (normal <50 μM) and subnormal plasma arginine concentrations (normal 62 ± 9 μM). In addition, a constellation of specific biochemical abnormalities occurs in each disorder. Deficiency of argininosuccinic-acid lyase is associated with massive accumulations of argininosuccinate in plasma and urine and modest (fivefold to tenfold) increases in plasma citrulline (normal 22 $\pm$ 6 μM). Deficiency of argininosuccinic-acid synthase is associated with a 100- to 200-fold increase in plasma and urine citrulline. Deficiency of either carbamyl-phosphate synthase I or ornithine transcarbamylase is associated with subnormal values of plasma citrulline, and patients with the latter excrete excessive amounts of orotic acid in their urine because of deficient utilization of carbamyl phosphate.[21]

The intact urea cycle synthesizes urea

$$H_2N - \overset{\displaystyle O}{\overset{\displaystyle \|}{C}} - NH_2$$

from the carbon and oxygen in bicarbonate and the nitrogens donated by ammonia and aspartic acid (Fig. 38-6). The latter two compounds ultimately derive their nitrogen from glutamate, which in turn is formed by transamination reactions involving α-ketoglutarate as the amino acceptor; several different amino acids are the amino donors. Ornithine serves as the chemical foundation on which the urea molecule is assembled and not consumed in these reactions, since each molecule converted to citrulline eventually is reformed when urea is cleaved from arginine. If dietary intake of arginine is less than that required for protein accretion, the enzymes of the urea cycle serve as the only synthetic pathway for this nonessential amino acid. Thus an inborn error affecting any of enzymes *1* to *4* in Fig. 38-6 not only interferes with urea production but also makes arginine an essential amino acid.

The pathophysiology of the acute symptoms of the urea cycle disorders appears to be related to hyperammonemia (precursor toxicity) and arginine deficiency (product deficit). Arginine deficiency results in growth failure, excessive protein catabolism, and skin rash; hyperammonemia is closely correlated with acute neurologic symptoms. Plasma ammonia concentrations in the range of 100 to 300 μM are associated with nausea, vomiting, headache, and lethargy whereas higher values produce somnolence and coma. Accumulation of specific precursors such as argininosuccinate or citrulline does not seem to be of major pathophysiologic significance.

In view of the proposed pathophysiologic mechanisms, the aims of therapy for these disorders are to supply the deficient product, arginine, and to reduce the toxic precursor, ammonia. Correction of arginine deficiency is accomplished by supplying 100 to 200 mg of arginine/kg body weight/day. For some of the defects, much higher pharmacologic doses of arginine are indicated. Correction of hyperammonemia is more difficult. Previously, the approach to this problem involved extreme limitation of protein intake, thereby minimizing the requirement for waste nitrogen excretion. Results were discouraging, however, with severe growth failure and/or relentless hyperammonemia and death the usual outcome.

Research[21,45] has greatly improved the prospects for these patients. New therapeutic approaches limit protein intake and exploit alternative pathways of waste nitrogen excretion.

Such an alternate pathway is shown in Fig. 38-6. In humans benzoate is conjugated with glycine to form hippurate, which is excreted rapidly in the urine. For each mole of benzoate converted to hippurate, 1 mole of nitrogen (derived from glycine) is lost from the body. Glycine is synthesized readily and derives its nitrogen from the same pool as ammonia. Similarly, phenylacetate, which is converted to phenylacetylglutamine, can be utilized for waste nitrogen excretion.

Additional excretion of waste nitrogen can be promoted in certain patients by utilizing the accumulated precursor. For example, argininosuccinate contains the two waste nitrogen atoms that normally would appear in urea. If patients with argininosuccinate lyase deficiency are provided with sufficient carbon skeletons for the synthesis of argininosuccinate (by increasing their intake of arginine and/or ornithine), this compound constitutes an acceptable alternate method of waste nitrogen excretion. Citrulline provides a means of waste nitrogen excretion in patients with argininosuccinic-acid synthase deficiency. Although this approach results in accentuated accumulation of the precursor (argininosuccinate or citrulline), such accumulations appear to be well tolerated, as predicted by the belief that the major toxic precursor is ammonia.

The promising results obtained with a combination of protein restriction and alternate pathway utilization for waste nitrogen excretion have emphasized the importance of early diagnosis of patients with inborn errors of the urea cycle. Neonates presenting with lethargy, vomiting, and coma can be screened for these disorders by measuring plasma ammonia and amino acids. The differential diagnosis of hyperammonemia includes the urea cycle defects, organic acidemias (usually distinguished by metabolic acidosis), liver failure, and transient hyperammonemia of the newborn.[43] Early therapy of such infants includes eliminating protein intake, providing 80 to 100 kcal/kg of body weight/day as carbohydrate and fat, providing arginine, reducing ammonia accumulation by peritoneal dialysis or preferably hemodialysis, and administering benzoate and phenylacetate.[43] Long-term management includes providing an amount of dietary protein just sufficient to support growth, providing benzoate and phenylacetate, and utilizing alternate pathways of waste nitrogen excretion suitable for the specific defect.[21]

INBORN ERRORS OF CARBOHYDRATE METABOLISM

Carbohydrates, like amino acids, are essential components of structural macromolecules (nucleic acids, glycosaminoglycans, glycosylated proteins). They also function as energy substrates in brain and muscle. Unlike amino acids, all simple carbohydrates can be synthesized in the body either from other carbohydrates or from amino acids. Thus, despite the fact that typical Western diets contain 40% or more carbohydrate calories, no dietary carbohydrates are required.[46] The major dietary carbohydrates include the glucose polymers, starch and glycogen, and the disaccharides sucrose (glucose-fructose) and lactose (glucose-galactose). Since the major blood sugar is glucose, a central aspect of carbohydrate metabolism is the conversion of nonglucose sugars to glucose. A second aspect of carbohydrate metabolism is the requirement to maintain blood glucose concentrations within relatively narrow limits to provide adequate energy substrates for the central nervous system. A complex homeostatic system, involving several hormones (insulin, glucagon, epinephrine) and organs (muscle, liver, small intestine), functions in a coordinated fashion to maintain almost constant levels of blood glucose. Numerous inborn errors of carbohydrate metabolism have been described. Two examples will be discussed: one involves the interconversion of sugars; the other involves maintenance of normal blood glucose concentrations. Nutritional therapy plays an important role in both.

Glycogen Storage Disease, Type I, or von Gierke's Disease

The most prominent clinical features of glycogen storage disease, Type I (GSD-I), are neonatal onset growth failure, massive hepatomegaly, and a peculiar distribution of subcutaneous fat that gives the patient a "chubby-cheeked" or "angelic" appearance. Older patients may have xanthomas over the extensor surfaces and gouty tophi. Adenomas are often demonstrable by radionuclide scanning of the livers of patients in the second decade of life. The adenomas occasionally undergo malignant transformation. Biochemically, affected individuals exhibit severe hypoglycemia, often without overt symptoms, and do not have a normal hyperglycemic response to parenteral glucagon. They also have metabolic acidosis, with increased plasma concentrations of lactate, cholesterol, triglycerides, and uric acid.[20]

The primary enzymatic lesion responsible for this autosomal recessively inherited disorder is a deficiency of glucose-6-phosphatase activity. This enzyme normally is found in the membranes of the endoplasmic reticulum of hepatic, small intestinal mucosal and kidney cells and catalyzes the conversion of glucose-6-phosphate to glucose, a reaction that is essential for glucose release from liver. About 10% of patients with the typical clinical and biochemical phenotype have normal hepatic glucose-6-phosphatase activity in frozen specimens but are unable to transport glucose-6-phosphate across the membrane of the endoplasmic reticulum to the enzyme.[47] In vivo, the phenotypic consequences are similar to those in glucose-6-phosphatase deficiency.

The disturbance in glucose homeostasis that results from this block in hepatic glucose production is shown schematically in Fig. 38-7. Within 3 to 4 hours following ingestion of a meal, hepatic glucose production becomes increasingly important in the maintenance of blood sugar concentrations. In patients with GSD-I, the blood glucose falls to subnormal levels and homeostatic mechanisms come into play, including the secretion of epinephrine and glucagon and the suppression of insulin release. The former two hormones stimulate hepatic glycogenolysis and gluconeogenesis and increase the formation of glucose-6-phosphate. Since the enzymatic de-

ficiency blocks hydrolysis of this substrate, alternate pathways of glucose-6-phosphate metabolism are utilized in excess. These include glycolysis, which leads to increased formation of lactate and acetyl-CoA; glycogen synthesis; and the pentose phosphate shunt, with resultant increased formation of phosphoribosylpyrophosphate, a precursor of purines.

The pathophysiologic mechanisms in this disorder are complex and include product deficiency (glucose) and alternate pathway overproduction (lactate, acetyl-CoA). The goals of nutritional therapy are to prevent hypoglycemia and to interrupt the homeostatic mechanisms that lead to alternate pathway overproduction. Fructose and galactose, which must be converted to glucose-6-phosphate in order to form glucose, are avoided because they only increase glucose-6-phosphate and accentuate lactic acidosis.

The early nutritional management of GSD-I patients requires frequent feeding with an infant formula in which glucose (dextrose) and/or glucose polymers are the sole carbohydrates (e.g., a mixture of RCF plus Polycose [Ross Labs]). Blood glucose levels should be maintained above 70 mg/dl, and plasma lactate concentration should be less than 2 mM (normal <1 mM). The interval between feedings may vary with each patient and can be determined by fasting the patient under controlled conditions. Generally, feeding every 2½-3 hours throughout the day is required. Hypercholesterolemia and hypertri-

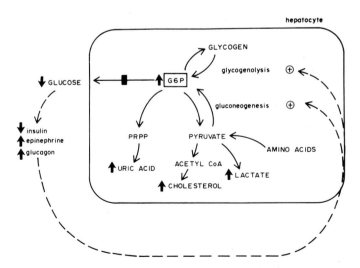

Figure 38-7 The metabolic derangements in Type I glycogen storage disease. *Solid vertical bar* denotes the deficiency of glucose-6-phosphatase; *dashed arrows,* the regulatory interactions; *G6P,* glucose-6-phosphate; *PRPP,* phosphoribosyl pyrophosphate; +, stimulation.

glyceridemia improve if hypoglycemia is prevented. Linear growth is improved, and some decrease in liver size may occur. Solid foods can be started as indicated as long as they do not interfere with formula intake.

After the first year, it becomes increasingly difficult to maintain this frequent feeding regimen. Intermittent hypoglycemia, metabolic acidosis, and poor linear growth are common. Nasogastric infusions of a mixture of glucose, glucose polymers, and protein have been used throughout the night (10-12 hr) in an amount that supplies 33% to 40% of the daily caloric needs.[48] This maintains the blood sugar during the night and prevents lactic acidosis. Patients treated in this fashion have exhibited improvement of their biochemical abnormalities and an increased linear growth rate. Preliminary results also suggest a decrease in the number and size of hepatic adenomas. Provision of a slowly hydrolyzable glucose polymer (cornstarch) to the diet has been shown[49] to be very useful in prolonging the interval between feedings and reducing the need for nasogastric infusions in these patients.

The ability of GSD-I patients to tolerate profound hypoglycemia at the time of their initial diagnosis is remarkable. This probably results from utilization by the central nervous system of ketone bodies in place of glucose as an energy source. This adaptation is in response to chronic hypoglycemia. When nutritional therapy is effective and hypoglycemia is prevented, the central nervous system quickly loses this adaptive mechanism and becomes normally sensitive to acute hypoglycemia. Successfully treated patients are therefore susceptible to symptomatic hypoglycemia with the risk of neurologic damage. Parents should be instructed in the use of Dextrostix (Ames) and in the treatment of acute hypoglycemia.

The long-term outlook for these patients is good. As they grow older, they often learn to manage their own diet. Intellectual performance is usually normal as long as symptomatic hypoglycemic attacks have not occurred.

Galactosemia

Infants with galactosemia most commonly present with poor feeding, vomiting, diarrhea, failure to thrive, jaundice with abnormal liver function, hyperchloremic metabolic acidosis, and mild hemolytic anemia. The symptoms begin within a few days after introduction of a formula containing lactose. The frequency of sepsis, particularly with *Escherichia coli,* seems to be greatly increased in these infants. Although cataracts occasionally are observed in infancy, they usually are not present until the infant is a few months old. As with other inborn errors, there is great variability in the clinical severity, and some patients have only mild symptoms in the neonatal period. They may be diagnosed at the age of several months with failure to thrive, hepatomegaly, developmental delay, and cataracts. A few patients have been entirely without symptoms but may still have an increased risk for cataracts. This milder appearance may be more common in blacks. Primary or secondary ovarian failure is a recognized long-term complication of galactosemia in females.[50]

The primary abnormality in this autosomal recessive disorder is a deficient activity of galactose-1-phosphate uridyl transferase, the second enzyme in the pathway by which galactose is converted to glucose (Fig. 38-8). Galactose, derived from the hydrolysis of the disaccharide lactose (glucose and galactose), and galactose-1-phosphate both accumulate. Galactitol, the end product of an alternative pathway for galactose, also accumulates in some tissues. An inherited deficiency of the first enzyme in the pathway (galactokinase) has also been described. These patients are normal during infancy but usually develop perinuclear cataracts in the second decade of life.

The frequency of galactosemia is about

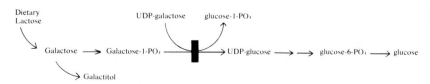

Figure 38-8 The metabolism of galactose in galactosemia. *Vertical bar* denotes the site of the metabolic block caused by the deficiency of galactose-1-phosphate uridyl transferase.

1:40,000 live births. The diagnosis can be suspected in sick neonates with nonglucose-reducing substance in the urine. Several neonatal screening techniques are also available. Confirmation of the diagnosis requires enzymatic analysis of the patient's erythrocytes or fibroblasts. Genetic variability is well documented. Several mutant alleles of the galactose-1-phosphate uridyl transferase gene have been identified on the basis of electrophoretic mobility and residual enzyme activity. The product of the Duarte allele has an activity intermediate between those of the normal allele and the usual galactosemic allele. Genetic compounds with one Duarte allele and one galactosemic allele have about 25% of normal activity and may require therapy if the erythrocyte galactose-1-phosphate level is high.

The pathogenesis of these disorders is thought to involve the toxic effects of accumulated galactose metabolites. The cataracts result from an accumulation of galactitol in the lens. Aldose reductase within the lens converts galactose to galactitol. The lens epithelium is relatively impermeable to galactitol and large amounts accumulate, causing lens swelling and cataract formation. The pathophysiology of mental retardation and of liver and renal disease in galactosemia is not well understood. Since these are not features of galactokinase deficiency and are prevented by a low-galactose diet, the major toxic agent is thought to be galactose-1-phosphate.

The manifestations of this disorder are due to toxic effects of accumulated precursors, and thus elimination of galactose is the goal of nutritional therapy. Dietary lactose is the major source of galactose and the predominant sugar in both cow's milk and human milk. Therefore milk and milk products are eliminated from the diet. In infancy this is accomplished easily by utilizing one of the soy-based formulas that contain no lactose. These formulas can continue to be substituted for milk in the diets of older children. Cow's milk, as well as processed foods containing milk, are avoided. The parents and eventually the child should be instructed to read product labels and to exclude foods listing milk, cheese, cream, milk solids, or lactose.

Children treated optimally for galactosemia should have a good outcome. Intellectual damage suffered before diagnosis cannot be corrected, however, and some[18] have suggested that the best outcome requires maternal avoidance of galactose during the pregnancy. Increased galactose intake at any time will lead to cataract formation.

INBORN ERRORS OF FAT METABOLISM

Fats, like amino acids and carbohydrates, have important roles as energy substrates and structural molecules. Many inborn errors involving structural lipids are included in the general heading of lysosomal storage diseases (e.g., sphingolipidoses, Gaucher's disease). Since these structural molecules are synthesized endogenously, these disorders are not amenable to nutritional therapy.

A few examples of effective nutritional therapy for inborn errors of lipid metabolism are known. Refsum's disease is a neurodegenerative inherited disorder in the catabolism of phytanic acid, a lipid of exogenous origin.[51] Experimental diets low in phytol and phytanic acid (mainly found in green vegetables) have been noted to lower plasma and tissue phytanic acid levels and to improve nerve conduction velocity. A second example has been proposed for the treatment of adrenoleukodystrophy. This neurodegenerative disorder is characterized by defective breakdown of very long-chain fatty acids in peroxisomes.[52] The possibility of nutritional therapy with a diet low in long-chain (C_{26}) fatty acids is under investigation.[53]

Dietary therapy is important in many of the inherited disorders of plasma lipoprotein metabolism associated with premature atherosclerosis and is discussed elsewhere in this volume.

Several hereditary disorders of fatty acid catabolism have been described recently that block complete oxidation of fatty acids.[54] Fasting hypoglycemia with subnormal plasma ketone levels, possibly associated with coma, cardiomyopathy, skeletal myopathy, or myoglobinuria, has been a common finding in this group of patients.

Primary defects have been found at several sites along the pathway between fatty acids and energy production, including carnitine-mediated transport of fatty acids into the mitochondrion and deficiencies of various enzymes of beta-oxidation and of the respiratory chain (Table 38-1). Carnitine is essential for the mitochondrial entry of C_{12} fatty acids (which have chains containing 12 or more carbon atoms) that form the major fatty acid fuels of the body. Carnitine can also compete with intracellular coenzyme A for binding of small toxic organic acids that accumulate in fatty acid oxidation disorders and other organic acidemias. These carnitine esters are relatively membrane permeable and are excreted. Qualitative analysis is useful in their diagnosis.[54]

Primary carnitine deficiency appearing as hypoglycemia, as skeletal muscle disorders, or as cardiomyopathy has become a well-described entity. In most cases pharmacologic doses of L-carnitine (50-100 mg/kg/da) have led to complete reversal of symptoms.[55] Furthermore, secondary carnitine deficiency has been observed in the numerous organic acidemias in which acylcarnitine esters are excreted. Carnitine depletion in these disorders can be severe, and some patients with organic acidemias may be misdiagnosed as having systemic carnitine deficiency.[56] L-Carnitine replacement (50-100 mg/kg/da) is frequently used as an ancillary therapy in the acute and chronic treatment of disorders with secondary carnitine deficiency, both to promote excretion of the accumulated toxic organic acid and to prevent the consequences of carnitine deficiency.[57]

In contrast to long-chain fatty acids, medium-chain fatty acids enter the mitochondria independently of carnitine. They can be useful in dietary therapy of disorders in which the metabolic block is confined exclusively to long-chain fatty acids (primary carnitine deficiency, carnitine palmityl transferase deficiency, and probably also long-chain fatty acyl–CoA dehydrogenase deficiency). However, they would be extremely toxic if administered to patients in whom medium- and/or short-chain fatty acid metabolism was impaired. Because these patients may resemble those with the long-chain defects clinically and may have similar urinary organic acid profiles and carnitine deficiency, great caution must be exercised before administering medium-chain triglycerides in cases of presumed fatty acid oxidation defects.

REFERENCES

1. Garrod A: Inborn errors of metabolism (Croonian lectures), Lancet **2**:1-7, 73-79, 142-148, 214-220, 1908.
2. LaDu BN, et al: The nature of the defect of tyrosine metabolism in alcaptonuria, J Biol Chem **230**:251-260, 1958.
3. Rosenberg LE: Inborn errors of metabolism. In Bondy PK, Rosenberg LE, editors: Metabolic control and disease, Philadelphia, 1980, WB Saunders Co, pp 73-102.
4. McKusick VA: Mendelian inheritance in man, ed 7, Baltimore, 1986, Johns Hopkins University Press.
5. Batshaw ML, et al: Cerebral dysfunction in asymptomatic carriers of ornithine transcarbamylase deficiency, N Engl J Med **302**:482-485, 1980.
6. Antonarakis SE, et al: DNA polymorphism and molecular pathology of the human globin gene clusters, Hum Genet **69**:1-14, 1985.
7. DiLella AG, et al: Tight linkage between a splicing mutation and a specific DNA haplotype in phenylketonuria, Nature **322**:799-803, 1986.
8. Guttler F, et al: Correlation between polymorphic DNA haplotypes at phenylalanine hydroxylase locus and clinical phenotypes of phenylketonuria, J Pediatr **110**:68-71, 1987.
9. Stout JT, Caskey CT: HPRT: gene structure, expression, and mutation, Ann Rev Genet **19**:127-148, 1985.
10. Myerowitz R, Hogikyan ND: Different mutations in Ashkenazi Jewish and non-Jewish French Canadians with Tay-Sachs disease, Science **232**:1646-1648, 1986.
11. Myerowitz R, Proia RL: cDNA clone for the α-chain of human β-hexosaminidase: deficiency of α-chain mRNA in Ashkenazi Tay-Sachs fibroblasts, Proc Natl Acad Sci USA **81**:5394-5398, 1984.
12. Beaudet AL, et al: The human argininosuccinate synthetase locus and citrullinemia, Adv Hum Genet **15**:161-196, 1986.
13. Nussbaum RL, et al: New mutation and prenatal diagnosis in ornithine transcarbamylase deficiency, Am J Hum Genet **38**:149-158, 1986.
14. Dancis J, Levitz M: Abnormalities of branched chain amino acid metabolism (hypervalinemia, maple syrup urine disease, isovaleric acidemia, and β-methylcrotonic aciduria). In Stanbury JB, et al, editors: The metabolic basis of inherited disease, New York, 1978, McGraw-Hill International Book Co, pp 397-410.
15. Mudd SH, Levy HL: Disorders of transulfuration. In Stanbury JB, et al, editors: The metabolic basis of inherited disease, New York, 1983, McGraw-Hill International Book Co, pp 522-559.
16. Harris H: Enzyme variants in human populations, Johns Hopkins Med J **138**:245-252, 1976.
17. Scriver CR, Clow CL: Phenylketonuria: epitome of human biochemical genetics, N Engl J Med **303**:1336-1342, 1394-1400, 1980.
18. Segal S: Disorders of galactose metabolism. In Stanbury JB, et al, editors: The metabolic basis of inherited disease, New York, 1983, McGraw-Hill International Book Co, pp 167-191.
19. Wolf B, et al: Phenotypic variation in biotinidase deficiency, J Pediatr **103**: 233-237, 1983.
20. Howell RR, Williams JC: The glycogen storage diseases, In Stanbury JB, et al, editors: The metabolic basis of inherited disease, New York, 1983, McGraw-Hill International Book Co, pp 141-166.
21. Brusilow SW: Inborn errors of urea synthesis. In Lloyd JK, Scriver CR, editors: Genetic and metabolic disease in pediatrics, New York, 1985, Butterworth & Co (Publishers) Inc, pp 140-165.
22. Holtzman NA, et al: Genetic aspects of human nutrition.

In Goodhart RS, Shils ME, editors: Modern nutrition in health and disease, Philadelphia, 1980, Lea & Febiger, pp 1193-1219.

23. Scriver CR, Rosenberg LE: Amino acid metabolism and its disorders, Philadelphia, 1973, WB Saunders Co.

24. Irwin MI, Hegstead DM: A conspectus of research on amino acid requirements of man, J Nutr **101:**539-566, 1971.

25. Jervis GA: Phenylpyruvic oliogophrenia: deficiency of phenylalanine-oxidizing system, Proc Soc Exp Biol Med **82:**514-515, 1953.

26. Guthrie R, Susi A: A simple phenylalanine method for detecting phenylketonuria in large populations of newborn infants, Pediatrics **32:**338-343, 1963.

27. Bartholome K, et al: Determination of phenylalanine hydroxylase activity in patients with phenylketonuria and hyperphenylalaninemia, Pediatr Res **9:**899-903, 1975.

28. Dhont JL: Tetrahydrobiopterin deficiencies: Preliminary analysis from an international survey, J Pediatr **104:**501-508, 1984.

29. Curtius H, et al: Atypical phenylketonuria due to tetrahydrobiopterin deficiency. Diagnosis and treatment with tetrahydrobiopterin, dihydrobiopterin, and sepiapterin, Clin Chim Acta **93:**251-262, 1979.

30. Milstein S, et al: Hyperphenylalaninemia due to dihydropteridine reductase deficiency: diagnosis by measurement of oxidized and reduced pterins in urine, Pediatrics **65:**806-810, 1980.

31. Bickel H, et al: Influence of phenylalanine intake on the chemistry and behavior of a phenylketonuric child, Acta Pediatr **43:**64-77, 1954.

32. Acosta PB, Wenz E: Diet management of PKU for infants and preschool children, USDHEW Publ 77-5209, Washington DC, 1977, Government Printing Office.

33. Products for dietary management of inborn errors of metabolism and other special feeding problems, New York, 1983, Mead-Johnson Nutritional Division.

34. Fomon SJ: Infant nutrition, Philadelphia, 1974, WB Saunders Co.

35. Acosta PB, Elsas LJ: Dietary management of inherited metabolic disease: phenylketonuria, galactosemia, tyrosinemia, homocystinuria, maple syrup urine disease, Atlanta, Ga, 1976, ACELMU Publishers Inc.

36. Williamson ML, et al: Correlates of intelligence test results in treated phenylketonuric children, Pediatrics **68:**161-167, 1981.

37. Holtzman NA, et al: Effect of age at loss of dietary control on intellectual performance and behavior of children with phenylketonuria, N Engl J Med **314:**593-598, 1986.

38. Levy HL, Waisbren SE: Effects of untreated maternal phenylketonuria and hyperphenylalaninemia on the fetus, N Engl J Med **309:**1269-1274, 1983.

39. Levy HL, et al, editors: Maternal PKU: proceedings of a conference, Washington DC, 1981, Department of Health and Human Services.

40. Menkes JH: The physician-scientist: past, present, and future, Johns Hopkins Med J **148:**175-178, 1981.

41. Committee for Improvement of Hereditary Disease Management: Management of maple syrup urine disease in Canada, Can Med Assoc J **115:**1005-1009, 1976.

42. Clow CL, et al: Outcome of early and long-term management of classical maple syrup urine disease, Pediatrics **68:**856-862, 1981.

43. Brusilow SW, Valle DL: Symptomatic inborn errors of metabolism in the neonate. In Nelson NM, editor: Current therapy in neonatal-perinatal medicine, New York, 1985, Marcel Dekker Inc. pp 207-212.

44. Rowe PC, et al: Natural history of symptomatic partial ornithine transcarbamylase deficiency, N Engl J Med **314:**541-547, 1986.

45. Brusilow SW, et al: New pathways of waste nitrogen excretion in inborn errors of urea synthesis, Lancet **2:**452-454, 1979.

46. Felig P: Disorders of carbohydrate metabolism. In Bondy, PK, Rosenberg LE, editors: Metabolic control and disease, Philadelphia, 1980, WB Saunders Co, pp 276-392.

47. Beaudet AL, et al: Neutropenia and impaired neutrophil migration in type 1B glycogen storage disease, J Pediatr **97:**906-910, 1980.

48. Greene HL, et al: Type I glycogen storage disease: five years of management with nocturnal intragastric feeding, J Pediatr **97:**590-595, 1980.

49. Chen YT, et al: Cornstarch therapy in type I glycogen storage disease, N Engl J Med **310:**171-175, 1984.

50. Kaufman FR, et al: Hypergonadotropic hypogonadism in female patients with galactosemia, N Engl J Med **304:**994-998, 1981.

51. Steinberg D: Phytanic acid storage disease: Refsum's syndrome. In Stanbury JB, et al, editors: The metabolic basis of inherited disease, New York, 1983, McGraw-Hill International Book Co, pp 731-747.

52. Singh I, et al: Lignoceric acid is oxidizid in the peroxisome: implications for the Zellweger cerebro-hepato-renal syndrome and adrenoleukodystrophy, Proc Natl Acad Sci USA **81:**4203-4207, 1984.

53. Moser AB, et al: A new dietary therapy for adrenoleukodystrophy: biochemical and preliminary clinical results in 36 patients, Ann Neurol **21:**240-249, 1987.

54. Roe CR, et al: Diagnostic and therapeutic implications of acylcarnitine profiling in organic acidurias associated with carnitine insufficiency. In Borum PR, editor: Clinical aspects of human carnitine deficiency, New York, 1986, Pergamon Press Inc, pp 97-107.

55. Waber JL, et al: Carnitine deficiency presenting as a familiar cardiomyopathy: a treatable defect in carnitine transport, J Pediatr **101:**700-705, 1982.

56. Coates PM, et al: Systemic carnitine deficiency simulating Reye syndrome [letter], Pediatrics **105:**679, 1984.

57. Chalmers RA, et al: Urinary excretion of L-carnitine and acylcarnitines by patients with disorders of organic acid metabolism: evidence for secondary insufficiency of L-carnitine, Pediatr Res **18:**1325-1328, 1984.

CHAPTER 39

Diabetes Mellitus

Alan Chait
Edwin L. Bierman

Diabetes mellitus represents a spectrum of inherited and acquired disorders, all of which are characterized by elevated circulating blood glucose levels. Nutritional management has long been considered the cornerstone of therapy in both main groups of diabetes, insulin-dependent diabetes (IDD) and non–insulin-dependent diabetes (NIDD).[1] In IDD, the onset frequently occurs at a young age, and patients are prone to ketosis. Patients with NIDD often are obese, are not prone to ketosis, but may require insulin to control symptoms related to hyperglycemia. With increased understanding of diabetes and its consequences, nutritional recommendations for diabetic persons have varied through the years, often on the basis of negligible scientific evidence.

As new scientific data lead to an increased understanding of the role of diet in the prevention or delay of the complications of diabetes, nutritional recommendations will no doubt continue to change. Although many questions remain unanswered, current nutritional management of the diabetic patient should be directed toward reducing the untoward short-term and long-term consequences. The regimen adopted should minimize symptoms and complications related to either hyperglycemia or hypoglycemia and should aim to prevent the devastating macrovascular and microvascular complications to which diabetics are prone. Any beneficial effect of diabetes therapy requires that the patient understand and comply with these dietary recommendations. To achieve this end and to facilitate compliance, the dietary regimen prescribed needs to be acceptable to the patient and should be individualized according to personal preferences in addition to requirements dictated by the disease state. This implies flexibility within predetermined guidelines. Finally, because of the long-term nature of diabetes, patient education and participation in a team approach to dietary therapy are of paramount importance.

PRINCIPLES OF THERAPY

1. The diet should meet all the nutritional needs compatible with good health practice in the general population. The use of special "diabetic foods" appears to offer no advantage, since dietary prescriptions can be met with commonly used foods.

2. Hyperglycemia and its consequences should be avoided by an attempt to maintain blood glucose levels as near the physiologic range as possible. For patients who have NIDD and are obese, the emphasis is on weight reduction to reduce hyperglycemia. For patients taking insulin, special attention must be given to the timing of meals and the distribution of foods to avoid large excursions in blood glucose levels. Hypoglycemic episodes are harmful to brain function and should be avoided at all costs in patients receiving insulin or oral agents to lower blood glucose levels.

3. To achieve compliance, the patient should receive thorough education and be a member of a tripartite team that consists also of physician and dietary counselor. The dietary regimen adopted should be individualized for the patient's needs, as dictated by the nature of his or her disease, its complications, and such factors as personality, life-style, eating habits, and food preferences. Once the regimen is adopted, the patient must be consistent in following it. Most persons are unlikely to comply successfully with a fixed "diabetic dietary formula" for all diabetic patients.

GOALS OF DIETARY MANAGEMENT

Diabetes represents a heterogeneous group of disorders for which the precise causes of much of the morbidity and mortality are unknown.

Nonetheless, it is useful to consider the long-term benefits that ideally might be achieved by dietary management of diabetics and then, through knowledge of what can be accomplished by diet, translate them into practical short-term goals on which to base dietary recommendations.

Ideal (Long-Term) Goals

1. Provide optimum nutrition throughout the diabetic patient's life, including times of increased requirements (e.g., growth and adolescence, pregnancy and lactation, infection and stress).
2. Prevent the atherosclerotic sequelae (coronary artery, peripheral vascular disease) that account for much morbidity and mortality in diabetics today.[2,3]
3. Prevent microvascular complications manifesting as eye disease (retinopathy) or renal disease (nephropathy).
4. Prevent nerve degeneration (neuropathy).
5. Avoid the consequences of recurrent hypoglycemia.

It is not yet known whether any of these long-term microvascular and macrovascular complications can be prevented or ameliorated by tight control of the blood glucose level or appropriate dietary management. However, years of clinical and research experience have demonstrated that diet can influence several aspects of the diabetic state, some of which are likely to relate to these long-term complications.

Variables that can be influenced by dietary treatment include blood glucose concentration, urinary glucose excretion, plasma triglyceride level, plasma cholesterol level, and body weight. The relationship between hyperglycemia and the development of complications remains vigorously disputed.[4] The resolution of this issue awaits a greater understanding of the pathogenesis of the different types of diabetes and adoption of newer modes of intensive therapy (e.g., the new insulin delivery systems) that for the first time allow good metabolic control to be achieved. A large multicenter study is now underway (the Diabetes Control and Complications Trial) that should provide insight into whether intensive efforts to lower blood glucose will reduce complication rates. With these considerations in mind, a practical set of goals can be derived in light of the realization that they are likely to change as our understanding of the pathogenesis of diabetes and its complications, and of the effect of tight hyperglycemic control on these complications, increases.

Practical (Short-Term) Goals

1. Maintain plasma glucose as near the physiologic range as possible without causing hypoglycemia.
2. Achieve and maintain ideal body weight.
3. Reduce the intake of saturated fat and cholesterol, which are believed to be major dietary risk factors contributing to the development of atherosclerosis in the population at large and may be of particular importance in the diabetic patient.
4. Provide extra nutrients and calories for times of increased need (e.g., stress, infection, growth, pregnancy, lactation).
5. Modify the diet as required for diabetic complications (e.g., nephropathy, which may require protein restriction) or other disease unrelated to diabetes (e.g., hypertension, for which salt intake should be restricted).
6. Allow sufficient flexibility so the diet is acceptable to the patient's needs and life-style.
7. Engage in a program of education, support, and follow-up to achieve long-term compliance.

CALORIC INTAKE

Although most aspects of dietary management discussed here are for diabetes mellitus in general, the approach to young lean diabetics taking insulin (in whom the timing and distribution of meals are of primary importance) differs substantially from the approach to obese middle-aged patients with NIDD, in whom caloric restriction may be all that is required to normalize plasma glucose and lipid levels. Therefore caloric intake is discussed separately for NIDD and IDD.

Non–Insulin-Dependent Diabetes

Since most patients with NIDD tend to be overweight, caloric restriction to effect weight reduction and achieve ideal body weight is the desired goal. This measure alone usually will result in a marked improvement in blood glucose levels and glucose tolerance because of increased insulin sensitivity. In many instances, reduction to ideal weight and maintenance at this new level will result in complete normalization of blood glucose levels in NIDD. In more severe cases of NIDD, weight reduction often allows insulin therapy or oral agents to be discontinued or their doses reduced drastically. In addition to correcting hyperglycemia and glycosuria, weight reduction is associated with reduced plasma triglyceride and cholesterol levels and reduced hypertension, all of which may be important in preventing or delaying the development of atherosclerotic complications.

Since weight reduction alone improves all the metabolic disturbances that can be influenced by diet, this becomes a logical goal of therapy in obese diabetic patients. However, sustained weight loss is difficult to achieve in practice. With traditional methods, long-term results are uniformly disappointing; more than 90% of patients regain their starting weight 5 to 10 years later. This underscores the necessity of continuous follow-up by a team that can provide encouragement and long-term psychologic support. More moderate weight loss may be easier to achieve and sustain and may benefit blood glucose levels and insulin tolerance significantly.

Weight loss can be achieved only by reducing caloric intake below caloric expenditure. The composition of the weight reduction diet is of little importance as long as it meets nutritional needs. Limiting the intake of simple sugars may be helpful in patients during phases of symptomatic hyperglycemia, but has little proven benefit otherwise. Total caloric restriction with a balanced diet engenders the best long-term compliance. Vitamin and mineral supplements should be provided in cases of severe and prolonged caloric restriction.

Insulin-Dependent Diabetes

Caloric intake also is important in IDD, although in these patients the emphasis should be on providing enough calories rather than on reducing calories. Adequate caloric intake is important for normal growth and development in young patients with IDD, particularly during the adolescent growth spurt. Sufficient calories for energy expenditure need to be provided for IDD patients with physically demanding jobs and for those actively participating in strenuous exercise. Thus caloric restriction generally should not be recommended in most young, lean patients with IDD.

Patients with IDD also have an increased caloric requirement during pregnancy and lactation and during catabolic states associated with stress, surgery, trauma, or infection. Good diabetic control during pregnancy is important to minimize fetal loss. A careful balance must be achieved between attaining optimum control and preventing hypoglycemia or fasting ketosis, yet ensuring adequate calories spread throughout the day to meet the needs of the growing fetus.

• • •

In summary, diet therapy in diabetes mellitus aims primarily at control of caloric intake: caloric restriction in adults with NIDD and provision of adequate calories for normal growth and development in patients with IDD. In young patients with NIDD, sufficient calories should be given for optimum growth and development, with special attention to preventing obesity. For the diabetic person already at the desirable weight, the objective is total caloric control to provide a nutritionally adequate diet for maintaing weight and avoiding weight gain with age.

Carbohydrate
Low Versus High Carbohydrate Content

No facet of dietary management in diabetes has been more controversial or oscillated more than the question of whether to restrict dietary carbohydrate in diabetic patients. Abundant scientific evidence from past and recent studies strongly supports the position that marked restriction of carbohydrate content within the framework of the caloric recommendation is of little benefit to the diabetic patient and might be detrimental. Current recommendations from the Food and Nutrition Committee of the American Diabetes Association[5] state that 50%-60% of total calories should be derived from carbohydrates (compared to 45% for the average nondiabetic American). This moderately higher carbohydrate intake facilitates blood glucose control by increasing insulin sensitivity and thus enhancing glucose clearance, as long as sufficient insulin (exogenous insulin in IDD, endogenous insulin in NIDD) is available. Difficulty in handling an increased carbohydrate load becomes a problem only when insufficient insulin is available in the untreated IDD patient.

The other major advantage of the current recommendation is that by increasing the percentage of total calories provided as carbohydrate, fat calories are reduced. This may be important in preventing the accelerated atherosclerosis seen so often in diabetes. However, diabetics, especially those with NIDD, should be closely observed for persistent hypertriglyceridemia in response to the increased carbohydrate content of the diet, since hypertriglyceridemia appears to be an important risk factor for atherosclerosis.

Two additional considerations largely determine the extent of blood glucose fluctuations: (1) the type of carbohydrate (simple or complex), and (2) the timing of carbohydrate consumption in relation to available insulin.

Glycemic Index for Various Carbohydrates

Many studies showing that increased carbohydrate intake had no adverse effect on diabetic control were performed on metabolic wards using liquid-formula diets that consisted mainly of glucose and its polymers. Until recently, however, there was general agreement that consumption of simple sugars should be limited and that diabetic patients should avoid table sugar and glucose in their diets. These were assumed to be more rapidly absorbed, thus leading to more hyperglycemia than complex carbohydrates. However, the effect of hyperglycemia and its control on complications of diabetes remain uncertain. The belief that simple sugars resulted in greater fluctuation in the blood glucose level than complex carbohydrates was based on scant and inconclusive data and has been challenged recently. Much recent scientific evidence,[6] based on the glycemic indices of foods, has demonstrated that carbohydrates are not absorbed and assimilated in a simple manner that can easily predict their effect on blood glucose levels. The glycemic index is defined as the blood glucose response to the consumption of a foodstuff relative to consumption of an equivalant amount of glucose or white bread. In general, carbohydrate foodstuffs can be classified as falling into low-, intermediate-, or high-glycemic index categories, but considerable variability in response can result for many reasons.[6,7] The foodstuff containing the carbohydrate, the physical state of the food and its preparation, its fiber content, the composition of the rest of the meal, and several other factors can influence the glycemic response to a particular food containing carbohydrate. Even though it is possible to apply glycemic indices to mixed meals, this approach often fails to predict the glycemic response in an individual patient. Because of the wide spectrum of responses to different complex and simple carbohydrates, the overlap present in each person, especially diabetic patients, does not allow carbohydrates to be easily classified into clinically useful groups.

Fiber

An increase in specific types of dietary fiber, such as the unrefined soluble fibers, guar, pectin, and some hemicelluloses, and the consumption of fiber supplements can help decrease the blood glucose response to meals.[8] However, the amount of fiber required to achieve these effects often causes gastrointestinal side effects that make the meal unpalatable. Also, basal (or fasting) glucose is not affected, and the long-term benefits of increased dietary fiber in diabetic patients have not been demonstrated. Thus the widespread clinical use of high-fiber diets or fiber supplements is premature in the management of patients with diabetes.

Fat

During caloric restriction in overweight subjects with NIDD, the macronutrient composition of the diet is not of major importance if adequate nutrients are provided. In diabetic patients at ideal weight or on weight maintenance diets, the fat content of the diet should be moderately restricted in the hope of preventing or slowing the development of atherosclerosis. Most diabetic adults die prematurely from atherosclerotic cardiovascular/renal disease, which is preceded by much morbidity.[2,3] Therefore more recent approaches to the diabetic diet reach beyond the short-term objective of preventing hyperglycemia and glycosuria and attempt to delay and minimize these macrovascular complications. Since diabetic persons are considerably more prone to develop atherosclerosis earlier and more severely than nondiabetic individuals, it seems prudent to restrict dietary fat and cholesterol by substituting carbohydrates.

Saturated fat intake in particular should be restricted along with foods rich in cholesterol. Saturated fats and cholesterol are usually found together in the same food, that is, animal fats and dairy products. These should be replaced partly by foods rich in polyunsaturated fatty acids, partly by monounsaturated fatty acids, and partly by carbohydrates. The average nondiabetic American consumes approximately 40% of total calories as fat. Thus a practical and yet palatably acceptable goal in both diabetic and nondiabetic persons is for fat to account for approximately 30% of total calories. Saturated fat content should be less than 10%, the remaining 20% being divided almost equally between polyunsaturated and monounsaturated fatty acids. The remaining caloric deficit resulting from fat restriction can be compensated by the increased carbohydrate intake recommended. Increasing the polyunsaturated fatty acid content of the diet above that recommended is not advised in view of uncertainties about long-term effects of a diet rich in polyunsaturated fatty acids.

Hyperlipidemia occurs frequently in diabetic patients of all types.[2,3] If present, hypertriglyceridemia and hypercholesterolemia may further predispose the person to develop atherosclerosis. Thus the presence of hyperlipidemia in a diabetic patient deserves particular attention, with perhaps further dietary restriction of cholesterol and saturated fat.

Protein

In the diabetic patient, as in the nondiabetic individual, protein should be of high quality and provide all the amino acids necessary for adequate nutrition. Approximately 15% of total calories should be derived from protein; apart from the avoidance of foods rich in both protein and saturated fat, no dietary recommendations regarding proteins are specific for diabetic patients. Vegetarian diets are suitable as long as they are nutritionally adequate and provide enough high-quality protein and other nutrients.

Vitamins and Minerals

Both diabetic and nondiabetic persons should receive a diet that contains adequate amounts of micronutrients. Since some insulin effects depend on certain B vitamins, administering a single daily vitamin supplement that provides the recommended daily allowance of the major vitamins is advised.

Although minerals such as potassium, calcium, and chromium have been reported to influence insulin secretion and glucose metabolism, their role in diabetes and their minimum daily requirements for diabetics are not known. Several reports suggest that osteopenia occurs more often in diabetic than in nondiabetic persons. Thus an adequate intake of calcium should be provided in an attempt to prevent osteoporosis. Supplementary calcium may be needed. An intake of 1.5 g of calcium/day should be the goal, taken either in the form of low-fat or nonfat milk or as a calcium supplement.

Nutritional recommendations for diabetes are summarized in Table 39-1.

TIMING OF MEALS

The release of insulin from its subcutaneous depot site occurs continuously and cannot be reg-

Table 39-1 Nutritional Recommendations for Diabetics

	Non–Insulin-Dependent Diabetes (NIDD)	Insulin-Dependent Diabetes (IDD)
Calories	↓ If overweight	Ensure adequate intake for growth and development
	Timing of meals critical if taking insulin	Timing of meals critical
Macronutrients		
Carbohydrate	↓ As part of caloric restriction if overweight	↑ To 50%-60% of total calories
	50%-60% of total calories if at ideal body weight (IBW)	Limit simple sugars
Fat	↓ As part of caloric restriction if overweight	↓ To 30% of total calories:
	30% of total calories if at IBW	10% saturated, 10% polyunsaturated; 10% monounsaturated
	↓ Intake of cholesterol	↓ Intake of cholesterol
Protein	No special recommendations	No special recommendations
Micronutrients		
Vitamins	Single daily multivitamin supplement	Single daily multivitamin supplement
Calcium	Ensure adequate intake	Ensure adequate intake

ulated in response to physiologic needs. For this reason timing of food intake is critical for all diabetics taking insulin injections. Inadequate attention to this aspect of the diet is widespread among both physicians and patients. Improper timing of food intake almost certainly causes the appearance of some "brittle" diabetes and the occurrence of many hypoglycemic episodes. By merely spreading the caloric content more evenly over the day, the physician can avoid wide excursions in blood glucose levels. Alternatively, more intensive insulin regimens in which multiple doses of regular insulin are administered with meals, over and above the administration of long-acting insulin or a constant insulin infusion (to mimic basal insulin output), also are likely to reduce blood glucose excursions.

Therefore all diabetic patients receiving conventional insulin therapy (i.e., once or twice daily) should consume some carbohydrate at least every 3 to 4 hours during the day when they are awake. In addition to their three main meals, they should have a midmorning and an afternoon snack as well as a snack before going to bed. The distribution of calories among these meals and snacks must be tailored to the individual patient's needs. Factors such as the timing, type, and dose(s) of insulin need to be considered, along with the patient's life-style, work, and physical activity habits. In view of recent reports of frequent asymptomatic and unsuspected nocturnal hypoglycemia, the bedtime snack is of special importance, particularly for patients on twice-daily insulin regimens.

In obese NIDD patients who take neither insulin nor oral agents, the timing of meals is far less important than careful attention to reduced caloric intake.

SPECIAL CONSIDERATIONS
Alcohol

Alcohol may be consumed in limited amounts by diabetic patients within the confines of their caloric allowances.[9] It provides 7 kcal/g (i.e., an intermediate value between fat and carbohydrate) but is of no other nutritive value. Therefore its use clearly should be limited in an overweight diabetic person whose prime goal is weight reduction. Before permitting the consumption of alcohol, attention should be paid to the plasma triglyceride level, since some hypertriglyceridemic individuals, including diabetic patients, may be extremely sensitive to the effects of alcohol in raising triglyceride levels. A further problem is that alcohol can cause hypoglycemia in nondiabetics who have low glycogen stores. Diabetic patients may be even more vulnerable to this effect of alcohol. Thus, the diabetic should not consume alcohol on an empty stomach. Abnormal behavior in a diabetic who recently has consumed alcohol should not automatically be equated with drunkenness; hypoglycemia also should be considered. Despite these potential problems, moderate alcohol intake in the setting of a mixed meal is not contraindicated in diabetes. Allowing such flexibility in the diet may enhance patient compliance with a dietary regimen.

Exercise

Rigorous exercise is never contraindicated in diabetics who are otherwise fit, and participation in a regular exercise program is a valuable adjunct to therapy. Regular exercise increases caloric expenditure and may be of value in achieving weight loss in overweight patients.[10] Also, plasma triglyceride levels tend to be lower with concomitant increases in high-density lipoprotein cholesterol levels, both of which may be beneficial in preventing atherosclerosis. Some caution is required when vigorous exercise is undertaken by diabetic patients receiving insulin therapy, since exercise accelerates glucose disposal and causes a more rapid release of insulin from subcutaneous depots, thereby predisposing the individual to hypoglycemia. Although reducing the insulin dose on days when vigorous exercise will be undertaken is of value to some patients, most respond more favorably to an increase in carbohydrate intake in anticipation of the increased needs. A carbohydrate-rich snack containing rapidly absorbable simple sugars just before exercise (or even during it when the period is prolonged) probably is the simplest way of preventing exercise-induced hypoglycemia. Once an appropriate exercise regimen has been determined for an individual patient, consistency of application is desirable to avoid wide fluctuations in diabetic control.

Sugar Substitutes

No general agreement yet exists as to the amount and/or the acceptability of nutritive or nonnutritive sugar substitutes. The nutritive sweeteners fructose, xylitol, and sorbitol have been used in diabetic diets to replace glucose and sucrose. Their main advantage is that blood glucose levels do not rise substantially after their use; however, all have side effects at high doses, and the effect of their long-term use is uncertain.[11] Aspartame appears to be a safe low-calorie sweetener that does not affect blood glucose levels. The efficacy of all these sweeteners in weight reduction has not been demonstrated. Similarly, the status and long-term safety of the nonnutritive sweetener saccharine currently is in doubt. Therefore recommendations about the use of nutritive or nonnutritive sugar substitutes must be somewhat guarded and must await further studies. Perfectly acceptable dietary regimens for all types of diabetic patients can be designed without their use, but some patients demand the increased palatability offered by sweeter-tasting foods that are low in calories and will not influence blood glucose levels.

EDUCATION AND INDIVIDUALIZATION

Since the dietary regimen recommended for an individual diabetic patient requires lifelong practice, the approach adopted must offer the best chance for adherence to the dietary plan. It is of little value for a physician to hand a patient a preprinted diet sheet and expect compliance.

A prime factor in adherence is that the patient understand the principles and goals involved in the diet. This education is best achieved by a team consisting of the physician, a diet counselor, and the patient. The patient's active participation in the education process is necessary for good compliance and for tailoring the diet to the patient's personal needs. Adherence is more likely if the dietary regimen does not constitute a major disruption to the diabetic patient's lifestyle and is not considered too restrictive by the patient. Therefore the patient's life-style, eating and social habits, and food preferences need to be considered when designing a dietary regimen. Ethnic and socioeconomic factors also are of great importance, as are the patient's personality and psychologic makeup. The level of regular physical activity and other modes of treatment

(e.g., insulin, oral hypoglycemics) must be considered so a meal plan can be devised that integrates these variables. Complications of diabetes or associated conditions also must be taken into account. These factors need to be integrated into a practical plan, which will vary greatly from patient to patient.

Although some individuals clearly prefer rigidly defined meal plans with exchange sheets, the majority prefer more flexibility. In most cases a wide choice within a set framework is desirable in developing a diet that is acceptable, palatable, and economical. Time spent at the outset of treatment ultimately will be of great value in improving the poor compliance with dietary regimens recently documented by several authorities. Since lifelong adherence to a dietary regimen is required, constant reinforcement and encouragement are necessary. The physician frequently has neither the time nor the expertise to advise on the practical details, and the diet counselor should provide such support.

REFERENCES

1. Wood FC, Bierman EL: Is diet the cornerstone in management of diabetes? N Engl J Med 315:1224-1228, 1986.
2. Bierman EL, Brunzell JD: Atherosclerosis, abnormal lipid metabolism, and diabetes. In Katzen HM, Mahler RJ, editors: Advances in modern nutrition, vol 2, New York, 1978, John Wiley & Sons Inc, pp 187-210.
3. Chait A, et al: Diabetic macroangiopathy. In Alberti KG, Krall LP, editors: Diabetes annual. I, New York, 1985, Elsevier Science Publishing Co Inc, pp 323-348.
4. Skyler JS: Complications of diabetes mellitus, Diabetes Care 2:499-504, 1979.
5. American Diabetes Association: Special report. Principles of nutrition and dietary recommendations for individuals with diabetes mellitus, Diabetes 28:1027-1030, 1979.
6. Crapo PA: Carbohydrate in the diabetic diet, J Am Coll Nutr 5:31-43, 1986.
7. Wolever TM, Jenkins DJ: The use of the glycemic index in predicting the blood glucose response to mixed meals, Am J Clin Nutr 43:167-172, 1986.
8. Anderson JW, et al: Fiber and diabetes, Diabetes Care 2:369-379, 1979.
9. McDonald J: Alcohol and diabetes, Diabetes Care 3:629-637, 1980.
10. Vranic M, Berger M: Exercise and diabetes mellitus, Diabetes 28:147-163, 1979.
11. Brunzell JD: Use of fructose, xylitol, or sorbitol as a sweetener in diabetes mellitus, Diabetes Care 1:223-230, 1978.

CHAPTER 40

Obesity

William Dietz

Obesity is a major medical problem in the United States. Few diseases are so difficult for the physician to treat, and few so often result in failure and frustration for the patient. The reasons appear to be rooted primarily because we have a poor understanding of this complex disease and because obesity is caused by a mixture of medical, psychologic, and environmental factors. Clearly, obesity is not a single disorder with a common etiologic basis. It is the clinical expression of a heterogeneous group of disorders; less than 5% of cases have an identifiable medical etiology. Successful treatment therefore rests on understanding the multifaceted origins of the patient's obesity and developing a rational approach to treatment and support.

ESTABLISHING ENERGY REQUIREMENTS

Adequate energy intake is required to maintain physical activity, growth, and body temperature. Allowances are expressed in terms of the physiologically available or metabolizable energy content of foods consumed.

In contrast to recommended nutrient allowances, which are set at levels that meet the needs of 97.5% of the healthy population, the recommended *energy* (caloric) allowance is set for an average person in each age/sex group and activity category. Recommendations for energy intakes are probably best defined as the energy intake required to maintain ideal body weight. Obesity therefore results from an energy intake that has been in excess of energy expenditure. Daily consumption of an extra 84 kcal (3% of the average daily energy intake for a grown man) will produce several pounds of body fat over a year.[1]

Food energy values and allowances are expressed in kilocalories. The accepted international unit of energy, the *joule (J)*, has begun to replace the kilocalorie. To convert energy allowances from kilocalories to kilojoules (kJ), the factor 4.2 may be used (1 kcal = 4.184 kJ). The energy conversion factors of 4 kcal (17 kJ)/g of protein and carbohydrate, 9 kcal (38 kJ)/g of fat, and 7 kcal (30 kJ)/g (5.6 kcal/ml) of alcohol (ethanol) may be used to compute the energy of typical diets in the United States.[2]

Age, sex, exercise, body size, and climate influence the amount of energy required. The age-, sex-, and weight-specific recommended energy intakes published by the National Research Council in 1980 are presented in Table 40-1. The basal metabolic rate accounts for 60%-75% of total daily energy expenditure and correlates with lean body mass. The greatest proportion of the BMR is determined by energy requirements of the brain, heart, kidneys, liver, and lungs. Although muscle accounts for the largest fraction of lean body mass, the energy requirement of resting muscle is low relative to that of the other major organ systems. This relationship accounts for the higher metabolic rates observed in infants and the progressive decline in metabolic rate with advancing age, estimated at approximately 2% per decade in adults.[3] The decrease in energy requirements with age may be further influenced by a decline in physical activity. Persons 45 to 75 years of age require approximately 200 kcal/day less than do individuals 20 to 45 years of age, whereas those above 75 need 500 kcal/day less than persons in the 20-to-45-year age group[4,5] (Fig. 40-1).

BMRs have a strong familial component. Nonetheless, obesity is not more prevalent among individuals from families with low metabolic rates.[6] Furthermore, because lean body mass is frequently increased in obesity, particularly among those with obesity of childhood or adolescent onset, metabolic rates among the obese are frequently elevated compared to metabolic rates among nonobese individuals of the same height.

Table 40-1 Mean Heights and Weights and Recommended Energy Intake*

Category	Age (yr)	Weight kg	Weight lb	Height cm	Height in	Energy Needs (with Range) kcal		Energy Needs (with Range) MJ
Infants	0.0-0.5	6	13	60	24	kg × 115	(95-145)	kg × 0.48
	0.5-1.0	9	20	71	28	kg × 105	(80-135)	kg × 0.44
Children	1-3	13	29	90	35	1300	(900-1800)	5.5
	4-6	20	44	112	44	1700	(1300-2300)	7.1
	7-10	28	62	132	52	2400	(1650-3300)	10.1
Males	11-14	45	99	157	62	2700	(2000-3700)	11.3
	15-18	66	145	176	69	2800	(2100-3900)	11.8
	19-22	70	154	177	70	2900	(2500-3300)	12.2
	23-50	70	154	178	70	2700	(2300-3100)	11.3
	51-75	70	154	178	70	2400	(2000-2800)	10.1
	76+	70	154	178	70	2050	(1650-2450)	8.6
Females	11-14	46	101	157	62	2200	(1500-3000)	9.2
	15-18	55	120	163	64	2100	(1200-3000)	8.8
	19-22	55	120	163	64	2100	(1700-2500)	8.8
	23-50	55	120	163	64	2000	(1600-2400)	8.4
	51-75	55	120	163	64	1800	(1400-2200)	7.6
	76+	55	120	163	64	1600	(1200-2000)	6.7
Pregnancy						+300		
Lactation						+500		

From Committee on Dietary Allowances, Food and Nutrition Board, National Research Council: Recommended dietary allowances, ed 9, Washington DC, 1980, National Academy of Sciences.

*The energy allowances for the young adults are for men and women doing light work. The allowances for the two older age groups represent mean energy needs over these age spans, allowing for a 2% decrease in basal (resting) metabolic rate per decade and a reduction in activity of 200 kcal/day for men and women between 51 and 75 years, 500 kcal for men over 75 years, and 400 kcal for women over 75 years. The customary range of daily energy output is shown in parentheses for adults and is based on a variation in energy needs of ±400 kcal at any one age, emphasizing the wide range of energy intakes appropriate for any group of people. Energy allowances for children through age 18 are based on median energy intakes of children of these ages followed in longitudinal growth studies. The values in parentheses are 10th and 90th percentiles of energy intake, to indicate the range of energy consumption among children of these ages.

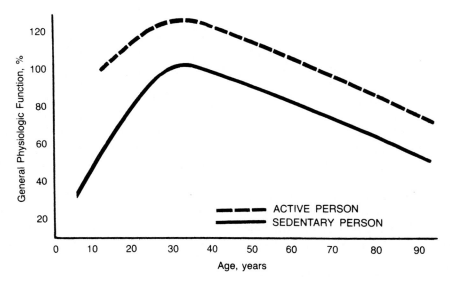

Figure 40-1 Generalized curve to illustrate changes in physiologic function with age. All comparisons are made against the 100% value achieved by a 20-to-30-year-old sedentary person.

From Katch FI, McArdle WD: Nutrition, weight control, and exercise, ed 2, Philadelphia, 1983, Lea & Febiger, p 240.

Table 40-2 Energy Expenditures of Adult Women and Men

	Time (hr)	Man, 70 kg		Woman, 58 kg	
		Rate (kcal/min)	Total (kcal [kJ])	Rate (kcal/min)	Total (kcal [kJ])
Sleeping, reclining	8	1.0-1.2	540 (2270)	0.9-1.1	440 (1850)
Very light	12	up to 2.5	1300 (5460)	up to 2.0	900 (3780)
Sitting and standing, painting, driving, laboratory work, typing, playing musical instruments, sewing, ironing					
Light	3	2.5-4.9	600 (2520)	2.0-3.9	450 (1890)
Walking on level (2.5-3 mph), tailoring, pressing, garage work, electrical trades, carpentry, restaurant trades, cannery workers, washing clothes, shipping with light load, golf, sailing, table tennis volleyball					
Moderate	1	5.0-7.4	300 (1360)	4.0-5.9	240 (1010)
Walking 3.5-4 mph, plastering, weeding and hoeing, loading and stacking bales, scrubbing floors, shopping with heavy load, cycling, skiing, tennis, dancing					
Heavy	0	7.5-12.0		6.0-10.0	
Walking with load uphill, tree felling, working with pick and shovel, basketball, swimming, climbing, football					
Total	24		2740 (11,500)		2030 (8530)

From Committee on Dietary Allowances, Food and Nutrition Board, National Research Council: Recommended dietary allowances, ed 9, Washington DC, 1980, National Academy of Sciences; and Durnin JVGA, Passmore R: Energy, work, and leisure, London, 1967, William Heinemann Ltd, p 166.

Physical activity is also a determinant of energy requirements in children and adults. The individual involved in sedentary activities and limited exercise obviously has a different energy need from someone of the same age and sex who is engaged in strenuous activities, whether at work or play or both. Athletics, construction work, and other similar activities mean higher levels of energy output (Table 40-2). Therefore excess body fat results from an imbalance between energy intake and energy output.

DEFINING AND MEASURING OBESITY

There are no clear cutoffs separating lean, normal, and obese individuals. In all populations, body fat and weight are distributed on a continuum. Optimum body weight and fat for any individual are a function of many variables, including genotype, environment, disease state, psyche, culture, and self-image. There are few quantitative data on which to develop firm guidelines for the most appropriate levels of body fat or weight.

The normal proportions of body weight as fat are 15%-20% of body weight for men and 20%-25% for women. In frankly obese individuals as much as 50% of body mass may be adipose tissue. By using standard tables, deviations in weight can be expressed as percentage overweight; 20% overweight indicates obesity.* Desirable weights for heights in adult males and females are shown in Table 40-3.[7]

Because obesity is defined as an excess accumulation of adipose tissue, its diagnosis depends on demonstrating excess body fat content. Measuring body fat and deciding what is "excessive" adiposity present certain clinical dilemmas. Techniques developed for estimating the gross composition of body fat include determinations of total body water (^{2}H, ^{18}O, ^{3}H, anti-

---

*More recently a body mass index (BMI) (weight [kg]/height squared [m]) in excess of 26.9 for women and 27.2 for men, based on the 1983 Metropolitan Life Insurance tables, has become rather widely accepted. These figures differ from prior actuarial data (1959).

Table 40-3 Desirable Weights for Heights

Height*		Weight†					
		Men				Women			
in	cm	lb		kg		lb		kg	
58	147	—		—		102	(92-119)	46	(42-54)
60	152	—		—		107	(96-125)	69	(44-57)
62	158	123	(112-141)	56	(51-64)	113	(102-131)	51	(46-59)
64	163	130	(118-148)	59	(54-67)	120	(108-138)	55	(49-63)
66	168	136	(124-156)	62	(56-71)	128	(114-146)	58	(52-66)
68	173	145	(132-166)	66	(60-75)	136	(122-154)	62	(55-70)
70	178	154	(140-174)	70	(64-79)	144	(130-163)	65	(59-74)
72	183	162	(148-184)	74	(67-84)	152	(138-173)	69	(63-79)
74	188	171	(156-194)	78	(71-88)	—		—	
76	193	181	(164-204)	82	(74-93)	—		—	

From Committee on Dietary Allowances, Food and Nutrition Board, National Research Council: Recommended dietary allowances, ed 9, Washington DC, 1980, National Academy of Sciences; and Bray GA, editor: Obesity in perspective. Fogarty International Center Series on Preventive Medicine, vol 2, part 1, USDHEW 75-708, Washington DC, 1975, Government Printing Office, p 107.
*Without shoes.
†Without clothes. (Ranges are given in parentheses.)

pyrine, conductance, impedance), lean body mass (whole body ^{40}K), total body fat (Xe, Kr, cyclopropane), body density (hydrostatic weighing), and body volume (water and gas displacement). Unfortunately, many of these techniques cannot be applied practically in infancy and early childhood. Some require levels of cooperation that are unachievable. Others pose biologic hazards that are unacceptable. Although these laboratory methods can provide a good estimate of adiposity, their clinical applications are limited.

Calipers and radiography have been used as clinical tools to estimate the thickness of subcutaneous fat and to determine its relative distribution. A detailed explanation of these techniques are found in Chapters 9 and 10. There are few data documenting the proportion of total body fat that is subcutaneous. Studies in experimental animals indicate that changes in the level of nutrition have little effect on the relative contribution of subcutaneous fat to total body fat. The few analyses of infants and adults who have died suddenly or after varying periods of malnutrition show that between 27% and 42% of body fat is located in subcutaneous tissue. Taking age, sex, and endocrine status into account, it appears that thickness of subcutaneous fat reflects long-term net energy balance. These observations justify the measure of subcutaneous fat as an estimate of total body fat.

It is difficult to measure skinfold thickness with calipers in an infant, and there are no appropriate reference data for the first 2 years of life. Thus weight and length measurements should be used as indicators of body leanness or fatness during early childhood. Thereafter, until the preadolescent age, periodic measurement of skinfold thickness (triceps or subscapular) is recommended along with weight and height. Such serial determinations aid in detecting trends and may be helpful in interpreting skinfold thickness, as well as weight and height measurements during the adolescent years.

Body weight, adjusted for patient height and sex, is the standard criterion for determining obesity. However, these data indicate very little about body fat, and they frequently presume that overweight and obesity are identical, which may not always be true. Using body weight as an index of obesity means comparing an individual's weight to an assumed average, ideal, or desirable weight derived from age- and sex-specific standard tables. These tables may be clinically misleading.[8] Percentiles of triceps and subscapular skinfold thickness for males and females 2-18 years of age are based on data collected by the National Center for Health Statistics (Fig. 40-2).[9] Skinfold thickness is therefore a useful and readily available clinical index of adiposity.

Skinfold values exceeding the 85th percentile

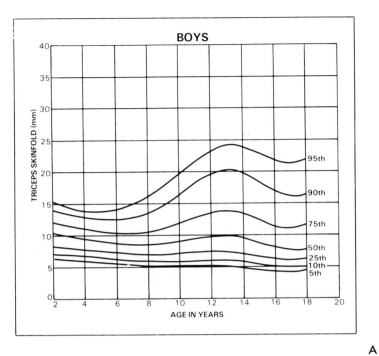

A

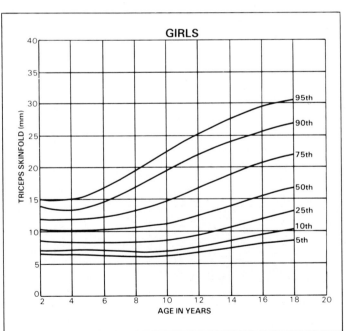

Figure 40-2 A, Smoothed percentiles of triceps skinfold for boys *(top)* and girls *(bottom)* 2 to 18 years of age, United States, 1963-65, 1966-70, and 1971-74.

From National Center for Health Statistics, Public Health Service: Vital Health Stat [II], 219, 1981.

Continued.

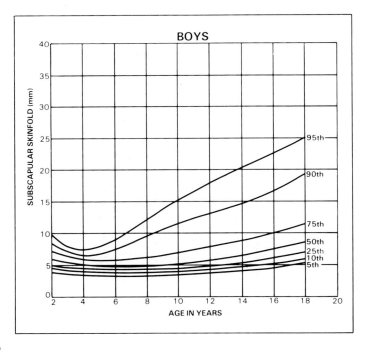

B

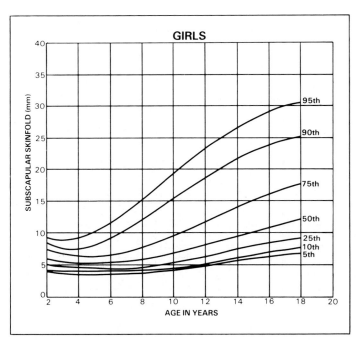

Figure 40-2, cont'd B, Smoothed percentiles of subscapular skinfold for boys *(top)* and girls *(bottom)* 2 to 18 years of age, United States, 1963-65, 1966-70, and 1971-74.

From National Center for Health Statistics, Public Health Service: Vital Health Stat [II], 219, 1981.

for age and sex are considered indicative of obesity. Weight-for-length or weight-for-height figures exceeding the 95th percentile of the National Center for Health Statistics growth chart have been equated with obesity in the preadolescent child. Similarly, a weight value exceeding 120% of the median weight for a given height has been used to define obesity throughout childhood and adolescence. A diagnosis based on weight for height requires a supportive measure of skinfold thickness because lean body mass is increased in childhood obesity. However, these are arbitrary definitions of obesity. At our present level of knowledge, it is not possible to specify a particular percentile or number that signifies a health risk.

DETERMINANTS OF OBESITY

Genetics, environment, and physical activity dictate how each person processes food, derives energy, and either expends or stores that energy. These events, in turn, influence the level of risk and potential biologic hazards associated with overeating.

Fat Cell Production

Childhood obesity is usually characterized by a rise in the number of fat cells (adipocytes) in the body whereas adult obesity is characterized by an increase in adipocyte size and number. During the first 18 months of life the amount of body fat increases, from an average 16% to 28% of body weight. This reflects primarily an enlargement of the adipocytes (from birth to 18 mo) and then an increase in their number (from 12 to 18 mo). These findings contrast with earlier suggestions that the increase in body fat during early infancy reflected predominantly an elevation in the number of cells.

The number of adipocytes is determined from estimates of total body fat and measures of adipocyte size. Measuring adipocyte size and number represents a major problem. The specimen examined may not be representative of the entire body, or the adipocytes may not contain fat and thus may not be included in the count. The disagreement over whether increased body fat during infancy is due to an increase in adipocyte number or in the size of the adipocyte is therefore understandable. Most likely both increase simultaneously. Although in the past it was argued that there was no increase in the number of fat cells after childhood, experimental data suggest that the number of adipocytes may not be fixed even during adult life. It is generally agreed, however, that the number of measurable adipocytes increases about 40 times from birth to adulthood, with most changes occurring in the first 13 to 14 years. At best, these are inexact estimates because of errors in estimating total body fat and variability in the size of adipocytes within a given sample of subcutaneous fat and in different sites.[10]

Little is known about mechanisms governing number and size of fat cells. During early infancy and early adolescence, excess energy may augment the normal increase in the number of adipocytes. An implied assumption, not yet proved, is that obesity associated with an increased number of adipocytes is somehow more resistant to treatment (dietary intervention) than obesity associated with increased cell size. At present there is no evidence that the type of obesity (increased cell number or increased cell size) in late childhood or early adolescence makes any difference as to treatment outcome. This problem is confounded by the frequent association of adolescent obesity, increased fat cell number, and severity of the condition. Nevertheless, early-onset obesity appears to have more serious social and emotional implications than does adult-onset obesity.

Brown Adipose Tissue

Studies in experimental animals suggest that thermogenesis controlled by the sympathetic nervous system in brown adipose tissue plays an important role in energy expenditure and thus in overall energy balance. At one extreme, the mouse becomes obese when, because of a genetic defect, its brown adipose tissue does not function. At the other extreme, the rat fed ad libitum remains lean because its brown adipose tissue grows and hyperfunctions, disposing of the excess fuel by burning it. In normal animals brown adipose tissue appears to serve as a caloric buffer disposing of energy excess when food intake is high and conserving energy when food intake is low.[11]

Diet-Induced Thermogenesis in Humans

In adult human subjects the rise in metabolic rate that follows a meal (diet-induced thermogenesis) accounts for approximately 10% of the energy ingested. Studies have investigated the possibility that obese persons may have a reduction in diet-induced thermogenesis, particularly in response to overfeeding. However, these studies have varied widely in the source of excess calories and have only rarely overfed calories in proportion to metabolic rate or lean body mass. Although a reduction in dietary-induced thermogenesis has been observed among obese adults, variations in lean body mass and failure to account for those differences during overfeeding may have therefore produced spurious inferences.

Adaptive increases or decreases in resting metabolic rate allow for energy balance despite wide variations in food intake.[12] The range of food intake that can be balanced by energy expenditure may depend on the individual's genetic makeup. Convincing data have yet to demonstrate that significant differences in adaptive thermogenesis cause obesity, or that such differences are attributable to brown adipose tissue.

Genetic Component

In the nonhomogeneous human population there is wide variation in the degree to which the so-called thrifty genotype[13] and its converse, the improvident genotype, occur. The thrifty genotype, which stores and conserves food efficiently, must have had an adaptive advantage when food availability was uncertain. Yet this genotype is no longer an advantage in affluent Western societies, given the current availability of food and the adverse effects of obesity. Because of modern day feeding practices, many individuals are virtually never hungry. For those of the thrifty genotype, such practices undoubtedly lead to obesity. In an affluent society the improvident genotype confers an advantage in avoiding the risks of obesity despite a large food intake. This advantage could be reversed if the pattern of food supply and feeding practices were to change.[14]

Early-onset obesity. The causes of childhood obesity are summarized in the box. Less than 1% of obese children have an identifiable disease state.

A study by Eid in 1970[15] showed positive correlations between obesity at 6 months of age and the weight status of the child at 5 to 7 years. Data from Rochester, N.Y., in 1976, suggested an association between obesity in infants and children and obesity in adults.[16] Johnson and Mack[17] then found 2 years later a significant association between relative weight, the weight/height ratio, the ponderal index, and the Quetelet index at ages 12 months and 5 years. However, only 30% of the variances at 5 years could be accounted for by the same indices at 1 year. Nevertheless, the risk of obesity in adolescents appears to be greater in children who are heaviest for length at 1 year of age,[17] even though this group accounts for a minority of obese adolescents.

There are often problems associated with design and interpretation of long-term studies of obesity. One problem is that weight and height data collected during routine pediatric visits are of uncertain quality. Various "obesity" indices (size at birth, weight gain during first yr, relative weight at age 1 yr) observed in longitudinal growth studies correlate poorly with subcutaneous adipose tissue thickness at 7, 10, and 16 years of age. Similarly, very low correlations are found in either sex between various skinfold measures at age 10 months and the same measures at 15 years. Altogether, available data provide no convincing evidence that the obese infant has more than a slight tendency to become an obese adolescent or adult.

However, childhood fatness appears to be the most important predictor of adolescent fatness.[18] These conclusions are based on skinfold measurements of 2177 children made between 6 and 11 years of age and again 2 to 6 years later, when the children were 12-17 years of age. This relation, found for each race and sex group, was independent of stature, economic status, and

---

CAUSES OF OBESITY IN CHILDHOOD

Congenital
Myelodysplasia

Endocrine
Cushing's syndrome
Frölich's syndrome
Mauriac syndrome
Pseudohypoparathyroidism

Rare Conditions
Alström's syndrome
Down's syndrome
Klinefelter's syndrome
Laurence-Moon-Biedl syndrome
Multiple X chromosomes
Prader-Labhart-Willi syndrome
Turner's syndrome
Vasquez' disease

skeletal or sexual maturation. Three fourths of the children whose skinfold thickness (triceps plus subscapular) was in the upper quintile at the younger age were still in the upper quintile as adolescents. Although the period over which these studies were conducted was short, the data suggest that increased canalization of fatness occurs with advancing age.

Prevalence in Adults

A higher proportion of women than men are obese. Racial and economic differences are noted in obese adults. In those 20 to 74 years of age, 14% of the men and 24% of the women are 20% or more overweight. A higher percentage of men than women are 10% to 19% overweight; the reverse is true in the cases of those 20% or more overweight. The percentage of women and men aged 25 to 44 years who are 20% or more overweight has increased over the past decade.

Racial and economic differences are noted in these obese adults. Black women are more likely to be obese than white women, regardless of age or income level. In adults 45 to 64 years of age whose incomes are below the poverty level, 49% of black women and 26% of white women are obese whereas 4% of black men and 5% of white men are obese. In adults of similar age who are above the poverty level, 40% of black women and 28% of white women are obese whereas 12% of black men and 13% of white men are.[19]

This uneven distribution of obesity may reflect different underlying attitudes toward eating and obesity in different strata of society. The degree of fatness and the proportion of obese individuals in a population also appear to be determined by food availability and cost. Psychologic, social, and cultural factors also may contribute to obesity. In Western cultures, an inverse relationship exists between the level of fatness in adult females and levels of education, income, and occupation.[18]

Biosocial Factors

Lifelong trends in fatness differ in males and females. Males are leaner than females from the first year through the ninth decade of life. During the preschool years the average male loses subcutaneous fat while the average female maintains subcutaneous fat (triceps and subscapular) and continues to deposit fat subcutaneously throughout adolescence. The prepubertal increase in subcutaneous fat is less in boys than in girls.

During adolescence, when there are differences in relative fatness among individuals of the same sex, chronologic age, race, and socioeconomic status, one must be cautious in interpreting measurements such as skinfold thickness. These differences in relative fatness reflect differences in maturation and in the start of the preadolescent "fat growth spurt." Adolescent girls have a significantly large absolute amount of body fat, a significantly greater percentage of body fat, and significantly larger adipocytes than do boys. Girls also have a considerably greater number of adipocytes than do boys during the adolescent years.

There are, furthermore, racial differences in subcutaneous fat thickness during childhood. White males and females are fatter than their black counterparts from the third year through adolescence. These racial differences persist when socioeconomic status is taken into account.

Family Patterns

Fatness follows family lines: obese parents tend to have obese children, and an obese child tends to have obese siblings. The children of obese parents become fatter with increasing age, while children of lean parents generally do not. The resemblance in fatness between parents and adopted children does not differ significantly from the resemblance in fatness between parents and biologic children in the same families.[20] Furthermore, there is evidence that obese mothers may have more children than may lean mothers.[8]

If one accepts arbitrary definitions of obesity, a child has an 80% chance of being obese when both parents are obese, a 40% probability when just the mother or just the father is obese, and a 7% probability when neither parent is obese. Family eating and physical activity patterns appear to be more important than genetic factors in explaining these observations. The association between relative fatness of parents and that of their offspring was amply demonstrated in the Ten-State Nutrition Survey. Adopted children and genetically unrelated "siblings" living together tended to be similarly fat.[21] The genetic contributions to this multifactorial problem remain unclear, however. Without doubt, the genetic profile can influence weight gain and body composition.

Studies of identical twins may provide some insight into genetic contributions to relative fatness. Among 78 monozygotic and 144 dizygotic same-sex twins,[22] heritability was significant for limb and trunk fat after age 10 years. Before this age, environmental factors appeared to have a greater influence on body fat. Two disadvantages of such studies are that the number of children involved usually has been small and most children have had normal body composition.

Early studies of monozygotic and dizygotic twins, as well as of age-paired siblings, indicated a genetic influence on body weight, with variance in weight decreasing dramatically as genetic backgrounds of paired subjects became closer. Although it is becoming clear that genetic factors are more important than generally thought, the many unanswered questions indicate a continuing need for investigation.

MEDICAL COMPLICATIONS OF OBESITY
Diabetes Mellitus

Obesity has long been associated with abnormal carbohydrate metabolism and diabetes mellitus, although the etiology of this relationship remains unclear. The distribution of body fat may be a more important determinant of abnormal glucose tolerance than the degree of adiposity. Among women, increases in the waist/hip circumference ratio are directly related to the area under the glucose and insulin curves in response to an oral glucose tolerance test.[23]

Obesity may be part of the complex disease diabetes mellitus or a primary factor responsible for abnormalities in insulin secretion and carbohydrate metabolism. An improvement in hyperinsulinemia and a resulting improvement in glucose metabolism are often seen with loss of weight in the obese patient. As shown in Fig. 40-3, obesity is the disorder most often associated with adult onset of diabetes.[23-25]

Increased pancreatic insulin secretion and blood levels both in the resting state and in response to glucose intake are associated with obesity. Insulin resistance, or the inability of insulin

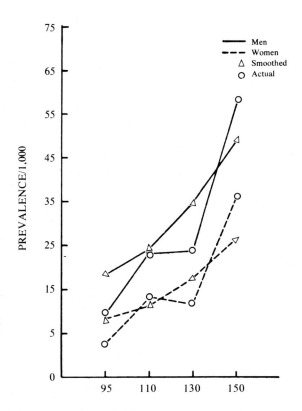

Figure 40-3 Prevalence of diabetes at relative weights. Framingham study, examination 2, men and women (age-adjusted rates), 45-65.

From Kannell WB, et al: Am J Clin Nutr **32:**1238-1245, 1979.

to effect glucose uptake and metabolism in the liver, skeletal muscle, and adipose tissue of obese patients, is the generally accepted explanation. Resistance to insulin has been thought to lead first to hyperglycemia and second to hyperinsulinemia. In fact, the action of insulin is impaired in adipose tissue, muscle, and liver in these patients.[26] The mechanism of insulin resistance in obesity remains unclear. Chapter 39 discusses additional aspects of the association between obesity and diabetes mellitus.

Hyperlipoproteinemia and Hypercholesterolemia

The association of obesity and hyperlipoproteinemia indicates a possible relationship between obesity and lipid metabolism. Obese patients frequently have elevated plasma triglyceride and/or plasma triglyceride, serum cholesterol, and low-density lipoprotein levels and low serum high-density lipoproteins.[27] Obesity and hypertriglyceridemia appear to have the clearest association. The hyperinsulinemia of obesity may be responsible for accelerated synthesis of hepatic triglyceride, and hence for increased plasma triglyceride in the form of very-low-density lipoprotein. Despite this postulated association, hypertriglyceridemia is not noted in all patients with insulin excess, so other causes must be considered.

Fat distribution may also have an effect on hypercholesterolemia. For example, subscapular skinfold thickness correlates better with serum total cholesterol, HDL-cholesterol, triglycer-

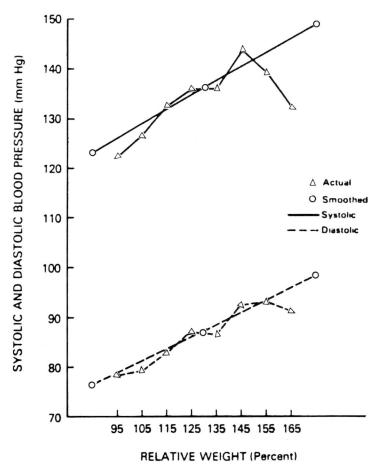

Figure 40-4 Regression of systolic and diastolic pressures against relative weight. Framingham study, examination 5, men ages 45-54.

From Kannell WB, Gordon T: In Bray GA, editor: Obesity in America, NIH Publ 79-359, Washington DC, 1979, Public Health Service, USDHEW, pp 125-143.

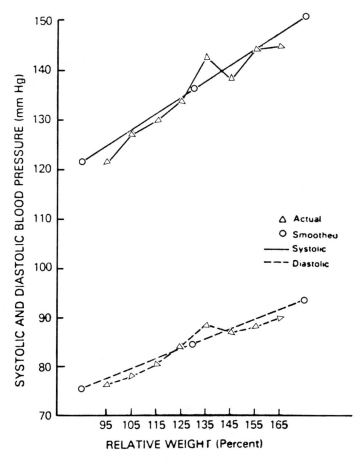

Figure 40-5 Regression of systolic and diastolic blood pressure against relative weight. Framingham study, examination 5, women ages 45-54.

From Kannell WB, Gordon T: In Bray GA, editor: Obesity in America, NIH Publ 79-359, Washington DC, 1979, Public Health Service, USDHEW, pp 125-143.

ides, and blood pressure than does the triceps skinfold. Obesity as a risk factor in cardiovascular disease is reviewed in Chapter 14.

Hypertension

A clear association between hypertension and obesity has been demonstrated in women,[28] and the rate of hypertension rises with increasing obesity. These data are complemented by blood pressure data in men and women reported from the Framingham study,[29] which found a linear association between systolic and diastolic pressures and relative weights (Figs. 40-4 and 40-5).

Gout and Arthritis

Weight loss in obese patients appears to reduce symptoms of gout and arthritis, especially in weight-bearing joints. Arthritis and gout are reported to be 1.5 times more common in obese individuals than in those with the lowest relative weight.[27]

Reproductive Cycle

Fat deposition in females increases at puberty. Some investigators consider that a minimum level of fat is necessary to initiate menarche and maintain a normal menstrual cycle (Chapters 4 and 18). On the other end of the spectrum, obesity may be associated with heavy menstrual flow, menstrual cycle irregularities, cycles of 36 days or more, and increased facial hair. Pathologic ovarian changes in women with marked obesity suggest an association between obesity and ovarian function, but the etiology remains unclear. Although it is rare for obesity to result from hormonal imbalance or hypothalamic damage, both have been implicated as possible

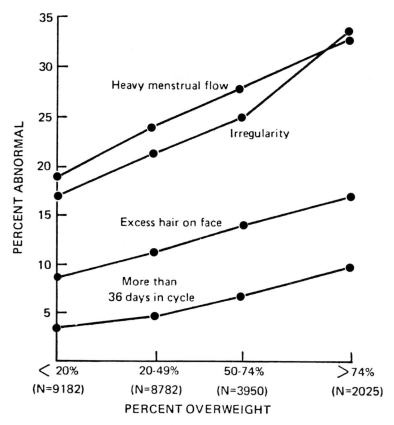

Figure 40-6 Relationship of weight to menstrual abnormalities.
From Hartz A, et al: Int J Obes **3:**57-73, 1979.

causes. Perhaps more convincing is the suggestion that emotional problems resulting in obesity may also influence the menstrual cycle.

Obesity may cause anovulatory cycles and polycystic ovaries by influencing estrogen storage or synthesis. Ovulation may be prevented by suppressed follicle-stimulating hormone if estrogen does not fall at the end of a menstrual cycle. Higher estrogen levels may sensitize the pituitary to gonadotropin-releasing hormone, thereby increasing the circulating levels of luteinizing hormone, stimulating androstenedione and testosterone in the ovary, and possibly inhibiting follicular maturation (Fig. 40-6).[30]

Other investigators report an association between adolescent-onset obesity and latent development of endometrial carcinoma.[31] This supports the hypothesis that prolonged estrogen stimulation, perhaps associated with obesity, may lead to cystic glandular hypoplasia of the endometrium, which may precede endometrial cancer. Additional information on the role of fat in the reproductive health of the adolescent and mature female is found in Chapters 4, 6, and 18.

Gallbladder Disease

Obesity and gallbladder disease have been linked at all age levels, but the association is more notable with increasing age, level of obesity, and parity in women.

Mortality

Mortality rates are higher in individuals who are overweight or obese. Adult males 20% above average weight have a 25% higher mortality rate than do those of the same age but average weight. Weights 40% and 60% above average were associated with mortality rates 67% and 150% higher than the norm. In one study[32] young obese men (200% of ideal body weight) had mortality rates that were 11 times greater than expected. Overweight women, however, had a lower rise in mortality. Other medical complications and smoking contributed to their risk.[33] Additional discussion of obesity as a risk factor and its role in cardiovascular disease is found in Chapter 14.

TREATMENT OF OBESITY
Patient Understanding

Understanding the psychodynamics of obese patients and their families is a prerequisite to successful treatment. It serves as a basis for correctly assessing the patient's needs and targeting the therapeutic approach. Overeating can be both a defensive mental pattern and a conditioned reflex. The patient may fear that too much will be demanded of his or her thinner self and overeat as a defense against unwanted activities and responsibilities. Prolonged deprivation or restriction of too many foods may in turn lead to excessive eating caused by self-hate or self-punishment.

Patients who have unrealistic expectations and are insufficiently motivated to lose weight are often emotionally unstable. Unsatisfied sexual urges, frustrations in achievement, and feelings of boredom, loneliness, fear, hostility, insecurity, and inadequacy all influence the nonnutritional need for food. Psychotic and even aggressive behavior is not uncommon in the psychologically maladjusted individual under pressure to reduce. Thus, for example, marital problems, mood disorders, and extreme anxiety must be treated before actual weight reduction can take place. After psychologic treatment is underway, the patient's reasons for wanting to lose weight can be explored. By the time actual treatment for obesity begins, the patient should have realistic goals and a sense of individual responsibility.[34]

It should be recognized that for some obese patients the body image is a deterrent to weight reduction. Childhood obesity often carries a negative body image into adulthood, and weight loss can provoke sudden disturbances in the individual's attitudes or feelings about his or her body.[35] The physician must realize that for some patients overweight may be the most suitable means of coping successfully. Loss of weight, although perhaps more esthetic and healthful, can produce emotional trauma and unhealthy physical effects in such patients.

Patient Interview

Motivation and adherence often depend on the physician's approach at the initial interview. To understand the pathogenic factors in the individual's condition and to select an appropriate and successful treatment strategy, a thorough physical examination and medical/dietary history are essential. In addition to the usual evaluation appropriate to age and sex, the medical examination should include an assessment of endocrine and cardiac status. Laboratory examination should include urinalysis for the presence of glucose and protein. A lipid screen and glucose tolerance test also may be considered. This information not only guides the physician to understand the patient but also helps the patient recognize reasons for being overweight and establishes initial confidence in the physician's concern and support.

An empathetic physician can begin to build an individualized program designed to alter longstanding eating habits and to heighten the patient's self-esteem. Ongoing interaction and support are essential if the patient is to remain in treatment and to achieve more than transient success with weight loss. Throughout diet therapy, the patient must be made to feel comfortable about expressing his or her feelings about the program. It should be made clear that, although the physician's role is to offer guidance and support, success in following the regimen is completely the patient's responsibility.

Setting Realistic Goals

The patient and physician should establish mutually acceptable realistic goals. Overly optimistic programs usually lead to failure and yet another blow to the obese patient's self image.

Substantial alterations in the morbid effects of obesity, such as improved glucose tolerance and reductions in blood pressure and hyperlipidemia, can be achieved with modest weight reduction. Therefore the selection of a diet should be oriented toward safe weight reduction. Although achievement of ideal body weight is a cosmetic ideal, the importance of some reduction in weight should not be discounted or ignored.

A reducing regimen should be predicated on the relationship between weight loss and energy deficit. In planning a treatment regimen, it is useful to consider energy stores as located in three body compartments: adipose tissue, lean body mass, and a small and labile pool of glycogen and water.

Adipose tissue is approximately 83% fat, 2% protein, and the remainder water. Fat represents some 9 kcal/g, and protein 4 kcal/g; water has no energy value. One kilogram of adipose tissue represents roughly 7550 kcal. Lean body mass and glycogen reserves are 25% protein and 25% glucose, respectively, and the remainder water. Lean body mass and glycogen reserves therefore represent an energy equivalent of practically 1000 kcal/kg.

Higher levels of weight loss are achieved early in a dieting regimen because initial losses result from glycogen mobilization and losses of lean body mass. This may be observed with a reducing regimen designed to achieve an energy deficit of 1000 kcal/24 hours. At the end of 1 week the deficit equals 7000 kcal. In a patient with maximum glycogen stores initially, greater weight loss will result because of initial glycogen depletion. With continued deficits in energy intake, reducing adipose tissue will require a deficit of approximately 7550 kcal/kg of weight to be lost. Therefore, given an energy deficit of 1000 kcal/day, weight loss after the first week will be considerably slower, approximately 0.5 to 1 kg/week (see box).

Both physician and patient should be prepared for the early higher level of weight loss and slower long-term weight loss that result from identical levels of caloric reduction (Fig. 40-7).[36]

Dietary Therapy

Weight reduction regimens can be divided into two dietary approaches: (1) manipulation of dietary patterns without specific caloric restriction to achieve a natural decrease in calories or (2) caloric restriction.[37]

Diet Modification

The dietitian can assist the patient in menu planning to achieve the desired weight by assessing and monitoring nutritional status and evaluating the many factors that may contribute to obesity. The dietitian may assess the patient's attitudes toward dietary modification, develop with the patient a realistic plan for modifying the diet, and instruct the patient on how to achieve these goals. A detailed diet history be-

---

CALORIC DEFICIT TO LOSE 1 POUND (454 g) PER WEEK
1 g of body fat = 7.7 kcal
454 g × 7.7 (kcal/g) = 3496 kcal
Thus reducing one's intake by 500 kcal/da will approximate a decrease of 3500 kcal in 7 days, or 454 g of body fat

---

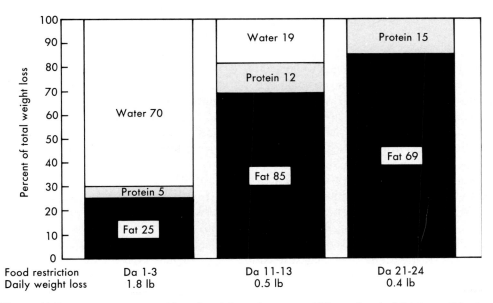

Figure 40-7 Percentage composition of weight at the start, middle, and end of 24 days of food restriction (1000 kcal/da) plus enforced exercise of 2.5 hours per day.

From Grande F: Nutrition and energy balance in body composition. Studies in techniques for measuring body composition, Washington DC, 1961, National Research Council, National Academy of Sciences.

gins with a review of all available objective clinical data (physical, anthropometric, laboratory) and requires effective communication between the physician and dietitian for interpretation. The patient interview, a critical aspect of the assessment process, provides the dietitian with information about patient attitudes, dietary habits, life-style, and environment. It permits the dietitian to assess what patients know about their condition and whether they believe that dietary modification will improve their health status.

The dietitian may use a variety of techniques (e.g., 24 hr recall, food frequency lists, 3 da record, food diary) to obtain information about the patient's food habits and eating patterns. Additional discussion of these instruments is found in Chapter 11. This information will make it possible to evaluate the nutritional adequacy of the current food intake and assess the magnitude of change necessary. Information about the patient's social and economic situation and ethnic and religious background will often reveal factors that the dietitian must take into account in developing an appropriate plan.

The overall evaluation should be discussed with the patient. In instances when someone else regularly prepares the meals, this person should participate in the discussions. Major problem areas should be identified. Changes occur slowly, and attempts to make too many changes simultaneously usually lead to failure. Thus the dietitian should stress changes believed to be of highest priority.

Sound judgment is required. If long-term dietary compliance is essential, it may be important to deal first with a patient's negative attitude toward change. This is especially important in working with patients who have failed in earlier attempts to change their eating habits. If these patients can achieve a few modest successes during the first weeks and can be supported and reinforced in their efforts, they may be stimulated to work toward more ambitious goals.

The following techniques may help the patient apply the information given during the diet-planning phase. Review a tray of food models representing items of high, moderate, and low caloric value. This permits the patient to become familiar with the caloric levels of foods typically consumed. Review menus and menu patterns to identify problem areas and permit the patient to become familiar with them. Encourage the patient to plan meals for several days and monitor his or her understanding and compliance. Identify differences in caloric content for alternative meals, patterns, and food preparation techniques. Review the net effect of different caloric intakes on weight gain and loss.

Very few people will permanently alter life-long food habits on the basis of a short-term encounter with any health professional. To effect change, follow-up instruction, support, and reinforcement are essential.[37-38]

Fad diets. Before seeking medical advice, the patient frequently will have elected a dietary approach that is considered popular or workable. Some diets promise rapid, painless weight loss with little sacrifice and even fewer changes in life-style; others may be nutritionally unbalanced without vitamin or mineral supplements. In view of their popularity, it is important for the physician to understand the profile of each "fad diet," including its advantages, disadvantages, and potential hazards. (See Appendix II for an analysis of popular reducing diets.)

Diets with an emphasis on one food are likely to be nutritionally unbalanced and therefore unsafe. The once-popular grapefruit diet has given way to yogurt and ice-cream diets, which, in addition to being nutritionally inadequate, can lead dieters to consume more calories than they thought. Vegetarian diets, however, if nutritionally balanced, may be used safely when planned by a qualified nutritionist who considers the individual's health needs.

Claims that "calories don't count" and that one "has to eat fat to burn fat" remain a part of the lure of high-fat diets, despite serious challenges. High-fat diets are nutritionally suspect and can pose health hazards, such as hyperlipidemia, atherosclerosis, increased blood uric acid, ketosis, and fatigue.

Restrictive Diets

Low-calorie balanced diets of 600 or more calories per day can be employed for a period with careful and experienced physician supervision. Protein intake in adults following such diets should be approximately 1.5 g/kg body weight/day. Other components of these diets include a vitamin tablet containing minerals that provide the RDA of all vitamins and minerals, 5 g of sodium chloride, 25 mEq of potassium, 800 mg of calcium, and a minimum of 1500 ml of fluids daily. In addition, these diets must be accompanied by a substantial behavior modification program.[39,40]

Hypocaloric low-carbohydrate ketogenic diets have potential side effects; weakness, apathy, fatigue, nausea, vomiting, dehydration, postural hypotension, and occasional exacerbation of preexisting gout may be associated with the dietary regimen. Therefore such diets must be monitored frequently for evidence of protein undernutrition or electrolyte abnormalities.[34]

Whether ketogenic regimens improve adherence remains controversial. Hunger may be blocked by ketogenesis, but hunger is rarely the only factor affecting adherence. Under hypocaloric regimens, protein alone appears to spare more body protein than carbohydrate. After maintenance protein is supplied, however, the merits of additional carbohydrate or protein remain unsettled.

The use of low-quality protein as a protein source is clearly dangerous. There have been reports of serious illness and death associated with use of commercial liquid-protein diets. By the end of 1977, the Food and Drug Administration had received reports of more than 40 deaths attributed to the use of these diets. A large proportion were attributed to cardiac arrhythmias caused either by the absence of electrolyte supplementation or by cardiac cachexia.

Highly structured restrictive diets may be especially appropriate for individuals with chronic weight problems stemming from poor eating habits. The lack of choice in menus can become monotonous in regimens that are rigidly prescribed and offer little or no choice. Other diets are designed for a limited period (e.g., 14 da). These are suitable only as short-term means of losing weight whereas plans that offer appropriate long-term maintenance programs may be followed over an extended period. Self-help groups are an integral component of several popular weight control programs. Other approaches may incorporate psychologic guidance, behavior modification, or exercise guidance in their published literature.

Physical Exercise

Physical fitness should be an integral part of diet therapy, and most obese patients need special urging to combine adequate exercise with restriction of caloric intake. Body image may

Table 40-4 Energy Estimates in Adults

Approximate Requirements	Kilocalories/24 hours	
	Reference Male (70 kg)	Reference Female (55 kg)
Basal requirements		
1 kcal/kg/hr	1680	1320
Additional requirements		
Very sedendatry activity (+20%)		
1.2 kcal/kg/hr	2016	1584
Sedentary activity (+30%)		
1.3 kcal/kg/hr	2184	1716
Moderately active (+40%)		
1.4 kcal/kg/hr	2352	1848
Very active (+50%)		
1.5 kcal/kg/hr	2520	1980

deter participation in activities such as swimming and aerobic dancing but may not be as critical a factor in walking or doing isometric or muscle tone exercises at home. Educating the patient in activity/caloric exchange values can help reinforce the need for regular exercise (Table 40-4).

Increased physical activity has benefits beyond those of increased caloric expenditure. A few cautions, however, should precede a general prescription. The emphasis should be on increasing *activity* rather than on exercise, which carries connotations of boredom and strenuous work. Activity described in the broader sense helps dispel the normal resistance to habit changes. The goal is to find activities that are enjoyable and therefore more likely to be self-motivating. Because many obese persons are in poor physical condition, the activity program must be carefully graded to prevent exercise from becoming another failure. The extra weight obese people are attempting to move can overload joints and muscles to the point of injury. Heavy lifting should be avoided by those with hypertension. Regular, graded activity should be sought. The clinician must realize that learning to enjoy what usually would be considered normal levels of activity constitutes an important success.

In conjunction with an activity program, the clinician may have to counter strongly ingrained notions that increased activity leads to increased appetite. If activity is regular and increasingly vigorous, the opposite can be expected. In addition, enjoyable physical activities may lead the individual away from an environment full of eating cues.

Behavior Modification

One of the major advances in the treatment of obesity has been the use of behavior modification. Because eating is a learned behavior, the reeducation techniques of behavior modification are especially well suited to the treatment of obesity. Two schools of thought on the relationship between personality and obesity have developed. One argues that obesity is caused by an underlying personality disorder that triggers eating responses; the other views emotional disturbances as the result of obesity. Regardless of this unresolved cause-and-effect relationship, motivational, situational, and sensory cues clearly dictate the selection of foods, location and time of eating, and amount of food ingested. To modify detrimental eating behaviors, specific cues that trigger individual eating patterns must first be identified. Only then can positive methods be devised for altering behavior.

Behavior modification techniques currently involve self-monitoring, stimulus control, family intervention, slowing the act of eating, reinforcement, and cognitive restructuring. The food diary is the basic tool of self-monitoring. With the food diary, the subject records daily the time and location of all eating, amount of food and how it is prepared, reason for eating and with whom, degrees of hunger and appetite, and level of stress. The diary provides specific information about the client's eating patterns on which to base and evaluate behavior changes. It is important to provide a convenient form on which patients can record the diary and to encourage them to record information immediately after or before eating events. If events are recorded hours or days later, the diary loses its power of bringing unnoticed patterns to awareness.

After eating cues are known, the slow step-by-step process of reshaping behavior begins. The first step is to use the diary to find the strongest eating cues and then design a creative and systematic reward program to eliminate or control them. A variety of eating cues or stimuli can be expected in most patients. Developing specific

techniques requires ingenuity on the part of both therapist and patient. The first goal in many cases is to limit the accessibility and visibility of high-calorie foods. This aim is often accomplished by having the client go through the house and throw away these foods. A parallel move is to expand the accessibility of low-calorie foods. Food shopping should be done with a list and after the client has had a satisfying meal to avoid impulse buying. Convenience foods should be avoided because they increase quick accessibility to food.

Foods that require preparation should be encouraged. This will increase the time between the desire to eat and the act of eating. Food preparation can also be an enjoyable food-related activity that helps the patient become more aware of food choices. Finally, eating environments should be defined and limited. For example, the patient will make a commitment to eat and snack in only one room of the house, with certain utensils and without distractions such as television. All these examples indicate how the eating environment can be changed to make the act of eating a conscious, controllable choice as opposed to a continued response to an environment in which the individual feels helpless and even victimized.

Pharmacologic Agents

The role of anorectic drugs in weight control has been a controversial subject. The use of amphetamines to treat obesity is now illegal in most states. The use of diuretics have no role in the management of uncomplicated obesity.

Of the nonamphetamines, fenfluramine (Pondimin) holds the greatest promise. Fenfluramine may act by enhancing serotonin release, thereby decreasing carbohydrate intake. Fenfluramine is therefore a logical drug for individuals with documented high-carbohydrate intake. Rigorous clinical trials in this population have yet to be performed, however, and application of fenfluramine to the general obese population has not yet been examined.

Surgery

Surgery must be reserved for patients with severe obesity (>200% ideal body weight, or less if a significant complication of obesity exists) in whom all more conservative approaches to weight reduction have been unsuccessful. Intestinal bypass is accompanied by such long-term morbidity that it can no longer be recommended. Gastric bypass surgery, which involves stapling the fundus of the stomach and creation of a Roux-en-Y anastomosis to the proximal jejunum, is currently the procedure of choice. Although surgical deaths are rare, complications such as wound infection, a leak at the anastomosed site, or laceration of the spleen occur in 5%-10% of patients. If the procedure is performed correctly and is accompanied by a vigorous ongoing program of behavior modification, weight losses average approximately 45 kg and continue for 18 months following surgery. Long-term successful weight reduction occurs in approximately 50% of patients, and less than 20% regain their former weight.

A gastric balloon, inserted and inflated through a gastroscope, is a recent addition to the surgical approaches to obesity. Current experience seems to indicate, however, that there has been an unacceptably high frequency of ulceration, along with occasional obstruction, following its deflation. So this approach must still be considered experimental.

Additional Determinants of Weight Loss

Psychologic screening of the obese patient can reveal underlying emotional problems that need to be resolved for optimum weight loss. Techniques such as relaxation therapy, assertiveness training, and role playing can help obese patients cope with such common problems as stress, noncompliance, negative body image, or low self-esteem. Group therapy appears to be especially effective to manage obese patients who otherwise might drop out of treatment or be noncompliant. If professionally directed group therapy is not available, self-help groups may be considered. Caution is advised in referring patients to such groups because they can vary greatly in quality. For the patient undergoing a drug or emotional crisis or with severe depression, psychotherapy must precede any weight reduction program.

Family involvement and support can be a major determinant in patient management. All too often the family, especially a spouse, can sabotage a carefully planned diet program through direct opposition, jealousy, lack of understanding, or unwillingness to modify established dietary practices. One must understand the patient and spouse, parent, or significant other persons to be able to alter negative dietary practices, attitudes, and behavior and reach the desired goal of weight reduction and maintenance.

REFERENCES

1. Garrow JS: Energy balance and obesity in man, ed 2, New York, 1978, Elsevier/North Holland Inc, p 243.
2. Committee on Dietary Allowances, Food and Nutrition Board, National Research Council: Recommended dietary allowances, ed 9, Washington DC, 1980, National Academy of Sciences, p 16.
3. Durnin JVGA, Passmore R: Energy, work, and leisure, London, 1967, William Heinemann Ltd, p 166.
4. McGandy RB, et al: Nutrient intakes and energy expenditure in men of different ages, J Gerontol **21**:581-587, 1966.
5. Katch FI, McArdle WD: Nutrition, weight control, and exercise, ed 2, Philadelphia, 1983, Lea & Febiger, p 240.
6. Bogardes C, et al: Familial dependence of resting metabolic rate, N Engl J Med **315**:96-100, 1986.
7. Bray GA, editor: Obesity in perspective. Fogarty International Center series on preventive medicine, vol 2, part 1, USDHEW 75-708, Washington DC, 1975, Government Printing Office, p 107.
8. Salans LB: Natural history of obesity. In Bray GA, editor: Obesity in America, NIH Publ 79-359, Washington DC, 1979, Public Health Service, pp 69-94.
9. National Center for Health Statistics, Public Health Service: Basic data on anthropometry and angular measures of the knee and hip for selected age groups, 1-74 years of age: United States, 1971-1975, Vital Health Stat [2], 219, 1981.
10. Hirsch J, Batchelor B: Adipose tissue cellularity in human obesity, Clin Endocrinol Metab **5**:299-311, 1976.
11. Himms-Hagen J: Obesity may be due to a malfunctioning of brown fat, Can Med Assoc J **121**:1361-1364, 1979.
12. Miller DS: Thermogenesis and obesity, Bibl Nutr Dieta **27**:25-32, 1979.
13. Mann GV: The influence of obesity on health, N Engl J Med **291**:178-185, 1974.
14. Himms-Hagen J: Determinants of human obesity. In Paige DM, et al, editors: Manual of clinical nutrition, Pleasantville NJ, 1982, Nutrition Publications Inc.
15. Eid EE: Follow-up study of physical growth of children who had excessive weight gain in first six months of life, Br Med J **2**:74-76, 1970.
16. Charney E, et al: Childhood antecedents of adult obesity, N Engl J Med **295**:6-9, 1976.
17. Johnston FE, Mack RW: Obesity in urban black adolescents of high and low relative weight at 1 year of age, Am J Dis Child **132**:862-864, 1978.
18. Zack PM, et al: A longitudinal study of body fatness in childhood and adolescence, J Pediatr **95**:126-130, 1979.
19. Bray GA: Obesity in America: an overview. In Bray GA, editor: Obesity in America, NIH Publ 79-359, Washington DC, 1979, Public Health Service, pp 1-19.
20. Garn SM, et al: Fatness similarities in adopted pairs, Am J Clin Nutr **29**:1067, 1976.

21. Garn SM, Clark DC: Trends in fatness and the origins of obesity, Pediatrics **57:**443-456, 1976.

22. Brooks CGD, et al: Influence of heredity and environment in the determination of skinfold thickness in children, Br Med J **2:**719-721, 1975.

23. Evans DJ, et al: Relationship of body fat topography to insulin sensitivity and metabolic profits in premenopausal women, Metabolism **33:**68-75, 1984.

24. National Commission on Diabetes report, vol 3, part 1, DHEW Publ 76-104, Washington DC, 1975, Government Printing Office.

25. Kannell WB, et al: Obesity, lipids, and glucose intolerance. The Framingham study, Am J Clin Nutr **32:**1238-1245, 1979.

26. Salans LB, Cushman SW: The role of adiposity and diet in the carbohydrate and lipid metabolic abnormalities of obesity. In Katzen HK, Mahler RJ, editors: Advances in modern nutrition, obesity, diabetes, and vascular disease, Washington DC, 1978, Hemisphere Publishing, pp 267-302.

27. Nestel P, Goldrick B: Obesity: changes in lipid metabolism and the role of insulin, Clin Endocrinol Metab **5:**313-335, 1976.

28. Rimm AA, et al: Relationship of obesity and disease in 73,532 weight conscious women, Public Health Rep **90:**44-51, 1975.

29. Kannell WB, Gordon T: Physiological and medical concomitants of obesity: The Framingham study. In Bray GA, editor: Obesity in America, NIH Publ 79-359, Washington DC, 1979, Public Health Service, pp 125-143.

30. Hartz A, et al: The association of obesity with infertility and related menstrual abnormalities in women, Int J Obes **3:**57-73, 1979.

31. Rimm AA, White PL: Obesity: its risks and hazards. In Bray GA, editor: Obesity in America, NIH Publ 79-359, Washington DC, 1979, Government Printing Office, p 105.

32. Drenick EJ, et al: Excessive mortality and causes of death in morbidly obese men, JAMA **243:**443-445, 1980.

33. Garrow JH: How to treat and when to treat. In Munro JF, editor: The treatment of obesity, Baltimore, 1979, University Park Press, p 8.

34. Bruch H: Eating disorders, anorexia nervosa, and the person within, New York, 1979, Basic Books Inc.

35. Pearlson G, et al: Body image in adults, Psychol Med **11:**147-154, 1981.

36. Grande F: Nutrition and energy balance in body composition. Studies in techniques for measuring body composition, Washington DC, 1961, National Academy of Sciences.

37. VanItallie TB: Conservative approaches to treatment. In Bray GA, editor: Obesity in America, NIH Publ 79-359, Washington DC, 1979, Public Health Service, pp 165-178.

38. MacCuish AC, Ford MJ: Dietary management of obesity and obesity related diseases. In Munro JF, editor: The treatment of obesity, Baltimore, 1979, University Park Press, pp 19-21.

39. Bistrian BR: Clinical use of a protein-sparing modified fast, JAMA **240:**2299-3304, 1978.

40. Hoffer LJ, et al: Metabolic effects of very low caloric weight reduction diets, J Clin Invest **73:**750-758, 1984.

CHAPTER 41

Adverse Reactions to Foods

S. Allan Bock
Noel W. Solomons

REACTIONS DUE TO IMMUNOLOGIC MECHANISMS

S. Allan Bock

The subject of food allergy has long been viewed with confusion by both the medical and the nutrition professions. This circumstance is no longer necessary if one carefully examines the scientific information that has accumulated in this field in recent years.[1] Much of the confusion surrounding the use of the term allergy when applied to foods has been eliminated. The double-blind food challenge has evolved as the "gold standard" for the objective confirmation of histories of adverse reactions to foods. Investigations of skin testing and other laboratory tests have demonstrated the usefulness as well as the limitations of these techniques. Proper evaluation of controversial techniques has pointed out their deficiencies. Long-term studies have taught us new things about the natural history of adverse reactions to foods in children, and procedures have been derived for the ongoing management of persons with confirmed histories of adverse reactions to foods. There are a number of frontiers in this area that make it both exciting and challenging to study. It is these concepts and the information derived from the studies of various investigators to which this chapter addresses itself.

Definitions

In an area in which there has been a great deal of controversy, it is important at the outset to define certain terms clearly. The reader may need to be reminded about some basic immunologic principles. The first of these concerns the access of antigens to the sensitized host. Sensitization means that a person's immune system has previously experienced exposure to a given protein and has made a specific response. This response may be "remembered" over a long period and thus sensitization may persist for many years. It is uncertain whether continuing exposure at some low level or exposure to a cross-reacting protein is required to maintain the sensitization indefinitely. There are persons who have persistently detectable sensitization to specific proteins in the absence of known exposure to those proteins, be they ingested, injected, or inhaled. Once a recognized antigen reaches the immune system, a sequence of events occurs involving cellular events, biochemical events such as the release and interaction of mediators, and stimulation of end organs to produce clinical manifestations. This is a fairly orderly sequence and may be interrupted at any point by an inadequate stimulus (Fig. 41-1).

The basic principle of the stimulus-response or dose-response relationship is applicable at each of the steps in the sequence depicted. The progression of reactions may be interrupted at any step if the stimulus is inadequate to exceed the threshold for the next reaction to proceed to a response. Therefore it should not be surprising that in certain instances food antigens ingested by a sensitized person do not produce symptoms, because the quantity ingested is insufficient.

The term allergy has been badly used (even abused) over the last several decades in connection with adverse food reactions. However, it should not be so employed. The designation adverse food reaction is more appropriate for discussing symptoms that have been observed and associated with food ingestion but for which no mechanism has been found and the association

□ I acknowledge the seminal participation of Charles D. May, M.D. in the development of the concepts in this chapter and the acquisition of the data in all of the studies from our institution. His wisdom in opening a scientific inquiry into the field of food allergy should serve as a beacon for all those who approach it in the future.

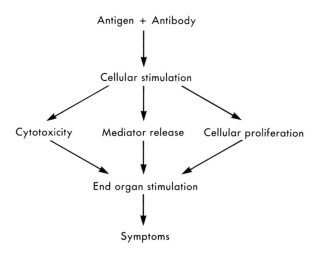

Figure 41-1   Antigen interacting with antibody in a sensitized host.

is only suspected. In this discussion "allergy" means that specific immunologic events are involved wherein there are (1) symptoms that drive the patient to seek help from the physician and/or nutritionist and (2) manifestations of antibody or antigen-reactive components of the immune system. When a person has detectable antibodies or antigen-reactive components of the immune system and symptoms caused by a foreign substance, whether ingested, injected, or inhaled, he may be said to have *symptomatic sensitivity* or *symptomatic sensitization*. This is a straightforward circumstance, and the most obvious example would be the child who eats peanuts and breaks out with an urticarial rash and has vomiting accompanied by breathing difficulty.

The confusion arises in circumstances in which sensitization is detectable but symptoms cannot be objectively reproduced on exposure of the individual to the putative antigen. Then one is tempted to confusion by disregarding the antibodies that have been detected as irrelevant and referring to their detection as "false positive." The sensitization is real, and this can be proved by exposing the individual to the antigen in such a way that the immune system is certain to recognize a sufficient quantity, such as an intravenous injection which would result in impressive symptoms. If the test which has detected the sensitization has been properly performed, then one may say that the patient has *asymptomatic sensitivity* or *asymptomatic sensitization*.

APPROACH TO PATIENTS WITH
ADVERSE FOOD REACTIONS

Obtain a complete history and physical examination.
Consider differential diagnoses.
Undertake food challenges (open and double blind).
Perform appropriate laboratory measurements (skin tests, etc.).
Prescribe an elimination diet.
Repeat challenges at appropriate intervals.

Approach to the Patient
History and Physical Examination

The basic approach to the patient complaining of adverse reactions to foods (see box) is to begin with a thorough history. If the patient is complaining about a specific food or foods, one must obtain a description of the symptoms accompanied by information as to the time of onset of the reaction following ingestion, the most recent occurrence, the quantity of food required to produce the symptoms, and the number of occasions on which the problem occurred. The physical examination is directed toward the systems in which food reactions are more likely, especially the gastrointestinal, cutaneous, and respiratory systems.

Differential Diagnoses

There are a number of mechanisms by which adverse reactions to foods can occur:

Deficiency of intestinal enzymes
Toxic reactions
Immunologic reactions
Undefined reactions from mediators of inflammation
Psychologic reactions

This chapter will concentrate on reactions due to immunologic mechanisms, although one should consider the others whenever a patient is seen who may be having symptoms due to another mechanism.

Probably the most common adverse reaction to food in the United States is disaccharidase deficiency. (The enzyme deficiencies are covered elsewhere in this manual.) Another adverse reaction, toxicity, has been reported, and the suggestion made that many physicians may be inadequately informed about food toxicology. Toxins in food can be either inadvertently added in the course of food processing or a natural constituent. Lists of these are available in toxicology tests. Furthermore, a number of adverse reactions to food have been hypothesized[2] as being due to biochemical mediators. This is an exciting area for research, especially as newer biochemical mediators are identified. Finally, a very important mechanism of adverse food reactions is psychologic reactions. Food occupies an important role in our society and culture. There are few areas of medicine about which more strongly held beliefs exist than what foods in our diet may do to us.

In our practice we have seen many patients who had strongly held beliefs that they wished to have confirmed and they were anywhere from mildly disappointed to totally furious when we were unable, by objective testing, to prove their beliefs. In fact, we have learned over the years that if adult patients have strongly held beliefs about adverse reactions to food and they seem to be coping well with food avoidance the best approach is to suggest to them that they do not require any evaluation. The situation with children is a different matter, about which we know too little. We often forget to ask children who have been prescribed an elimination diet, either appropriately or inappropriately, how they feel about the diet. Careful observation will usually reveal that they have strongly held feelings and beliefs about what is being done to them. They often feel that they are being placed in an awkward position with respect to their peers when certain foods are removed from their diet. In young children who spend their preschool years on very restricted diets because of severe food allergies, we have seen the development of decided food aversions as they grew older, even when with the passage of time certain foods could be tolerated either totally or in small quantities. Further observations are important so it can be determined whether these youngsters will sustain long-term eating disorders because of dietary prohibitions. It seems that this is a reasonable caution to raise, since American society has a propensity for food fads and dietary manipulations that are often inflicted on children without their agreement.

Manifestations of immunologic adverse reactions. Over the years of food allergy research at the National Jewish Center for Immunology and Respiratory Medicine we have heard complaints of almost every symptom that can occur in major bodily systems. The list is far too long to explore in depth in this discussion, but it is important to concentrate on the manifestations that are commonly reproduced in objective challenges.[1,3-5]

The most common adverse reactions to foods in children occur in the gastrointestinal tract and include nausea, diarrhea, vomiting, and abdominal pain. A small number of patients in our series[5] and in well-controlled studies of children in Scandinavia[6,7] had colic following ingestion of certain foods. This appeared to be a minority of the children, however.

The second most frequent symptoms are cutaneous manifestations and include urticaria, nonspecific erythematous macular eruptions, eczema, and angioedema. There has long been controversy between allergists and dermatologists about the ability of foods to produce atopic dermatitis. Studies at our institution and those of Sampson[8-11] show unequivocally that some children with atopic dermatitis have as one precipitating factor the ingestion of certain foods.

Respiratory symptoms have been the least common manifestations of food reactions to be confirmed, and in some studies have been most commonly associated with either gastrointestinal or cutaneous manifestations. In the group of asthmatics we have studied asthma as the sole manifestation of an adverse reaction to food has been distinctly uncommon.

Behavioral reactions constitute a major area of controversy in this field. The responsibility to investigate children's behavioral reactions objectively has frequently been ignored by people making vociferous claims about the relationship between various foods and food constituents and abnormal behavioral reactions. Based on properly controlled, rigorously performed, double-blind food challenges[12-15] it seems safe to say that behavioral symptoms as the sole manifestation of adverse reactions to foods are distinctly unusual. Although there have been some claims that behavioral reactions have been reproduced by double-blind challenges, these are often small numbers or have not been confirmed by other investigators. At present one is entitled to view with skepticism claims about the association between food elimination and behavioral improvements.

An area receiving increased attention is the association between food ingestion and migraine headache. There has long been anecdotal evidence to suggest that adverse reactions to foods may produce migraine headaches. Recently some patients undergoing double-blind food challenges[16-18] seem to have had an association between their headaches and food ingestion. These studies await confirmation and increased numbers, but it certainly would be helpful to the many migraine headache sufferers in the world if food elimination were identified as a source of their disability.

Food Challenges

The most important principle in the study of adverse reactions to foods is the double-blind food challenge. It has been referred to as the "gold standard" for studying food allergy. Before describing it, however, some comments on open food challenges are in order.

The open challenge. As mentioned earlier, once the patient's history has been carefully obtained it should be possible to administer a challenge that will reproduce the patient's symptoms. Unlike other areas of medicine, however, in which the history is usually the path that leads to the diagnosis, in the case of food allergy numerous studies at different institutions have demonstrated the inaccuracy of food histories. Many reasons have been proffered for this discrepancy, but it is sufficient to say that in most studies*

*References 3, 4, 5, 8, 9, 10, 11, 19, 20, 21.

less than 50% of the histories have been confirmed. It should be added that in many of these studies the patients were from a highly selected population likely to have the reaction.

Because histories are so often inadequate, open food challenges are fraught with danger. During open food challenges, the administration of the food to the patient is in a usual and customary fashion prepared in usual ways. The open challenge, therefore, allows the patient's bias to come into play. The greatest use of the open food challenge is the refutation of suspicions that particular foods are producing specific symptoms. It is particularly useful under circumstances in which the patient has avoided food for a long time but does not have a strongly held belief that the food is a problem or under circumstances in which food has been eliminated by a health care provider on flimsy grounds. If an open food challenge is negative and the patient can ingest the food, then the problem may be quickly eliminated. If the open challenge is positive, then in most circumstances a double-blind food challenge is required. Interestingly enough, this is also true for young children because the frequent association between symptoms and food ingestion by parents becomes a strongly held belief of the parents.

The double-blind challenge. In the double-blind food challenge both the patient receiving the food and the person providing it and making the observations are blind to the contents of the challenge. One should make the distinction between a blind challenge in which the patient has no idea that anything is happening and a blind challenge where the patient realizes that something different is occurring and that foods are being administered and hidden by some device.

Since dietitians and nutritionists often are asked to aid in the administration of double-blind food challenges, a few comments seem appropriate about the preparation of blind food challenges. Several vehicles can be used to hide foods:

Opaque capsules
Vivonex (iced and flavored)
Milkshakes
Applesauce
Tapioca-fruit mixtures
Hamburger

Our favorite has been opaque capsules into which we placed dried food. These have the virtue of completely obscuring the food that the patient is to ingest. Since foods are given in a dried form, large amounts can be placed in a relatively few capsules. Some investigators use milkshakes as the vehicle; but since dairy products are often under suspicion and some foods are easily detected in a milkshake, this is often not a suitable vehicle. An elemental diet (Vivonex) that can be iced and flavored with vanilla, orange, or grape is an excellent medium in which to hide liquids or fairly large quantities of certain foods. Most foods are well hidden and the flavor packets make a rather unpalatable taste more acceptable for food challenges. A tapioca-fruit mixture has been used by some investigators. We have found that in young children applesauce is an excellent vehicle in which to hide many foods. As long as the challenge tastes like applesauce, most young children do not raise strenuous objections. Our dietitian has also taught us that, at least for purposes of challenging children, hamburger is a readily accepted vehicle. When beef is the food under consideration, we have found in certain circumstances that if the quantity under suspicion is fairly small it may be hidden in tuna fish. There are numerous other possibilities for hiding or masking foods. The more completely the food is hidden, the more objective will be the results. Any deviation from absolute blinding must be appreciated and taken into consideration in the interpretation of results, which can be biased by either the patient or the observer.

The double-blind food challenge is generally begun at an amount approximately half that suspected by the patient of producing a reaction. The dose may be doubled at intervals determined by the patient's history. We have generally found that if a single challenge containing 8-10 g of a dried food does not reproduce the adverse reaction reported, then this should be reported to the patient and the food should be reintroduced into the diet openly and preferably under observation. (A single dose of 8 to 10 g may have been preceded by several smaller doses, thus making the total dose larger than 10 g.) Under the vast majority of circumstances, this has sufficed to eliminate the problem in patients not having a strongly held belief about what would happen when they ingested certain foods. The ability of the patient to eat the food eliminates all questions about preparation and the effects of cooking or heating and digestion. During the administration of a food challenge, a systematic record of manifestations is kept. The reason it is so important for the observer to be blind is that in single-blind settings the person making and recording the observations can actually tip the patient as to whether the challenge is active or placebo.

The placebo that we most commonly use is dextrose, which is readily available for human consumption. Dextrose is easy to place in capsules since it is available as a powder, and it can also be placed in many of the vehicles mentioned above. When capsules are in use, certain substances are hard to hide even in opaque capsules because the capsule may be discolored by the material it contains. This is often not a problem with children, who do not pay much attention to the capsules but consume them rapidly if the process is made to seem like a game. By contrast, adults frequently resist the ingestion of capsules and spend a great deal of time examining them. For a substance like chocolate, which does make certain opaque capsules appear darker than the placebo, we have found that carob is an excellent and unrelated placebo.

A perusal of the literature on food allergy will disclose numerous undocumented reports of "late" or "delayed" food reactions. Recent research in respiratory tract immunology has begun to uncover late-phase reactions and their mechanism, but these have not yet been documented in the gastrointestinal tract. Although a late-onset food reaction similar to the late asthma reaction appears eminently possible, a careful perusal of the published double-blind food challenges in which patients reported a delayed-onset reaction will reveal that these reactions generally have not been reproducible. An exception may be the gastroenteropathies, including gluten-sensitive enteropathy in young children. The well-known enteropathies in children include, besides the gluten-sensitive type, a cow's milk protein enteropathy and a soy protein enteropathy.[22-27] In both children and adults there have been reports[28,29] of other foods producing a flat intestinal lesion upon ingestion. Whether these reactions were primarily immunologic or whether the immunologic events associated with them were secondary to other mechanisms has yet to be determined. They would seem to be the best models in which to look for late-phase reactions; but since they occur most often in young children and are rather transient, there are limitations on research into them. A good alternative is the food-induced eczematous skin changes that Sampson is investigating (unpublished data). Some of these changes could be late-phase reactions, and this is a fertile area for research.

At present one is entitled to view with skepticism reports of late or delayed reactions due to food ingestion, especially in the production of vague symptoms. The notion that these may occur is certainly not out of the question, but claims that patients have had them should be studied under carefully controlled conditions. Rarely have these reactions studied up to the present time been found to be reproducible many hours to days after food ingestion.

Laboratory Measurements

There are several laboratory measurements to which attention should be drawn because they are in common use and have been subject to much misinterpretation.

Skin testing. The allergy skin test, when used for foods, has been condemned as useless and inaccurate. Careful investigation of food skin testing, however, has shown this to be an incorrect conclusion. If one understands the uses, limitations, and interpretations of allergy skin tests, they can be quite helpful in the evaluation of patients complaining of adverse reactions to foods.*

Like any other laboratory reagent, skin testing material must be verified. This means that the material must have been shown to be not irritating in normal persons and to be able to detect antibody in patients who are sensitized. Unfortunately, at present, many allergy extracts, especially those for foods, are not standardized and therefore it remains the responsibility of the individual practitioner to be sure that extracts in use are verified. Published studies demonstrate that allergy skin testing is particularly helpful in identifying patients who are unlikely to have positive reactions during a double-blind food challenge. Sampson has found the negative predictability of allergy skin tests to be in the range of 99%. However, the positive predictability of the allergy skin test is much lower. Some foods to which patients have detectable antibodies are almost never shown to correlate well with double-

*References 8, 9, 10, 19, 20, 21, 30, 31.

blind food challenges. Three often mentioned are corn, chocolate, and tomatoes. By contrast, peanuts, other nuts, eggs, milk, soy, and wheat are foods for which a positive skin test is more likely to be associated with a positive double-blind food challenge. The most efficacious method for skin testing is the prick/puncture technique using a 1:10 or 1:20 weight/volume concentration of extract. Intradermal skin tests for foods are more likely to identify patients who have clinically irrelevant antibodies. In other words, the patient has asymptomatic sensitization. At present, the puncture skin test can be used to identify people in whom a double-blind food challenge should be performed. If the skin test is negative, unless the patient has a strongly held belief about the reaction, an open food challenge may suffice; if the skin test is positive, a double-blind food challenge may be the proper tool.

Radioimmunoassays. The radioallergosorbent test (RAST) and a growing number of enzyme-linked immunoassays (ELISA) for detecting specific antibodies have become widely available. However, they are fraught with problems. There may be substantial variability in the detection of IgE, especially at low levels, among even highly sophisticated laboratories.[32] There has yet to be a widespread investigation of the proper performance of these tests in commercial laboratories, but discrepancies in test performance between scientific laboratories are disturbing. The tests are expensive, often in the range of 2-10 times the cost of a skin test. A number of factors can interfere with proper results; and despite apparent sophistication, the scoring systems currently in use are qualitative, not quantitative. The tests are excellent research tools but have obvious limitations as clinical implements for daily use.

It is presently the recommendation of the American Academy of Allergy and Immunology that the RAST and other similar tests not be used for routine clinical evaluation because they yield no more information than a properly performed skin test does and they increase the cost of medical care. There are some exceptions to this recommendation in special circumstances, however.

The ability to detect antibodies and antigen-antibody combinations (immune complexes) to foods is improving and also is becoming more widespread, but these tests should be regarded as primarily research tools until their clinical usefulness can be demonstrated in proper clinical studies.

A number of earlier comments alluded to symptoms in the gastrointestinal tract. In certain circumstances a biopsy of the small intestine or colon may be extremely helpful for evaluating a possible effect of foods on the intestinal mucosa. The protein-induced enteropathies are the most obvious example. There is also a condition called eosinophilic gastroenteritis that is most properly evaluated by the small bowel biopsy.[33,34]

Controversial tests. Over the years several controversial tests have appeared in the popular food allergy literature and subsequently disappeared. The most tenacious of these has been the cytotoxic food test, which until recently had a large commercial following. Close examination of the extravagant claims made for its ability to detect hundreds of food allergies, however, showed it to be rarely reproducible and rarely to correlate with the results of double-blind food challenge–proved food reactions. Numerous regulatory agencies (including the Federal Government) have been discouraging the use of this test, and it has been falling into disfavor.

The Elimination Diet

Once objective testing has identified patients with true adverse reactions to foods, the cornerstone of management is the elimination diet coupled with frequent careful rechallenge. Several principles, however, should be kept in mind:

1. When the patient presents with elimination diet recommendations, the dietitian or nutritionist needs to consider whether the history sounds plausible and the request reasonable. Remember that most patients who have true adverse reactions to foods, except young infants, react to one or at most two or three foods. Exceptions to this finding, as identified by blind food challenges, have been quite rare. Therefore the patient presenting with a long list of foods that must be eliminated for a prolonged time might need to obtain a second opinion before embarking on a prolonged elimination diet.

2. The use of very strict elimination of mulitple foods for short periods has been discussed. Once the elimination diet is in force, the foods to which the patient has had documented reactions should be challenged at intervals that may be as frequent as every month

or as infrequent as once every several years. Patients who have a long history of reactions to nuts in particular may never lose their clinical reactivity. Although rigorous longitudinal studies in adults are lacking, the food proteins that children have been least likely to tolerate over a prolonged period are peanuts and other nuts.

3. Recommendations for longitudinal food challenging include repeating the double-blind challenge in approximately the same fashion as used to produce symptoms in the most recent challenge. If the patient's symptoms are mild and the quantity of the tolerated food seems to be increasing, the challenges may be performed at 1-to-3-month intervals. When the symptoms are more impressive and a small quantity of food is sufficient to reproduce the reaction, the intervals should be longer, perhaps 6 to 12 months.

4. A number of medications have been used in the treatment of food allergy. These include oral disodium cromoglycate, antihistamines, and corticosteroids.

   a. Most of the patients studied with the first two medications have not received proper determination of the presence of a true food reaction prior to the administration of treatment. Therefore the putative success of cromolyn sodium and antihistamines often is due to an inaccurate diagnosis of the food reaction. At present, we suggest that these medications be viewed as experimental for the treatment of adverse reactions to foods. (Disodium cromoglycate is not currently licensed for oral use in the United States.)

   b. Corticosteroids have very specific applications and may be lifesaving in the treatment of secretory diarrheas in young children. They may also be extremely important in the successful management of eosinophilic gastroenteritis. For the chronic management of non–life-threatening food reactions, they are contraindicated because of their harmful long-term side effects.

5. Desensitization to foods is an excellent idea whose time has *not* arrived. Although there are many places in the United States where food injections are administered, properly controlled studies have never shown these in-

jections to be more efficacious than the placebo with which they have been compared. In a small number of studies, double-blind methodology has been claimed, and successful results attributed to food injections. However, many of these studies suffer from the fault that objective challenges were not used to demonstrate that the patient truly had the problem at the outset.

Repeat Challenges

Studies of the natural history of food reactions have involved a number of different patient populations. A few have been conducted on the general population, but they generally looked at the incidence or prevalence of food reactions with only a short period of longitudinal evaluation. Studies have been done on a limited number of children who had double-blind food-challenge–proved food sensitivity.[35] We also have had the opportunity to evaluate nine children with severe reactions to foods over a period of years.[36]

Studies on children in the general population[37] show that adverse reactions to foods are rather uncommon and usually disappear fairly promptly. The evidence supporting immunologic mechanisms for these reactions is somewhat limited. One conclusion has been that most foods incriminated as producing symptoms in young children should be retested at short intervals using open techniques initially. In a large majority of these children, food reactions will not be reproduced.

In children with double-blind food challenge–confirmed reactions, some of the problems are "outgrown." The physiology of the disappearance of these reactions is not understood. It may involve a number of physiologic and immunologic processes in the gastrointestinal tract where antigens may be excluded from the circulation and thus prevented from being recognized by antibodies or antigen-reactive cells. The foods studied in greater number and shown to be most likely to be outgrown as problems include egg, milk, and soy. As noted earlier, cow's milk and soy milk protein enteropathies seem to be transient conditions and most of the literature would support the notion that these reactions disappear by the third or fourth year of life. Gluten-sensitive enteropathy, by contrast, when accurately diagnosed, seems to be a lifelong condition in the majority of patients who have been studied.

In a study of nine young children with very severe adverse reactions to foods,[36] we were gratified to find that most lost their life-threatening reactions despite continuing to have some response (mild to moderate) for varying lengths of time. It was encouraging also to find that some of these children completely outgrew their symptoms and consumed the foods that had been a problem in customary amounts. It must be stressed again, however, that food challenges in children with life-threatening reactions are dangerous and potentially very harmful. They should be undertaken only in settings where emergency treatment is available and personnel experienced in treating severe allergic reactions are continuously present. The major justification for challenging these patients at all appears to be twofold: First, and especially with children, it is invariable that there will be accidental ingestion of foods to which the patient is markedly allergic (although our most recent scare occurred in an adult who ingested peanut butter from an unlikely source). Despite their obvious appearance, nuts are often hidden in foods that children, especially younger ones, eat without being aware of it.* The same is true of dairy products, which may be even harder to detect. The second justification for performing a food challenge under extremely controlled conditions is that if the reactions truly do disappear this is most comforting information for the parents of young children.

Prevention of Allergy in Young Children

The subject of prevention of allergy in young children by dietary manipulation has received a great deal of research attention. Unfortunately, we do not presently know the answer to this problem. Several studies have managed to show diametrically opposed results. Careful perusal of them suggests that this may be due to the fact that different populations were being studied and that many of the groups being compared were not controlled and thus only one variable was changed. An intriguing notion has been advanced[38] that mothers produce different amounts of IgA antibody, which may limit the ability of certain foreign proteins to reach beyond the intestinal lumen of breast-fed infants. It seems probable that the family history is related

---

*We were recently impressed by our ability to teach a 4-year-old that peanuts would cause him harm, but just as impressed by the inability of adults around him to notice the occult presence of peanuts in certain foods.

to the development of both food and inhalant allergy in young children. A well-controlled study by Zeiger and colleagues in San Diego is beginning to yield results as this chapter is being written. Some of their preliminary data have been presented. The reader may be well advised to watch for the most recent developments from these investigators. Also Zeiger et al.[39] have written a state of the art review that can easier be read than summarized in this chapter.

Some recommendations, which are not definitive, can be made. For most children, and especially those with a family history of food or inhalant allergy, prolonged breast-feeding without supplementation may prove to be preventive or to decrease symptoms in certain situations. Nevertheless, it is well known[4,40] that children may have adverse reactions to foods that their mothers have ingested. The most common of these in our experience have been milk, soy, eggs, and peanuts. For infants from highly atopic families who are having problems with proteins ingested by their mothers or who are not going to be breast-fed, one of the elemental formulas may be a useful way to prevent exposure to ingested foreign proteins in the first few months of life. A major drawback to this recommendation is the expense of these formulas.

Conclusion

It is clear that complaints of adverse reactions to foods may be approached in a logical and orderly fashion and that confusion is no longer necessary.[41] The reader should be persuaded that it is possible in almost all circumstances to determine by objective means whether an adverse reaction to a food is occurring as described by the patient. As more is learned about the natural history and immunology in this area, better laboratory techniques will be developed and increasingly accurate prognostications will be possible. In the meantime, the tools currently available will allow most patients to receive assistance with their problems, so long as proper diligence is undertaken in evaluation and treatment.

REACTIONS DUE TO NONIMMUNOLOGIC MECHANISMS

Noel W. Solomons

Adverse reaction to food not only encompasses immunologic reaction but may include any illness, or metabolic or biochemical abnormality, associated with the ingestion of a food or dietary component, whether the latter is a nutrient or a nonnutrient substance. Since a reaction can result from substances with nutritive

---

Food

Food is any nutrient or mixture of nutrients and other chemicals that is eaten and processed in the digestive system. This processing includes mastication, swallowing, digestion, absorption, intermediary metabolism, and excretion. Food may be relatively simple and pure chemically (e.g., sodium chloride, sucrose) or extremely complex and composed of a variety of substances not all of which are known (e.g., chocolate layer cake, milk, eggs, oranges). In addition to one or more nutrients, food may contain metabolites, nondigestible residues, endogenously produced substances (flavor- and aroma-producing extracts, caffeine, druglike additives), and exogenously added coloring agents, emulsifiers, antibiotics, or antioxidants. One must distinguish between nutrients and foods. Not all nutrients are foods—water and oxygen, for instance.

Nutrient

A nutrient is any chemical that is utilized by the body directly or indirectly to produce energy or a cellular structure. An essential nutrient is one that is not synthesized at all or is only partially synthesized by metabolic processes and leads to recognizable illness when totally excluded from the diet. A nonessential nutrient is one that can be synthesized by the metabolic processes of the body but also can be supplied by the diet. Total exclusion of a nonessential nutrient from the diet does not cause any recognizable illness. Both essential and nonessential nutrients are metabolites.

Pseudofood

Pseudofoods are certain food items that contain few if any nutrients. They may incorporate chemicals that have potent physiologic effects and may thus be considered drugs. In this category belong coffee, tea, chocolate, spices, and herbs.

From Herman RH, Hagler L: West J Med **130**:95-116, 1979.

value, such as carbohydrates, lipids, as well as proteins or amino acids, treatment as already noted usually depends on eliminating the offending agent. Water, oxygen, vitamins, and minerals, also vital nutrients, are similarly capable of inducing a reaction. (Precise definitions of terms are found in the box on p. 663.)

Food intolerance often produces an adverse response when the offending substance is eaten. The level of individual susceptibility to the offending nutrient varies. Some patients are capable of identifying the association between a specific food and the physical response; others do not recognize a connection.

A secondary adverse restriction is common when an acute illness, such as anorexia, alters normal function so severely that the individual rejects certain foods. Such reactions usually disappear if the primary disease is cured and the patient returns to normal health. Smell and taste disorders also may cause food rejection. Other causes of secondary food reaction include cultural practices, personal idiosyncrasies, religious beliefs, and psychologic problems. Some individual aversions or toxic responses to certain foods cannot be explained. The food intolerances associated with diarrhea, gastrointestinal disorders, and anorexia nervosa are discussed elsewhere in this manual.

Several basic mechanisms produce clinical manifestations of primary adverse reactions (Table 41-1). Metabolic or biochemical abnormalities can alter the intermediary metabolism of a substance. Inborn errors of metabolism, amino acid disorders such as phenylketonuria and tyrosinemia, and galactosemia all can have this effect. The failure to absorb macronutrients, specifically fats and carbohydrates, leads not only to inefficient utilization of the diet but also to disordered gastrointestinal physiology. Thus the dietary lipids not absorbed in abetalipoproteinemia or the carbohydrates malabsorbed in disaccharidase deficiencies reach the colon, where the action of bacterial enzymes produces harmful metabolites. Both nutrients in high doses (vitamin A, vitamin D, potassium) and nonnutrients (food toxins) can produce systemic toxicity. As previously discussed immunologically mediated hypersensitivity to a given protein (milk protein) or class of proteins (iodinated pro-

Table 41-1 Pathogenesis of Primary Adverse Reactions to Foods

Mechanism	Manifestation
Metabolic disturbance	Galactosemia, Type II hyperlipidemia (β-hyperlipoproteinemia)
Intestinal malabsorption and colonic fermentation	Lactase deficiency, abetalipoproteinemia
Systemic toxicity	Potassium overdose
Immunologically mediated hypersensitivity	True food allergies
Miscellaneous	Gluten-sensitive enteropathy

Table 41-2 Food Group(s) Avoided Because of Adverse Reactions in British Adults

	Number of Persons	Percentage of Reactors (185)	Percentage of Respondents (560)
Alcoholic beverages	36	19.4	6.4
Vegatables	30	16.2	5.4
Meat products	29	15.6	5.2
Cheese	27	14.6	4.8
Fish products	23	12.4	4.1
Other dairy products	13	7.0	2.3
Chocolate	14	7.6	2.5
Other sugar confectionary and sugar	8	4.3	1.4
Cereals	19	10.2	3.4
Fats and oils	10	5.4	1.8
Fruit	10	5.4	1.8
Eggs	5	2.7	0.9

From Bender AE, Matthews DR: Br J Nutr **45**:403-406, 1981.

teins) can produce the range of allergic manifestation on ingestion of offending foods. Finally, specific end-organ sensitivity often exists to a given food, as demonstrated most profoundly in gluten-sensitivity enteropathy.

Although information about the number of individuals who experience adverse reaction to classes of foods is limited, a report of a survey in Great Britain suggested that one third of a population of 560 London school faculty responding to a survey questionnaire suffered an adverse reaction to a food. Approximately twelve groups of foods were frequently cited in addition to caffeine products and red wine (Table 41-2).[42]

Carbohydrate-Induced Adverse Food Reactions

Monosaccharides

Frequently carbohydrate-induced food reactions may be traced specifically to an inability to metabolize the monosaccharides fructose and glucose. In normal individuals, monosaccharide consumption increases the activity of jejunal epithelial glycolytic enzymes and decreases that of fructose diphosphatase.[43] In those whose normal enzyme adaptive responses are impaired, glucose and fructose consumption can bring on chronic intermittent diarrhea or a dumping-like syndrome. Although the etiology of the condition is unknown, the symptoms often disappear on a low-carbohydrate diet. Tropical sprue also is characterized by histologic abnormalities of the small intestine, but in this case the normal adaptive response returns once the primary gastrointestinal disorder is treated.

Fructose intolerance. In hereditary fructose intolerance the individual has severely reduced levels of the enzyme fructose-1-phosphate aldolase in many tissues, particularly the liver. When fructose or sucrose is ingested, fructose-1-phosphate accumulates in the liver and other tissues, producing hypoglycemia, and, in severe responses, sometimes leading to shock and death. Consumption of both fructose and sucrose must be restricted in such cases. Fructose-1-phosphate aldolase activity may be increased by the oral administration of pharmacologic doses of folic acid,[44] but enzyme activity cannot be restored to normal levels. Fructose-1,6-diphosphate aldolase activity also is diminished in such individuals, although not sufficiently to prevent

normal function. The activity of both enzymes is found in a single polypeptide chain but in different locations.

Individuals with fructose-diphosphatase deficiency are intolerant of fructose, sucrose, ethanol, glycerol, or a ketotic diet and fasting.[45] Since the enzyme is essential to the function of the gluconeogenic pathway in the liver, such individuals may suffer from chronic ketotic hypoglycemia or (in rare cases) reactive hypoglycemia. The hypoglycemia is provoked by a ketotic diet or fasting as well as by sucrose, fructose, glycerol, and ethanol. Restriction of these provocative agents, along with frequent glucose feedings, is appropriate therapy for the chronic hypoglycemic form of the disease. Folic acid may induce fructose-diphosphatase activity and thereby improve blood glucose levels; it therefore can protect patients with milder forms of the disease.

Galactose intolerance. In galactosemia, a hereditary disorder of galactose metabolism, the enzyme uridyltransferase is deficient. When galactose is ingested, galactose-1-phosphate accumulates in the liver, kidney, lens of the eye, and other sites. If consumption is chronic, hypoglycemia, cataracts, mental retardation, poor weight gain, hepatic and renal damage, and ultimately death will follow. Thus, in galactosemia all products containing milk must be avoided.[46]

Another rare condition involving galactose intolerance is glucose-galactose intolerance. It occurs primarily in infants and is due to a defect in the glucose-galactose carrier protein in the small intestine's mucosal epithelial cells. The infant is intolerant to large amounts of both glucose and galactose.[47] Symptoms of osmotic diarrhea and renal glycosuria may be relieved by restricting dietary glucose and galactose (milk is the primary source) and substituting fructose as the source of carbohydrate.

Disaccharides and Polysaccharides

The prevalence of intolerance to the complex carbohydrates varies widely, with lactose intolerance being quite common. As with the monosaccharides, intolerance to the disaccharides and polysaccharides results from deficiencies in the enzymes needed to metabolize these sugars.

Lactose intolerance. The jejunal brush-border enzyme lactase is needed to hydrolyze milk into glucose and galactose. Lactase activity

Table 41-3 Prevalence of Lactose Intolerance Among Adults

<15%	60%–80%	>80%
White population of northwest European background (U.S.)	Blacks (U.S.)	Full-blooded Indians (U.S.)—Pima, Papago, Hopi, Apache
Scandinavians	Mixed-ancestry Indians (U.S.)	Eskimos
Western Europeans	Jews (U.S.)	Japanese
White Australians	Mexican-Americans	Formosans
Nomadic Fulani		South Nigerians
Tussi		

From Paige DM, Bayless TM: Lactose digestion: clinical and nutritional implications, Baltimore, 1981, Johns Hopkins University Press.

is deficient in a majority of the world's adult population, which therefore is unable to consume milk without experiencing diarrhea and other gastrointestinal symptoms.[48] Lactose intolerance may rarely be evident in very young children. It is more commonly recognized clinically when lactase activity declines even further in adolescence and adulthood. It is commonly identified in many adult populations (Table 41-3). Treatment entails restricting or avoiding milk and milk products. Many lactose-intolerant individuals can consume small quantities of milk (one glass with a meal) without symptoms. Milk products such as cheese in which the lactose has been hydrolyzed and yogurt may be tolerated more readily than regular cow's milk. Lactase additives and lactose-hydrolyzed milk are available for lactose-intolerant individuals who want to continue to drink milk.

Sucrose and starch intolerance. In rare cases sucrose-starch intolerance is caused by deficiencies in the activity of the two jejunal brush-border enzymes sucrase isomaltase and maltase. As a result the individual cannot hydrolyze the disaccharide products of the ingested starch. Osmotic diarrhea may be relieved by restricting both sucrose and starch and feeding fructose to induce sucrase and maltase activity.

Pure starch intolerance has been identified in individuals with alpha-amylase deficiency. Diarrhea resulting from colonic fermentation of undigested starch may be relieved by eliminating starch from the diet.

Intolerance to other disaccharides and oligosaccharides. In one family[49] intolerance to the disaccharide trehalose was traced to a deficiency in the jejunal enzyme trehalase. The family suffered vomiting and diarrhea after eating mushrooms, which contain trehalose normally hydrolyzed by the enzyme.

The oligosaccharides raffinose, stachyose, and verbascose, found in some plants, are not digested easily in the small intestine. Instead of being hydrolyzed, they are fermented by *Clostridium perfringens,* producing flatulence and discomfort. The major food sources of these polysaccharides include sugar beets, cottonseed meal, legumes, and the roots and rhizomes of plants in the mint family.

High-Carbohydrate Diet Reactions

Diets high in carbohydrate may be associated with reactive hypoglycemia and related to a variety of medical problems. These may include diabetes and hormonal (hypothyroid, Addison's disease), alimentary, or idiopathic diseases. In some patients with Type IV hyperlipoproteinemia, a high-carbohydrate diet may be responsible for panhyperlipemia. This may be reversed with a restriction in carbohydrate intake. A diet high in carbohydrate is also associated with maturity-onset diabetes, which results easily in an abnormal glucose tolerance and hyperinsulinemia. Obesity is frequently associated with this set of events.

In some normal individuals, glucose and fructose feedings increase the activity of jejunal epithelial glycolytic enzymes and decrease fructose diphosphatase activity. Such individuals may exhibit a dumping syndrome (e.g., diathesis, diarrhea) that is chronic and intermittent in character; clinical studies fail to demonstrate any disease. These individuals frequently show improvement when they are provided with a low-carbohydrate diet.

Individuals who are ingesting a low-carbohydrate diet or are subsisting or starving demonstrate a reduction in jejunal glycolytic enzyme activity. Carbohydrate administered as glucose may provoke gastrointestinal symptoms and diarrhea. Feeding after gastric resection will result in the so-called dumping syndrome, with rapid intestinal transit time and diarrhea. A comprehensive listing of carbohydrate-induced food intolerance is as follows*:

Glucose-galactose intolerance from glucose-galactose malabsorption

Lactose intolerance from lactase deficiency

Sucrose-starch intolerance from sucrase-isomaltase deficiency

Sucrose-fructose intolerance (hereditary fructose intolerance) from fructose-1-phosphate aldolase deficiency

Sucrose-fructose-glycerol intolerance caused by fructose-diphosphatase deficiency

Galactose intolerance

Galactosemia caused by uridyltransferase deficiency

Cataracts caused by galactokinase deficiency

Galactose intolerance after ethanol ingestion

Trehalose intolerance caused by trehalase deficiency

Starch intolerance caused by α-amylase deficiency

Adverse carbohydrate reactions

Reactive hypoglycemia

Hyperlipoproteinemia (Type IV)

Glucose intolerance and hyperinsulinemia

Obesity

Precipitation of paralysis in familial hypokalemic periodic paralysis, especially after exercise

Gastrointestinal maladaption syndrome related to failure of jejunal glycolytic enzyme adaptation to dietary carbohydrate

Primary

Secondary

Postoperative dumping syndrome

Lactic acidosis due to pyruvate dehydrogenase deficiency

Dental caries related to sucrose and *Streptococcus mutans*

Raffinose-stachyose-verbascose intolerance due to indigestibility

Protein-Induced Reactions

Protein and amino acid induced adverse food reactions are listed below.* A comprehensive discussion of this topic is included in the section "Reactions Due to Immunologic Mechanisms."

*From Herman RH, Hagler L: West J Med **130**:95-116, 1979.

Protein-induced

Gluten reactions

Celiac disease (gluten enteropathy)

Dermatitis herpetiformis

IgA deficiency and diarrhea

Mastocytosis

Adverse protein reactions

Food allergy

Milk protein allergy

Soybean protein toxicity

Hepatic encephalopathy in cirrhosis, especially in portosystemic shunting

Renal failure

Pancreatic insufficiency

Enterokinase deficiency

Urea cycle enzyme defects

Ornithine transcarbamylase deficiency

Argininosuccinic acid synthase deficiency

Argininosuccinate lyase deficiency

Carbamyl phosphate synthase deficiency

Arginase deficiency

Lysine-ornithine-arginine malabsorption

Cystine-lysine-arginine-ornithine transport defect (cystinuria)

Homocystinuria

Succinyl-CoA—3-ketoacid—CoA-transferase deficiency

Avidin binding of biotin

Amino acid—induced

Tryptophan

Hartnup disease

Tryptophan malabsorption (blue diaper syndrome)

Phenylalanine (phenylketonuria)

Leucine-isoleucine-valine (maple syrup urine disease)

Valine (hypervalinemia)

Leucine-isoleucine (hyperleucine isoleucinemia)

Lysine (persistent hyperlysinemia)

Methionine (methionine malabsorption syndrome or oasthouse urine disease)

Leucine-induced hypoglycemia

Monosodium glutamate reaction (Chinese restaurant syndrome)

Valine-isoleucine-threonine-methionine-thymine-propionate adverse reaction

Propionic acidemia

Methylmalonic aciduria

Isovaleric acidemia

β-Methylcrotonylglycine and β-hydroxyisovaleric acidurias

α-Methylacetoacetic and α-methyl-β-hydroxybutyric acidurias

Hereditary tyrosinemia

Histidinemia

Hyperprolinemia

Lipid-Induced Reactions

Adverse reactions to lipids are common in America, where the fat composition of the average diet often exceeds 40% of total caloric intake. The many forms of lipid-induced food reactions are listed below.*

Malabsorption syndromes
Pancreatic insufficiency
    Cystic fibrosis
    Pancreatitis
    Carcinoma
    Other causes
Small intestinal disease
    Tropical sprue
    Celiac disease
    Regional enteritis
    Scleroderma
    Lymphoma
    Collagenous sprue
    Mastocytosis
    Multiple small intestinal diverticula
    Amyloidosis
    Immunoglobulin deficiency with lymphoid nodular
      hyperplasia
    Macroglobulinemia with infiltration of the bowel
      wall
    Short bowel syndrome
    Other causes
Hepatobiliary disease
Lymphatic disease
    Whipple disease
    Lymphangiectasia
    Lymphatic obstruction
    Other causes
Vascular disease
Pancreatic endocrine disease
    Diabetes mellitus
    Zollinger-Ellison syndrome
Nonpancreatic endocrine disease
    Carcinoid
    Thyrotoxicosis
    Medullary carcinoma of the thyroid
    Hypoparathyroidism
Sitosterol intolerance
Alpha-hydroxylase deficiency
(Refsum's disease)
Hyperlipoproteinemia and hyperchylomicrone-mia
Type I hyperlipoproteinemia
    Lipoprotein lipase deficiency
    Apolipoprotein C-II deficiency
Type V hyperlipoproteinemia

*From Herman RH, Hagler H: West J Med **130:**95-116, 1979.

Rhabdomyolysis (carnitine palmityltransferase deficiency)
Tangier disease

Malabsorption Syndromes

Lipid malabsorption accompanies many illnesses and invariably causes steatorrhea. This may be seen in pancreatic insufficiency, various types of small intestinal disease, hepatobiliary disease, and lymphatic obstruction, as well as other disease states. Usually this abnormally high fat content in the feces disappears when the primary disease is cured and the patient's metabolism returns to normal. A low-fat diet is advised when lipid malabsorption is evident. Additional discussion of lipid-induced food intolerance will be found in the chapters on gastrointestinal disorders and on liver and biliary disease.

Sitosterol

A rare disorder, beta-sitosterolemia and xanthomatosis, has been diagnosed in individuals unable to metabolize the plant steroid sitosterol, found primarily in soybean oil and cacao butter.[61] There is increased absorption of sitosterol in the small intestine. Accumulation of sitosterol is found in red blood cells, adipose tissue, tendon xanthomas, and skin surface lipids. Lesser amounts of campesterol and stigmasterol are also present. Serum cholesterol levels are usually normal, but in one case hypercholesterolemia was reported. Sitosterol accumulations in plasma and tissues decreased on a sitosterol elimination diet.

Alpha-Hydroxylase (Refsum's disease)

Refsum's disease, the inability to metabolize the branched-chain lipid phytanic acid because of a deficiency of the enzyme α-hydroxylase, is an inherited chronic disorder characterized by slow but progressive neurologic deterioration. Serum phytanic acid levels may be controlled and symptoms alleviated by restricting phytanic acid intake. The lipid, found primarily in dairy and ruminant fats, is derived from the phytol of chlorophyll.

Hyperlipoproteinemia and Hyperchylomicronemia

In Type I hyperlipoproteinemia one observes a severe hyperchylomicronemia in the fasting state along with an increase in plasma triglycerides. Eruptive xanthomas of the skin and episodes of recurrent abdominal pain due to pancreatitis are characteristic. A congenital absence of lipoprotein lipase is responsible for the disease. A diet low in fat can control the disease process. The symptoms for Type V hyperlipoproteinemia parallel those for Type I. Treatment entails a weight reduction diet that is low in fat and in calories.[58] A more extensive discussion of this complex disorder is found in Chapter 14.

Rhabdomyolysis. A rare disorder characterized by muscle disintegration, excess accumulation of triglycerides in the blood, and recurring excretion of myoglobin in the urine, rhabdomyolysis is caused by a deficiency of the enzyme carnitine palmityltransferase, needed for fat oxidation.[59] Acute symptoms may be brought on by exercise, especially if the subject is fasting, and by a diet low in carbohydrates. Clinical management entails a low-fat diet comparable to that used in Type I hyperlipoproteinemia.

Tangier disease. In Tangier disease, normal high-density lipoproteins are deficient in the blood, and cholesterol esters accumulate in the tonsils, cornea, peripheral nerves, spleen, bone marrow, lymph nodes, thymus, intestinal mucosa, and skin. As a result of defective chylomicron metabolism, abnormal high-density lipoproteins appear in the plasma. Their production can be limited by restricting dietary fat.[60]

Mineral-Induced Reactions

In general, healthy people are not intolerant of the amounts of major or trace minerals that are usually consumed. Various chronic conditions or a predisposition to them may alter metabolism, however, and mineral ingestion then aggravates or precipitates the condition.

Sodium

Hypertension. Although sodium may be an important pathogenic factor in those genetically predisposed to hypertensive vascular disease, the exact relationship between sodium intake and the development of hypertension remains in dispute. In obese hypertensives an energy-sufficient low-sodium diet returns blood pressure to normal whereas a high-sodium low-energy diet leads to weight loss but no change in blood pressure. Weight reduction and decreased hypertension have also been found with no change in dietary sodium intake.[62] Hypertension and strokes are common in the population of northern Japan, where the diet is extremely high in sodium.[63]

In primary or essential hypertension, sodium balance determines the extent to which the renin-angiotensin system will sustain high blood pressure. Even hypertensives of the low-renin type can become renin-dependent with sufficient sodium depletion. A diet low in sodium or diuretic therapy often can control mild to moderate hypertension.

Conditions in which sodium is retained are closely associated with hypertension. These include Cushing's syndrome, primary hyperaldosteronism, and other conditions in which there is hypersecretion of adrenocortical steroids, as well as chronic licorice ingestion. In hypertension associated with secondary aldosteronism, the extraadrenal stimulus that elevates aldosterone also activates the renin-angiotensin system.[64]

Edema. Sodium consumption often aggravates edema resulting from renal failure, cirrhosis with ascites, congestive heart failure, and cyclic or metabolic edema. Obese patients who fast to lose weight may experience edema when they begin eating again. This phenomenon appears to be associated with the suppression of hyperglucagonemia that occurs with fasting.[65] Elevated glucagon levels result in the excretion of abnormal amounts of sodium in the urine, but this effect disappears with the resumption of normal eating patterns.

Potassium

Potassium can be toxic in certain situations. In renal failure, ingesting potassium may exacerbate hyperkalemia and lead to death. In cases of familial hyperkalemic periodic paralysis, potassium ingestion may bring on the paralysis. Potassium also may cause hyperkalemia in individuals with Addison's disease or selective hypoaldosteronism or in those on diuretic therapy in which a potassium-sparing agent such as triamterene is used.

Calcium

Calcium may be toxic in pseudoxanthoma elasticum, a rare skin disease characterized by swollen and calcified elastic fibers, skin lesions, progressive loss of vision, and arterial disease. In vitro studies have shown that the abnormal elastic fibers have an increased affinity for calcium.[66] Progression of calcification can be curtailed, and lesions prevented, by administering a low-calcium diet. In renal failure, a high-phosphate diet may aggravate already existing hyperphosphatemia and hypocalcemia. Neuromuscular irritability and parathyroid hyperplasia occur as a result of the hypocalcemia. The persistent chronic hyperphosphatemia and hypocalcemia then lead to stimulation of parathyroid hormone secretion and consequent bone resorption. In chronic renal failure, serum phosphate is elevated because of the fact that the kidney cannot excrete phosphate.[67] In hypercalcemia, plasma calcium levels may be decreased by administering phosphate orally or intravenously. Phosphate absorption can be controlled with phosphate-binding gels; use of vitamin D and calcium will decrease serum phosphate and increase serum levels of calcium. Orally given phosphate has produced extraskeletal calcification. Infants fed cow's milk may experience tetany. Since the phosphate/calcium ratio in cow's milk (1:1) is higher than that in human (1:2), phosphate consumption may exceed the level filtered by the normal infant kidney, producing hyperphosphatemia, hypocalcemia, and tetany. The tetany and leg cramps that some women experience during pregnancy are attributed to increased milk consumption (hence higher phosphate intake) and to the calcium drain produced by the growing fetus.

Iron

Disorders of iron metabolism may be hereditary (idiopathic hemochromatosis) or induced by excessive dietary consumption of iron (hemosiderosis). In hemochromatosis, iron accumulates in the tissues, especially the liver and pancreas, heart and testes. The skin becomes bronze in color, and patients develop cirrhosis, diabetes, cardiac and pituitary disorders, and hypogonadism.[68] The most effective treatment is phlebotomy.

Iodine

Although its mechanism is not understood, it appears that iodine consumption can bring on hyperthyroidism. Such increases may occur with iodide medication or iodine-supplemented foods, or when an individual from a region where iodine is deficient relocates to an area where iodine levels are higher.[69] Other times the chronic ingestion of large amounts of iodine can lead to

hypothyroidism. Pregnant women who consume iodides, often as medication, can produce offspring with goiter and hypothyroidism.[70] Patients with diffuse toxic goiter rendered euthyroid by radioiodine or surgical treatment have experienced myxedema when given small pharmacologic doses of iodide.

Copper

The accumulation of copper in patients with Wilson's disease leads to progressive cirrhosis, cerebral degeneration, or both, and results in a fatal neurologic disorder. Although treatment with a low-copper diet is impractical, penicillamine combines with copper, thereby halting or preventing excess copper accumulation and the attendant symptoms.

Fluoride

Excessive fluoride consumption usually is due to high fluoride levels in the water supply. Moderately high levels produce dental fluorosis, a harmless white mottling of the teeth. In some countries, like India, where in certain regions unusually large amounts of fluoride are consumed, the mineral can cause endemic skeletal fluorosis. The disease is characterized by osteosclerosis, periosteal bone deposits, ossified tendons and ligaments, osteophyte formation, and fragile bones. Symptoms, including skeletal pain, stiffness, and limited movement, may improve on a low-calcium diet. A comprehensive review of fluoride is found in the chapter on the mouth.

Vitamin-Induced Reactions

Vitamin-induced reactions will be noted with the excess ingestion of certain vitamins. Excess ingestion of vitamin A causes hair loss, pigmentation, desquamation, hepatomegaly, and bone pain. In infants and children, excess vitamin D intake leads to hypercalcemia, nausea, anorexia, vomiting, and azotemia. Adults manifest polyuria, dehydration, hypokalemia, mental confusion, bone resorption, and metastatic calcification.

Nicotinic acid in large doses has been associated with pruritus, abdominal discomfort, hyperuricemia, hyperglycemia, and postural hypotension. These findings are probably chemical effects and unrelated to the function of nicotinic acid as a vitamin. Some patients with hyperlipoproteinemia (Types II, IV, and V) treated with nicotinic acid in pharmacologic doses have developed vasodilatation of skin capillaries, resulting in flushing and increased skin temperature. In individual patients, pharmacologic levels of nicotinic acid have also been associated with central vision loss and macular edema, which are resolved with discontinuation of nicotinic acid.

Nonspecific and Idiopathic Adverse Food Reactions

A number of physiologic factors may cause nonspecific multiple food reactions. In malabsorption syndromes, many kinds of foods can increase such symptoms as diarrhea and steatorrhea. Gastrointestinal ischemia and splanchnic vascular insufficiency can cause abdominal pain after eating, regardless of the specific foods contained in the meal. Acute or chronic infectious and inflammatory conditions or neoplasias often are accompanied by anorexia and intolerance. Although the mechanism of anorexia is not known, in the case of neoplasia the cancer cells produce anorexigenic peptides. Primary disorders of taste (dysgeusia) or the absence of smell (anosmia) may be factors leading to food rejection. Zinc sulfate has been used in treating these disorders, but it is not effective in all cases.

Individuals who have been fasting or starving will become ill if they quickly resume a normal food intake. They will often experience abdominal swelling and fluid accumulation, enlargement of the liver and spleen, eosinophilia, nausea, vomiting, and other symptoms. This nutritional recovery syndrome is unrelated to the type of food ingested. Some people, particularly patients with diabetic autonomic neuropathy, experience facial sweating after eating certain foods. Cheese ingestion in particular may result in gustatory sweating; atropine and oral cholinergic drugs may control the condition.[71]

Multiple food reactions also have been reported in adults with a rare formiminotransferase deficiency. The enzyme transforms tetrahydrofolate into a formimino derivative. Resulting intolerance to dietary carbohydrates induces anorexia, nausea, vomiting, diarrhea, lightheadedness, and fainting.

Since food preferences are conditioned by social, economic, cultural, and religious factors, certain reactions may be explained by these influences. Psychological disturbances, in turn, may explain food faddism or rejection, compulsive eating that results in obesity and other abnormal eating patterns. Some foods cause illness for unknown reasons. It is difficult to identify what component of the food causes the difficulty. Some foods that have been identified as causing problems include liver, chicken, beets, cucumbers, Worcestershire sauce, fish, nuts, and curry. These are among the foods commonly reported to cause idiopathic food reactions. Many people dislike liver and report that it causes nausea, vomiting, or diarrhea. One patient apparently suffered shock at the appearance of beet pigment in the urine. Some feel that heavy use of Worcestershire sauce and curry can lead to renal disorders. Many reports of such food tolerance are anecdotal and poorly documented. Clearly "one man's meat is another man's poison."

REFERENCES

1. Bock SA, May CD: Adverse reactions to foods caused by sensitivity. In Middleton E, editor: Allergy. Principles and practice, ed 2, St. Louis, 1983, The CV Mosby Co, p 1415.
2. Dodge JA, et al: Prostaglandin induced diarrhea, Arch Dis Child **52:**800, 1977.
3. May CD: Objective clinical and laboratory studies of immediate hypersensitivity reactions to foods in children, J Allergy Clin Immunol **58:**500, 1976.
4. Bock SA, et al: Studies of hypersensitivity reactions to foods in infants and children, J Allergy Clin Immunol **62:**327, 1978.
5. Bock SA: A critical evaluation of clinical trials in adverse reactions to foods in children, J Allergy Clin Immunol **78** (Suppl 1, Pt 2):165, 1986.
6. Lothe L, et al: Cow's milk formula as a cause of infantile colic: a double-blind study, Pediatrics **70:**7, 1982.
7. Jakobsson I, Lindberg T: Cow's milk proteins cause infantile colic in breast-fed infants: a double-blind crossover study, Pediatrics **71:**268, 1983.
8. Sampson HA: Role of immediate food hypersensitivity in the pathogenesis of atopic dermatitis, J Allergy Clin Immunol **71:**473, 1983.
9. Sampson HA, Albergo R: Comparison of results of skin tests, RAST, and double-blind, placebo-controlled food challenges in children with atopic dermatitis, J Allergy Clin Immunol **74:**26, 1984.
10. Sampson HA, McCaskill RN: Food hypersensitivity and atopic dermatitis, J Pediatr **107:**669, 1985.
11. Sampson HA, Jolie PL: Increased plasma histamine concentrations after food challenges in children with atopic dermatitis, N Engl J Med **311:**372, 1984.
12. Harley JP, et al: Hyperkinesis and food additives: testing the Feingold hypothesis, Pediatrics **61:**818, 1978.
13. Harley JP, et al: Synthetic food colors and hyperactivity in children: a double-blind challenge experiment, Pediatrics **62:**975, 1978.

14. Behar D, et al: Sugar challenge testing with children considered behaviorally "sugar reactive," Nutr Behav **1**:277, 1984.

15. Mahan LK, et al: Sugar "allergy" and children's behavior (Abstr), J Allergy Clin Immunol **75**:177, 1985.

16. Egger J, et al: Is migraine food allergy? Lancet **1**:865, 1983.

17. Mansfield LE, et al: Food allergy and adult migraine: double-blind and mediator confirmation of an allergic etiology, Ann Allergy **55**:126, 1985.

18. Vaughan TR, et al: Food and migraine headache: a controlled study (Abstr), Ann Allergy **56**:522, 1986.

19. Bernstein M, et al: Double-blind food challenge in the diagnosis of food sensitivity in the adult, J Allergy Clin Immunol **70**:205, 1982.

20. Atkins FM, et al: Evaluation of immediate reactions to foods in adult patients. I. Correlation of demographic, laboratory, and prick skin tests data with response to controlled oral food challenge, J Allergy Clin Immunol **75**:348, 1985.

21. Atkins FM, et al: Evaluation of immediate adverse reactions to foods in adult patients. II. A detailed analysis of reaction patterns during oral food challenge, J Allergy Clin Immunol **75**:356, 1985.

22. Strober W, et al: The pathogenesis of gluten-sensitive enteropathy, Ann Intern Med **83**:242, 1975.

23. Falchuk ZM, et al: Gluten-sensitive enteropathy: genetic analysis and organ culture study in 35 families, Scand J Gastroenterol **13**:839, 1978.

24. Falchuk ZM, Strober W: Gluten-sensitive enteropathy: synthesis of antiglobular antibody in vitro, Gut **15**:947, 1974.

25. Ament ME, Rubin CE: Soy protein—another cause of the flat intestinal lesion, Gastroenterology **62**:227, 1972.

26. Perkkiö M, et al: Morphometric and immunohistochemical study of jejunal biopsies from children with intestinal soy allergy, Eur J Pediatr **137**:63, 1981.

27. Bock SA, et al: Immunochemical localization of proteins in the intestinal mucosa of children with diarrhea, J Allergy Clin Immunol **72**:262, 1983.

28. Vitoria JC, et al: Enteropathy related to fish, rice, and chicken, Arch Dis Child **57**:44, 1982.

29. Baker AL, Rosenberg IH: Refractory sprue: recovery after removal of nongluten dietary proteins, Ann Intern Med **89**:505, 1978.

30. Bock SA, et al: Proper use of skin tests with food extracts in diagnosis of hypersensitivity to food in children, Clin Allergy **7**:375, 1977.

31. Bock SA, et al: Appraisal of skin tests with food extracts for diagnosis of food hypersensitivity, Clin Allergy **8**:559, 1978.

32. Helm RM, et al: Variability of IgE protein measurement in all culture supernatants: results from a multicenter collaborative study, J Allergy Clin Immunol **77**:880, 1986.

33. Katz AJ, et al: Gastric mucosal biopsy in eosinophilic (allergic) gastroenteritis, Gastroenterology **73**:705, 1977.

34. Katz AJ, et al: Milk-sensitive and eosinophilic gastroenteropathy: similar clinical features with contrasting mechanisms and clinical course, J Allergy Clin Immunol **74**:72, 1984.

35. Bock SA: The natural history of food sensitivity, J Allergy Clin Immunol **69**:173, 1982.

36. Bock SA: The natural history of severe reactions to foods in young children, J Pediatr **107**:676, 1985.

37. Bock SA: A prospective study of the natural history of adverse reactions to food in children during the first three years of life, Pediatrics **76**:683, 1987.

38. Machtinger S, Moss R: Cow's milk allergy in breast fed infants: the role of allergen and maternal secretory IgA antibody, J Allergy Clin Immunol **77**:341, 1986.

39. Zeiger RS, et al: Effectiveness of dietary manipulations in the prevention of food allergy in infants, J Allergy Clin Immunol **78**(Suppl):224, 1986.

40. Lake AM, et al: Dietary protein-induced colitis in breast-fed infants, J Pediatr **101**:906, 1982.

41. May CD: Are confusion and controversy about food hypersensitivity really necessary? J Allergy Clin Immunol **75**:392, 1985.

42. Bender AE, Matthews DR: Adverse reaction to foods, Br J Nutr **45**:403, 1981.

43. Rosensweig NS, et al: Dietary regulations of glycolytic enzymes. VI. Effect of dietary sugars and oral folic acid on human jejunal pyruvate kinase, phosphofructokinase, and fructosediphosphatase activities, Biochim Biophys Acta **208**:373, 1970.

44. Greene HL, et al: Hereditary fructose intolerance—treatment with pharmacologic doses of folic acid, Clin Res **20**:275, 1972.

45. Greene HL, et al: "Ketotic hypoglycemia" due to hepatic fructose-1,6-diphosphatase deficiency—treatment with folic acid, Am J Dis Child **124**:415, 1972.

46. Segal S: Disorders of galactose metabolism. In Stanbury JB, et al, editors: The metabolic basis of inherited disease, ed 3, New York, 1972, McGraw-Hill Book Co Inc, p 174.

47. Winberley PD, et al: Congenital glucose-galactose malabsorption, Proc R Soc Med **67**:755, 1974.

48. Paige DM, Bayless TM: Lactose digestion: clinical and nutritional implications, Baltimore, 1981, Johns Hopkins University Press.

49. Madzarovova-Noheilova J: Trehalase deficiency in a family, Gastroenterology **65**:130, 1973.

50. Katz AJ, Falchuk ZM: Current concepts in gluten sensitive enteropathy (celiac sprue), Pediatr Clin North Am **22**:767, 1975.

51. Ament ME: Immunodeficiency syndromes and gastrointestinal disease, Pediatr Clin North Am **22**:807, 1975.

52. Broitman SA, et al: Mastocytosis and intestinal malabsorption, Am J Med **48**:382, 1970.

53. Freier S, Berger H: Disodium cromoglycate in gastrointestinal protein intolerance, Lancet **1**:913, 1973.

54. Ament ME, Rubin CE: Soy protein—another cause of the flat intestinal lesion, Gastroenterology **62**:227, 1972.

55. Walser M, et al: The effect of ketoanalogues of essential amino acids in severe chronic uremia, J Clin Invest **52**:678, 1973.

56. Graham DY: Enzyme replacement therapy of exocrine pancreatic insufficiency in man, N Engl J Med **296**:1314, 1977.

57. Lebanthal E, et al: Enterokinase and trypsin activities in pancreatic insufficiency and diseases of the small intestine, Gastroenterology **70**:508, 1976.

58. Fredrickson DS, et al: The familial hyperlipoproteinemias. In Stanbury JB, et al, editors: The metabolic basis of in-

herited disease, ed 4, New York, 1978, McGraw-Hill International Book Co, p 604.

59. Bank WJ, et al: A disorder of muscle lipid metabolism and myoglobinuria—absence of carnitine palmityl transferase, N Engl J Med **292**:443, 1975.

60. Herbert PN, et al: Tangier disease—one explanation of lipid storage, N Engl J Med **299**:519, 1978.

61. Shulman RS, et al: β-Sitosterolemia and xanthomatosis, N Engl J Med **294**:282, 1976.

62. Reisin E, et al: Effect of weight loss without salt restriction on the reduction of blood pressure in overweight hypertensive patients, N Engl J Med **298**:1, 1978.

63. Dahl LK: Possible role of excess salt consumption in the pathogenesis of essential hypertension, Am J Cardiol **8**:571, 1961.

64. Biglieri EG: Mineralocorticoids and hypertension. In Davis JO, et al, editors: Hypertension—mechanisms, diagnosis, and management, New York, 1977, HP Publishing Co Inc, p 100.

65. Spark RF, et al: Renin, aldosterone and glucagon in the natriuresis of fasting, N Engl J Med **292**:1335, 1975.

66. Gordon SG, et al: In vitro uptake of calcium by dermis of patients with pseudoxanthoma elasticum, J Lab Clin Med **86**:638, 1975.

67. Bricker NS: On the pathogenesis of the uremic state, N Engl J Med **286**:1093, 1972.

68. Feller ER, et al: Familial hemochromatosis: physiologic studies in the precirrhotic stage of the disease, N Engl J Med **296**:1422, 1977.

69. Sobrinho LG, et al: Thyroxine toxicosis in patients with iodine induced thyrotoxicosis, J Clin Endocrinol Metab **45**:25, 1977.

70. Carswell F, et al: Congenital goitre and hypothyroidism produced by maternal ingestion of iodides, Lancet **1**:1241, 1970.

71. Bronshvag MM: Spectrum of gustatory sweating, with especial reference to its presence in diabetics with autonomic neuropathy, Am J Clin Nutr **31**:307, 1978.

72. Herman RH, Hagler L: Food intolerance in humans, West J Med **130**:95, 1979.

VII

EXERCISE, DIET, AND COUNSELING

CHAPTER 42

Nutrition and Exercise

E. David Wright

Despite the persistence of energy-intensive practices in the economies of Third World countries, developed nations have largely transcended the need for strenuous activity in daily living. Within these societies diet and exercise bear an entirely different relationship to one another. The emergence of leisure time and with it new cultural norms regarding beauty and health has precipitated an epidemic of exercise. Individuals striving to overcome the physical and psychologic factors associated with a sedentary lifestyle exercise to offset the deleterious effects attributed to this pattern of living. In addition, the intense competition within elite athletic circles now subsidizes industries devoted to improving athletic performance. On a more pragmatic level many individuals now recognize how their patterns of diet and physical activity may alter the onset and progression of aging[1] and disease.[2] In short, an enormous amount of interest and research are now focused on the synergism between nutrition and exercise.[3] This chapter examines the relationship between diet and physical performance, with particular attention to how exertion may influence requirements for nutrients and energy substrates. With this frame-

work one may then design a prudent eating strategy to meet the needs of individuals engaging in a variety of different sports and exercise.

METABOLIC FUELS

From an evolutionary standpoint humans are designed as migratory animals. Although compared to other terrestrial mammals they may run slowly, they are endowed with noteworthy endurance. This latter feature is consistent with certain attributes of all migratory creatures, paramount among which is the combination of a highly fatigue-resistant musculature and abundant endogenous fuel stores to support continuous movement.

The relative deposition of potential metabolic fuels in a 70 kg "reference" man is displayed in Table 42-1.[6] In this context *carbohydrate* refers to glucose and its storage polymer, glycogen. Correspondingly, *fat* refers to fatty acids and their storage form, triacylglycerol (triglyceride). The striking feature of this breakdown is that fat reserves far outweigh carbohydrate reserves. Weiss-Fogh[5] explained the significance of this disparity in 1967. Fat is roughly 8 times more efficient as a fuel source than carbohydrate (gly-

Table 42-1 Fuel Stores in the Average Man

			How Long They Last (min)	
	Grams	Kilojoules	Walking*	Marathon Running*
Adipose tissue triglyceride	9000	337,500	15,500	4018
Liver glycogen	100	1660	86	20
Muscle glycogen	350	5800	288	71
Blood glucose	3	48	2	<1

From Newsholme EA, Leech AR: The runner, New York, 1983, Fitness Books.
*It is assumed that the energy expenditure during walking is about 22 kJ per minute and during marathon running (elite runner) is 84 kJ per minute. The amount of adipose tissue triglyceride will be much less in many elite marathon runners (perhaps 4000 g).

cogen) is, because fat is stored in anhydrous form and on a dry weight basis is more energy-dense (9 kcal/g [35 kJ/g]) than glycogen, the principal form of cellular carbohydrate storage (4 kcal/g [16 kJ/g]). Although carbohydrate is burned at a lower oxygen cost than fat, it is stored in mammals with approximately 2.7 times its weight in water.[4] On this basis, Weiss-Fogh[5] concludes that "the enormous range of land and sea covered by migrating birds and insects is a direct consequence of their ability to utilize fat for heavy sustained work." This observation is entirely consistent with the evolutionary success of human beings engaged in a hunting and gathering life-style.

Perhaps because of its disproportionately low representation within total body energy stores, carbohydrate is the most precious metabolic fuel. In the form of blood glucose (and the hepatic glycogen that provides it) carbohydrate is the primary respiratory fuel for the brain, which oxidizes glucose, and for the so-called "anaerobic" tissues (retina, renal medulla, skin, blood cells), which metabolize glucose to lactate via anaerobic glycolysis. Carbohydrate is essential to the provision of energy in these tissues, since under normal circumstances they cannot oxidize fat. Fatty acid oxidation (beta-oxidation) provides the bulk of cellular energy for all tissues besides those just cited. This occurs when acetyl-CoA, the end product of beta-oxidation, is terminally oxidized to water and CO_2 via the tricarboxylic acid (Krebs) cycle. In this regard, carbohydrate becomes essential to fatty acid oxidation by providing a constant supply of Krebs cycle intermediates. Carbohydrate is also necessary for the synthesis of glycoproteins and glycolipids.

Body protein is also a potentially large source of fuel, especially under fasting conditions. Some work has suggested that even in the well-nourished state exercise promotes a net degradation of body protein[7] and a substantial increase in the oxidation of certain essential (branched-chain) amino acids.* Although the quantitative contribution of these nitrogenous fuels to the overall energy cost of exercise is minimal (roughly 5%-10%), such losses may occur at the expense of the body's structural integrity. Protein is unique in this regard because it serves a dual role, as the major structural component of tissues

*References 8, 9, 9a, 9b, 9c, 9d, 9e.

and as a qualitatively important metabolic fuel. Thus although not a primary fuel for muscular activity under normal conditions, it is of potentially great significance.

The biochemical properties, relative abundance and accessibility of these fuels places definite limitations upon human performance. This is particularly true for carbohydrates, the metabolic fuel that is always in shortest supply but essential to the energy needs of intense exercise. The diet, training state, and genetic makeup of the individual as well as the intensity and duration of the exercise all influence the supply and demand of these fuels. Because skeletal muscle is the end organ or effector of exercise, an appreciation of its metabolic characteristics is crucial to predicting nutrient requirements during and after exercise.

MUSCLE STRUCTURE AND FUNCTION

Muscle is highly active metabolically and abundant, representing 45% of the body weight in young adults. As shown in Table 42-2,[20] it is a major contributor to resting metabolic rate and the primary determinant of energy expenditure during exercise. Human muscle is composed of three morphologically and biochemically distinct fiber types[11]: They are shown in Table 42-3 and can be broadly classified as slow-twitch (slow-oxidative [SO] or Type I), fast-twitch oxidative-glycolytic (FOG or Type IIa), and pure fast-twitch (FT or Type IIb).[11]

In general, *slow-twitch* fibers develop the least contractile speed and force but are most resistant to fatigue. Their neuromuscular innervation consists of small motor neurons, slow-conducting nerve axons, and few motor endplates. Consequently, these fibers contract slowly. Metabolically, they derive most of their energy from fatty acid oxidation. To facilitate this, they are abundantly supplied with blood capillaries, myoglobin, mitochondria, and intracellular deposits of glycogen and triglyceride.

The *fast-twitch* fibers are different, in being adapted more to rapid contraction and peak force development. They are innervated by large motor neurons, via rapidly conducting axons and numerous large motor endplates. These fibers display near complete reliance on anaerobic glycolysis for their respiratory energy, have few mitochondria, and are easily fatigued (apparently because of the rapid accumulation in them of protons released during the conversion of gly-

Table 42-2 ATP Turnover

Tissue	Oxygen Consumption (liters/da)	Glucose Oxidation (g/da)	ATP Turnover (kg/da)
Brain	76	103	10.3
Heart	43	57	5.7
Kidneys	64	88	8.8
Liver	81	108	10.8
Skeletal muscle (at rest)	74	98	9.8
Skeletal muscle (marathon running)	5757	7710	771

From Newsholme EA, Leech AR: The runner, New York, 1983, Fitness Books.
Since the ATP yield from different fuels is known, it becomes possible to calculate the rate of ATP turnover in a tissue from its fuel and oxygen uptake, which are relatively easily measured. This has been done on the assumption that all the energy is provided by the oxidation of glucose (although this is certainly not so in all instances). Note that at rest the rate of energy utilization by the whole of the skeletal musculature is similar to that of other tissues; however, on the basis of 1 g of tissue the rate in muscle would be very much smaller. Nevertheless, this rate increases dramatically in exercise; and during a marathon race, for example, a runner consumes at least 500 liters of oxygen, corresponding to about 700 g of glucose, although in practice he is more likely to use about 350 g of glucose and 150 g of triglyceride.

Table 42-3 Types of Human Skeletal Muscle Fibers

	Type I (slow twitch)	Type IIa (fast-twitch oxidative)	Type IIb (slow-twitch glycolytic)
ATPase activity after preincubation at pH 10.3	—	Pronounced	Pronounced
ATPase activity after preincubation at pH 10.3 and 4.6-4.8	—	—	Pronounced
Speed of contraction	Slow	Fast	Fast
Glycolytic capacity	Low	Moderate	High
Oxidative capacity	High	Moderate	Low
Glycogen store	Moderate to high	Moderate to high	Moderate to high
Triacylglycerol (triglyceride) store	High	Moderate	Low
Capillary supply	Good	Moderate	Poor

Modified slightly from Saltin B, et al: Ann NY Acad Sci **301**:3-29, 1977.

cogen and glucose to lactate via the cytoplasmic enzymes of glycolysis). To support their enormous demands for carbohydrate fuels, FT fibers store vast quantities of intracellular glycogen.

The *FOG,* also known as intermediate, fibers display most of the rapid speed and force of contraction characteristic of FT fibers yet have considerable fatigue resistance. This appears to be related to their increased mitochondrial content and an aerobic capacity intermediate between those of FT and SO fibers.

A person's fiber type distribution is primarily genetically determined and relatively balanced (50% SO versus 50% FT and FOG) in untrained muscle groups. Some muscles, such as the soleus and triceps, may have a predominance of one basic fiber type. No sex- or age-related differ-

ences in fiber distribution exist; however, individual variation may be great, particularly among men.[12] Since fiber types do correlate with speed and endurance, there is some truth to the maxim that the elite athlete "must pick his parents carefully." This is evident from histologic examination of the muscles of speedy animals such as the American racing quarterhorse and the greyhound. In these animals natural selection and animal husbandry have produced a particular pattern of muscle structure and function. Indeed, the greyhound, which can sustain speeds exceeding 1000 meters/min over a 400 m distance, has a muscle mass comprising 57% of its body weight and composed of nearly 100% Type II fibers in the active limb musculature.[10] Similar, but less exaggerated, adaptations can be seen in the musculature of conditioned athletes. Even so, an elite fiber type profile does not accurately predict winning performance; coordination, motivation, biomechanics, and other variables are also important determinants thereof.

Although genetic factors are likely the predominant determinants of athletic performance, the powerful physiologic and psychologic impact of training must not be discounted. Training mediates both peripheral and central physiologic adaptations. *Peripheral* adaptations are changes induced in skeletal muscle and its neurovascular supply in response to specific contractile events.* *Central* adaptations are changes in the endocrine, cardiovascular, pulmonary, and nervous systems that, despite being less activity-specific than their peripheral counterparts, are especially critical in limiting physical performance.

This chapter discusses only those training-related adaptations that directly influence the use of metabolic fuels. A brief overview of skeletal muscle adaptations will introduce this fascinating subject. In general, skeletal muscle responds to exercise in two ways: (1) by changing its size and (2) by altering its composition. These changes may occur together or be totally independent of one another.

Specific training alters the relative proportions of fiber types within the muscle groups involved.[13] Endurance training has little effect on the size of muscle fibers but induces profound changes in their content of oxidative enzymes. The trained muscles of endurance athletes show a preponderance of Type I fibers whereas those of speed/power athletes contain a higher percentage of Type II fibers. There is no consensus among exercise physiologists as to whether Type II fibers can be completely transformed into Type I fibers by training, but it seems clear that the opposite does not occur. It is believed that endurance training may induce a complete reversion of Type IIb (pure fast-twitch) to Type IIa (FOG, intermediate) fibers. In addition, endurance exercise results in relatively greater increments of mitochrondrial content of Type II than of Type I fibers. Consequently, distinctions in mitochondrial enzyme content between SO and

FT fibers are largely or totally obscured in highly trained athletes.[14] Recent evidence from cross-innervation experiments in animals indicates that neural input to muscle fibers may be the primary stimulus for such morphologic changes. Indeed, Type I and Type II muscle fibers can be interconverted in vivo by simply switching their motor neuronal input.

Commensurate increases in the ability to store and oxidize fatty acids accompany the increases in aerobic capacity of endurance-trained muscle. Similarly, endurance training both reduces lactic acid production and enhances lactate metabolic clearance. The tissue acidosis that accompanies high rates of flux through anaerobic glycolysis has been implicated as a cause of muscle fatigue. Thus, to the extent that high circulating levels of blood lactate reflect muscle acidification, lower levels of lactate may be said to be associated with better endurance.

In contrast to endurance training, whose primary effect is to alter muscle enzyme content, speed/strength training principally increases muscle size. This is accomplished primarily by hypertrophy (i.e., enlargement of the cross-sectional area of preexisting fibers). The increase in cross-sectional area reflects remodeling of the cell to accommodate additional contractile machinery (myofibrillar proteins), with a resultant dilution of mitochrondrial density. Such hypertrophy may be extensive, as evidenced by the 45% larger cross-sectional area of muscle fibers in weight lifters compared to those of sedentary or endurance-trained persons.[15] Despite the fact that current data suggest high-intensity training promotes a modest increase in muscle fiber number (hyperplasia), the wider consensus is that *hypertrophy* explains most of the training-induced increase.

Although different forms of exercise may share some common beneficial effects on the cardiovascular and other organ systems, the adaptive changes seen in skeletal muscle are specific for the type of exercise performed and occur only in the muscles undergoing chronic use. Thus, although an Olympic-caliber cyclist may have a higher exercise tolerance in general than nonathletes, he may swim rather poorly in comparison to even a recreational swimmer who trains regularly. Elite athletic ability in one sport does not ensure comparable performance in another.

---

*For example, the interosseous muscles in the fingers of both a concert pianist and a world-class rock climber may be highly trained, but they are morphologically distinct on a functional basis.

Because of the specificity of these exercise-related alterations in fiber composition, they quickly revert to baseline when the appropriate exercise stimulus is withdrawn. Such regression is seen in detraining[16] and in limb immobilization.[17] A major determinant of these changes is the withdrawal and/or alteration in quality of nervous input to the affected muscles.

Indeed, animal experiments[18] have demonstrated that Type I fibers can be changed to Type II fibers and vice versa by cross innervation. Because training brings about changes in fiber type, and hence in the composition of motor units, it also alters the fuel requirements of exercise. Endurance training enhances the relative contribution of oxidative metabolism to overall energy needs. Specifically it fosters fatty acid oxidation, thereby reducing the relative contribution of carbohydrate to fuel economy at all exercise intensities. Conversely, speed/strength training tends to emphasize the use of glycogen and glucose by fostering growth and recruitment of large motor units.

In view of the structural makeup and functional organization of skeletal muscle, it is appropriate to consider how contractile activity influences energy expenditure during different types of human movement. The ability to quantitate athletes' exercise capacity and hence to estimate their energy requirements is an essential foundation for sensible dietary counseling. As will be seen, those activities that are ostensibly the most strenuous may, in fact, contribute least to total daily energy expenditure and to nutritional requirements.

ENERGY EXPENDITURE

A keen intellect and capacity for abstract thinking allow the human being to expend energy in a multitude of ways not shared by other members of the animal kingdom. Admittedly, homo sapiens will never run as speedily as a cheetah or fly with impunity around the summit of Mt. Everest as does the bar-headed goose; however, motivated humans have bicycled and submarined around the world, flown in outer space, written music, and surgically implanted artificial organs! Indeed, the human's system for energy production and transduction must be elegantly diversified to perform all the functions expected of them.

Earlier discussion of muscle fiber types has laid the groundwork for understanding how speed and endurance are achieved. The present subsection will discuss the biochemistry of the energy-producing systems used by humans and how knowledge thereof allows for accurate prediction of energy expenditure and, hence, of energy/nutrient requirements.

Energy Systems

Adenosine triphosphate (ATP) is the ultimate source of metabolic fuel for humans and other animals. Despite the enormous energy content of its phosphate bonds, it is stored in only minute and easily depleted quantities within human tissues. Consequently, two independent but coordinately controlled biochemical systems exist to ensure a continuous supply of ATP in human muscle[12,23]: (1) anaerobic or non–oxygen requiring processes and (2) aerobic or oxygen-dependent processes. An overview of this complex topic appears in Chapter 2. A complete discussion may be found in the report of Newsholme and Leech.[20]

Anaerobic Systems

Two sources of anaerobic energy are used to fuel the needs of muscular exercise: (1) the phosphocreatine-ATP (PC-ATP) or phosphagen system, also known as the alactic or alactacid system, and (2) anaerobic glycolysis, the lactic or lactacid system. The enzymes for these reactions are localized in the muscle cell cytoplasm. It has been suggested, however, that the term anaerobic is no longer strictly applicable to the lactic acid system because this system also supplies energy to muscular contraction during fully aerobic conditions.* Nevertheless, "anaerobic" continues to be used in the exercise physiology literature to describe lactic acid production.

Human muscle is functionally diversified by the presence of slow-twitch and fast-twitch fiber types. Movement that demands great force or speed of contraction or that must occur immediately without any warmup is primarily subserved by Type II, or fast-twitch, fibers. These are biomechanically well suited to the task because they rely almost totally on anaerobic energy systems, which, though finite in capacity,

---

*Connett RJ, et al: Lactate efflux is unrelated to intracellular Po_2 in a working red muscle in situ, J Appl Physiol **61**:402-408, 1986.

can respond instantaneously under conditions of limited availability of oxygen and blood-borne fuels. Indeed, most of these fibers have a poor blood supply and minimum mitochondrial content but are richly endowed with glycogen stores, glycolytic enzymes, and creatine kinase, the key enzyme of the PC-ATP system. Both the phosphagen and the lactic systems are present in slow-twitch fibers but are not nearly as important for energy production in them as the aerobic processes are.

Of the systems that provide rapid energy to muscle cells, the phosphagen system is the fastest and most immediate means of replenishing ATP. Within the muscle cell, contraction is initiated by calcium-dependent activation of a myofibrillar ATPase that splits stored ATP via the following reaction:

$$ATP^{-4} + H_2O \rightarrow ADP^{-3} + P_i^{-2} + H^+$$

Because ATP stores are finite, they must be continuously replenished if contraction is to continue. This function is performed by the creatine kinase or Lohmann reaction using phosphocreatine to regenerate ATP from ADP:

$$H^+ + ADP^{-3} + \text{Phosphocreatine}^{-2} \rightarrow ATP^{-4} + \text{Creatine}$$

Because it operates at near equilibrium conditions in vivo, this reaction affords an energy buffer to the myocyte, providing ATP when needed and using excess ATP to maintain adequate phosphocreatine stores in anticipation of future need. In theromodynamic terms the phosphagen system has great *power* (the ability to perform work per unit time) but limited *capacity* (total amount of energy produced). In humans it is the "first responder" to the demand for muscle energy, but it has the capacity to support less than 10 seconds of continuous maximum muscular contraction. Consquently, the other two energy systems are already at work (albeit at reduced capacity) even before this time expires. The question then remains "how do the other systems provide the ATP for regenerating phosphocreatine?"

The ATP for regenerating PC from creatine may come from either aerobic or anaerobic systems depending on the urgency of the need and the availability of oxygen. If ATP is being consumed faster than it can be provided by aerobic means, the body uses anaerobic glycolysis to make "rapid" ATP from the transformation of glycogen or blood glucose to lactate. The initial conversion of glucose or glycogen carbon to pyruvate is common to both aerobic and anaerobic glycolyses. In aerobic glycolysis pyruvate is transported from the cell cytoplasm into the mitochondria and converted to acetyl-CoA for subsequent oxidation in the tricarboxylic acid cycle. In contrast, during anaerobic glycolysis pyruvate is reduced by the cytosolic enzyme lactate dehydrogenase (LDH) as indicated below:

$$\text{Glycogen or free glucose} \rightarrow \text{Pyruvate} \overset{\text{LDH}}{\rightleftarrows} \text{Lactate} + 3 \text{ ATP}$$

As shown in Table 42-4, this process, though expedient, is extraordinarily wasteful of energy.[20] Anaerobic glycolysis provides a maximum of 3 ATP per molecule of glucose derived from glycogen whereas aerobic glycolysis of the same molecule provides 39 ATP. Thus aerobic glycolysis is preferable when the demand for ATP can be met by this slower to respond, but more efficient, means. Although quite powerful, the lactacid energy system is metabolically extravagant and inferior in its capacity for generating large quantities of fuel. It can support maximum rates of muscle contraction for only about 120 seconds. Despite these limitations, the lactacid system is critical to muscle function because

Table 42-4 Yield of ATP from Various Fuels under Aerobic and Anaerobic Conditions.

Fuel	Conditions	ATP Per Mole of Fuel Utilized
Glucose	Aerobic, complete oxidation	38
Glucose	Anaerobic, conversion to lactate	2
Glycogen	Aerobic, complete oxidation	39
Glycogen	Anaerobic, conversion to lactate	3
Palmitate	Aerobic, complete oxidation	129
Acetoacetate	Aerobic, complete oxidation	24

From Newsholme EA, Leech AR: Biochemistry for the medical sciences, New York, 1983, John Wiley & Sons Inc.

it bridges the gap between the readily available but finite phosphagen fuels and those derived from the slow-responding aerobic system, which takes several minutes to begin functioning well.

Aerobic Systems

Aerobic fuels are those that are oxidized with molecular oxygen as the final proton acceptor. The hydrogen atoms removed during this oxidation are transferred to the respiratory or electron transport chain, which uses them to form water from oxygen and synthesize ATP from ADP. Aerobic metabolism is quantitatively the most important supplier of human energy because of its enormous capacity to provide energy. Indeed, aerobic metabolism can support continuous running and cycling at race pace for 36 hours or more in well-trained endurance athletes. The great capacity of the aerobic system resides in its highly efficient conversion of the chemical energy in foodstuffs to ATP.

In humans the most important aerobic energy pathway is the tricarboxylic acid (TCA) or Krebs cycle, whose enzymes are localized exclusively within mitochondria.[21] The major aerobic fuels—carbohydrates, fats, proteins—are oxidized following entry into the TCA cycle as either acetyl-CoA or cycle intermediates. Acetyl-CoA is oxidized to CO_2, with simultaneous reduction of the electron carriers NAD^+ and FAD, and hydrogen atoms are removed in the process. When the resultant NADH and $FADH_2$ donate their hydrogen to the electron transport chain, ATP is synthesized. Cycle intermediates can also be oxidized and in analogous fashion.[21]

Carbohydrates and lipids are the principal aerobic fuels, and the main energy substrates for the body. Carbohydrates are transformed via aerobic glycolysis to pyruvate and then to acetyl-CoA. Fatty acids derived from the hydrolysis of triglycerides are also degraded to the common end product acetyl-CoA via a sequential process known as beta oxidation. Ketone bodies (acetoacetate and beta-hydroxybutyrate), derivatives of fatty acid oxidation, may also be used as oxidative fuels but are thought to be quantitatively unimportant during conventional muscular exercise. This is also true in long-term starvation, in which ketone bodies become quantitatively significant supplements to glucose as fuels for the brain but provide little energy to muscle.

Ethanol too can be an important, but metabolically disruptive, aerobic fuel if it becomes a significant part of the diet. It is converted in the liver, via specific alcohol and aldehyde dehydrogenases, to acetate, with the formation of excessive hydrogen ions. This accumulation alters the normal intracellular redox potential, favoring a more reduced state. Consequently pyruvate, which is essential for gluconeogenesis, is reduced to lactate (which cannot contribute to gluconeogenesis). Thus de novo glucose formation may be impaired.

Amino acids derived from protein turnover are being increasingly recognized as important oxidative fuels. They may enter the TCA cycle via acetyl-CoA (e.g., leucine) or one of the cycle intermediates such as oxaloacetate (e.g., aspartate). Amino acid oxidation is not a quantitatively significant fuel source for exercise, however, although it serves a number of critical qualitative functions in sustaining muscle contraction.

The potential contribution of an aerobic fuel to the energy needs of exercise is a function of the relative hydrogen atom content of the molecule (e.g., how reduced it is) and the extent to which this potential energy is recovered. In terms of energy content, fat is a better fuel than alcohol, which in turn is better than carbohydrate. Furthermore, aerobic glycolysis, which uses the full oxidative potential of the glucose molecule to form acetyl-CoA, is nearly 20 times more efficient in supplying ATP than is anaerobic glycolysis to lactate (Table 42-4).[20] These data clearly demonstrate the advantages of employing oxidative metabolism, especially of fatty acids, to meet the fuel requirements of exercise. In view of the potentially great contribution of aerobic metabolism to the energy needs of exercise, it is not surprising that elite endurance athletes display a remarkable capacity for storing, mobilizing, and oxidizing fats.

Integration of Fuel Systems During Exercise

The body's transition from rest to vigorous exercise occurs via a highly integrated continuum of events. The goal of these biochemical as well as physiologic adjustments is to attain a new steady state in which the enhanced fuel requirements of working tissues are adequately met. The exact nature of this response is a function of not only the intensity and duration of the ex-

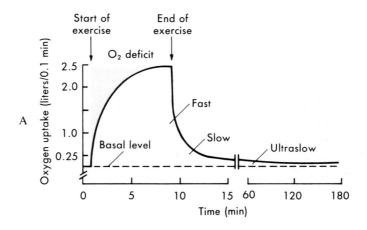

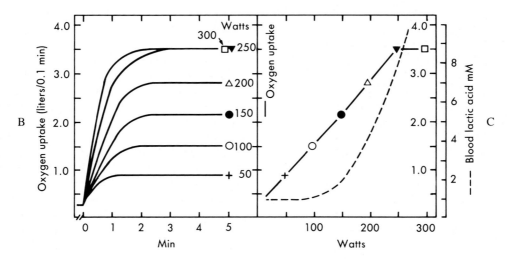

Figure 42-1 A, During the first minutes of exercise there is an oxygen deficiency while oxygen uptake increases to a level adequate to meet the demands of the tissues. At the cessation of exercise, there is a gradual decrease in oxygen uptake and several components can be identified. Note the change in time scale. **B,** Schematic of the increase in oxygen uptake during exercise on a cycle ergometer within different intensities (noted within the *shadowed area*) performed during 5 to 6 minutes. **C,** Oxygen uptake in these experiments, measured after 5 min. and plotted in relation to rate of exercise. Note that 250 watts (1500 kpm min[-1]) brought the oxygen uptake up to this subject's maximum and that 300 watts did not further increase the oxygen update; the increased rate of exercise was possible thanks to anaerobic processes. Maximum aerobic power = 3.5 liters/min[-1]. (For simplicity, the work rate that is sufficient to bring the oxygen uptake to the subject's maximum, in this case 250 watts, may be written $WL_{max}\dot{V}O_2$.) Peak lactate concentrations in the blood at each experiment have been included (blood samples secured immediately after exercise and every other minute up to 10 min following recovery).

A modified from Newsholme EA, Leech AR: Biochemistry for the medical sciences, New York, 1983, John Wiley & Sons Inc; **B** and **C** from from Åstrand P-O, Rodahl K: Textbook of work physiology: physiological bases of exercise, New York, 1986, McGraw-Hill International Book Co.

ercise but also the individual's genetic makeup and physical condition.

When exercise begins, a complex cascade of neuroendocrine adjustments commences. It is characterized by early reliance on anaerobic energy systems in muscle, and concomitant initiation of physiologic adjustments that will subsequently facilitate oxidative metabolism. At rest, aerobic metabolism supports all of muscle's energy need and some aerobic metabolism and is possible at the onset of exercise because of oxygen stored in blood (hemoglobin primarily) and muscle (myoglobin); but these O_2 stores are small and thus, initially, most energy must come from the phosphagens and anaerobic glycolysis using muscle glycogen stores.

While the anaerobic processes are hard at work, the body is rapidly increasing pulmonary ventilation, cardiac output, and muscle blood flow so the badly needed oxygen and fuels for aerobic metabolism will soon be available. These changes in cardiopulmonary output and vascular resistance are primarily effected by increased input from the sympathetic nervous system; however, local changes in metabolite concentration also cause vasodilation in muscle capillaries.

At the same time sympathetic nervous outflow enhances release of the counterregulatory hormones, especially the catecholamines (epinephrine and norepinephrine), cortisol, and glucagon. Insulin secretion from the pancreas is accordingly diminished. These changes cause an inversion of the normal insulin/glucagon ratio associated with the fed (anabolic) state. The body, consequently, assumes a catabolic hormonal state, which initiates lipolysis and glycogenolysis, thereby mobilizing free fatty acids and glucose, respectively, into the bloodstream. The resultant higher circulating levels of these blood-borne substrates ensures that contracting muscle will ultimately have an abundant fuel supply. It appears that muscle initially relies on its own endogenous stores of glycogen and lipids to fuel contraction. Later, as these stores dwindle, blood-borne (exogenous) fuels become increasingly important.

The net result of these early circulatory, hormonal, and pulmonary compensations is a relatively precise matching of energy supply to demand within about 5 minutes of the onset of exercise.

The body attempts to use aerobic metabolism to the fullest extent possible during any given exercise, and thus the uptake of O_2 increases linearly with exercise intensity until either the demand is met or the ability to supply it is exceeded. The latter is referred to as the maximum oxygen uptake, aerobic capacity, or $\dot{V}O_2max$, and it represents an individual's maximum capability to transport and deliver oxygen to working tissues. As such, it is the major index of a person's ability to perform sustained work or exercise.

At exercise intensities below $\dot{V}O_2max$ (submaximum exercise) an end point is reached at which oxygen transport, tissue uptake, and fuel utilization are theoretically constant. This condition is referred to as a steady state and corresponds to the plateau in oxygen consumption seen in Fig. 42-1. Physiologically it is characterized by constancy of cardiac output, heart rate, and minute ventilation. The contribution of anaerobic metabolism at steady state is fixed, and lactic acid concentrations do not rise in the blood. At intensities above $\dot{V}O_2max$ (supramaximum exercise) a steady state cannot exist; lactate accumulates and (in that it reflects muscle acidification) contributes to muscle failure.

Until steady state condition prevail, the overall demand for energy greatly outstrips what can be supplied aerobically. This is because the demand for contractile energy is instantaneous once exercise begins whereas the availability of aerobically produced energy increases over a more gradual time course. Such a lag period, seen as the shaded area in Fig. 42-1, *B*, represents the energy that must be supplied by anaerobic means until oxygen uptake becomes either adequate or maximal. Thus, a so-called "oxygen debt" is accumulated. At the end of exercise, oxygen consumption remains disproportionately elevated above resting tissue requirements. During this "repayment" phase the oxygen debt is being resolved. Precisely what the oxygen debt corresponds to is being debated. Åstrand and Rodahl[22] as well as di Prampero[23] provide excellent discussions thereof.

The relative contributions of aerobic and anaerobic processes to the energy needs of maximal exercise of varying duration are summarized in Fig. 42-2.[12] As intensity of exercise increases (thereby decreasing duration), so does the need for anaerobically supplied energy.

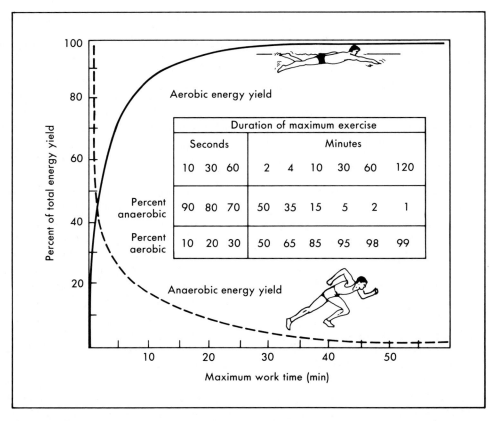

Figure 42-2 Relative contributions of aerobic and anaerobic energy during maximum physical activity of varying durations. Note that 1½-2 minutes of maximum effort requires 50% of the energy from aerobic and anaerobic processes.

From McArdle WD, et al: Exercise physiology: energy, nutrition, and human performance, Philadelphia, 1986, Lea & Febiger; modified from Åstrand P-O, Rodahl K: Textbook of work physiology, New York, 1977, McGraw-Hill International Book Co.

This reflects primarily the increased participation of Type II fibers as larger motor units are recruited; however, it may also reflect increased lactate production by Type I fibers striving to augment their aerobic power output from beta-oxidation with additional energy from anaerobic glycolysis.

The key point is that intensity serves as the primary determinant of how energy metabolism will be partitioned between anaerobic and aerobic systems. Specific training of any one or all of the energy systems in muscle will also augment the corresponding system's influence on fuel needs.

Oxygen Uptake as an Index of Energy Expenditure

From earlier discussions on muscle architecture and energy systems it can be seen that all types of physical exercise are not created equal. Different fiber populations and energy systems subsidize differing forms of exercise in unique but predictable fashion. Consequently, by examining the type of exercise and its intensity and duration, one can predict its physiologic and nutritional impact on the individual, and by identifying the energy cost of exercise and the metabolic fuels required to support it, one may then construct an appropriate dietary intake to meet these needs.

Selection of appropriate energy intake is a key dietary adjustment to supporting optimum human performance. With few exceptions, even the most strenuous exercise does not mandate vitamin/mineral supplementation or other major reconfigurations of dietary nutrient content; reather, it demands the prudent selection of regular whole foods so the dietary supply of energy and nutrients will be congruent with metabolic need. For these reasons a sound knowledge of how energy expenditure is quantitated will prevent some common pitfalls.

Energy expenditure in humans can be quantitated by several calorimetric methods. Nutritionists and other health scientists are familiar with the bomb calorimeter used to estimate the energy content of foodstuffs. The foods are combusted in an insulated chamber and their energy content calculated from the net heat released. Precisely analogous methods (albeit without complete combustion!) are used to estimate human energy expenditure. Subjects are confined to a large insulated chamber and the change in heat content of the system is used to assess energy expended. Although extremely accurate, such direct calorimetry is too costly and time consuming for regular application and thus newer, indirect, methods have been developed that are more useful.[24,25]

When using indirect calorimetry, one assumes that the majority of energy production is due to aerobic metabolism. Energy expenditure is calculated by measuring oxygen uptake, ignoring the contribution of anaerobic processes. Thus the caloric value of 1 liter of O_2 is taken to be roughly 5 kcal or 21 kJ (kilojoules). For practical applications this oxygen equivalent is satisfactory although its exact value is known to vary according to the metabolic fuel being oxidized.

The caloric value of metabolized oxygen is a function of the relative hydrogen and oxygen contents of the fuels being oxidized. The higher the hydrogen content of a fuel or foodstuff, the more respiratory oxygen is required to oxidize it and the more energy is released from it in the process. In biochemical terms these variations are reflected by the *respiratory quotient* or RQ, which is the ratio of the volumes of carbon dioxide produced to oxygen consumed at the tissue level during aerobic respiration (liters of CO_2/ liters of O_2).* The RQ associated with com-

busting pure carbohydrates is 1.0; with pure fats, 0.70; with pure protein, 0.82.[26]

Because the RQ actually reflects simultaneous combustion of all three energy substrates, it must be corrected for the contribution of protein before fat and carbohydrate combustion can be factored out. This correction is accomplished by subtracting out the gaseous equivalents of the urinary nitrogen excreted during the time period measured. The resulting *nonprotein RQ* closely approximates the relative contributions of carbohydrate and fat to the fuel mix. Details of these and other pertinent calculations may be found in McArdle et al.[12] These authors suggest that by using a median value of RQ = 0.82 and the corresponding 4.825 kcal/liter of O_2 energy equilavent for a mixed diet, it is possible to minimize the error in estimating energy expenditure to 4%.

Quantitating Energy Expenditure

Although numerous technologies, ranging from the wearing of a pedometer to radar tracking, have been used to assess human energy expenditure, measurement of oxygen uptake ($\dot{V}O_2$) remains the method of choice. Oxygen uptake is measured easily using open- or closed-circuit spirometry[12] while the subject is resting comfortably in the postabsorptive state; and under these conditions it ranges between 160 and 290 ml of O_2 per minute (0.8-1.43 kcal/min). This *basal metabolic rate* (BMR) reflects basal heat production from ongoing metabolic and homeostatic processes not including those associated with meal feeding (thermic effect of food, TEF, or specific dynamic action, SDA). As such, the BMR is a function of lean body mass (metabolically active tissue), which in turn is closely correlated with body surface area.

From knowledge of an individual's height and weight, the body surface area (BSA) (m^2) is rapidly calculated by use of existing nomograms. Tables show metabolic rate as a function of BSA (kcal/m^2/da), and the BMR can be closely approximated without measuring oxygen uptake directly. Men and women of the same BSA differ in metabolic rate, these differences reflecting the relatively greater leanness of males (especially after puberty), but the variance can be largely resolved when metabolic rate is expressed per unit of lean body mass.[27]

Energy expenditure during exercise and the maximum capacity for it ($\dot{V}O_2$max) are also ac-

---

*NOTE: The RQ is quite different from the RER (or R) (respiratory exchange ratio), which is the ratio of the volumes of carbon dioxide expired to oxygen inspired at the *pulmonary* level. Consequently R is a composite of the RQs of all body tissues as well as of nonmetabolic CO_2 production occurring when non–steady state changes in acid-base balance develop. For example, a hyperventilating endurance athlete could easily generate an R value of 1.0 when, in reality, his tissue-level RQ was 0.78, indicating reliance on fatty acid oxidation rather than on carbohydrate oxidation.

curately estimated from oxygen consumption and the respiratory exchange ratio. In the laboratory this process (referred to as ergometry) is usually performed on a treadmill or stationary cycle, which allows the subject to breathe into an automated gas analyzing system.[28]

Although it cannot precisely quantitate energy production via anaerobic processes, measurement of $\dot{V}O_2$ (including any accumulated "oxygen debt") provides an accurate assessment of energy expended in aerobic processes. It not only estimates power production at any time (kcal or mJ/min, Watts) but, when compared to either the resting or the maximum oxygen uptake of an individual, $\dot{V}O_2$ shows the relative intensity of any activity. Several methods of describing exercise intensity are shown in Table 42-5.[12]

Although $\dot{V}O_2$max is predominantly genetically determined, it is also influenced by age, sex, body composition, aerobic training, and disease. Maximum aerobic capacity peaks at age 18-20 and declines thereafter, largely because of age-related losses in lean body mass. This dependence of $\dot{V}O_2$max on lean body mass is logical, for it is muscle that consumes most of the excess oxygen required during exercise. Lean body mass is virtually identical in prepubertal males and females of comparable body size but increases rapidly in males after puberty. This increment is attributed to the anabolic effects of testosterone, which induces and maintains muscle mass. Precisely why lean body mass (and hence $\dot{V}O_2$max) declines from early adulthood onward is not understood; however, age-dependent declines in protein metabolism have been documented.

Aerobic training positively affects $\dot{V}O_2$max in individuals of all ages. The magnitude of the increase is 15%-20% at most, with the largest training-related changes seen in previously sedentary persons. In view of these parameters, the lowest values for maximum oxygen consumption would be observed in sedentary elderly women with significant cardiac or pulmonary disease; intermediate values would be seen in healthy active individuals; and the highest recordings would occur in elite male endurance athletes. $\dot{V}O_2$max averages about 45 ml/kg/min in active subjects and is proportionally higher in better-conditioned athletic persons.[12] The highest recorded $\dot{V}O_2$max values to date have been found in elite cross-country skiers (94 ml/kg/min in a male, 77 ml/kg/min in a female).[6] Two excellent reviews[28,29] discuss the changing role of $\dot{V}O_2$max in sports performance.

Energy Expenditure: Practical Applications

How can knowledge of maximum oxygen uptake be related to optimum nutrition for the physically active person? The answer lies primarily in the fact that it predicts an individual's capacity to expend energy. Consider, for example, the elite runner who can complete a marathon at a 6-minute/mile pace. If he weighs 70 kg, his energy cost at this pace is 112 kcal (469 kJ)/mile.[12] On this basis the metabolic cost of the marathon is 2900 kcal (12,139 kJ) over the course of 156 minutes, for an average energy

Table 42-5 Classification of Physical Activity in Terms of Exercise Intensity

	kcal/min^{-1}	Liters/min^{-1}*	ml/kg^{-1}/min^{-1}	METS
		Men		
Light	2.0-4.9	0.40-0.99	6.1-15.2	1.6-3.9
Moderate	5.0-7.4	1.00-1.49	15.3-22.9	4.0-5.9
Heavy	7.5-9.9	1.50-1.99	23.0-30.6	6.0-7.9
Very heavy	10.0-12.4	2.00-2.49	30.7-38.3	8.0-9.9
Unduly heavy	12.5-	2.50-	38.4-	10.0-
		Women		
Light	1.5-3.4	0.30-0.69	5.4-12.5	1.2-2.7
Moderate	3.5-5.4	0.70-1.09	12.6-19.8	2.8-4.3
Heavy	5.5-7.4	1.10-1.49	19.9-27.1	4.4-5.9
Very heavy	7.5-9.4	1.50-1.89	27.2-34.4	6.0-7.5
Unduly heavy	9.5-	1.90-	34.5-	7.6-

From McArdle WD, et al: Exercise physiology: energy, nutrition, and human performance, Philadelphia, 1986, Lea & Febiger.
*Liters/min^{-1} based on 5 kcal per liter of O_2; ml/kg^{-1}/min^{-1} based on a 65 kg man and a 55 kg woman; 1 MET is equivalent to 250 ml O_2 per minute, or the average resting oxygen consumption.

expenditure of 18.6 kcal or 78 kJ/min. If the runner has a $\dot{V}O_2$max of 80 ml/kg/min, his maximum rate of aerobic power production is 70 kg × 0.08 liter/kg/min × 4.825 kcal/liter of O_2 = 28 kcal (117 kJ)/min. On this basis he is working at only 18.6/27 or 69% of his maximum capacity, a relatively comfortable pace. What level of effort does this "comfortable pace" represent for a sedentary 70 kg individual with a $\dot{V}O_2$max of 45 ml/kg/min? Such a person's maximum aerobic power would be 70 kg × 0.045 liter/kg/min × 4.825 = 15.2 kcal/min, less than that required to run a single 6-minute mile. Clearly, this individual could not race at a 6-minute pace, unless perhaps on a motor-scooter!

It is clear that knowledge of both an individual's $\dot{V}O_2$max and those of representative athletes in different sports can help predict potential energy expenditures. This information, along with knowing the age, body size, type of physical activity, and duration of daily sports participation, will then allow for accurate estimation of total daily energy expenditure. Table 42-6 displays the energy needs for a variety of sports and representative athletes.[30] When the energy needs of this population (50 kcal [200 kJ]/kg/da or more) are compared to those of sedentary persons (30-35 kcal [126-147 kJ]), a large discrepancy can be seen to exist. What factors are responsible for these differences?

A brief discussion of energy balance will help clarify how predictions of energy need are made and further explain the broad range of energy expenditures observed among athletes of differing size and athletic focus.

The components of energy expenditure during weight maintenance are *resting metabolic rate* (RMR), *thermic effect of exercise* (TEE), *thermic effect of food* (TEF), and *adaptive thermogenesis* (AT).[31] *RMR* is the energy expended to maintain normal body function, homeostasis, and sympathetic nervous system activity. For practical purposes it is the same as *BMR,* which it has now largely replaced in the literature. *TEE* represents the energy expended during muscular exercise. *TEF* (also called *specific dynamic action* [SDA]) is the increase in energy expenditure above *RMR* because of the digestion and assimilation of food. *AT* is best viewed as the change in *RMR* associated with adaptation to environmental stress, which could include alterations in

dietary intake, ambient temperature, or emotional status.

Because the RMR correlated with body size, big athletes tend to need more energy. Their energy needs may also be greater because the sports in which they participate usually are weight bearing or involve overcoming wind/water resistance and these are more energetically costly for larger persons. This generalization should be applied cautiously, however, because it may prejudice such persons against competing successfully in sports like distance running and bicycle racing, in which aerobic energy expenditure is greatest. Furthermore, the RMR may vary as much as 30% between individuals, thereby potentially obscuring the expected variations in resting energy expenditure among persons of different age or size. Training status seems to be yet another important contributor to RMR. Quite recent work by Poehlman et al.* indicates that highly conditioned endurance athletes have a small but significantly higher RMR than do untrained individuals.

Exercise energy expenditure (TEE) is governed by many factors—the type, intensity, and duration of exercise, the athlete's skill and level of training, and the prevailing environmental conditions. Endurance athletes who require superior aerobic capacity and long training hours at a high percentage of their $\dot{V}O_2$max will burn more energy per kilogram of body weight than will athletes in more intense but intermittent activities like sprinting or weight lifting. Even so, the relatively light body weight of most endurance athletes precludes their having the highest overall energy needs.

The highest needs for energy are seen in sports such as hammer throw, shotput, and discus that require *both* large muscle mass and exhaustive training. Competitors in these events, paradoxically, have the highest daily energy requirements of all despite the fact that their time in actual competition is but a few minutes or less.[12]

Some authors[33] have suggested that energy expenditure among American football players is higher than among the heavy track athletes just mentioned and may reach 10,000-14,000 kcal (42-58.6 mJ) as the result of 4 to 5 hours

*Poehlman ET, et al: Resting metabolic rate and postprandial thermogenesis in highly trained and untrained males, Am J Clin Nutr **47**:793-798, 1988.

Table 42-6 Median Energy Consumption and Corresponding Daily Food Requirements of Groups of Elite Male Athletes

Selected Sports Category	Expenditure of Energy Per kg of Body Weight Per Day (kcal)	Average Body Weight (kg)	Normative Daily Net Needs Based on Computed Energy Requirements (column 1 × column 2) (kcal)	Optimum Daily Gross Requirements, with 10% added for SDA Effect (kcal)
Group A				
Cross-country skiing	82.14	67.5	5550	6105
Crew racing	69.21	80.0	5550	6105
Canoe racing	72.72	75.0	5450	5995
Swimming	69.87	76.0	5300	5830
Bicycle racing	80.39	68.0	5450	5995
Marathon racing	79.07	68.0	5400	5940
AVERAGE VALUES			5450	5995

Rounded-off norm: 6000 kcal

Also belonging to Group A are skiing (Norwegian combination), middle-distance racing, walking, ice racing, modern pentathlon, equine sports (military), and touring (alpine climbing)

Group B				
Soccer	72.28	74.0	5350	5885
Handball	68.06	75.0	5100	5610
Basketball	67.93	75.0	5100	5610
Field hockey	69.18	75.0	5200	5720
Ice hockey	71.87	68.0	4900	5390
AVERAGE VALUES			5130	5643

Rounded-off norm: 5600 kcal

Also belonging to Group B are rugby, water polo, volleyball, tennis, polo, and bicycle polo

Group C				
Canoe slalom	67.16	68.0	4550	5005
Shooting	62.71	72.5	4550	5005
Table tennis	59.96	74.0	4450	4895
Bowling	62.69	75.0	4700	5170
Sailing	63.77	74.0	4700	5170
AVERAGE VALUES			4590	5049

Rounded-off norm: 5000 kcal

Also belonging to Group C are circuit cycle racing (1000-4000 m), fencing, ice sailing, and gliding

Group D				
Sprinting	61.77	69.0	4250	4675
Running short to middle distances	65.62	65.0	4250	4675
Pole vault	57.83	73.0	4200	4620
Diving	69.24	61.0	4200	4620
Boxing (middle- and welterweight, to 63.5 kg)	67.25	63.0	4250	4675
AVERAGE VALUES			4230	4653

Rounded-off norm: 4600 kcal

Also belonging to Group D are hurdle races, broad- and high-jump, hop-skip-and-jump, ballet swimming, figure skating, figure roller skating, skiing, ski jump, bobsled, and tobogganing

From American College of Sports Medicine: Encyclopedia of sport sciences and medicine, New York, 1971, Macmillan Publishing Co.

Table 42-6 Median Energy Consumption and Corresponding Daily Food Requirements of Groups of Elite Male Athletes—cont'd

Selected Sports Category	Expenditure of Energy Per kg of Body Weight Per Day (kcal)	Average Body Weight (kg)	Normative Daily Net Needs Based on Computed Energy Requirements (column 1 × column 2) (kcal)	Optimum Daily Gross Requirements, with 10% added for SDA Effect (kcal)
Group E				
Subgroup I				
Judo (lightweight)	72.92	62.5	4550	5005
Weightlift (light-weight)	69.15	67.5	4650	5115
Javelin	56.95	76.0	4350	4785
Gymnastics with apparatus	67.14	65.0	4350	4785
Steeplechase	63.96	68.0	4350	4785
Ski Alpine competition	71.29	67.5	4800	5280
AVERAGE VALUES			4508	4959
		Rounded-off norm: 5000 kcal		
Subgroup II				
Hammerthrow	62.46	102.0	6350	6985
Shotput and discus	62.47	102.0	6350	6985
		Rounded-off norm 7000 kcal		

Also belonging to Group E I are wrestling, automobile rallies, motor racing, gymnastics, acrobatics, parachute jumping, equine sports, decathlon, and bicycle gymnastics

of daily training. These data must be seriously questioned on logical grounds. Consider the energy needs of a 25-year-old lineman 6'5" (195.6 cm) tall and weighing 315 pounds (143 kg). Based on his age and a total body surface area of 2.7 m², he would have a BMR of 2430 kcal. If this amount is subtracted from 10,000 kcal, then the remaining 7570 kcal represents TEE + AT + TEF. A conservative estimate for the energy cost of AT + TEF would be 10% of 7570 or 757 kcal. If this were factored out, the remaining 6800 kcal would represent TEE, most of which would be occurring in 5 hours of intense football practice. Well, just how intense does the practice have to be to burn 6800 kcal in 300 minutes of nonstop (unlikely) activity? This represents a power output of 6800/300 = 23 kcal/min or, at 5 kcal/liter of O_2, a continuous $\dot{V}O_2$ of 4.6 liters/minute. Such energy production corresponds to the limit of aerobic power that can be sustained by a world-class cross-country skier racing for 2 hours. It is not

likely that any football player could or would work this hard!

Environmental conditions also have a potentially great impact on energy expenditure. It is well recognized that better marathon times are recorded in relatively cool low-humidity weather, in which the energy cost of thermoregulation is minimal. The cyclist racing into a 20 mph headwind expends considerably more energy to maintain pace than under windless conditions. Finally, the high-altitude mountaineer climbing Mt. Everest encounters extreme hypoxia and can work at only a fraction of his sea level $\dot{V}O_2$max. The topic of energy expenditure in athletes is complex and fascinating. The interested reader is referred to several classic works in this field for further information.[12,22,33]

Summary

Muscle displays structural and functional adaptations enabling it to provide the speed, strength, precision, and endurance required for the diverse physical activities that humans undertake. The basic "currency" of muscular energy is ATP, which is ultimately derived from the oxidation of carbohydrates, fats, proteins, and other foodstuff by either aerobic or anerobic energy systems. Aerobic energy metabolism requires oxygen, anaerobic does not. The immediate source of ATP under all circumstances is the phosphagen system, an anaerobic pathway that is itself fueled by either anaerobic glycolysis (lactic acid system) or the aerobic tricarboxylic acid cycle depending on the magnitude and urgency of the demand for ATP.

The anaerobic systems provide energy for all muscle fibers when oxygen is not available and when the need for ATP is urgent. They have great power to provide energy, but limited capacity. The anaerobic phosphagen and lactic acid systems are especially important in fast-twitch fibers, which furnish most of the power for high-speed and high-intensity exercise using stored glycogen or blood glucose as fuel.

In contrast, aerobic metabolism is the predominant fuel source in the fatigue-resistant slow-twitch fibers that provide muscular endurance. These fibers display limited power production but have enormous capacity to generate ATP over the long term. They can combust all fuels but rely on fatty acid oxidation for most of their energy needs.

The relative contribution of these systems to whole-body exercise fuel needs can be assessed by measuring the respiratory exchange ratio (R). A high R value and high blood lactate levels indicate the use of carbohydrates as fuel whereas low R values indicate fat oxidation. Measurement of oxygen uptake using R allows energy expenditure to be quantitated. In turn, an individual's maximum oxygen uptake reflects his capacity for aerobic exercise, and hence his potential for energy expenditure. Knowledge of the $\dot{V}o_2$max, the type of physical activity, and the intensity and duration of training will allow accurate prediction of the energy needs of different athletes.

CARBOHYDRATE NUTRITION AND EXERCISE

Carbohydrate availability and utilization during exercise are critical determinants of human performance. The storage of carbohydrates in the form of blood glucose, hepatic glycogen, and muscle glycogen is minimal relative to the energy needs imposed by prolonged exercise.[20] A metabolic conflict may appear in which the demands of contracting muscle and those of glucose-requiring tissues cannot be met simultaneously.

High-intensity activities, such as sprinting or power lifting, create little conflict since they can last only a few seconds or minutes before fatigue sets in. Fatigue occurs rapidly despite ample carbohydrate stores in liver and muscle. By contrast, endurance related activities requiring continuous muscular contraction for 1 hour or more jeopardize carbohydrate homeostasis. Such activities become limited as muscle glycogen dwindles and the liver is unable to supply the brain, anaerobic tissues, and muscle with blood-borne glucose. As carbohydrate stores dwindle, there is a progressive drop in the respiratory exchange ratio (R), reflecting a reversion from carbohydrate to fatty fuels.[34] This metabolic "default" necessitates a deterioration in performance, since fatty acid oxidation alone will not support exercise at intensities above 50%-60% of an individual's $\dot{V}o_2$max.[35]

Hypoglycemia, a potential serious consequence of the disparity between glucose availability and its requirement for normal CNS function, may also occur during endurance exercise. Although the precise contribution of low blood sugar to impaired performance remains highly controversial, some athletes seem particularly susceptible to its untoward effects. Symptoms may range from feeling slightly "off" to ataxia and other manifestations of severe central nervous system dysfunction. With profound hypoglycemia, coma and even death may result. Although the latter are rare, lesser degrees of hypoglycemia are prevalent during endurance events and may impair nearly 40% of competitors.[36] Indeed, such symptomatic hypoglycemia is well recognized (and feared) among elite runners, who refer to it as "bonking."

One approach to increasing carbohydrate availability during exercise is to enhance the body's glycogen stores is by so-called "glycogen loading" or "supercompensation" techniques. Another is to train one's muscles to rely more heavily on fat for energy. Yet another is to supplement endogenous stores with dietary carbohydrates (liquids or solids) immediately before as well as during competition. The value of these approaches will be considered in the ensuing discussion of carbohydrates and energy production.

Whole Body Carbohydrate Homeostasis

Carbohydrates, despite their prevalence in our foodstuffs, are not a requisite in the human diet. Indeed, the native Eskimo diet, largely devoid of carbohydrate, is well tolerated by those previously accustomed to a mixed fare.[37] This ketogenic diet's adequacy is due to its generous protein content, which provides ample quantities of amino acids for both protein synthesis and gluconeogenesis. In the absence of dietary carbohydrate, the so-called glycogenic amino acids* are easily converted to glucose in the liver. This occurs during starvation when gluconeogenesis synthesizes carbohydrate for the brain and other tissues from amino acids released into the bloodstream by proteolysis.

Since dietary carbohydrates are both inexpensive and highly palatable, they constitute 40% or more of the American diet. Following their digestion they are absorbed as monosaccharides (glucose and fructose) and are metabolized, converted to fat, or stored as glycogen (a branched

*The *levo* configurations of alanine, arginine, aspartate, cystine, glutamate, glycine, histidine, hydroxyproline, methione, proline, serine, threonine, and valine. (Harper HA, et al: Review of physiological chemistry, ed 17, Los Altos Calif, 1979, Lange Medical Publications.)

polymer of glucose). Although most if not all body tissues have the capacity to store intracellular glucose as glycogen, the largest amounts are found in liver and muscle. Glycogen can either supply glucosyl carbon to the cell, where it is stored, or provide free glucose to the bloodstream. In muscle and most other tissues glycogen serves exclusively as a source of local fuel, since only the liver and kidney contain glucose-6-phosphatase, the critical enzyme that forms free glucose from glucose-6-phosphate released during glycogenolysis.

Glucoregulatory Mechanisms During Exercise

When exercise begins, muscle fuel utilization is optimized through an orderly sequence of events (Fig. 42-3). Complex hormonal and neural glucoregulatory mechanisms ensure that the simultaneous fuel demands of different tissues will be met (Fig. 42-4).[22] Exercise-related stress leads to increased sympathetic nervous activity with an associated rise in secretion of the counterregulatory hormones—epinephrine, norepinephrine, glucagon, growth hormone, cortisol. Collectively these changes cause hepatic glucose output (initially almost entirely from glycogenolysis) to increase 2 to 5 times, depending on the intensity of the exercise.[38] Simultaneously a

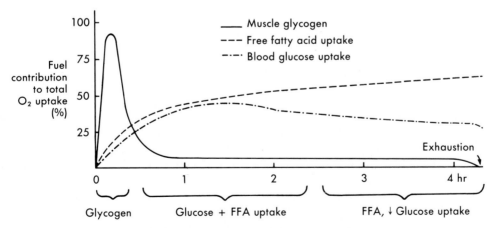

Figure 42-3 Three phases of fuel consumption during exercise. In the first few minutes, muscle glycogen is the main fuel used to generate energy (ATP). Beyond 5-10 minutes, blood glucose and free fatty acids become increasingly important. If exercise is extended beyond 120 minutes (as with marathon runners), the muscle displays an increasing dependence on free fatty acids with lesser uptake of blood-borne glucose. Although muscle glycogen contributes only a small proportion of the fuel requirements during prolonged exercise, its depletion is associated with exhaustion.

From Calles-Escandon J, Felig P: In Loke J, editor: Symposium on exercise: physiology and clinical appication, Clin Chest Med **5**(1):3-11, 1984.

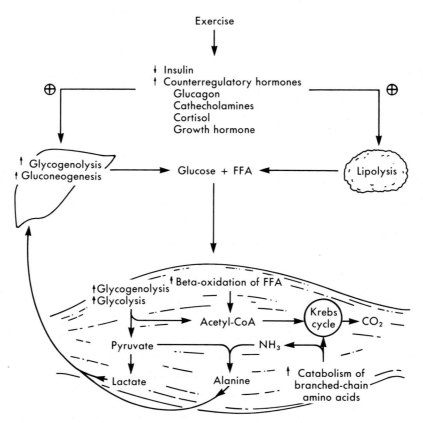

Figure 42-4 Exercise-induced hormonal and metabolic changes. The hormonal changes during exercise create a metabolic milieu that increases the fuel supply (glucose and free fatty acids) to the working muscles while maintaining the fuel supply to vital tissues (e.g., glucose delivery to brain). The hormonal changes induced by exercise (decreased insulin, increased counterregulatory hormones) enhance glucose delivery by stimulating glycogenolysis and gluconeogenesis in the liver and elevate free fatty acid delivery by stimulating lipolysis in the fat cell.

From Calles-Escandon J, Felig P: In Loke J, editor: Symposium on exercise: physiology and clinical application, Clin Chest Med **5**(1):3-11, 1984.

decrease in pancreatic islet cell output causes plasma insulin levels to fall. As a result the peripheral tissue utilization of glucose (R_d, rate of disappearance) becomes more selective during exercise, facilitated by the combined effects of diminished insulin and elevated hormone concentrations, which antagonize the glucose transporting effects on the periphery.

Ostensibly these changes would nearly eliminate peripheral glucose uptake altogether. However, exercise itself selectively increases muscle glucose uptake. The present consensus among exercise endocrinologists is that insulin is not required for this exercise-mediated augmentation of glucose uptake.[69] Consequently, hormonal changes may ultimately facilitate the availability

of glucose to the CNS and active muscles without unnecessarily subsidizing less critical tissues (resting muscles and fat).

Because normal liver glycogen stores are limited to roughly 90 g, gluconeogenesis gradually replaces glycogenolysis as the principal source of blood glucose during prolonged activity (>90 min).[40] The significance of the liver's gluconeogenic capacity during prolonged exercise is "underscored" by the estimation that 50-60 g of liver glycogen is mobilized during 4 hours of mild exercise, corresponding to about 57% of the hepatic glycogen reserve.[41]

With prolonged exercise a disparity between glucose production (R_a [rate of appearance], which equals the sum of glycogenolysis and glucogenesis) and glucose disappearance (R_d) develops, and blood glucose levels fall. This happens because gluconeogenesis, the major contributor to R_a late in exercise, provides glucose less rapidly than does the breakdown of preformed glycogen. The fall in blood sugar during prolonged exercise does not necessarily precipitate either diminished performance or symptomatic hypoglycemia. Some athletes are remarkably resistant to the development of hypoglycemia and its symptoms (others are much more prone). Hypoglycemia cannot be consistently linked to impaired performance, nor can steps taken to obviate low blood sugar predictably prevent impairment.[36] Although endurance exercise may be limited by muscle glycogen depletion, muscle fatigue is a complex and multifactorial process in which one or several defects can appear within the "chain of command" linking the brain to muscle power production.[42] It seems logical that the CNS would discontinue muscular activity before the latter could seriously compromise glucose availability to the brain or other vital organs. The precise role played by carbohydrate availability in the development of fatigue remains an intriguing question.

Initial Stage

Regardless of the nature of the exercise that follows, the initial period of muscular contraction is fueled by endogenously stored (local) energy substrates. Although local (intramuscular) triacylglycerol stores are used during this period, glycolysis from glycogen provides most of the needed energy and this initial reliance on carbohydrate is reflected by a high respiratory exchange ratio ($R > 0.9$). After this initial period of reliance on local stores, the intensity of subsequent exercise determines what fuels will be used.

Lipids are the predominant muscle fuel during low- to moderate-intensity aerobic activity, but their relative contribution to the fuel mix decreases with increasing exercise intensity. Above 55%-60% $\dot{V}O_2$max, at which level fat and carbohydrate are consumed in equal amounts, there is a progressive need for more carbohydrate. If exercise is intense ($> 65\%$ $\dot{V}O_2$max), the R will remain high until muscle glycogen depletion becomes prominent. This reliance on carbohydrate fuels reflects the recruitment of large motor units (containing many Type II [fast-twitch] fibers)

and the need for slow-twitch fibers to maximize power output via aerobic glycolysis. Why carbohydrates also become a preferred aerobic fuel remains unclear. Two likely reasons include easy availability and the fact that carbohydrate oxidation produces about 5% more energy per liter of oxygen consumed than does fat oxidation. Thus, when available, glycogen is a more efficient fuel than fatty acids. Indeed, the highest rates of carbohydrate utilization are seen when the needs for sustained maximum power are greatest. This extreme reliance on CHO fuels is seen during sprinting events (e.g., the 400- and 800-meter runs),* which generate the highest recorded blood lactate levels (25 mM).[43]

Low-Intensity Exercise

Carbohydrate also is important to the fuel needs of low- to moderate-intensity exercise of long duration (e.g., ultradistance running and cycling) because of its involvement in fatty acid oxidation, ongoing aerobic lactate production, and the maintenance of blood glucose homeostasis. Davies and Thompson[35] examined the time course of changes in fuel metabolism in four elite ultradistance runners racing for 24 consecutive hours. The athletes began the race with full glycogen stores and an oxygen consumption equaling 90% of their previously determined $\dot{V}O_2$max. With racing time both oxygen consumption (power output) and R declined in parallel until a plateau was reached at approximately 12-16 hours. Presumably, muscle glycogen was spent by that time and virtually all fuel requirements were being met by fatty acid oxidation. Indeed, the R at plateau was 0.7, confirming this observation.

Diet also has a profound influence on the selection of fuels during exercise. This is true for the athlete's habitual diet as well as for what he consumes immediately prior to and during competition. In a sense the body is metabolically programmed by the customary diet. Both carbohydrates and fats are metabolized in greater quantities when the regular dietary intake of these respective substrates is high. This is true

---

*It might be recalled that although lactate production is associated with poor muscle performance (to the extent that it reflects local muscle acidification) it is an important source of fuel for all muscle and for the liver, which scavenges lactate from the bloodstream.

both at rest and during exercise. In the present context, it means that if generous quantities of dietary carbohydrate are available the body becomes "addicted" to them. This being the case, muscle becomes dependent on readily available carbohydrates, which require less oxygen to burn than fats, which preference reflects the relative abundance of muscle and liver glycogen when dietary carbohydrate is high as well as the enhanced enzymatic capacity to use these fuels.[44]

Just as a high-carbohydrate diet fosters dependence on glycogen and glucose, so a low CHO diet deemphasizes these fuels. This is well illustrated by the innovative studies of Fisher et al.,[45] utilizing the eucaloric ketogenic diet designed by Steven Phinney,[37,39] showing that when the diet contains minimum carbohydrate glucose oxidation and muscle glycogen utilization are decreased accordingly. This down-regulation is due in part to decreased preexercise muscle glycogen concentration. Similar observations are seen when exercise rather than diet is used to deplete glycogen. When glycogen is low, the body conserves it.

Training Status

Training status is yet another important determinant of fuel utilization. If an athlete trains regularly for a high-intensity activity, such as power lifting or sprinting, he selectively cultivates the function of his fast-twitch fiber populations. This would likely not result in a larger dietary carbohydrate requirement but would allow him to use more of his stored glycogen and blood glucose to generate increased power. If the athlete became so fit or motivated that he began to work out for a much longer time, he might conceivably require additional dietary carbohydrate to ensure minimum adequate levels of muscle glycogen.

It should be recalled that endurance-trained athletes exercise at a lower R than the untrained, indicating a greater reliance on fatty acid oxidation for energy at any exercise intensity. This ability to "spare" carbohydrate stems directly from the enhanced ability of these athletes to use oxygen and fatty acids at the muscle cell level for oxidative metabolism.

Inherited and acquired physiologic needs also influence the choice of fuels during exercise. An example is the inheritance of a particular muscle fiber phenotype. Since there is considerable truth in the statement that the elite athlete must pick his parents wisely, it is reasonable to assume that a particular fiber type profile predisposes the individual toward competing in sports in which it confers an advantage. A child born with a predominance of Type II fibers who can easily outsprint all of his schoolmates but tires easily is less likely to become an elite marathoner and more likely to become a basketball player or 100-yard dash man. On this basis, carbohydrate usage may ultimately be determined by the genetic "choice" between sprinting and an endurance-type sport along with the physiologic necessities each dictates.

In similar fashion, individuals with either congenital or acquired metabolic disease may also display different fuel requirements.[46] The patient with McArdle's disease,[47] a congenital deficiency of the enzyme myophosphorylase, cannot mobilize muscle glycogen. Hence a carbohydrate-rich diet might be imprudent for this individual. Similarly, the metabolic impact of therapeutic drugs must be taken into account. Consider, for example, the active individual being treated with nicotinic acid for hyperlipidemia. Nicotinic acid is a potent inhibitor of adipose tissue lipolysis. This person would be forced to utilize more carbohydrate during exercise because the availability of free fatty acids for beta-oxidation was dramatically reduced.

Supplying Carbohydrate Needs During Exercise

The amounts of carbohydrate fuel used during exercise are determined by a complex interplay between the many previously identified variables. On balance, however, exercise duration and intensity emerge as the single most important determinants thereof. This "reductionist" approach stems from the realization that only *submaximal* or *intermittent maximal* exercise can persist long enough for glycogen supplies to limit performance. In this light the following discussion will focus on the importance of carbohydrate fuels for prolonged exercise and how dietary manipulation may potentially influence performance. The interested reader is referred to several excellent reviews for further information.[44,48,49]

In practice there are two types of endurance exercise, those lasting several hours and those continuing much longer. The marathon provides a familiar example of shorter more intense endurance activity. In elite circles this race is run in under 130 minutes at an average caloric cost of about 20 kcal/minute. Running at 85%-90% of $\dot{V}O_2$max for this time interval is sufficiently stressful to preclude eating during the race; thus the athlete must begin competition with an in situ metabolic capability to sustain such a high power output for the entire distance (42.2 km). To do so, he must store and use glycogen in the most efficient way possible.

By contrast, the truly prolonged duration and associated energy costs of ultraendurance events require considerably more carbohydrate than the body can store. An interesting example is the Race Across America (RAAM) in which bicyclists ride from Huntington Beach, California, to Atlantic City, New Jersey. In 1985 the winner rode 20-22 hours per day throughout the event, at an average speed of 15 mph (*Official Race Manual*, RAAM). Based on the maximum oxygen uptake of elite riders (5 liters of O_2/min), cycling at 15 mph represents a relative intensity of 50%-60% $\dot{V}O_2$max and an energy expenditure of 15,000 kcal (63,000 kJ)/day. If protein oxidation accounts for 5% of energy needs and fat and carbohydrates are burned in equal proportion, the winner required roughly 1700 g of CHO each day to maintain energy balance. Indeed, participants in a competition such as this must eat continuously throughout the race and still fail to maintain energy balance. In practice, they focus on consuming as much carbohydrate as possible since protein and fat are far less palatable under race conditions.

Glycogen Supercompensation (carbohydrate loading): The Rationale

Although few endurance events require such massive energy expenditure as the RAAM, any endurance activity for 1 hour or longer duration is potentially limited by the availability of hepatic and muscular glycogen stores. In view of this metabolic constraint, exercise physiologists have examined potential ergogenic (performance-improving) benefits of dietary manipulations before, during, and after exercise. A brief examination of the rationale and pertinent experiments behind current recommendations in this exciting area may be useful in advising athletes how to eat sensibly.

In the late 1930s Swedish exercise physiologists Christensen and Hansen[50] demonstrated that a diet rich in carbohydrate could prolong endurance. Postulating that this beneficial effect was due to altered muscle glycogen levels, two younger colleagues, Bergström and Hultman,[51] later demonstrated that the duration of exercise at 75% $\dot{V}O_2$max was linearly correlated with initial muscle glycogen content. If muscle glycogen levels were boosted by a carbohydrate-rich diet prior to exercise, the time to exhaustion was demonstrably prolonged.[52] Extensions of this research demonstrated that liver glycogen behaved in much the same manner as muscle glycogen, becoming severely depleted after either 1 hour of vigorous exercise or 24 hours of starvation. Following depletion, 2 days of a high-carbohydrate diet actually boosted hepatic glycogen content to twice that observed under normal conditions.[51] Follow-up experiments have confirmed these pioneering observations, and a major review article on this subject[44] concluded that evidence to date "has clearly shown that performance in prolonged severe exercise is improved by eating a CHO (carbohydrate)-rich diet to elevate the liver and muscle glycogen stores."

In view of these data, several dietary strategies designed to boost the body's glycogen stores are commonly used. Known as "carbohydrate loading" or "glycogen supercompensation" diets, these regimens are now recognized as reproducible phenomena. Proper glycogen loading is contingent on the additive effects of depletion exercise to empty preexisting stores and a carbohydrate-rich postexercise diet to overfill them. Both conditions are necessary, with neither alone sufficient to achieve the desired results. In particular, a CHO-rich diet alone will not induce supercompensation, since exercise appears necessary to "prime" glycogen synthesis for the storage of supranormal amounts of dietary carbohydrate. In the absence of such an exercise stimulus, excessive dietary carbohydrate is simply stored as triglyceride.

Two established regimens for carbohydrate loading exist: the "classic" approach[52] (box) and the more modern "modified" approach[53] (Fig. 42-5). Each utilizes exhaustive exercise to deplete glycogen stores, but they differ in regard to the carbohydrate content and timing of the ensuing diet. The *classic* approach involves a bout of exhaustive exercise followed by a 3-day interim of low-carbohydrate intake (<5% of calories) and moderate training. On day 5 a second bout of depletion exercise is completed, after which the subject consumes a 95% CHO diet for 2-3 days and rests until competition. The *modified* approach involves a depletion-taper sequence: The athlete consumes a mixed diet containing 50% CHO (350 g of CHO/da) for days 1-3. Then during the remaining 3 days prior to competition, a higher-carbohydrate diet (70% or 550 g/da) is eaten. Daily exercise is begun on day 1 with a 90-minute bout of exercise at 70%-75% $\dot{V}O_2$max and tapered through day 5. Day 6

(the day before competition) allows for complete rest. Carbohydrate loading must occur within the context of a nutritionally complete diet that includes generous amounts of water.

Both methods achieve comparable results. Muscle biopsy data confirm that glycogen levels may reach nearly 300 mM of glucosyl units/kg ww (wet weight).[*] Because of the more serious nature of hepatic needle biopsy, there are fewer comparable data on the liver, but existing studies[†] show relative glycogen elevations similar to those in muscle.

The classic and the modified methods share putative benefits of delaying the onset of hypoglycemia and improving muscle performance through increased availability of body water for thermoregulatory purposes. This is possible because glycogen is stored with three to four times its weight in intracellular water.

Although the diets yield comparable results, they may differ considerably as to their side ef-

---

TWO-STAGE DIETARY PLAN FOR INCREASING MUSCLE GLYCOGEN STORAGE

Stage 1—Depletion
  Day 1: Exhausting exercise performed to deplete specific muscles of glycogen
  Days 2, 3, 4: Low-carbohydrate food intake (high percentage of protein and fat in daily diet)
Stage 2—Carbohydrate Loading
  Days 5, 6, 7: High-carbohydrate food intake (normal percentage of protein and fat in daily diet)
Competition day
  High-carbohydrate preevent meal

From Bergström J, et al: Acta Physiol Scand **71**:140-150, 1967.

---

[*]Bergström J, Hultman E: Synthesis of muscle glycogen in man after glucose and fructose ingestion, Acta Med Scand **182**:93-107, 1967.

[†]Nilsson LH, et al: Carbohydrate metabolism of the liver in normal man under varying dietary conditions, Scand J Lab Invest **32**:331-337, 1973.

Nilsson LH, Hultman E: Liver glycogen in man: the effect of total starvation or a carbohydrate-poor diet followed by carbohydrate refeeding, Scand J Lab Invest **32**:325-330, 1973.

MUSCLE GLYCOGEN SUPERCOMPENSATION

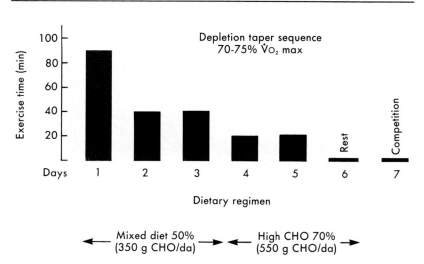

Figure 42-5 A modified sequence of depletion-tapering exercise and dietary manipulation that results in supercompensated levels of muscle glycogen.

From Sherman WM, et al: Int J Sports Med **2**:114-118, 1981.

fects and their acceptance by the athlete.[54] The disadvantages associated with glycogen loading can include the following:

1. Excessive weight gain from both water retention (potentially several kilograms) and/or excessive CHO intake
2. Gastrointestinal distress, particularly if refined CHO sources are a mainstay of the diet
3. Untoward effects of having the exhaustive exercise bout(s) so close to competition day
4. Malaise associated with the carbohydrate deprivation (ketotic) phase: hypoglycemia, weakness, postural hypotension, etc.
5. Malaise associated with carbohydrate excess (e.g., drowsiness, lethargy, muscle stiffness)
6. Lack of palatability of high-carbohydrate diets (Many athletes find the isocaloric substitution of CHO for fat needed to achieve an intake of 2000 + kcal of CHO/day to be extremely uncomfortable. One actually reported feeling "stuffed like a Strasbourg goose" [from which goose liver pate is made] while eating this diet!)
7. Laboratory test abnormalities: elevated blood glucose, lipids, and BUN along with ECG alterations

Despite the numerous potential side effects, glycogen loading is considered safe for the majority of individuals. Questions have been raised concerning its suitability for individuals with renal disease, muscle enzyme deficiencies, or predisposition to arteriopathy from diabetes or the hyperlipidemias.[55] However, a study of blood lipid and ECG responses to carbohydrate loading failed to detect any clinically significant changes in these variables.[56] In general, individuals who may be at risk should be followed by their physician.

Given that many of the side effects of glycogen loading are associated with the classic regimen, this protocol has been largely replaced by its less taxing modern counterpart. A discussion of the particulars of CHO loading will follow later under the heading "Methods" on p. 701.

Carbohydrate Ingestion Immediately Prior to Exercise

Whereas substantial data exist to support the use of carbohydrate loading in the days prior to a race, the practice of ingesting CHO immediately before competition remains controversial. For years athletes have ingested concentrated sugar solutions or solid foods immediately before competing. The principal arguments leveled against these feedings were that they predispose the athlete to reactive hypoglycemia and accelerate the utilization of glycogen stores. We shall examine briefly the data supporting and refuting these allegations. The interested reader may consult Hultman and Spriet.*

Following the ingestion of carbohydrate-containing solutions there is a rise in blood glucose levels in direct proportion to the rate of absorption of the simple sugars. Since such solutions are usually hyperosmolar, they delay gastric emptying and may even cause gastrointestinal distress as they await dilution within the stomach. Once in the intestine, they are rapidly absorbed, inducing a commensurate rise in plasma insulin and reduction in peripheral lipolysis. Solid carbohydrate feedings will elicit similar absorption kinetics and insulin secretion depending on their glycemic index and the physiochemical properties of food (e.g., fiber and fat content). Within minutes of the onset of exercise, the combined effects of the insulin and muscle contraction may cause blood sugar to fall rapidly.

Until recently there was a consensus that carbohydrate feedings immediately prior to exercise had a deleterious effect on performance by inducing hypoglycemia and accelerating muscle glycogen utilization.† Whereas it appears that such feedings (glucose in particular) may predispose certain individuals to hypoglycemia, new studies from our laboratory have produced different results. Devlin et al.‡ demonstrated that a candy bar given ½ hour before submaximal exercise at 70% $\dot{V}O_2$max did not influence either the use of metabolic fuels during exercise or the rate of glycogen utilization. Furthermore, blood

*Hultman E, Spriet LL: Dietary intake prior to and during exercise. In Horton ES, Terjung RL, editors: Exercise, nutrition, and energy metabolism, New York, 1988, Macmillan Publishing Co.

†Costill DL: Carbohydrate nutrition before, during, and after exercise, Fed Proc **44:**364-368, 1985.

‡Devlin JT, et al: Effects of preexercise snack feeding on endurance cycle exercise, J Appl Physiol **60:**980-985, 1986.

glucose levels were better maintained during exercise, although the overall endurance times were not prolonged.

In a slightly different study design, Coyle et al.[58] fed trained subjects a meal containing 142 g of glucose exactly 4 hours prior to 105 minutes of cycling at 70% $\dot{V}O_2$max. They found total carbohydrate utilization and muscle glycogen utilization to be increased relative to those in fasted subjects performing comparable exercise. Curiously, however, although the increased glycogen utilization could be entirely accounted for by a 43% elevation of muscle glycogen prior to exercise, by 105 minutes the muscle glycogen levels in the fed and fasted groups were indistinguishable.

Great controversy exists as to the effects of low blood sugar on performance. Some studies[57] report that hypoglycemia limits performance. Others[36] conclude that it is inconsistent in causing impairment and that performance can be limited even when hypoglycemia is prevented. Whereas hypoglycemia may impair performance, its detrimental effects cannot be predicted from the blood sugar alone. Indeed, in normal subjects, lowering plasma glucose concentration to within or slightly below physiologic range activates glucose-elevating (counterregulatory) systems to restore normoglycemia before symptoms occur.* Just as there are clearcut differences with regard to the plasma glucose concentration at which hypoglycemia symptoms will occur,† so there can be considerable differences among normal athletes with regard to respiratory thresholds. Although one person may have no symptoms with a plasma glucose level as low as 30-40 mg/dl (normal fasting range 70-110), another (e.g., a poorly controlled diabetic) may have a severe reaction at 100 mg/dl if his blood glucose falls precipitously from a much higher level (say 300 mg/dl).[59] Thus the athlete's response to lowered blood glucose must be considered on an individual basis.

It may be concluded that carbohydrate feedings as early as 4 hours prior to exercise increase insulin secretion and may increase carbohydrate oxidation for 6 or more hours afterward. Glucose feedings result in higher peak and trough blood levels than do feedings containing fructose. This stabilizing effect on blood sugar occurs because fructose elicits less insulin secretion and is largely metabolized by the liver. The precise influence of preexercise CHO feedings on performance depends on the individual, but mounting evidence suggests that carbohydrate feedings before exercise cause a transient exchange of CHO for fatty fuels, which will not adversely affect performance in most persons. However, since preexercise feeding (particularly of glucose) can predispose certain persons to hypoglycemia, the effiency of such ingestion should be thoroughly evaluated by field testing prior to any serious competition.

Carbohydrate Supplementation During Exercise

The rationale for carbohydrate supplementation during exercise (CSDE) is the same as for such supplementation given prior to exercise. Endurance athletes in particular wish to maintain muscle power output, prevent symptomatic hypoglycemia, and ward off fatigue. CSDE therefore is considered important in events requiring more carbohydrate for optimum performance than the body is capable of storing. This is particularly true in view of the fact that racing distances and the popularity of ultraendurance events have dramatically increased. These competitions last from as little as 4-5 hours (bicycle road races, cross-country ski marathons), to 24 hours (Western States 100 [a footrace across California's Sierra Nevada mountains]), to 10 days or more (the Sri Chinmoy Ultramarathon [a 1000-mile foot-race, won in 1988 by Yiannis Kouros, of Greece, in 10 da, 10 hr, 30 min, 35 sec!*]).

---

*Schwartz NS, et al: Glycemia thresholds for activation of glucose counterregulatory systems are higher than the threshold for symptoms, J Clin Invest **79:**777-781, 1987.
†Boyle PJ, et al: Plasma glucose concentrations at the onset of hypoglycemic symptoms in patients with poorly controlled diabetes and in nondiabetics, N Engl J Med **318:**1487-1492, 1988.

*Thomas RM Jr: Racing in the footsteps of his ancestors. Sports Section of *The New York Times*, Monday, June 6, 1988, p 21.

Given these demanding circumstances, continuous eating and drinking to maintain energy and hydration are essential even to finish the race, much less to be competitive.

Carbohydrate supplementation during exercise differs from that given prior to activity in not inducing a delayed decline in blood sugar. On the contrary, blood sugar levels tend to remain higher than they would be without any supplementation. High ambient levels of insulin are not present when exercise begins. Consequently neuroendocrine adjustments can be more appropriate, thereby allowing local changes in muscle glucose uptake to control blood glucose levels. Does this normalization of blood sugar and increased availability of carbohydrate offer any particular benefits or disadvantages?

During prolonged exercise (i.e., activity lasting over 90 min) both liver glycogen and muscle glycogen become limiting to performance. Even with prerace carbohydrate loading, glycogen levels will be sufficient for optimum performance only in events lasting up to 3 or possibly 4 hours. Beyond this time blood sugar, R, and power output decline inexorably since neither available glycogen nor ongoing gluconeogenesis (nor muscle lactate recycling) can support the previous high rates of carbohydrate utilization. It makes intuitive sense that CSDE would have a beneficial effect on performance. How might this occur?

It is well established that glycogen is the primary substrate for lactate production and that as glycogenolysis increases during exercise lactate turnover exceeds that of glucose.[62] Since most lactate produced during exercise is oxidized by contracting muscle, it now appears that muscle glycogen, and not blood glucose, is the predominant carbohydrate fuel during exercise.[63] In view of this crucial role of glycogen, it is noteworthy that, except at very high work loads, which preclude the use of exogenous fuels, muscle glucose uptake during contraction is enhanced in proportion to the prevailing degree of muscle glycogen depletion. Furthermore, net glycogen synthesis has been demonstrated in glycogen-depleted muscle *during* ongoing moderate exercise provided an adequate blood glucose supply existed.[64] There is clear evidence, however, that large quantities of exogenous glucose can be oxidized during submaximal exercise. Using stable isotope methodology, Pallikarakis et

al.* demonstrated that when ^{13}C glucose was given in divided doses during 285 minutes of treadmill running at 45% $\dot{V}O_2max$ its oxidation was dose dependent. Indeed, at higher intake levels exogenous glucose oxidation could account for up to 88% of total-body carbohydrate oxidation during the run! At present the mechanisms by which this occurs remain obscure. In toto, these data indicate the potentially great contribution of exogenous carbohydrate feeding to the maintenance of glucose and glycogen homeostasis during prolonged activity.

Methods. Given the need for CSDE during prolonged competitions and the nonfeasibility of eating solid food during them (especially running), athletes have traditionally ingested sugar-containing solutions of varying composition. Until recently the only solutions available were homemade sugar-water preparations or commercial ones combining simple sugars with electrolytes. Unfortunately, the osmolarity of such solutions had to be unacceptably high if they contained enough sugar to be an effective energy source. Solutions with osmolarity greater than 200 mOsm/liter empty slowly from the stomach and may cause significant GI distress (bloating, nausea, osmotic diarrhea, cramps). With these limitations in mind, scientists sought a more acceptable method for carbohydrate delivery and found it in the form of glucose polymers.

Glucose polymers, formed by the partial enzymatic digestion of starch, consist of glucose molecules joined in a variety of configurations. Because of their macromolecular nature, they appear to offer some distinct advantages over simple sugars. Being assimilated more evenly, they produce less fluctuation in blood sugar levels. They also offer lower osmolarity and higher energy density at any given concentration. As a result an isotonic (isosmolar) solution of glucose polymers emptys more rapidly from the stomach and delivers more glucose per unit of time than does a comparable solution of free glucose. Glucose polymers are now the mainstay of most commercial ergogenic drinks.

Although seasoned athletes usually have found by trial and error what type of CSDE they

---

*Pallikarakis N, et al: Remarkable metabolic availability of oral glucose during long-duration exercise in humans, J Appl Physiol **60**:1035-1042, 1986.

tolerate best, several guidelines may be helpful in facilitating this process:

1. Supplementary carbohydrate is necessary for ultradistance events but is unlikely to be of significant value in exercise of less than 2 hours' duration. A well-trained athlete consuming adequate dietary carbohydrate stores sufficient glycogen to cover his needs during the above time period.

2. CSDE may be either liquid or solid depending on the sport and individual preference. In general, solid foods are better tolerated by cyclists and cross-country skiiers than by runners.

3. Whether the CSDE be liquid or solid, it should be "tested" by the athlete well in advance of competition to ascertain its palatability and tolerance under "race" conditions.

4. Solid feedings should be high in CHO but low in fiber and fat so they will not delay gastric emptying. Bananas, peaches, and other succulent fruits are ideal since they are moist enough to taste good even when the athlete's mouth is parched.

5. Carbohydrate solutions can be composed of either simple sugars such as fructose or glucose, glucose polymers, or admixtures thereof. Avoid high-osmolarity solutions (>200 mOsm), which tend to cause gastrointestinal upset unless the athlete has clearly demonstrated tolerance of them.

   Some useful guidelines for formulating such solutions might be as follows[65]:

   a. In general, free glucose/fructose solutions should not exceed 2%-3% in concentration and glucose polymers should be less than 5% to avoid delays in gastric emptying. To make such solutions, no more than 2.5 g of sugar should be added per 100 ml of water.

   b. Alternatively, fruit juices can be diluted with 5 parts water, and soft drinks (colas, etc.) with 3 parts water, adjusting for individual taste. Most commercial solutions need dilution, so read labels carefully. See Table 42-7 for the sugar content of several popular commercial solutions.[66]

6. When environmental conditions make fluid replacement critical (heat, high altitude), lower-concentration solutions should be employed to maximize the rate of gastric emptying.

Table 42-7 Sugar Content of Replacement Fluids (based on nutritional information on the package)

Product	Glucose (g/100 ml)
A.I.D.	8.0
Competition II	1.6
Gatorade	5.6
Lasco	6.0
Pripps Pluss	6.8
Soft Drinks	10.1
ACSM Recommendation	2.5 (15-40 g/100 ml in cold environment)

From Parr RB: In Butts NK, et al, editors: The elite athlete, New York, 1985, Spectrum Publications.

Carbohydrate Metabolism During Recovery

When exercise ceases, the body returns slowly from its energy mobilizing (catabolic) mode to an energy storage and rebuilding mode. This transition to anabolic conditions is issued in by a fall in the levels of circulating counterregulatory hormones and a restitution of the elevated insulin/glucagon ratio. Under these conditions dietary carbohydrate is directed toward restoring muscle and liver glycogen stores and boosting blood glucose levels. During this recovery the importance of adequate dietary carbohydrate cannot be underestimated, for it will determine the time frame of and extent to which glycogenesis occurs. Glycogenesis is critical to any endurance athlete's daily performance.

The great majority of glycogen resynthesis results from carbohydrates fed during recovery. Dietary starches and sugars are digested to simple sugars (glucose and fructose), which are then available for glycogen formation. Until recently it was believed that most glycogen was synthesized from free glucose extracted from the circulation and trapped intracellularly after conversion to glucose-6-phosphate by glucokinase in the liver and hexokinase in muscle. We now know that glycogenesis from dietary carbohydrate is a far more complex process.

A growing body of evidence has accumulated to show that dietary glucose serves only as a direct precursor for glycogen synthesis in muscle. It appears that liver glycogen is restored primarily by ongoing gluconeogenesis using lactate, glycerol, alanine, and other three-carbon fragments.[60,67] In fact, most absorbed glucose bypasses the liver and is used for preferential early resynthesis of muscle glycogen. This is in addition to the contribution of whatever three-carbon fragments (lactate in particular) are still available within the muscle or circulating in the blood.

During muscle glycogenesis peripheral glucose utilization is selectively targeted toward previously contracting muscle. Because of the combined effects of enhanced plasma insulin and residual exercise-induced muscle sensitivity to glucose, glycogen-depleted muscle stands "first in line" for plasma glucose. Interestingly, high levels of glucose and insulin in the portal circulation have little effect in promoting hepatic glycogenesis. Instead, most glucose in portal blood evades hepatic extraction and is metabolized by skeletal muscle and other tissues to lactate, which recirculates in venous blood to the liver. In view of this circuitous process, it is noteworthy that high levels of blood lactate generated during strenuous exercise ultimately facilitate renewal of both liver glycogen and muscle glycogen. Furthermore, fructose, which is metabolized to lactate by the liver, is nearly four times as efficient as glucose in restoring liver glycogen.[68]

The biochemistry of glycogenesis in the postexercise period is a fascinating, but poorly understood, process. One thing is clear: The body carefully prioritizes metabolism to ensure adequate restitution of glycogen. Hence the restitution proceeds even during the fasting state. A detailed description of glycogenesis is beyond the scope of this discussion, but information is available.[19]

Following exercise, tissue sensitivity to glucose is enhanced. In rat muscle, enhanced glucose uptake can be demonstrated in the complete absence of insulin, suggesting a direct effect of exercise on cell membrane permeability.[69] With meal feeding, a high insulin/glucagon ratio is reestablished along with its anticipated anabolic effects on muscle and other peripheral tissues. This high ratio not only promotes glucose uptake into cells but also converts glycogen synthase, the rate-limiting enzyme for glycogen synthesis, from its inactive to its active form. The resulting increase in glucose transport and glycogen synthase activity allows glycogenesis to proceed rapidly, so long as sufficient dietary carbohydrate is available.

The time for glycogenesis varies according to both diet and degree of depletion. With moderate depletion a mixed diet usually restores liver glycogen within several meal feedings. In contrast, muscle glycogen content is normalized much more slowly and may require 48 hours to be complete. When depletion is profound (e.g., after a marathon or ultramarathon), muscle glycogen levels may require more than a week to reach baseline.

Kinetics of Glycogen Restitution

The kinetics of glycogen restitution are nonlinear and vary according to preexercise (starting) levels, degree of depletion, diet, and training state. Studies[49,70,71] have indicated that muscle glycogen resynthesis is highly dependent on the degree of depletion induced by exercise. When levels are normal to start with (80-130 mM/kg ww), depletions of less than 50-55 mmol/kg ww can be restored within 24 hours on a CHO-rich diet. By contrast, when depletion is greater than 70-80 mM/kg wet weight, resynthesis is incomplete by 24 hours.[44]

The absolute carbohydrate content of the athlete's diet also appears to be an important determinant of glycogen restitution. Studies by Sherman[48] imply that glycogen resynthesis during postexercise refeeding is proportional to the carbohydrate content of the diet until that reaches 500-600 g/day. Above this intake, no further gains in muscle glycogen content are observed, suggesting that synthetic pathways are saturated. In fact, some data indicate that feeding excessive carbohydrate in the early period following exercise will prematurely diminish glycogen synthase activity and prevent optimum glycogenesis.

Although the key to optimum glycogen restoration is adequate dietary CHO content, the type of carbohydrate consumed may also influence this process. A study by Costill et al.[71] compared the relative efficacies of simple sugars versus complex carbohydrates in restoring muscle glycogen following submaximal exercise. The two carbohydrate sources were equally effective within the first 24 hours; however, the starch diet resulted in significantly higher muscle glycogen levels by 48 hours postexercise. Another case in which a specific type of carbohydrate may improve glycogenesis involves restoration of liver supplies by dietary fructose, which appears to be a more efficient substrate than glucose.

Endurance training is the final variable that may significantly influence glycogen storage. Endurance-trained muscle relies more heavily on fatty acid oxidation for its fuel needs than does untrained muscle. Thus, at the same relative or absolute exercise intensity, muscle glycogen utilization in trained muscle is lower than in its untrained counterpart. Paradoxically, such adaptation is accompanied by increased muscle content of glycogenic enzymes (glycogen synthase in particular) and hence of stored glycogen. With this in mind we shall consider how glycogen stores influence performance.

Does Extra Muscle Glycogen Improve Performance?

Present thinking holds that performance in events of less than 1-1.5 hours' duration is not limited by glycogen availability. However, numerous laboratory and several field studies document that endurance performance is limited by muscle glycogen stores when competition extends beyond this time frame. Since most athletes are reluctant to undergo pre- and post-race muscle biopsy, data regarding the efficacy of glycogen supercompensation under true race conditions are conspicuously absent from the literature. Nevertheless, the majority of existing information supports a true ergogenic effect for this practice. If so, how does it actually improve performance?

This issue was elegantly addressed by Karlsson and Saltin,[72] who queried whether or not glycogen supercompensation allowed competitors to race at faster speeds. These authors scrutinized the speeds in two separate 18.6-mile footraces of trained runners whose prerace meals were either glycogen supercompensating or not. Subjects served as their own controls and ran two races each. At no time in the races were the speeds of the supercompensated runners faster than those to which they were previously accustomed. In fact, running speeds were identical in both groups up to mile 9 of the race, at which point the average speeds of the uncompensated runners began to decline faster than did those of the runners who had loaded glycogen. The gly-

cogen-loaded runners finished faster by maintaining their normal speed more consistently throughout the race.

It is also frequently stated that glycogen loading improves performance in hot weather by providing extra water for cooling. This thinking stems from the observation that glycogen is stored with roughly three times its weight in water and produces additional water when fully oxidized. Research to date is unable to substantiate such claims for thermoregulatory benefits.

How Much Dietary Carbohydrate is Necessary to Maintain Optimum Glycogen Levels?

When athletes train at carbohydrate-dependent intensities (65%-90% $\dot{V}O_2max$) on a daily basis, they incur muscle and liver glycogen losses that must be offset by a proper diet. This is particularly true of ultraendurance competitors such as triathletes who train at least 20 hours per week and expend 4000 kcal (16.7 MJ) or more each day.[73] When athletes train at such intensities and habitually consume a high-carbohydrate diet, they are creating an unfortunate metabolic dependency on carbohydrate fuels. This being the case, failure to replenish glycogen stores adequately will predictably result in premature fatigue and diminished performance. In view of this necessity for glycogen repletion and the kinetics of the process, the successful athlete must approach his diet with the same discipline that he applies to his training.[74]

Although high-carbohydrate diets are currently viewed as the gold standard for endurance athletes, the reader should be aware of an alternative line of thinking regarding the optimum choice of fuels. The gist of this argument is "Why train the body to prefer carbohydrate over fatty fuels when it is carbohydrates that inevitably are in shorter supply during competition. Why not condition the body to rely more heavily on its own abundant adipose tissue stores?" Phinney et al.[75] tested and proved their hypothesis that just as a high-carbohydrate diet emphasizes the use of CHO fuels so a high–fat/protein diet will program the body to oxidize fats in preference to carbohydrates. As described under "Lipid Metabolism and Exercise," these authors tested endurance performance and $\dot{V}O_2max$ during elite cycling races before and after the competitors were adapted to an iscaloric ketogenic (negligible CHO) diet. Interestingly, $\dot{V}o_2$max was maintained on the ketogenic diet; and when the men were ridden to exhaustion during cycle ergometry at 64% $\dot{V}o_2$max, their endurance (time to failure) was also preserved. When on the ketogenic diet, the athletes uniformly exercised at a lower R value and finished their endurance trial with higher muscle glycogen levels than when they consumed the mixed diet. Muscle glycogen depletion during the trial was 90 mM/kg ww on the normal mixed diet as opposed to 20 mM/kg on the ketogenic diet. This represented a 78% decrease in muscle glycogen utilization. During the trial blood glucose was more stable in the ketoadapted subjects and hypoglycemia was never observed.

Whether such low-carbohydrate diets could support the fuel needs of exercise intensities known to be highly carbohydrate-dependent (>65% $\dot{V}o_2$max) remains to be seen. Following ketoadaptation the athletes in Phinney's study (personal communication) complained of difficulty during hill climbing and sprinting. Clarification of this fascinating question is still forthcoming, but it is clear that any such studies must be carefully supervised. Athletes attempting the ketogenic diet by themselves are at serious risk of life-threatening electrolyte abnormalities.

So far two opposing points of view regarding dietary manipulation to optimize endurance performance have been presented. Although physiologically sound, the ketogenic diet remains only a research tool. Even so, several of its key features may be used in designing a diet that is both sparing of glycogen and practical.

The essence of such a diet would be to deemphasize reliance on carbohydrate by not consuming large quantities on a daily basis and by conducting one of each day's training sessions in the postabsorptive condition (e.g., 8-10 hr postprandially). Such training would encourage the body to rely on endogenous fuel sources rather than on glucose from a recent or currently digesting meal. In the absence of a recent feeding the body is hormonally poised by a high glucagon/insulin ratio for optimum fatty acid oxidation and gluconeogenesis. If a significant amount of the athlete's training were done under these conditions, the body might be trained to be more carbohydrate independent than otherwise. A carbohydrate-rich diet could then be included in the days immediately prior to competition to optimize glycogen stores. However, despite anecdotal evidence suggesting that it works, such a diet has not been evaluated in controlled trials.

Table 42-8 A 4000 kcal Diet Containing 600 g of Carbohydrate

Meal	ADA Exchanges	Kilo-calories
Breakfast		1035
2 cups of 2% milk	2 low fat milk	
2 cups bran flakes	6 bread	
1 banana	8 fruit	
2 slices wheat toast	1 fat	
1 tsp butter/margarine		
½ cantaloupe		
2 cups orange juice		
Lunch		1521
2 cups of 2% milk	2 lowfat milk	
2 sandwiches each with	6 bread	
2 slices wheat bread	2 medium	
1 oz Swiss cheese	meats	
½ tomato	9 vegetables	
½ cup bean sprouts	6 fruits	
1 tsp mayannaise	4 fats	
Medium baked potato		
with 1 tsp sour cream		
Spinach salad made with		
1 cup spinach, ½ cup		
mushrooms, 1 tomato		
1 Tbsp salad dressing		
1 large apple		
Dinner		1470
2 cups of 2% milk	2 lowfat milk	
4 oz fish broiled in 1 tsp	4 lean meats	
butter	9 breads	
1½ cups cooked broc-	4 fruits	
coli	3 fats	
2 ears corn each with ½	3 vegetables	
tsp butter		
2 wheat rolls		
4 graham crackers		
½ cup icemilk with 1		
cup raspberries		

Formulated by N. Yaron, M.S., using published guidelines from American Dietetic Association: Handbook of clinical dietetics, New Haven Conn, 1981, Yale University Press.

Practical Aspects of Dietary Carbohydrate Administration

1. Athletes desiring optimum daily glycogen replacement require 550-600 g of dietary carbohydrate. This corresponds to 60% of a

4000 kcal diet and should preferably be obtained from liberal intake of complex high–nutrient density carbohydrates like vegetables, fruits, pasta, and whole grain breads. A sample menu is shown in Table 42-8.

When daily energy expenditure is great, consumption of refined carbohydrates and fats may have to be increased so energy balance and glycogen restitution can be achieved without the athlete's having to eat too frequently or feel uncomfortably full. In many ultraendurance events energy balance simply cannot be attained. Under these circumstances the athlete's goal becomes eating as much carbohydrate as possible so as to maintain power output and minimize lean tissue losses. Any caloric deficit must then be covered by fat stores.

2. Recommendations for carbohydrate loading (glycogen supercompensation) are summarized as follows[54]:

   a. Loading should be practiced only before events in which it may confer an advantage. These are usually endurance competitions held at high aerobic intensity over prolonged time intervals. Loading is theoretically advantageous in competitions lasting 90 minutes or longer.

   b. If a depletion episode is used, it should involve the same exercise as the anticipated competition. Furthermore, it should be conducted 7 days prior to competition to allow sufficient recovery time.

   c. The athlete should taper both the intensity and the duration of his workouts during the 6 days prior to racing; 1 or even 2 full days of rest might be considered within this sequence.

   d. It appears that the classic period of high–fat/protein diet is unnecessary. Instead, a well-balanced diet containing 500-600 g of carbohydrate should provide optimum nourishment and palatability.

   e. The last big "loading meal" should be ingested 14-16 hours before competition, with a high-carbohydrate bedtime snack also recommended. A comparable light breakfast eaten about 3 hours before competition may help offset prerace hunger.

3. If sugar solutions are to be used, they should be of low enough osmolarity (<200 mOsm/liter) to exit the stomach quickly. It appears that glucose polymers can deliver more glu-

cose per unit time to the gut than simple sugar solutions of comparable osmolarity can. As such they may be preferable to simple sugar solutions.

Nevertheless, some athletes tolerate relatively concentrated simple sugar solutions quite well. It is reported that Scandinavian cross-country skiers habitually ingest solutions in the 5%-40% range without untoward effects.[22] Of course, tolerance to such drinks must be established well in advance of competition.

More concentrated solutions are preferred and better tolerated during colder weather, when fluid needs for maximum hydration are less urgent.

LIPID METABOLISM AND EXERCISE

With the exception of minute quantities of the essential fatty acid linoleic, and possibly also of linolenic[27] (2%-4% of daily needs), the human's only requirement for dietary fat is to act as a facilitator of the intestinal absorption of fat-soluble vitamins. Aside from these trace amounts, the body has no need for exogenous fat and makes what is necessary from excess dietary carbohydrates and proteins.

Lipid Fuels

Triacylglycerols (triglycerides, TGs) are the most important storage form of fatty fuel in the body. TGs are so named because they consist of a single glycerol backbone to which three fatty acid molecules of varying chain length and saturation have been esterified. These esterified FAs are released from TG as so-called free fatty acids (FFAs) via enzymes, called lipases, in response to a number of well-coordinated neuroendocrine stimuli. Since FFAs are insoluble in water, most are circulated in the blood bound to the soluble plasma protein albumin. Thus TGs are not used directly as fuel; they simply serve as a reservoir for fatty acids, which are the principal lipid fuels at the cellular level.

Triacylglycerol is stored in the body in three ways: as depot, intercellular, and intracellular fat.

Depot fat consists of aggregates of specialized fat storage cells called adipocytes, which are approximately 90% TG in anhydrous form. Depot TG is destined for export to other tissues following its release as FFA into the bloodstream.

Intercellular fat is stored "locally" within adipocytes residing adjacent to metabolically active tissues. A good example is the fat seen between muscle fibers, presumably for use as fuel therein.

Intracellular fat, by contrast, is stored within muscle and other active cells. In the form of cytoplasmic lipid droplets, it becomes an immediately available energy source.

The composition of TG in body stores is heterogeneous with regard to fatty acid content and reflects a person's dietary fatty acid intake as well as endogenous synthesis.

Lipoproteins and Storage of Lipid Fuels

Distribution of lipid via the bloodstream is mediated by two analogous but independent transport systems, an endogenous and an exogenous one.[77] A common feature of these systems is that they overcome the problem of poor lipid/water solubility by packaging the lipids along with protein molecules (called apoproteins) into complex lipoproteins. The apoproteins not only facilitate miscibility in aqueous solution (blood and lymph), they also function as receptors to ensure specific delivery and disposal of the lipoproteins' cargo to different body loci.

The lipoproteins are subdivided on the bases of size, composition, density, and electrophoretic mobility[77] into five major classes as follows: (1) chylomicrons, (2) very low density, (3) low density, (4) intermediate density, and (5) high density.

Lipid Fuel Reserves in Humans

The contribution of adipose tissue to body weight in a 70 kg reference male is 10.5 kg or 15%, and in a 56.8 kg reference female 15.4 kg or 27%.[12] Fat is functionally distributed within the body in two sites or depots: *Essential* fat, stored in bone marrow, heart, lungs, liver, spleen, kidneys, intestines, muscles, and tissues of the nervous system, plays both a structural and a functional role. It is necessary for maintaining normal physiologic function and includes the so called "sex-specific" or "sex-characteristic" fat in a female. *Storage* fat, which resides in adipose tissue, constitutes the larger of the fatty reserves and includes both subcutaneous fat (which serves as insulation) and omental and perinephric fat (protecting the viscera).

In the aforementioned reference male, essential fat comprises 3% of body weight, and storage fat 12%. In the reference female essential fat constitutes 12%, including 5% to 9% "sex-specific" fat (breasts, pelvis, thighs). The woman's storage fat accounts for 15% of her body weight. Thus storage fat in men and women is roughly comparable but essential fat reserves are four times greater in women.

In the average man adipose tissue represents some 90,000 kcal (or 522 MJ) of stored energy, enough for 34 days of starvation, 10.8 days of walking, or 30 fast-paced marathons.[6] In a woman there are correspondingly more lipid stores. However, whether essential fat is an accessible energy source in either sex is unclear. Indeed, there is evidence that the fat cells in different body regions show a differential response to the hormones of lipid storage and mobilization. Apparently adipocytes in the gluteal-femoral regions of women not only are larger than those in men but also are blunted in their lipolytic response relative to other adipocytes.[78] Although no experimental data support the regional or "spot" losses of adipose tissue from exercise, region-specific differences in adipose tissue metabolism do make this theoretically possible.[78]

Parenthetically the differential between the sexes regarding adipose tissue stores may reflect a physiologic "awareness" of the enhanced energy needs of childbearing. Female endurance athletes and women afflicted with eating disorders (anorexia nervosa, bulimia) frequently become amenorrheic when their adipose tissue stores drop below 16%-17% of body weight and generally return to the eumenorrheic state upon regaining adequate levels of body fat.

Metabolism

When exercise begins, changes in pulmonary ventilation, cardiac output, and lipolysis begin to provide exercising muscle with additional oxygen and circulating free fatty acids in anticipation of prolonged need for fuel. Because the increases in cardiopulmonary output occur more rapidly than do those in lipolysis, the ability of muscle to oxidize FA momentarily outstrips the prevailing supply of blood-borne FFAs. As a result the FFA levels in blood drop during the initial 10-20 minutes of aerobic exercise and subsequently recover. As time progresses, rates of adipose tissue lipolysis meet and exceed the demand for FFA and plasma FFA levels rise accordingly.

Because lipid stores are far greater than carbohydrate (glycogen) stores, blood-borne and intramuscular FFA supplies remain adequate despite a continuous time-dependent depletion of liver and muscle glycogen. Consequently the relative contribution of FA to a muscle's fuel supply increases with exercise duration. This trend is seen as a progressive decrease in the respiratory exchange ratio (R) with exercise duration and reflects both an exercise-mediated increase in FA turnover and a progressive diminution in glycogen supply and utilization.[79] Concomitant with the drop in R is a decrease in muscle power output; this inevitable decrease in performance forms the basis for prerace carbohydrate loading (glycogen supercompensation) to improve endurance performance.

Determinants of Lipid Metabolism

The degree to which lipids are used as fuel during exercise is determined by five variables: (1) exercise intensity, (2) exercise duration, (3) diet, (4) degree of endurance training, and (5) presence of an altered metabolic state. Each will be addressed briefly.

Exercise intensity is an important determinant of fat utilization, for it reflects the muscle fiber populations being recruited. Low-intensity exertion ($< 50\%$ $\dot{V}O_2$max) involves predominantly Type I fibers, which rely heavily on FFA oxidation for fuel. As exercise intensity increases, Types IIa and IIb are progressively recruited, explaining why FFA oxidation is the principal fuel source for exercise at 50% $\dot{V}O_2$max and below. Carbohydrate fuels play an increasingly important role in energy provision at intensities above this level.[22] At 60% $\dot{V}O_2$max, fat and carbohydrate contribute equally whereas at 100%, fat contributes 10% of energy at most.

The latter concept is particularly clear within the context of exercise of long duration, such as the marathon. In the absence of carbohydrate feedings, the R values of marathon runners progressively decrease with racing time. This decline is largely in parallel with the decline in muscle glycogen reserves, reflecting the reliance on fats when available carbohydrate is gone. As mentioned earlier, this inevitable reversion to lipid oxidation with glycogen loss causes a reduction in running speed and is thought to underlie the dreaded sense of fatigue experienced when runners "hit the wall."

Just as human musculature adapts to chronic exercise, so it adapts to diet. Although skeletal muscle apparently favors the use of carbohydrate fuels, it will revert to oxidizing lipid fuels when dietary carbohydrates are unavailable. Indeed, when muscle RQ is measured in the postabsorptive condition (overnight fast) it is found to be roughly 0.7, a numerical value corresponding to near complete reliance on lipids for fuel.

In keeping with this observation, early investigators became interested in how the Eskimo[80] enjoyed vigorously good health on a diet that was virtually carbohydrate-free. To assess the validity of historical evidence documenting that the Eskimos tolerated hard physical labor quite well and traditionally survived as hunters and gatherers, several studies on the effects of dietary composition on exercise metabolism were undertaken.[81,82] They revealed that a diet high in fat enhanced the contribution of fat as a fuel during muscular exercise but resulted in a decreased exercise capacity as compared to a high-carbohydrate diet.

Later studies by Christensen and Hansen[83] investigated the influence of variations in dietary carbohydrate content on endurance performance. Results of these experiments in non-Eskimo subjects are summarized in Fig. 42-6.[22] When subjects ate a 93% carbohydrate-free diet for 3 days, fat supported 70%-99% of the energy during 90 minutes of submaximum exercise to exhaustion on a cycle ergometer. In contrast, when subjects consumed a diet containing 90% of calories as carbohydrate, they could tolerate 4 hours of cycling before exhaustion; and energy derived from fatty acid oxidation ranged from 30% (hour 1) to 60% (hour 4) as glycogen stores progressively dwindled. When a mixed diet was provided, the reliance on lipid fuels and the subjects' exercise tolerance were intermediate to those observed with the other regimens.

Even more dramatic evidence of poor exercise tolerance following an acute change from a mixed to a high–fat/protein diet has come from field trials of different rations during World War II.[84,85] These studies, conducted in winter by the Canadian Department of National Defense, involved an acute change from the normal diet of infantry soldiers to one consisting entirely of pemmican, a traditional North American Indian food that contains 70% fat and 30% protein. No acclimatization period was allowed, nor were

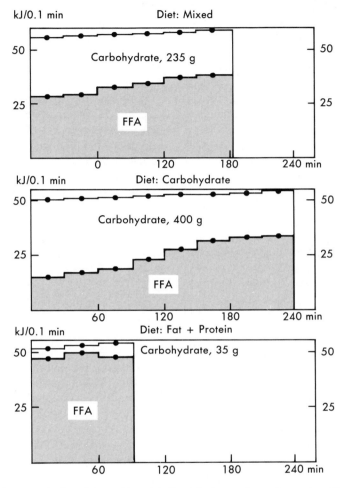

Figure 42-6 Increase in free fatty acid metabolism during prolonged exercise. One well-trained subject exercising on a cycle ergometer produced 183 Watts after a mixed diet and than 176 W after a carbohydrate-rich diet for 3 days. In another experiment 176 W was produced by an individual whose performance was preceded by a 3-day period on fat and protein, excluding carbohydrate from the diet. This subject exercised until exhausted. The total energy output was calculated from the measured oxygen uptake and respiratory quotient (R) during 15-minute periods; the energy yield from carbohydrate and free fatty acids (FFA), respectively was estimated from the R values. The calculated total carbohydrate consumption (g) is presented. Note how exercise time and the diet affect the choice of substrate. At a given rate of exercise the endurance time varied from 93 to 240 minutes depending on the diet. (The subjects' maximum oxygen uptakes were not determined.)

From Åstrand P-O, Rodahl K: Textbook of work physiology: physiological bases of exercise, New York, 1986, McGraw-Hill International Book Co; data from Christensen and Hausen, 1939.

supplementary salt, vitamins, or minerals provided. After 3 days of field maneuvers, all the
highly conditioned experienced troops became
physically incapacitated, complaining of extreme weakness and malaise with nausea and
dehydration. Physical performance, as assessed
by the Harvard Step Test, was reduced by 50%
in the soldiers studied. Symptoms and functional
deficits were rapidly reversed by refeeding of
carbohydrate-containing foods. In view of these
and other studies documenting the untoward effects of rapidly instituted high-fat diets, the traditional consensus has been that such diets are
to be avoided.

Dietary Adaptation to Exercise Conditions

More contemporary scientific as well as historic empirical evidence clearly demonstrates
that if a proper period of dietary adaptation (usually with vitamin-mineral supplementation) is allowed a high fat-protein (ketogenic) intake is
both well tolerated and supportive of substantial
submaximum exercise capacity. Indeed, Phinney
et al.[39,86] have shown both in obese normal subjects and in highly-trained racing cyclists that
both $\dot{V}O_2$max and exercise capacity (time to exhaustion at 60% of $\dot{V}O_2$max during cycle ergometry) were maintained durring 4-6 weeks of a
eucaloric ketogenic diet (EKD). Adaptation to
the EKD was accompanied by a lowering of exercise R to 0.72 and a profound decrease in both
glucose oxidation and muscle glycogen utilization during exercise. No evidence of either cardiac dysrhythmias or hypoglycemia during exercise could be found; however, the trained cyclists complained of poor tolerance for hill
climbing during their daily training rides in Boston (personal communication, Steven Phinney).

The key differences between these successful
trials with the ketogenic diet and those that failed
are the presence of a sufficient adaptation period
and medical supervision of fluid and electrolyte
status. Because the acute withdrawal of dietary
carbohydrate is associated with massive ketonuria and diuresis, careful attention must be paid
to replacement of cations (e.g., K^+, Na^+). In
addition to being required for normal cardiac and
nervous system function, these positively
charged ions are used by the kidney to neutralize excreted ketoanions (acetoacetate$^-$, beta-
hydroxybutyrate$^-$), thereby facilitating the ex-

cretion of electrochemically neutral urine. If cation replacement is inadequate, life-threatening
alterations in nerve transmission, cardiac function, and circulating blood volume may result.
Furthermore, hypokalemia is sufficient by itself
to precipitate rhabdomyolyis (whole body muscle dissolution), with an associated risk of acute
renal failure. Thus the use of ketogenic diets
remains largely a research tool and should be
attempted only with expert medical supervision.

Although the physiologic consequences of endurance training include recognizable changes in
body composition and morphology, an equally
important increase in the capacity for oxidative
metabolism also occurs. This is reflected in the
trained individual's capacity to maintain a given
intensity (absolute or as a percent of $\dot{V}O_2$max)
of submaximum exercise for a longer period than
before training. The difference relates to a higher
maximum oxygen uptake ($\dot{V}O_2$max) and, more
important, an enhanced ability to oxidize lipid
fuels. Indeed, morphologic and biochemical
analyses of endurance-trained muscle demonstrate greater mitochondrial number and protein
content with commensurate increases in the activities of citric acid cycle enzymes, fatty acid
oxidation, and oxidative phosphorylation. The
importance of enhanced lipid oxidation is preem-
inent, for the changes in endurance capacity and
in the ability to burn fat are considerably more
impressive than those in maximum oxygen uptake.[87]

This increased reliance on lipid fuels following endurance training is manifested in four distinct ways[87]: (1) lower R at the same exercise
intensity, (2) lower RQ in trained muscle, (3)
decreased rate of glycogen utilization in working
muscle, and (4) diminished production and release of lactate from working muscle.

These metabolic modifications result from a
number of training-induced alterations in the
storage, mobilization, muscular uptake, and oxidation of fats. However, a complete discussion
of these is beyond the scope of this chapter. The
interested reader is referred to several current
reviews on the subject.[19,87,88]

The presence of an altered metabolic state
may also influence lipid utilization during exercise. In this regard, any pathologic condition
that diminishes or prevents muscle from using
carbohydrate energy substrates will foster in-

creased reliance on lipid fuels. Some specific examples include diabetes mellitus and McArdle's disease. (See "Carbohydrate Supplementation During Exercise," p. 700.)

In analogous fashion, any disease or pharmacologic intervention that impairs lipid mobilization or utilization will also predictably interfere with fatty acid oxidation. Thus, the ingestion of nicotinic acid (an inhibitor of hormone-sensitive lipase, and hence of lipolysis) will substantially impair lipid mobilization. As mentioned previously, this compound is a routine medication for hyperlipidemic patients but may also be consumed inadvertently by athletes who take nutritional yeast products (which may contain large amounts of this substance) prior to competition. A similar inhibition of lipolysis has been attributed to high plasma levels of lactic acid as well as of ketone bodies.

Congenital deficiency of muscle enzymes (e.g., carnitine palmityl transferase) also impairs fatty acid oxidation. Afflicted patients have symptoms of muscle cramping and weakness that worsen with lengthening duration of exercise or a high-fat diet.[89]

Potential Advantages and Disadvantages of Lipid Oxidation During Exercise

The chief advantages attributed to the use of lipid fuels are (1) their greater fuel/weight efficiency and relative abundance compared to glycogen, and (2) the role of fatty acid oxidation in "sparing" glycogen utilization (e.g., the glucose–fatty acid cycle).

Fatty acid oxidation is the mainstay of endurance exercise, because of the great efficiency and relative abundance of energy stored as lipid. Because lipids cannot provide significant energy for Type II muscle fibers, however, the use of lipid fuels declines in proportion to exercise intensity. One mechanism by which training fosters increased use of lipid fuels is by transforming pure fast-twitch glycolytic fibers to "intermediate" FOG (fast-oxidative glycolytic) fibers, thereby permitting fatty acids to substitute for glycogen as the major contractile fuel.

Implications for the Athlete's Diet

Is the athlete's requirement for dietary fat altered by his or her pattern of daily activity? In most circumstances probably not; however, fat intake may be altered by the athlete's choice of foods.

In view of the magnitude of fat stores in even the leanest individual and the ease of synthesis of all but the essential fatty acids, the availability of lipid fuels will probably never become rate-limiting for the athlete on a eucaloric diet. Given the equivalence of dietary energy from different food sources, even the endurance athlete who requires extra dietary carbohydrate will maintain ample depot fat on a diet containing adequate energy content.

There are several circumstances that can alter fat intake. The most common of these relates to the need to maintain optimum body weight and composition for a given sporting event. Wrestlers, rowers, and other weight-conscious athletes (particularly competitive body builders) diet regularly and may eschew fatty foods, because of their energy density, to eat carbohydrate. Similarly the triathlete or endurance runner may exclude fats so as to ensure ample carbohydrate intake. At high altitude, climbers develop a distaste for dietary fat and a craving for carbohydrate despite evidence for increased metabolic reliance on fatty fuels under hypoxic conditions.[90,91]

Alternatively, there are circumstances in which the dietary preference for fats is increased. Endurance athletes who expend enormous amounts of energy may dislike the sensation of fullness that accompanies high-carbohydrate diets and will "fill in" the energy deficit with fat to avoid discomfort. In comparable fashion, climbers often increase their fat intake in winter because of the high energy/weight ratio of fats, the tendency for fruits and other carbohydrate sources to freeze, and the beneficial effects of fatty foods in maintaining body warmth. Indeed, a high–fat/protein diet has been reported to be optimal for both sled dogs and humans[93] during extended winter expeditioning.

The question of whether changes in dietary fat can improve human exercise performance remains unanswered. A crucial aspect of this argument is the issue of whether ketogenic diets may support exercise at intensities above 65% of $\dot{V}O_2$max, when muscle power output is dependent on glycogen consumption. Although anecdotal reports from the racing cyclists in Phinney's experiments suggest this is not the case, definitive studies remain to be conducted.

FLUID AND ELECTROLYTES

Even under ideal environmental conditions exercise imposes substantially upon fluid and electrolyte economy. Sports and physical work often necessitate exercising in extremes of temperature, and high or low humidity may add even greater stresses to the system. Alternatively, rules may be imposed limiting fluid intake during competition, forcing athletes to resort to drastic fluid restriction.

Water homeostasis in humans is maintained by counterbalancing fluid intake and output. The term dehydration has been used to describe the process by which body water and electrolytes are lost. The resulting state of negative water balance is commonly referred to as hypohydration. In practice the two terms are often used interchangeably. Both obligatory and elective components contribute to the balance, and large alterations of water intake or loss are usually compensated by the kidney or by behavioral changes (thirst, satiety). The same type of balance exists regarding electrolytes. In the presence of an adequate diet the body retains electrolytes it requires and, after adjustment for ongoing fecal and sweat-related losses, discards any excess via the urine.

Water Balance and Exercise

The turnover of body water and electrolytes is greatly stimulated by strenuous physical activity. The respiratory tract accounts for substantial losses (through exercise hyperventilation and the attendant increased evaporation of water) to humidify the incoming air and dissipate heat. This is particularly true at high altitude, where low relative humidity and hypoxic ventilatory drive prevail. Aerobic exercise, which is fueled by the oxidation of carbohydrates, fats, and proteins, results in a metabolic production of CO_2 and water. Furthermore, since each gram of glycogen is stored intracellularly with approximately 3 g of water, glycogenolysis releases this "sequestered" H_2O. Additional water (and possibly electrolytes) may be provided by oral fluid intake secondary to thirst, but in virtually all instances the exercise-induced losses of water and ions generally exceed any intake.

To help compensate for this physiologic water loss, urinary output is reduced. Whereas during light exercise renal function is largely preserved, during more intense efforts renal plasma flow, the glomerular filtration rate, and free water clearance are all diminished.[94] These reductions stem directly from vasoconstriction within the blood vessels supplying the splanchnic organs (liver, spleen, pancreas, gut). Indeed, splanchnic blood flow appears to vary inversely with exercise intensity, expressed as either heart rate or percentage of $\dot{V}O_2$max.* This shunting of cardiac output away from the digestive organs and toward working muscles can be impressive, accounting for up to an 80% reduction in splanchnic blood flow during maximal exercise. In view of these changes, it is hardly surprising that the body's reaction to exercise (particularly in the heat) is analogous to the reaction observed during hypovolemic shock. Antidiuretic hormone (ADH or arginine-vasopressin) is released from the posterior pituitary, and the renin-angiotensin axis is activated to increase plasma aldosterone. Collectively these neuroendocrine adjustments lead to a reduction in urinary losses of both water and electrolytes.

Of all potential routes for water and ion loss during exercise, sweating is the most significant. Regrettably, the composition of sweat is difficult to quantitate since it is influenced by a number of variables. Among these are secretion rate, body region, stimulus (thermal [exercise] versus metabolic), and degree of heat acclimatization. The Na^+ and Cl^- content of human sweat far outweighs that in other species. Human perspiration contains more than 99% water, and its osmolarity varies between 80 and 185 mOsm/liter.[96] Thus it is always hypotonic with respect to the blood and extracellular fluid as a whole. Rates of sweat loss during exercise may exceed 30 times those observed at rest. Indeed, rates of 1.5-2.0 liters/hour are common during intense exercise in the heat, and daily losses as high as 14 liters have been reported.[97]

In all cases electrolyte losses represent small percentages of exchangeable body stores. Acutely losses of Na^+ and Cl^- in sweat far outweigh those of other ions (Ca^{+2}, Mg^{+2}, K^+), but with chronic exercise whole-body content of NaCl increases as the plasma volume is expanded. Although some of these losses may ac-

---

*Rowell LB, et al: Splanchnic vasomotor and metabolic adjustments to hypoxia and exercise in humans, Am J Physiol **247**:H251-H258, 1984.

count for substantial percentages of the mean daily intake of certain electrolytes, they are compensated by a nutritious diet in the majority of cases.

Exercise creates, aside from these irreversible losses of H_2O and ions, a transient loss in the intravascular fluid volume via redistribution of body water. When exercise begins, an immediate 15%-20% reduction in plasma volume occurs. This extravasation results from increased vascular hydrostatic pressure combined with new osmotic forces due to the local appearance of muscle metabolites in the intracellular and interstitial fluid.

Water Loss

Initially plasma volume loss is proportional to exercise intensity. With time protein accumulates in the intravascular space and the balance between hydrostatic and osmotic forces is restored. So where do water losses come from during hypohydration? Evidence indicates that both the intracellular and the interstitial compartments contract as water is lost. This results in a relative sparing of the intravascular volume. Thus the plasma volume tends to remain stable and hypohydration appears to have little influence on circulating blood volume until the subject has lost 4%-5% of total body weight.* Nevertheless, when hypohydration occurs it has a profoundly detrimental effect on performance at both submaximum and maximum intensities.[106]

Water loss equal to or greater than 2% of body weight will diminish cardiovascular and thermoregulatory capacity during exercise. Heart rate and body temperature progressively increase in parallel with hypohydration, reflecting decreased plasma volume and increased osmolality of body fluids.[98]

Although hypohydration generally decreases exercise capability, it exerts differential effects.[106] For example, local muscle strength and endurance are relatively preserved during dehydration up to 5% of body weight. A similar conservation of Vo_2 max is seen, although exercise performance (speed and endurance) is impaired. This disparity is curious but not unpredictable, since Vo_2 max has less value in predicting endurance performance than do blood lactate and other biochemical variables.

Fluid Intake

Fluid intake during exercise is a key determinant of hydration status. In view of the magnitude and detrimental effects of fluid loss during heavy exercise, every attempt must be made to optimize fluid replacement. Since thirst does not accurately reflect physiologic needs for fluid, all humans tend toward voluntary hypohydration during exercise. In other words, they drink far less fluid than necessary to restore losses. This undershoot is less pronounced in trained and heat-acclimatized persons; even so water loss may not be restored until 24 hours after exercise. On this basis it is clear that adequate fluid replacement is a learned phenomenon. What factors influence intake and subsequent assimilation of ingested fluids?

As with food, the intake of fluid may be influenced by its palatability and thirst-quenching properties. Plain water is a suitable replacement for exercise-induced fluid losses, and indeed many athletes prefer it because it is a potent thirst quencher and leaves no residual taste in the mouth. However, other athletes will prefer the taste and visual appearance of commercial sugar-electrolyte replacement drinks. Whereas plain water is recommended by many authorities as the optimum replacement, there are those who disagree. Bar-Or[99] believes water's potency as a thirst quencher is undesirable and he recommends flavored drinks, which tend to stimulate further drinking.

Once fluid is ingested, a number of variables influence the rate at which it is absorbed. Since bowel absorption of fluid and solutes is quite fast and remains unimpaired until 75% of Vo_2max or greater,[101] gastric emptying becomes rate limiting under most circumstances. Factors intrinsic to the fluid that dictate gastric emptying include composition, osmolality, temperature, and volume. Whereas certain solutes (e.g., simple sugars, potassium) inhibit gastric emptying in proportion to their concentration, others have minimum effects. Sodium promotes gastric emptying to a certain degree. For example, a solution containing 20 mEq of salt is emptied faster than water.[99] Glucose polymers, being higher in molecular weight than free glucose, also exhibit

---

*Senay LC Jr, Pivarnik JM: Fluid shifts during exercise, Exerc Sport Sci Rev **13**:335-387, 1985.

lower osmolality and higher caloric density. At low concentration (5%), the polymers appear to have little effect on gastric emptying; thus, relative to a comparable glucose-bolus, they can deliver more fluid and carbohydrate per unit of time. The differences between the polymers and free glucose disappear at higher concentrations. Cold fluids ($<20°$ C, $60°$ F) are also emptied more rapidly from the stomach and are more palatable in hot weather.[101]

Exercise intensity exerts an effect on gastric emptying. At intensities below 65%-70% of $\dot{V}o_2$max there is little diminution in emptying. Above this level, however, impairment is evident.[101]

Practical Considerations for Fluid Electrolyte Replacement

Fluid before competition. Baseline hydration status can be optimized by careful attention to water intake and awareness of the diuretic effects of caffeine and alcohol. Excessive dietary protein can also impair hydration via obligatory water losses due to urea excretion.

Hyperhydration or water loading prior to competition seems to exert a beneficial effect on exercise, especially in the heat. Several studies[102] have documented lower heart rates and core temperatures and significantly higher sweat rates when subjects took extra water prior to exercise. Although water supplementation during exercise reduces core temperature more than hyperhydration alone, when both are used together thermoregulation is optimized.[103]

Hyperhydration should involve drinking 0.5 to 1 liter of cold fluid (water or isotonic sugar/electrolyte drink) 20-30 minutes prior to exercise. If fluid is consumed much earlier, diuresis may necessitate untimely urination.

Fluid during competition. Ambient temperature and humidity dictate hydration priorities. When heat stress is high, delivery of water to the gut takes precedence over delivery of ions or glucose. Regular ingestion of cold water at 10-15 minute intervals will provide adequate hydration during events lasting 2 to 5 hours. However, if a sugar-electrolyte solution is desired, it should be one with gastric emptying characteristics comparable to (or better than) those of water. The suggested volume of fluid taken at each ingestion is 150-250 ml; however, the exact amount should be dictated by prior individual experience. In cold weather higher-concentration sugar solutions are better tolerated and physiologically "affordable" since body cooling is less of a priority.

During prolonged endurance events (5 hr), especially those in hot conditions, participants must be aware of the possibility of dilutional hyponatremia posed by overdrinking.[104,105] Danger is highest for slower runners and those unacclimated to the heat (e.g., anyone with disproportionately large NaCl losses in sweat), who may consume fluids far in excess of their sweat and urine losses. In these events consumption of glucose-electrolyte solutions may be preferable to drinking water. Even so, care must be taken since most commercial electrolyte-containing drinks are still considerably hypotonic with respect to sweat. During some such events participants are weighed and screened for orthostatic changes in blood pressure to ensure that they have neither gained nor lost water in hazardous quantities.

Fluid after competition. Rehydration should begin immediately. In single-day events a normal diet and ample water will restore fluid balance within 24 hours. In multiday competitions the athlete may have to "push" both fluids and food to facilitate nutritional repletion prior to the next day's events. Regardless of the urgency of repletion, the diet should include fruits and vegetables high in potassium. Generous use of the salt shaker at meals should suffice to replenish NaCl levels in all but the most extreme conditions. There are two specific instances when salt tablets may be advisable[54]: (1) during the first 1 or 2 weeks of heat acclimatization when salt losses in sweat are much higher than afterward and (2) in sports activities when large water losses (over 5-6 lb/da) are routine. Weight loss can be determined by using pre- and postexercise weighings and electrolyte replacement begun only when the loss is more than 5-6 pounds per day. One 7 gr NaCl tablet should be consumed with 1 pint of water for each pound of weight loss over 6 pounds.

Current research indicates that potassium supplementation is not necessary as long as the diet contains adequate amounts of potassium-rich fruits and vegetables (i.e., citrus, bananas).

SUMMARY

Exercise can lead to large losses of fluid and less substantial losses of electrolytes. If the resulting hypohydration is equal to or greater than

2% of body weight, decreased cardiovascular and thermoregulatory capacity during exercise will follow. In the worst instance such losses can result in heat stroke and death. At the very least, exercise performance will be impaired, although V_{O_2} max and local muscle strength are relatively preserved. In general, electrolyte losses during exercise are minimal and easily replaced, possibly with extra salting of food, via a good diet. Exception to this may occur during early acclimatization to heat and during strenuous training when daily fluid losses of 6 liters or more are anticipated. In this case supplementary NaCl tablets should be given. Drinking appropriate fluids before, during, and after exercise will replace or at least offset the losses of fluid during exercise.

Forced drinking of fluids is necessary in most cases, since the thirst mechanism will not effect adequate replacement. During long endurance events fluid replacement is critical, but it should be closely monitored (ideally by measuring body weight) to prevent the dangers posed by either dehydration or excessive fluid intake with subsequent hyponatremia and hypochloremia.

REFERENCES

1. Paffenbarger RS, et al: Physical activity, all-cause mortality, and longevity of college alumni, N Engl J Med **314**:605-613, 1986.
2. Frisch RE, et al: Lower lifetime occurrence of breast cancer and cancers of the reproductive system among former college athletes, Am J Clin Nutr **45**:328-335, 1987.
3. Wretlind A: Nutritional problems in healthy adults with low activity and low caloric consumption. In Blix G, editor: Nutrition and physical activity. Symposia of the Swedish Nutrition Foundation, ed 5, Uppsala, 1967, Almquist & Wiksell, Bookseller, Printers, & Publishers.
4. McBride JJ, et al: The storage of the major liver components; emphasizing the relationship of glycogen to water in the liver and the hydration of glycogen, J Biol Chem **139**:943-952, 1941.
5. Weiss-Fogh T: Metabolism and weight economy in migrating animals, particularly birds and insects. In Blix G, editor: Nutrition and physical activity. Symposia of the Swedish Nutrition Foundation, ed 5, Uppsala, 1967, Almquist & Wiksell, Booksellers, Printers, & Publishers.
6. Newsholme EA, Leech AR: The runner, Roosevelt NJ, 1983, Fitness Books.
7. Dohm GL, et al: Protein metabolism during endurance exercise, Fed Proc **44**:348-352, 1985.
8. Wright ED: Whole body leucine metabolism: effects of physical exercise. Unpublished thesis for Master of Science degree in nutritional biochemistry and metabolism, Massachusetts Institute of Technology, Cambridge Mass, 1981.
9. Hoerr RA, et al: Protein metabolism and exercise. In

White PL, Mondeika T, editors: Diet and exercise: synergism in health maintenance, Chicago, 1982, American Medical Association.
9a. Rennie MJ, et al: Exercise induced increase in leucine oxidation in man and the effect of glucose. In Walser M, Williamson JR, editors: Metabolism and clinical implications of the branched chain amino and keto acids, New York, 1981, Elsevier/North Holland, pp 361-366.
9b. Millward DJ, et al: Effect of exercise on protein metabolism in humans as explored with stable isotopes, Fed Proc **41**:2686-2691, 1982.
9c. Kasperek GJ, et al: Activation of branched-chain keto acid dehydrogenase by exercise, Am J Physiol **248**:R166-R171, 1985.
9d. Lemon PWR, Nagle FJ: Effects of exercise on protein and amino acid metabolism, Med Sci Sports Exerc **13**(3):141-149, 1981.
9e. Goodman MN: Amino acid and protein metabolism. Chapter 6 in Horton ES, Terjung RL: Exercise, nutrition, and energy metabolism, New York, 1988, Macmillan Publishing Co.
10. Snow DH: The horse and dog, elite athletes—why and how? Proc Nutr Soc **44**:267-272, 1985.
11. Saltin B, et al: Fiber types and metabolic potentials of skeletal muscles in sedentary man and endurance runners, Ann NY Acad Sci **301**:3-29, 1977.
12. McArdle WD, et al: Exercise physiology. Energy, nutrition, and human performance, Philadelphia, 1986, Lea & Febiger.
13. Jansson E, et al: Changes in muscle fiber type distribution in man after physical training, Acta Physiol Scand **104**:235-237, 1978.
14. Holloszy JO, Coyle EF: Adaptations of skeletal muscle to endurance exercise and their metabolic consequences, J Appl Physiol **56**:831-838, 1984.
15. Edström L, Ekblom B: Differences in sizes of red and white muscle fibres in vastus lateralis of musculus quadriceps femoris of normal individuals and athletes. Relation to physical performance, Scand J Clin Lab Invest **30**:175-181, 1972.
16. Chi M M-Y, et al: Effects of detraining on enzymes of energy metabolism in individual human muscle fibers, Am J Physiol **244**:C276-C287, 1983.
17. Eriksson E: Rehabilitation of muscle function after sport injury—a major problem in sports medicine, Int J Sports Med **2**:1-6, 1981.
18. Perry SV: The biochemistry and physiology of the muscle cell, Proc Nutr Soc **44**:235-243, 1985.
19. Durnin JVGA: The energy cost of exercise, Proc Nutr Soc **44**:273-282, 1985.
20. Newsholme EA, Leech AR: Biochemistry for the medical sciences, New York, 1983, John Wiley & Sons Inc.
21. Martin DW, et al, editors: Harper's review of biochemistry, Los Altos Calif, 1981, Lange Medical Publications.
22. Åstrand P-O, Rodahl K: Textbook of work physiology: physiological bases of exercise, New York, 1986, McGraw-Hill International Book Co.
23. di Prampero PE: Energetics of muscular exercise, Rev Physiol Biochem Pharmacol **89**:143-222, 1981.
24. Consolazio CF, et al: Physiological measurements of metabolic functions in man, New York, 1963, McGraw-Hill Book Co Inc.
25. Consolazio CF, Johnson HL: Measurement of energy cost in humans, Fed Proc **30**:1444-1453, 1971.

26. Frayn KN: Calculation of substrate oxidation rates in vivo from gaseous exchange, J Appl Physiol **55**:628-634, 1983.

27. Alpers DH, et al: Manual of nutritional therapeutics, Boston, 1983, Little Brown & Co.

28. Snell PG, Mitchell JH: The role of maximal oxygen uptake in exercise performance, Clin Chest Med **5**:51-62, 1984.

29. Sjodin B, Svedenhag J: Applied physiology of marathon running, Sports Med **2**:83-99, 1985.

30. American College of Sports Medicine: Encyclopedia of sports sciences and medicine, New York, 1971, Macmillan Publishing Co.

31. Woo R, et al: Regulation of energy balance, Ann Rev Nutr **5**:411-433, 1985.

32. Short SH, Short WR: Four-year study of university athletes' dietary intake, J Am Diet Assoc **82**:632-645, 1983.

33. Durnin JVGA, Passmore R: Energy, work, and leisure, London, 1967, William Heinemann Ltd.

34. Rahkila P, et al: Lipid metabolism during exercise, Eur J Appl Physiol **44**:245-254, 1980.

35. Davies CTM, Thompson MW: Aerobic performance of female marathon and male ultramarathon athletes, Eur J Appl Physiol **41**:233-245, 1979.

36. Felig P, et al: Hypoglycemia during prolonged exercise in normal men, N Engl J Med **306**:895-900, 1982.

37. Phinney SD, et al: The human metabolic response to chronic ketosis without caloric restriction: physical and biochemical adaptation, Metabolism **32**:757-768, 1983.

38. Wahren J, et al: Glucose metabolism during leg exercise in man, J Clin Invest **50**:2715-2725, 1971.

39. Phinney SD: The eucaloric ketogenic diet: human metabolic response with rest and exercise. Thesis for the degree of Doctor of Philosophy in nutritional biochemistry with metabolism, Massachusetts Institute of Technology, September 1980.

40. Winder WW: Regulation of hepatic glucose production during exercise, Exerc Sport Sci Rev **13**:1-31, 1985.

41. Wahren J, et al: Physical exercise and fuel homeostasis in diabetes mellitus, Diabetolog **14**:213-222, 1978.

42. Gibson H, Edwards RHT: Muscular exercise and fatigue, Sports Med **2**:120-132, 1985.

43. Jacobs I: Blood lactate: implication for training and sports performance, Sports Med **3**:10-25, 1986.

44. Costill DL: Carbohydrate nutrition before, during, and after exercise, Fed Proc **44**:364-368, 1985.

45. Fisher EC, et al: Changes in skeletal muscle metabolism induced by a eucaloric ketogenic diet. In Knuttgen HG, et al, editors: Biochemistry of exercise. International series on sports sciences, vol 13, Champaign Ill, 1983, Human Kinetics Publishers Inc.

46. Berger M: Metabolic diseases and exercise performance. In Knuttgen HG, et al: Biochemistry of exercise. International series on sports sciences, vol 13, Champaign Ill, 1983, Human Kinetics Publishers Inc.

47. Lewis SF, Haller RG: The pathophysiology of McArdle's disease: clues to regulation in exercise and fatigue, J Appl Physiol **61**:391-401, 1986.

48. Sherman WM: Carbohydrates, muscle glycogen, and muscle glycogen supercompensation. In Williams MH, editor: Ergogenic aids in sport, Champaign Ill, 1983, Human Kinetics Publishers Inc.

49. Sherman WM, Costill DL: The marathon: dietary manipulation to optimize performance, Am J Sports Med **12**:44-51, 1984.

50. Christensen E-H, Hansen O: Arbeitsfähigkeit und Ehrnährung, Scand Arch Physiol **81**:160-171, 1939.

51. Bergström J, Hultman E: Nutrition for maximal sports performance, JAMA **221**:999-1006, 1972.

52. Bergström J, et al: Diet, muscle glycogen, and physical performance, Acta Physiol Scand **71**:140-150, 1967.

53. Sherman WM, et al: Effects of exercise-diet manipulation on muscle glycogen and its subsequent utilization during performance, Int J Sports Med **2**:114-118, 1981.

54. Williams MH: Nutritional aspects of human physical and athletic performance, Springfield Ill, 1985, Charles C Thomas Publisher.

55. Jetté M, et al: The nutritional and metabolic effects of a carbohydrate-rich diet in a glycogen supercompensation training regimen, Am J Clin Nutr **31**:2140-2148, 1978.

56. Blair S, et al: Blood lipid and ECG responses to carbohydrate loading, Physician Sportsmed, vol 8, no 7, 1980.

57. Pruett EDR: Glucose and insulin during prolonged work stress in men living on different diets, J Appl Physiol **28**:199-208, 1970.

58. Coyle EF, et al: Carbohydrate feeding during prolonged strenuous exercise can delay fatigue, J Appl Physiol **55**:230-235, 1983.

59. Cahill GF: Hypoglycemia. In Rubenstein E, Federman DD, editors: Medicine, New York, 1987, Scientific American Books.

60. Foster D: From glycogen to ketones—and back, Diabetes **33**:1188-1199, 1984.

61. Katz J, McGarry JD: The glucose paradox: Is glucose a substrate for liver metabolism? J Clin Invest **74**:1901-1909, 1984.

62. Stanley WC, et al: Lactate extraction during net lactate release in legs of humans during exercise, J Appl Physiol **60**:1116-1120, 1986.

63. Brooks GA: The lactate shuttle during exercise and recovery, Med Sci Sports Exerc **18**:360-368, 1986.

64. Constable SH, et al: Glycogen resynthesis in leg muscles of rats during exercise, Am J Physiol **247**:R880-R883, 1984.

65. American College of Sports Medicine: Position statement: Prevention of heat injuries during distance running, Med Sci Sports **7**:7, 1975.

66. Parr RB: Nutrition and performance: carbohydrates, fluids, and pregame meal. In Butts NK, et al, editors: The elite athlete, New York, 1985, SP Medical & Scientific Books.

67. Devlin JT, et al: Effects of preexercise snack feeding on endurance cycle exercise, J Appl Physiol **60**:980-985, 1986.

68. Nilsson LH, Hultman E: Liver and muscle glycogen in man after glucose and fructose infusion, Scand J Clin Lab Invest **33**:5-10, 1974.

69. Richter EA, et al: Increased muscle glucose uptake after exercise. No need for insulin during exercise, Diabetes **34**:1041-1048, 1985.

70. Piehl K: Time course for refilling of glycogen stores in human muscle fibres following exercise induced glycogen depletion, Acta Physiol Scand **90**:297-302, 1974.

71. Costill DL, et al: The role of dietary carbohydrates in muscle glycogen resynthesis after strenuous running, Am J Clin Nutr **34**:1831-1836, 1981.

72. Karlsson J, Saltin B: Diet, muscle glycogen, and endurance performance, J Appl Physiol **31:**203-206, 1971.

73. Burke LM, Read RSD: Diet patterns of elite Australian male triathletes, Physician Sportsmed **15:**157-164, 1987.

74. Costill DL, Miller JM: Nutrition for endurance sports: carbohydrate and fluid balance, Int J Sports Med **1:**2-14, 1980.

75. Phinney SD, et al: The human response to chronic ketosis without caloric restriction: preservation of submaximal exercise capability with reduced carbohydrate oxidation, Metabolism **32:**769-776, 1983.

76. American Dietetic Association: Handbook of clinical dietetics, New Haven Conn, 1981, Yale University Press.

77. Arky RA, Perlman AJ: Hyperlipoproteinemia. In Rubenstein E, Federman DD, editors: Medicine, New York, 1987, Scientific American Books.

78. Björntorp P: Interrelation of physical activity and nutrition on obesity. In White PL, Mondeika T, editors: Diet and exercise, Chicago, 1982, American Medical Association.

79. Rahkila P, et al: Lipid metabolism during exercise. II. Respiratory exchange ratio and muscle glycogen content during 4 h bicycle ergometry in two groups of healthy men, Eur J Appl Physiol **44:**245-254, 1980.

80. Krogh A, Krogh M: A study of the diet and metabolism of Eskimos, Copenhagen, 1913, Bianco Luno.

81. Krogh A, Lindhard J: Relative value of fat and carbohydrate as sources of muscle energy, Biochem J **14:**290-317, 1920.

82. Marsh ME, Murlin JR: The muscular efficiency of high-carbohydrate and high-fat diets, J Nutr **1:**105-137, 1928.

83. Christensen EH, Hansen O: Zur Methodik der Respiratorischen Quotient-Bestimmungen in Ruhe und bei Arbeit. Scand Arch Physiol **81:**137-151, 1939.

84. Kark R, et al: Defects in pemmican as an emergency ration for infantry troops, War Med **8:**345-352, 1946.

85. Consolazio CF: Nutrition and performance, Prog Food Nutr Sci **7:**1-187, 1983.

86. Phinney SD, et al: Capacity for moderate exercise in obese subjects after adaptation to a hypocaloric, ketogenic diet, J Clin Invest **66:**1152-1161, 1980.

87. Gollnick PD: Metabolism of substrates: energy substrate metabolism during and as modified by training, Fed Proc **44:**353-357, 1985.

88. Holloszy JO, Coyle EF: Adaptations of skeletal muscle to endurance exercise and their metabolic consequences, J Appl Physiol **56:**831-838, 1984.

89. Reza MJ, et al: Recurrent myoglobinuria due to muscle carnitine palmityl transferase deficiency, Ann Intern Med **88:**610-615, 1978.

90. Sutton JR, et al: Exercise at altitude, Ann Rev Physiol **45:**427-437, 1983.

91. Hannon JP: Nutrition at high altitude. In Horvath SM, Yousef MK, editors: Environmental physiology: aging, heat, and altitude, New York, 1981, Elsevier/North-Holland.

92. Kronfeld DS: Diet and the performance of racing sled dogs, J Am Vet Med Assoc 162:470-473, 1973.

93. Stefansson V: The fat of the land, New York, 1956, The Macmillan Co.

94. Casstenfors J, et al: Effect of prolonged heavy exercise on renal function and urinary protein excretion, Acta Physiol Scand **70:**194-206, 1967.

95. Poortmans JR: Postexercise proteinuria in humans, JAMA **253:**236-240, 1985.

96. Costill F, et al: Acid-base balance during repeated bouts of exercise: influence of HCO_3, Int J Sports Med **5:**228-231, 1984.

97. Shephard RJ: Effects of cardiac disease upon pulmonary function during exercise, J Sports Med Phys Fitness **22:**314-322, 1982.

98. Gisolfi CV, Wenger CB: Temperature regulation during exercise: old concepts, new ideas, Exerc Sport Sci Rev **12:**339-372, 1984.

99. Bar-Or O: Pediatric sports medicine for the practitioner: from physiologic principles to clinical applications, New York, 1983, Springer-Verlag New York Inc, pp 1-65.

100. Åstrand PO, et al: Disposal of lactate during and after strenuous exercise in humans, Bethesda, 1986, American Physiological Society, pp 338-343.

101. Costill DL, Saltin B: Factors limiting gastric emptying rest and exercise, J Applied Physiol **37:**679-683, 1974.

102. Williams LR, et al: Effects of exercise on choice reaction latency and movement speed, Percept Mot Skills **60:**67-71, 1985.

103. Gisolfi CV, Copping JR: Thermal effects of prolonged treadmill exercise in the heat, Med Sci Sports Exerc **6:**108-113, 1974.

104. Noakes TD, et al: Physiological and biochemical measurements during a 4-day surf-ski marathon, S Afr Med J **67:**212-216, 1985.

105. Frizzell RT, et al: Hyponatremia and ultramarathon running, JAMA **255:**772-774, 1986.

106. Williams B: Nutritional aspects of exercise-induced fatigue, Proc Nutr Soc **44:**245-256, 1985.

CHAPTER 43

Nutritional Value of Foods and the Elements of an Adequate Diet

Johanna T. Dwyer

The nutritional management of a patient depends on a knowledge of the nutritional value of diets, the standards employed, and the patient's specific requirements.

The nutritional value of diets depends primarily on amount and quality in matching human needs for the 45 required nutrients with the nutrients provided by foods in the diet. Besides meeting these criteria, foods must be wholesome and safe (i.e., free from microbial or chemical hazards) and palatable enough that they are eaten.

The food groups differ in two major ways. First, the energy value of foods in each group varies. Fruits and vegetables average about 50 calories per serving; breads and cereals about 100 calories; milk and milk substitutes about 150 calories; and meat, poultry, fish, and eggs about 250 calories. Even when foods are compared on a weight basis for their caloric contributions, their caloric densities are quite different. Second, the groups differ in their nutrient densities—the ratio of nutrients to the energy they supply. Fruits and vegetables have relatively high nutrient densities for carbohydrate, ascorbic acid, and vitamin A but are relatively low in protein and fat. Breads and cereals have high nutrient densities for carbohydrate, several of the B vitamins, iron, and protein but are low in fat. Milk is relatively high in nutrient density for calcium, riboflavin, protein, fat, niacin, and vitamin B_{12}. Meat, poultry, fish, eggs, and beans are relatively high in nutrient density for protein, vitamin B_6, and other macronutrients.

CALORIC DENSITY

Caloric density describes the energy value of food in relation to its weight. For example, the caloric density of sugar is 4 kcal/g, of cooking fat 9 kcal/g, of purified protein 4 kcal/g, and of breast milk 0.7 kcal/g. Because most foods contain substantial amounts of water, other noncaloric or indigestible substances such as dietary fiber, and macronutrients, caloric densities vary widely, from 0.1 to 9 kcal/g depending upon their composition.[1,2]

People do not require diets of specific caloric density. We eat for energy not for bulk; and within the normal range of caloric density in diets, it is possible to meet energy needs by adjusting the quantity of foods eaten. However, caloric density does have practical significance in cases of extremes. For example, on very dilute weaning diets such as maize-based paps (a dietary staple for infants in developing countries), stomach capacity may be reached quickly. Unless feedings are frequent, the amount eaten may fall short of energy requirements. At the other extreme, diets of very high caloric density often are fed to patients too weak to eat usual foods so as to limit the effort required to take in enough to meet energy needs.

Depending on the combination of food groups chosen (and the caloric density of individual foods within these groups), the caloric density of overall diets can vary considerably. In an affluent society, people eat not only because of hunger but also because of habit and for social and situational reasons. Since the volume of high–caloric density foods is lower than that of low–caloric density foods, it is easier to exceed energy needs on such regimens, especially if the foods are also high in sensory appeal. For this reason foods high in caloric density are especially perilous to those who have problems controlling their weight.

It has recently been suggested[3] that diets high in fiber and bulk and low in caloric density may improve regulation of the amount of food eaten, thus helping to prevent obesity in adults; however, this remains to be demonstrated conclusively.

NUTRIENT DENSITY

Nutrient density is the ratio of nutrients to energy in a food. It is a simplified way of comparing the nutritive values in foods.

U.S. Recommended Dietary Allowances

The usual standards for describing human nutrient needs are the Recommended Dietary Allowances (RDAs).[4] Because so many nutrients are involved, interrelationships among amounts of the nutrients also may be important. As a result, succinct statements about nutrient needs are difficult to make using these tables. In addition, recommendations for nutrient needs vary by age, sex, and physiologic group. Some of these variations are not meaningful from the statistical standpoint, because estimates of requirements for most macronutrients are imprecise and margins of error by age and sex groups are large. To formulate a reference standard that would assure coverage of the group with the highest needs for each nutrient of interest, the highest recommended level of each nutrient can be used in a composite profile of nutrient needs. Such a reference profile currently is used for the standard of comparison on foods labeled for their nutrient content; it is referred to as the U.S. Recommended Dietary Allowance (USRDA). The USRDA for adults is based on the 1968 RDAs for men, which represent the highest nutrient recommendations. The only exception is iron, for which a higher recommendation for women is used. Currently food labeling includes percentages of the USRDAs for protein, vitamins A and C, riboflavin, niacin, calcium, and iron. For purposes other than labeling, comparisons of additional nutrients can be made.

Index of Nutritional Quality

The Index of Nutritional Quality (INQ) is the ratio of the nutrient composition of a diet or a specific food to the nutrient needs of people insofar as such needs are known. The common denominator of these comparisons is energy. The standard for nutrient needs is usually the USRDA, which normally is expressed per 1000 calories (kcal). Further simplification is possible if nutrient needs are expressed simply in terms of nutrient density, but this assumes that energy

supplies are adequate. From the nutritional standpoint, energy needs are particularly important because virtually all bodily functions require energy, and health cannot be sustained without it. In addition, the need for some nutrients, such as protein and thiamine, depends on the extent to which energy needs are met.

Healthy Americans normally fulfill their energy requirement easily, since hunger and satiety are driven automatically by energy need and appetite functions to achieve this outcome. Although the amounts of energy required to maintain good health vary among different groups in the population, the U.S. minimum average energy needs normally are met. When this assumption is made, needs for other nutrients can be expressed per kilocalorie of energy required. This procedure is helpful in comparing nutrient needs of various physiologic groups and in assessing how well diets or individual foods meet nutrient needs.

It is reasonable from the physiologic standpoint to express the nutrient content of foods and diets in relation to energy, since people eat primarily for energy and obtain other nutrients incidentally in the process. When energy needs are not met, there is usually a shortage of other nutrients. Moreover, the individual's need for energy is a minimum average requirement sufficient for energy balance or growth, and deviations from this requirement can be ascertained easily at the clinical level. Recommendations for other nutrients cover a somewhat broader range between the points at which sufficiency and excess are reached. Finally, linking nutrient needs to energy ensures that protein/calorie ratios will be sufficient for protein to be utilized for its unique functions rather than solely as a source of energy.

NUTRIENT DENSITIES OF FOOD GROUPS AND INDIVIDUAL FOODS

The practical use of nutrient density calculations lies in the fact that there is no guarantee that when energy needs are met, other nutrients in the diet will be adequate. Neither diets nor individual foods necessarily supply nutrients in the exact ratios to the body's energy needs. Nutrient density calculations can help identify shortages of specific nutrients. For example, the amount of a nutrient such as iron is calculated per kcal and compared to the USRDA stated in the same units. If all of the RDA for iron is met, the nutrient density will be exactly 1. If the diet provides more than the RDA per kcal, the nutrient density is greater than 1; if the diet provides less than the RDA per kcal, the nutrient density is less than 1.

Estimates of nutrient density for each nutrient for which there is an RDA also can be calculated for individual foods or groups of foods. By grouping foods with similar nutrient density profiles, some foods emerge as especially rich sources of certain nutrients in relation to the calories they provide, while others do not.

Low–Nutrient Density Foods

Food groups with densities of less than 1 for most nutrients do not "carry their weight" compared to the calories they provide. Low–nutrient density foods include sweets, soft drinks, alcoholic beverages, most fats and oils, sugar, gum, and many candies.

High–Nutrient Density Foods

Very few foods have "perfect" nutrient profiles of 1 for every nutrient. Foods with density ratios higher than 1 for many nutrients or those that are particularly rich sources of a few key nutrients are referred to as high–nutrient density foods. Examples include many items in the basic four food groups (milk and milk products; breads and cereals; meat, poultry, fish, eggs, and beans; fruits and vegetables). When such foods are consumed in a form close to their natural state, without added high-calorie recipe alterations, they are especially likely to be of high nutrient density.

COMPOSITE INDICES OF NUTRITIONAL QUALITY

There is no generally agreed-upon procedure for combining the nutrient density scores for the nutrients in foods into a composite index of nutritional quality. For a more detailed picture of a given food's overall benefits in meeting nutrient needs, it is necessary to consider the food's caloric contribution, how often it is eaten, the amount eaten, and the nutrient contributions of the rest of the diet. Other criteria, such as availability, cost, and likeability of the food, are also important, since even the most theoretically perfect foods are of no nutritional significance until people eat them.

"Junk" Foods

Foods that are relatively high in caloric density but low in nutrient density sometimes are referred to as "junk" foods. Although they may have redeeming sensory or aesthetic attributes, from the standpoint of nutritional value there is little basis for recommending them to a population whose major diet-related difficulty is getting too many calories. Examples include soft drinks, alcoholic beverages, most fats and oils, sugar, most candies, and sweets.

"Protective" Foods

Foods that are particularly high in nutrient density for specific nutrients or groups of nutrients not distributed uniformly in most dietary items sometimes are referred to as "protective" foods, because they protect against dietary inadequacy. Examples include dark green and deep yellow vegetables, which are good sources of vitamin A; citrus fruits, which are good sources of vitamin C; and milk and milk products, which are rich sources of riboflavin, calcium, and vitamin D. Their caloric densities vary from high to low. It should be noted that nutritionists do not apply this term automatically to "health," "natural," or "organic" foods, which may or may not possess such properties.

Bulky Foods

Solid foods that are relatively low in caloric density and contain large amounts of fiber or other indigestible components and water sometimes are referred to as bulky foods. They may be high or low in nutrient density.

DIETARY CONSIDERATIONS

Since the usual American diet consists of hundreds of items rather than a few staple foods, the overall nutrient profile of diets in comparison to human needs rather than the profiles of specific foods of high- or low-nutrient density is important in determining nutritional health. "Health" or "natural" foods that may be high in nutrient density, megadoses of nutrients, or nutritional remodeling of specific foods by fortification, enrichment, or alterations in their nutrient composition are not synonymous with nutritional improvement. Improvement is likely only when an unfilled nutrient need exists and such foods (food vehicles chosen to carry the additional nutrients) are consumed in sufficient amount often enough to provide levels of the nutrient that meet human needs better than ordinary diets. All too often one or more of these preconditions is not met, and alternative diets fail to achieve their objectives.

In the past decade health scientists have become more sophisticated in assessing the nutritional adequacy of diets and in developing better methods for nutritional surveillance.[5,6] At the same time the realization has grown that nutrient adequacy alone is not enough, that balance, variety, and moderation to avoid consuming excessive amounts of nutrients also are needed. A number of guides can be used to help patients achieve nutrient adequacy while avoiding excess in their food choices.[7-10]

REFERENCES

1. Merrill AL, Watt BK: Human Nutrition Research Branch, United States Department of Agriculture: Energy value of foods; basis and derivation, Agriculture Handbook 74, Washington DC, 1955, Government Printing Office.
2. Southgate DAT, Durnin JVGA: Calorie conversion factors; an experimental reassessment of the factors used in calculation of the energy value of human diets, Br J Nutr **24:**517-535, 1970.
3. Bray GA: Obesity: a disease of nutrient or energy balance? Nutr Rev **45:**33-43, 1987.
4. Committee on Dietary Allowances, Food and Nutrition Board, National Research Council: Recommended dietary allowance, ed 9, Washington DC, 1980, National Academy of Sciences.
5. Subcommittee on Criteria for Dietary Evaluation, Coordinating Committee on Evaluation of Food Consumption Surveys, Food and Nutrition Board, National Research Council: Nutrient adequacy: assessment using food consumption surveys, Washington DC, 1986, National Academy of Sciences.
6. Mason JB, et al: Nutritional surveillance, Geneva, 1984, World Health Organization.
7. United States Department of Agriculture and Department of Health and Human Services: Nutrition and your health: dietary guidelines for Americans, Washington DC, 1985, Government Printing Office.
8. Science and Education Administration, Human Nutrition, United States Department of Agriculture: Ideas for better eating: menus and recipes to make use of the dietary guidelines, Washington DC, 1981, Government Printing Office.
9. American National Red Cross: Better eating for better health; participant's guide, Washington DC, 1984, The American Red Cross.
10. Eat better, live better: a commonsense guide to nutrition and good health, Pleasantville NY, 1982, The Reader's Digest Association.

CHAPTER 44

Behavioral, Cultural, and Environmental Influences on Dietary Practices

Phyllis L. Fleming

Eating always involves choices, often from an array of alternatives. People can choose to eat or not to eat, to use butter or margarine, to order prime rib or broiled fish. To understand eating behavior, health professionals must know what the alternatives are, identify the pressures and influences at work in a situation, and recognize the factors that motivate and drive a person. The purpose of this chapter is to provide health professionals with a framework for clarifying the elements involved in eating behavior.

LIFE-STYLE AND ITS RELATIONSHIP TO EATING BEHAVIOR

Eating behavior is embedded in life-style. A health professional who advises a patient to lose weight quickly learns that changing energy balance is not simply a matter of eating less. It is linked to other life-style components, including whether and how much the patient exercises, expends energy on the job, socializes, cooks, eats others' cooking, smokes, drinks alcoholic beverages, and uses leisure time for sedentary activities.

Eating behavior evolves as a result of environmental, cultural, social, and personal influences. These influences act as a series of screens through which potentially edible substances must pass to reach the point of consumption. The screens are diagrammed in the model of food consumption in Fig. 44-1.

Like other life-style components, eating behavior is stable because it serves the individual in some way. For example, potato chips may be an available quick breakfast for a teenager late for school. Gelatin dessert requires little chewing

for an elderly person having trouble with dentures. Frankfurters are a popular alternative for a busy parent facing hungry children after a full day at work. A beautiful array of cheeses served at a cocktail party for corporate officers poses a strong temptation for a junior executive trying to control lipid intake. In each case the nutrition or healthfulness of the food may be secondary to a more important function the food serves.

Because eating behavior is functional, stable, and connected to other aspects of a patient's life, it can be difficult to change to healthier habits. However, understanding eating behavior in terms of a person's life-style and its influences can provide the key to successful nutrition management.

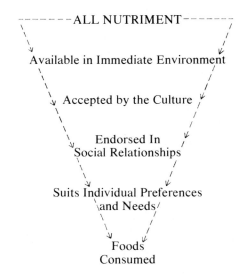

Figure 44-1 Factors that influence individual food choices.

ENVIRONMENT

Environment determines the availability of food. In hunting and gathering cultures and in famine-stricken areas of the world, environment limits alternatives and therefore dictates eating behavior. Environmental factors influence eating behavior in wealthier societies as well. Supermarkets, restaurants, and fast-food outlets offer an array of alternatives from which to choose.

The availability of food in the home is also an issue, and responsible weight reduction programs recognize this; dieters are cautioned not to allow unhealthy ready-to-eat foods or snacks in the house and to keep low-calorie alternatives on hand. What is available may get eaten.

The cost of food also influences its availability. Food choices fluctuate with food prices. In a national survey the most frequently mentioned problem facing families was coping with the high cost of food. Some families said they had to postpone or cut back on buying high quality food, on serving meat at every meal, and on serving fresh fruits or vegetables.[1] For these families, then, cost prevented some foods from reaching the table.

The amount of time that must be spent shopping for and preparing food influences its availability as well. Some diet regimens are difficult to follow, such as the Feingold diet for hyperactive children. Some programs require foods not readily available in supermarkets and restaurants; others call for nutrients disguised behind complicated nutrition labeling or for lengthy and involved preparation techniques.

Environment also influences eating by presenting cues that stimulate the desire to eat, and sometimes to eat specific foods. Advertisements concoct tantalizing images of food, of pleasant situations in which food is eaten, and of good feelings that come with eating. Cues in the immediate environment trigger eating behavior more directly. For a child, arriving home from school may signal a peanut butter sandwich, just as watching a ball game on television may trigger his father's desire for popcorn and beer.

Behavior modification programs designed for weight reduction recognize the impact of environment on eating behavior. The guiding principle of these programs, which is applicable to other diet modification regimens, is to change the environmental cues to eating in the hope of changing the eating behavior as well. Sugges-

tions for changing cues include portioning food on plates in the kitchen rather than serving family-style at the table (which allows second helpings); reducing the amount of time spent in the kitchen; avoiding making the kitchen a family room; eating only when the table is completely set; storing food in opaque containers and out of sight; shopping for and preparing food only when the impact of cues to eat is likely to be minimal (e.g., shopping for food soon after eating and preparing food for the next meal just after eating the previous meal); and, when the urge to eat strikes, starting an activity that makes it impossible to eat, such as taking a shower.[2]

CULTURAL FACTORS

Americans eat beyond hunger. With estimates of obesity among adult Americans as high as 40%, it is apparent that eating is a response to more than a physiologic need. Yet, although we may eat more food than our bodies require, we do not eat all edible foods. Culture intervenes to define which foods are acceptable and appropriate. It also may define what times of the day we feel hungry.[3]

Eating is a cultural phenomenon, part of an interwoven cultural fabric. A useful example of food's interrelationship with other cultural phenomena comes from work in the Pholela Health Center, which is located on a Zulu reserve in the Republic of South Africa. Among the Zulus the diets of mothers and children consisted primarily of corn supplemented with dried beans, small amounts of meat, milk, wild greens, potatoes, and pumpkins—a diet too low in some nutrients to promote adequate growth, development, and good health. The supply of milk was limited. When girls reached puberty, they drank no milk at all because it was believed that during menstruation and pregnancy, women exerted evil influences on cattle if they had any contact with them, including drinking milk. Although the precise reasons for the milk taboo were lost, cattle were thought to be a link between a man and his ancestors. Nothing was to interfere with that link. Therefore members of a kin group could drink milk only from cattle owned by the kin group. At marriage a woman left her own kin group to live with her husband's group, where she could not drink the milk.

Health workers recognized that women during their reproductive years, as well as their children, would benefit from drinking more milk. The challenge was to introduce milk without ripping the cultural fabric. This was achieved by encouraging the people to drink powdered milk made from cows belonging to people outside the community. Over a 12-year period, the demand outstripped the supply. In a number of more educated families on the reserve, women eventually were allowed to drink milk from family cows without marked reaction from the community.[4]

Closer to home, the "Americanization" of ethnic families pointed up the interwoven nature of cultural phenomena. As young people adopted American ways, they also adopted middle-class values. Traditional life-styles gave way to the pursuit of job advancement, accompanied by work-related stress, and to bigger homes away from the ethnic enclave. This led to weakened family support systems. Health problems expected with the life-style changes also appeared.[5]

Broad cultural values, standards, and norms influence how Americans eat and when and why they eat. Food is used to express friendship and hospitality. The apple for the teacher, the potluck social, the box of chocolates for a special valentine, and the pot of coffee "always on the stove" are accepted gestures of friendship. Food is also used to express sympathy during an illness or death. It accompanies the celebration of holidays like Thanksgiving, Christmas, and Passover.

Food can also reflect wealth, power, and status. Exclusive restaurants, prime cuts of meat, fresh fruits and vegetables out of season, and exotic ingredients associated with gourmet cooking convey images of sophistication, affluence, and influence. As these images emerge, social boundaries are delineated. Just as food patterns can define high status, they can stigmatize low-status groups on the periphery of the community. A study of the food patterns in a rural Illinois community showed that headcheese for a German-American subgroup and fish for poor people who lived by the river symbolized their low status.[6] In this community, members of a low-status subcultural group tried to eat the same kinds of foods as a higher-status group. Implicit in this was the notion that people who eat like the group to which they aspire have the right to identify with that group. Similar observations have been made among people who changed to vegetarian or food-fad eating patterns. Eating like the group

to which persons aspire provides a psychologic entree into the group.

A cursory look at current food patterns leads to the tentative conclusion that the American diet is fairly consistent throughtout the country. Judging from the appearance of major thoroughfares, it is easy to conclude that the American diet consists uniformly of hamburgers, colas, french fries, fried chicken, and pizza. The more than $19 billion spent on fast foods each year reinforces this conclusion. The results of the 1977 Household Food Consumption Survey also support the impression of increasing similarity. The survey showed that the gap between the diets of high-income groups and low-income groups narrowed considerably between 1965 and 1977.[7]

Assumptions about homogeneity for each individual should not be made too quickly, however. Even though more people than ever before are eating in regular and fast-food restaurants, between 40% and 60% of all meals are eaten at home. These meals are more likely to bear the imprint of subcultural differences, if they exist. Nevertheless, a study of food habits among low-income black families in Milwaukee[8] showed that despite apparent homogeneity of this subcultural group, there were differences in the amount of money spent on food, in the consumption of certain kinds of foods, particularly citrus fruits and green vegetables, and in the maintenance of rural Southern food patterns.

From a cultural point of view, an adequate diet is one that recognizes and respects culturally determined classifications of edible and inedible substances. An adequate diet does not require a Moslem to eat pork or a Hindu to eat beef; nor does it impose milk on groups that don't drink milk or strange new foods on a group unfamiliar with them.

More subtly, an adequate diet adapts to existing culturally guided food patterns. The seeming uniformity of the American diet is partly an illusion. To be sure, consumption of fast foods, convenience foods, and soft drinks is high and increasing; however, the role of food in defining group boundaries and distinctiveness should not be overlooked. This is especially true in planning dietary changes.

A low-calorie diet for a Greek American, for example, would take advantage of several common group preferences, such as including raw vegetable salads as important parts of every meal, using fruit for dessert and snacks, and avoiding butter on bread or cream in coffee. Yogurt made with nonfat dry milk might be recommended as a substitute for higher-fat dairy products. Reducing the amount of butter and oil used in cooking vegetables might be encouraged.[9] Similarly, counseling aimed at Spanish-speaking people should carefully distinguish among Mexicans, Puerto Ricans, Cubans, and Central and South Americans, since dietary patterns for each group are distinct.[10]

Uniformity should not be assumed; if nutrition counseling is to succeed, the possibility of cultural distinctions must be examined carefully.

SOCIAL FACTORS

The health professional usually encounters an individual patient who needs nutrition counseling. This individual becomes the focus of a nutrition management and counseling program, and appropriately so. Nutrition counseling is more effective, however, when the individual's involvement in social networks is recognized as well. Social networks can influence when and why a person eats, and they represent potent sources of support or resistance for proposed changes.

From infancy, food serves as a significant means of communication. For a howling, hungry infant, food initially assuages hunger pains and provides a sense of relief and well-being. When food is accompanied by snuggling with another warm person who coos, strokes, and rocks, food begins to represent the security, love, and comfort that comes with social interaction. From the parental point of view, offering an abundance of good food to a child can express concern, responsibility, and affection as well. Food marketers exploit the expressive capacities of food to sell all kinds of products, from vitamin-fortified soft drinks to commercially baked cupcakes. Typically the message is: Parents who love their children will give them product X.

Food is an important means of relating within families.[11,12] It is offered as an incentive or disincentive in some relationships. Proposing candy, ice cream, or snack food as a reward for desired behavior is seen as an effective incentive for some children. The parent who sends a child to bed without dinner is expressing very clearly a power differential in the family. It is not uncommon to hear stories of parents supplying their children with fast-food feasts to assure the children that they are loved and to compensate for the lack of time and attention spent on them.

Food and its capacity to communicate take on excessive importance in some families. In psychologic observations of obese adolescents undergoing starvation treatment, mothers spoke of the gratification they felt when their children ate well and indicated they made certain that ample amounts of food were available. Gifts of food, particularly sweets, were used as rewards and expressions of attention.[13]

Food is a vehicle for communicating and expressing relationships outside the family as well. Gifts of food and invitations to share food can express thanks, friendship, interest, and caring. Such gifts and invitations are ways of building and supporting social networks. For the health professional, these networks may influence how a person defines and describes symptoms and responds to diagnosis and recommendations for treatment. Family, friends, and neighbors often help a person decide whether prescribed changes in eating habits—for example, to cut back on foods high in fat or to increase foods high in fiber—make sense and are appropriate. When recommendations coincide with network norms and values, the networks become important sources of social support and help to enforce the recommendations. When recommendations run counter to network norms and values, the networks become equally important sources of sabotage.[14]

If those in a patient's social network are not supportive, ad hoc support groups may provide valuable reinforcement for prescribed changes in behavior. The success of support groups in encouraging and promoting eating behavior has varied, but certainly the popularity of groups such as Weight Watchers and Overeaters Anonymous attests to the value of social support. People involved in diet modification have shown varying levels of dependence on support groups. Sincere statements of, "I owe it all to the group," suggest that successful maintenance of diet changes may require a group weaning process, allowing the individual to attribute success to his or her own efforts as well.

The patient in the health professional's office may represent only the tip of a social iceberg. The probability of successfully changing eating behavior is enhanced by taking into account the influences of important social relationships and networks.

PERSONAL PREFERENCES AND MOTIVATIONS

When people are asked why they eat the foods they do, the most frequent response is that the food tastes good. For many people, eating is an obvious source of pleasure, which may take precedence over good nutrition. An adequate diet, even if it involves some deprivation, such as cutting calories or decreasing salt, must be appetizing if it is to become part of a habitual change in life-style.

Taste preferences are probably environmental, cultural, and social in origin. For example, research has linked children's preferences with the availability of food[15] and the preferences of their parents.[16] Once these preferences are in place, they exert an influence that must be dealt with in efforts to change behavior.

Besides satisfying tastebuds, food can serve other functions for an individual. People who are ill or have symptoms of illness have reason to heed recommendations for changes in eating behavior.[17,18] They may turn optimistically to those changes as ways of solving their problems. Even with strong motivation and expert guidance, changing comfortable, established, pleasant eating behaviors is not easy. The environmental, cultural, social, and personal pressures remain.

For people who are at risk of future problems or for whom a preventive, healthy life-style would be prudent, the motivation for making recommended changes is less clear. Why should a healthy 25-year-old women worry about calcium or fiber? Why should a 40-year-old man who feels fine bother about taking off the 15 pounds that began accumulating 10 years ago? For these people the link between sound nutrition and good health may not be compelling; for them, other functions of food and eating may take precedence.

Because eating habits serve other functions besides satisfying hunger and supporting health, they often resist change. Eating patterns are a means of expressing a sense of self. Foods must not only satisfy hunger, they must also be congruent with a person's sense of identity. Whether the connotation is a fine palate or concern for world hunger expressed by eating lower on the food chain, we know more about a person by associating him or her with the label "gourmet" or "vegetarian" than if we had no label at all. People may also try to convey messages about their identity by adopting food patterns that express satisfaction or dissatisfaction with food producers' politics; for example, boycotting foods or products marketed by companies with whose actions they disagree. Some people may reject the eating patterns of their subcultural group or the "typical" American diet in a mood of rebellion.

People also may turn to food as a source of health or even superhealth, as a defense against the aging process or the threats of environmental hazards or carcinogens (e.g., oat fiber, amaranth flour, fish oil, bee pollen). Dietary regimens or particular foods in these cases may provide a sense of security and stability or serve as defense mechanisms in a threatening world.

Nutrition counselors must understand that sound nutrition information may be unpleasant, threatening, promising, or supportive. An array of values competes with the value of health. A patient's perceptions of recommendations to change eating behavior may range from panacea to doom. Logical arguments and factual presentation of the information may not work if the patient responds by protecting his or her personal needs and the food patterns that fulfill those needs.

To succeed in their efforts, nutrition counselors must also recognize that even with strong motivation to change, some people have trouble changing because they doubt their ability to do so. Research on successful attempts to change health behaviors, including eating, exercise, and smoking, has shown consistently the importance of people believing in their ability to make the changes required of them. This personal conviction has been labeled self-efficacy.[19-21] The nutrition counselor must develop and reinforce the patient's sense that the recommended changes in eating behavior not only are possible but also that the patient can make them.

REFERENCES

1. American family report, 1978-1979: family health in an era of stress, Minneapolis, 1979, General Mills Inc.
2. Bellack AS: Behavioral treatment of obesity: appraisal and recommendations, Prog Behav Modif **4:**1-18, 1977.
3. Foster GM: Medical anthropology, New York, 1978, John Wiley & Sons Inc, p 266.
4. Cassel J: Social and cultural implications of food and food habits, Am J Public Health **47:**732-740, 1957.
5. Greenberg J: The americanization of Roseto, Sci News **113:**378-782, 1978.
6. Bennett JW: Food and social status in a rural society, Am Sociol Rev **8:**561-569, 1943.
7. Gap narrowing between diets of rich and poor, Commun Nutr Institute Newsletter **9:**6-7, 1979.
8. Jerome N: Food consumption patterns in relation to life style of in-migrant Negro families [discussion paper], Madison Wisc, Institute for Research on Poverty, 1971.
9. Valassi KV: Food habits of Greek-Americans, Am J Clin Nutr **11:**240-248, 1962.
10. Yohai F: Dietary patterns of Spanish-speaking people living in the Boston area, J Am Diet Assoc **71:**273-275, 1977.
11. Frankle RT: Obesity a family matter: creating new behavior, J Am Diet Assoc **85:**597-601, 1985.
12. Schafer RB, Keith PM: Influences on food decisions across the family life cycle, J Am Diet Assoc **78:**144-147, 1981.
13. Nathan S, Pisula D: Psychological observations of obese adolescents during starvation treatment, J Am Acad Child Psychiatry **9:**722-740, 1970.
14. Friedson E: Client control and medical practice, Am J Sociol **65:**374-383, 1960.
15. Davis CJ: Self-selection of diet experiments: its significance for feeding in the home, Ohio State Med J **34:**862-868, 1938.
16. Olson CM, et al: Parent-child interaction: its relation to growth and weight, J Nutr Ed **8:**67-70, 1972.
17. Eraker SA, et al: Smoking behavior, cessation techniques, and the health belief model, Am J Med **78:**817, 1985.
18. Ockene JK, Camic PM: Public health approaches to cigarette smoking cessation, Ann Behav Med **7:**14-18, 1985.
19. O'Leary A: Self-efficacy and health behavior, Behav Res Ther **23:**437-451, 1985.
20. Supnick JA, Coletti G: Relapse coping and problem solving training following treatment for smoking, Addic Behav **9:**401-404, 1984.
21. Rosenstock IM: Understanding and enhancing patient compliance with diabetic regimens, Diabetes Care **8:**610-616, 1985.

CHAPTER 45

Vegetarianism and Other Alternative Dietary Practices

Johanna T. Dwyer

VEGETARIANISM

Interest in vegetarianism is high today, not because it represents a widespread eating style but because many people see it as a healthy way to eat and a means to reduce their risk of some diseases, such as atherosclerosis and hypertension. Many vegetarians tend to be vigorous advocates of this way of eating. However, vegetarian diets require careful planning if health risks are to be minimized and health benefits maximized. Some vegetarians fail to plan their diets using sound nutritional principles, or they put undue emphasis on diets while neglecting health care. Physicians who are unfamiliar with the special characteristics of vegetarian regimens may fail to recognize untoward effects on nutritional health status. Thus they must be equipped to provide dietary advice, encourage ongoing health supervision, and recognize diet-related difficulties that may arise among vegetarians.

Types of Vegetarians

Vegetarianism is the consumption of a diet composed predominantly of plant foods. In Western countries the reasons for eating in this manner are most frequently philosophic, religious, or health-related rather than primarily cultural or economic. Although vegetarianism has grown in the United States in the past decade, particularly among young adults, it still involves probably less than 1% of the total population. Vegans, who avoid all animal foods, constitute a tiny minority of vegetarians.

The term vegetarianism suggests a uniformity of diet that does not exist among the disparate groups eating in this manner. Nutritionists therefore describe the extent to which vegetarians avoid animal foods by the types of animal foods left in their diets.[1] *Vegans* abstain from all forms of animal foods (e.g., red meat, poultry, fish and seafood, eggs, dairy products). *Lactovegetarians,* such as Trappist monks, add only milk. *Lactoovovegetarians,* such as Seventh Day Adventists, add milk and eggs. Other new vegetarian patterns almost always involve abstinence from red meat and poultry but may incorporate some other animal foods. These include lactovegetarianism as practiced by the Hare Krishnas and certain yogic groups, and vegan-like vegetarianism using small amounts of animal foods as condiments (e.g., that practiced by macrobiotics).[2,3]

However, a classification that concentrates solely on the kinds of animal foods eaten or the lack thereof does not adequately describe other alterations that influence the diets and nutritional status of American vegetarians. In one study of vegetarian adults,[4] fully 92% claimed that they also avoided some foods (animal and other) which they considered "processed," not "natural," or not organically grown. The extent of these other food avoidances, as with the animal food avoidances, appears to range from the extremists (who consume only raw plant foods or reject certain plant foods [cereals, legumes, fruits, vegetables] if not organically grown) to moderates (who avoid such products as refined sugar or commercially formulated foods). These preferences appear to be especially common among people who have but recently adopted vegetarianism. Their diets usually include health foods that they believe have special potencies to promote health or prevent disease (miso, ginseng, tofu, tempeh, herbal teas). A smaller but also sizable group of vegetarians, including many Seventh-Day Adventists, use vitamin-mineral supplements or specially fortified products on a regular basis.[5] New vegetarians vary from totally avoiding supplements to using megadoses of one or more nutrients.[6]

Vegetarians also vary in the extent and strength of their dietary group affiliations with various philosophic, religious, or quasireligious sects or cults that have disparate views and practices related to health. Traditional vegetarian groups, such as the Seventh-Day Adventists and Trappist monks, generally differ little from nonvegetarians except in not using tobacco, alcohol, and caffeine and in their religious commitment. In contrast, membership in groups (e.g., macrobiotics, Zen buddhists, Hare Krishnas, raw food eaters, some yogics) is associated not only with religious fervor and avoidance of tobacco, alcohol, caffeine, and drugs but also with negative attitudes toward orthodox or "Western" health care services and reliance on homeopaths or lay healers for all but the most serious illnesses.[2,3,7,8] Although these new vegetarian groups may be quite different from more traditional vegetarian groups in their life-styles, they are so heterogeneous that even within some dietary groups generalization is hazardous.

Other Americans periodically or habitually adopt semivegetarian eating styles. They consume some but not all groups of animal foods other than meat but usually in rather limited amounts. In the strict sense they are not vegetarians, since they eat flesh foods, but they often regard themselves as vegetarians. The dietary practices of semivegetarians often differ in other respects from those of traditional vegetarians.[1] Semivegetarians frequently are motivated solely by a desire to achieve a "healthy" diet; therefore they adopt a diet that is low in red meat and other animal foods in the belief that it will be low in fat, saturated fat, and cholesterol and high in dietary fiber.[9-12]

Health Effects

Mortality among some groups of vegetarians is lower than among nonvegetarians, especially for disorders caused by smoking and alcohol. It is likely that, rather than vegetarianism per se, the healthy life-styles associated with many vegetarian patterns account for a number of the observed differences in mortality.[13-15] Although some vegetarian life-styles and diets appear to be healthier than those of nonvegetarians, others seem less so.[16,17] Summaries of the current state of knowledge with respect to the health effects of vegetarian diets[2,6,18-22] are available, and major findings from them will be discussed.

Traditional vegetarian diets and moderate avoidance of animal foods pose fewer risks than do some of the newer regimens or vegan diets that involve extensive food avoidances and self-treatment of health problems.[2,6,18-22] Because different types of vegetarian diets predispose a person to different risks and benefits, the physician must establish exactly what is being eaten before deciding what to investigate further. Some factors useful in evaluating the vegetarian's health status are presented in the box on p. 730.

The basic problem with diets based largely on plants is that sources of some essential nutrients are extremely limited unless the diet is carefully planned.[23-25] When, in addition, "processed" foods or vitamin-mineral supplements are avoided, the probability decreases that all nutrient needs will be met. When such people also fail to seek medical care, health problems may not come to the attention of health professionals until they are serious. Vegans' philosophies and life-styles often differ from those of the general population, and they may experience dietary inadequacies and ill health.[26-29] Lactoovovegetarians or lactovegetarians appear to be less susceptible to such deficiencies, but it is difficult to evaluate dietary adequacy or inadequacy without a dietary history and knowledge of the person's habits as outlined in the box.* If a vegetarian patient shows clinical problems or abnormal laboratory values for which no plausible explanation is available, further probing of diet is warranted.

Risks of Deficiency Disease

Dietary difficulties among vegetarians usually are related to insufficiency rather than to excess. Thus the physician must ascertain the patient's nutritional status and explain how to ensure adequate nutrition on vegetarian diets before searching for rare metabolic or behavioral difficulties to explain unusual findings. Since dietary deficiency diseases are rare today, it is easy to discount them as possibilities in making differential diagnoses. The risks of deficiency diseases are greatest on a vegan diet that is combined with (1) self-imposed restriction to only

*References 14, 30, 31, 32, 33.

"natural," "organically grown," or unprocessed foods, and (2) avoidance of fortified or enriched foods and appropriate vitamin-mineral supplements. This may be compounded by negative attitudes toward Western medicine. Such dietary practices are particularly hazardous among pregnant or lactating women, infants, growing children or adolescents, and those who are sick or recovering from disease. Nutrient inadequacies are of greatest concern for energy, protein, vitamins B_{12}, B_2, and D (among infants and children), iron, and possibly other minerals, such as calcium, zinc, magnesium, and iodine.[34-42] Besides the amount and foods eaten, nutrient bioavailability must be considered.[43-45]

Energy and protein. While as a group vegetarians are leaner than nonvegetarians, sufficiency of energy intake rarely poses a problem among adults. Reports on infants and children in some of the new vegetarian groups indicate that because of the bulk of the diet, parental feedings practices, or related illness, growth velocities and size differ from those of vegetarians on less extreme diets and from nonvegetarians.[46-52] Frank protein-energy malnutrition is exceedingly rare but has been reported and differentiated from simple neglect leading to starvation.[53]

If energy intake is adequate and several cereals and legumes are combined for amino acid balance and supplementation, diets restricted solely to plant foods can be satisfactory for the growth of infants and young children. When some animal food (e.g., breast milk) is included, the higher quality of these proteins helps to ensure the overall value of the protein mixture and hence normal growth. For young children it is especially important that the diet include a variety of plant-food sources of protein; vegetarians should be cautioned against monodiets based on only one cereal grain for young children.[54-56] Another concern about vegan diets for children is the diets' bulk. When stomach capacity is limited and feedings are infrequent, it may not be possible for children to eat enough of a very bulky diet to meet their energy or protein needs.[52]

Vitamin B_{12}. Cases of vitamin B_{12} deficiency

FACTORS INFLUENCING HEALTH STATUS OF VEGETARIANS

Diet	Extensiveness of animal-food avoidances
	Extensiveness of other food avoidances (Note: pay attention to frequency and amount of foods eaten rather than simply to whether they are eaten at all)
	Willingness to use special foods (enriched, fortified, or naturally occurring sources rich in nutrients) or specific vitamin-mineral supplements
	Length of time person has subsisted on diet
	Knowledge of scientific principles of diet planning
	Groups with especially high needs (e.g., adolescents during their growth spurt, pregnant or lactating women, children, infants)
	Family dietary patterns (e.g., nonvegetarian or vegetarian)
Related health practices	Use of tobacco, alcohol, or any drugs
	Use of "Western" medical advice—on a regular basis or only as a last resort in acute crisis
	Use of vitamin, mineral, or other dietary supplements
	Use of techniques (e.g., fasting, enemas, purgatives, self-induced vomiting) that may affect absorption or metabolism
Coexisting disease states	Use of special therapeutic diets or supportive therapy
Other social characteristics	Living arrangements (e.g., with or without family, on or off campus, single person, shared or communal household)
	Socioeconomic status
	Affiliation with groups having special teachings about diet or other aspects of life-style
	Intelligence

continue to appear among vegans and very strict vegetarians and are frequent among Hindu Indian immigrants to the United Kingdom and Canada, who subsist on lactovegetarian diets that include only very small amounts of milk products.[57-59] Vitamin B_{12} is not found in most plant foods, so vegans are likely to have depleted stores of the vitamin, as shown by lowered serum levels of the nutrient. More serious sequelae, such as subacute combined degeneration of the spinal cord or death, are reported rarely although the prevalence of these disorders is higher among vegans than among nonvegetarians. Fortunately, vitamin B_{12} is reabsorbed more efficiently from the bile when intake is low than when it is high. Nevertheless, clinicians should closely monitor patients whose body stores have been depleted by a long-term diet deficient in B_{12} (e.g., 5-10 yr), patients whose stores are abnormal initially, and those suspected of having genetic or acquired abnormalities of vitamin B_{12} metabolism. Vegetarians' high folic acid intake may mask the megaloblastic anemia of vitamin B_{12} deficiency, and biochemical tests for vitamin B_{12} may show falsely high values unless carefully standardized.[60]

Since milk and eggs are relatively high in vitamin B_{12}, deficiencies rarely occur among lactoovovegetarians. Recently a number of infants fed exclusively at the breast by mothers who ate strict vegetarian diets have been reported to suffer from vitamin B_{12} deficiency.[61] The syndrome appears to be due to a combination of low fetal stores, low vitamin B_{12} in the breast milk of vegan mothers, and lack of supplementary vitamin B_{12} sources rather than to prolonged breastfeeding, since breast-fed infants generally do not develop such difficulties.[62]

Vitamin B_{12} supplements are mandatory for vegans and for the breast-fed infants of vegans or strict vegetarians. If the patient refuses to take vitamin supplements, vitamin B_{12}–fortified soy products may be suggested as alternatives. The root nodules from leguminous plants and seaweeds also contain vitamin B_{12} of microbic origin. Some vitamin B_{12} may be ingested accidentally on a vegan diet if foods are heavily contaminated with insect residues or soil, but these sources are too unreliable. Also, some of these sources contain forms of the vitamin that cannot be used by people. The problem is to ensure that the vitamin comes from a reliable source. Some fermented foods, such as tempeh or miso, contain variable but unknown amounts of vitamin B_{12}, and all the vitamin that is present may not be utilizable. Brewer's yeast and spirolina, a blue-green alga, also contain the vitamin, but it now appears that the forms and availability of the vitamin are questionable. For infants a safe alternative is the fortified soy formulas produced commecially. More research on the content of usable forms of the vitamin must be done before supplements consisting of yeasts grown on a vitamin B_{12}–enriched medium can be recommended with assurance.[6,25,56]

Calcium. Studies show that calcium nutriture of lactovegetarians is usually satisfactory, since milk products are high in the nutrient. Vegans should include ample servings of plant foods high in calcium, such as leafy dark green vegetables, legumes, fortified soy milks, filberts, almonds, and sesame seeds to ensure adequate supplies of calcium. During pregnancy and periods of rapid growth, calcium and vitamin D supplements are advisable.[63,64]

Iron. The prevalence of iron deficiency anemia or indices of low iron stores is higher among vegans than nonvegetarians. People with high iron needs (e.g., infants, young children, adolescents, pregnant women) and those who refuse to take iron supplements are particularly vulnerable. In such people iron bioavailability may be decreased further by phytates in cereals.[65] These phytates bind iron, whereas animal foods enhance iron absorption. In contrast to vegans, lactoovovegetarians appear to be in a more favorable situation in their iron nutritional status. Milk and eggs enhance iron absorption even though they provide relatively little iron themselves.[66,67] The relatively high ascorbic acid content of most vegan and vegetarian diets promotes iron absorption by keeping the dietary iron in a reduced form.[68] Routine iron supplementation is in order for vulnerable groups and vegans. Other vegetarians should be encouraged to eat foods fortified with iron to keep iron stores high.

Folic acid. Foods high in folic acid, such as fresh green leafy vegetables, are plentiful in most vegetarian diets; therefore megaloblastic anemia caused by folic acid deficiency is rare. However, vegans who eat diets based largely on grains and very well cooked vegetables may have folic acid deficiency.

Vitamin D. Most vegetarian adults are outdoors enough or obtain sufficient vitamin D from milk products to meet needs for the vitamin, and deficiencies are rare. However, infants and rapidly growing children, owing to their higher needs, require a dietary source of vitamin D. There have been several reports[2,69-71] of nutritional rickets among macrobiotic infants and children subsisting on vegan diets nearly devoid of milk products. Rickets also has been reported among vegetarian adolescents and osteomalacia in a vegan lactating woman of high parity.[72,73] Water-soluble vitamin D preparations, cod-liver oil, and liberal amounts of vitamin D–fortified dairy products can prevent such disorders.

Other vitamins. Vegan or vegetarian diets that do not contain milk products are low in riboflavin (vitamin B_2), although usually not so inadequate as to produce clinical deficiency disease. Milk and milk products, dark green leafy vegetables, legumes, and whole grains are relatively rich sources of the nutrient and should be stressed in the diet. Extremely restrictive vegetarian diets consisting exclusively of grains may be deficient in vitamins A and C and lead to disease such as xerophthalmia or scurvy.

Zinc. Risk of zinc inadequacy is increased among vegans and vegetarians because of low intakes of animal foods high in zinc, and because plant foods contain dietary fiber and phytates that may bind zinc and lower its bioavailability.[74] Low serum zinc values have been reported[31,75] among vegetarians in Western countries, but there appears to be no correlation between hair or serum zinc values and growth failure among vegetarian infants and children.[76] In several other studies,[77-80] vegetarians' intakes were low but did not appear to be associated with biologically significant functional abnormalities. Zinc supplementation does not seem warranted, but plant sources high in zinc, such as nuts, dried peas and beans, and whole grain or fortified cereals should be stressed. If small amounts of animal foods such as hard cheeses are acceptable, these can be helpful as well. As fiber and phytate levels in diets rise, greater care in selecting foods high in zinc is necessary, since bioavailability may be adversely affected. Tofu, cheese, and other foods with highly available zinc are preferred sources.[74]

Risks of Chronic Degenerative Diseases

Diet-related risk factors for several chronic degenerative diseases are lower among vegetarians than among nonvegetarians. As previously mentioned, vegetarians, and especially vegans, are usually leaner than nonvegetarians.* When nonvegetarians eat semivegetarian diets, their blood pressure drops, especially when the diet is combined with an active life-style and weight loss.[84,85] The drop in blood pressure is not caused by dietary protein levels[86] or levels of saturated fat and cholesterol[87] or sodium.[88-90] However, the higher potassium/sodium ratios of vegetarian diets may be important.[89] The role of high dietary fiber in lowering blood pressure is not well supported,[91] and the effects of potassium and calcium intakes continue to be explored.[92-96] Clearly life-style factors, such as not smoking plus a physically active life and leanness, as well as diet, are important.

Atherosclerosis and heart disease. Vegetarians generally have lower serum cholesterol and low-density lipoprotein (LDL) cholesterol levels, along with lower triglyceride levels, than do nonvegetarians but slightly higher serum cholesterol and high-density lipoprotein (HDL) cholesterol:apoprotein A-1 ratios. Vegans tend to have lower levels than do less strict vegetarians.† The incidence of atherosclerosis has been found to be lower and the first heart attack to occur later among Seventh-Day Adventists, who are predominantly lactoovovegetarians or vegans, than in the general population.[99] Studies of Western Europeans whose rations during World Wars I and II amounted to a lactovegetarian diet have also shown a decreased incidence of circulatory diseases and diabetes mellitus.[100] The lower saturated fat and cholesterol content of the vegetarian diet may not be the only factor in reducing these risks. The fiber content of leguminous seeds, the low content of animal protein, or the high content of complex carbohydrates and/or phytosterols may play important roles. The prevalence of diabetes mellitus, hypertension, obesity, and smoking also may be lower among vegetarians. In the past few years individual animal foods and food constituents have been assessed for their risk-reducing effects. When vegetarians follow nonvegetarian diets, or vice versa, the effects seem to be due mostly to alterations in specific constituents rather than to vegetarianism per se.[101-107]

---

*References 2, 20, 80, 81, 82, 83, 84.
†References 2, 18, 97, 98.

Diverticular disease. Both symptomless and frank diverticular disease are less prevalent among vegetarians than among nonvegetarians. Vegetarians' high intake of dietary fiber, especially from cereals, increases the bulk of the excreta reaching the lower bowel, thereby reducing abnormally high intrasigmoid pressures and altering intestinal transit times.[108-112]

Kidney stones. Vegetarian diets are associated with decreased incidence of kidney stones containing calcium oxalate.[113,114] Three of the six major urinary risk factors for calcium stone formation—increased urinary excretion of calcium, oxalate, and uric acid—are increased on diets high in animal protein. These risks are lower on vegetarian diets.

Cancer. Positive correlations have been found between the risk of breast and colon cancers and diets high in animal protein, fat, and refined carbohydrate but low in dietary fiber.* Vegetarians living in Western countries have lower rates for cancers of the lung, mouth, and some other sites.[120-122] Body size and energy balance may be involved. Some of these differences may be explained by characteristics other than diet (e.g., abstinence from tobacco and alcohol), but others may be due to diet. Vegetarian diets alter levels of some hormones, even in the absence of weight loss.† These alterations may be the mechanism whereby diet plays a role in the etiology of breast and prostate cancers. Diet-induced endocrine effects, as well as changes in the gut flora or the physical characteristics of the excreta, have been postulated as explanations for the lower rates of colon cancer among vegetarians.[130]

Other disorders. It has been suggested that because of their diets, vegetarians have less dental disease and are less susceptible to adult-onset diabetes mellitus of the nonketosis-prone type, but there are few data on these issues.[131-133] Because of high intake of cereal fibers, vegetarians are seldom constipated. Usually they have greater stool frequency, softer and larger stools, and sometimes more rapid transit times than do nonvegetarians.[134-139] Differences between vegetarians and nonvegetarians in other diseases are more poorly documented but nevertheless are worthy of further study.[2,18]

*References 10, 115, 116, 117, 118, 119.
†References 18, 125, 126, 127, 128, 129.

Mental Health

There is no evidence that vegetarians differ from the general population in their mental health or that their diets either cause or cure emotional disorders.[140] Most of those who adopt "alternative" diets are informed and intelligent people who do not proselytize but may sway others to their eating practices by example.[141] Most are not followers of irrational or subversive cults who want to convert the world to their ways by force. Therefore they should be treated as rational people, not eccentrics. However, exceptions do exist. The possibility of a concurrent emotional disorder should be considered when the diet is extreme and the individual also has made many other changes in life-style.[141]

Nutrition Counseling

In many respects vegetarians have different value systems from nonvegetarians. They are often highly knowledgeable about nutrition, contrary to popular opinion, which casts them as nutritional ignoramuses; nor are physicians necessarily well-informed about nutritional issues applying to vegetarians.[142,143]

To help vegetarians attain the best possible nutritional health, counseling must be based on respect for the patient's dietetic individualism with minimum disruption of existing eating habits unless they are clearly harmful. With careful planning based on sound nutritional principles, vegetarian diets can be followed with no risk of malnutrition and without violating the individual's philosophic and religious beliefs.

Vegetarian diets for adults. Planning adequate vegetarian diets for adults poses few problems. Guidance is available to the clinician in several publications.[1,2,16,29,144-147]

For those following lactoovovegetarian diets, the *first* step is to reduce high-calorie low–nutrient density foods and substitute unrefined foods that are higher in nutrient density for the calories they supply; the *second* step is to replace the protein-rich (meat) group with plant proteins from legumes, seeds, nuts, or meat analogues; and *third*, it may be necessary to increase the amount of nonfat or low-fat milk products in the diet. Fruits and vegetables should be used liberally, and ascorbic acid–rich foods should be eaten at each meal to enhance iron absorption.

Besides the previous steps, vegans must pay particular attention to adequate energy intake. A variety of legumes and whole grains, with seeds and nuts, should be included in meals to complement plant proteins. Since vegans do not use milk products, other foods must supply the nutrients in which milk products are rich. Vitamin D supplements are helpful unless sunlight is ample, and vitamin B_{12} supplements should be provided unless foods fortified with the vitamin are eaten.

During pregnancy or other special times of adult life in which nutrient needs are elevated, further dietary adjustments are necessary.[62-64]

Vegetarian diets for children. Recent reports on the ill effects of poorly planned vegetarian diets on children illustrate the importance of understanding the complicated eating practices vegetarians adopt.* Vegan diets limited to a few foods post the greatest risks; especially when the infant or child is not under regular pediatric care. The dietary modifications necessary to achieve nutritional adequacy while not violating parental beliefs or compromising the child's health are summarized in several publications.[54,143,148]

ORGANICALLY GROWN FOODS

The major reasons for concern about organically grown foods are their high cost and the fact that differences in nutrient content are not demonstrable. Foods labeled organic or organically grown purportedly are cultivated by organic gardening and farming methods. The soil's own organic materials, animal manures, and crop residues such as humus and compost are used to fertilize the plants and maintain the consistency, fertility, moisture content, and temperature of the soil. Commercial inorganic salt fertilizers, pesticides, fungicides, and herbicides generally are not used. Highly mechanized production techniques sometimes are avoided as well.[149,150]

Health Effects

Those who eat organically grown vegetables or other foods often do so because they believe such foods are more nutritious and healthful. These claims have little basis. Organic foods do not differ appreciably in nutrient composition from similar varieties grown in other ways. The major contribution of organic fertilizer is to improve soil texture; it possesses no inherent superiority as a source of nutrients for the plants. If the soil is depleted of nutrients, yields are

reduced but the nutritional quality of the harvest remains constant.[149,151]

The health effects of organically grown foods are no different from those of their more conventional counterparts. Most organic food advocates assume that indirect additives, environmental contaminants, and natural contaminants of microbial or compositional origin are eliminated in these products. Actually, while pesticide, herbicide, and fungicide residues may be slightly lower, there is no guarantee that other potentially toxic substances are absent.[152-154] Environmental contaminants, such as polybrominated biphenyls (PBBs), polychlorinated biphenyls (PCBs), and Kepone may enter the food supply regardless of cultivation techniques.[155] Microbial contaminants such as the spores of *Clostridium botulinum* recently were discovered in samples of organically grown honey.[156] Mycotoxins such as aflatoxin sometimes appear on rye, corn, and peanuts, while naturally occurring toxic constituents of the food itself are just as likely to occur with organically grown as conventional products.[157] Monitoring and regulation of all food sold at retain outlets protect the consumer from foods containing these substances in levels high enough to have known adverse effects upon health. The organic food consumer thus has no health advantage in this respect.

Economic Considerations

Organically grown foods are more costly than their conventional counterparts largely because production costs are higher. Organic farming techniques are relatively expensive, and economies of scale are more difficult to achieve, since the farms tend to be smaller. Organic foods also may be higher in price because profit margins are higher at retail.

The premium paid for these foods is not justifiable on nutritional and health grounds, but some consumers prefer organically grown varieties. These may differ from the varieties grown with inorganic fertilizers, since certain types of plants grow best in organically manured soil rich in humus.

Counseling

There is no reason for the physician to prohibit organic foods, but the patient should not be misled into assuming that organically grown foods have an inherent nutritional or health advantage.

---

*References 1, 2, 47-52, 56, 69, 144.

Some products even are dishonestly labeled as organic by unscrupulous promoters when in fact they are not.

"NATURAL" FOOD DIETS

"Natural" foods have not been processed at all or have been subjected only to traditional techniques. Canning, freezing, dehydrating, using food additives, and milling are regarded as processing; smoking, drying, salting, roasting, pasteurizing, and fermenting are considered natural. The term "natural" usually is applied to fresh or unprocessed foods, although the definitions vary. Examples include whole grain breads and cereals, foods rich in dietary fiber, molasses, brown sugar, fresh fruits, and vegetables. People cite several reasons for preferring natural foods, including nostalgia, quality, variety, and taste, but the dominant reason for using "fresh," "natural," and "whole" foods is that they are considered healthier than ordinary foods. "Natural" foods have an image of being uncontaminated by agricultural chemicals, food additives, or the supposedly deleterious effects of processing. However, little evidence supports the belief that such foods have superior effects on health or diet quality.[154-161]

Reasons for Concern

Diets high in "natural" foods pose little risk to health. The major concern is consumer misinformation about the superiority of these foods. No definitive statements can be made about the nutritional superiority of "natural" as opposed to processed foods. Contrary to popular opinion, some processed foods are superior to their unprocessed equivalents in vitamin and mineral content, especially if the supposedly fresh versions have been stored improperly.[150] "Natural" foods are not necessarily lower in fat, sugar, cholesterol, sodium, or energy, as many assume. Better labeling of processed foods is helping consumers to distinguish the nutritional characteristics of processed foods and to realize that nutritious diets can be constituted solely from natural or processed foods, or from a combination of the two. None of these alternatives is clearly superior from the nutritional standpoint.

Another reason for concern is cost. "Natural" products that are heavily advertised and promoted are often more expensive than conventional foods.[150] Consumers need to exercise judgment in buying these foods.

A third concern is that advertising often implies that "natural" foods are healthier. Actually, "natural" vitamins are no more efficacious than their synthesized counterparts, and "natural" snacks are as cariogenic as their processed counterparts.[162]

Health Effects

"Natural" foods have no intrinsic nutritional or health advantage over processed foods. The overall healthfulness of the diet depends chiefly upon appropriate selections. The belief that diets made up largely of "processed" foods predispose a person to subclinical vitamin deficiencies is erroneous, as is the notion that risks of inadequacy are eliminated on diets consisting predominantly of "natural" foods. Indeed the classic nutritional deficiency diseases were discovered first among populations whose diets consisted of "natural" foods.

The contention that the American food supply would be healthier if processed food were eliminated also is erroneous. In fact, if all food processing were abandoned, much of the food supply would spoil before it reached urban consumers, and they would face imminent starvation.[150] The solution lies not in abandoning food processing but in emphasizing human nutrition considerations with the increased use of highly processed, preprepared convenience foods.[158] There are legitimate reasons to pay more attention to these issues.[163] First, food engineering skills have been used to greatly enhance the sensory appeal and convenience of these items, and it is easy to overeat. Nutritional considerations have not always been given the same emphasis. Second, vigilance is required to assure that processing techniques are properly controlled to preserve the nutritive quality of the products. Third, analogues or formulated foods for farm-produced or home-recipe items are produced from highly purified ingredients, and care must be taken to assure that overall nutrient intakes are not radically altered as more items of this type enter the food supply.

Recommendations for prudent food selection are discussed under "Prudent Dietary Changes," p. 741. With sensible guidelines, both those who wish to include "organic," "natural," and "health" foods in their diets and those who do not can make wise food choices.

HEALTH FOODS AND SUPPLEMENTS

Dietary practices that involve adding foods or nutrients to either conventional or unconventional diets are of concern for three reasons. First, and most important, the health foods chosen often are thought to be homeopathic remedies with special health-promoting, disease-preventing, or curative properties that obviate the need for conventional medical supervision and treatment. Second, some of these items may cause pharmacologic effects detrimental to health. Third, the use of health foods often is combined with other alternative dietary styles. As a result, the individual's nutritional status profile may include nutrient deficiencies, imbalances, and excesses.

Health foods are self-prescribed items that users believe have special properties to promote health or prevent or cure disease. The specific foods vary, but representative items include kelp, ginseng, mineral water, royal jelly, buckwheat, yogurt, molasses, tiger's milk, herbal teas, garlic, sea salt, demarara sugar, honey, bean sprouts, miso (a fermented soup paste), granola, and bran. These foods also may be used conventionally by those who do not share the health-food enthusiast's views about their efficacy. This complicates the professional's task, since consumption alone is not enough to ascertain whether a client regards an item as a health food. The client's views about the food and evidence of alterations in attitudes toward or use of health services are also necessary.

Because of the way they are regarded by users, some supplements also can be categorized as health foods. Such preparations include "natural" vitamins, mineral salt mixtures, sea salt, protein supplements, nutritional yeasts, herbal tablets, yeast extract, wheat bran or germ, other forms of dietary fiber, laetrile, rutin, bioflavonoids, marine fish oils, essential fatty acids, omega-3 fatty acid supplements, and megadoses of vitamin or mineral supplements.[161-163] Reviews of the latest fads are produced periodically by an authoritative source.[164]

Characteristics of Health Foods and Supplements

Health foods have special characteristics that set them apart from other items in the diet and from therapeutic supplements or diets prescribed by health professionals. First, they are exotic and unpopular in the larger community. The very fact that they are unpopular is claimed by health-food proponents as the reason why the larger population suffers from certain ills, although there is no evidence that this is the case. Second, health foods are promoted as having special homeopathic or health-promoting properties. Their efficacy usually is attributed to some protective or accessory food factor necessary for health but absent from usual foods. In fact, there is no evidence that such deficiencies exist in the general population, and reports of better health resulting from such foods undoubtedly are placebo effects. Third, the claims employed in marketing health foods, especially at the point of purchase, often are exaggerated. Many of these products are sold by direct mail, in health-food stores, or by door-to-door salesmen. Salesclerks are often "believers," and they frequently stress unproven and dramatic properties of the preparations. Illegitimate claims may be made on labels or in advertising, although these are kept in check by federal regulatory agencies. Fourth, the exotic and unusual qualities of health foods are emphasized because they are sold under different brand names and in special retail outlets (such as health, natural, or organic food and drug stores). Fifth, the prices of health foods and supplements usually are much higher than those of the same foods not marketed with this emphasis or of similar nutrient preparations sold under generic or national brands by large pharmaceutical houses.

Dose levels for nutrient supplements are frequently higher, and nutrient combinations as well as doses are irrational from the medical standpoint. Claims for the superiority of "natural" as opposed to "artificial" nutrient sources are totally without scientific foundation. The major reason for price differentials appears to be the higher markups on these items rather than high production costs. Finally, because of the way health foods and supplements are marketed and in some cases because of their inherent nutrient composition, the dangers of misuse and overdosage are high.

Patterns of Use

People who use health foods regularly often believe that many disorders are caused by undiagnosed nutritional deficiencies and that there is little nutritional value in processed foods.

To avoid these hazards, they eat health foods thought to remedy these deficits in their diets.[164-169]

Some health-food users adopt vegetarian, "natural," or "organic" eating styles; others simply add health foods or supplements to conventional diets. Health-food users probably are older, less well educated, and in poorer health than the American public as a whole. They may persist in using these remedies even though severely ill and often seek treatment only late in the course of an illness.

Nutrient supplement use also is widespread in the United States; between 25% and 50% of American adults use some vitamin or mineral supplement. When such supplements are advised or prescribed by a physician for a legitimate preventive or therapeutic reason, there is little risk to health. Examples of such use include parenteral vitamin B_{12} for patients suffering from pernicious anemia, iron supplements for pregnant women or young infants, and fluoride supplements for infants and children living in areas with unfluoridated water supplies. Other patterns of nutrient supplement use may be ineffective but harmless. Physicians may prescribe nutrient supplements as placebos, or consumers themselves may decide to use small doses of nutrients sold in drugstores. Of greatest concern is the extravagant use of large doses of nutrients for purposes with no physiologic rationale. The regular use of megadoses of vitamins, minerals, protein, or other nutrients (e.g., pharmacologic doses of 10 to 100 times the RDAs) can produce effects quite different from those at physiologic dose levels. The unsupervised use of amounts larger than the RDAs and nutrient ranges judged safe is imprudent and uneconomic, confers no known health advantage, and may be harmful.[161,162]

Health effects

There is no objective evidence that people who eat health foods or those who take unusually large doses of nutrient supplements enjoy improved health as a result.[163,164] The major risk in such practices is that these people often delay seeking sounder preventive, diagnostic, or treatment services from health professionals.

Harmful effects such as toxicities and hypervitaminoses may result from the use of some health foods and supplements. The difficulties that may result from the use of specific health foods[170,171] are summarized in the box on p. 738.

Hypervitaminoses and nutrient imbalances are a particular risk for people who choose to use megadoses of vitamins, minerals, or nutrient supplements or for whom such supplements have been prescribed for inappropriate reasons. Specific hazards can result from misuse of currently popular nutrient supplements.[172-185]

Vitamin D. Chronic intakes of 3000 to 4000 international units (IU) of vitamin D (about 10 times the RDA) can cause idiopathic hypercalcemia in infants whereas 100,000 IU (1000 to 3000 IU/kg) produces toxicity.[179-181] Doses of this magnitude increase bone resorption and intestinal absorption of calcium, which in turn leads to hypercalcemia, increased renal excretion, and possibly kidney stones. Clinical signs of toxicity include anorexia, constipation, vomiting, polydypsia, polyuria, muscular hypotonia, bradycardia, and cardiac arrhythmias. If hypercalcemia persists, metastatic calcification of soft tissues, especially in the kidney, may result in nephrocalcinosis and irreversible renal tubular damage. Idiopathic hypercalcemia, sometimes coupled with mental retardation and osteosclerosis, is more prevalent in populations using exceptionally high doses of vitamin D.[180,181,182]

Toxicity rarely results from dietary sources alone; usuallly oversupplementation with vitamin D, vitamin pills, or cod-liver oil is involved as well. The clinician should make sure that if such supplements are used, doses are physiologic and the patient is aware of the serious effects of misuse. Vitamin D toxicity is difficult to treat. The first step is to withdraw the vitamin and reduce calcium intake while dehydrating the patient if necessary. Some physicians also use prednisone to block the intestinal action of vitamin D. Intravenous or intramuscular diphosphate has been administered on a trial basis to correct hypercalcemia, and this approach shows some promise.

Vitamin A. Toxicity has been reported among adults who chronically ingest 50,000 IU of vitamin A per day* and among infants ingesting 20,000 IU daily for 1 to 2 months.[184] It is almost impossible to develop vitamin A toxicity from food sources alone, but occasional cases have

---

*References 181, 182, 183.

HEALTH FOODS AND HERBAL REMEDIES WITH TOXIC EFFECTS

Effect	Cause
Diuretic	Teas made with juniper berries, shave grass, or horsetail plant are most violent and potent; other teas (e.g., buchu, quack grass, dandelion, Chinese or green) also have approximately equivalent weak diuretic effects
Cathartic	Buckhorn, senna, dock, and aloe teas are all strong irritant cathartics
Anticholinergic or psychogenic	Burdock-root tea has been reported to produce blurred vision, dry mouth, bizarre behavior and speech, hallucinations, and inability to void because of either a contaminant or high levels of atropine-like alkaloids
	When catnip, juniper, hydrangea, lobelia, jimson weed, or wormwood is used in teas or smoked, euphoric, stimulant, or hallucinogenic effects have been reported from the anticholinergics present
	Nutmeg can cause severe headaches, cramps, and nausea and is hallucinogenic in large doses
Hormonal	Ginseng has small amount of estrogens
	Mandrake root (often sold as ginseng) contains scopolamine; snakeroot contains reserpine
Gastroenteritis	Mistletoe leaves, stems, and berries contain toxic amines and proteins that have phytotoxic effects
	Poke (pokeweed or inkberry) in small quantities can cause gastroenteritis, and in large quantities may cause death from respiratory failure
Cyanosis	Large doses of the seeds, pits, bark, or leaves of apricot, bitter almond, cassova bean, cherry, chokecherry, peach, pear, apple, or plum cause cyanide poisoning because of cyanogenetic glycosides (e.g., amygdalin or prunasin, which may liberate hydrogen cyanide after ingestion)
Allergens	Camomile teas often provoke contact dermatitis in persons allergic to Compositae (ragweed, asters, chrysanthemums) or to goldenrod, marigold, and yaupon; anaphylaxis and severe hypersensitivity also have been reported in those highly allergic to these substances
	Saint-John's-wort tea can cause delayed hypersensitivity or photodermatitis
Cardiovascular toxicity	Licorice in large amounts can cause sodium and water retention, hypokalemia, hypertension, heart failure, and cardiac arrest
Possible carcinogenicity	Sassafras oil is at least 70% safrole, a hepatocarcinogen in experimental animals
	Unprocessed cassava (tapioca) plant eaten on a regular basis produces chronic cyanide intoxication and such signs as goiter, tropical ataxic neuropathy, and tropical amblyopia
Salmonellosis	Edible beef-liver powder sold in health-food stores is sometimes contaminated with salmonella; usually heating and drying processes are sufficient to prevent this
High risk of dental caries	Health-food snacks can produce dental caries unless good oral hygiene is followed

developed from bizarre food habits.[185] More commonly, massive doses of vitamin A are taken in hopes of preventing or curing acne, some form of cancer, or other diseases.[186-191] Carotenemia can develop if very large quantities of foods containing carotene (e.g., carrots, carrot juice) are consumed daily or if beta-carotene supplements sold in health-food stores are used on a chronic basis. Use of carotene supplements has become popular recently because of the publicity given to an as-yet-uncompleted clinical trial to test its efficacy in preventing cancer of the lung. Blood levels of carotene and the yellow cast of the skin disappear rapidly when intake is reduced.[192] The usual cause of toxicity with vitamin A is megadoses of vitamin A given by mothers to their infants to keep them healthy, doses taken by teenagers to cure acne, or self-medication by adults to "protect themselves against cancer." However, current objective evidence does not support the effectiveness of these uses. Only under medical supervision should infants be ingesting more than 10,000 IU daily or adults more than 25,000 IU. It goes without saying that any of the vitamin A–like derivatives used to treat acne and psoriasis should be given only under the close supervision of a dermatologist, since toxic side effects are often present.

Vitamin E. The effects of vitamin E on reproductive capacity in experimental animals have made it a favorite of health enthusiasts. In fact there is no evidence that it has any effect whatsoever upon sexual potency or that it prevents mental retardation, heart disease, or cancer.[193,194] Vitamin E is so widely distributed in vegetable oils and cereal grains that usual diets are unlikely to be low in this nutrient, except in some cases of prematurity and intestinal malabsorption.

The risks associated with megadoses of vitamin E are fewer than those seen with vitamins A and D; some people show signs of toxicity at 400 to 1000 IU daily, but most tolerate these doses.[195] Large doses of vitamin E interfere with vitamin K metabolism, thus increasing prothrombin time and predisposing the individual to bleeding. Creatinuria and gastrointestinal disturbances may result. Large doses of alphatocopherol given to anemic children can suppress the normal hematologic response to parenteral iron.[196]

Ascorbic acid. Factors such as age, sex, drug use, smoking, and oral contraceptive use affect ascorbic acid metabolism.[197] Evidence shows that low serum ascorbic acid values in the elderly can be raised by supplementation[198]; however, lowered serum levels may be a normal concomitant of aging, and no health benefits of supplementation have been demonstrated. Therefore there is little reason to encourage the elderly to take ascorbic acid supplements. The findings on how serum levels of ascorbic acid are altered by these factors have received widespread publicity. Advertising claims that subclinical, "biochemical" vitamin deficiencies exist when serum levels are lower than usual have convinced people to supplement their diets with the vitamin. The significance of the alterations in ascorbic acid metabolism induced by these factors is unclear, and the health benefits of ascorbic acid supplements for such people are questionable. Although the use of vitamin C supplements in amounts approximating the Recommended Dietary Allowances by people in these categories is not known to be harmful, the positive health effects are not documented.

The use of megadoses (e.g., 1 g or more) of ascorbic acid became popular shortly after Nobel Laureate Linus Pauling advocated megadoses of ascorbic acid for prevention of the common cold.[199] Since then several carefully controlled clinical trials have been carried out to ascertain if the hypothesis is valid. Large doses of ascorbic acid have not been demonstrated to be an effective cold remedy. The effects are generally negative, and in the few cases in which positive effects were noted, they involved severity and duration of symptoms rather than the number of colds.[200-202] Claims also have been made that high doses of vitamin C benefit advanced cancer[203,204]; that has been disproved in well-conducted clinical trials.[205-207]

Megadoses of ascorbic acid can be dangerous. Harmful side effects include uricosuria,[208] excessive absorption of food iron,[209] impaired bactericidal activity of leukocytes,[210] and other difficulties.

Vitamin B₆. Megadoses of pyridoxine have been suggested as useful in relieving premenstrual tension syndrome, but existing studies[211] do not rule out the role of placebo effects. Megadoses for any purpose should be avoided, because severe and possibly irreversible neuropathies have been reported among those who take megadoses of vitamin B_6, including several women who took doses ranging from 500 to 6000 mg per day to remedy premenstrual symptoms. The vitamin's effectiveness in relieving such symptoms has not been established.[212,213]

Other vitamins and minerals. Several recent reviews* detail evidence that excessive amounts or megadoses of other vitamins and minerals pose health hazards rather than provide any purported health benefits.

Dietary fiber. Dietary fiber currently is widely used as a health food. It is the part of plant foods that resists digestion in the gastrointestinal tract.[215] Tables giving the dietary fiber content of foods are not readily available. Most tables of food composition list crude fiber, the cellulose and lignin materials associated with the cell wall, but do not analyze other poorly digested polysaccharides, such as dextrins, starch gums, mucilages, algae, pectins, and hemicellulose. Newer analytic methods now permit analysis of all these substances, and up-to-date tables should be available shortly.[216]

The water-soluble fibers (e.g., pectins, gums, storage polysaccharides, hemicelluloses) have a relatively minor effect on fecal bulk but a considerable effect on metabolism. In contrast, water-insoluble fiber (e.g., cellulose, lignin, certain hemicelluloses) have a considerable effect on gastrointestinal transit time and fecal bulk although little impact on metabolism.[217-220]

Dietary fiber has positive effects on laxation and, depending on the type of fiber consumed, on fecal bulk. The soluble polysaccharides such as pectins and gums are ineffective as fecal bulking agents because they are completely broken down in the intestine. They may have other positive effects, however, such as those of oat bran in reducing serum lipids. By contrast, cereal fiber, which is only slightly degraded by the colonic microflora, holds water and increases fecal bulk considerably.[221] Thus 1 g of cereal fiber, particularly if it is in a coarse form, increases stool bulk by 3-9 g whereas a 1 g increase in dietary fiber from fruits and vegetables produces only a 2 g increase in stool bulk. The use of food sources of dietary fiber or fiber supplements such as bran or wheat germ in moderate amounts (e.g., 20-35 g/da) is not harmful and may be beneficial to laxation. If very large amounts of purified dietary fibers such as bran or wheat germ are consumed (200-400 g) and fluid intake is low, obstruction may occur.

The benefits of fiber also have been touted for other diseases. Since the types of fiber vary in their physiologic and metabolic effects, it is difficult to generalize about their health effects. High-fiber diets do appear to help in the treatment of diverticular disease of the colon and possibly in irritable bowel syndrome.[222-225] The hypothesis that eating large amounts of plant foods high in dietary fiber reduces risks of colon cancer has received some support from recent epidemiologic and case-control studies,* but fiber intake has not been conclusively demonstrated to be involved. Other hypotheses point to the positive correlations between colon cancer and increasing amounts of dietary fat, cholesterol, and meat, the effects of calcium and other nutrients, and genetic factors, such as the predisposition to adenomatous polyps. Diets high in fiber and complex carbohydrates have also been suggested for the control of diabetes mellitus.[230,231]

The current consensus is that an increase in varied food sources of dietary fiber is not harmful and may be beneficial to health. Clearly, increasing dietary fiber can relieve constipation in many cases, and if a moderate amount is eaten, mineral bioavailability is not adversely affected. Eating more dietary fiber also may alleviate symptoms or reduce risks of certain diseases, but large amounts of fiber supplements should be used only under medical supervision.

Nutritional Counseling

The patient who uses health foods or supplements deserves an objective discussion of the risks, benefits, and costs. If there is reason to suspect that such use will be prejudicial to health, efforts should be made to dissuade the patient. When there are no clear contraindications, the choice is best left up to the patient. Counseling time is best spent stressing effective measures to promote health and prevent disease. The clinician should urge the patient not to neglect health problems by relying too much on health foods or supplements.

*References 164, 165, 214, 215.

*References 115, 226, 227, 228, 229.

There is no need to use multivitamin or mineral supplements on a regular basis if a food guide such as the basic four or basic seven is used. Once body stores have been filled, excesses of these nutrients either are not absorbed or are excreted. Food contains ample amounts of most nutrients. People whose stores of a specific nutrient are depleted require much larger doses of the deficient nutrient than the amount provided in these supplements. Vitamin and mineral supplements do not ensure adequate nutrition if the diet is haphazard. Although multiple vitamin–mineral supplements taken in amounts less than or equal to the RDAs for these nutrients pose little risk, they are neither a substitute for careful diet selection nor an alternative to regular health care. Patients who take multivitamin or mineral supplements in amounts that exceed the RDAs should be warned of the hazards of the practice.

People who take megadoses of supplements often develop a strong preference for a particular nutrient or nutrients and are likely to take very large doses of it. If the health professional fails to comment on such use, that often is taken as tacit approval. It is especially important that the health professional point out the hazards of such practices, especially with the fat-soluble vitamins.

PRUDENT DIETARY CHANGES

Most Americans do not follow the differing eating practices discussed so far, but many health professionals and patients feel the need to adjust their diets in a more prudent direction. Indeed evidence is now available that suggests such changes may be advisable to avoid both dietary inadequacy and excess.[232-239]

Several publications[240-244] summarize prudent recommendations for Americans. In brief, they are

1. Maintain desirable body weight or alter diet and physical activity to achieve it.
2. Eat a variety of foods to obtain adequate but not excessive amounts of protective nutrients. The U.S. Department of Agriculture daily food guide emphasizes the inclusion of at least the following number of servings from these food groups: vegetables and fruits (4); breads and cereals (4); milk and cheese (2 for adults, 3 for pregnant women and children, 4 for lactating women); meat, poultry, fish, and beans (2); fats, sweets, and alcohol (to be consumed only after recommended servings from other groups are eaten.
3. When making choices from the food groups, remember:
   Avoid too much fat, saturated fat, and cholesterol
   Eat foods with adequate starch and fiber
   Avoid too much sugar
   Avoid too much sodium
   Drink alcoholic beverages only in moderation
   Those who wish more quantitatively oriented goals may refer to publications by the American Dietetics Association, other recognized nutritional organizations, and the U.S. Government.
4. Make any adjustments for age or special physiologic condition only after consulting a health professional.

These recommendations are better grounded in current nutrition knowledge than are "health," "natural," and "organic" diets and can be followed even by vegetarians.

REFERENCES

1. American Dietetic Association: Position paper on the vegetarian approach to eating, J Am Diet Assoc **77**:61-69, 1980.
2. Dwyer JT: Nutritional status and alternative life style diets, with special reference to vegetarianism in the U.S. In Rechcigl M, editor: CRC handbook of nutritional supplements. Vol 1. Human use, Boca Raton Fla, 1983, CRC Press, pp 343-410.
3. Freeland Graves JH, et al: A demographic and social profile of age and sex matched vegetarians and nonvegetarians, J Am Diet Assoc **86**:907-913, 1986.
4. Dwyer JT, Kandel RF, Mayer J: The new vegetarians: Group affiliation and dietary strictures related to attitudes and life styles, J Am Diet Assoc **64**:376-382, 1974.
5. Read MH, Thomas DC: Nutrient and food supplement practices of lactoovo vegetarians, J Am Diet Assoc **83**:402-404, 1982.
6. Sanders T: Vegetarianism: dietetic and medical aspects, J Plant Foods **5**:3-14, 1983.
7. Freeland Graves JH, et al: Health practices, attitudes, and beliefs of vegetarians and nonvegetarians, J Am Diet Assoc **86**:913-918, 1986.
8. Erhard D: The new vegetarians. I. Vegetarianism and its medical consequences, Nutr Today **8**:4, November-December 1973.
9. Liebman B: Are vegetarians healthier than the rest of us? Natl Forum **64**:8-10, 1984.
10. Kune GA, Kune S: The nutritional causes of colorectal cancer: an introduction to the Melbourne study, Nutr Cancer **9**:1-4, 1987.
11. Connor SL, Connor WE: The new American diet, New York, 1986, Simon & Schuster.
12. Roe DA: History of promotion of vegetable cereal diets, J Nutr **116**:1355-1363, 1986.

13. Hirayama T: Mortality in Japanese with life-styles similar to Seventh Day Adventists.' Strategy for risk reduction by life-style modification, Natl Cancer Inst Monogr **69:**143-153, 1985.

14. Kahn HA, et al: Association between reported diet and all-cause mortality. Twenty-one-year follow-up on 27,530 adult Seventh Day Adventists, Am J Epidemiol **119:**775-787, 1984.

15. Burr M, Sweetnam P: Vegetarianism, dietary fiber, and mortality, Am J Clin Nutr **36:**873-877, 1982.

16. Register UD, Crooks H: Nutritionally adequate vegetarian diets. In Rechcigl M, editor: CRC handbook of nutritional supplements. Vol I. Human use, Boca Raton Fla, 1983, CRC Press, pp 331-342.

17. Slone C: Disease epidemiology of vegetarians. In Anderson JJB, editor: Nutrition and vegetarianism, Chapel Hill NC, 1982, Health Sciences Consortium, pp 124-133.

18. Dwyer J: Health implications of vegetarian diets, Compr Ther **9:**23-28, 1983.

19. Robson JRK: Zen macrobiotic diets. In Jelliffe EFP, Jelliffe DB, editors: Adverse effects of foods, New York, 1982, Plenum Press Inc.

20. Dwyer JT: Vegetarian diets: health aspects. In Proceedings of the First International Congress on Vegetarian Nutrition, Am J Clin Nutr. (In press, 1988.)

21. Committee on Nutrition, American Academy of Pediatrics: Nutritional aspects of vegetarianism, health foods, and fad diets, Pediatrics **59:**460-464, 1977.

22. Dwyer JT: Wonderful world of vegetarianism: benefits and disadvantages. In Anderson JJB, editor: Nutrition and vegetarianism, Chapel Hill NC, 1982, Health Sciences Consortium, pp 5-25.

23. Roe DA: Nutrient deficiencies in naturally occurring foods. In Jelliffe EFP, Jelliffe DB, editors: Adverse effects of foods, New York, 1982, Plenum Press Inc, pp 407-426.

24. The vegetarian diet: food for us all, Chicago, 1981, American Dietetic Association.

25. Truesdell DD, et al: Nutrients in vegetarian foods, J Am Diet Assoc **84:**28-35, 1984.

26. Ellis FR, Montegriffo VM: Veganism; clinical findings and investigations, Am J Clin Nutr **23:**249-255, 1970.

27. McKenzie J: Profile on vegans, Plant Foods Hum Nutr **2:**79, 1971.

28. Kurtha AN, Ellis FR: The nutritional, clinical, and economic aspects of vegan diets, Plant Foods Hum Nutr **2:**123, 1970.

29. Miller DS, Mumford P: The nutritive value of Western vegan and vegetarian diets, Plant Foods Hum Nutr **2:**201, 1972.

30. Taber LAL, Cook RA: Dietary and anthropometric assessment of adult omnivores, fish eaters, and lactoovovegetarians, J Am Diet Assoc **76:**21-29, 1980.

31. Harland BF, Peterson M: Nutritional status of lactoovo vegetarian Trappist monks, J Am Diet Assoc **72:**259-264, 1978.

32. Armstrong BK, et al: Hematological, vitamin B_{12} and folate studies on Seventh Day Adventist vegetarians, Am J Clin Nutr **27:**712, 1983.

33. McEndress LS, et al: Iron intake and iron nutritional status of lactoovo vegetarian and omnivore students eating in a lactoovovegetarian food service, Nutr Rep Int **27:**200, 1983.

34. Hanning RM, Zlotkin SH: Unconventional eating practices and their health implications, Pediatr Clin North Am **32:**429-445, 1985.

35. Sklar R: Nutritional vitamin B_{12} deficiency in a breast fed infant of a vegan diet mother, Clin Pediatr **25:**219-221, 1986.

36. James JA, et al: Screening Rastafarian children for nutritional rickets, Br Med J (Clin Res) **290:**899-900, 1985.

37. Rider AA, et al: Diet, nutrient intake, and metabolism in populations at high and low risk for colon cancer. Selected biochemical parameters in blood and urine, Am J Clin Nutr **40:**917-920, 1984.

38. Calkins BM, et al: Diet, nutrient intake, and metabolism in populations at high and low risk for colon cancer. Nutrient intake, Am J Clin Nutr **40:**896-905, 1984.

39. Abdulla M, et al: Nutrient intake and health status of lactovegetarians: chemical analyses of diets using a duplicate portion sampling technique, Am J Clin Nutr **40:**325-338, 1984.

40. Shinwell ED, Gorodischer R: Totally vegetarian diets and infant nutrition, Pediatrics **70:**582-586, 1982.

41. Kramer L, et al: Mineral and trace element content of vegetarian diets, J Am Coll Nutr **3:**3-11, 1984.

42. Lockie A, et al: Comparison of four types of diet using clinical, laboratory, and psychological studies, J R Coll Gen Pract, pp 333-335, July 1985.

43. McNeill D, et al: Mineral analyses of vegetarian, health and conventional foods: magnesium, zinc, copper and manganese content, J Am Diet Assoc **85:**569-572, 1985.

44. Anderson BM, et al: The iron and zinc status of long-term vegetarian women, Am J Clin Nutr **34:**1042-1048, 1981.

45. King JC, et al: Effect of vegetarianism on the zinc status of pregnant women, Am J Clin Nutr **34:**1049-1055, 1981.

46. Brown PT, Bergan JG: The dietary status of the "new" vegetarians, J Am Diet Assoc **67:**455-459, 1975.

47. Fulton JR, et al: Preschool vegetarian children, J Am Diet Assoc **76:**360-365, 1980.

48. Shull, MW, et al: Velocities of growth in vegetarian preschool children, Pediatrics **60:**410-417, 1977.

49. Dwyer JT, et al: Growth of "new" vegetarian preschool children using the Jenss Bayley curve fitting technique, Am J Clin Nutr **37:**815-827, 1983.

50. Dwyer JT, et al: Size, obesity and leanness in vegetarian preschool children, J Am Diet Assoc **77:**734-739, 1980.

51. Sanders TAB, Purves R: An anthropometric and dietary assessment of the nutritional status of vegan preschool children, J Hum Nutr **35:**349, 1981.

52. Dietz WH, Dwyer JT: Nutritional implications of vegetarianism for children. In Suskind RM, editor: Textbook of pediatric nutrition, New York, 1981, Raven Press, pp 179-188.

53. Lozoff B, Finaroff AA: Kwashiorkor in Cleveland, Am J Dis Child **129:**710-711, 1975.

54. Vhymeister IB, et al: Safe vegetarian diets for children, Pediatr Clin North Am **24:**203-210, 1977.

55. Dwyer JT, et al: Preschoolers on alternative life-style diets, J Am Diet Assoc **72:**264-270, 1978.

56. Truesdell DD, Acosta PB: Feeding the vegan infant and child, J Am Diet Assoc **85:**837-840, 1985.

57. Matthews JH, Wood, JK: Megaloblastic anaemia in vegetarian Asians, Clin Lab Haematol **6:**1-7, 1984.

58. Murphy MF: Vitamin B_{12} deficiency due to a low-cholesterol diet in a vegetarian, Ann Intern Med **94:**57-58. 1981.

59. Chanarin I, et al: Megaloblastic anaemia in a vegetarian Hindu community, Lancet **2:**1168-1172, 1985.

60. Long A: Vitamin B_{12} for vegans, Br Med J **2:**192, 1977.

61. Higginbottom MC, et al: A syndrome of methylmalonic aciduria, homocystinuria, megaloblastic anemia, and neurologic abnormalities of a vitamin B_{12}–deficient breast-fed infant of a strict vegetarian, N Engl J Med **299:**317-323, 1978.

62. Dwyer JT: Vegetarian diets in pregnancy and lactation: recent studies of North Americans, J Can Diet Assoc **44:**26-35, 1983.

63. Thomas J, Ellis FR: The health of vegans during pregnancy, Proc Nutr Soc **36:**46A, 1977.

64. Dwyer JT: Vegetarian diets in pregnancy. In Committee on Nutrition of the Mother and Preschool Child, Food and Nutrition Board, Commission on Life Sciences, National Research Council: Alternative dietary practices and nutritional abuses in pregnancy: proceedings of a workshop, Washington DC, 1982, National Academy Press, pp 61-63.

65. International Nutritional Anemia Consultative Group: The effects of cereals and legumes on iron availability, Washington DC, 1982, The Nutrition Foundation.

66. Cook JD: Determinants of nonheme iron absorption in man, Food Tech, pp 124-126, October 1983.

67. Clydesdale FM: Psychicochemical determinants of iron bioavailability, Food Tech, pp 133-138, October 1983.

68. Hallberg L, et al: Effect of ascorbic acid on iron absorption from different types of meals. Studies with ascorbic acid–rich foods and synthetic ascorbic acid given in different amounts with different meals, Hum Nutr Appl Nutr **40A:**97-113, 1986.

69. Dwyer JT, et al: Risk of nutritional rickets among vegetarian children, Am J Dis Child **133:**134-140, 1979.

70. Curtis JA, et al: Nutritional rickets in vegetarian children, Can Med Assoc J **128:**150-152, 1983.

71. Belton NR: Rickets: not only the English disease, Acta Paediatr Scand (suppl) **323:**68-75, 1986.

72. Moncreiff MW, et al: Nutritional rickets at puberty, Arch Dis Child **48:**221-224, 1973.

73. Elinson P, et al: Nutritional osteomalacia, Am J Dis Child **134:**427, 1980.

74. Freeland Graves JH, et al: Zinc and copper content of foods used in vegetarian diets, J Am Diet Assoc **77:**648-654, 1980.

75. Treuherz J: Zinc and dietary fiber: observations on a group of vegetarian adolescents, Proc Nutr Soc **39:**10A, 1980.

76. Dwyer JT, et al: Nutritional status of vegetarian children, Am J Clin Nutr **35:**204-216, 1982.

77. Freeland Graves JH, et al: Zinc status of vegetarians, J Am Diet Assoc **77:**655-661, 1980.

78. Abraham R, et al: Diet during pregnancy in an Asian community in Britain—energy, protein, zinc, copper, fiber, and calcium, Hum Nutr Appl Nutr **39A:**23-35, 1985.

79. Gibson RS, et al: The trace metal status of a group of postmenopausal vegetarians, J Am Diet Assoc **82:**246-250, 1983.

80. Latta D, Liebman M: Iron and zinc status of vegetarian and nonvegetarian males, Nutr Rep Int **30:**141-149, 1984.

81. Armstrong B, et al: Urinary sodium and blood pressure in vegetarians, Am J Clin Nutr **32:**2472-2476, 1979.

82. Anholm AC: The relationship of a vegetarian diet to blood pressure, Prev Med **7:**35, 1978.

83. Armstrong B, et al: Blood pressure in Seventh Day Adventist vegetarians, Am J Epidemiol **105:**444-449, 1977.

84. Acheson RM, Williams DRR: Does consumption of fruit and vegetables protect against stroke? Lancet **1:**1191-1193, 1983.

85. Barnard RJ, et al: Effects of diet and exercise on blood pressure and viscosity in hypertensive patients, J Cardiac Rehabil **5:**185-190, 1985.

86. Sacks FM, et al: Stability of blood pressure in vegetarians receiving dietary protein supplements, Hypertension **6:**199-201, 1984.

87. Sacks FM, et al: Lack of an effect of dietary saturated fat and cholesterol on blood pressure in normotensives, Hypertension **6:**193-198, 1984.

88. Rouse IL, et al: Blood pressure lowering effect of a vegetarian diet: controlled trial in normotensive subjects, Lancet **1:**5-9, 1983.

89. Ophir O, et al: Low blood pressure in vegetarians: the possible role of potassium, Am J Clin Nutr **37:**755-762, 1983.

90. Margetts BM, et al: A randomized control trial of a vegetarian diet in the treatment of mild hypertension, Clin Exp Pharmacol Physiol **12:**263-266, 1985.

91. Brussaard JH, et al: Blood pressure and diet in normotensive volunteers: absence of an effect of dietary fiber, protein, and fat, Am J Clin Nutr **34:**2023-2029, 1981.

92. Kesteloot H, Geboers J: Calcium and blood pressure, Lancet **2:**813-815, 1982.

93. Ackley S, et al: Dairy products, calcium, and blood pressure, Am J Clin Nutr **38:**457-461, 1983.

94. Khaw KT, Barrett-Connor E: Dietary potassium and blood pressure in a population, Am J Clin Nutr **39:**963-968, 1984.

95. Reed D, et al: Diet, blood pressure, and multicolinearity, Hypertension **7:**405-410, 1985.

96. Staessen J, et al: Four urinary cations and blood pressure, Am J Epidemiol **117:**676-687, 1983.

97. Sacks FM, et al: Plasma lipids and lipoproteins in vegetarians and controls, N Engl J Med **292:**1148-1151, 1975.

98. Lock DR, et al: Apoprotein E levels of vegetarians, Metabolism **31:**917-921, 1982.

99. Phillips RL, et al: Coronary heart disease mortality among Seventh Day Adventists with differing dietary habits: a preliminary report, Am J Clin Nutr **31:**(suppl)191-198, 1978.

100. Hindhede M: The effect of food restriction during war on mortality in Copenhagen, JAMA **74:**381-382, 1920.

101. Sacks FM, et al: Effects of a low-fat diet on plasma lipoprotein levels, Arch Intern Med **146:**1573-1577, 1986.

102. Fisher M, et al: The effect of vegetarian diets on plasma lipid and platelet levels, Arch Intern Med **146:**1193-1197, 1986.

103. Cooper RS, et al: The selective llipid lowering effect of vegetarianism on low density lipoproteins in the crossover experiment, Atherosclerosis **44:**293-305, 1982.

104. Masarei JRL, et al: Effects of a lactoovo vegetarian diet on serum concentrations of cholesterol, triglyceride,

HDL-C, HDL2-C, HDL3-C, apoprotein B, and Lp(a), Am J Clin Nutr **40:**468-479, 1984.

105. Sacks FM, et al: Effect of ingestion of meat on plasma cholesterol of vegetarians, JAMA **246:**640-644, 1981.

106. Sacks FM, et al: Ingestion of egg raises plasma low density lipoproteins in free living subjects, Lancet **1:**647-649, 1984.

107. Liebman M, Bazzarre TL: Plasma lipids of vegetarian and nonvegetarian males: effects of egg consumption, Am J Clin Nutr **38:**612-619, 1983.

108. Gear JS, et al: Symptomless diverticular disease and intake of dietary fibre, Lancet **1:**511-514, 1979.

109. Gear JAA: Dietary fiber and asymptomatic diverticular disease of the colon, J Plant Foods **3:**57-62, 1978.

110. Miettinin TA, Tarpila S: Fecal beta sitosterol in patients with diverticular disease of the colon and in vegetarians, Scand J Gastroenterol **13:**573-576, 1978.

111. Ohi G, et al: Changes in dietary fiber intake among Japanese in the 20th century: a relationship to the prevalence of diverticular disease, Am J Clin Nutr **38:**115-121, 1983.

112. Heaton KW: Diet and diverticulosis: new leads, Gut **26:**541-543, 1985.

113. Robertson WG, et al: Should recurrent calcium oxalate stone formers become vegetarians? Br J Urol **51:**427-431, 1979.

114. Robertson WG, et al: Prevalence of urinary stone disease in vegetarians, Eur Urol **8:**334-339, 1982.

115. McKeown-Eyssen GE, Bright-See E: Dietary factors in colon cancer: international relationships, Nutr Cancer **6:**160-170, 1984.

116. Wynder EL, Rose DP: Diet and breast cancer, Hosp Pract **19:**73-88, 1984.

117. Goldin BR: The metabolism of the intestinal microflora and its relationship to dietary fat, colon and breast cancer. In Ip C, et al, editors: Dietary fat and cancer, New York, 1986, Alan R Liss Inc, pp 655-685.

118. Bingham SA, et al: Dietary fibre consumption in Britain: new estimates and their relation to large bowel cancer mortality, Br J Cancer **52:**399-402, 1985.

119. Wynder E: Reflections on diet, nutrition, and cancer, Cancer Res **43:**3024-3027, 1983.

120. Phillips RL, Snowdon DA: Association of meat and coffee use with cancers of the large bowel, breast, and prostate among Seventh Day Adventists: preliminary results, Cancer Res **43:**2403-2408, 1983.

121. Phillips RL, et al: Mortality among California Seventh Day Adventists for selected cancer sites, J Natl Cancer Inst **65:**1097-1107, 1980.

122. Phillips RL: Role of lifestyle and dietary habits in risk of cancer among Seventh Day Adventists, Cancer Res **35:**3513-3522, 1975.

123. Graham S: Fats, calories, and caloric expenditure in the epidemiology of cancer, Am J Clin Nutr **45:**342-346, 1987.

124. Micozzi M: Nutrition, body size, and breast cancer, Yearbook Phys Anthropol **28:**175-206, 1985.

125. Hill PB, Wynder EL: Effect of a vegetarian diet and dexamethasone on plasma prolactin, testosterone, and dehydroepiandrosterone in men and women, Cancer Lett **7:**273-282, 1979.

126. Armstrong BK, et al: Diet and reproductive hormones: a study of vegetarian and nonvegetarian postmenopausal women, J Natl Cancer Inst **67:**761-767, 1981.

127. Howie BJ, Shultz TD: Dietary and hormonal interrelationships among vegetarian Seventh Day Adventists and nonvegetarian men, Am J Clin Nutr **42:**127-134, 1985.

128. Shultz TD, Leklem JE: Nutrient intake and hormonal status of premenopausal vegetarian Seventh Day Adventists and premenopausal nonvegetarians. Nutr Cancer **4:**247-259, 1983.

129. Goldin BR, et al: Estrogen excretion patterns and plasma levels in vegetarian and omnivorous women, N Engl J Med **307:**1542-1547, 1982.

130. Gorbach SL: Estrogens, breast cancer, and intestinal flora, Rev Infect Dis **6**(suppl):S85-S90, 1984.

131. Snowdon DA, Phillips RL: Does a vegetarian diet reduce the occurrence of diabetes? Am J Public Health **75:**507-512, 1985.

132. Wolever TMS, Jenkins DJA: The glycaemic index: implications of dietary fibre and the digestibility of different carbohydrate foods in the management of diabetes, J Plant Foods **4:**127-138, 1982.

133. Kinmonth AL, et al: Whole foods and increased dietary fibre improve blood glucose control in diabetic children, Arch Dis Child **57:**187-194, 1982.

134. Davies GJ, et al: Bowel function measurements of individuals with different eating patterns, Gut **27:**164-169, 1986.

135. Burkitt DP, et al: Effect of dietary fibre on stools and transit times, and its role in the causation of disease, Lancet **2:**1408-1412, 1972.

136. Gear JSS, et al: Fibre and bowel transit times, Br J Nutr **45:**77-82, 1981.

137. Goldberge MJ, et al: Comparison of the fecal microflora of Seventh Day Adventists with individuals consuming a general diet. Ann Surg **186:**97-100, 1977.

138. Kuhnlein U, et al: Mutagens in feces from vegetarians and nonvegetarians, Mutat Res **85:**1-12, 1981.

139. Drossman DA, et al: Bowel patterns among subjects not seeking health care, Gastroenterology **83:**529-534, 1982.

140. Dwyer JT, et al: The new vegetarians: the natural high? J Am Diet Assoc **65:**529-536, 1974.

141. Freeland Graves JH, et al: Nutrition knowledge of vegetarians and nonvegetarians, J Nutr Ed **14:**21-26, 1982.

142. Strobl CM, Groll L: Professional knowledge and attitudes on vegetarianism: implications for practice, J Am Diet Assoc **79:**568-574, 1981.

143. Sims LS: Food related value orientations, attitudes, and beliefs of vegetarian, Ecol Food Nutr **7:**23-35, 1978.

144. Jacobs C, Dwyer JT: Vegetarian diets for children: appropriate and inappropriate. Proceedings, First International Congress on Vegetarian Nutrition, Am J Clin Nutr. (In press 1987.)

145. Williams ER: Making vegetarian diets nutritious, Am J Nurs **75:**2168-2173, 1975.

146. Seventh Day Adventist Dietetic Association: Diet manual: utilizing a vegetarian diet plan, ed 5, Loma Linda Calif, 1979, The Association.

147. Smith EB: A guide to good eating the vegetarian way, J Nutr Ed **7:**109-111, 1975.

148. MacLean WC Jr, Graham GG: Vegetarianism in children, Am J Dis Child **134:**513-519, 1980.

149. Bender AE: Health foods, Proc Nutr Soc **38:**163-171, 1979.

150. Gussow JD, Thomas PR: Health, natural, and organic: foods or frauds? In Gussow JD, Thomas PR: The nutrition

debate: sorting out some answers, Palo Alto, 1986, Bull Publishing Co, pp 208-267.

151. Leverton RM: Organic, inorganic: what they mean. In Yearbook of agriculture, Washington DC, 1974, Government Printing Office, pp 70-73.

152. Mustafa MG: Agricultural chemicals. In Jelliffe EFP, Jelliffe DB: Adverse effects of foods, New York, 1982, Plenum Press Inc, pp 111-128.

153. Hambraeus L: Naturally occurring toxicants in food. In Jelliffe EFP, Jelliffe DB: Adverse effects of foods, New York, 1982, Plenum Press Inc, pp 13-36.

154. Srikantia SG: An outbreak of aflatoxicosis in man. In Jelliffe EFP, Jelliffe DB: Adverse effects of foods, New York, 1982, Plenum Press Inc, pp 45-50.

155. Lindsay DG, Sherlock JC: Environmental contaminants. In Jelliffe EFP, Jelliffe DB: Adverse effects of foods, New York, 1982, Plenum Press Inc, pp 85-110.

156. Andrews WH, et al: Bacteriological survey of 60 health foods, Appl Environ Microbiol **37:**559-566, 1979.

157. Mislivec PB, et al: Mycological survey of selected health foods, Appl Environ Microbiol **37:**567-571, 1979.

158. Southgate, DAT: Natural or unnatural foods? Br Med J **288:**881-882, 1984.

159. Hiscoe HB: Does being natural make it good? N Engl J Med **308:**1474-1475, 1983.

160. Yetiv J: Natural foods, food additives, and food intolerances. In Yetiv J: Popular nutrition practices: a scientific appraisal, Toledo, 1985, Popular Medicine Press, pp 51-67.

161. Dwyer JT: Commercial additives. In Jelliffe EFP, Jelliffe DB: Adverse effects of foods, New York, 1982, Plenum Press Inc, pp 163-194.

162. Martin JB, Berry CW: Cariogenicity of selected processed machine vended and health food snacks, J Am Diet Assoc **75:**159-161, 1979.

163. Gussow JD, Thomas PR: Food safety: is it really safe at the plate? In Gossow JD, Thomas PR: The nutrition debate: sorting out some answers, Palo Alto, 1986, Bull Publishing Co, pp 342-405.

164. Yetiv J: Multivitamins and megavitamins: are they megahealthy? In Yetiv J: Popular nutritional practices: a scientific appraisal, Toledo, 1986, Popular Medicine Press, pp 159-197.

165. Yetiv J: And what about megaminerals? In Yetiv J: Popular nutritional practices: a scientific appraisal, Toledo, 1986, Popular Medicine Press, pp 196-216.

166. Yetiv J: Should you eat like a Bantu? (or the role of dietary fiber). In Yetiv J: Popular nutritional practices: a scientific appraisal, Toledo, 1986, Popular Medicine Press, pp 239-247.

167. Nutrition forum, Philadelphia, 1986, George F Stickley Co.

168. Margolis S: Health foods: facts and fakes, New York, 1973, Walter Press Inc.

169. Barret S, Knight G, editors: The health robbers, Philadelphia, 1975, George F Stickley.

170. Nutrition as therapy. Consumer Reports books: Health quackery, New York, 1980, Holt Rinehart Winston, pp 218-237.

171. Herbert V: Nutrition cultism: facts and fictions, Philadelphia, 1980, George F Stickley Co.

172. Taktor D: The great vitamin hoax, New York, 1973, Macmillan Publishing Co.

173. Toxic reactions to plant products sold in health food stores, Med Lett Drugs Ther **21:**29-30, 1979.

174. Thomason BM, et al: Salmonellae in health foods, Appl Environ Microbiol **34:**602-603, 1977.

175. Hodges RS: Megavitamin therapy, Primary Care **9:**605-619, 1982.

176. Truswell AS: ABC of nutrition. Vitamins I, Br Med J **291:**1033, 1985.

177. Truswell AS: ABC of nutrition. Vitamins II, Br Med J **291:**1103, 1985.

178. McClaren DS: Excessive nutrient intakes. In Jelliffe EFP, Jelliffe DF: Adverse effects of foods, New York, 1982, Plenum Press Inc, pp 367-404.

179. Food and Nutrition Board, Division of Biological Sciences, Assembly of Life Sciences, National Research Council: Vegetarian diets, Washington DC, 1974, National Academy of Sciences.

180. Committee on Nutrition, American Academy of Pediatrics: The relationship between infantile hypercalcemia and vitamin D: public health implications in North America, Pediatrics **40:**1050-1061, 1967.

181. Committee on Nutrition, American Academy of Pediatrics: The prophylactic requirement and the toxicity of vitamin D, Pediatrics **31:**512-525, 1963.

182. Forbes GH, Woodruff CW: Nutritional aspects of vegetarianism, health foods, and food diets. In Forbes G, Woodruff CW, editors: Pediatric nutrition handbook, Elk Grove Village Ill, 1983, American Academy of Pediatrics, pp 298-310.

183. Korner WF, Vollm J: New aspects of the tolerance of retinol in humans, Int J Vitam Nutr Res **45:**363-372, 1975.

184. Committee on Nutrition and Committee on Drugs, American Academy of Pediatrics: The use and abuse of vitamin A, Pediatrics **48:**655-665, 1977.

185. Selhorst JB, et al: Liver lover's headache: pseudotumor cerebri and vitamin A intoxication, JAMA **252:**3365, 1984.

186. Maldonado RR, Tamayo L: Retinoids in keratinizing diseases and acne, Pediatr Clin North Am **30:**721-734, 1983.

187. Herbert V: Toxicity of 25,000 IU vitamin A supplements in "health" food users, Am J Clin Nutr **36:**185-186, 1982.

188. Goodman DS: Vitamin A and retinoids in health and disease, N Engl J Med **310:**1023-1031, 1984.

189. Bollag W: Vitamin A and retinoids: from nutrition to pharmacotherapy in dermatology and oncology, Lancet **1:**860-863, 1983.

190. Vitamin A and cancer [editorial], Lancet **2:**325-326, 1984.

191. Willett WC, et al: Relation of serum vitamins A and E and carotenoids to the risk of cancer, N Engl J Med **310:**430-434, 1984.

192. Kemmann E, et al: Amenorrhea associated with carotenemia, JAMA **249:**926-929, 1983.

193. Horwitt MK: Therapeutic uses of vitamin E in medicine, Nutr Rev **38:**105-113, 1980.

194. Bieri JG, et al: Medical uses of vitamin E, N Engl J Med **308:**1063-1071, 1983.

195. Committee on Dietary Allowances, Food and Nutrition Board, National Research Council: Recommended dietary allowances, ed 9, Washington DC, 1980, National Academy of Sciences.

196. Melhorn DK, Gross S: Relationship between iron dextran and vitamin E in iron deficiency anemia in children, J Lab Clin Med **74:**789-802, 1969.

197. Irwin MI, Hutchins BK: A conspectus of research on vitamin C requirements of man, J Nutr **106:**823-879, 1976.

198. Burr ML, et al: Vitamin C supplementation of old people with low blood levels, Gerontol Clin **17:**236-243, 1975.

199. Pauling L: The significance of the evidence about ascorbic acid and the common cold, Proc Natl Acad Sci USA **68:**2678-2681, 1971.

200. Anderson TW: Large scale trials of vitamin C, Ann NY Acad Sci **258:**498-504, 1975.

201. Karlowski TR, et al: Ascorbic acid for the common cold: a prophylactic and therapeutic trial, JAMA **231:**1038-1042, 1975.

202. Chalmers TC: Effects of ascorbic acid on the common cold: an evaluation of the evidence, Am J Med **58:**532-536, 1975.

203. Cameron E, Pauling L: Supplemental ascorbate in the supportive treatment of cancer: prolongation of survival times in terminal human cancer, Proc Natl Acad Sci USA **73:**3685-3689, 1976.

204. Pauling L: Vitamin C therapy of advanced cancer, N Engl J Med **302:**694, 1980.

205. Creagan ET, et al: Failure of high dose vitamin C (ascorbic acid) therapy to benefit patients with advanced cancer. A controlled trial, N Engl J Med **301:**687-690, 1979.

206. Moertel CG, et al: High dose vitamin C versus placebo in the treatment of patients with advanced cancer who have had no prior chemotherapy. A randomized double blind comparison, N Engl J Med **312:**137-141, 1985.

207. Wittes RE: Vitamin C and cancer, N Engl J Med **312:**178-179, 1985.

208. Stein HG, et al: Ascorbic acid induced uricosuria: a consequence of megavitamin therapy, Ann Intern Med **84:**385-388, 1976.

209. Cook JD, Monsen ER: Vitamin C, the common cold, and iron absorption, Am J Clin Nutr **30:**235-241, 1977.

210. Shilotri PG, Bhat KS: Effects of megadoses of vitamin C on bactericidal activity of leukocytes, Am J Clin Nutr **30:**1077-1081, 1977.

211. Barr W: Pyridoxine supplements in the premenstrual syndrome, Practitioner **228:**425-427, 1984.

212. Schaumburg H, et al: Sensory neuropathy from pyridoxine abuse, N Engl J Med **309:**445-448, 1983.

213. Berger A, Schaumburg H: More on neuropathy from pyridoxine abuse, N Engl J Med **311:**986-987, 1984.

214. Allen LH: The role of nutrition in the onset and treatment of metabolic bone disease. In Weininger J, Briggs GM, editors: Nutrition update, vol 1, New York, 1983, John Wiley & Sons Inc, pp 263-284.

215. Spiller GA, Freeman HJ: Dietary fiber in human nutrition. In Weininger J, Briggs GM, editors: Nutrition update. Vol 1, New York, 1983, John Wiley & Sons Inc, pp 163-178.

216. Lanza E, Butrum RR: A critical review of food fiber analysis and data, J Am Diet Assoc **86:**732-743, 1986.

217. Munoz J: Fiber and diabetes, Diabetes Care **7:**297-298, 1984.

218. Crapo PA: Simple versus complex carbyhydrate use in the diabetic diet, Ann Rev Nutr **5:**95-114, 1985.

219. Kay RM: Dietary fiber, J Lipid Res **23:**221-242, 1982.

220. Roth C, Leitzmann C: Fiber and the large gut. In Leeds AR, editor: Dietary fiber perspectives, London, 1985, John Libbey & Co Ltd, pp 1-22.

221. Eastwood MA: Measurement of water holding properties of fiber and their faecal bulking ability in man, Br J Nutr **50:**539-547, 1983.

222. Ornstein MH, et al: Are fibre supplements really necessary in diverticular disease of the colon? A controlled clinical trial, Br Med J **282:**1353-1356, 1981.

223. Broadribb AJM: The treatment of diverticular disease with dietary fiber, J Plant Foods **3:**63-73, 1978.

224. Leahy AL, et al: High fibre diet in symptomatic diverticular disease of the colon, Ann Coll Surg Engl **67:**173-174, 1985.

225. Heaton KW: Role of dietary fiber in irritable bowel syndrome. In Read NW, editor: Irritable bowel syndrome, New York, 1985, Grune & Stratton Inc, pp 203-218.

226. International Agency for Research on Cancer: Dietary fibre, transit time, faecal bacteria, steroids, and colon cancer in two Scandanavian populations, Lancet **2:**207-211, 1977.

227. Bingham SA, et al: Dietary fiber consumption in Britain; new estimates and their relation to large bowel cancer mortality, Br J Cancer **52:**399-402, 1985.

228. Kune S, et al: Case control study of dietary and etiological factors: the Melbourne colorectal cancer study, Nutr Cancer **9:**21-42, 1987.

229. Hara N, et al: Statistical analyses of the pattern of food consumption and digestive tract cancers in Japan, Nutr Cancer **6:**220-228, 1985.

230. Mann JI: Fiber and diabetes, Diabetes Care **8:**192-193, 1985.

231. Munoz J: Fiber and diabetes: a reply, Diabetes Care **8:**193-194, 1985.

232. Ahrens EH, Connor WE: Report of the task force on the evidence relating six dietary factors to the nation's health, Am J Clin Nutr **32**(suppl):2621-2626, 1979.

233. Nutrition Statistics Branch, Division of Health Examination Statistics, National Center for Health Statistics: Diet, nutrition, disease, and the dietary goals in health, United States, DHEW Publ (PHS) 80-132, Washington DC, 1979, Department of Health, Education, and Welfare, pp 31-44.

234. Abraham S, Carroll MD: Fats, cholesterol, and sodium intake in the diet: United States. In Beecher GA, editor: Beltsville symposia in agricultural research. 4. Human nutrition research, Totowa NJ, 1981, Allanheld Osmun Inc, pp 75-94.

235. Mertz W: Vitamins and minerals. In Beecher GA, editor: Beltsville symposia in agricultural research. 4. Human nutrition research, Totowa NJ, 1981, Allanheld Osmun Inc, pp 49-56.

236. Nestle M, et al: Nutrition policy update. In Weininger J, Briggs GM, editors: Nutrition update, vol 1, New York, 1983, John Wiley & Sons Inc, pp 285-314.

237. Dwyer J: Dietary recommendations and policy implications: the U.S. experience. In Weininger J, Briggs GM,

editors: Nutrition update, vol 1, New York, 1983, John Wiley & Sons Inc, pp 315-356.

238. Food and Nutrition Board, National Reserach Council: Toward healthful diets, Washington DC, 1980, National Academy of Sciences.

239. Palmer S: Public health policy on diet, nutrition, and cancer, Nutr Cancer **6:**273-283, 1984.

240. United States Department of Agriculture and Department of Health and Human Services: Nutrition and your health: dietary guidelines for Americans, ed 2, Washington DC, 1985, Government Printing Office.

241. United States Department of Agriculture, Science and Education Administration: Food. House and Garden Bulletin, 228, Washington DC, 1979, Government Printing Office.

242. Science and Education Administration/Human Nutrition, United States Department of Agriculture: Ideas for better eating: menus and recipes to make use of the dietary guidelines, Washington DC, 1981, Government Printing Office.

243. Better eating for better health, Washington DC, 1984, The American National Red Cross.

244. United States Department of Health and Human Services: Diet, nutrition, and cancer prevention: a guide to food choices, NIH Publ 85-2711, Bethesda, 1984, National Cancer Institute, National Institutes of Health.

CHAPTER 46
Nutrition Education and Counseling

Phyllis L. Fleming

People smoke cigarettes, drive without seat belts, eat too many calories, and avoid exercise if they can. Yet all these behaviors are hazardous to their health. If promoting good health and preventing and treating disease were the primary motivations of most people, we would have a smoke-free, seat-belted, normal weight, and fit population. The fact that we do not represents a challenge for health professionals. When a person's condition calls for changes in life-style, what tools, strategies, and techniques are available to initiate and facilitate those changes? This chapter presents guidelines for helping a client successfully change his or her life-style through nutrition education and counseling.

When necessary changes are related to health, it seems obvious to develop rationales around the premises, "It's good for you," or, "I'm the health expert, and I am asking you to do this." These strategies are simple, straightforward, and, unfortunately, ineffective for the most part. A person's behavior is comfortable and in some way functional for him or her. People who put a high priority on personal health may respond to an appeal for change for health's sake, yet empirical data suggest that health ranks behind taste, cost, and preferences of family and friends as a reason for selecting foods.[1] Clearly, just prescribing a diet and expecting compliance oversimplifies the complex task of changing eating behavior. Similarly, a client has trouble seeing the health professional's expertise as a reason for change when the influences of environment, culture, social situation, and personal motivation pressure the individual to eat as always.

Nutrition educators traditionally have elaborated upon the "it's good for you" strategy to include "why it's good for you." It was assumed that once a person had the facts linking eating behavior to health outcome, his or her behavior would change. A lot of time and money have been spent trying to make this knowledge-attitude-behavior model work. Pamphlets, posters, fliers, media presentations, books, lectures, small-group presentations, and face-to-face consultations have been devoted to teaching food groups, nutrient requirements, recommended dietary intakes, physiology, diet-disease links, and similar cognitively oriented concepts. The impact these efforts have had is difficult to assess, but neither research nor practice significantly supports a direct relationship between knowledge and behavior.[2-4]

The knowledge-attitude-behavior sequence oversimplifies the problems of behavior change. In some cases a positive attitude change may occur first and stimulate an interest, which leads to greater knowledge, which then guides behavior change. In other cases behavior change may precede changes in both attitude and knowledge. For example, an unexpectedly pleasant encounter with vegetarian food may lead to a positive attitude toward and pursuit of information about the benefits of the vegetarian diet and food preparation techniques. In contrast, a lecture in the health professional's office on the physiology of osteoporosis may not be enough to persuade a 40-year-old woman to rearrange her eating pattern to include calcium sources.

NUTRITION EDUCATION

Although some research on behavior change has indicated a correlation between knowledge and behavior, the incidence, without exception, is too small to be useful.[2-4] In most of this research, knowledge accounts for approximately 4% to 8% of the variance in eating behavior, leaving 92% to 96% of the behavior to be accounted for by other influences. Effective strategies for changing behavior require that other influences be identified and pursued. In practice, knowledge and behavior seem to be only weakly related. Indeed if knowing were related to doing, those in the health field would be robust, trim, and vigorous. Unfortunately that is frequently not the case.

Research in the areas of health behavior change and education suggests an expansion of the knowledge-attitude-behavior sequence to conform more closely to the process of behavior change. The health belief model, for example, proposes that compliance with health-related recommendations depends upon perceptions of personal relevance. Other research highlights the importance of (1) obtaining a commitment or statement of intent from the client that he or she will try the recommended change, and (2) showing the client how to make the change.

The impact of building nutrition management and counseling programs on the weak link between knowledge and behavior is telling. Health professionals to date have been unsuccessful for the most part in converting growing interest in nutrition to a change in nutrition behavior.[5-8] Part of the problem has been the reliance on ineffective communication efforts. Another part of the problem is the use of traditional educational strategies, such as recommended dietary allowances or food groups, which are more suitable for education addressing problems of undernutrition than problems related to the complexity and diversity of the American diet. Still another part of the problem is that educational strategies have been developed from the perspective of the health professionals rather than the clients.

The task of using nutrition information to persuade a client to change his or her life-style encompasses more than a pamphlet, poster, or 5-minute discussion about recommended amounts of nutrients. It involves capturing the attention of a client distracted by nutrition messages from many sources and with different levels of credibility and legitimacy. It means motivating a client to shift away from comfortable but questionable eating patterns. It requires teaching the client to discriminate among the 16,000 supermarket items, the array of foods presented on restaurant and fast-food menus, and the spectrum of legitimate and quack nutrition messages. If nutrition management and counseling are to be effective, they must be heard above the din of all the other nutrition noise. Health professionals must acquire the sophisticated communication skills and strategies of their competitors.

Strategies for Client Motivation

National marketing data can provide valuable clues about how to approach clients effectively to help change nutrition behavior. Recent national surveys indicate that there is considerable consumer interest in nutrition, although not necessarily for health reasons.

The fairly extensive interest in nutrition revealed by these surveys may be surprising. It may be for the sake of beauty, improved appearance, more energy to work or play, or a more satisfying sex life rather than for health. Whatever the motivation, marketers would build on these interests to develop and promote successful products and services. Following the lead of marketing strategies that are strongly consumer-oriented, nutrition management strategies should be client-centered. What does the client value? What is his or her current life-style? How can proposed modifications fit into that life-style? How much change can the client comfortably make at one time? How much change is he or she willing to try? A thorough history and diagnosis of life-style for each client can reveal the motivational and informational foundations on which an effective program of dietary change can be built.

Clients cannot necessarily be told what they want to hear; calorie restrictions and substitutions for favorite foods do not come as welcome news. However, nutrition counselors can work to link what they tell each client and how they tell him or her to the clients' personal concerns, life-style, and objectives. In essence, the client should be given the lead in indicating how to meet nutritional needs, how to shape the content of the message, what kind of appeal to use, and which strategy to implement for changing behavior.

Behavior Modification

Another approach to patient management is behavior modification. This approach has been used extensively in managing the obese client. Programs of behavior modification for weight reduction acknowledge the impact of environment on eating behavior. The stimulus-response-reinforcer model is the cornerstone of these programs. The model emanates from the animal research of I.P. Pavlov and B.F. Skinner. Basically, it proposes that eating behavior is a learned response to many environmental and emotional stimuli. Just as Pavlov's dogs learned to salivate (response) when a light was turned on or a bell rung (stimuli), so humans learn to eat (response), when they go to the movies, see a bag of potato chips, or have nothing else to do (stimuli). Skinner's work contributed the concept of a reinforcer, a consequence that makes behavior more likely to occur. Thus a hungry pigeon presses a bar (response) more frequently when initially grain (reinforcer) followed a random press of the bar. Similarly, according to Skinner's model, humans will eat more frquently if they discover that eating provides relief from boredom, makes them feel comfortable, or pleases an important other person. From a behavior modification point of view, changing nutrition behavior involves breaking learned and established stimulus-response-reinforcer links that are associated with maladaptive behavior (e.g., overeating or eating foods high in sodium) and teaching and establishing new links to take their places.

Changing nutrition behavior also involves motivation and commitment. The client is an active participant in the effort, while the health professional helps develop strategies to establish adaptive links between stimuli, responses, and reinforcers in place of previous maladaptive ones.

In the area of weight loss, behavior modification programs generally appear to be more effective than any other current programs (with the exception of surgical intervention). Dropout rates are lower, and dieting has fewer negative emotional effects. However, people vary greatly in the amount of weight they lose and in their ability to maintain the loss. Average weight loss is modest, and often some relapse occurs after a year.

Client education depends on an alliance between health professional and client. Information must be exchanged, a rapport established, and a mutual, satisfactory strategy developed. These considerations form the basis of nutrition education and counseling.

GUIDELINES FOR NUTRITION EDUCATION AND COUNSELING

The following guidelines have been distilled from the previously discussed considerations and from research on changing health behavior reported in the behavioral medicine literature. The guidelines are drawn from a range of theoretical perspectives and from research dealing with several health behaviors, most of which concern eating and smoking. These guidelines represent issues that should be considered throughout the process of behavior change.

Form a partnership with the client

There is growing agreement among nutritionists that nutrition education and counselors must pay more attention to the perspectives and interests of the client.[9-11] Food marketers have known for a long time that it is easier to promote a product for which there is an exciting consumer need or demand than to persuade people that they want a product for which they do not feel a need.[12]

This same orientation has been recognized in health care. It is called a therapeutic alliance between health professional and client. Through this alliance, the two identify the need to change, potential sources of resistance to change, and strategies for change that are both possible and acceptable.[13] The client takes an active role in specifying current eating patterns, food preferences, and the social, cultural, and environmental contexts that surround his or her eating behavior. The health professional integrates nutritional expertise with the client's information to define an adequate diet.

Know the patient well

For therapeutic alliance to exist, the health professional must know and respect the client's point of view. The personal, social, cultural, and environmental contexts of the client's eating patterns must be assessed, and appropriate and relevant motivation for changing must be identified.

For a person who is sick or has symptoms of illness, an appeal to health may be effective.[14,15] However, compliance with health recommendations depends on the person's conviction that the existing or anticipated health problem is worth heeding and that it could have personal repercussions. According to the health belief model, people will change a behavior for health reasons only if they believe that the change will truly deal with the problem. The client must be convinced that compliance is important to future health and must see the recommendations as leading to the desired health state. For example, a middle-aged man who is not convinced that he is at risk for cardiovascular disease and that reduction of cholesterol decreases that risk is not likely to give up prime ribs and cheese.

For the person who has no symptoms of illness—say, a 40-year-old woman with no sign of osteoporosis—effective change strategies may have to include other motivational bases. These can include the desire to look good, to fulfill responsibilities as spouse or parent, to enjoy life to its fullest, or to take dream vacations. Specifications of the motivational base must come from the client.

Specify a diet that is adequate from the client's point of view

An adequate diet can be defined from many perspectives. In physiologic terms, it provides sufficient nutrients to promote and maintain normal physiologic functioning and weight. It also coincides with the meanings the individual or culture assigns to food and the benefits besides physiologic well-being that the individual expects to derive from eating. Culturally determined classifications of edible and inedible substances are respected. The diet also respects individual taste preferences, because taste is an important determinant in food selection. The diet must include foods that the client considers acceptable and desirable to eat. It must taste good and be generally a source of pleasure; it must be affordable and accessible and allow the client to maintain normal social functioning; it also must match existing cultural norms and patterns.

This requires nutritional expertise along with a sensitivity to individual and cultural cues and sufficient ingenuity to keep the two integrated. When a diet or eating pattern cannot accommodate all these factors, the health professional and the client must decide, as partners in the alliance, which ones to ignore.

Address client needs specifically

Information and change strategies should be tailored to each client rather than passed along as standard clinic information.[16] Research has shown that with pregnant women who smoked, health education methods relating directly to their condition were more effective than the general advice to quit smoking that is typically used in a clinic.[17]

Develop a plan of change and set goals as partners

The development of a plan and the kinds of goals set are critical to the success or failure of efforts to change behavior.[18] The plan must be realistic in terms of effort, money, and expectations. Goals must be short-term with imme-

diate outcomes. When the desired outcome is a weight loss of 40 pounds, goals must be segmented to specify behavior that will produce it. For example, goals might be framed in terms of replacing whole milk with skim milk, substituting fresh fruit for doughnuts at coffee breaks, or using stairways rather than escalators and elevators at least twice a day.

Whatever the goals, the client must be convinced that he or she will be able to accomplish them. If a client lacks confidence or is insecure, the health professional and the client must work together to establish conviction. The importance of this conviction, known as self-efficacy, has been documented frequently.[19-22]

Have the client make a definite commitment and a statement of intention to pursue the goals

Nutrition counselors must obtain from their clients a commitment or statement of intention to pursue the plan and achieve the goals. This commitment may take the form of a written contract, an oral agreement, a handshake, or even earnest money. The statement of intent or commitment was found to be effective in World War II experiments designed to increase consumption of organ meats, and it is still critical in strategies to change nutrition behavior.[23] Intention has predicted behavior in the extensive research of Schifter and Ajzen[18] and Ajzen and Fishbein.[24,25]

Help the client develop appropriate skills to achieve the goals

Showing the client how to make a requested change is essential for following up on a statement of intent.[15] Necessary skills may include reading food labels, calculating diabetic exchanges, planning menus, or shopping for food or preparing it. For example, a diabetic adolescent who is told to eat six small meals a day may need some help figuring out how to do that. This help may include how to incorporate snacks into the school day, how to handle popular fast foods, and perhaps how to deal with friends who are puzzled by the youngster's lack of conformity to adolescent food ways.

Use rewards to initiate and support the behavior change

Changing familiar eating patterns is difficult and at times unpleasant. The client is likely to experience a reinforcement or reward imbalance. The immediate consequences of eating favorite foods are positive; the immediate consequences of giving them up or replacing them with something less desirable are negative. The benefits of these sacrifices are distant and remote.

Nutrition counselors may have to help clients restore the reinforcement balance. Rewards for achieving goals may be built into the plan for behavior change. Such rewards are defined by the client. They may include despositing a sum of money at the start of the program that the client earns back through achieving goals; depositing a small amount of money each time a goal is achieved until enough money has accumulated for a special purchase; or earning free time to read or take a walk.

Systems of rewards have proved particularly effective in initiating new health behavior. To maintain the behavior over time, all the contexts in which it occurs must be dealth with.[26]

Identify sources of social support for the behavior change

Other people can lend support in a variety of ways. They can help alter environmental influences, particularly the availability of food. They can reinforce achievement of goals and sanction deviation from goals. They can represent a source of pressure to comply with the behavior-change plan.

Nutrition counselors can help clients identify and involve family members, coworkers, and friends who will support the change process. If support is not available in these settings, support groups may be formed.

The effectiveness of support in the social setting has been discussed extensively in the literature.[13,27,29]

Involve the client in monitoring his or her success and difficulties

Monitoring success or failure in achieving goals is useful for many reasons. Records of success are reinforcing and serve to support the behavior change. They indicate to the client that he or she is in fact efficacious; that is, able to make the changes. Records of difficulties point out the need to examine the plan and may help to troubleshoot and revise the plan. Monitoring also actively involves the client in controlling the process and paves the way for turning over increasing responsibility for the change process and its outcome to him or her.

Compliance with the self-monitoring process has been related to long-term weight loss[30] and metabolic control in diabetes.[31]

The partnership between health professional and client provides an effective model for nutrition education and counseling. The critical two-way flow of information assures that the client's life-style, culture, needs, and interests will be respected. It allows the health professional to integrate these with specific dietary information and strategies and, in cooperation with the client, to develop successful strategies for changing eating behavior.

REFERENCES

1. Schafer RB: Factors affecting food behavior and the quality of husbands' and wives' diets, J Am Diet Assoc **72**:138-143, 1978.
2. Sims LS: Dietary status of lactating women, J Am Diet Assoc **73**:147-154, 1978.
3. Fusillo AE, Beloian AM: Consumer nutrition knowledge and self-reported food shopping behavior, Am J Public Health **67**:846-850, 1977.
4. Eppright ES, et al: The North Central regional study of diets of preschool children. 2. Nutrition knowledge and attitudes of mothers, J Home Economics **62**:327, 1970.
5. Report on task force on nutrition education for the general public, Federal Register **44**:46929-46933, 1979.
6. Report on task force on nutrition education for pregnant women, children and adolescents, Federal Register **44**:46933-46937, 1979.
7. Richmond FW: The role of the federal government in nutrition education, J Nutr Ed **9**:150-151, 1977.
8. Robinson CH: Nutrition education—What comes next? J Am Diet Assoc **69**:126-132, 1976.
9. Dunlap BJ: Marketing in the health care arena: a preventive approach, J Am Diet Assoc **86**:31-32, 1986.
10. Parks SC, Moody DL: Marketing: a survival tool for dietetic professionals in the 1990's, J Am Diet Assoc **86**:33-36, 1986.
11. Fleming PL: Applications of the marketing perspective in nutrition education, J Am Diet Assoc **87**:64-68, 1987.
12. Evans RI, Hall Y: Social-psychologic perspective in motivating changes in eating behavior, J Am Diet Assoc **72**:378-383, 1978.
13. Eraker SA, et al: Smoking behavior, cessation techniques, and the health belief model, Am J Med **78**:817, 1985.
14. Ockene JK, Camic PM: Public health approaches to cigarette smoking cessation, Ann Behav Med **7**:14-18, 1985.
15. Becker MH, editor: The health belief model and personal health behavior, Health Educ Monogr **2**:326-473, 1974.
16. Lorish CD, et al: Effective patient education: A quasi experiment comparing an individualized strategy with a routinized strategy, Arthritis Rheum **28**:1289-1297, 1985.
17. Windsor RA, et al: The effectiveness of smoking cessation methods for smokers in public health maternity clinics: a randomized trial, Am J Public Health **75**:1389-1392, 1985.
18. Schifter DE, Ajzen I: Intention, perceived control and weight loss: an application of the theory of planned behavior, J Pers Soc Psychol **49**:843-851, 1985.
19. Supnick JA, Colletti G: Relapse coping and problem solv-

ing training following treatment for smoking, Addict Behav **9:**401-404, 1984.

20. Mitchell C, Stuart RB: Effect of self-efficacy on dropout from obesity treatment, J Consult Clin Psychol **52:**1100-1101, 1984.

21. O'Leary A: Self-efficacy and health behavior research, Behav Res Ther **23:**437-451, 1985.

22. Rosenstock IM: Understanding and enhancing patient compliance with diabetic regimens, Diabetes Care **8:**610-616, 1985.

23. Lewin K: Group decision and social change. In Maccoby EE, Readings in social psychology, New York, 1952, Henry Holt & Co, pp 197-211.

24. Ajzen I, Fishbein M: Attitude-behavior relations: a theoretical analysis and review of empirical research, Psychol Bull **84:**888-918, 1977.

25. Ajzen I, Fishbein M: Understanding attitudes and predict-ing social behavior, New York, 1980, Prentice-Hall Inc.

26. Lund AK, Kegeles SS: Rewards and adolescent health behavior, Health Psychol **3:**351-369, 1984.

27. Frankle RT: Obesity a family matter: Creating new behavior, J Am Diet Assoc **85:**597-601, 1985.

28. Coppotelli HC, Orleans CT: Partner support and other determinants of smoking cessation maintenance among women, J Consult Clin Psychol **53:**455-460, 1985.

29. Etringer BD, et al: Influence of group cohesion on behavioral treatment of smoking, J Consult Clin Psychol **52:**1080-1086, 1984.

30. Wing RR, et al: Intermittent low calorie regimen and booster sessions in the treatment of obesity, Behav Res Ther **22:**445-449, 1984.

31. Kaplan RM, et al: Social learning intervention to promote metabolic control in type I diabetes mellitus: pilot experimental results, Diabetes Care **8:**152-155, 1985.

APPENDICES

APPENDIX I
U.S. Dietary Standards

RECOMMENDED DIETARY ALLOWANCES

Recommended dietary allowances (RDAs) represent the average daily nutrient intake that population groups should consume over a period of time. They do not represent requirements for a specific individual. The RDA, except for energy, are estimates that *exceed* the requirements of most individuals in order to ensure that the needs of nearly all in the population are met. Levels of nutrient intake below recommended allowances do not necessarily represent inadequate nutrient intake. However, the risk of inadequate intake does increase to the extent that intake is less than the recommended safe level.

Conditions that may modify the RDA include physical activity, climate, aging, chronic diseases, and drug intake.

The allowance indicated for energy should be considered differently from allowances for specific nutrients. The energy values listed are estimates of the average needs of age- and sex-specific population groups and are not recommended intakes for individuals. Individual needs vary greatly and cannot be predicted with any certainty in the absence of detailed information on a variety of individual characteristics, including activity.

RECOMMENDED DAILY DIETARY ALLOWANCES,[a] REVISED 1980

Designed for the maintenance of good nutrition of practically all healthy people in the U.S.A.

	Age (yr)	Weight (kg)	Weight (lb)	Height (cm)	Height (in)	Energy (average needs)	Protein (g)	Fat-Soluble Vitamins — Vitamin A (μg RE)[b]	Vitamin D (μg)[c]	Vitamin E (mg α-TE)[d]	Water-Soluble Vitamins — Vitamin C (mg)	Thiamine (mg)	Riboflavin (mg)	Niacin (mg-NE)[e]
Infants	0.0-0.5	6	13	60	24	kg × 115	kg × 2.2	420	10	3	35	0.3	0.4	6
	0.5-1.0	9	20	71	28	kg × 105	kg × 2.0	400	10	4	35	0.5	0.6	8
Children	1-3	13	29	90	35	1300	23	400	10	5	45	0.7	0.8	9
	4-6	20	44	112	44	1700	30	500	10	6	45	0.9	1.0	11
	7-10	28	62	132	52	2400	34	700	10	7	45	1.2	1.4	16
Men	11-14	45	99	157	62	2700	45	1000	10	8	50	1.4	1.6	18
	15-18	66	145	176	69	2800	56	1000	10	10	60	1.4	1.7	18
	19-22	70	154	177	70	2900	56	1000	7.5	10	60	1.5	1.7	19
	23-50	70	154	178	70	2700	56	1000	5	10	60	1.4	1.6	18
	51+	70	154	178	70	2400[f]	56	1000	5	10	60	1.2	1.4	16
Women	11-14	46	101	157	62	2200	46	800	10	8	50	1.1	1.3	15
	15-18	55	120	163	64	2100	46	800	10	8	60	1.1	1.3	14
	19-22	55	120	163	64	2100	44	800	7.5	8	60	1.1	1.3	14
	23-50	55	120	163	64	2000	44	800	5	8	60	1.0	1.2	13
	51+	55	120	163	64	1800	44	800	5	8	60	1.0	1.2	13
Pregnant						+300	+30	+200	+5	+2	+20	+0.4	+0.3	+2
Lactating						+500	+20	+400	+5	+3	+40	+0.5	+0.5	+5

[a]The allowances are intended to provide for individual variations among most normal persons as they live in the United States under usual environmental stresses. Diets should be based on a variety of common foods in order to provide other nutrients for which human requirements have been less well defined.

[b]Retinol equivalents. 1 retinol equivalent = 1 μg retinol or 6 μg β carotene.

[c]As cholecalciferol, 10 μg cholecalciferol = 400 I.U. vitamin D.

[d]α-Tocopherol equivalents. 1 mg *d*-α-tocopherol = 1 α-TE.

[e]1 NE (niacin equivalent) is equal to 1 mg of niacin or 60 mg of dietary tryptophan.

[f]Over 75 years of age, energy needs are 2050 kcal in males and 1600 kcal in females.

	Age (yr)	Weight (kg)	Weight (lb)	Height (cm)	Height (in)	Water-Soluble Vitamins — Vitamin B₆ (mg)	Folacin[g] (µg)	Vitamin B₁₂ (µg)	Minerals — Calcium (mg)	Phosphorus (mg)	Magnesium (mg)	Iron (mg)	Zinc (mg)	Iodine (µg)
Infants	0.0-0.5	6	13	60	24	0.3	30	0.5[h]	360	240	50	10	3	40
	0.5-1.0	9	20	71	28	0.6	45	1.5	540	360	70	15	5	50
Children	1-3	13	29	90	35	0.9	100	2.0	800	800	150	15	10	70
	4-6	20	44	112	44	1.3	200	2.5	800	800	200	10	10	90
	7-10	28	62	132	52	1.6	300	3.0	800	800	250	10	10	120
Men	11-14	45	99	157	62	1.8	400	3.0	1200	1200	350	18	15	150
	15-18	66	145	176	69	2.0	400	3.0	1200	1200	400	18	15	150
	19-22	70	154	177	70	2.2	400	3.0	800	800	350	10	15	150
	23-50	70	154	178	70	2.2	400	3.0	800	800	350	10	15	150
	51+	70	154	178	70	2.2	400	3.0	800	800	350	10	15	150
Women	11-14	46	101	157	62	1.8	400	3.0	1200	1200	300	18	15	150
	15-18	55	120	163	64	2.0	400	3.0	1200	1200	300	18	15	150
	19-22	55	120	163	64	2.0	400	3.0	800	800	300	18	15	150
	23-50	55	120	163	64	2.0	400	3.0	800	800	300	18	15	150
	51+	55	120	163	64	2.0	400	3.0	800	800	300	10	15	150
Pregnant						+0.6	+400	+1.0	+400	+400	+150	i	+5	+25
Lactating						+0.5	+100	+1.0	+400	+400	+150	i	+10	+50

From Committee on Dietary Allowances, Food and Nutrition Board, National Research Council:: Recommended dietary allowances, ed 9, Washington DC, 1980, National Academy of Sciences.

[g]The folacin allowances refer to dietary sources as determined by *Lactobacillus casei* assay after treatment with enzymes (conjugases) to make polyglutamyl forms of the vitamin available to the test organism.

[h]The recommended dietary allowance for vitamin B₁₂ in infants is based on average concentration of the vitamin in human milk. The allowances after weaning are based on energy intake (as recommended by the American Academy of Pediatrics) and consideration of other factors, such as intestinal absorption.

The increased requirement during pregnancy cannot be met by the iron content of habitual American diets nor by the existing iron stores of many women; therefore, the use of 30-60 mg of supplemental iron is recommended. Iron needs during lactation are not substantially different from those of nonpregnant women, but continued supplementation of the mother for 2-3 months after parturition is advisable in order to replenish stores depleted by pregnancy.

RDA LISTED NUTRIENTS

Selected Summary of Availability, Digestion, and Function

	Protein	Vitamin A	Vitamin D (calciferol)

Food Source	8 g in
	  30 g meat, fish, poultry
	  30 g cheese; 1 c milk
	7 g in
	  1 egg
	  ½ c cooked dry beans
	  2 Tbsp peanut butter
	3 g in
	  ½ c ice cream
	2 g in
	  1 serv bread or cereal
	  ½ c vegetables
		15,000 IU in
		  30 g beef liver
		4000 IU in
		  ½ c carrots or
		    cooked spinach
		2000 IU in
		  ¼ c cantaloupe melon
		  ½ c broccoli, cooked
		    cabbage, canned apricots
		1000 IU in
		  ½ c tomatoes or tomato
		    juice, apricot nectar
		500 IU in
		  1 Tbsp butter or fortified
		    margarine
		250 IU in
		  1 c whole or fortified milk
		  30 g cheddar cheese
		  ½ c ice cream
			400 IU in
			  1 quart fortified milk
			  1 tsp natural-form cod-liver oil
			Also produced by ultraviolet
			  radiation of 7-dehydrocholes-
			  terol in the skin

Stability	A browning reaction may occur with heating or long storage in which certain amino acids (particularly lysine) are destroyed, thus decreasing nutritive value	Gradual destruction by exposure to air; more rapid at high temperatures	Stable to heat, oxidation, acid and alkali; destroyed by excess ultraviolet irradiation
Absorption	Amino acids absorbed mainly in upper gastrointestinal tract by specific carrier mechanisms	Absorbed in duodenum and upper jejunum in presence of bile; decreases when diet is unusually low in fat; some intestinal provitamin A converted to vitamin A within intestinal mucosal cell	Absorbed in presence of bile, primarily in jejunum; decreased with fat malabsorption
Function	Maintains structural integrity of cells; regulates colloid osmotic pressure of body fluids; synthesis of cell proteins, protein hormones, enzymes, antibodies and circulating or storage molecules of essential body compounds; protein will be oxidized for energy with insufficient carbohydrate or fat kilocalories or converted to fat when protein and energy requirements are exceeded	Constituent of visual pigments; maintains normal epithelial tissue; provides for normal bone development and influences normal tooth formation; promotes normal growth	Increases calcium absorption from intestine; facilitates reabsorption of phosphate in kidney tubule and maintains plasma calcium in conjunction with parathyroid hormone and calcitonin
Deficiency Effects	Weakness, apathy, anorexia, underweight, dermatitis, hepatomegaly, edema, stunted growth, kwashiorkor	Night blindness, follicular hyperkeratosis, growth failure of bones, xerophthalmia, blindness	Osteomalacia (adults), rickets (children)
Toxic Effect	Elevated blook nitrogenous wastes in (some) infants and individuals with impaired renal function; may aggravate liver and kidney disturbances	Swelling over long bones, dry scaly rough skin, bone and joint pain, decalcification of bones	Loss of weight, anorexia, vomiting, calcification of soft tissue

From Utah Dietetic Association: Handbook of clinical dietetics, ed 2, Salt Lake City, 1977, Birkco Graphic

Vitamin E (tocopherol)	Ascorbic Acid (vitamin C)	Thiamine (vitamin B₁)

5 IU in
  1 tsp cottonseed, corn, soybean, safflower, wheat germ oil or shortening
  2 tsp margarine, mayonnaise, or vegetable oil (other than above)
2 IU in
  ½ c cooked cabbage, asparagus, spinach, or dark green vegetables
1 IU in
  ½ c fruit or other vegetable
  90 g meat, fish or poultry
  1 egg
  2 slices whole grain breads
	70 mg in
	  ½ c cooked broccoli or brussels sprouts
	  1 medium orange
	60 mg in
	  ½ c orange juice
	40 mg in
	  ½ c green pepper, grapefruit, or ½ c grapefruit juice
	  ½ c strawberries
	30 mg in
	  ½ c cooked cauliflower
	  ¼ c cantaloupe
	20 mg in
	  ½ c cooked or raw cabbage, cooked asparagus, canned tomatoes or tomato juice
	  1 medium potato, baked or boiled
	10 mg in
	  ½ c squash, spinach, pineapple, or pineapple juice
	  1 small banana
		1.25 mg in
		  1 Tbsp brewer's yeast
		0.2 mg in
		  30 g pork, ½ c cooked peas, enriched or whole grain cereal products and pastas
		0.1 mg in
		  1 c milk
		  ½ c cooked dry beans
		0.06 mg in
		  30 g meat (except pork)
		  1 egg
		  1 slice whole grain or enriched bread
		  ½ c cooked greens

Stable to heat and acids; destroyed by oxidation, alkali, lead and iron salts, and UV light	Unstable to heat and oxidation, except in acid media	Unstable to heat, alkali, and oxygenation; heat stable in acid solution
Absorbed in upper part of small intestine in presence of bile	Readily absorbed from upper part of small intestine	Readily absorbed in upper small intestine
Functions as an antioxidant; protects unsaturated fatty acids and vitamin A from oxidation; participates in hemoglobin synthesis and maintains cell membrane integrity	Provides for wound healing, resistance to infections and maintains capillary integrity as an essential for proline hydroxylation in collagen synthesis; enhances iron absorption and facilitates conversion of folic to folinic acid	Forms thiamin pyrophosphate which acts as coenzyme in oxidative decarboxylation and transketolase reactions
Increased hemolysis of red blood cells in vitro; macrocytic anemia and dermatitis in infants	Sore and bleeding gums; tendency to bruise easily because of weak capillary walls and impaired wound healing; scurvy	Anorexia, fatigue, constipation, burning-feet syndrome, foot and wrist drop, cardiomegaly, beriberi
Numerous toxic effects reported, but data inconclusive	Adaptation of fetus to higher levels, with resultant increased requirement postpartum; acidic urine may promote oxalate stone formation; may interfere with anticoagulant therapy and urine-glucose tests or tests for stool-blood (as a false negative)	Variety of pharmacologic effects when administered in doses thousands of times the RDA level

Specialities, pp 1-9.

Continued.

Selected Summary of Availability, Digestion, and Function—cont'd

	Pyridoxine (vitamin B$_6$)	Vitamin B$_{12}$ (cyanocobalamin)	Folacin (folic acid)

Food Source	0.5 mg in
	  90 g beef liver
	  1 small banana
	0.3 mg in
	  90 mg meat, fish, poultry
	0.2 mg in
	  1 medium potato
	  ½ c tomato juice or cooked corn
	0.1 mg in
	  1 c milk (any)
	  ¾ c 40% bran flakes
	  ½ c broccoli, Brussels sprouts, cauliflower, spinach, pineapple or pineapple juice
	0.05 mg in
	  60 g cheddar cheese
	  1 egg
	  30 g raisins
	  2 slices whole grain bread
	  ½ c cottage cheese
		50 µg in
		  60 fried beef liver
		2 µg in
		  90 g beef or lamb
		  30 g crab, salmon, other fish or shellfish
		1 µg in
		  90 g chicken
		  1 egg
		  ½ c cottage cheese
		  1 c milk (any)
		0.5 µg in
		  90 g pork
		  60 g cheddar cheese
			(These values are for total folacin)
			300 µg in
			  1 Tbsp brewers yeast
			70 µg in
			  60 g liver
			  1 medium orange
			  ½ c orange juice
			  ½ c peanuts
			  ½ c cooked beets or spinach
			50 µg in
			  1 c cooked dry beans
			  ½ c cooked broccoli
			  ¼ cantaloupe
			25 µg in
			  1 egg
			  1 c lettuce
			  ½ c peas
			  ½ c grapefruit juice or tomato juice

Stability	Stable to heat, acid, and alkali but destroyed by ultraviolet light and oxidation	Slowly destroyed by acid, alkali, light and oxidation	Unstable to heat and oxidation
Absorption	Readily absorbed by simple diffusion	Absorption in ileum; requires intrinsic factor from gastric secretions to complex with B$_{12}$ in presence of ionic calcium	Absorbed primarily from proximal third of small intestine, but capable of being absorbed from entire length of small bowel
Function	Forms coenzyme pyridoxal phosphate, which functions in nearly all reactions involved in nonoxidative degradation of amino acids; transamination, deamination, desulfhydration, and decarboxylation; active in conversion of tryptophan to niacin and linoleic acid to arachidonic acid	Involved in metabolism of single carbon units, DNA synthesis, myelin synthesis, red blood cell maturation	Forms coenzyme, tetrahydrofolic acid, which transfers one-carbon units to various compounds in the synthesis of DNA, RNA, cystine; essential for formation and maturation of red and white blood cells in bone marrow
Deficiency Effects	Depression, nausea, vomiting, seborrheic dermatitis, peripheral neuritis, anemia, renal calculi	Macrocytic (megaloblastic) anemia, glossitis, other GI disturbances, neurologic syndromes, pernicious anemia	Megaloblastic (macrocytic) anemia, weakness, glossitis, gastrointestinal disturbances
Toxic Effect	Sleepiness, reduces clinical benefit of levodopa therapy in Parkinson's disease	Not known	Not known

Niacin (nicotinic acid)	Riboflavin (vitamin B$_2$)	Iron

8 mg in
  60 g beef liver
  ⅓ c peanuts
7 mg in
  90 g chicken or salmon
  60 g tuna
3 gm in
  90 g meat (other than above)
  1 Tbsp brewer's yeast
  2 Tbsp peanut butter
1.5 mg in
  1 c enriched macaroni products
  2 slices enriched or whole grain bread
  1 medium potato
  ½ c green peas
	1 mg in
	  30 g liver
	0.4 mg in
	  1 c milk or yogurt
	0.3 mg in
	  ½ c cottage cheese
	  1 Tbsp brewer's yeast
	0.2 mg in
	  90 g meat
	  ½ c custard
	0.15 mg in
	  30 g cheddar cheese
	  1 egg
	  ½ c broccoli, asparagus, or winter squash
	0.1 mg in
	  1 medium orange or ½ c orange juice
	0.05 mg in
	  1 slice enriched or whole grain bread
	  ½ c pineapple, pineapple juice
	  ½ c cooked dry beans
		5 mg in
		  60 g beef liver
		  ½ c prune juice or 40% Bran Flakes
		3 mg in
		  90 g lean beef, pork (except ham) or turkey
		  ½ c raisins
		2 mg in
		  90 g ham
		  ½ c cooked dry beans, split peas, asparagus, spinach and other greens
		1 mg in
		  90 g fish or chicken
		  1 egg
		  1 c enriched or whole grain cereal, 1 slice whole wheat bread, or 1 medium potato
		  ½ c green beans

Stable to heat, light, oxidation, acid, and alkali	Stable to heat, acids, and oxidation; unstable to light and alkali	
Absorbed in upper small intestine	Readily absorbed by simple diffusion in upper small intestine	5–20% absorbed primarily in upper duodenum; increased by need, reducing agents, adequate calcium; decreased by achlorhydria, high cellulose, steatorrhea, precipitation by phosphates, phytates, oxalates, alkalinization, ingested alkaline clays and antacid preparations
Forms coenzymes NAD and NADP, which transfer hydrogen ions in oxidation-reduction reactions during energy metabolism	Forms coenzymes FMN and FAD, which transfer hydrogen ions in oxidation-reductions during energy metabolism	Involved in transport of oxygen as constituent of hemoglobin; involved in tissue respiration as myoglobin; part of various enzymes that catalyze oxidative reductive processes in cell
Anorexia, indigestion, nervous depression, neuritis, pellagra (dermatitis, dementia, diarrhea, death)	Glossitis, seborrheic dermatitis, eye sensitivity, cheilosis	Pallor, fatigue, hypochromic, microcytic anemia
Flushing reaction, gastrointestinal irritation	None clearly documented	Idiopathic hemochromatosis, transfusional hemosiderosis with tissue cirrhosis and fibrosis resulting

Continued.

Selected Summary of Availability, Digestion, and Function—cont'd

	Magnesium	Zinc	Calcium
Food Source	70 mg in ½ c cooked dry beans or dark leafy greens 50 mg in 30 g nuts 2 Tbsp peanut butter 30 mg in 90 g fish or shellfish 1 Tbsp wheat germ 1 c cooked macaroni or spaghetti 1 c milk 20 mg in 1 slice whole wheat bread 15 mg in 90 g meat 30 g cheddar cheese ½ c most vegetables	2 mg in 30 g in pork liver or roast beef 1 mg in 30 g other meats, shellfish, poultry, or peanuts 1 egg 1 c milk 0.5 mg in 30 g cheese 1 slice whole grain bread ½ c cooked rice or peas	350 mg in 1 c 2% of fortified skim milk 300 mg in 1 c buttermilk, whole milk or yogurt 250 mg in 30 g swiss cheese ½ c red salmon (with bone) 200 mg in 30 g cheddar cheese 1 c ice cream or ice milk 175 mg in ½ c milk puddings or baked custard 150 mg in 30 g American processed cheese ½ c dark greens except beet greens, spinach, or chard
Stability			
Absorption	25–85% absorbed primarily in upper intestine; enhanced or depressed by same factors that affect calcium absorption except that vitamin D has no effect	30–50% absorbed; readily absorbed in upper small intestine; decreased by presence of phytic acid and by high dietary calcium	Only 20–30% absorbed; absorbed in duodenum in acid medium; enhanced by need, acid pH, lactose, adequate vitamin D, adequate protein; decreased by chronic renal insufficiency, steatorrhea, phytic acid, oxalates, immobilization
Function	Essential for normal metabolism of calcium and phosphorus; constituent of phosphokinase; activator for enzymes of carbohydrate and amino acid metabolism; important in neuromuscular activity and impulse transmission	Most important as a component of metalloenzyme; participates in RNA metabolism; associated with the hormone insulin; plays role in stimulating wound healing	Essential for bone and tooth formation; acts as a catalyst in conversion of prothrombin to thrombin; regulates muscle contractibility, including heartbeat and normal nerve transmission; activates enzymes and controls permeability of cell membrane to various nutrients
Deficiency Effects	Hypomagnesemia, hypocalcemia, hypokalemia, anorexia, nausea, apathy, neuromuscular irritability	Defective wound healing, iron deficiency anemia, hypogonadism, dwarfism	Muscle cramping and tetany, osteomalacia, rickets, stunted growth (possibly) osteoporosis
Toxic Effect	Possible hypermagnesemia with renal insufficiency, central nervous system depression, anesthesia, paralysis of skeletal muscle	Nausea, vomiting, abdominal cramps, diarrhea and fever; decreased absorption of iron and copper (may result in hypochromic microcytic anemia)	Idiopathic hypercalcemia in infants; milk alkali syndrome, hypercalciuria, kidney stones; calcification of soft tissues

Phosphorus	Iodine

300 mg in
  60 g sardines or beef
    liver
200 mg in
  90 g turkey
  30 g cheese
  1 c milk or yogurt
  100 g cauliflower
150 mg in
  6 Tbsp cottage cheese
  ¾ c 40% Bran Flakes
  1 large artichoke
100 mg in
  1 egg
  2 Tbsp peanut butter
  1 serving whole grain
    cereal
50 mg in
  1 slice bread
  1 average serving
    other fruit
  1 average serving
    other fruit or vege-
    table
	(varies greatly with season
	  and location)
	300 mg in
	  90 g haddock
	150 mg in
	  90 g cod
	  ½ tsp iodized salt
	125 mg in
	  90 g lobster
	50 mg in
	  90 g other shellfish,
	    herring or halibut
	30 mg in
	  90 g other marine fish
	    or shrimp
	  1 c milk
	20 mg in
	  ½ c spinach

Enhanced when calcium and phosphorus in 1:1 ratio, in presence of vitamin D; decreased by same factors that decrease calcium ab- sorption	Dietary iodine converted to iodide in intestinal tract; then absorption is rapid and complete
Essential for bone and tooth formation; acts as constituent of DNA, RNA, phospholipids, phosphate buffer sys- tem; forms high-en- ergy phosphate com- pounds (ATP, ADP for muscle and tissue ac- tivity, creatine phos- phate)	Necessary for formation of thyroxine and related compounds synthesized by thyroid gland; thy- roxine controls rate of metabolism
Weakness, anorexia, malaise, bone pain	Goiter
None reported	Certain individuals not able to adapt to high doses, with resultant hypothyroidism, iodide myxedema, or iodide goiter

SELECTED VITAMINS AND MINERALS[a]: ESTIMATED SAFE AND ADEQUATE DAILY DIETARY INTAKES IN INFANTS, CHILDREN, AND ADULTS

	Age (yr)	Vitamins		
		Vitamin K (μg)	Biotin (μg)	Pantothenic Acid (mg)
Infants	0-0.5	12	35	2
	0.5-1	10-20	50	3
Children and adolescents	1-3	15-30	65	3
	4-6	20-40	85	3-4
	7-10	30-60	120	4-5
	11+	50-100	100-200	4-7
Adults		70-140	100-200	

	Age (yr)	Trace Elements[b]					
		Copper (mg)	Manganese (mg)	Fluoride (mg)	Chromium (mg)	Selenium (mg)	Molybdenum (mg)
Infants	0-0.5	0.5-0.7	0.5-0.7	0.1-0.5	0.01-0.04	0.01-0.04	0.03-0.06
	0.5-1	0.7-1.0	0.7-1.0	0.2-1.0	0.02-0.06	0.02-0.06	0.04-0.08
Children and adolescents	1-3	1.0-1.5	1.0-1.5	0.5-1.5	0.02-0.08	0.02-0.08	0.05-0.1
	4-6	1.5-2.0	1.5-2.0	1.0-2.5	0.03-0.12	0.03-0.12	0.06-0.15
	7-10	2.0-2.5	2.0-3.0	1.5-2.5	0.05-0.2	0.05-0.2	0.10-0.3
	11+	2.0-3.0	2.5-5.0	1.5-2.5	0.05-0.2	0.05-0.2	0.15-0.5
Adults		2.0-3.0	2.5-5.0	1.5-4.0	0.05-0.2	0.05-0.2	0.15-0.5

	Age (yr)	Electrolytes		
		Sodium (mg)	Potassium (mg)	Chloride (mg)
Infants	0-0.5	115-350	350-925	275-700
	0.5-1	250-750	425-1275	400-1200
Children and adolescents	1-3	325-975	550-1650	500-1500
	4-6	450-1350	775-2325	700-2100
	7-10	600-1800	1000-3000	925-2775
	11+	900-2700	1525-4575	1400-4200
Adults		1100-3300	1875-5625	1700-5100

From Committee on Dietary Allowances, Food and Nutrition Board, National Research Council: Recommended dietary allowances, ed 9, Washington DC, 1980, National Academy of Sciences.

[a]Because there is less information on which to base allowances, these figures are provided in the form of ranges of recommended intakes.

[b]Since the toxic levels for many trace elements may be only several times usual intakes, the upper levels for the trace elements given should not be habitually exceeded.

WATER AND ELECTROLYTES

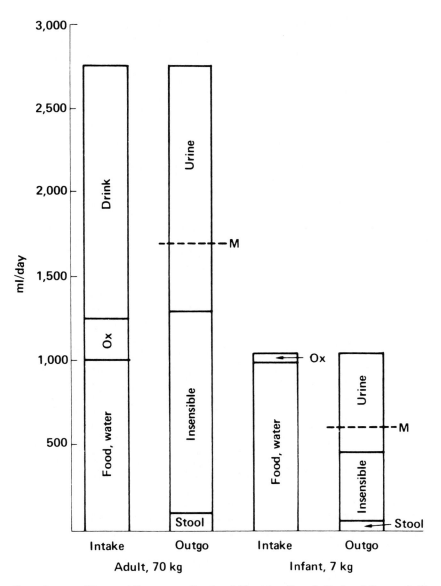

From Committee on Dietary Allowances, Food and Nutrition Board, National Research Council: Recommended dietary allowances, ed 9, Washington DC, 1980, National Academy of Sciences. Routes and approximate magnitude of water intake and outgo without sweating. *M,* Minimal urine volume at maximal solute concentration; *Ox,* water oxidation.

UNITED STATES RECOMMENDED DAILY ALLOWANCES

The United States recommended daily allowances (USRDAs) are for use in nutrition labeling of foods, including vitamin and mineral supplements. They are a consumer guide and are far less precise than the more detailed age-specific National Research Council Recommended Dietary Allowances. The USRDAs commonly used on food labels indicate nutrient requirements for adult men, since their requirements are highest. (In the case of iron, however, the requirement shown is that for women, who have the greater requirements.) There are actually four sets of USRDAs, but the other three are designed for special population groups: infants, preschoolers, pregnant and lactating women. As an example, baby foods will carry the USRDAs for infants under 13 months. Similarly, junior foods and foods designed for pregnant women will carry the group-specific USRDAs.

United States Recommended Daily Allowances

	Population							
	Adults and Children over 4 yr		Children under 4 yr		Infants under 13 mo		Pregnant or Lactating Women	
Protein	65	g*	28	g*	25	g*	65	g*
Vitamin A	5000	IU	2500	IU	2500	IU	8000	IU
Vitamin C	60	mg	40	mg	40	mg	60	mg
Thiamine	1.5	mg	0.7	mg	0.7	mg	1.7	mg
Riboflavin	1.7	mg	0.8	mg	0.8	mg	2.0	mg
Niacin	20	mg	9.0	mg	9.0	mg	20	mg
Calcium	1.0	g	0.8	g	0.8	g	1.3	g
Iron	18	mg	10	mg	10	mg	18	mg
Vitamin D	400	IU	400	IU	400	IU	400	IU
Vitamin E	30	IU	10	IU	10	IU	30	IU
Vitamin B_6	2.0	mg	0.7	mg	0.7	mg	2.5	mg
Folacin	0.4	mg	0.2	mg	0.2	mg	0.8	mg
Vitamin B_{12}	6	μg	3	μg	3	μg	8	μg
Phosphorus	1.0	g	0.8	g	0.8	g	1.3	g
Iodine	150	μg	70	μg	70	μg	150	μg
Magnesium	400	mg	200	mg	200	mg	450	mg
Zinc	15	mg	8	mg	8	mg	15	mg
Copper	2	mg	1	mg	1	mg	2	mg
Biotin	0.3	mg	0.15	mg	0.15	mg	0.3	mg
Pantothenic acid	10	mg	5	mg	5	mg	10	mg

*If the protein efficiency ratio of a protein is equal to or better than that of casein, the USRDA is 45 g for adults and pregnant or lactating women, 20 g for children under 4 years of age, and 18 g for infants.

DIETARY GUIDELINES FOR HEALTHY AMERICANS

General guidelines have been developed by the U.S. Departments of Agriculture and Health, Education, and Welfare that attempt to synthesize in straightforward language a consensus position with respect to a vast number of research and other scientific reports on diet and health. This statement, released in 1980, acknowledges great heterogeneity within the population, but stresses the fact that good eating habits based on moderation and common sense will provide a foundation for maintaining good health.

Dietary Guidelines for Americans*

1. *Eat a variety of foods daily.* Include selections of
   Fruits
   Vegetables
   Whole grain and enriched breads, cereals and grain products
   Milk, cheese, and yogurt
   Meats, poultry, fish, eggs
   Legumes (dry peas and beans)
2. *Maintain ideal weight.*
   Improve eating habits
   Eat slowly
   Prepare smaller portions
   Avoid "seconds"
   Maintain a balanced program of physical activity
   Eat less sugar and sweets
   Avoid too much alcohol
3. *Avoid too much fat, saturated fat, and cholesterol.*
   Choose lean meat, fish, poultry, dry beans and peas as your protein sources
   Moderate the use of eggs and organ meats (e.g., liver)
   Limit the intake of butter, cream, hydrogenated margarines, shortenings, and coconut oil, as well as foods made from such products
   Trim excess fat off meats
   Broil, bake, or boil rather than fry
   Read labels carefully to determine both amount and types of fat contained in foods

4. *Eat foods with adequate starch and fiber.*
   Substitute starches for fats and sugars
   Select foods that are good sources of fibers and starch, such as whole-grain breads and cereals, fruits and vegetables, beans, peas, and nuts
5. *Avoid too much sugar.*
   Use less of all sugars, including white sugar, brown sugar, raw sugar, honey, and syrups.
   Eat less of foods containing these sugars, such as candy, soft drinks, ice cream, cakes, cookies
   Select fresh fruits or fruits canned without sugar or with light syrup rather than heavy syrup
   Read food labels for clues on sugar content—if the words sucrose, glucose, maltose, dextrose, lactose, fructose, or syrups appear first, then there is a large amount of sugar
   How often one eats sugar is as important as how much sugar is eaten
6. *Avoid too much sodium.*
   Learn to enjoy the unsalted flavors of foods
   Cook with only small amounts of added salt
   Add little or no salt to food at the table
   Limit the intake of salty foods, such as potato chips, pretzels, salted nuts and popcorn, condiments (soy sauce, steak sauce, garlic salt), cheese, pickled foods, cured meats
   Read food labels carefully to determine the amounts of sodium in processed foods and snack items
7. *Drink alcohol in moderation.*
   Alcohol is high in calories and low in nutrients
   Heavy drinkers will suffer appetite loss
   Vitamin and mineral deficiencies are common in heavy drinkers
   Pregnant women should sharply limit or restrict their alcohol intake

---

*From United States Department of Agriculture and Department of Health, Education, and Welfare: Dietary guidelines for Americans, Washington DC, 1980, Government Printing Office.

Selected Reference Diets

REPRESENTATIVE DIET FOR BREAKFAST, LUNCH, DINNER, AND SNACKS

A representative diet is provided for breakfast, lunch, dinner, and snacks. This "typical" diet is partitioned into a lower (1551 kcal) and higher (2200 kcal) caloric pattern by modification, reduction, or elimination of only a limited number of foods while leaving the core menu intact. Energy and selected nutrient values are provided for each food. In addition, the food code as it appears in the Department of Agriculture handbook is provided for reference. The menu plan outlined will serve not only to illustrate a reference diet, but also to instruct individuals about how relatively minor adjustments

in food preparation and selection will result in different levels of energy intake. To plan for the lower level, 1551 kcal, of energy intake, use the food values that are on the line with the food listed (e.g., bran muffin [1] [104 kcal]). To adjust the diet for the higher level (2207 kcal) of energy intake, use the food amounts and values given in parentheses (e.g., bran muffin [2] [208 kcal]). In some cases a food is not intended to be provided on the lower-caloric pattern; then the first line opposite the food is filled with dashes, while the second line, in parentheses, indicates the portion and the nutrient values for the food as it is used in the higher-calorie diet. Foods that do not change between diets have only one line of information in the table.

REPRESENTATIVE DIET

	Amount	kcal	Protein (g)	Fat (g)	Carbohydrate (g)	Calcium (mg)	Iron (mg)	Sodium (mg)	Vitamin A (IU)	Thiamine (mg)	Riboflavin (mg)	Niacin (mg)	Vitamin C (mg)	Reference Number
Breakfast														
Grapefruit	½	40	0.5	0.1	10.3	16	0.4	1	80	.04	.02	0.2	37	1053b
Bran muffin	1	104	3.1	3.9	17.2	57	1.5	179	90	.06	.10	1.6	t	1346b
	(2)	(208)	(6.2)	(7.8)	(34.4)	(114)	(3.0)	(358)	(180)	(.12)	(.20)	(3.2)	(t)	
Egg (soft cooked)	1	82	6.5	5.8	.5	27	1.2	61	590	.05	.15	t	—	968b
Butter	—													505d
	(2 tsp)	(68)	(t)	(7.6)	(t)	(2)	—	—	(320)	—	—	—	—	
Jelly	(1 Tbsp)	(49)	(t)	(t)	(12.7)	(4)	(0.3)	(3)	(t)	(t)	(.01)	(t)	(1)	1149e
Milk	1 c skim	88	8.8	0.2	12.5	296	0.1	127	10	.09	.44	0.2	2	1322b
	(1 c whole)	(159)	(8.5)	(8.5)	(12.0)	(288)	(0.1)	(122)	(350)	(.07)	(.41)	(0.2)	(2)	(1320b)
Coffee	6 oz	2	t	t	t	4	0.2	2	—	—	t	0.5	—	800b
TOTAL		316 (608)	18.9 (21.7)	10 (29.8)	40.5 (69.9)	400 (455)	3.4 (5.2)	370 (639)	770 (1520)	.24 (.28)	.71 (.79)	2.5 (4.1)	39 (40)	
Lunch														
Chicken	2 oz	103	18.3	2.8	—	6.3	0.7	37	63	.05	.06	6.7	—	728c
Swiss cheese	1 oz	105	7.8	7.9	0.5	262	0.3	201	320	t	.11	t	—	652f
Lettuce	1 leaf	3	0.2	t	0.6	4	0.1	2	70	.01	.01	.1	1	1258c
Mayonnaise	—													1938b
	(1 Tbsp)	(101)	(0.2)	(11.2)	(0.3)	(3)	(0.1)	(84)	(40)	(t)	(.01)	(t)	(—)	
Whole-wheat bread	2 slices	112	4.8	1.4	22	46	1.4	242	t	.12	.06	1.2	t	471c
Yogurt	1 c skim	123	8.3	4.2	12.7	294	0.1	125	170	.10	.44	0.2	2	2481b
	(1 c whole)	(152)	(7.4)	(8.3)	(12.0)	(272)	(0.1)	(115)	(340)	(.07)	(.39)	(0.2)	(2)	(2482b)
Strawberries	½ c	28	0.5	0.4	6.3	16.0	0.8	0.5	45	.02	.05	0.5	44	2217e
TOTAL		474 (604)	39.9 (39.2)	16.7 (32.0)	42.1 (41.7)	628.3 (609.3)	3.4 (3.5)	607.5 (681.5)	668 (878)	.30 (.27)	.73 (.69)	8.7 (8.7)	47 (47)	

Food	Amount													Code
Dinner														
Vegetable soup	1 c	160	4.5	4.3	26.5	40	2.0	1710	5750	.08	.08	1.8	—	2107
Baked fish with butter	3 oz	171	25.5	6.9	—	21	1.2	201	—	.06	.06	2.1	3	1019d
Broccoli	½ c	20	2.4	0.3	3.5	68	0.6	8	1940	.07	.15	0.6	70	484d
Brown rice	½ c	116	2.5	0.6	24.9	11.5	0.5	275	—	.09	.02	1.4	—	1870a
Iceberg lettuce	1 leaf	3	0.2	t	0.6	4	0.1	2	70	.01	.01	0.1	1	1258c
Spinach	½ oz	4	0.5	—	0.6	13	0.4	10	1148	.01	.03	0.08	7	2169d
Green onion	1 Tbsp	3	0.1	t	0.6	2	t	t	t	t	t	t	2	1416c
Cucumbers	6 slices	4	0.3	t	1.0	7	0.3	2	70	.01	.01	0.1	3	942d
Lemon juice	1 Tbsp	4	0.1	t	1.2	1	t	t	t	t	t	t	7	1245b
(Italian salad dressing)	(1 Tbsp)	(83)	(t)	(9.0)	(1.0)	(2)	(t)	(314)	(t)	(t)	(t)	(t)	(—)	1936b
Butter	(2 tsp)	(68)	(t)	(7.6)	—	(2)	(—)	—	(320)	(—)	(—)	(—)	(—)	
Grapes	½ c	54	0.5	0.3	13.9	9.5	0.3	2.5	80	.04	.03	.25	3	505d
TOTAL		539	36.6	12.4	72.8	177	5.4	2221	6058	.37	.39	6.43	96	1085b
		(686)	(36.5)	(29.0)	(72.6)	(180)	(5.4)	(2617)	(6378)	(.37)	(.39)	(6.43)	(89)	
Total Meals		1329	95.4	39.1	155.4	1205.3	12.2	3188.5	7496	0.91	1.83	17.63	182	
		(1898)	(97.4)	(90.8)	(184.2)	(1244.3)	(14.1)	(3937.5)	(8776)	(0.95)	(1.87)	(19.23)	(176)	
Snacks														
Watermelon	2 slices	222	4.2	1.8	54.6	60	4.2	8	5020	0.26	0.26	1.8	60	2424b
Wine	(3.5 oz)	(87)	(0.1)	(—)	(4.3)	(9)	(0.4)	(5)	(—)	(.01)	(.01)	(0.1)	(—)	
Total		1551	99.6	40.9	210	1265.3	16.4	3196.5	12516	1.17	2.09	19.43	242	
Daily		(2207)	(101.7)	(92.6)	(243.1)	(1313.3)	(18.7)	(3937.5)	(13796)	(1.21)	(2.14)	(21.13)	(236)	
% of kcal			24.8	22.9	52.3									
			(18.3)	(37.7)	(44.0)									

Based on data from Adams CF: Nutritive value of American foods in common units. Agriculture Handbook 456, USDA. Washington DC, 1975, Government Printing Office.

Table prepared by K. E. Andrup, M.S., Nutritionist, Johns Hopkins University.

*Parentheses indicate higher caloric intake (explanation on p. 771).

t, Trace.

KILOCALORIE-RESTRICTED DIET

1200 kcal (approximate)
  65 g protein (approximately 20% of calories)
  130 g carbohydrate (approximately 44% of calories)
  50 g fat (approximately 37% of calories)

Sample Meal Plan	Sample Menu
AM	AM
1 fruit exchange	½ c orange juice
1 medium fat meat exchange	1 soft-cooked egg
1 bread exchange	1 slice toast
1 fat exchange	1 tsp butter or fortified margarine
Coffee or tea	Coffee or tea
Noon	Noon
2 lean meat exchanges	2 oz sliced turkey
1 bread exchange	1 slice enriched bread
2 fat exchanges	2 tsp butter or fortified margarine
1 vegetable exchange	½ c broccoli
1 fruit exchange	2 unsweetened whole apricots
1 milk exchange	1 c skim milk
Coffee or tea	
PM	PM
2 lean meat exchanges	2 oz round steak
1 bread exchange	1 small baked potato with skin
2 fat exchanges	2 tsp butter or fortified margarine
2 vegetable exchanges	½ c carrots
	½ c lettuce and cucumber salad with
1 fat exchange	1 Tbsp Italian dressing
1 fruit exchange	¼ cantaloupe
Coffee or tea	Coffee or tea
Between Meals	Between Meals
1 milk exchange	1 c skim milk
1 bread exchange	2 graham crackers

Modified from American Dietetic Association: Handbook of clinical dietetics, New Haven Conn, 1981, Yale University Press, p F31.

DIETARY MODIFICATION OF CALORIC AND/OR CARBOHYDRATE INTAKE

The dietary objective is to modify or reduce caloric intake to achieve weight reduction while maintaining adequate nutrition. Generally, a weight loss of 1-2 pounds per week is desirable. (See Chapter 38.) Clearly, attention to physical exercise and dietary modification must accompany any dietary approach to weight modification.

An initial estimate of kilocalories required can be made as follows:

1. Estimate kilocalories required for an adult patient at ideal weight and general level of activity:

Energy Need	kcal/hour	kcal/24 hours /kg BW
Basal level	1.0	24.0
Very sedentary (20%)	1.2	28.8
Sedentary (30%)	1.3	31.2
Moderately active (40%)	1.4	33.66
Very active (50%)	1.5	36.0

   Multiply energy required by weight in kilograms for daily requirement (e.g., for a very active 70 kg man: 1.5 kcal/hr, or 36 kcal/24 hr $\times$ 70 = 2520 kcal/ 24 hr)

2. Set the desired and agreed upon level of weight loss (usually 1-2 lb/wk). Multiply this figure by 3500 kcal (the energy loss necessary to lose 1 pound per week beyond the first week [see Chapter 38, Table 38-5]) and divide by 7 (da/wk) to determine the kilocalorie reduction per day.
   Object: Loss of 1 pound/week
     1 (lb) $\times$ 3500 (kcal) = 3500 kcal deficit/wk
     3500 $\div$ 7 (da/wk) = 500 kcal reduction per day

3. Reduce the usual requirement as determined in step 1 by the above figure to arrive at a new estimate of kilocalorie intake to achieve weight reduction, e.g., a 55-kg sedentary female (31.2 kcal/kg/24 hr) requires 1716 kcal/24 hr minus 500 kcal, approximately 1200 kcal, to achieve weight reduction of 1 pound per week.

4. The converse approach may be utilized for patients who would benefit from weight gain.

5. Kilocalorie requirements per day may be divided into 15%-20% protein, 50% carbohydrate, and 30%-35% fat.

6. Food exchange lists have been prepared to facilitate menu planning. A guide to these substitutions is outlined in the next section.

FOOD EXCHANGE LISTS FOR CONTROLLED-CALORIE AND MODIFIED-FAT DIETS

Exchange lists for dietary planning prepared by the American Diabetes Association and the American Dietetic Association in 1976 are designed to provide ease of substitution of foods within a specific carbohydrate, protein, energy category. The reference tables facilitate menu planning, enhance variety, and permit individualization of menu planning for those patients who require controlled-calorie and modified-fat diets by substitution, elimination, or reduction of exchange categories or specific foods therein.

Exchange tables 1 to 8: The Exchange Lists are the basis of a meal planning system designed by a committee of the American Diabetics Association and The American Dietetic Association. While designed primarily for people with diabetes and others who must follow special diets, the Exchange Lists are based on principles of good nutrition that apply to everyone. © 1976 American Diabetes Association, Inc., American Dietetic Association.

1. MILK EXCHANGES

Type of Milk	Measure	Weight (g)
Non-fat fortified milk		
Carbohydrate—12 g, Protein—8 g		
Calories—80		
Skim or non-fat milk	1 c	240
Powdered (non-fat dry, before adding liquid)	⅓ c	35
Canned, evaporated-skim milk	½ c	120
Buttermilk made from skim milk	1 c	240
Yogurt made from skim milk (plain, unflavored)	1 c	240
Low-fat fortified milk		
Carbohydrate—12 g, Protein—8 g, Fat—2.5 g, Calories—105		
Fat—2.5 g, Calories—105		
†1% fat-fortified milk	1 c	240
Carbohydrate—12 g, Protein—8 g, Fat—5 g, Calories—125		
†2% fat-fortified milk	1 c	240
†Yogurt made from 2% milk (plain, unflavored)	1 c	240
1 slice regular ice cream	½ c	66
Whole Milk		
Carbohydrate—12 g, Protein—8 g, Fat—10 g, Calories—170		
†Whole milk	1 c	240
†Powdered whole milk (dry, before adding liquid)	⅓ c	35
†Canned, evaporated whole milk	½ c	120
†Buttermilk made from whole milk	1 c	240
†Yogurt made from whole milk (plain, unflavored)	1 c	240

Adjustments may include 1 cup of skim milk plus two fat exchanges for 1 cup of whole milk. Foods indicated with a † should be avoided when fat control is indicated.

2. VEGETABLE EXCHANGES

Asparagus	Greens: Kale
Bamboo shoots	Mustard
Bean sprouts	Spinach
Beets	Turnip
Broccoli	Mushrooms
Brussels sprouts	Okra
Cabbage	Onions
Carrots	Rhubarb
Cauliflower	Rutabaga
Celery	Sauerkraut
Chinese vegetables, canned	String beans, green or
Chop suey vegetables,	yellow
canned	Summer squash
Cucumbers	Tomatoes
Eggplant	Tomato juice
Green pepper	Turnips
Greens: Beet	Vegetable juice cocktail
Chards	Zucchini
Collards	
Dandelion	

Carbohydrate—5 g; Protein—2 g; Calories—28
One exchange is ½ c (100 g)
The following *raw vegetables* may be used as desired:

Chicory
Chinese cabbage
Endive
Escarole
Lettuce
Parsley
Radishes
Watercress

3. FRUIT EXCHANGES

	Measurement	Weight (g)
Apple	1 small	80
Apple cider	⅓ c	80
Apple juice	⅓ c	80
Applesauce (unsweetened)	½ c	100
Apricots, fresh, canned	2 medium	100
Apricots, dried	4 halves	20
Banana	½ small	50
Blackberries	½ c	70
Blueberries	½ c	70
Cantaloupe	¼ (6″ dia)	150
Cherries	10 large	75
Cranberry juice, sweetened	¼ c	60
Dates	2	15
Figs, fresh	1	50
Figs, dried	1	15
Fruit cocktail	½ c	100
Grapefruit	½	100
Grapefruit juice	½ c	120
Grapes	12	75
Grape juice	¼ c	60
Guava	1 small	80
Honeydew melon	⅛ medium	150
Mango	½ small	70
Nectars	½ c	120
Nectarines	1 small	70
Orange	1 small	100
Orange juice	½ c	120
Papaya	¾ c	100
Peach, fresh, canned	1 medium	100
Pear, fresh, canned	1 small	100
Persimmon, native	1 medium	30
Pineapple	½ c	80
Pineapple juice	⅓ c	80
Plantain	⅓ small	35
Plums	2 medium	100
Pomegranate	1 small	100
Prunes, dried, cooked	2 medium	40
Prune juice	¼ c	60
Raisins	2 Tbsp	15
Raspberries	½ c	70
Strawberries	¾ c	100
Tangerine	1 medium	100
Watermelon	1 cup	175

All fruits to be fresh, frozen, or canned *without sugar*.
Carbohydrate—10 g; Calories—40

4. BREAD EXCHANGES

	Measure		Measure
Bread		Lima beans	½ c
White (including French and Italian)	1 slice	Parsnips	⅔ c
Whole wheat	1 slice	Peas, green (canned or frozen)	½ c
Rye or pumpernickel	1 slice		
Raisin	1 slice	Potato, white	1 small
Bagel, small	½	Potato (mashed)	½ c
English muffin, small	½	Pumpkin	¾ c
Plain roll, bread	1	Winter squash, acorn, or butternut	½ c
Frankfurter roll	½		
Hamburger bun	½	Yam or sweet potato	¼ c
Dried bread crumbs	3 Tbsp	**Prepared Foods**	
Tortilla, 6″	1	†*Biscuit 2″ diameter	1
Cereal and Cereal Products		†*Corn bread, 2″ × 2″ × 1″	1
Bran flakes	½ c	†*Corn muffin, 2″ diameter	1
Other ready-to-eat unsweetened cereal	¾ c	†*Muffin, plain small	1
		†*Potatoes, french fried, length 2″ to 3½″	8
Puffed cereal, unfrosted	1 c		
Cereal (cooked)	½ c	†**Potato or corn chips	15
Grits (cooked)	½ c	†*Pancake, 5″ × ½″	1
Rice or barley (cooked)	½ c	Poultry stuffing	⅓ c
Pasta (cooked) spaghetti, noodles, macaroni	½ c	†*Waffle, 5″ × ½″	1
		Ice Cream and Desserts	
Popcorn (popped, no fat added)	3 c	†**Ice cream, 16% fat	½ c
Cornmeal (dry)	2 Tbsp	†*Ice cream, 10% fat	½ c
Flour	2½ Tbsp	Ice milk, 5% fat (omit ½ fat)	½ c
Wheat germ	¼ c	Sherbet	¼ c
Tapioca	2 Tbsp	†*Soft-serve French vanilla ice cream	⅓ c
Crackers			
†*Crackers, round, butter type (Ritz)	5	Soft-serve vanilla ice milk (omit ½ fat)	⅓ c
Graham, 2½″ square	2	Flavored gelatin	½ c
Matzoth, 4″ × 6″	½	#Ice cream cone, plain	1
Oyster	20	Ice cream cone, sugar	1
Pretzels, 3⅛″ long × ⅛″ diameter	25	**Cakes and Cookies**	
		Angel Food	1½″ cube
Pretzel, Dutch	1	†**Doughnut, plain cake	1 small
Melba toast	4 rectangular or 8 round	†**Doughnut, plain raised	1 avg.
		†Plain cake (mix) (2 bread exchanges)	3″ × 3″ × 1″
Pilot cracker	1		
Rye wafers, 2″ × 3½″	3	†**Pound cake	½″ slice
Saltines	6	†Sponge cake	1½″ cube
Soda, 2½″ square	4	Animal crackers	7
Zwiebach	3	Arrowroot	3
Starchy Vegetables		†*Chocolate chip, 2⅓″ dia.	2
Beans, peas, lentils (dried and cooked)	½ c	Ginger or lemon snaps, small	5
		Lorna Doones	3
Baked beans, no pork (canned)	¼ c	†*Oatmeal	2
Corn	⅓ c	Vanilla wafers	5
Corn on cob	1 small		

Carbohydrate—15 g; Protein—2 g; Calories—68

Modifications of Bread Exchanges

*Omit 1 fat exchange

**Omit 2 fat exchanges

½ bread exchange

† Avoid on saturated fat-controlled diet

5. MEAT EXCHANGES

	Measure	Weight (g)
Lean Meat: Protein—7 g; Fat—3 g; Calories—55		
Beef: Baby beef (very lean), chipped beef, chuck, flank steak, tenderloin, plate ribs, plate skirt steak, round (bottom, top), rump (all cuts), spare ribs, tripe	1 oz.	30
Lamb: leg, rib, sirloin, loin (roast and chops), shank, shoulder	1 oz	30
Pork: leg (whole rump, center shank), ham, smoked (center slices)	1 oz	30
Veal: leg, loin, rib, shank, shoulder, cutlets	1 oz	30
Poultry: chicken, turkey, cornish hen, guinea hen, pheasant (skin removed)	1 oz	30
Fish: any fresh or frozen	1 oz	30
canned salmon, tuna, mackerel, crab, lobster	¼ c	30
clams, oysters, scallops, shrimp	5 or 1 oz	30
sardines drained	3	30
Cheeses containing less than 5% butterfat	1 oz	30
Cottage cheese: dry and 2% butterfat	¼ c	45
Dried beans and peas (omit 1 bread exchange)	½ c	45

	Measure	Weight (g)
Medium-Fat Meat: For each exchange of medium-fat meat, omit ½ fat exchange		
Note: On a saturated fat–controlled and cholesterol-restricted diet, limit egg yolk and cheese to 3 servings per week.		
Beef: Ground (15% fat), corned beef (canned), rib eye, round (ground commercial)	1 oz	30
Pork: Loin (all cuts tenderloin), shoulder arm (picnic), shoulder blade, Boston butt, Canadian bacon, boiled ham	1 oz	30
Organ meats: Liver, heart, kidney, sweetbreads (THESE ARE HIGH IN CHOLESTEROL)	1 oz	30
Cottage cheese, creamed	¼ c	45
Cheese: Mozzarella, ricotta, farmer's cheese, Neufchatel	1 oz	30
Parmesan	3 Tbsp	15
Egg (HIGH IN CHOLESTEROL)	1	50
Peanut butter (omit 2 additional fat exchanges)	2 Tbsp	30

	Measure	Weight (g)
High-Fat Meat: For each exchange of high-fat meat, omit 1 fat exchange		
Note: Avoid high-fat meats on a saturated fat–controlled diet.		
Beef: Brisket, corned beef (brisket), ground beef (more than 20% fat), hamburger (commercial), chuck (ground commercial), roasts (rib), steaks (club and rib)	1 oz	30
Lamb: Breast	1 oz	30
Pork: Spare ribs, loin (back ribs), pork (ground), country style ham, deviled ham	1 oz	30
Veal: Breast	1 oz	30
Poultry: Capon, duck (domestic), goose	1 oz	30
Cheese: Cheddar types	1 oz	30
Cold cuts	4½″ × ⅛″ slice	30
Frankfurter	1 small	50

6. ALCOHOLIC BEVERAGES

		Exchange Values Reduction Diabetic			
	Measure	Caloric Value	Fat Only	Bread	Fat
Malt Liquors					
Ale	8 oz	150	2	½	2
American	12 oz	225	3½	1	3½
Mild	8 oz	100	5	½	½
Mild	12 oz	150	2	1	2
Beer, Lager	8 oz	113	2½	⅔	1½
Lager	12 oz	175	4	1	2½
Distilled Liquors					
Brandy (Calif)	1 oz	75	1½		1½
Cognac	1 brandy pony	75	1½		1½
Gin					
Dry	1½	105	2½		2½
Sloe	3 oz	75	1½	⅓	1
Whiskey					
Rye, bourbon, or Scotch	1½	120	2½		2½
Rum (Bacardi)	1 oz	75	1½		1½
	1½ oz	110	2⅓		2½
	⅔ oz	65	1½		1½
Vodka	1½ oz	150	3½		3½
Wines					
Champagne, domestic	4 oz	83	2		2
dry	3½ oz	95	2		2
sweet	3½ oz	130	2½	⅔	1½
Muscatelle or port	3½ oz	130	3½	1	2
Sauterne (Calif)	3½ oz	83	2	⅓	1½
Sherry, domestic	2 oz	85	2	⅓	1½
Vermouth					
French	3½ oz	103	2½		2½
Italian	3½ oz	165	3½	⅔	2½
Burgundy	3½ oz	75	1½		1½
Cocktails					
Manhattan	3½ oz	165	3½	½	3
Martini	3½ oz	140	3		3

Mixers used should be unsweetened (soda water) or artificially sweetened carbonated beverages.

7. FAT EXCHANGES

	Measure	Weight (g)		Measure	Weight (g)
Avocado	⅛ (4″ dia.)	25	Nuts—cont'd		
†Bacon, crisp	1 slice	10	Filberts	5	7
†Butter	1 tsp	5	Peanuts		
†Cream, light 20%	2 Tbsp	30	Spanish	20 whole	10
†Cream, heavy 40%	1 Tbsp	15	Virginia	10 whole	10
†Cream cheese	1 Tbsp	15	Pecans	2 large	7
†Cream cheese spread	1 Tbsp	15		whole	
†Cream substitute, dry	4 tsp	8	Pinon	1 Tbsp	7
French dressing	1 Tbsp	15	Pistachio	20	10
†Gravy	2 Tbsp	30	Walnuts	6 small	8
Italian dressing	2 tsp	10	Oil, cooking	1 tsp	5
Mayonnaise	1 tsp	5	Olives	5 small	50
Nuts			Margarine	1 tsp	5
Almonds	10 whole	10	Salad dressing,	2 tsp	10
Brazil	2	7	mayonnaise type		
†Cashews	5	10	†Salt pork	¾″ cube	10
			†Sour cream	2 Tbsp	30

Fat—5 g; Calories—45

† Avoid on saturated fat-controlled and cholesterol-restricted diets.

Gravy and salad dressing allowed in saturated fat-controlled diet if made with acceptable margarine or oil.

8. FOODS CONSIDERED ACCEPTABLE IN UNLIMITED AMOUNTS

Sugar substitutes

Coffee

Decaffeinated coffee

Fat-free broth

Bouillon

Consommé

Sugar-free carbonated beverages

Unsweetened gelatin

Unsweetened pickles

Vinegar

Spices and herbs

Mustard

Dietetic catsup

Horseradish

Fruits (sweetened with sugar substitutes)

    Cranberries

    Lime

    Lemon

VEGETARIAN DIET

When appropriately planned, vegetarian diets can adequately meet individual energy and nutrient requirements. Four basic types of vegetarian diets have been defined: (1) the lactoovovegetarian diet includes milk, cheese, and eggs in addition to an all-vegetable diet; (2) the lactovegetarian diet omits eggs; (3) vegan, or strict vegetarian, diet is more restrictive than the other two; it specifically excludes all foods of animal origin, including fish, eggs, and all dairy products, as well as meat and poultry*; and (4) the Zen macrobiotic diet is a dietary regimen composed of ten basic diets that increase, at the highest level, to an intake that is 100% cereals; at the highest level, this is highly restrictive and is considered grossly inadequate; it should be discouraged and avoided.

*Very careful planning is required to achieve adequate protein, essential amino acid, and vitamin B_{12} intake with this diet. In children, vegetarianism brings an added and increased risk of calcium deficiency due to the elimination of milk products, and of vitamin D deficiency if the child is not exposed to sunlight at regular intervals.

Diet planning should originate with a modified version of the basic food groups, individual requirements, and personal food preferences. Specific attention should be given to protein-rich foods. Eggs, legumes, nuts, seeds, and meat analogues from the lists below may be substituted for meat, poultry, and fish. Meat analogues are not necessary, but they do provide for ease of meal planning and variety in the diet. Four or more servings of whole-grain breads and cereals should be included daily. A minimum of 2 cups of milk and other dairy products should be included as well as four or more servings of vegetables and fruits daily. In the lactovegetarian diet, eggs will be eliminated.

Individuals should be instructed to use high–nutrient density foods, a wide variety of foods, adequate intakes of milk products, and vegetable proteins with complementary amino acid patterns. The following vegetarian diet plan notes the quantity of food from each category to be consumed each day. The two protein food equivalent lists provide examples of generally available foods and commercial meat analogues in each category. Nut and seed equivalents, as well as legume equivalents, are also provided.

VEGETARIAN DAILY DIET PLAN

Food Category	Quantity
Milk or equivalent	2 c or more
Protein food	5 equivalents
Nuts and seeds	1 or more equivalents
Vegetable and fruits	4 or more servings
Cereals and breads (unrefined)	5 or more servings
Fats and oils	1 Tbsp or more

VEGETARIAN DAILY DIET PLAN

Protein Food Equivalents (75 kcal, 7 g protein, 5 g fat)		
Generally Available Foods	**Quantity**	**Weight**
Cottage cheese	¼ c	45 g
Cheddar cheese	1 oz	30 g
Egg	1	50 g
Soy cheese (tofu)	¼ c	40 g
Peanut butter	2 Tbsp (omit 2 fat)	30 g
Commercially Prepared Foods		
Loma Linda Foods		
Big Franks	1 frankfurter	1½ oz
Chili with Beans	⅓ c	3 oz
Dinner Cuts	1 cut (add 1 fat)	1½ oz
Linketts	1 linkett	1¼ oz
Little Links	2 links	1½ oz
Nuteena	1 slice (⅜″ thick) (omit 1 fat)	2 oz
Proteena	1 slice (¼″ thick)	1¼ oz
Redi-Burger	1 slice (¼″ thick)	1¼ oz
Sandwich Spread	6 Tbsp (omit ½ fat and ½ bread)	2½ oz
Stew-Pac	¼ c	1½ oz
Soybeans, Boston	¼ c (omit ½ bread, add 1 fat)	2 oz
Soybeans, green	⅓ c (omit ½ bread, add 1 fat)	2½ oz
Tenderbits	4 bits	2½ oz
Tender Rounds	2 rounds	1½ oz
VegeBurger	3 Tbsp (add 1 fat)	1¼ oz
Vegelona	1 slice (¼″ thick) (add ½ fat)	1¼ oz
VitaBurger (reconstituted)	¼ c (add 1 fat)	2 oz
Worthington Foods		
Beef Style	1 slice (add ½ fat)	1 oz
Chicken Style	1 slice	1 oz
Choplets	½ chop (add 1 fat)	1 oz
Choplet Burger	3 Tbsp (add 1 fat)	1½ oz
Corned Beef Style	3 slices (omit ½ fat)	1½ oz
Cutlets	½ piece (add 1 fat)	1 oz
Fillet	¾ fillet	20 g
Fried Chicken Style	1½ pieces (omit ½ fat)	1½ oz
Granburger (rehydrated)	¼ c (add 1 fat)	2 oz
Non-meat Balls	2 balls	1 oz
Prosage	1 slice (⅜″)	1 oz
Salisbury Steak Style	1 patty (omit ½ bread)	2 oz
Saucettes	2 links	1 oz
Smoked Beef Style	5 slices (add ½ fat)	1 oz
Smoked Turkey Style	2 slices	40 g
Vegetable Skallops	1½ pieces (add 1 fat)	1½ oz
Vegetarian Burger	⅓ c (add 1 fat)	70 g
Veja-Links	2 links	70 g
Wham	¼ c diced (add 1 fat)	1 oz

Include 1 citrus fruit, 1 legume equivalent, and 1 serving dark green or yellow vegetable. Increase portions for the vegan diet.
Modified from American Dietetic Association: Handbook of clinical dietetics. New Haven, 1981, Yale University Press, pp A36-A37.

VEGETARIAN DAILY DIET PLAN—cont'd

Protein Food Equivalents (reduced fat; 55 kcal, 7 g protein, 3 g fat)

Generally Available Foods	Quantity	Weight
Egg whites	3 whites	1½ oz
Count Down (Fisher)	1 slice	1½ oz
Low-fat cottage cheese	¼ c	45 g

Commercially Prepared Foods
Loma Linda Foods

Chili with Beans	⅓ c (omit 1 bread)	3 oz
Dinner Cuts	1 cut (add ½ fat)	1½ oz
Soybeans, Boston	¼ c (omit ½ bread)	2 oz
Soybeans, green	⅓ c (omit ½ bread)	2½ oz
Tender Rounds	1 round	
VegeBurger	3 Tbsp (add ½ fat)	1¼ oz
Vegelona	1 slice (¼" thick)	1½ oz
VitaBurger (reconstituted)	¼ c (add ½ fat)	2 oz

Worthington Foods

Beef Style	1 slice	1 oz
Choplets	½ chop (add ½ fat)	1 oz
Choplet Burger	3 Tbsp (add ½ fat)	1½ oz
Corned Beef Style	3 slices	1½ oz
Cutlets	½ piece (add ½ fat)	1 oz
Granburger	¼ c (add ½ fat)	2 oz
Vegetable Skallops	1½ pieces	1½ oz
Vegetarian Burger	⅓ c (add ½ fat)	70 g
Wham	¼ c diced	1 oz

Note: Other protein foods may be used if the fat is adjusted in the day's menu.

Nut and Seed Equivalents (6 g protein, 16 g fat, 6 g carbohydrates)

Nuts*

Brazil nuts	10 nuts
Cashew nuts	12-16 nuts
Peanuts	2 Tbsp
Peanut butter	2 Tbsp
Pistachio nuts	1 oz or 30 g
Walnuts, black	16-20 nuts

*Almonds, English walnuts, and pecans may also be added to the diet occasionally. However, they contain more kcal and/or fat than other nuts.

Seeds

Pumpkin and squash seeds	2 Tbsp
Sesame seeds	3 or 4 Tbsp meal
Sunflower seeds	3 or 4 Tbsp meal

Legume Equivalents

(approximately 12 g protein, 1 g fat, 30 g carbohydrates)
One equivalent = ¼ to ⅓ dry beans (makes ¾-1 c cooked)

Black beans	Mung beans
Broad beans	Pea beans or dried peas
Chickpeas or garbanzos	Pinto beans
Cowpeas, including black- eyed peas	Red beans
Lentils	Soybeans
Lima beans	White beans

SODIUM-RESTRICTED DIET

A sodium-restricted diet is designed to restrict sodium to a therapeutic level without unduly altering the diet, so that it remains consistent with the nutrient requirements of the patient.

500 mg Sodium Diet (approximately 1600 calories,* 70 g protein)

AM	Noon	Dinner
Grapefruit (½) 1 egg Rolled wheat cereal with milk and sugar	Sliced chicken sandwich with lettuce, tomato, and spread Sliced tangerine Milk	Cantaloupe (¼) Veal (1 oz edible portion) Green beans and cauliflower Hot roll with spread (no sodium added) Milk
Alternatives	**Alternatives**	**Alternatives**
Oatmeal (½ c), Flake cereal (¾ c), Farina, rolled oats, puffed rice, shredded wheat Low-sodium, enriched, or whole-grain bread or toast	Cooked beef, veal, lamb, poultry or fish (1 oz—no salt added) Cucumber salad (tomatoes, summer squash, cauliflower, radishes, and eggplant)	Strawberries (1 c) Red raspberries (1 c) See noon alternatives

Modified from Turner D: Handbook of diet therapy, ed 5, Chicago, 1970, University of Chicago Press, p 110.

*To increase caloric intake, add 45 kcal/tsp fat or oil, 20 kcal/tsp sugar, jelly, or honey.

FOODS GROUPED BY SODIUM CONTENT PER SERVING

500 mg	250 mg	200 mg	100 mg	50 mg
Scant ¼ tsp salt	1 oz canned tuna	1 slice regular bakery bread or roll	½ c unsalted vegetables: beet greens, frozen mixed peas and carrots, Swiss chard	½ c fresh, frozen, or canned vegetables, without salt: Artichoke, edible base and leaves
¾ tsp monosodium glutamate	2 oz canned sardines or salmon	2 thin slices bacon, crisp and drained	1 oz fresh kosher meat	Beets
½ bouillion cube	⅔ c buttermilk	3 oz canned shrimp cooked in salted water	1 oz frozen fish fillets	Carrots
1 c tomato juice	½ c canned or regularly sea-	½ c canned or regularly sea-		Celery
1 average serving ½ c cooked rice, spaghetti, noodles, hominy, etc., seasoned with salt	soned carrots, spinach, beets, celery, kale, or white turnips	soned vegetables not listed elsewhere		Dandelion greens Kale
½ c drained sauerkraut	5 salted crackers (2″ square)	1 day's supply of drinking water if it contains 100 mg Na/qt		Mustard greens Peas, black-eyed
1 average frankfurter (1½ oz)	¾ c tomato juice	½ c frozen peas or lima beans		Spinach Succotash
1 day's supply of drinking water if it contains 220 mg Na/qt	1 day's supply of drinking water if it contains 120 mg Na/qt	1 oz natural cheddar cheese		Turnip greens Turnip, white
		1 Tbsp catsup		1 day's supply of drinking water if it contains 40 mg Na/qt

Modified from American Dietetic Association: Handbook of clinical dietetics, New Haven, Conn, 1981, Yale University Press, p G8.

LACTOSE-FREE DIET

Foods Allowed	Foods Excluded
Beverages	**Beverages**
Isomil,* Prosobee,† Pregestimil,† Mocha Mix,‡ meat base formulas used as milk substitutes, carbonated drinks, coffee, freeze-dried coffee, fruit drinks, some instant coffees (check labels), Lidalac§ and other lactose-free milks or those treated with lactase enzymes; lactose-free products (e.g., Ensure,* Ensure Plus Citrotein,* Nutramigen,† Nutri 1000 LF⊥)	All untreated milk of any species and all products containing milk, except lactose-free milk, such as skim, dried, evaporated, or condensed milk; yogurt; cheese; ice cream; sherbet; malted milk; Ovaltine;° hot chocolate; some cocoas and instant coffees (read labels); powdered soft drinks with lactose curds; whey and casein milk that has been treated with lactobacillus/acidophilus culture rather than lactase (e.g., Nutrish●)
Breads and cereals	**Breads and cereals**
Breads and rolls made without milk, Italian bread, some cooked cereals and prepared cereals (read labels), macaroni, spaghetti, soda crackers	Prepared mixes, such as muffins, biscuits, waffles, pancakes; some dry cereals such as Total,†† Special K,‡‡ and Cocoa Krispies‡‡ (read labels carefully); Instant Cream of Wheat;§§ commercial breads and rolls to which milk solids have been added; zwieback; French toast made with milk
Desserts	**Desserts**
Water and fruit ices; gelatin; angel food cake, homemade cakes, pies, cookies made from allowed ingredients; puddings made with water	Commercial cakes and cookies and mixes, custard, puddings, sherbets, ice cream made with milk; any containing chocolate, pie crust made with butter or margarine, gelatin made with carrageen
Eggs	**Eggs**
All	Omelets and soufflés containing milk
Fats	**Fats**
Margarines and dressings that do not contain milk or milk products, oils, shortening, bacon, Rich's Whip Topping,** some nondairy creamers (read labels), nut butters, nuts	Margarines and dressings containing milk or milk products, butter, cream, cream cheese, peanut butter with milk solids fillers, salad dressings containing lactose
Fruits	**Fruits**
All fresh, canned, or frozen that are not processed with lactose	Any canned or frozen processed with lactose

*Ross Laboratories, Columbus, OH 43216.
†Mead Johnson and Co., Evansville, IN 47721.
‡Presto Food Products, Los Angeles, CA 90021.
§Lidano Co., Kalunborg, Denmark.
⊥Cutter Laboratories, Berkeley, CA 94710.
°Ovaltine Products, Villa Park, IL 60181.
●Knudsen Bros., North Haven, CT 06473.
**Rich Products Corp., Buffalo, NY 14212.
††General Mills, Minneapolis, MN 55435.
‡‡Kellogg Co., Battle Creek, MI 49016.
§§Nabisco, Inc., East Hanover, NJ 07936.
⊥⊥G. D. Searle and Co., Skokie, IL 60076.
°°NIFDA (National Institutional Food Distributor Associates, Inc.), Atlanta, GA 30325.
***Domino Amstar Corporation, New York, NY 10020

LACTOSE-FREE DIET—cont'd

Foods Allowed	Foods Excluded
Meat, fish, poultry, etc.	**Meat, fish, poultry, etc.**
Plain beef, chicken, fish, turkey, lamb, veal, pork, and ham; strained or junior meats and vegetables and meat combinations that do not contain milk or milk products; kosher frankfurters	Creamed or breaded meat, fish, or fowl; sausage products, such as weiners, liver sausage, cold cuts containing nonfat milk solids; cheese
Soups	**Soups**
Clear soups, vegetable soups, consommés, cream soups made with Mocha Mix‡ or nondairy creamers	Cream soups unless made with allowed ingredients, chowders, commercially prepared soups containing lactose
Vegetables	**Vegetables**
Fresh, canned, or frozen; artichokes, asparagus, broccoli, cabbage, carrots, cauliflower, celery, chard, corn, cucumber, eggplant, green beans, kale, lettuce, mustard, okra, onions, parsley, parsnips, pumpkin, rutabagas, spinach, squash, tomatoes, white and sweet potatoes, yams, lima beans, beets	Any to which lactose is added during processing; peas; creamed, breaded, or buttered vegetables; instant potatoes, corn curls, and frozen French fries if processed with lactose
Miscellaneous	**Miscellaneous**
Soy sauce, carob powder, popcorn, olives, pure sugar candy, jelly or marmalade, sugar, corn syrup, carbonated beverages, gravy made with water, baker's cocoa, pickles, pure seasonings and spices, wine, molasses (beet sugar), pure monosodium glutamate, instant coffees that do not contain lactose	Chewing gum; chocolate; some cocoas; toffee; peppermint; butterscotch; caramels; some instant coffees, dietetic preparations (read labels); certain antibiotics and vitamin and mineral preparations; spice blends if they contain milk products; monosodium glutamate extender; artificial sweeteners containing lactose, such as Equal,⊥⊥ Sweet n' Low,°° Wee Cal;*** some nondairy creamers (read labels)

SAMPLE MENU

AM	Noon	Between Meals	PM	Bedtime
½ c orange juice	3 oz roast beef	1 slice angel cake with sliced peaches	4 oz round steak	½ c apricot nectar
1 egg, soft cooked	½ c rice		1 small baked potato	
2 slices Vienna bread, toasted	½ c green beans		2 tsp milk-free margarine	
2 tsp milk-free margarine	1 pear		½ c spinach	
1 Tbsp grape jelly	2 slices Vienna bread		2 slices Vienna bread, toasted	
2 tsp sugar	2 tsp milk-free margarine		½ c fruit cocktail	
Coffee or tea	1 tsp sugar		1 tsp sugar	
	Coffee or tea		Coffee or tea	

Reprinted from American Dietetic Association: Handbook of clinical dietetics, New Haven, Conn, 1981, Yale University Press, pp D15-D16.

FAT-RESTRICTED DIET

Foods Allowed	Foods Excluded
Beverages Skim milk or buttermilk made with skim milk, coffee, tea, Postum, fruit juice, soft drinks, cocoa made with cocoa powder and skim milk	**Beverages** Whole milk, buttermilk made with whole milk, chocolate milk, cream in excess of amounts allowed under fats
Bread and Cereal Products Plain, nonfat cereals, spaghetti, noodles, rice, macaroni; plain whole-grain or enriched bread	**Bread and Cereal Products** Biscuits, breads, egg or cheese bread, sweet rolls made with fat, pancakes, doughnuts, waffles, fritters, popcorn prepared with fat, muffins, natural cereals and breads to which extra fat is added.
Cheese Cottage, ¼ c to be used as substitute for an ounce of cheese, or specially processed American cheese containing less than 5% butterfat	**Cheese** Whole milk cheeses
Desserts Sherbet made with skim milk; fruit ice; gelatin; rice, bread, cornstarch, tapioca, or Junket pudding made with skim milk; fruit whips with gelatin, sugar, and egg white; fruit; angel food cake; meringues	**Desserts** Cake, pie, pastry, ice cream, or any dessert containing shortening, chocolate, or fats of any kind, unless especially prepared using part of fat allowance
Eggs 3 per week prepared only with fat from fat allowance; egg whites as desired; low fat egg substitutes	**Eggs** More than 1/day unless substituted for part of the meat allowed
Fats Choose up to the limit allowed on diet among the following (1 serving in the amount listed equals 1 fat choice): 1 tsp butter or fortified margarine 1 tsp shortening or oil 1 tsp mayonnaise 1 Tbsp Italian or French dressing 1 strip crisp bacon ⅓ avocado (4″ diameter) 2 T light cream 1 T heavy cream 6 small nuts 5 small olives	**Fats** Any in excess of amount prescribed on diet; all others

Reprinted from American Dietetic Association: Handbook of clinical dietetics, New Haven, Conn, 1981, Yale University Press, pp E4-E5.

FAT-RESTRICTED DIET—cont'd

Foods Allowed	Foods Excluded
Fruits	**Fruits**
As desired	Avocado in excess of amount allowed on fat list
Lean meat, fish poultry	**Meat, fish poultry**
Choose up to the limit allowed on diet among the following: poultry without skin, fish, veal (all cuts), liver, lean beef, pork, and lamb, with all visible fat removed—1 oz cooked weight equals 1 equivalent; ¼ c water-packed tuna or salmon equals 1 equivalent	Fried or fatty meats, sausage, scrapple, frankfurters, poultry skins, stewing hens, spareribs, salt pork, beef unless lean, duck, goose, ham hocks, pig's feet, luncheon meats, gravies unless fat free, tuna and salmon packed in oil, peanut butter
Milk	**Milk**
Skim, buttermilk or yogurt made from skim milk	Whole, chocolate, buttermilk made with whole milk
Seasonings	**Seasonings**
As desired	None
Soups	**Soups**
Bouillon, clear broth, fat-free vegetable soup, cream soup made with skimmed milk, packaged dehydrated soups	All others
Sweets	**Sweets**
Jelly, jam, marmalade, honey, syrup, molasses, sugar, hard sugar candies, fondant, gumdrops, jelly beans, marshmallows	Any candy made with chocolate, nuts, butter, cream, or fat of any kind
Vegetables	**Vegetables**
All plainly prepared vegetables	Potato chips; buttered, au gratin, creamed, or fried vegetables unless made with allowed fat; commercially frozen vegetables, casseroles, or frozen vegetables in butter sauce

DIETS FOR TYPES I–V HYPERLIPOPROTEINEMIA

	Type I	Type IIa	Type IIb or III	Type IV	Type V
Incidence	Very rare	Common	Relatively uncommon	Common	Uncommon
Diet prescription	Low fat, 25–35 g	Low cholesterol Polyunsaturated fat increased	Low cholesterol Approximately: 20% kcal protein 40% kcal fat 40% kcal CHO	Controlled CHO Approximately 45% of kcal Moderately restricted cholesterol	Restricted fat, 30% of kcal Controlled CHO, 50% of kcal Moderately restricted cholesterol
Kilocalories	Not restricted	Not restricted	Achieve and maintain "ideal" weight, i.e., reduction diet if necessary	Achieve and maintain "ideal" weight, i.e., reduction diet if necessary	Achieve and maintain "ideal" weight, i.e., reduction diet if necessary
Protein	Total protein intake is not limited	Total protein intake is not limited	High protein	Not limited, other than control of patient's weight	High protein
Fat	Restricted to 25–35 g Type of fat not important	Saturated fat intake limited Polyunsaturated fat intake increased	Controlled to 40% of kilocalories (polyunsaturated fats recommended in preference to saturated fats)	Not limited other than control of patient's weight (polyunsaturated fats recommended in preference to saturated fats)	Restricted to 30% of kcal (polyunsaturated fats recommended in preference to saturated fats)
Carbohydrate	Not limited	Not limited	Controlled—concentrated sweets are restricted	Controlled—concentrated sweets are restricted	Controlled—concentrated sweets are restricted

Cholesterol	Not restricted	As low as possible; the only source of cholesterol is the meat in the diet	Less than 300 mg—the only source of cholesterol is the meat in the diet	Moderately restricted to 300-500 mg	Moderately restricted to 300-500 mg
Alcohol	Not recommended	May be used with discretion	Limited to 2 servings (substituted for carbohydrate)	Limited to 2 servings (substituted for carbohydrate)	Not recommended
Clinical Findings					
Age of detection	Early childhood	Early childhood (in severe cases)	Adulthood (over age 20)	Adulthood	Early adulthood
Origin and possible mechanism	Genetic recessive; deficiency in lipoprotein lipase	When genetic, dominant, sporadic; decreased catabolism of β-lipoprotein	When genetic, recessive; sporadic?	When genetic, dominant, sporadic; excessive endogenous glyceride synthesis or deficient glyceride clearance?	Probably genetic, dominant, sporadic
Cholesterol	Normal or elevated	Elevated	Elevated	Normal or elevated	Elevated or normal
Triglyceride	Markedly elevated	Normal or slightly elevated	Usually elevated	Elevated	Elevated to markedly elevated
Lipoprotein family	Elevated chylomicrons	Increased LDL	IIb Increased LDL and VLDL, III increased ILDL	Increased VLDL	Increased chylomicrons and VLDL

Modified from American Dietetic Association: Handbook of clinical dietetics. New Haven, Conn, 1981, Yale University Press, pp E24-25.

CLEAR LIQUID DIET

A clear liquid diet is restricted to foods that, at room temperature, are liquid. Examples include tea, bouillon, fat-free broth, gelatin, carbonated beverages, and strained fruit juices. The diet is of little nutritional benefit, and should be used for only very brief periods.

AM	Midmorning	Noon	Midday	Evening	Bedtime
Apple juice (4 oz) Flavored gelatin (1c) Ginger ale (8 oz) Coffee or tea (sugar may be added)	Flavored gelatin (½ c)	Bouillon or fat-free broth (1 c) Strained fruit (4 oz) Flavored gelatin (½ c) Coffee or tea (sugar may be added)	Ginger ale (8 oz)	Repeat AM/noon pattern Mix and vary foods and flavors per preferences	Flavored gelatin (½ c)

Modified from Turner D: Handbook of diet therapy, ed 5, Chicago, 1970, University of Chicago Press, pp 35-47.

FULL LIQUID DIET

A variety of foods may contribute to a full liquid diet. The single criterion is that the food is liquid or will liquefy at room temperature. Examples include available dietary gruel, pasteurized eggs, frozen desserts, and milk.

AM	Midmorning	Noon	Midday	Evening	Bedtime
Fruit juice (½ c) Cereal (1 c—with margarine, sugar, and milk) Coffee or tea (with sugar) Eggnog (1 c)	Eggnog (1 c)	Apricot nectar (½ c) Cream of potato soup (1 c) Milk (1 c) Soft custard	Milkshake (include malt, syrup, and ice cream)	Juice (½ c) Egg substitutes Coffee or tea Fruit ices	Plain ice cream

Modified from Turner D: Handbook of diet therapy, ed 5, Chicago, 1970, University of Chicago Press, pp 35-47.

APPENDIX III
Food Tables

*The following sources were used in compiling this table:

Adams C: Nutritive Value of American Foods in Common Units. Agriculture Handbook 456. Washington, D.C.: USDA, Nov. 1975.

Adams C, Richardson M: Nutritive Value of Foods. Rev. USDA Home & Garden Bull. No. 72. Washington, D.C.: USDA, 1978.

Anderson B: Comprehensive evaluation of fatty acids in foods. Pork products. J Am Diet Assoc 69:44–49, 1976.

Anderson B, Fristrom G, Weihrauch J: Comprehensive evaluation of fatty acids in foods. Lamb and veal. J Am Diet Assoc 70:53–58, 1977.

Anderson B, Kinsella J, Watt B: Comprehensive evaluation of fatty acids in foods. Beef products. J Am Diet Assoc 67:35–41, 1975.

Church C, Church H: Food Values of Portions Commonly Used. 12th ed. Philadelphia: Lippincott, 1975.

Exler J, Avena R, Weihrauch J: Comprehensive evaluation of fatty acids in foods. Leguminous seeds. J Am Diet Assoc 71:412–15, 1977.

Exler J, Weihrauch J: Comprehensive evaluation of fatty acids in foods. Finfish. J Am Diet Assoc 69:244–48, 1976.

Exler J, Weihrauch J: Comprehensive evaluation of fatty acids in foods. Shellfish. J Am Diet Assoc 71:518–21, 1977.

Feeley R, Criner P, Watt B: Cholesterol content of foods. J Am Diet Assoc 61:134–49, 1972.

Fristrom G, Stewart B, Weihrauch J, Posati L: Comprehensive evaluation of fatty acids in foods. Nuts, peanuts and soup. J Am Diet Assoc 67:351–55, 1975.

Marsh A: Composition of Foods. Soups, Sauces and Gravies. Rev. USDA Handbook 8–6. Washington, D.C.: USDA, 1980.

Marsh A, Klippstein R, Kaplan S: The Sodium Content of Your Food. USDA Home & Garden Bull. No. 233. Washington, D.C.: USDA, 1980.

Posati L: Composition of Foods. Poultry Products. Rev. USDA Handbook 8–5. Washington, D.C.: USDA, 1979.

Posati L, Orr ML: Composition of foods. Rev. Dairy and Egg Products. USDA Handbook 8–1. Washington, D.C.: USDA, 1979.

Reeves J, Weihrauch J: Composition of Foods. Rev. Fats and Oils. USDA Handbook 8–4. Washington, D.C.: USDA, 1979.

Richardson M, Posati L, Anderson B: Composition of Foods. Rev. Sausages and Lunchmeats: USDA Handbook 8–7. Washington, D.C.: USDA, 1980.

Watt B, Merrill A: Composition of Foods—Raw, Processed, Prepared. Rev. USDA Agriculture Handbook No. 8. Washington, D.C.: USDA, 1963.

ENERGY, FAT, AND SELECTED NUTRIENT COMPONENTS OF FOODS COMMONLY EATEN IN THE UNITED STATES

Food*	Portion Size	Energy (kcal)	Carbohydrate (g)	Protein (g)	Total Fat (g)	Saturated Fat (g)	Polyunsaturated Fat (g)	Cholesterol (mg)	Sodium (mg)	Potassium (mg)	Iron (mg)	Magnesium (mg)
Apple (medium)	1	96	24		1				2	182	0.5	14
Apple juice	4 oz	60	15							124	0.8	5
Applesauce (sweetened)	4 oz	103	27						2	74	0.6	5
Asparagus (frozen)	4 oz	26	4	4					1	270	1.0	16
Avocado	½	188	7	2	19	6	5		5	680	0.7	56
Bacon	4 oz	673	4	30	56	21	6	105	1157	267	4.0	28
Baking powder	1 tsp	4	1						329	5	†	†
Banana (medium)	1	101	26	1					1	440	0.8	58
Beans												
Navy (dry)	4 oz	133	24	9	1				8	467	3.0	†
Lima (frozen)	4 oz	112	22	7					115	483	2.0	54
Snap (frozen)	4 oz	30	7	2					2	154	0.8	24
Beef												
Chuck arm steak (trimmed)	4 oz	219		36	8	3	1	103	61	277	4.0	20
Porterhouse (trimmed)	4 oz	254		34	12	5	1	103	84	384	4.0	33
Round steak (trimmed)	4 oz	214		36	7	3		103	87	398	4.0	33
Ground beef (19% fat)	4 oz	371		29	26	9	1	103	52	236	4.0	24
Beets (canned)	4 oz	42	10	1					268	190	0.8	17
Beverages (alcoholic)												
Beer	12 oz	151	14	1					25	90		20
Gin, rum, vodka, whiskey (80 proof)	1 oz	65		?	?					1	†	†
Wine	1 oz	25	1						1	27	0.1	3
Beverages (nonalcoholic)												
Pepsi Cola	8 oz	106	28						35	7	†	†
Gingerale	8 oz	80	21						18	1	†	†
Biscuit (baking powder with vegetable shortening)	1 oz	103	13	2	5	1	1‡		175	33	0.4	6
Blueberries (fresh)	4 oz	70	17	1	1				1	92	1.0	7
Bouillon cube	1	5		1					960	4	†	†
Bread												
Rye	1 slice	61	13	2					139	36	0.4	11
White	1 slice	63	12	2					114	28	0.6	5
Whole wheat	1 slice	61	12	3	1				132	68	0.8	20
Broccoli (frozen)	4 oz	30	5	4					14	250	0.8	24
Brussels sprouts (frozen)	4 oz	38	7	4					16	336	0.9	24

Continued.

Food	Serving										
Butter	1 tsp	36			4	3	11	41	1	0.01	1
Cabbage (fresh)	4 oz	23	10					16	185	0.4	15
Candy											
Butterscotch	1 oz	113	27		3			19		0.4	
Jelly beans	1 oz	104	26					3	1	0.3	†
Carrots (fresh)	4 oz	35	8	1				38	252	0.7	26
Cashews	4 oz	636	33	20	52	10		17	526	4.0	303
Cauliflower	4 oz	21	4	2				11	235	0.6	27
Celery	1 stalk	7	2					50	136	0.1	1
Cheese											
American	1 oz	106	1	6	9	6	27	406	46	0.11	6
Blue	1 oz	100	1	6	8	5	21	396	73	0.09	7
Cheddar	1 oz	114		7	9	6	30	176	28	0.19	8
Cottage (4% fat)	1 oz	29	1	4	1	8	4	114	24	0.05	
Cream	1 oz	99	1	2	10	6	31	84	34	0.34	2
Swiss	1 oz	95	1	7	7	5	24	388	61	0.2	10
Cherries	4 oz	80	20	1				2	217	0.5	16
Chicken (light meat without skin)	4 oz	196		35	5	1	96	87	279	2.0	33
Clams (hardshell)	4 oz	91	7	13	1		57	233	353	9.0	54
Coconut	4 oz	392	11	4	40	31		26	290	2.0	52
Cod	4 oz	88		20	1		57	80	433	0.5	32
Coffee											
Regular	1 tsp	1						26			4
Freeze-dried instant	1 tsp	1						29		0.1	†
Collards (frozen)	4 oz	34	6	3				18	268	1.0	40
Corn (medium)	1 ear	70	16	3	1				151	‡	48
Cornflakes	1 c	97	21	2				251	30	0.6	4
Crab, blue (canned)	4 oz	113		20	2		113	1134	125	0.9	39
Crackers											
Graham	1	55	10	1	1			95	55	0.2	7
Saltine	4	48	8	1	1			123	13	0.1	3
Cream											
Light	8 oz	469	9	6	46	29	159	95	292	0.10	21
Heavy	8 oz	821	7	5	88	55	326	89	179	0.07	17
Cucumber (pared)	6 slice (1 oz)	4	1					2	45	0.1	3

Compiled by Nancy Cusack, R.D., Chief Nutritionist, Baltimore Center of the Multiple Risk Factor Intervention Trial (MRFIT), and Roger Sherwin, M.B., B. Chir.

*Values are for cooked food unless otherwise stated.

†No reliable data available.

‡Linoleic fatty acid available only.

ENERGY, FAT, AND SELECTED NUTRIENT COMPONENTS OF FOODS—cont'd

Food*	Portion Size	Energy (kcal)	Carbohydrate (g)	Protein (g)	Total Fat (g)	Saturated Fat (g)	Polyunsaturated Fat (g)	Cholesterol (mg)	Sodium (mg)	Potassium (mg)	Iron (mg)	Magnesium (mg)
Dates (without pits)	4 oz	270	72	2	1				1	639	3.0	66
Egg (boiled)	1	79	1	6	6	2	1	274	69	65	1.0	6
Eggplant (fresh)	4 oz	22	5	1					1	170	0.7	18
Flounder (raw)	4 oz	90		19	1			57	88	387	0.9	34
Fruit cocktail (sweetened)	4 oz	86	22	1					6	183	0.5	8
Gelatin (sweetened)	4 oz	71	17	2					61	?	†	†
Grapefruit (fresh)	½	40	10	1					1	132	0.4	22
Grapefruit juice (unsweetened)	4 oz	52	12	1						200	0.4	10
Grapes (fresh)	4 oz	52	12	1					2	118	0.3	15
Haddock (raw)	4 oz	90	21	1				68	69	345	0.8	27
Halibut (raw)	4 oz	113	24	1				57	61	509	0.8	26
Honey	1 Tbsp	64	17						1	11	0.1	2
Horseradish	1 tsp	2	1						5	15		
Ice cream (10% fat)	4 oz	135	16	2	7	4		30	58	129	0.6	16
Ice milk	4 oz	92	14	3	3	2		9	53	133	0.9	15
Ices (flavored)	4 oz	123	31							6		
Jams	1 Tbsp	54	14						2	18	0.2	†
Kale (frozen)	4 oz	35	6	3	1				24	219	1.0	36
Lamb, rib chop (trimmed)	4 oz	240		32	8	3	1	113	76	348	2.0	25
Lard	1 Tbsp	116			13	5	1	12			†	†
Lemon juice (fresh)	1 Tbsp	4	1						1	21		
Lemonade (frozen)	8 oz	107	28						2	40	0.1	
Lentils	4 oz	120	22	9					2	282	2.0	91
Lettuce (iceberg)	4 oz	15	3	1					10	199	0.6	12
Liver (fried with margarine)	4 oz	260	7	29	12	3	1‡	497	208	431	10.0	20
Lobster (raw)	4 oz	103	1	19	1		1	96	238	204	0.7	25
Macaroni	4 oz	168	34	6	1				1	90	1.0	23
Margarine												
Stick	1 tsp	34			4	1	1		44	2	†	
Tub (corn oil)	1 tsp	34			4	1	2		51	2	†	
Milk												
Whole	8 oz	150	11	8	8	5		33	120	370	0.1	33
Skim	8 oz	86	12	8				4	126	406	0.1	28
Buttermilk	8 oz	99	12	8	2	1		9	257	371	0.1	28
Chocolate (whole)	8 oz	208	26	8	8	5		30	149	417	0.6	33
Evaporated (whole)	8 oz	336	25	17	19	12	1	72	264	760	0.5	60
Condensed	8 oz	982	166	24	27	17	1	104	389	1136	0.6	78

Mushrooms (raw)	4 oz	32	4	3					17	470	0.9	15
Muskmelons												
Cantaloupe	4 oz	34	9	1					13	285	0.5	18
Honeydew	4 oz	38	9	1					14	285	0.5	11
Mustard (prepared)	1 tsp	4							63	7	0.1	2
Noodles (egg)	4 oz	142	26	5	2			31	2	50	1.0	60
Oatmeal	4 oz	62	11	2	2				247	69	0.7	24
Oils												
Corn	1 Tbsp	120			14	2	8					
Olive	1 Tbsp	119			14	2	1				0.05	
Peanut	1 Tbsp	119			14	2	1					
Safflower	1 Tbsp	120			14	1	10					
Soybean-cottonseed (blend)	1 Tbsp	120			14	2	7					
Okra (frozen)	4 oz	43	10	3					2	186	0.6	60
Olives (green)	4 med	15	1		2				323	7	0.2	4
Onion (raw)	1 Tbsp	4	1						1	16	0.1	1
Orange (medium)	1	64	16	1					1	263	0.5	20
Orange juice (frozen, unsweetened)	1	61	14	1					1	252	0.1	11
Oysters (raw)	4 oz	76	4	9	2	1	1	57	151	137	6.0	30
Parsley (fresh)	1 Tbsp	2							2	25	0.2	2
Parsnips (fresh)	4 oz	75	17	2	1				9	430	0.7	36
Peach (medium)	1	58	15	1					2	308	0.8	18
Peaches (canned and sweetened)	4 oz	88	23						2	148	0.3	7
Peanuts (roasted, salted)	4 oz	663	21	29	56	11	17		474	765	0.2	198
Peanut butter	1 Tbsp	94	3	4	8	2	2		97	100	0.3	28
Pear (medium)	1	86	22		1				3	183	0.4	11
Pears (canned and sweetened)	4 oz	86	22						1	95	0.2	6
Peas (frozen)	4 oz	77	13	6					130	153	2.0	27
Pepper (sweet)	1	93	4						10	157	0.5	16
Pickle (dill)	1	7	1						928	130	0.7	8
Pies (9″ diameter)												
Apple	⅙	404	60		18	5	4‡		476	126	0.5	9
Custard	⅙	331	36	9	17	6	3‡	160	436	208	0.9	20
Pineapple (fresh)	4 oz	59	16						1	166	0.6	15
Pineapple (canned and sweetened)	4 oz	84	22						1	109	0.4	9
Pizza (cheese, 10″ diameter)	⅐	139	20	5	4	2	1‡	27	367	65	0.5	3
Plum (fresh, medium)	1	32	8						1	112	0.3	6
Plum (canned and sweetened)	4 oz	90	23			2			1	153	1.0	6
Popcorn (popped in coconut oil, with salt)	1 c	40	5	1	2				175	?	0.2	?
Pork												
Ham (trimmed, sliced, baked)	4 oz	208	4		12	5	1	64	1492	376	1.0	20
Chop, loin (trimmed)	4 oz	300			16	5	1	100	82	374	4.0	36

Continued.

ENERGY, FAT, AND SELECTED NUTRIENT COMPONENTS OF FOODS—cont'd

Food*	Portion Size	Energy (kcal)	Carbo-hydrate (g)	Protein (g)	Total Fat (g)	Satu-rated Fat (g)	Poly-unsatu-rated Fat (g)	Cho-lesterol (mg)	Sodium (mg)	Potassium (mg)	Iron (mg)	Magne-sium (mg)
Potato (baked in skin)	1	145	33	4					6	782	1.1	?
Potato chips	4 oz	644	57	6	45	12	23‡		1134	1280	2.0	54
Pretzels Dutch	1	62	12	2	1				269	21	0.2	?
Prunes (uncooked, without pits)	4 oz	289	76	2	1				9	787	4.0	45
Prune juice	4 oz	99	24	1					3	301	5.0	11
Pudding (chocolate, from mix)	4 oz	140	26	4	3	2		13	146	154	0.3	16
Radishes	4 oz	19	4	1					21	365	1.0	17
Raisins	4 oz	328	88	3					32	864	4.0	40
Rice	4 oz	124	27	2					424	32	1.0	9
Rolls												
Brown and serve	1	84	14	2	2		1‡		136	25	0.5	6
Hamburger/hot dog	1	119	21	3	2		1‡		202	38	0.3	9
Hard	1	156	30	5	2	1	1‡		313	49	1.0	12
Salad dressings												
Blue cheese	1 Tbsp	77	1	1	8	2	4	†	164	6		
French	1 Tbsp	67	3		6	2	3	†	219	13	0.1	
Italian	1 Tbsp	69	2		7	1	4	†	116	2		
Mayonnaise	1 Tbsp	99	0.4		11	2	6	8	78	5	0.1	1
Thousand Island	1 Tbsp	59	2		6	1	3	†	109	18	0.1	
Salmon (sockeye, canned, solids and liquids)	4 oz	193		23	8	1	4	40	439	409	0.9	33
Salt	1 tsp								2132			7
Sardines (drained) (Atlantic herring)	4 oz	230		27	19	3	3	159	932	668	3.0	27
Sauerkraut (canned)	4 oz	21	4	1					847	159	0.6	†
Sausage												
Bologna (beef)	1 oz	89	1	3	8	3		16	284	44	0.4	3
Braunschweiger	1 oz	102	1	4	9	3	1	44	324	57	3.0	3
Frankfurter (beef)	1	184	1	6	17	7	1	27	584	90	0.8	6
Pork link	1	265	1	15	22	8	3	46	1020	228	0.8	2
Scallops (raw)	4 oz	92	4	17	1			40	289	449	2.0	43
Sherbet (orange)	4 oz	135	29	1	2	1		7	44	99	0.2	†

Food	Measure										
Shrimp (raw)	4 oz	103	2	21	1		170	159	249	2.0	48
Syrup (cane and maple)	1 Tbsp	50	13						5		
Soup (canned)											
Beef noodle (with water)	8 oz	84	9	5	3	1	5	952	99	1.0	6
Cream of mushroom (with water)	8 oz	129	9	2	9	4	2	1031	101	0.5	5
Vegetable (with water)	8 oz	72	12	2	2	1		823	209	1.0	7
Soy sauce	1 Tbsp	25	4	2				2666	138	2.0	?
Spaghetti	4 oz	126	26	4	1			1	69	1.0	40
Spinach (frozen)	4 oz	26	4	3	1			59	378	2.0	74
Squash											
Summer (fresh)	4 oz	16	4	1				1	160	0.5	18
Winter (fresh)	4 oz	72	17	2				1	523	0.9	19
Strawberries (fresh)	4 oz	42	10	1				1	186	1.0	14
Strawberries (frozen, sweetened)	4 oz	104	27	1				1	118	0.7	6
Sugar	1 tsp	15	4								
Sweet potatoes (baked)	1	161	37	2		5		14	342	1.0	35
Sweet potatoes (candied, canned)	4 oz	129	31	1		8		55	136	0.8	19
Tomato (fresh, medium)	1	27	6	1				4	300	0.6	14
Tomatoes (canned)	4 oz	24	5	1				148	246	0.6	3
Tomato catsup	1 Tbsp	16	4					156	54	0.1	11
Tomato juice	4 oz	24	5	1	1			244	276	1.0	36
Trout, rainbow (raw)	4 oz	221		24	5	1	62	89	?	?	?
Tuna in water (solids and liquid)	4 oz	144		32	1	2	71	384	317	2.0	32
Turkey (light meat without skin)	4 oz	177		34	4	1	79	73	345	2.0	23
Turnips (fresh)	4 oz	26	6	1				39	213	0.5	20
Veal cutlet	4 oz	245		31	13	1	115	75	344	4.0	149
Walnuts (shelled)	4 oz	712	17	23	72	47		4	512	4.0	9
Watermelon	4 oz	30	7	1				1	114	0.6	60
Wheat germ	1 Tbsp	23	3	2	1				57	0.5	19
Wheat (puffed)	1 c	54	12	2				1	51	0.6	33
Wheat (shredded)	1 biscuit	89	20	3	1			1	87	0.9	26
Yogurt (whole milk, plain)	8 oz	139	11	8	7	5	29	105	351	0.1	40
Yogurt (low fat, plain)	8 oz	144	16	12	4	2	14	159	531	0.2	40
Yogurt (low fat, fruit varieties)	8 oz	225	42	9	3	2	10	121	402	0.1	30

DIETARY FIBER CONTENT OF FOODS

	Total dietary fiber (g/100)	Noncellulose polysaccharides (g/100)	Cellulose (g/100)	Lignin (g/100)	Common Serving Size	Weight (g)	Total dietary fiber/serving
Fruits							
Apples (flesh only)	1.42	0.94	0.48	0.01	1 med	141	2.00
(peel only)	3.71	2.21	1.01	0.49	1 med	11	0.41
Bananas	1.75	1.12	0.37	0.26	One 6″	100	1.75
Cherries (flesh and skin)	1.24	0.92	0.25	0.07	25 sm/med 15 lg	100	1.24
Grapefruit (canned)	0.44	0.34	0.04	0.55	½ c	120	0.53
Guavas (canned)*	3.64	1.67	1.17	0.80	1 med	10	3.64
Mandarin oranges (canned)*	0.29	0.22	0.04	0.03	½ c	100	0.29
Mangoes (canned)*	1.00	0.65	0.32	0.03	½ c	83	0.83
Peaches (flesh and skin)	2.28	1.46	0.20	0.62	1 med	100	2.28
Pears (flesh only)	2.44	1.32	0.67	0.45	½ med	87	1.12
(peel only)	8.59	3.72	2.18	2.67	½ med	11	0.95
Plums (flesh and skin)	1.52	0.99	0.23	0.30	2 med	100	1.52
Rhubarb (raw)	1.78	0.93	0.70	0.15	½ c	60	1.07
Strawberries (raw)	2.12	0.98	0.33	0.81	10 lg	100	2.12
(canned)*	1.00	0.48	0.20	0.33	⅜ c	100	1.00
Sultanas	4.40	2.40	0.83	1.17			
Nuts							
Brazils	7.73	3.60	2.17	1.96	¼ c	35	2.71
Peanuts	9.30	6.40	1.69	1.21	1 Tbsp	9	0.84
Preserves							
Jam, plum	0.96	0.80	0.14	0.03	1 Tbsp	20	0.19
strawberry	1.12	0.85	0.11	0.15	1 Tbsp	20	0.22
Lemon curd	0.20	0.18	0.02	tr			
Marmalade	0.71	0.64	0.05	0.01	1 Tbsp	20	0.14
Mincemeat	3.19	2.09	0.60	0.50			
Peanut butter	7.55	5.64	1.91	tr	1 Tbsp	15	1.13
Pickles	1.53	0.91	0.50	0.12			
Dried soups							
Minestrone	6.61	4.60	1.91	0.10			
Oxtail	3.84	2.89	0.94	0.01			
Tomato	3.32	1.95	1.33	0.04	1 serv	16	0.53
Beverages							
Cocoa	43.27	11.25	4.13	27.90	1 oz	28	12.12
Chocolate drink	8.20	2.61	1.16	4.43	1 oz	28	2.30
Coffee and chicory essence	0.79	0.73	0.02	0.04			
Instant coffee	16.41	15.55	0.53	0.33	1 serv	2	0.33
Extracts							
Bovril	0.91	0.85	0.03	0.03			
Marmite	2.69	2.60	0.03	0.06			
Leafy vegetables							
Broccoli tops (boiled)	4.10	2.92	0.85	0.03	½ c	73	2.99
Brussels sprouts	2.86	1.99	0.80	0.07	½ c	70	2.00
Cabbage	2.83	1.76	0.69	0.38	½ c	73	2.07
Cauliflower	1.80	0.67	1.13	tr	½ c	63	1.13
Lettuce (raw)	1.53	0.47	1.06	tr	½ c	55	0.84
Onions (raw)	2.10	1.55	0.55	tr	one 2¼″	100	2.10

Adapted from Southgate DAT, et al: A guide to calculating intakes of dietary fiber. J Hum Nutr **30**:303, 1976. Reprinted from American Dietetic Association: Handbook of Clinical Dietetics. New Haven, Conn, 1981, Yale University Press, pp 811–812.
*Fruit and syrup.
†Drained.

DIETARY FIBER CONTENT OF FOODS—cont'd

	Total dietary fiber (g/100)	Noncellulose polysaccharides (g/100)	Cellulose (g/100)	Lignin (g/100)	Common Serving Size	Weight (g)	Total dietary fiber/serving
Legumes							
Beans (baked) canned	7.27	5.67	1.41	0.19	⅓ c	85	6.18
Beans (runner) boiled	3.35	1.85	1.29	0.21	½ c	50	1.67
Peas, frozen (raw)	7.75	5.48	2.09	0.18	½ c	73	5.66
garden (canned)†	6.28	3.80	2.47	0.01			
processed (canned)†	7.85	5.20	2.30	0.35	½ c	67	5.26
Root vegetables							
Carrots, young (boiled)	3.70	2.22	1.48	tr	½ c	75	2.78
Parsnips (raw)	4.90	3.77	1.13	tr	½ lg	100	4.90
Swedes (raw)	2.40	1.61	0.79	tr			
Turnips (raw)	2.20	1.50	0.70	tr	⅔ c	86	1.89
Potato							
Main crop (raw)	3.51	2.49	1.02	tr	one 2¼″	100	3.51
French fries	3.20	2.05	1.12	0.03	10 pcs	20	0.64
Chips	11.90	10.60	1.07	0.32	3½ oz	10	11.90
Canned (solid and liquid)	2.51	2.23	0.28	tr	⅔ c	10	2.51
Peppers (cooked)	0.93	0.59	0.24	tr	½ c	68	0.63
Tomatoes (fresh)	1.40	0.65	0.45	0.30	1 small	10	1.40
Tomatoes (canned)†	0.85	0.45	0.37	0.03	½ c	12	1.02
Sweet corn cooked	4.74	4.31	0.31	0.12	½ ear	83	2.37
canned†	5.69	4.97	0.64	0.08	½ c	83	4.72
Flours							
White, breadmaking	3.15	2.52	0.60	0.03	½ c	60	1.89
Brown	7.87	5.70	1.42	0.75			
Whole meal	9.51	6.25	2.46	0.80	½ c	67	6.28
Bran	44.0	32.70	8.05	3.23	½ c	30	13.20
Breads							
White	2.72	2.01	0.71	tr	1 slice	23	0.63
Brown, Boston	5.11	3.63	1.33	0.15	1 slice	35	1.79
Whole meal	8.50	5.95	1.31	1.24	1 slice	23	1.96
Breakfast cereals							
All Bran	26.70	17.82	6.01	2.88	¾ c	42	11.20
Cornflakes	11.00	7.26	2.42	1.32	¾ c	19	2.09
Grapenuts	7.00	5.14	1.28	0.58	⅔ c	84	5.88
Rice Krispies	4.47	3.47	0.78	0.22	¾ c	21	0.94
Puffed wheat	15.41	10.35	2.59	2.47	¾ c	9	1.39
Sugar Puffs	6.08	4.00	0.99	1.09			
Shredded wheat	12.26	8.79	2.63	0.84	1 biscuit	22	2.70
Special K	5.45	3.68	0.72	1.05	¾ c	12	0.65
Swiss breakfast	7.41	5.31	1.36	0.74			
Miscellaneous							
Choc. digestine ½ coated	3.50	2.13	0.59	0.78			
Choc. fully coated	3.09	1.36	0.42	1.31	1 cookie	11	0.34
Crispbread, rye	11.73	8.33	1.66	1.74	2 crax	13	1.48
Crispbread, wheat	4.83	3.34	0.94	0.55			
Ginger biscuits	1.99	1.45	0.30	0.24	1 snap	4	0.08
Matzo	3.85	2.72	0.70	0.43	1 pc	20	0.77
Oatcakes	4.00	3.16	0.40	0.44			
Short-sweet	1.66	1.42	0.11	0.13	1 cookie	7	0.12
Wafers (filled vanilla)	1.62	1.08	0.47	0.07	1 wafer	3	0.05

NUTRITIONAL ANALYSES OF FAST FOODS*

	Wt (g)	Energy (kcal)	Protein (g)	Carbo-hydrate (g)	Fat (g)	Choles-terol (mg)	Vitamins A (IU)	B₁ (mg)	B₂ (mg)	Nia-cin (mg)
ARBY'S®										
Roast Beef	140	350	22	32	15	45	X	0.30	0.34	5
Beef and Cheese	168	450	27	36	22	55	X	0.38	0.43	6
Super Roast Beef	263	620	30	61	28	85	X	0.53	0.43	7
Junior Roast Beef	74	220	12	21	9	35	X	0.15	0.17	3
Ham & Cheese	154	380	23	33	17	60	X	0.75	0.34	5
Turkey Deluxe	236	510	28	46	24	70	X	0.45	0.34	8
Club Sandwich	252	560	30	43	30	100	X	0.68	0.43	7

Source: Consumer Affairs, Arby's, Inc., Atlanta, Georgia. Nutritional analysis by Technological Resources, Camden, New Jersey.

	Wt (g)	Energy (kcal)	Protein (g)	Carbo-hydrate (g)	Fat (g)	Choles-terol (mg)	A (IU)	B₁ (mg)	B₂ (mg)	Nia-cin (mg)
BURGER CHEF®										
Hamburger	91	244	11	29	9	27	114	0.17	0.16	2.7
Cheeseburger	104	290	14	29	13	39	267	0.18	0.21	2.8
Double Cheeseburger	145	420	24	30	22	77	431	0.20	0.32	4.4
Fish Filet	179	547	21	46	31	43	400	0.23	0.22	2.7
Super Shef® Sandwich	252	563	29	44	30	105	754	0.31	0.40	6.0
Big Shef® Sandwich	186	569	23	38	36	81	279	0.26	0.31	4.7
Funmeal® Feast	—	545	15	55	30	27	123	0.25	0.21	4.6
Rancher® Platter*	316	640	32	33	42	106	1750*	0.29	0.38	8.6
Mariner® Platter*	373	734	29	78	34	35	2069*	0.34	0.23	5.2
French Fries, small	68	250	2	20	19	0	0	0.07	0.04	1.07
Vanilla Shake (12 oz)	336	380	13	60	10	40	387	0.10	0.66	0.5
Hot Chocolate	—	198	8	23	8	30	288	0.93	0.39	0.3

Includes salad. Source: Burger Chef Systems, Inc., Indianapolis, Indiana. Nutritional analysis from *Handbook No. 8*. Washington: US Dept of Agriculture.

	Wt (g)	Energy (kcal)	Protein (g)	Carbo-hydrate (g)	Fat (g)	Choles-terol (mg)	A (IU)	B₁ (mg)	B₂ (mg)	Nia-cin (mg)
CHURCH'S FRIED CHICKEN®										
White Chicken Portion	100	327	21	10	23	—	160	0.10	0.18	7.2
Dark Chicken Portion	100	305	22	7	21	—	140	0.10	0.27	5.3

Source: Church's Fried Chicken, San Antonio, Texas. Nutritional analysis by Medallion Laboratories, Minneapolis, Minnesota.

	Wt (g)	Energy (kcal)	Protein (g)	Carbo-hydrate (g)	Fat (g)	Choles-terol (mg)	A (IU)	B₁ (mg)	B₂ (mg)	Nia-cin (mg)
DAIRY QUEEN®										
Frozen Dessert	113	180	5	27	6	20	100	0.09	0.17	X
DQ Cone, regular	142	230	6	35	7	20	300	0.09	0.26	X
DQ Dip Cone, regular	156	300	7	40	13	20	300	0.09	0.34	X
DQ Sundae, regular	177	290	6	51	7	20	300	0.06	0.26	X
DQ Malt, regular	418	600	15	89	20	50	750	0.12	0.60	0.8
DQ Float	397	330	6	59	8	20	100	0.12	0.17	X
DQ Banana Split	383	540	10	91	15	30	750	0.60	0.60	0.8
DQ Parfait	284	460	10	81	11	30	400	0.12	0.43	0.4
DQ Freeze	397	520	11	89	13	35	200	0.15	0.34	X
Mr. Misty® Freeze	411	500	10	87	12	35	200	0.15	0.34	X
Mr. Misty® Float	404	440	6	85	8	20	100	0.12	0.17	X
"Dilly"® Bar	85	240	4	22	15	10	100	0.06	0.17	X
DQ Sandwich	60	140	3	24	4	10	100	0.03	0.14	0.4
Mr. Misty Kiss®	89	70	0	17	0	0	X	X	X	X

From Young EA, Perspective on fast foods. Publ Health Curr, vol 21(3) Ross Laboratories, Columbus, Ohio, 1981.

*For space consideration, some items or sizes of items have been eliminated from this Appendix. For full tables, see the issue of *Public Health Currents* cited.

Dashes indicate no data available; X, less than 2% USRDA; *tr,* trace.

	Vitamins				Minerals								Mois-ture (g)	Crude Fiber (g)
B₆ (mg)	B₁₂ (µg)	C (mg)	D (IU)	Ca (mg)	Cu (mg)	Fe (mg)	K (mg)	Mg (mg)	P (mg)	Na (mg)	Zn (mg)		

B₆ (mg)	B₁₂ (µg)	C (mg)	D (IU)	Ca (mg)	Cu (mg)	Fe (mg)	K (mg)	Mg (mg)	P (mg)	Na (mg)	Zn (mg)	Moisture (g)	Crude Fiber (g)
—	—	X	—	80	—	3.6	—	—	—	880	—	—	—
—	—	X	—	200	—	4.5	—	—	—	1220	—	—	—
—	—	X	—	100	—	5.4	—	—	—	1420	—	—	—
—	—	X	—	40	—	1.8	—	—	—	530	—	—	—
—	—	X	—	200	—	2.7	—	—	—	1350	—	—	—
—	—	X	—	80	—	2.7	—	—	—	1220	—	—	—
—	—	X	—	200	—	3.6	—	—	—	1610	—	—	—
0.16	0.26	1.2	—	45	0.08	2.0	208	9	106	—	1.6	41	0.2
0.17	0.36	1.2	—	132	0.08	2.2	218	9	202	—	1.9	46	0.2
0.31	0.73	1.2	—	223	0.10	3.2	360	15	355	—	3.6	67	0.2
0.04	0.10	1.0	—	145	0.04	2.2	271	19	302	—	1.2	72	0.4
0.45	0.87	9.3	—	205	0.21	4.5	578	25	377	—	4.5	143	0.5
0.31	0.63	1.0	—	152	0.05	3.6	382	14	280	—	3.4	80	0.3
0.16	0.26	12.8	—	61	0.24	2.8	688	26	183	—	1.6	70	0.8
0.61	1.01	23.5	—	66	0.38	5.3	1237	53	326	—	5.6	209	1.3
0.09	0.56	23.5	—	63	0.32	3.3	996	49	397	—	1.2	195	1.8
—	0	11.5	—	9	0.16	0.7	473	16	62	—	<0.1	29	0.6
0.1	1.77	0	—	497	—	0.3	622	40	392	—	1.3	—	—
0.1	0.79	2.1	—	271	0.09	0.7	436	50	245	—	1.1	—	—
—	—	0.7	—	94	—	1.00	186	—	—	498	—	45	0.10
—	—	1.0	—	15	—	1.3	206	—	—	475	—	48	0.20
—	0.6	X	—	150	—	X	—	—	100	—	—	—	—
—	0.6	X	X	200	—	X	—	—	150	—	—	—	—
—	0.6	X	X	200	—	0.4	—	—	150	—	—	—	—
—	0.6	X	X	200	—	1.1	—	—	150	—	—	—	—
—	1.8	3.6	100	500	—	3.6	—	—	400	—	—	—	—
—	0.6	X	X	200	—	X	—	—	200	—	—	—	—
—	0.9	18	X	350	—	1.8	—	—	250	—	—	—	—
—	1.2	X	8	300	—	1.8	—	—	250	—	—	—	—
—	1.2	X	X	300	—	X	—	—	250	—	—	—	—
—	0.12	X	X	300	—	X	—	—	200	—	—	—	—
—	0.6	X	X	200	—	X	—	—	200	—	—	—	—
—	0.5	X	X	100	—	0.4	—	—	100	—	—	—	—
—	0.2	X	X	60	—	0.4	—	—	60	—	—	—	—
—	X	X	X	X	—	X	—	—	X	—	—	—	—

Continued.

NUTRITIONAL ANALYSES OF FAST FOODS—cont'd

	Wt (g)	Energy (kcal)	Protein (g)	Carbo-hydrate (g)	Fat (g)	Choles-terol (mg)	Vitamins			
							A (IU)	B₁ (mg)	B₂ (mg)	Nia-cin (mg)
DAIRY QUEEN—cont'd										
Brazier® Chili Dog	128	330	13	25	20	—	—	0.15	0.23	3.9
Brazier® Dog	99	273	11	23	15	—	—	0.12	0.15	2.6
Fish Sandwich	170	400	20	41	17	—	tr	0.15	0.26	3.0
Super Brazier® Dog	182	518	20	41	30	—	tr	0.42	0.44	7.0
Super Brazier® Dog w/Ch	203	593	26	43	36	—	—	0.43	0.48	8.1
Brazier® Fries, small	71	200	2	25	10	—	tr	0.06	tr	0.8
Brazier® Onion Rings	85	300	6	33	17	—	tr	0.09	tr	0.4

Source: International Dairy Queen, Inc., Minneapolis, Minnesota. Nutritional analysis by Raltech Scientific Services, Inc. (formerly WARF), Madison, Wisconsin. (Nutritional analysis not applicable in the state of Texas.)

	Wt (g)	Energy (kcal)	Protein (g)	Carbo-hydrate (g)	Fat (g)	Choles-terol (mg)	A (IU)	B₁ (mg)	B₂ (mg)	Nia-cin (mg)
JACK IN THE BOX®										
Hamburger	97	263	13	29	11	26	49	0.27	0.18	5.6
Cheeseburger	109	310	16	28	15	32	338	0.27	0.21	5.4
Jumbo Jack® Hamburger	246	551	28	45	29	80	246	0.47	0.34	11.6
Super Taco	146	285	12	20	17	37	599	0.10	0.12	2.8
Moby Jack® Sandwich	141	455	17	38	26	56	240	0.30	0.21	4.5
Breakfast Jack® Sandwich	121	301	18	28	13	182	442	0.41	0.47	5.1
Apple Turnover	119	411	4	45	24	17	—	0.23	0.12	2.5
Vanilla Shake	314	342	10	54	9	36	440	0.16	0.47	0.5
Ham & Cheese Omelette	174	425	21	32	23	355	766	0.45	0.70	3.0
Ranchero Style Omelette	196	414	20	33	23	343	853	0.33	0.74	2.6
French Toast	180	537	15	54	29	115	522	0.56	0.30	4.4
Pancakes	232	626	16	79	27	87	488	0.63	0.44	4.6
Scrambled Eggs	267	719	26	55	44	259	694	0.69	0.56	5.2

Source: Jack-in-the-Box, Foodmaker, Inc., San Diego, California. Nutritional analysis by Raltech Scientific Services, Inc. (formerly WARF), Madison, Wisconsin.

	Wt (g)	Energy (kcal)	Protein (g)	Carbo-hydrate (g)	Fat (g)	Choles-terol (mg)	A (IU)	B₁ (mg)	B₂ (mg)	Nia-cin (mg)
KENTUCKY FRIED CHICKEN®										
Original Recipe® Dinner*										
Wing & Rib	322	603	30	48	32	133	25.5	0.22	0.19	10.0
Wing & Thigh	341	661	33	48	38	172	25.5	0.24	0.27	8.4
Drum & Thigh	346	643	35	46	35	180	25.5	0.25	0.32	8.5
Extra Crispy Dinner®										
Wing & Rib	349	755	33	60	43	132	25.5	0.31	0.29	10.4
Wing & Thigh	371	812	36	58	48	176	25.5	0.31	0.35	10.3
Drum & Thigh	376	765	38	55	44	183	25.5	0.32	0.38	10.4
Mashed Potatoes	85	64	2	12	1	0	<18	<0.01	0.02	0.8
Gravy	14	23	0	1	2	0	<3	0.00	0.01	0.1
Rolls	21	61	2	11	1	1	<5	0.10	0.04	1.0
Corn (5.5-inch ear)	135	169	5	31	3	X	162	0.12	0.07	1.2

*Includes two pieces of chicken, mashed potato and gravy, cole slaw, and roll. Source: Kentucky Fried Chicken, Inc., Louisville, Kentucky. Nutritional analysis by Raltech Scientific Services, Inc. (formerly WARF), Madison, Wisconsin.

	Vitamins							Minerals						
B₆ (mg)	B₁₂ (µg)	C (mg)	D (IU)	Ca (mg)	Cu (mg)	Fe (mg)	K (mg)	Mg (mg)	P (mg)	Na (mg)	Zn (mg)	Mois- ture (g)	Crude Fiber (g)

B$_6$ (mg)	B$_{12}$ (µg)	C (mg)	D (IU)	Ca (mg)	Cu (mg)	Fe (mg)	K (mg)	Mg (mg)	P (mg)	Na (mg)	Zn (mg)	Moisture (g)	Crude Fiber (g)
0.17	1.29	11.0	20	86	0.13	2.0	—	38	139	939	1.8	—	—
0.08	1.05	11.0	23	75	0.79	1.5	—	21	104	868	1.4	—	—
0.16	1.20	tr	40	60	0.08	1.1	—	24	200	—	0.3	—	—
0.17	2.09	14.0	44	158	0.18	4.3	—	37	195	1552	2.8	—	—
0.18	2.34	14.0	44	297	0.18	4.4	—	42	312	1986	3.5	—	—
0.16	—	3.6	16	tr	0.04	0.4	—	16	100	—	tr	—	—
0.08	—	2.4	8	20	0.08	0.4	—	16	60	—	0.3	—	—
0.11	0.73	1.1	20	82	0.10	2.3	165	20	115	566	1.8	43	0.2
0.12	0.87	<1.1	20	172	0.10	2.6	177	22	194	877	2.3	47	0.2
0.30	2.68	3.7	42	134	0.22	4.5	492	44	261	1134	4.2	139	0.7
0.22	0.77	1.6	9	196	0.18	1.9	415	53	235	968	2.1	92	1.0
0.12	1.1	1.4	24	167	0.08	1.7	246	30	263	837	1.1	57	0.1
0.14	1.1	3.4	51	177	0.11	2.5	190	24	310	1037	1.8	59	0.1
0.03	0.17	<1.2	1	11	0.06	1.4	69	10	33	352	0.2	45	0.2
0.18	1.1	3.5	44	349	0.06	0.4	536	48	318	263	1.0	238	0.3
0.18	1.44	<1.7	64	260	0.14	4.0	237	29	397	975	2.3	94	0.2
0.18	1.51	<2.0	78	278	0.14	3.8	260	29	372	1098	2.0	117	0.4
0.47	1.62	9.2	22	119	0.11	3.0	194	27	256	1130	1.8	78	0.9
0.19	0.56	<26.2	23	105	0.12	2.8	237	36	633	1670	1.9	104	0.7
0.34	1.31	<12.8	80	257	0.24	5.0	635	55	483	1110	3.0	137	1.3
—	—	36.6	—	—	—	—	—	—	—	—	—	—	—
—	—	36.6	—	—	—	—	—	—	—	—	—	—	—
—	—	36.6	—	—	—	—	—	—	—	—	—	—	—
—	—	36.6	—	—	—	—	—	—	—	—	—	—	—
—	—	36.6	—	—	—	—	—	—	—	—	—	—	—
—	—	36.6	—	—	—	—	—	—	—	—	—	—	—
—	—	4.9	—	—	—	—	—	—	—	—	—	—	—
—	—	<0.2	—	—	—	—	—	—	—	—	—	—	—
—	—	0.3	—	—	—	—	—	—	—	—	—	—	—
—	—	2.6	—	—	—	—	—	—	—	—	—	—	—

Continued.

NUTRITIONAL ANALYSES OF FAST FOODS* —cont'd

	Wt (g)	Energy (kcal)	Protein (g)	Carbo-hydrate (g)	Fat (g)	Choles-terol (mg)	Vitamins A (IU)	B₁ (mg)	B₂ (mg)	Nia-cin (mg)
LONG JOHN SILVER'S										
Fish w/Batter (2 pc)	136	366	22	21	22	—	—	—	—	—
Treasure Chest	143	506	30	32	33	—	—	—	—	—
Chicken Planks (4 pc)	166	457	27	35	23	—	—	—	—	—
Peg Legs w/Batter (5 pc)	125	350	22	26	28	—	—	—	—	—
Ocean Scallops (6 pc)	120	283	11	30	13	—	—	—	—	—
Shrimp w/Batter (6 pc)	88	268	8	30	13	—	—	—	—	—
Breaded Oysters (6 pc)	156	441	13	53	19	—	—	—	—	—
Breaded Clams	142	617	18	61	34	—	—	—	—	—
Fish Sandwich	193	337	22	49	31	—	—	—	—	—
French Fries	85	288	4	33	16	—	—	—	—	—
Cole Slaw	113	138	1	16	8	—	—	—	—	—
Hushpuppies (3)	45	153	3	20	7	—	—	—	—	—
Clam Chowder (8 oz)	170	107	5	15	3	—	—	—	—	—

Source: Long John Silver's Food Shoppes, Lexington, Kentucky. Nutritional analysis by L. V. Packett, PhD. The Department of Nutrition and Food Science, University of Kentucky.

	Wt (g)	Energy (kcal)	Protein (g)	Carbo-hydrate (g)	Fat (g)	Choles-terol (mg)	A (IU)	B₁ (mg)	B₂ (mg)	Nia-cin (mg)
McDONALD'S										
Egg McMuffin	138	327	19	31	15	229	97	0.47	0.44	3.8
English Muffin, Buttered	63	186	5	30	5	13	164	0.28	0.49	2.6
Hotcakes w/Butter & Syrup	214	500	8	94	10	47	257	0.26	0.36	2.3
Sausage (Pork)	53	206	9	tr	19	43	<32	0.27	0.11	2.1
Scrambled Eggs	98	180	13	3	13	349	652	0.08	0.47	0.2
Hashbrown Potatoes	55	125	2	14	7	7	<14	0.06	<0.01	0.8
Big Mac	204	563	26	41	33	86	530	0.39	0.37	6.5
Cheeseburger	115	307	15	30	14	37	345	0.25	0.23	3.8
Hamburger	102	255	12	30	10	25	82	0.25	0.18	4.0
Quarter Pounder	166	424	24	33	22	67	133	0.32	0.28	6.5
Quarter Pounder w/Ch	194	524	30	32	31	96	660	0.31	0.37	7.4
Filet-O-Fish	139	432	14	37	25	47	42	0.26	0.20	2.6
Regular Fries	68	220	3	26	12	9	<17	0.12	0.02	2.3
Apple Pie	85	253	2	29	14	12	<34	0.02	0.02	0.2
Cherry Pie	88	260	2	32	14	13	114	0.03	0.02	0.4
McDonaldland Cookies	67	308	4	49	11	10	<27	0.23	0.23	2.9
Vanilla Shake	291	352	9	60	8	31	349	0.12	0.70	0.3
Hot Fudge Sundae	164	310	7	46	11	18	230	0.07	0.31	1.1
Caramel Sundae	165	328	7	53	10	26	279	0.07	0.31	1.0
Strawberry Sundae	164	289	7	46	9	20	230	0.07	0.30	1.0

Source: McDonald's Corporation, Oak Brook, Illinois. Nutritional analysis by Raltech Scientific Services, Inc. (formerly WARF), Madison, Wisconsin.

	Wt (g)	Energy (kcal)	Protein (g)	Carbo-hydrate (g)	Fat (g)	Choles-terol (mg)	A (IU)	B₁ (mg)	B₂ (mg)	Nia-cin (mg)
TACO BELL®										
Bean Burrito	166	343	11	48	12	—	1657	0.37	0.22	2.2
Beef Burrito	184	466	30	37	21	—	1675	0.30	0.39	7.0
Beefy Tostada	184	291	19	21	15	—	3450	0.16	0.27	3.3
Bellbeefer®	123	221	15	23	7	—	2961	0.15	0.20	3.7
Burrito Supreme®	225	457	21	43	22	—	3462	0.33	0.35	4.7
Combination Burrito	175	404	21	43	16	—	1666	0.34	0.31	4.6
Enchirito®	207	454	25	42	21	—	1178	0.31	0.37	4.7
Pintos 'N Cheese	158	168	11	21	5	—	3123	0.26	0.16	0.9
Taco	83	186	15	14	8	—	120	0.09	0.16	2.9
Tostada	138	179	9	25	6	—	3152	0.18	0.15	0.8

Sources: 1) *Menu Item Portions,* San Antonio, Texas; Taco Bell Co., July 1976. 2) Adams CF: Nutritive value of American foods in common units in *Handbook No. 456.* Washington: USDA Agricultural Research Service, November 1975. 3) Church EF, Church HN (eds), *Food Values of Portions Commonly Used,* ed. 12, Philadelphia. JB Lippincott Co., 1975. 4) Valley Baptist Medical Center, Food Service Department: *Descriptions of Mexican-American Foods,* Fort Atkinson, Wisconsin, NASCO.

	Vitamins				Minerals								Mois- ture (g)	Crude Fiber (g)
B_6 (mg)	B_{12} (μg)	C (mg)	D (IU)	Ca (mg)	Cu (mg)	Fe (mg)	K (mg)	Mg (mg)	P (mg)	Na (mg)	Zn (mg)			
—	—	—	—	—	—	—	—	—	—	—	—	—	—	
—	—	—	—	—	—	—	—	—	—	—	—	—	—	
—	—	—	—	—	—	—	—	—	—	—	—	—	—	
—	—	—	—	—	—	—	—	—	—	—	—	—	—	
—	—	—	—	—	—	—	—	—	—	—	—	—	—	
—	—	—	—	—	—	—	—	—	—	—	—	—	—	
—	—	—	—	—	—	—	—	—	—	—	—	—	—	
—	—	—	—	—	—	—	—	—	—	—	—	—	—	
—	—	—	—	—	—	—	—	—	—	—	—	—	—	
—	—	—	—	—	—	—	—	—	—	—	—	—	—	
—	—	—	—	—	—	—	—	—	—	—	—	—	—	
—	—	—	—	—	—	—	—	—	—	—	—	—	—	
—	—	—	—	—	—	—	—	—	—	—	—	—	—	
—	—	—	—	—	—	—	—	—	—	—	—	—	—	
—	—	—	—	—	—	—	—	—	—	—	—	—	—	
0.21	0.75	<1.4	46	226	0.12	2.9	168	26	322	885	1.9	70.7	0.1	
0.04	0.02	0.8	14	117	0.69	1.5	71	13	74	318	0.5	21.7	0.1	
0.12	0.19	4.7	5	103	0.11	2.2	187	28	501	1070	0.7	97.8	0.2	
0.18	0.53	0.5	31	16	0.05	0.8	127	9	95	615	1.5	22.9	0.1	
0.19	0.93	1.2	65	61	0.06	2.5	135	13	264	205	1.7	68.1	<0.1	
0.13	0.01	4.1	<1	5	0.04	0.4	247	13	67	325	0.2	30.9	0.3	
0.27	1.8	2.2	33	157	0.18	4.0	237	38	314	1010	4.7	100.4	0.6	
0.12	0.91	1.6	13	132	0.11	2.4	156	23	205	767	2.6	108.4	0.2	
0.12	0.81	1.7	12	51	0.10	2.3	142	19	126	520	2.1	48.0	0.3	
0.27	1.88	<1.7	23	63	0.17	4.1	322	37	249	735	5.1	83.7	0.7	
0.23	2.15	2.7	25	219	0.18	4.3	341	41	382	1236	5.7	96.0	0.8	
0.10	0.82	<1.4	25	93	0.10	1.7	150	27	229	781	0.9	59.5	0.1	
0.22	<0.03	12.5	<1	9	0.03	0.6	564	27	101	109	0.3	25.4	0.5	
0.02	<0.04	<0.8	2	14	0.05	0.6	39	6	27	398	0.2	38.3	0.3	
0.02	<0.02	<0.8	<2	12	0.06	0.6	35	7	27	427	0.2	38.9	0.1	
0.03	0.03	0.9	10	12	0.07	1.5	52	11	74	358	0.3	2.2	0.1	
0.12	1.19	3.2	26	329	0.09	0.2	422	31	314	201	1.2	211.3	<0.3	
0.13	0.7	2.5	16	215	0.13	0.6	410	35	236	175	1.0	97.9	0.2	
0.05	0.6	3.6	14	200	0.09	0.2	338	30	230	195	0.9	93.2	<0.2	
0.05	0.6	2.8	16	174	0.11	0.4	290	28	80	96	0.8	101.0	0.2	
—	—	15.2	—	98	—	2.8	235	—	173	272	—	—	—	
—	—	15.2	—	83	—	4.6	320	—	288	327	—	—	—	
—	—	12.7	—	208	—	3.4	277	—	265	138	—	—	—	
—	—	10.0	—	40	—	2.6	183	—	140	231	—	—	—	
—	—	16.0	—	121	—	3.8	350	—	245	367	—	—	—	
—	—	15.2	—	91	—	3.7	278	—	230	300	—	—	—	
—	—	9.5	—	259	—	3.8	491	—	338	1175	—	—	—	
—	—	9.3	—	150	—	2.3	307	—	210	102	—	—	—	
—	—	0.2	—	120	—	2.5	143	—	175	79	—	—	—	
—	—	9.7	—	191	—	2.3	172	—	186	101	—	—	—	

Continued.

NUTRITIONAL ANALYSES OF FAST FOODS* — cont'd

	Wt (g)	Energy (kcal)	Protein (g)	Carbo-hydrate (g)	Fat (g)	Choles-terol (mg)	Vitamins A (IU)	B$_1$ (mg)	B$_2$ (mg)	Nia-cin (mg)
WENDY'S®										
Double Hamburger	285	670	44	34	40	125	128	0.43	0.54	10.6
Double w/Cheese	325	800	50	41	48	155	439	0.49	0.75	11.4
Chili	250	230	19	21	8	25	1188	0.22	0.25	3.4
French Fries	120	330	5	41	16	5	40	0.14	0.07	3.0
Frosty	250	390	9	54	16	45	355	0.20	0.60	X

Source: Wendy's International, Inc., Dublin, Ohio. Nutritional analysis by Medallion Laboratories, Minneapolis, Minnesota.

	Wt (g)	Energy (kcal)	Protein (g)	Carbo-hydrate (g)	Fat (g)	Choles-terol (mg)	Vitamins A (IU)	B$_1$ (mg)	B$_2$ (mg)	Nia-cin (mg)
BEVERAGES										
Coffee*	180	2	tr	tr	tr	—	0	0	tr	0.5
Tea*	180	2	tr	—	tr	—	0	0	0.04	0.1
Orange Juice	183	82	1	20	tr	—	366	0.17	0.02	0.6
Chocolate Milk	250	213	9	28	9	—	330	0.08	0.40	0.3
Skim Milk	245	88	9	13	tr	—	10	0.09	0.44	0.2
Whole Milk	244	159	9	12	9	27	342	0.07	0.41	0.2
Coca-Cola®	246	96	0	24	0	—	—	—	—	—
Fanta® Ginger Ale	244	84	0	21	0	—	—	—	—	—
Fanta® Grape	247	114	0	29	0	—	—	—	—	—
Fanta® Orange	248	117	0	30	0	—	—	—	—	—
Fanta® Root Beer	246	103	0	27	0	—	—	—	—	—
Mr. Pibb®	245	95	0	25	0	—	—	—	—	—
Mr. Pibb® w/o Sugar	236	1	0	tr	0	—	—	—	—	—
Sprite®	245	95	0	24	0	—	—	—	—	—
Sprite® w/o Sugar	236	3	0	0	0	—	—	—	—	—
Tab®	236	tr	0	tr	0	—	—	—	—	—
Fresca®	236	2	0	0	0	—	—	—	—	—

Sources: 1) Adams CF: Nutritive value of American foods in common units, In *Handbook No. 456*. Washington: USDA Agricultural Research Service, November 1975; 2) The Coca-Cola Company, Atlanta, Georgia, January 1977; 3) *American Hospital Formulary Service,* Washington, American n Society of Hospital Pharmacists, Section 28:20, March 1978.

*6-oz serving; all other data are for 8-oz serving.

†Caffeine content depends on strength of beverage.

‡Value when bottling water with average sodium content (12 mg/8 oz) is used.

Vitamins				Minerals								Mois-ture (g)	Crude Fiber (g)
B₆ (mg)	B₁₂ (μg)	C (mg)	D (IU)	Ca (mg)	Cu (mg)	Fe (mg)	K (mg)	Mg (mg)	P (mg)	Na (mg)	Zn (mg)		
—	—	1.5	—	138	—	8.2	—	—	364	980	8.4	162.1	1.1
—	—	2.3	—	177	—	10.2	—	—	489	1414	10.1	179.2	1.3
—	—	2.9	—	83	—	4.4	—	—	168	1065	3.7	195.9	2.3
—	—	6.4	—	16	—	1.2	—	—	196	112	0.5	54.9	1.2
0	X	0.7	—	270	—	0.9	—	—	278	247	1.0	1.0	0.0

Vitamins				Minerals								Caf-feine (mg)	Sac-char. (mg)
B₆ (mg)	B₁₂ (μg)	C (mg)	D (IU)	Ca (mg)	Cu (mg)	Fe (mg)	K (mg)	Mg (mg)	P (mg)	Na (mg)	Zn (mg)		
—	—	0	—	4	—	0.2	65	—	7	2	—	100†	0
—	—	1	—	5	—	0.2	—	—	4	—	—	40†	0
—	—	82.4	—	17	—	0.2	340	18	29	2	—	0	0
—	—	3.0	—	278	—	0.5	365	—	235	118	—	—	0
—	—	2.0	—	296	—	0.1	355	—	233	127	—	—	0
—	—	2.4	100	188	—	tr	351	32	227	122	—	—	0
—	—	—	—	—	—	—	—	—	40	20‡	—	28	0
—	—	—	—	—	—	—	—	—	0	30‡	—	0	0
—	—	—	—	—	—	—	—	—	0	21‡	—	0	0
—	—	—	—	—	—	—	—	—	0	21‡	—	0	0
—	—	—	—	—	—	—	—	—	0	23‡	—	0	0
—	—	—	—	—	—	—	—	—	29	23‡	—	27	0
—	—	—	—	—	—	—	—	—	28	37‡	—	38	76
—	—	—	—	—	—	—	—	—	0	42‡	—	0	0
—	—	—	—	—	—	—	—	—	0	42‡	—	0	57
—	—	—	—	—	—	—	—	—	30	30‡	—	30	74
—	—	—	—	—	—	—	—	—	0	38	—	0	54

CALORIC VALUE OF SELECTED SNACK FOODS

Food	Approximate measure	Calories
Beverages		
Carbonated, cola type	1 bottle, 6 oz	70
Malted milk	1 regular (1½ c)	420
Chocolate milk (made with skim milk)	1 c	190
Cocoa	1 c	235
Soda, vanilla ice cream	1 regular	260
Cake		
Angel food	2-inch sector	110
Cupcake, chocolate, iced	1 cake, 2¾″ diameter	185
Fruit cake	1 piece, 2″ by 2″ by ½″	115
Candy and popcorn		
Butterscotch	3 pieces	60
Candy bar, plain	1 bar	295
Caramels	3 medium	120
Chocolate coated creams	2 average	130
Fudge	1 piece	115
Peanut brittle	1 oz	125
Popcorn with oil added	1 c	65
Cheese		
Camembert	1 oz	85
Cheddar	1 oz	105
Cream	1 oz	105
Swiss (domestic)	1 oz	105
Cookies		
Brownies	1 piece, 2″ by 2″ by ¾″	140
Cookies, plain and assorted	1 cookie, 3″ diameter	120
Crackers		
Cheese	5 crackers	85
Graham	2 medium	55
Saltines	4 crackers	70
Rye	2 crackers	45
Dessert type cream puff and doughnuts		
Cream puff—custard filling	1 average	245
Doughnut, cake type, plain	1 average	125
Doughnut, jelly	1 average	225
Doughnut, raised	1 average	120
Miscellaneous		
Hamburger and bun	1 average	330
Ice cream, vanilla	3½ oz container	130
Sherbet	½ c	120
Jams, jellies, marmalades, preserves	1 Tbsp	55
Syrup, blended	¼ c	240
Waffles	1 waffle, 4½″ by 5½″ by ½″	210
Nuts		
Mixed, shelled	8–12	95
Peanut butter	1 Tbsp	95
Peanuts, shelled, roasted	1 c	840

From Williams SR: Nutrition and diet therapy, ed 4, Appendix E, St. Louis, 1981, The CV Mosby Co, pp 781–782.

CALORIC VALUE OF SELECTED SNACK FOODS—cont'd

Food	Approximate measure	Calories
Pie		
Apple	4″ sector	345
Cherry	4″ sector	355
Custard	4″ sector	280
Lemon meringue	4″ sector	305
Mince	4″ sector	365
Pumpkin	4″ sector	275
Potato chips	10 chips, 2″ diameter	115
Sandwiches		
Bacon, lettuce, tomato	1 sandwich	280
Egg salad	1 sandwich	280
Ham	1 sandwich	280
Liverwurst	1 sandwich	250
Peanut butter	1 sandwich	330
Soups, commercial canned		
Bean with pork	1 c	170
Beef noodle	1 c	70
Chicken noodle	1 c	65
Cream (mushroom)	1 c	135
Tomato	1 c	90
Vegetable with beef broth	1 c	80

CAFFEINE CONTENT OF BEVERAGES

Beverage	Caffeine (mg/100 ml)	Beverage	Caffeine (mg/100 ml)
Carbonated		Coffee: decaffeinated	
Coca Cola*	17.97	Infused‡	1.00–3.00
Dr. Pepper*	16.92	Instant‡	0.50–1.50
Mountain Dew*	15.19	Decaf†	0.90
Diet Dr. Pepper*	15.06	Nescafe†	3.30–5.60
Tab*	13.72	Sanka†	1.80
Pepsi-Cola*	11.98	Tea, bagged	
RC Cola*	9.36	Black, 5 min brew*	33.00
Diet RC*	9.17	Black, 1 min brew*	20.00
Diet Rite*	8.81	Tea, loose	
Fanta Root Beer†	0	Black, 5 min brew*	29.00
Coffee		Green, 5 min brew*	25.00
Instant*	44.00	Green, Japan, 5 min brew*	15.00
Percolated*	73.00	Cocoa; chocolate*	6.00
Dripolated*	97.00	Ovaltine‡	0.00

From American Dietetic Association: Handbook of clinical dietetics, New Haven Conn, 1981, Yale University Press, p 149.
*Bunker ML, McWilliams M: Caffeine content of common beverages, J Am Diet Assoc 74:28, 1979.
†Nutritional analysis data supplied by the manufacturer.
‡Nagy M: Caffeine content of beverages and chocolate, JAMA 229:337, 1974.

CALCIUM, PROTEIN, AND CALORIC CONTENT OF SELECTED FOODS

Food	Quantity	Calcium (mg)	Protein (g)	kcal
Bran muffin	1	57	3.1	104
Brazil nuts	1 c	109	8.4	382
Bread, white (enriched)	1 slice	26	2.4	74
Bread pudding (with raisin)	½ c	145	7.4	248
Candy caramel	1 oz	42	1.1	113
Candy peanut bar	1 oz	12	5.0	146
Cashew nuts	14 large	11	4.9	159
Cheddar cheese	1 oz	213	7.1	113
Chocolate disk candy	1 oz	38	1.5	132
Coconut custard pie	⅛ pie	107	6.8	268
Cupcake (plain)	1	53	1.6	116
Flour, wheat (enriched self rising)	1 c	331	11.6	440
Ice cream	1 c	194	6.0	257
Kale, frozen	1 c	206	5.0	43
Maple syrup	2 Tbsp	40	0.0	100
Milk	1 c	288	8.5	159
Mustard greens (cooked, boiled)	1 c	193	3.1	32
Okra	1 c	147	3.2	46
Orange, navel	1	69	2.2	87
Orange juice (dilute)	1 c	19	1.5	84
Pancake (6″ diameter)	2	148	10.4	338
Pizza pie	⅛ pizza	144	7.8	153
Potatoes, scalloped au gratin	½ c	156	6.5	178
Pudding, chocolate	1 c	265	8.8	322
Pudding, vanilla	1 c	298	8.9	283
Salmon, sockeye (red)	3.9 oz	285	22.0	188
Sauerkraut	1 c	85	2.4	42
Scallops, steamed	7-10	115	23.0	112
Soup, minestrone Canned (equal volume of water)	1 c	37	4.9	105
Soup, pea Canned (equal volume of water)	1 c	44	5.6	130
Soybean (cooked)	1 c	131	19.8	234
Spinach (cooked)	1 c	232	6.2	47
Squash, butternut (cooked)	1 c	82	3.7	139
Strawberries (frozen)	1 c	36	1.3	278
Sweet potato (with skin)	1	52	2.8	185
Tapioca cream pudding	1 c	173	8.3	221
Turnip greens	1 c	267	3.2	29
Turnips (mashed)	1 c	81	1.8	53
Waffle (home recipe with enriched flour)	½ waffle	113	9.3	279
Watermelon	1 piece	30	2.1	111
Yogurt	1 c	272	7.4	152

COMPARISON OF HUMAN MILK AND INFANT FORMULAS

	Human Milk	SMA®*	Similac® w/Fe*	Enfamil® w/Fe*
Protein (w/v)	1.2%	1.5%	1.5%	1.5%
Casein	40%	40%	82%	82%
Whey protein	60%	60%	18%	18%
Fat (w/v)	3.6%	3.6%	3.6%	3.7%
% Polyunsaturated	11	14	25	50
% Monounsaturated	40	41	15	21
% Saturated	49	45	60	29
Total %	100	100	100	100
Vitamin E (IU/qt)	5	9	14.2	12
E: Linoleate (IU/g linoleate)	1.8	2.1	1.8	0.8
Minerals (mg/100 ml)				
Total (ash)	210	250	360	380
Na	16	15	25	25
K	55	56	78	65
Ca	34	44	51	52
P	14	33	39	52
Cl	37	37	53	46
Iron (per qt)	0.8 mg	12 mg†	12 mg†	12 mg†
Carbohydrate (w/v)	7.2%	7.2%	7.2%	7.0%
	(lactose)	(lactose)	(lactose)	(lactose)

Wyeth Laboratories, 1982. For additional information, see Chapter 29.

Note: All data for competitive products are derived from product labels, PDR®, or analyses.

*Concentrate.

†SMA® lo-iron, Enfamil® and Similac® contain 1.4 mg of iron per quart. Infants fed these formulas should receive supplemental dietary iron from an outside source to meet daily requirements.

PREMATURE FORMULAS COMPARISON CHART

	Minimum Recommendations (per 100 ml)	"preemie" SMA® (per 100 ml)	Similac® Special Care (per 100 ml)	Enfamil® Premature (per 100 ml)
Protein (g)	1.5	2.0	2.2	2.4
Whey protein:casein ratio	60:40	60:40	60:40	60:40
Fat (g)	2.7	4.4	4.4	4.1
MCT (medium-chain triglycerides)		12.5%	50%	40%
Oleo oil		20%	0%	0%
Corn oil		0%	30%	40%
Oleic oil		25%	0%	0%
Coconut oil		27%	20%	20%
Soy oil		18%	0%	0%
Carbohydrate (g)		8.6	8.6	8.9
Lactose		50%	50%	40%
Glucose polymers		50%	50%	60%
Minerals (ash) (total mg)		400	650	500
Calcium (mg)	41	75	144	94
Phosphorus (mg)	20	40	72	47
Sodium (mg)	16	32	35	31
Potassium (mg)	65	75	100	88
Chloride (mg)	45	53	65	68
Magnesium (mg)	5	7	10	8
Zinc (mg)	0.4	0.5	1.2	0.5
Iron (mg)	0.1	0.3	0.3	0.1
Copper (μg)	49	70	200	73
Manganese (μg)	4	20	20	21
Iodine (μg)	4	8.3	15	6
Vitamins	(per liter)	(per liter)	(per liter)	(per liter)
A (IU)	2030	3200	5500	2496
D (IU)	325	510	1200	499
E (IU)	2.4	15	30	16
K_1 (μg)	32	70	100	75
C (ascorbic acid) (mg)	65	70	300	68
B_1 (thiamine) (μg)	325	800	2000	624
B_2 (riboflavin) (μg)	487	1300	5000	728
B_6 (μg)	284	500	2000	500
B_{12} (μg)	1.22	2.0	4.5	2.5
Niacin (mg)	2.0	6.3	24.0	9.6
Folic acid (μg)	32	100	300	240
Pantothenic acid (μg)	2436	3600	15000	3744
Biotin (μg)	12.2	18	300	19
Choline (mg)	57	165	80	57
Inositol (mg)	32.4	40	45	38
Calories per liter		810	810	810
Calories per fl oz		24	24	24
Osmolality (mOsm/kg H_2O)	400 (maximum)	268	300	300
Potential renal solute load (PRSL) (mOsm/liter)		175.2	208.0	220.0
Ca:P ratio	1.1:1	1.9:1	2:1	2:1
$\dfrac{Na + K \text{ ratio}}{Cl}$	1.5	2.2	2.2	1.9

Wyeth Laboratories, 1982.

COMPARISON OF COW MILK PRODUCTS

	Whole Cow Milk	2% Fat Milk	Skim Milk
Protein (w/v)	3.3%	3.3%	3.4%
Casein	82%	82%	82%
Whey protein	18%	18%	18%
Fat (w/v)	3.7%	1.9%	0.18%
% Polyunsaturated	4	4	4
% Monounsaturated	30	30	30
% Saturated	66	66	66
Total %	100	100	100
Vitamin E (IU/qt)	1.3	0.67	0.06
E: Linoleate (IU/g linoleate)	1.8	1.8	1.8
Minerals (mg/100 ml)			
Total (ash)	720	763	787
Na	52	52	54
K	148	159	172
Ca	122	126	127
P	96	98	104
Cl	96	98t	112
Iron (per qt.)	0.05 mg	0.05 mg	0.04 mg
Carbohydrate (w/v)	4.8% (lactose)	5.0% (lactose)	5.0% (lactose)

Wyeth Laboratories, 1982.

COMPARISON OF SOY PROTEIN FORMULAS

	Nursoy®	Isomil®	Prosobee®	I-Soyalac®
Protein (w/v)	2.1%	2.0%	2.1%	2.1%
Casein	—	—	—	—
Whey protein	—	—	—	—
Fat (w/v)	3.6%	3.6%	3.6%	3.7%
% Polyunsaturated	14	26	50	62
% Monounsaturated	41	14	21	26
% Saturated	45	60	29	12
Total (%)	100	100	100	100
Vitamin E (IU/qt)	9	15	10	15
E: Linoleate (IU/g linoleate)	2.1	1.1	0.70	0.82
Minerals				
Total (ash)	350	380	400	400
Na	20	30	29	37
K	74	71	81	80
Ca	64	70	62	63
P	44	50	50	42
Cl	37	53	55	53
Iron (per qt)	12 mg	12 mg	12 mg	12 mg
Carbohydrate (w/v)	6.9%	6.8%	6.9%	6.6%
	(sucrose)	(corn syrup solids, sucrose)	(corn syrup solids)	(sucrose, tapioca, dextrins)

Wyeth Laboratories, 1982.

SELECTED ENTERAL FEEDINGS

	Polymeric (Meal Replacements)						
	Compleat B	Isocal	Osmolite	Portagen	Ensure	Sustacal	Precision LR
Calorie/cc	1	1	1	1	1	1	1
Carbohydrate source	Hydrolyzed cereal solid, green beans, peas, peach puree, non-fat dry milk, maltodextrin, orange juice	Glucose oligosaccharides	Corn syrup solids	Maltodextrin	Corn syrup solids, sucrose	Corn syrup solids, sucrose	Maltodextrin, sucrose
Protein source	Beef puree, non-fat dry milk	Sodium and calcium caseinate, soy protein isolates	Sodium and calcium caseinate, soy protein isolates	Sodium caseinate	Sodium and calcium caseinate, soy protein isolates	Sodium and calcium caseinate, soy protein isolates	Egg albumin
Fat source	Beef puree, corn oil	Soy oil, MCT	MCT, corn oil, soy oil	Corn oil, MCT	Corn oil	Soy oil	Soy oil, MCT
Carbohydrate (g/liter)	128 (48%)	130 (50%)	146 (55%)	115 (45%)	145 (55%)	138 (55%)	248 (89%)
Protein (g/liter)	43 (16%)	34 (13%)	37 (14%)	35 (14%)	37 (14%)	60 (24%)	26 (10%)
Fat (g/liter)	43 (36%)	44 (37%)	39 (34%)	48 (41%)	37 (32%)	23 (21%)	1.6 (1%)
Na/K (mEq/liter)	55/36	23/34	24/27	20/31	32/33	40/53	31/22
(mOsm/kg)	450	300	300	357	450	625	560
*Vitamin content	1600	2000	1900	1000	1900	1100	1700
Cost per 1000 kcal	3.73	2.83	2.37	3.29	1.79	3.00	4.17
Features	Tube feeding only, requires digestion and absorption, not lactose free, moderate sodium	Tube feeding, requires digestion and absorption, lactose free, low sodium, 20% MCT	Tube feeding, requires digestion and absorption, lactose free, low sodium, moderate potassium, 50% MCT	Tube feeding, requires digestion and absorption, high in MCT (86%), lactose free, low sodium	Tube feeding, oral supplement, requires digestion and absorption, lactose free	Tube feeding, oral supplement, requires digestion and absorption, lactose free, high protein	Tube feeding, oral supplement, lactose free, absorbed in upper gut, low fat, low potassium

SELECTED ENTERAL FEEDINGS—cont'd

| | Polymeric (high density) | | | | Monomeric (elemental) | |
	Ensure Plus	Magnacal	Pregestimil	Vital HN	Vivonex	Vivonex HN
Calorie/cc	1.5	2	1	1	1	1
Carbohydrate source	Corn syrup solids, sucrose	Maltodextrin, glucose, corn syrup solids	Glucose polymers, modified tapioca starch	Glucose oligosaccharides, sucrose	Glucose oligosaccharides	Glucose oligosaccharides
Protein source	Sodium and calcium caseinate, soy protein isolates	Sodium and calcium caseinate	Casein hydrolysate, amino acids	Whey, soy, and meat protein hydrolysate, free amino acid	Crystalline amino acids	Crystalline amino acids
Fat source	Corn oil	Soy oil	Corn oil, MCT	Safflower oil, MCT	Safflower oil	Safflower oil
Carbohydrate (g/liter)	200 (53%)	250 (53%)	137 (54%)	188 (74%)	230 (91%)	211 (81%)
Protein (g/liter)	55 (15%)	70 (14%)	29 (11%)	42 (17%)	21 (8%)	42 (18%)
Fat (g/liter)	53 (32%)	80 (36%)	41 (35%)	11 (9%)	1.5 (1%)	1 (1%)
Na/K (mEq/liter)	46/48	44/32	20/28	17/30	20/30	23/30
(mOsm/kg)	600	520	522	460	550	810
*Vitamin content	200	1000		1500	1800	3000
Cost per 1000 kcal	1.36	2.20	4.30	6.17	5.19	9.96
Features	Tube feeding, oral supplement, lactose free, requires digestion and absorption	Tube feeding, oral supplement, lactose free, requires digestion and absorption	Tube feeding, lactose free, 40% MCT	Tube feeding, oral supplement, lactose free, absorbed in upper gut, minimal residue, low sodium, 45% MCT	Tube feeding, oral supplement, lactose free, absorbed in upper gut, minimal residue, low fat, cal:N suitable for maintenance	Tube feeding, oral supplement, lactose free, absorbed in upper gut, minimal residue, low fat, cal:N suitable for anabolism, minimal pancreatic stimulation

This table is an abbreviated set of information on selected commercially used formula feedings available for use by the staff of the Johns Hopkins Hospital. A complete discussion of the formulas, along with a more comprehensive analysis, is found in Chapter 29.

From Department of Nutrition, The Johns Hopkins Hospital. Copyright JHH Nutrition August 1982.

*Volume required at standard dilution to meet 100% of the RDAs.

FOOD ADDITIVES

Additive	Function	Maintain/Improve Nutritional Quality	Maintain Product Quality	Aid in Processing or Preparation	Affect Appeal Characteristics
Acetic acid	pH control			X	
Acetone peroxide	Maturing and bleaching agents, dough conditioners			X	
Adipic acid	pH control			X	
Ammonium alginate	Stabilizers, thickeners, texturizers			X	
Annatto extract	Color				X
Arabinogalactan	Stabilizers, thickeners, texturizers			X	
Ascorbic acid	Nutrient, preservative, antioxidant	X	X		
Azodicarbonamide	Maturing and bleaching agents, dough conditioners				
Benzoic acid	Preservative		X		
Benzoyl peroxide	Maturing and bleaching agents, dough conditioners			X	
Beta-apo-8' carotenal	Color				X
Beta-carotene	Nutrient	X			
BHA (butylated hydroxyanisole)	Antioxidant		X		
BHT (butylated hydroxytoluene)	Antioxidant		X		
Butylparaben	Preservative		X		
Calcium alginate	Stabilizers, thickeners, texturizers			X	
Calcium bromate	Maturing and bleaching agents, dough conditioners			X	
Calcium lactate	Preservative		X		
Calcium phosphate	Leavening			X	
Calcium propionate	Preservative		X		
Calcium silicate	Anti-caking			X	
Calcium sorbate	Preservative		X		
Canthaxanthin	Color				X
Caramel	Color				X
Carob bean gum	Stabilizers, thickeners, texturizers			X	
Carrageenan	Emulsifier			X	
Carrot oil	Color				X
Cellulose	Stabilizers, thickeners, texturizers			X	

Substance	Function
Citric acid	Preservative, antioxidant, pH control
Citrus Red No. 2	Color
Cochineal extract	Color
Corn endosperm	Color
Corn syrup	Sweetener
Dehydrated beets	Color
Dextrose	Sweetener
Diglycerides	Emulsifier
Dioctyl sodium sulfosuccinate	Emulsifier
Disodium guanylate	Flavor enhancer
Disodium inosinate	Flavor enhancer
Dried algae meal	Color
EDTA (ethylenediaminetetraacetic acid)	Antioxidant
FD & C Colors	
Blue No. 1	Color
Red No. 3	Color
Red No. 40	Color
Yellow No. 5	Color
Fructose	Sweetener
Gelatin	Stabilizers, thickeners, texturizers
Glucose	Sweetener
Glycerine	Humectant
Glycerol monostearate	Humectant
Grape skin extract	Color
Guar gum	Stabilizers, thickeners, texturizers
Gum arabic	Stabilizers, thickeners, texturizers
Gum ghatti	Stabilizers, thickeners, texturizers
Heptylparaben	Preservative
Hydrogen peroxide	Maturing and bleaching agents, dough conditioners
Hydrolyzed vegetable protein	Flavor enhancer
Invert sugar	Sweetener
Iodine	Nutrient
Iron	Nutrient

From Food and Drug Administration, HEW Publication No. (FDA)79-2115, U.S. Department of Health, Education and Welfare, Public Health Service, U.S. Government Printing Office, Washington, D.C., 1979.

Continued.

FOOD ADDITIVES—cont'd

Additive	Function	Maintain/Improve Nutritional Quality	Maintain Product Quality	Aid in Processing or Preparation	Affect Appeal Characteristics
				Technical Use in Food Preparation	
Iron-ammonium citrate	Anti-caking			X	
Iron oxide	Color			X	X
Karaya gum	Stabilizers, thickeners, texturizers			X	
Lactic acid	pH control, preservative		X	X	
Larch gum	Stabilizers, thickeners, texturizers			X	
Lecithin	Emulsifier			X	
Locust bean gum	Stabilizers, thickeners, texturizers			X	
Mannitol	Sweetener, anti-caking, stabilizers, thickeners, texturizers			X	X
Methylparaben	Preservative		X		
Modified food starch	Stabilizers, thickeners, texturizers			X	
Monoglycerides	Emulsifier			X	
MSG (monosodium glutamate)	Flavor enhancer				X
Niacinamide	Nutrient	X			
Paprika (and oleoresin)	Flavor, color				X
Pectin	Stabilizers, thickeners, texturizers			X	
Phosphates	pH control			X	
Phosphoric acid	pH control			X	
Polysorbates	Emulsifiers			X	
Potassium alginate	Stabilizers, thickeners, texturizers			X	
Potassium bromate	Maturing and bleaching agents, dough conditioners			X	
Potassium iodide	Nutrient	X			
Potassium propionate	Preservative		X		
Potassium sorbate	Preservative		X		
Propionic acid	Preservative		X		
Propyl gallate	Antioxidant		X		
Propylene glycol	Stabilizers, thickeners, texturizers, humectant			X	
Propylparaben	Preservative		X		
Riboflavin	Nutrient	X			
Saccharin	Sweetener				X

Substance	Function				
Saffron	Color			X	
Silicon dioxide	Anti-caking			X	X
Sodium acetate	pH control			X	X
Sodium alginate	Stabilizers, thickeners, texturizers			X	X
Sodium aluminum sulfate	Leavening		X	X	
Sodium benzoate	Preservative		X		
Sodium bicarbonate	Leavening			X	X
Sodium calcium alginate	Stabilizers, thickeners, texturizers			X	X
Sodium citrate	pH control		X	X	
Sodium diacetate	Preservative		X		
Sodium erythorbate	Preservative		X		
Sodium nitrate	Preservative		X		
Sodium nitrite	Preservative		X		
Sodium propionate	Preservative		X		
Sodium sorbate	Preservative		X		
Sodium stearyl fumarate	Maturing and bleaching agents, dough conditioners			X	
Sorbic acid	Preservative		X		
Sorbitan monostearate	Emulsifier			X	X
Sorbitol	Humectant, sweetener			X	X
Spices	Flavor				X
Sucrose (table sugar)	Sweetener				X
Tagetes (Aztec Marigold)	Color				X
Tartaric acid	pH control				X
TBHQ (tertiary butyl hydroquinone)	Antioxidant		X	X	
Thiamine	Nutrient	X			
Titanium dioxide	Color			X	X
Toasted, partially defatted cooked cottonseed flour	Nutrient, antioxidant	X			X
Tocopherols (vit. E)	Nutrient, antioxidant		X	X	X
Tragacanth gum	Stabilizers, thickeners, texturizers			X	
Turmeric (oleoresin)	Flavor, color			X	X
Ultramarine blue	Color				X
Vanilla, vanillin	Flavor	X			X
Vitamin A	Nutrient	X			
Vitamin C (ascorbic acid)	Antioxidant, nutrient, preservative		X	X	
Vitamin D (D$_2$, D$_3$)	Nutrient	X		X	
Vitamin E (tocopherols)	Nutrient	X		X	
Yeast-malt sprout extract	Flavor enhancer				
Yellow prussiate of soda	Anti-caking		X		X

EFFECTS OF FOOD ON ABSORPTION OF ANTIBIOTICS

Antibiotic			
Generic Name	Brand Name	Effect of Food on Percent Absorption	Comments
Amoxicillin	Larocin Amoxil	None	
Ampicillin	Various	Decrease	Peak levels in one study decreased by about 40% (from 5 to 3 μg/ml) when given with food.
Cephalexin	Keflex	82%—fasting 73%—with food	Other authors reported 95% absorption when given with food or fasting.
Cephradine	Anspor Velosef	None	Absorption slightly more rapid when patient was fasting. However, the peak serum concentration and total amount of drug absorbed was not affected by food.
Clindamycin	Cleocin	None	Peak serum levels may be delayed if given with food, but total amount absorbed unchanged.
Demethy-chlortetra-cycline	Declomycin	Non-dairy food produced about a 50% decrease in absorption	Milk decreased absorption by about 70%.
Doxycyline	Vibramycin Doxy-11	None; non-dairy food did not affect absorption	Milk or other products containing calcium, zinc, iron or other divalent or trivalent cations may decrease absorption.
Erythromycin estolate	Illosone	None	Absorption with food comparable to that achieved while fasting.
Erythromycin base (enteric coated)	E-Mycin Erythrocin	Decrease	Peak serum concentrations when 500 mg given 2 hr before a meal about 2.3 μg, 1 hr before a meal about 1.00 μg/ml, immediately after a meal 1.7 μg/ml, 1 hr after a meal 1.71 μg/ml.
Erythromycin propionate		Decrease	Marked decrease in absorption when given with food.
Erythromycin stearate	Bristamycin Ethril SK-Erythromycin	Decrease	Marked decrease in absorption when given with food.
Hetacillin	Versapen	Decrease	Peak blood level decreased by 50% when taken with food.
Lincomycin	Lincocin	Decrease	Give the drug at least 2 hr before or after meals.
Minocycline	Minocin	None	Claim by Lederle (Minocin) and Parke-Davis (Vectrin) "food did not effect the absorption." No published clinical data available.
Oxytetracycline	Terramycin	None	No difference in serum levels 3 hr after an oral dose with or without food.
Penicillin G	Various	Decrease	Only about 35% absorption under optimal conditions. Gastric pH of 2.0 rapidly destroys drug. If used it should be given no later than ½ hr before a meal and no earlier than 2–3 hr after a meal.
Rifampin	Rifadin Ramactane	Decrease	Absorption was delayed by food and total amount and peak serum concentrations were decreased. However, the authors felt that food did not significantly decrease the time for which the serum rifampin levels remained above the MIC and therefore, it is not necessary to insist that rifampin be taken in the fasting state.
Triacetyl-oleando-mycin	TAO Cyclamycin	None	Delay in peak serum concentration when given with food. However, total amount absorbed appeared comparable to fasting state.

From Schweigert BS: Drug and Therapeutic Informatin Bulletin. Long Beach, California: Memorial Medical Center, 1974.

IRON ABSORPTION

Recent methods of calculating iron absorbed from food, while not yet fully field tested, may provide a more precise measure than the usual clinical estimates of 10% absorption of dietary iron. The improved methods reported by Monsen et al. (Am J Clin Nutr **31**:134-141, 1978) recognized the existence of two categories of iron in foods, heme and nonheme compounds, and of dietary factors, particularly ascorbic acid, influencing their absorption. An average of 40% of heme iron is found in all animal tissue, which includes not only meat and liver, but fish and poultry as well. The remaining 60% of iron in the above tissue and all of the iron of vegetable products are classified as nonheme iron. The absorption of nonheme iron is enhanced by the ascorbic acid level and the quantity of animal tissue present in each meal. The levels present serve to classify meals according to the low, medium, or high availability of their nonheme iron.

AVAILABILITY OF IRON IN DIFFERENT MEALS

Meal	Absorption of Iron Present in Meal (%)	
	Nonheme Iron	Heme Iron
Low-Availability Meal <30 g meat, poultry, fish <25 mg ascorbic acid	3	23
Medium-Availability Meal 30–90 g meat, poultry, fish or 25–75 mg ascorbic acid	5	23
High-Availability Meal >90 g meat, poultry, fish or >75 mg ascorbic acid; or 30–90 g meat, poultry, fish plus 25–75 mg ascorbic acid	8	23

National Academy of Sciences, Food and Nutrition Board, 1980. Adapted from Monsen et al., 1978.

EXAMPLES OF METHOD TO CALCULATE ABSORBABLE IRON FROM SINGLE MEALS

Meal	Weight (g)	Total Iron (mg)	Heme Factor	Heme Iron (mg)	Nonheme Iron (mg)	Ascorbic Acid (as served) (mg)
Meat, poultry, fish (26 g protein, 650 kcal)						
Beef-vegetable stew						
Beef, lean, raw, 3 oz	85	2.7	0.4	1.1	1.6	0
Potatoes, ½ c.	78	0.4			0.4	13
Carrots, 2 Tbsp.	20	0.1			0.1	1
Onions, 2 Tbsp.	15	0.1			0.1	2
Green pepper, raw, 2 slices	20	0.2			0.2	26
Bread sticks, 2 medium	35	0.3			0.3	Trace
Margarine, 2 tsp.	10	0			0	0
Peaches, canned, ½ c.	128	0.4			0.4	4
Gingerbread	63	1.0			1.0	Trace
Total		5.2		1.1	4.1	46
Evaluation: 30–90 g meat,		% absorbable iron		23%	8%	
25–75 mg ascorbic acid:		absorbable iron (mg)		0.25	0.33	
High availability.		total absorbable iron (mg)		0.58 mg		
Nonmeat, nonpoultry, nonfish (22 g protein, 730 kcal)						
Beans, navy, cooked, ½ c	95	2.6			2.6	0
Rice, brown, cooked, ½ c.	98	0.5			0.5	1
Cornbread, 1 piece	78	0.9			0.9	1
Margarine, 1 Tbsp.	14	0			0	0
Apple slices, ½ c.	55	1.1			1.1	1
Walnuts, black, raw, 1 Tbsp.	8	0.5			0.5	0
Almonds, raw, 1 Tbsp.	8	0.4			0.4	Trace
Yogurt, skim milk, 1 c	226	0.1			0.1	2
Total		5.1			5.1	4
Evaluation: No meat, poultry, fish less than 25 mg ascorbic acid:					3%	
		% absorbable iron				
		total absorbable iron (mg)		0	0.15	
Low availability.		total absorbable iron (mg)		0.15 mg		

From National Academy of Sciences, Food and Nutrition Board, 1980. Adapted from Monsen et al., 1978.

Growth Standards

Origin of Current Standards
Girls
    Length: Birth–36 months
    Weight: Birth–36 months
    Head circumference: Birth–36 months
    Stature: 2–18 years
    Weight: 2–18 years
    Weight by stature: Prepubescent
Boys
    Length: Birth–36 months
    Weight: Birth–36 months
    Head circumference: Birth–36 months
    Stature: 2–18 years
    Weight: 2–18 years
    Weight by stature: Prepubescent

ORIGIN OF CURRENT STANDARDS
National Center for Health Statistics (NCHS) Growth Curves for Children, Birth–18 years

In 1974, the National Academy of Sciences suggested that new growth charts be developed to replace the widely used but increasingly outdated Stuart-Meredith charts of the 1940s. The Academy suggested that the growth data collected in more recent studies, such as the Health and Examination Survey of the NCHS, and augmented by data from the Fels Research Institute and from an Ohio State University team, headed at that time by Dr. George Owen, be used. The objective was to construct growth curves that would more accurately reflect a current cross-section of the racial, ethnic, and socioeconomic composition of the United States. A task force of experts was formed that included R. Reed (Harvard University), A. Roche (Fels Research Institute), G. Owen (University of New Mexico), M. Lane, M. Nichaman, and J. Goldsby (CDC), and T. Drizd, J-P Habicht, C. Johnson, A. McDowell, and P. Hamill (representing NCHS), to achieve this objective. The resulting growth charts have been carefully developed, well received, and widely disseminated. They are reproduced in this appendix for clinical use.

GIRLS
Length: Birth–36 months

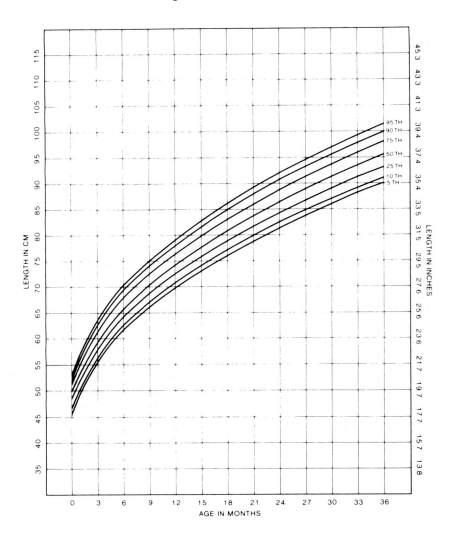

From National Center for Health Statistics, 1974.

GIRLS
Weight: Birth−36 months

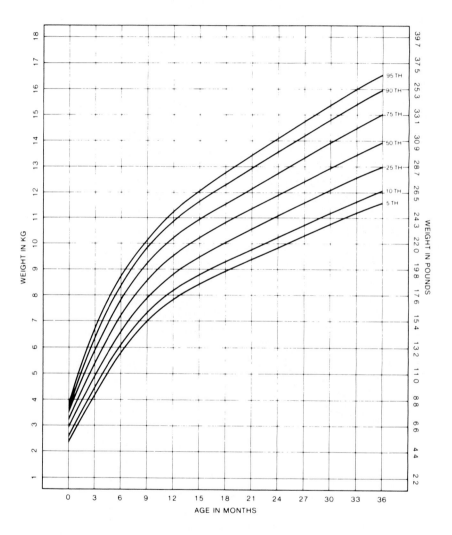

From National Center for Health Statistics, 1974.

GIRLS
Head circumference: Birth–36 months

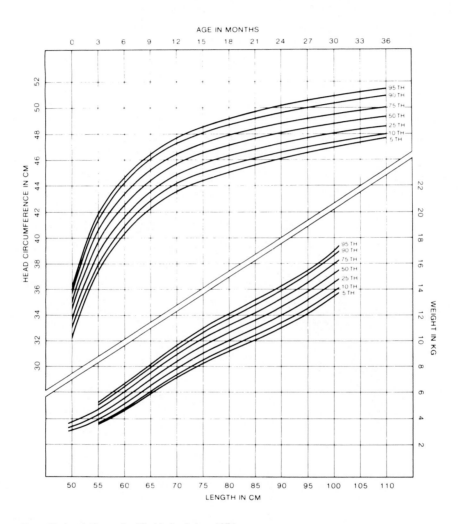

From National Center for Health Statistics, 1974.

GIRLS
Stature: 2–18 years

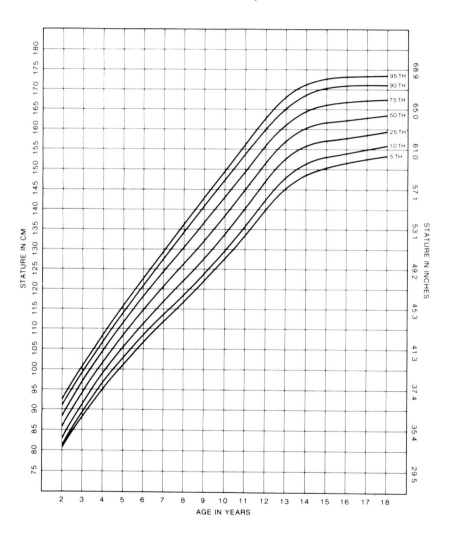

From National Center for Health Statistics, 1974.

GIRLS
Weight: 2–18 years

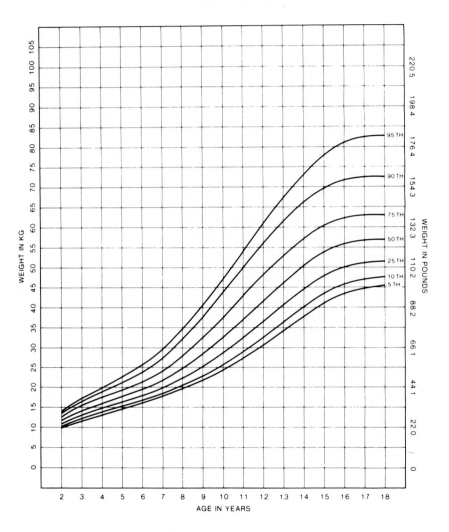

From National Center for Health Statistics, 1974.

GIRLS
Weight by stature: Prepubescent

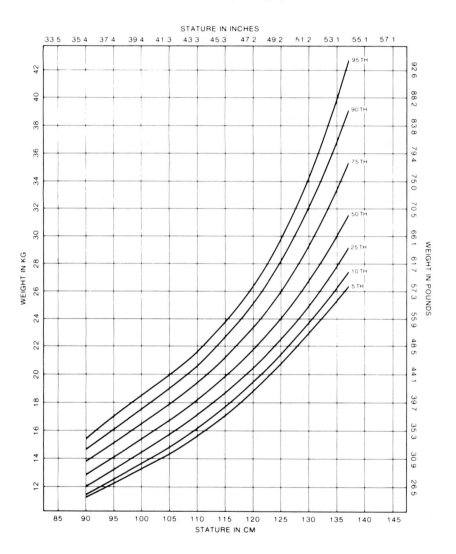

From National Center for Health Statistics, 1974.

BOYS
Length: Birth–36 months

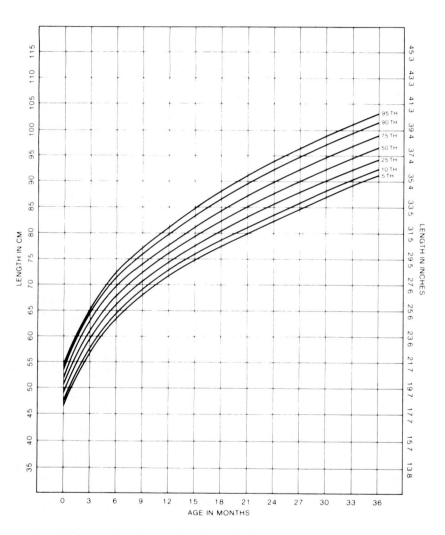

From National Center for Health Statistics, 1974.

BOYS
Weight: Birth—36 months

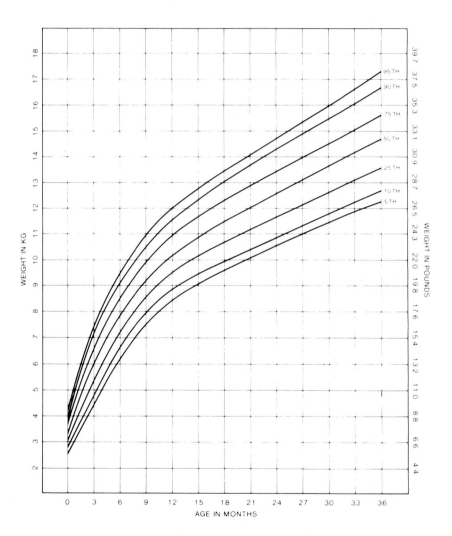

From National Center for Health Statistics, 1974.

BOYS
Head circumference: Birth–36 months

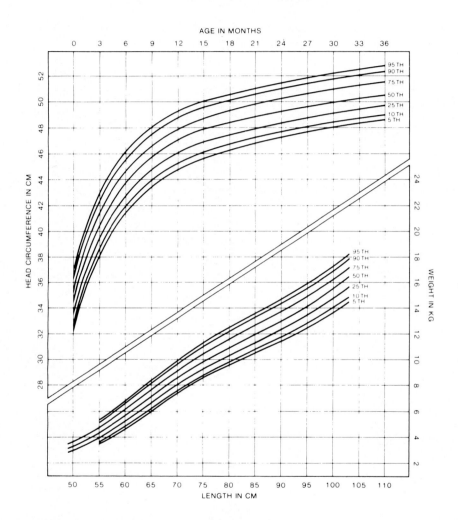

From National Center for Health Statistics, 1974.

BOYS
Stature: 2–18 years

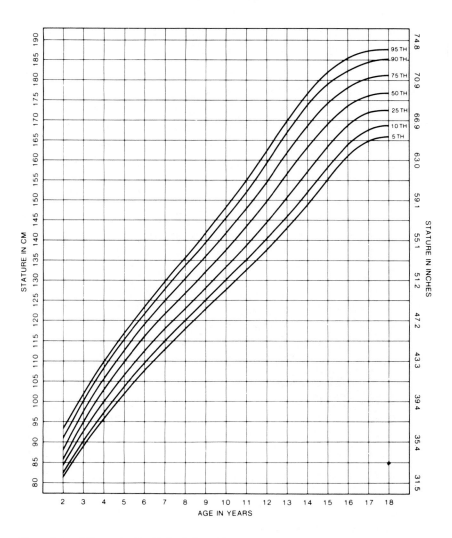

From National Center for Health Statistics, 1974.

BOYS
Weight: 2–18 years

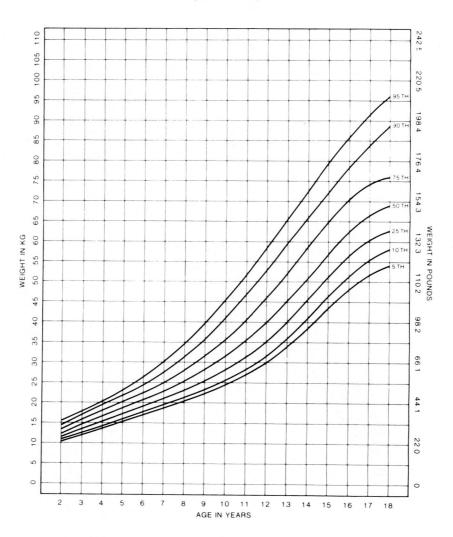

From National Center for Health Statistics, 1974.

BOYS
Weight by stature: Prepubescent

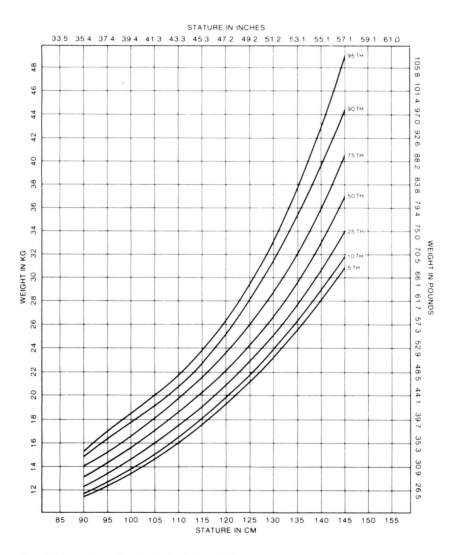

From National Center for Health Statistics, 1974.

Analyses of Popular Diets

Johanna T. Dwyer

ANALYSES OF SELECTED POPULAR DIETS

Name of Diet	Calories	Techniques Employed	Comments
*Kempner Rice Diet or Duke University Rice Diet (from McCall's Diet of the Month, McCall's Magazine, April 1970)	2200	Unspecified energy level, fixed menu; unbalanced energy sources (very low fat); low sodium; vitamin and mineral supplements required.	This diet consists of very large amounts of cooked rice, fruits and vegetables. It is virtually devoid of sodium and low in protein as well as vitamin A, riboflavin, calcium, and iron. No foods from the milk or meat groups of the Basic Four are permitted. The blandness and monotony are so great that most dieters reduce their food intakes far below the 2200 kcal level. If this is done, then fat may be lost. Otherwise, early weight loss is likely to be due chiefly to shifts in water balance. Vitamin-mineral supplements are needed. This diet is not necessarily approved by Duke University.
*Stillman Diet, also known as The Doctor's Quick Weight Loss Diet (IM Stillman and S Baker, Dell Publishing Company, New York, 1977)	2000	Unspecified energy level; unbalanced energy sources (very low carbohydrate); special conditions on eating (use of at least eight glasses of water a day).	Also known as the water diet, the diet works by specifying the types, but not the amounts, of foods permitted. Fails to meet the Basic Four for either fruits and vegetables or breads and cereals, since none of these foods are allowed. The diet consists of low-fat cheeses, lean meat, fish, poultry, eggs, and 8 glasses of water a day. Neither milk nor visible fats are permitted, but the contribution of the other foods makes the diet very high in fat, especially saturated fat, and protein and low in carbohydrate. Vitamins A, C, thiamine and iron are low in the diet. A multi-vitamin pill is suggested.

*Modified from Dwyer J: Sixteen popular diets. In Obesity, A Stunkard (ed). Philadelphia: WB Saunders, 1980, pp. 277–85.

†From Dwyer JT: In Hirsch J, Van Itallie T: Recent Advances in Obesity Research IV. Proceedings of the 4th International Congress on Obesity. John Libbey. New York, 1983, pp. 179–192.

‡From Nicholas P, Dwyer J: In Brownell KD, Forey† JP: Handbook of Eating Disorders: Physiology, Psychology, and Treatment of Obesity Anorexia and Bulimia. Basic Books, 1986 pp.122–144.

§Additional diet books and products that were reviewed and analyzed by J Dwyer, D.Sc., Director, and Ms. Elizabeth Patillo, Dietetic Intern at Frances Stern Nutrition Center, Boston, Massachusettes.

‖From Dazzi A, Dwyer J: Nutritional Analyses of Popular Weight Reduction Diets in Books and Magazines. International Journal of Eating Disorders **3**:61–80. 1984.   *Continued.*

ANALYSES OF SELECTED POPULAR DIETS—cont'd

Name of Diet	Calories	Techniques Employed	Comments
*Calories Don't Count (from the book by the same name by H Taller. Simon & Schuster, New York, 1961)	1800	Unspecified energy level, fixed menus; unbalanced energy sources (high fat); special supplement of polyunsaturated vegetable oil required as well as food; one hour walk also specified; other specifications on eating; low sodium.	This diet is extremely high in fat and quite high in protein. Particular emphasis is paid to consuming large amounts of meat and milk products, avoiding sugars and starches, including most fruits, breads, and cereals. One-third of a cup of vegetable oil high in polyunsaturated fat is consumed each day. It contributes 800 kcal. Many commonly eaten foods are forbidden. Weight loss is likely to be due in great measure to a temporary diuresis induced by the low carbohydrate/low sodium nature of the diet and the liberal use of black coffee, a weak diuretic.
*Behavioral Control Diet (from Eating is Okay by HA Jordan, LS Levitz, and GM Kimbrell, Rawson Associates Publishers, New York, 1976). (Note: Other books outlining similar self-directed diet change methods include: Permanent Weight Control: A Total Solution to the Dieter's Dilemma (M & K Mahoney, WW Norton, New York, 1976), Habits, Not Diets: The Real Way to Weight Control (JM Ferguson, Bull Publishing Co., Palo Alto, 1976), Learning to Eat: Behavioral Modification for Weight Control (JM Ferguson, Bull Publishing Co., Palo Alto, 1976), and Take It Off and Keep If Off (DB Jeffrey and R Katz, Prentice-Hall, Englewood Cliffs, 1977)	Variable, but approximately 1500	Unspecified energy level; balanced energy sources; special conditions on eating (keeping diet records, behavior modification); physical activity.	This diet is actually a self-administered course in behavior modification rather than a diet per se, written by clinicians with extensive experience in the field. If the instructions are followed, all nutrient needs other than energy should be met, and the dieter will gain insight into how to plan eating styles over the long term to maintain reduced weights. Most patients find that the assistance of a health professional knowledgeable in behavior therapy and nutrition helpful in following the directions.
The Diet Center Program (S Ferguson, Little Brown, Boston, 1983)	1400-1700	Gimmick marketing techniques, use of a famous name, "scientific" and biochemical claims, prophylactic claims, stimulate adherence by special menus, special foods or supplements, use of group and cognitive techniques.	A high protein relatively low fat diet which goes through four phases. Dieters can also enroll in Diet Center group classes. Provides less than the recommended number of servings of milk products, breads and cereals.

Diet	kcal	Characteristics	Analysis
Doctors' Calorie Plus Diet† (H Jordan and T Berland, Chicago, Contemporary Books, 1981)	1400	Famous name, gimmick of special foods, special conditions on eating, fixed menus, cognitive techniques.	A well planned reasonable diet. The "gimmick" is the "IQ" or intake quotient, which rates foods by caloric density, preparation time, amount of time it takes to eat foods. The diet starts out with fixed menus and then expands to offer wider choice using a food exchange list. Attitude, habit and behavior change are stressed.
*Pritikin Diet (from Live Longer Now: The First One Hundred Years of Your Life, by N Pritikin, Grosset & Dunlop, New York, 1974).	1400	Unspecified energy level; unbalanced energy sources (extremely low fat); special conditions on eating (portion size control); low sodium.	This diet is extremely low in fat (only about 10% of total calories) and also low in salt and carbohydrate, especially sugar. The diet pattern forbids butter, margarine, oils, grain-fed beef, sugar, and products containing them. While the types of foods allowed meet the Basic Four, particular emphasis is given to large amounts of fruits, vegetables, breads and cereals. Dairy products are forbidden unless they are made with skim milk. Slightly low in iron.
*The Fat Counter Guide (RM Deutsch, Hawthorne Books and Bull Publishing Co., Palo Alto, 1978).	1300	Specified energy level, balanced energy sources; special conditions on eating (use of fat counter to plan menus and analyze choices).	With the help of the so-called fat counter table, which lists the percent of protein, fat, and carbohydrate in foods, the dieter analyzes his food intake. Using the Basic Four and the fat counter guide, the dieter then plans a diet with a 500 kcal deficit to his or her individual tastes, which is somewhat lower in fat and higher in carbohydrate than usual, somewhat limiting the variety of foods. The nutrition information presented is sound.
*Dietary Goals Diet (from the analysis of B Peterkin, C Shone, and RL Kerr in Some diets that meet the dietary goals. J Amer Dietet Assoc 74:423, 1979).	1300	Specified energy level; fixed menus; balanced energy sources.	This is a reducing diet based on the U.S. Dietary Goals. It meets Recommended Dietary Allowances but provides very large amounts of breads, cereals, fruits, and vegetables and fewer servings from the meat and milk group than specified in the Basic Four. Variety of foods allowed is somewhat limited.
*Anti-Stress Diet (Dr. Neil Solomon, Harper's Bazaar, August 1976).	1300	Unspecified energy level (fixed menu); balanced energy sources; special conditions on eating.	This is a good reducing diet that is to be followed only three days a week. The diet is sensible. Simple relaxation techniques and exhortations to exercise to relieve stress are also included. Meets all nutrients needs.

Continued.

ANALYSES OF SELECTED POPULAR DIETS—cont'd

Name of Diet	Calories	Techniques Employed	Comments
The Diet That Lets You Cheat‡ (RB Parr, DC Bachman and H Bates Noble, Crown Publishers, New York, 1983)	1300	Gimmick marketing techniques, "scientific" and biochemical claims, fixed menus to stimulate adherence, reward and incentive foods.	This is a high protein low fat diet which is fairly reasonable. It is based on the authors' experiences in community weight control programs. After a rather rigid start with fixed menus, the dieter graduates to less restrictive menus. The dieter is also permitted to "cheat".
California Diet and Exercise Program‡ (P Wood Anderson, World Books, Mountain View, California, 1983)	1300	Use of a famous name, "scientific" and biochemical claims, prophylactic claims, special foods or supplements, reward and incentive foods, cognitive techniques.	This is a high fiber, relatively high protein, low fat diet. It is reasonable and well balanced. Vigorous physical activity is also stressed.
The Over 30 All Natural Health‡ and Beauty Plan (E Martin Bantam Books, New York, 1982)	1100-1500	Gimmick marketing techniques, use of a famous name, prophylactic claims, stimulate adherence by fixed menus, special foods or supplements and cognitive techniques.	High fat ketogenic diet very low in carbohydrates. Megadoses of vitamin B_6 are also recommended, which are likely to cause side effects. Low in milk products, breads and starches.
§Dr. Rader's No Diet Program for Permanent Weight Loss (W Rader, Warner Books, New York, 1981)	1300	Unspecified energy level; balanced energy sources if on the Basic Four menu.	Emphasizes behavior modification while following the Basic Four Diet program. The dieter is given flexibility by using an exchange list so the diet is not monotonous. The diet has fewer servings of bread and milk group than the Basic Four.
§Craig Claiborne's Gourmet Diet (Craig Claiborne, Ballantine Books, New York, 1980)	>1300	Unspecified energy levels; restricted sodium (2 g Na); menus are high in fat.	This diet is for dieters who have to restrict their sodium intake, and who also want to enjoy "haute cuisine." The menus given are high in fat and protein. The diet is balanced over all, but the servings of milk and bread vary day to day and are sometimes lower than the Basic Four. The book gives helpful hints on eating out in restaurants. Emphasizes a change in diet structure—less fatty meats and cholesterol, rich foods, fewer sweets, fewer salty and processed foods, and a switch over to more natural wholesome foods.
§The Atkins Diet from Dr. Atkins' Nutrition Breakthrough (Robert C Atkins, Bantam Books, New York, 1981)	>1200	Unspecified energy level; unbalanced energy sources (low CHO—20 g; high protein). Ketogenic diet. Vitamin and mineral supplements.	This diet is higher in the meat group, lower in the bread, milk, and fruit groups. The menu is restricted. Unlimited quantities of protein (except cheese), limited vegetables, and no milk are allowed. This diet is also high in fat; vitamin and mineral supplements are recommended. The diet excludes fruit, fruit juice,

Diet	Energy	Characteristics	Comments
§Beverly Hills Medical Diet (Arnold Fox, Bantam Books, New York, 1981)	1200 cal maximum (14-day everyday weight loss)	Specified energy level; high fiber, high complex carbohydrates, low fat (only fat is found in the foods, none used in recipes), vitamin, mineral supplements. Biochemical claims related to high-fiber diets.	This diet emphasizes "natural" foods. No cholesterol, no fats, no refined carbohydrates. Stresses the complex carbohydrate, and a high-fiber diet to decrease appetite, decrease weight, decrease stress. Set menus and recipes. High in fruits, vegetables and grains; protein is split between animal and plant sources. No fat is allowed on the diet except for naturally occurring fats. Recommends a vitamin/mineral supplement daily.
*Slim Chance in a Fat World (RB Stuart and B Davis. Research Press, Champaign, Illinois, 1972). [See also Act Thin, Stay Thin (R Stuart, WW Norton, New York, 1978.]	Variable, depending upon the food plan chosen, but usually 1200–1500 kcal for women, more for men.	Specified energy level; balanced energy sources; special conditions on eating (use of behavior modification techniques and environmental manipulation, record keeping); recommendations for exercise.	This diet places heavy emphasis on behavior modification techniques, but includes a good deal of information on diet planning from the nutritional standpoint. If instructions are followed, nutrient needs other than energy will be met. Most patients using this diet benefit from the simultaneous assistance of a health professional knowledgeable in behavior therapy and nutrition, since directions are many and rather complicated.
Complete University Medical Diet† (M Simonson and J Heilman, Rawson Associates, New York, 1983)	1200	Famous name, cognitive techniques.	Well balanced diet, emphasizes behavior, habits, attitudes and gaining insights into causes of obesity. A food exchange system helps individuals to choose menus sensibly.
§Orthocarbohydrate Diet. Diet from the Book "Mega-Nutrition" (Richard Kunin, New American Library, New York, 1981)	1200	Ketogenic diet; unspecified energy level. Unbalanced energy sources depending upon chosen CHO level (<100 g CHO & 60 g protein). Biochemical claims; vitamins and mineral supplements recommended.	This diet is very low in carbohydrates if one chooses the lower levels. Emphasizes the mechanism of ketosis. There is a basic menu, but does not give alternative menu based on carbohydrate level desired. Meals are lower in the milk and bread group, higher in the meat group, and sufficient in vegetable and fruit group.
§Dr. Solomon's Easy No-Risk Diet (Warner Books, New York, 1974)	1200	Specified energy level; no calorie counting based on exchange or "shares" list; balanced energy sources.	This diet uses exchange lists and follows the Basic Four plan. Unlimited amounts of vegetables of some types are allowed. It uses behavior modification techniques and is varied. All the four food groups are met if the person follows the Basic Easy No-Risk Diet, although the "carboholic" diet has more meat than bread servings when it is compared to the Basic Four and is also very high in fat.

Continued.

ANALYSES OF SELECTED POPULAR DIETS—cont'd

Name of Diet	Calories	Techniques Employed	Comments
*Wise Woman's Diet (Redbook, June 1979; repeated each season)	1200	Specified energy level; set menus; balanced energy sources.	This diet meets all of the Recommended Dietary Allowances and also the Basic Four guide. It is repeated with different menus several times a year in the same magazine along with behavior modification hints and a discussion of special problems dieters face. Some limited exchanges of one food for another are permitted.
Slendernow (RA Passwater, St. Martin's Press, New York, 1982)	1200-1500	"Scientific" and biochemical claims, special foods, prophylactic claims.	A high protein diet which is ketogenic. Attempts to sell a special food (milk shakes) made with a special protein powder. The diet is low in iron and thiamine.
Never Say Diet† (R Simmons, Warner Books, New York, 1981)	1200	Famous name, "scientific" and biochemical claims, prophylactic claims.	This is a three-part program of diet, exercise and attitude change. Many erroneous statements are made and diets are low in iron and calcium.
F Plan† (A Eyton, Crown Publishers, New York, 1980)	1200	Special foods, "scientific" and biochemical claims, prophylactic claims.	A questionable regimen, stressing very large amounts (35–50 g) of bran and other forms of dietary fiber. The diet is very high in complex carbohydrates and fiber, and low in protein.
§Weight Watchers	1000-2000	Restricted calories; self-help groups; exercise; nutrition education.	Wide choice of foods, comprehensive supplemental programs, fair to good source of most nutrients. Heavy emphasis on fish, exact weighing and measuring required.
§Diet Workshop	1200	Restricted calories; basic menus; nutrition education; exercise; behavior modification techniques.	Adaptable to individual needs; comprehensive supplemental programs; good course of vitamins A, D, C, B_{12}, calcium; fair source of minerals and vitamin E. Weight goals high, exact weighing and measuring required, poor source of B vitamins.
Beverly Hills Diet† (J Mazel, MacMillan, New York, 1982)	1100	"Scientific" and biochemical claims, special foods such as bran, brewer's yeast used.	A low protein, high carbohydrate diet fraught with mistaken notions of metabolism. The notion of "conscious combining" which entails eating only foods high in protein or carbohydrate makes little sense. Many nutrients are low, including protein, iron, calcium and riboflavin.

Diet	Calories	Techniques	Analysis
Carbohydrate Craver's Diet† (JJ Wurtman, Houghton Mifflin, Boston, 1982)	1100	"Scientific" and biochemical claims, famous name, gimmick of a special sweet reward.	Greatest emphasis is given to the role of dieter's carbohydrates in triggering neurotransmitter action. The diet is well balanced. The gimmick is a 200 calorie carbohydrate rich snack reward each day.
Aerobic Nutrition‡ (D Mannerberg and J Rohr, Berkeley Books, New York, 1981)	1100	Use of a famous name, "scientific and biochemical" claims, prophylactic claims, stimulate adherence by fixed menus.	High A has a high protein, very low fat diet written by a former director of the Prikkin Longevity Center. Aerobic exercises are also suggested. Low in milk products and breads and starches.
The Women Doctor's Diet for Women‖ (B Edelstein, Ballantine Books, New York, 1977)	1030	Specified intake, unbalanced energy sources, fixed menus, famous name, behavior modification, unproven scientific claims.	High protein. The diet is low in calcium, iron and thiamine.
I Love New York† (B Myerson and B Adler, William Morrow, New York, 1982)	1000–1900	"Scientific" and biochemical claims, gimmick, famous name, diet meals, rewards and incentives, crash phase.	A low-fat high-fiber diet. Both a low calories ketogenic "crash" diet and a 1900 calorie "eating holiday", are included, which alternate every week. Diet meals are available in restaurants that conform to the diet. The diet is nutritionally adequate.
§No Choice Diet	1000	Daily low-calorie menus for 5 weeks; exercise; relaxation; grooming.	Simple to follow; fair source of most vitamins and minerals. No weight maintenance or nutrition guidance; no substitutions; low in vitamin E and iron; low in essential fatty acids.
§Woman Doctor's Diet for Women	1000	Restricted calories; balanced fat, carbohydrate, and protein (40%–50% protein).	Simple to follow; little measuring; food added as diet progresses; good source of vitamin B_{12}; fair source of vitamins A, D, C, B_6, and minerals. No substitutions; portions not specified; poor source of vitamin E and thiamine, riboflavin, niacin.
*Protein Program Reducing Diet (from diet included with Health Brand Protein Powder, Republic Drug Co., Buffalo, New York)	1000	Unspecified energy level; fixed menu; unbalanced energy sources (low fat); use of special supplement required.	This diet involves the use of a protein powder "supplement" at one or two meals a day in addition to a regular meal and snack. The powder contains a mixture of soy protein, casein nad lactalbumin, along with Brewer's yeast. While the protein sources are somewhat better than those found in liquid protein formula diets, directions about meals are ambiguous, except for dinner. The diet is low in iron. It falls short of the Basic Four in the milk group and the breads and cereals group.

Continued.

ANALYSES OF SELECTED POPULAR DIETS—cont'd

Name of Diet	Calories	Techniques Employed	Comments
Dr. Abravanel's Body Type‡ and Lifetime Nutrition Plan (ED Abravand and EA King, Bantam Books, New York, 1983)	900-1400	Gimmick marketing techniques, "scientific" and biochemical claims, stimulate adherence by fixed menus, a crash phase, special foods and supplements, cognitive techniques.	Various diets are provided for different "body types". Each diet targets different foods which are wrongly assumed to cause weight gain. Several of the menus are ketogenic, and most of the diets are unbalanced.
The Delicious Quick Trim Diet‡ (SS Baker and S Schur, Villard Books, New York, 1983)	950-1200	Gimmick marketing techniques, use of a famous name, "scientific" and biochemical claims, stimulate adherence by fixed menus and use of crash phase, eating retrials, and cognitive techniques.	A very low fat high protein diet which is different in several nutrients, very low in breads and cereals, and replete with unproven claims.
*Snack Diet or Wisconsin Diet (from article by the same name in McCall's, October 1970)	950	Unspecified energy level (fixed menu); unbalanced energy sources (low carbohydrate); special conditions on eating.	The University of Wisconsin does not endorse this diet. While an eating regimen of 6 small meals a day is stressed, it is the low-calorie aspect of the diet that is crucial. The diet is ketogenic and relatively low in sodium, so that a diuresis would be likely to ensue in the first few days on the regime, which would lead to rapid weight loss. The pattern recommended is lower in the milk group and breads and cereals group than the Basic Four, and the diet is low in calcium and iron.
*The Doctor's Metabolic Diet (WL Kremer, Crown Publishers, New York, 1975)	900	Unspecified energy level (fixed menu alternating with a fast); unbalanced energy sources (low carbohydrate); special conditions on eating; low sodium.	The most unusual features of this diet are that it insists on no food intake before lunch and only two meals per day, with one day a week devoted to a total fast. The diet is ketogenic, low in sodium, and recommends weak tea and coffee—all measures which are likely to induce a diuresis in the first few days and rather rapid weight loss at first. Breads and cereals and the milk group fail to meet the Basic Four. The diet is low in riboflavin, thiamine, calcium and iron; the use of vitamin-mineral supplements is mentioned but not stressed. The very low calorie levels, periodic fasts, absence of a morning meal and lack of emphasis on selection of potassium-rich foods make medical supervision appropriate.

Diet	Energy (kcal)	Characteristics	Comments
Fabulous Fructose Diet† (JT Cooper and FP Hogon, M Evans & Co., New York, 1982)	900	"Gimmick" of special foods, "scientific" and biochemical claims.	A low carbohydrate, ketogenic diet, high in fat and protein. It is to be used in conjunction with fructose tablets. The diet is low in calcium.
Southhampton Diet† (S Berger, Simon & Schuster, New York, 1982)	900	"Scientific" and biochemical claims, famous name, prophylactic claims.	Another questionable diet. It claims that food constituents influence neurotransmitters and thus mood, and foods are categorized into "happy" and "sad". Low in phosphorus, iron and thiamin.
*Scarsdale Diet (Published as The Complete Scarsdale Medical Diet, Herman Tarnower and Samm Sinclair Baker. Bantam Books, New York, 1978)	750	Unspecified energy level; set or fixed menu; unbalanced energy sources (very low carbohydrate and fat); low sodium.	This diet requires medical supervision. This is one version of a popular new crash diet variously called the Scarsdale Diet and the Scarsdale Medical Group Diet, which is to be used for 14 days only and is "guaranteed" to cause a weight loss of 20 lbs. Because of its low carbohydrate (about 50 g) and energy content, this diet is ketogenic. Additional constraints on fluid intake, which is limited to black coffee or tea, both diuretics in themselves, and on salting, favor diuresis. The diet is low in iron, vitamin A, calcium, and riboflavin. The diet is low in the milk and bread and cereals groups. Dehydration is possible, since fluid intakes are not specified.
Nutraerobics‡ (Bland J, Harper & Row, San Francisco, 1983)	607	Gimmick marketing techniques, "scientific" and biochemical claims, prophylactic claims, stimulate adherence by a crash phase, use of special foods or supplements, monotonous or unpalatable foods.	This is a protein supplemented modified fast. A protein supplement is suggested to replace two meals. The diet is inadequate in vitamins A, D, C, B₆, B₁₂, folacin and several minerals (calcium, phosphorous, iron, zinc). Such fasts are not recommended without medical guidance and nutritional adequacy.
*Fasting Is a Way of Life (L Cott, Bantam Books, New York, 1977)	500	Specified energy level (fast followed by formula); unbalanced energy sources (low carbohydrate).	The type of fasting described in this diet requires medical supervision. This book suggests a total fast followed by a very low-calorie diet of liquid meals. The diet is very low in the meat group and breads and cereals compared to the Basic Four. It is lower than recommendations in protein, niacin, riboflavin, thiamine, calcium and iron. The diet is ketogenic because of the low carbohydrate levels.

Continued.

ANALYSES OF SELECTED POPULAR DIETS—cont'd

Name of Diet	Calories	Techniques Employed	Comments
*Last Chance Refeeding Diet (from "The Last Chance Diet" by R Linn, Bantam Books, New York, 1977)	500	Specified energy level; unbalanced energy sources (very low carbohydrate); special formula required as well as food.	This diet requires medical supervision. This diet follows a protein-supplemented fast, a high-protein powder, called ProLinn, is suggested for the fast itself. Such fasts may induce ketosis, hypokalemia, and other complications when attempted by persons not under skilled medical supervision. During the fast, vitamin and mineral supplements, potassium, and folic acid are also prescribed with at least 2 quarts of noncaloric fluids a day. Gradually, food is introduced—this is called the refeeding phase and is detailed here. The ProLinn powder must still be consumed twice a day. Dehydration, hypokalemia, etc. are possible if directions are not followed, intakes of vitamin A, riboflavin, thiamine, iron, and calcium are inadequate as the diet is stated.
§The Cambridge Diet (from the Cambridge Plan International, London)	330 (per module or can)	Specific energy level; unbalanced energy sources (low fat, high protein). Extremely low calorie, low sodium.	A formula diet supplemented with 100% of the RDA for vitamins and minerals. Diet is very low in calories and is low in all energy sources: protein, carbohydrate, and fat. Weight loss results from an extreme caloric deficit. This diet could be harmful to individuals with medical problems.
Fasting: The Ultimate Diet§ (A Cott, Bantam Books, New York, 1981)	0	Use of a famous name, "scientific" and biochemical claims, prophylactic claims, stimulate adherence by a "crash" phase. Special conditions on eating or foods in the environment and cognitive techniques.	This is a dangerous self-initiated total fast. Fasting wastes lean body mass. It is inadequate in vitamins, minerals and protein.

APPENDIX VI

U.S. Dietary Intake

Calories	Thiamine
Protein	Riboflavin
Carbohydrate	Preformed Niacin
Fat	Vitamin C
Calcium	Saturated Fatty Acid
Iron	Oleic Acid
Sodium	Linoleic Acid
Potassium	Serum Cholesterol Levels
Vitamin A	Cholesterol

Dietary Intake Patterns by Age, Sex, and Income Level: United States

The data in this section were collected by the National Center for Health Statistics through the Second National Health and Nutrition Examination Survey, conducted from 1976 through 1980 and reported in *Vital and Health Statistics,* Series 11, No. 231, in March 1983. Information was collected in 64 locations selected from 1924 primary sampling units that represented standard metropolitan statistical areas (a county, or two or three contiguous counties). The population sampled is representative of the civilian noninstitutionalized U.S. population. Two income levels are represented: (1) income below poverty level, as expressed by a poverty/income ratio of less than 1, and (2) income at and above poverty level, as represented by a ratio of 1 or more.

Persons who were examined but who had an unknown income are excluded from the income groups but are included in the total.

The 24-hour recall dietary interviews were done on a Tuesday through Saturday schedule, so the information represents foods eaten on weekdays only. The data base used to calculate the nutrient content was obtained from the U.S. Department of agriculture and from manufacturers. The resources included *Handbook* No. 8, sections 1-6, and *Handbook* No. 456. Items were updated appropriately with information from the food manufacturer. The dietary interviewer recorded the item(s) and the quantity(ies) of food or drink consumed during the previous day. The method used to obtain dietary intake data was the same as that used previously. Usual patterns of food consumption were determined. When the sample size was insufficient to provide a stable percentile estimate, a dash appears in the tabulated data.

Data from the National Health Survey, March 1983.

CALORIC INTAKE, AGES 6 MO–74 YR, UNITED STATES, 1976–80

| Income Level, Sex, and Age | No. Examined | Mean | Calories | | | | | | |
| | | | Percentile | | | | | | |
			5th	10th	25th	50th	75th	90th	95th
ALL INCOMES									
Male									
6 mo–74 yr	9983	2381	976	1193	1614	2187	2891	3721	4400
6-11 mo	179	1001	513	610	739	922	1194	1476	1740
1-2 yr	745	1311	653	788	973	1259	1560	1976	2204
3-5 yr	1219	1628	857	977	1249	1556	1933	2337	2667
6-8 yr	428	1981	1084	1267	1569	1915	2371	2754	2943
9-11 yr	457	2183	1154	1329	1705	2092	2592	3028	3454
12-14 yr	504	2430	1049	1305	1736	2324	2957	3670	4121
15-17 yr	535	2817	1133	1362	1906	2629	3386	4479	5575
18-24 yr	988	3040	1185	1456	2040	2731	3668	4805	5840
25-34 yr	1067	2734	1213	1495	1963	2577	3365	4172	4749
35-44 yr	745	2424	1073	1294	1753	2299	2931	3586	4211
45-54 yr	690	2361	1019	1226	1713	2224	2805	3613	4058
55-64 yr	1227	2071	948	1125	1529	1966	2554	3136	3481
65-74 yr	1199	1829	841	1015	1335	1723	2212	2725	3096
Female									
6 mo–74 yr	10,339	1578	683	825	1116	1493	1925	2408	2768
6-11 mo	177	991	530	639	762	949	1146	1525	1592
1-2 yr	672	1262	649	727	918	1170	1516	1822	2115
3-5 yr	1126	1508	807	947	1146	1433	1796	2172	2426
6-8 yr	415	1807	1010	1155	1424	1755	2142	2451	2789
9-11 yr	425	1857	1024	1166	1426	1768	2156	2667	2958
12-14 yr	487	1813	863	999	1337	1772	2217	2699	2899
15-17 yr	449	1731	710	888	1204	1636	2120	2682	3152
18-24 yr	1066	1687	670	804	1158	1593	2091	2578	3009
25-34 yr	1170	1643	677	837	1177	1547	2001	2546	2889
35-44 yr	844	1579	686	844	1140	1510	1909	2292	2708
45-54 yr	763	1439	632	767	1052	1377	1726	2155	2402
55-64 yr	1329	1401	606	735	1010	1308	1705	2131	2448
65-74 yr	1416	1295	607	745	972	1221	1570	1881	2172
INCOME BELOW POVERTY LEVEL*									
Male									
6 mo–74 yr	1539	2214	771	999	1442	2008	2755	3581	4296
6-11 mo	48	—	—	—	696	922	1198	—	—
1-2 yr	170	1296	602	669	909	1234	1605	1987	2156
3-5 yr	298	1688	880	964	1256	1577	2050	2509	2900
6-8 yr	82	1971	823	1234	1642	1911	2460	2941	3010
9-11 yr	88	1997	728	1042	1568	1971	2403	2906	3178
12-14 yr	89	2254	871	1106	1541	2209	2803	3644	3957
15-17 yr	89	2547	906	1210	1645	2303	3120	4438	4883
18-24 yr	178	2971	1059	1360	1912	2731	3685	4543	6470
25-34 yr	91	2573	1090	1214	1735	2302	3205	4242	4744
35-44 yr	63	—	—	—	1389	2051	2699	—	—
45-54 yr	46	—	—	—	1683	2360	2825	—	—
55-64 yr	129	1873	548	764	1263	1715	2431	3065	3456
65-74 yr	168	1602	667	871	1169	1495	1875	2404	2623

*Excludes persons with unknown income.

CALORIC INTAKE, AGES 6 MO–74 YR, UNITED STATES, 1976–80—cont'd

Income Level, Sex, and Age	No. Examined	Mean	Calories						
			Percentile						
			5th	10th	25th	50th	75th	90th	95th
INCOME BELOW POVERTY LEVEL— cont'd									
Female									
6 mo–74 yr	1910	1557	606	765	1076	1460	1900	2467	2850
6-11 mo	36	—	—	—	—	908	—	—	—
1-2 yr	153	1359	632	721	932	1298	1568	1963	2765
3-5 yr	272	1572	714	909	1113	1499	1928	2333	2596
6-8 yr	95	1858	1002	1121	1468	1832	2258	2570	2956
9-11 yr	102	1806	951	1056	1342	1680	2156	2668	2960
12-14 yr	104	1721	854	957	1212	1614	2149	2671	3073
15-17 yr	88	1771	765	977	1256	1650	2107	2683	3064
18-24 yr	253	1604	589	780	1102	1559	1992	2497	2877
25-34 yr	162	1711	621	787	1163	1575	2051	2667	3334
35-44 yr	119	1420	576	685	918	1327	1830	2270	2825
45-54 yr	82	1331	543	667	964	1293	1700	1962	2200
55-64 yr	188	1258	503	614	815	1204	1548	1991	2361
65-74 yr	256	1223	464	628	882	1163	1461	1865	2030
INCOME ABOVE POVERTY LEVEL*									
Male									
6 mo–74 yr	8084	2410	1005	1220	1638	2214	2916	3741	4431
6-11 mo	121	1013	507	619	764	914	1209	1500	1827
1-2 yr	551	1317	680	805	980	1259	1558	1978	2273
3-5 yr	892	1620	860	988	1254	1554	1911	2291	2589
6-8 yr	336	1989	1089	1273	1567	1918	2366	2712	2921
9-11 yr	356	2217	1189	1359	1723	2122	2622	3011	3452
12-14 yr	399	2469	1111	1337	1749	2361	3005	3721	4232
15-17 yr	418	2892	1155	1386	1996	2675	3446	4542	5612
18-24 yr	770	3063	1184	1478	2058	2732	3678	4918	5875
25-34 yr	945	2751	1277	1516	1974	2592	3374	4162	4788
35-44 yr	658	2468	1140	1313	1817	2324	2952	3620	4264
45-54 yr	603	2378	997	1236	1706	2226	2815	3676	4123
55-64 yr	1048	2087	978	1160	1543	1979	2555	3159	3521
65-74 yr	987	1858	859	1032	1367	1744	2245	2769	3137
Female									
6 mo–74 yr	8036	1582	695	843	1123	1501	1930	2407	2761
6-11 mo	135	979	530	639	762	950	1123	1524	1590
1-2 yr	505	1240	649	738	916	1163	1484	1804	2053
3-5 yr	815	1497	848	966	1156	1429	1777	2091	2369
6-8 yr	308	1794	1030	1178	1415	1755	2114	2436	2693
9-11 yr	307	1875	1040	1185	1487	1790	2165	2668	2956
12-14 yr	363	1846	919	1025	1384	1831	2240	2703	2912
15-17 yr	342	1692	699	872	1161	1595	2116	2655	3069
18-24 yr	771	1713	689	832	1169	1636	2119	2614	3010
25-34 yr	982	1632	683	838	1178	1545	1996	2544	2872
35-44 yr	702	1598	744	871	1149	1531	1924	2344	2709
45-54 yr	655	1451	643	784	1060	1377	1731	2162	2403
55-64 yr	1071	1428	623	780	1050	1352	1712	2172	2466
65-74 yr	1080	1312	649	766	993	1231	1587	1901	2191

PERCENT DISTRIBUTION OF CALORIC INTAKE, AGES 6–11 MO, UNITED STATES

Kcal	Both Sexes			Male			Female		
	All (356)	Below Poverty (84)	Above Poverty (256)	All (179)	Below Poverty*	Above Poverty (121)	All (177)	Below Poverty*	Above Poverty (135)
<500	3.8	3.8	3.5	4.3		4.6	2.9		2.4
500–599	8.3	7.5	8.7	9.3		9.9	7.3		7.4
600–699	17.3	26.3	15.2	17.8		14.0	16.8		16.4
700–799	32.2	38.6	31.2	32.9		29.7	31.5		32.8
800–899	46.5	47.1	46.8	48.2		49.2	44.8		44.4
900–999	57.5	60.1	57.3	58.4		58.6	56.5		56.1
1000–1099	69.8	67.9	70.1	68.1		66.9	71.5		73.4
1100–1199	77.2	76.6	77.1	76.1		74.8	78.3		79.5
1200–1299	81.8	79.8	82.4	80.3		79.1	83.5		85.6
1300–1399	85.0	84.5	85.4	84.0		83.1	86.1		87.6
1400–1499	89.4	91.8	89.1	90.9		89.8	87.8		88.4
1500–1599	93.7	93.3	93.9	92.4		91.8	95.1		96.0
≥1600	100	100	100	100		100	100		100

1976–80. National Center for Health Statistics, 1983.
*Data unavailable.

PERCENT DISTRIBUTION OF CALORIC INTAKE, AGES 1–2 YR, UNITED STATES

Kcal	Both Sexes			Male			Female		
	All (1417)	Below Poverty (323)	Above Poverty (1056)	All (745)	Below Poverty (170)	Above Poverty (551)	All (672)	Below Poverty (153)	Above Poverty (505)
>500	1.8	2.3	1.7	1.3	2.4	.9	2.3	2.2	2.4
500–749	9.7	11.7	9.2	8.6	11.3	7.9	10.9	12.1	10.6
750–799	12.4	13.4	12.2	10.4	13.6	9.7	14.5	13.2	14.8
800–999	29.5	29.7	29.5	27.6	32.0	26.8	31.4	27.3	32.4
1000–1099	39.8	40.7	37.3	37.3	38.1	37.3	42.4	34.6	44.2
1100–1249	52.3	48.0	53.3	49.4	50.2	49.3	55.4	45.6	57.5
1250–1399	65.6	60.7	66.7	64.1	59.9	65.3	67.1	61.5	68.1
1400–1499	72.7	68.3	73.5	71.1	69.0	71.4	74.3	67.6	75.6
1500–1599	79.2	75.0	80.0	77.8	74.8	78.1	80.7	75.4	81.9
1600–1749	85.3	83.4	85.4	84.0	83.3	83.6	86.6	83.7	87.2
1750–1999	92.3	90.3	92.6	91.0	90.3	91.0	93.6	90.3	94.3
2000–2249	25.8	95.1	95.9	95.4	97.1	94.9	96.1	93.0	96.9
≥2250	100	100	100	100	100	100	100	100	100

1976–80. National Center for Health Statistics, 1983.

PERCENT DISTRIBUTION OF CALORIC INTAKE, AGES 3–5 YR, UNITED STATES

Kcal	Both Sexes			Male			Female		
	All (2345)	Below Poverty (570)	Above Poverty (1707)	All (1219)	Below Poverty (298)	Above Poverty (892)	All (1126)	Below Poverty (272)	Above Poverty (815)
<750	3.2	4.1	2.7	2.8	1.8	2.8	3.7	6.3	2.7
750–999	12.2	13.0	11.5	10.7	10.9	10.3	13.8	15.1	13.0
1000–1099	18.3	19.7	17.4	15.4	15.4	14.9	21.4	23.8	20.2
1100–1249	29.4	28.8	29.0	25.1	24.4	24.4	33.9	33.0	33.9
1250–1399	41.1	38.2	41.2	35.8	33.8	35.4	46.5	42.5	47.4
1400–1499	50.1	47.2	50.4	45.5	43.8	45.3	55.0	50.6	56.0
1500–1599	57.6	53.7	58.1	53.2	50.8	53.4	62.3	56.5	63.2
1600–1749	68.8	64.0	69.5	65.5	61.0	66.0	72.4	66.9	73.3
1750–1999	81.5	76.0	82.8	78.5	73.4	79.5	84.7	78.6	86.3
2000–2249	89.6	84.5	90.9	87.5	83.0	88.5	91.9	85.9	93.5
2250–2499	94.3	91.4	95.0	92.9	89.9	93.6	95.8	92.2	96.6
2500–2749	96.8	94.7	97.3	95.4	93.4	95.9	98.2	95.9	98.8
≥2750	100	100	100	100	100	100	100	100	100

1976–80. National Center for Health Statistics, 1983.

PERCENT DISTRIBUTION OF CALORIC INTAKE, AGES 6–8 YR, UNITED STATES

Kcal	Both Sexes			Male			Female		
	All (843)	Below Poverty (177)	Above Poverty (644)	All (428)	Below Poverty (82)	Above Poverty (336)	All (415)	Below Poverty (95)	Above Poverty (308)
<1000	3.0	5.5	2.5	3.0	6.9	2.1	3.0	4.1	2.9
1000–1099	6.8	9.2	6.3	5.8	8.7	5.2	8.0	9.6	7.6
1100–1249	11.4	12.7	11.3	8.7	11.6	8.2	14.4	13.8	14.7
1250–1399	19.0	17.6	19.0	14.9	15.0	14.1	23.6	20.4	24.3
1400–1499	24.3	23.7	24.0	19.4	20.0	18.8	29.7	27.5	29.8
1500–1599	32.2	28.9	32.8	26.5	23.3	26.9	38.4	34.7	39.2
1600–1749	42.9	43.9	42.2	37.9	43.3	36.4	48.3	44.6	48.6
1750–1999	61.7	59.3	62.2	56.4	56.8	56.6	67.5	62.0	68.3
2000–2249	74.6	71.9	75.2	68.5	69.5	68.2	81.2	74.5	82.8
2250–2499	86.9	83.6	87.4	83.2	79.0	83.3	91.0	88.4	91.9
2500–2749	92.0	88.5	92.8	89.7	85.1	90.3	94.6	92.1	95.6
2750–2999	96.2	95.4	96.5	95.5	94.5	95.5	97.0	96.3	97.7
≥3000	100	100	100	100	100	100	100	100	100

1976–80. National Center for Health Statistics, 1983.

PERCENT DISTRIBUTION OF CALORIC INTAKE, AGES 9–11 YR, UNITED STATES

Kcal	Both Sexes			Male			Female		
	All (882)	Below Poverty (190)	Above Poverty (663)	All (457)	Below Poverty (88)	Above Poverty (356)	All (425)	Below Poverty (102)	Above Poverty (307)
<1000	3.3	6.9	2.5	2.5	7.8	1.6	4.0	6.2	3.6
1000–1099	6.0	10.5	5.0	4.0	10.2	2.8	7.9	10.8	7.5
1100–1249	10.3	15.2	9.3	7.5	11.1	6.8	13.0	18.4	12.0
1250–1399	17.5	23.9	15.9	12.3	14.3	11.6	22.6	31.2	20.4
1400–1499	22.3	29.4	20.0	15.6	18.3	14.9	29.0	37.9	25.5
1500–1599	28.5	37.4	25.8	19.3	26.2	18.0	37.6	46.0	34.1
1600–1749	38.4	48.0	35.5	28.6	36.2	27.1	48.1	57.0	44.5
1750–1999	55.7	58.9	54.5	44.4	52.2	43.0	66.8	64.1	66.7
2000–2249	68.4	74.3	66.8	58.2	69.5	56.3	78.4	78.0	78.1
2250–2499	78.4	82.8	77.4	71.3	81.5	69.7	85.3	83.8	85.6
2500–2749	86.8	89.7	86.2	82.0	88.0	81.1	91.5	91.1	91.6
2750–2999	92.8	94.1	92.7	89.5	90.6	89.5	96.1	96.8	96.1
3000–3249	95.2	96.9	95.0	92.9	96.1	92.6	97.4	97.6	97.6
3250–3499	96.8	97.5	97.0	95.4	96.1	95.8	98.2	98.5	98.3
≥3500	100	100	100	100	100	100	100	100	100

1976–80. National Center for Health Statistics, 1983.

PERCENT DISTRIBUTION OF CALORIC INTAKE, AGES 12–14 YR, UNITED STATES

Kcal	Both Sexes			Male			Female		
	All (991)	Below Poverty (193)	Above Poverty (762)	All (504)	Below Poverty (89)	Above Poverty (399)	All (487)	Below Poverty (104)	Above Poverty (363)
<1000	7.2	13.0	5.7	4.2	9.1	3.4	10.3	16.2	8.1
1000–1099	10.6	15.6	9.3	5.4	9.1	4.9	16.0	21.0	14.2
1100–1249	14.4	20.9	12.9	8.2	11.9	7.8	20.8	28.4	18.4
1250–1399	20.3	27.9	18.5	12.5	17.2	11.8	28.4	36.7	25.8
1400–1499	25.3	34.4	23.2	14.8	21.3	13.5	36.2	45.3	33.8
1500–1599	30.0	38.7	27.9	20.0	28.1	18.4	40.4	47.5	38.4
1600–1749	37.7	49.7	35.1	26.6	35.6	25.1	49.2	61.4	46.0
1750–1999	49.8	57.0	47.7	35.5	40.8	34.3	64.6	70.4	62.4
2000–2249	61.9	68.4	60.2	47.7	56.8	46.2	76.6	78.0	75.5
2250–2499	70.9	76.9	69.4	58.2	65.3	56.9	84.1	86.5	83.0
2500–2749	79.0	81.2	78.3	67.2	68.5	66.8	91.3	91.8	91.0
2750–2999	85.9	88.0	85.1	76.1	79.8	74.9	96.1	94.9	96.2
3000–3249	90.0	91.8	89.4	82.4	86.6	81.3	97.9	96.2	98.3
3250–3499	93.3	94.0	92.9	87.9	89.8	87.3	98.8	97.4	99.0
3500–3749	95.0	95.7	94.6	91.0	92.9	90.3	99.2	98.1	99.4
≥3750	100	100	100	100	100	100	100	100	100

1976–80. National Center for Health Statistics, 1983.

PERCENT DISTRIBUTION OF CALORIC INTAKE, AGES 15–17 YR, UNITED STATES

Kcal	Both Sexes All (984)	Below Poverty (177)	Above Poverty (760)	Male All (535)	Below Poverty (89)	Above Poverty (418)	Female All (449)	Below Poverty (88)	Above Poverty (342)
<1000	8.9	9.0	9.0	3.6	6.3	2.9	14.3	11.3	15.4
1000–1099	11.6	12.3	11.8	4.9	9.0	4.0	18.5	15.1	20.0
1100–1249	18.1	19.8	18.5	7.9	14.1	6.9	28.7	24.9	30.8
1250–1399	23.3	23.6	23.9	11.3	18.3	10.1	35.6	28.3	38.3
1400–1499	27.1	29.1	27.1	12.8	19.0	11.5	41.8	38.1	43.6
1500–1599	31.3	34.8	31.2	14.8	22.6	13.2	48.5	45.6	50.1
1600–1749	38.5	43.2	38.2	19.6	27.8	18.0	58.1	56.8	59.4
1750–1999	48.1	53.3	47.2	27.7	38.2	25.0	69.1	66.8	70.5
2000–2249	58.0	63.9	56.4	37.0	48.8	33.0	79.5	77.3	81.0
2250–2499	64.3	69.9	63.0	44.6	53.8	41.5	84.7	84.3	85.6
2500–2749	72.3	78.1	71.1	54.7	63.4	52.0	90.4	91.1	91.3
2750–2999	78.0	84.1	77.2	63.4	72.4	61.1	93.1	94.4	94.0
3000–3249	83.7	86.8	83.4	71.8	76.7	70.2	96.0	95.8	97.2
3250–3499	87.0	88.3	86.8	76.6	79.9	75.6	97.7	95.8	98.6
3500–3749	90.4	93.1	90.0	82.2	87.1	81.1	98.8	98.5	99.4
3750–3999	92.1	94.4	92.0	85.2	89.0	84.5	99.3	99.2	99.8
4000–4249	93.8	94.4	93.9	88.3	89.0	88.2	99.4	99.2	100
4250–4499	94.9	95.5	94.7	90.0	90.4	89.7	100	100	
≥4500	100	100	100	100	100	100			

1976–80. National Center for Health Statistics, 1983.

PERCENT DISTRIBUTION OF CALORIC INTAKE, AGES 25–34 YR, UNITED STATES

Kcal	Both Sexes All (2237)	Below Poverty (253)	Above Poverty (1927)	Male All (1067)	Below Poverty (91)	Above Poverty (945)	Female All (1170)	Below Poverty (162)	Above Poverty (982)
<1000	9.9	11.4	9.8	2.1	3.2	1.9	17.3	15.9	17.7
1000–1099	12.7	14.6	12.5	3.4	5.1	3.1	21.5	19.8	21.7
1100–1249	18.1	22.2	17.6	5.5	10.9	4.7	30.0	28.4	30.4
1250–1399	24.5	30.3	23.8	7.6	12.8	6.9	40.5	39.9	40.6
1400–1499	29.0	34.5	28.2	10.0	13.6	9.5	46.8	46.1	46.8
1500–1599	34.4	39.5	33.7	13.7	17.4	13.0	53.9	51.7	54.3
1600–1749	41.6	51.1	40.5	18.9	28.6	17.9	63.0	63.6	62.9
1750–1999	51.3	59.7	50.5	26.3	34.6	25.6	74.8	73.5	75.2
2000–2249	61.6	68.6	61.0	37.7	44.4	37.2	84.1	82.1	84.6
2250–2499	68.9	76.3	68.0	47.1	55.3	46.3	89.6	88.0	89.6
2500–2749	75.8	80.7	75.3	57.1	63.6	56.8	93.3	90.1	93.7
2750–2999	81.7	85.6	81.4	66.3	72.5	66.0	96.2	92.9	96.6
3000–3249	84.9	88.0	84.7	72.2	76.8	71.9	97.0	94.3	97.4
3250–3499	88.6	90.7	88.4	78.3	80.3	78.1	98.3	96.5	98.6
3500–3749	91.6	91.3	91.7	84.3	81.9	84.4	98.6	96.5	98.9
3750–3999	93.9	93.0	94.0	88.4	86.8	88.7	99.0	96.5	99.3
4000–4249	95.3	94.8	95.4	91.3	91.1	91.5	99.0	96.9	99.3
≥4250	100	100	100	100	100	100	100	100	100

1976–80. National Center for Health Statistics, 1983.

PERCENT DISTRIBUTION OF CALORIC INTAKE, AGES 65–74 YR, UNITED STATES

Kcal	Both Sexes			Male			Female		
	All (2615)	Below Poverty (424)	Above Poverty (2067)	All (1199)	Below Poverty (168)	Above Poverty (981)	All (1416)	Below Poverty (256)	Above Poverty (1080)
<750	7.3	11.8	6.5	3.3	5.4	3.2	10.3	15.7	9.1
750–799	9.4	16.0	8.3	3.9	7.2	3.6	13.6	21.5	12.0
800–999	19.3	26.5	18.0	9.0	14.4	8.4	27.2	33.9	25.8
1000–1099	26.9	34.9	25.3	13.6	21.7	12.5	37.1	43.0	25.8
1100–1249	38.8	48.2	37.0	21.0	33.5	19.1	52.5	57.1	51.7
1250–1399	49.5	59.2	47.6	29.4	42.4	27.6	64.8	69.4	63.9
1400–1499	56.0	67.7	53.9	36.0	51.2	34.2	71.3	77.7	70.0
1500–1599	62.2	71.3	60.3	43.0	56.0	41.4	76.8	80.6	75.8
1600–1749	70.7	77.5	69.3	51.9	62.8	50.7	85.2	86.5	84.6
1750–1999	80.6	88.3	79.0	65.6	80.5	63.5	92.1	93.0	91.6
2000–2249	87.5	93.3	86.3	76.7	87.4	75.3	95.1	96.8	95.3
2250–2499	91.9	96.1	91.1	84.4	93.0	83.4	97.6	98.1	97.5
2500–2749	94.9	97.6	94.4	90.4	96.3	89.6	98.3	98.4	98.3
2750–2999	96.9	98.0	96.7	93.9	96.3	93.6	99.2	99.0	99.2
≥3000	100	100	100	100	100	100	100	100	100

1976–80. National Center for Health Statistics, 1983.

PROTEIN INTAKE (g), AGES 6 MO–74 YR, UNITED STATES, 1976–80

Income Level, Sex, and Age	No. Examined	Mean	Percentile						
			5th	10th	25th	50th	75th	90th	95th
ALL INCOMES									
Male									
6 mo–74 yr	9983	92	33	42	58	82	114	154	186
6-11 mo	179	40	16	19	29	38	49	65	75
1-2 yr	745	49	21	25	34	46	58	75	88
3-5 yr	1219	58	26	32	42	55	70	87	98
6-8 yr	428	73	37	44	55	69	87	108	122
9-11 yr	457	81	36	45	58	74	97	129	141
12-14 yr	504	90	32	45	62	83	113	144	166
15-17 yr	535	111	36	46	69	98	135	189	238
18-24 yr	988	118	43	53	74	104	142	196	235
25-34 yr	1067	107	40	51	70	98	131	174	210
35-44 yr	745	95	38	47	63	87	118	151	186
45-54 yr	690	93	37	44	63	87	115	147	172
55-64 yr	1227	84	35	41	56	78	102	131	158
65-74 yr	1199	73	29	38	51	67	90	115	135
Female									
6 mo–74 yr	10,339	60	22	28	40	55	74	95	114
6-11 mo	177	39	15	20	26	38	48	60	68
1-2 yr	672	47	20	25	33	44	57	70	84
3-5 yr	1126	54	24	29	39	52	65	81	90
6-8 yr	415	64	31	39	48	61	77	91	100
9-11 yr	425	67	32	37	46	63	82	103	121
12-14 yr	487	65	26	32	45	60	81	104	116
15-17 yr	449	63	21	29	44	60	78	103	120
18-24 yr	1066	64	19	27	42	59	79	106	130
25-34 yr	1170	64	21	28	42	59	80	103	127
35-44 yr	844	62	22	29	41	57	76	100	118
45-54 yr	763	58	23	29	39	52	72	91	104
55-64 yr	1329	55	22	27	36	51	69	90	107
65-74 yr	1416	51	21	26	36	48	63	81	92

*Excludes persons with unknown income.

Continued.

PROTEIN INTAKE (g), AGES 6 MO–74 YR, UNITED STATES, 1976–80—cont'd

Income Level, Sex, and Age	No. Examined	Mean	5th	10th	25th	50th	75th	90th	95th
					Percentile				
INCOME BELOW POVERTY LEVEL*									
Male									
6 mo–74 yr	1539	84	25	33	51	73	104	144	167
6-11 mo	48	—	—	—	25	35	49	—	—
1-2 yr	170	50	20	26	35	49	60	80	91
3-5 yr	298	59	27	32	43	57	73	92	98
6-8 yr	82	71	27	40	59	70	83	102	112
9-11 yr	88	75	31	34	56	68	95	128	133
12-14 yr	89	81	26	34	56	80	104	131	143
15-17 yr	89	96	32	36	61	93	121	167	179
18-24 yr	178	118	31	48	65	103	149	181	222
25-34 yr	91	95	25	33	59	86	120	166	205
35-44 yr	63	—	—	—	49	76	99	—	—
45-54 yr	46	—	—	—	64	83	116	—	—
55-64 yr	129	67	23	29	45	60	82	121	131
65-74 yr	168	65	21	30	45	63	82	113	115
Female									
6 mo–74 yr	1910	57	19	25	37	53	72	93	110
6-11 mo	36	—	—	—	—	29	—	—	—
1-2 yr	153	51	18	25	37	46	60	86	104
3-5 yr	272	57	24	29	40	56	69	85	92
6-8 yr	95	64	32	39	48	67	76	86	100
9-11 yr	102	67	28	39	44	60	82	100	126
12-14 yr	104	59	22	26	34	54	75	106	116
15-17 yr	88	63	24	26	45	60	79	100	111
18-24 yr	253	59	18	22	35	55	70	90	113
25-34 yr	162	66	18	26	42	57	84	112	141
35-44 yr	119	53	14	19	34	49	67	93	103
45-54 yr	82	48	21	25	32	48	58	80	91
55-64 yr	188	48	21	23	28	43	57	78	98
65-74 yr	256	48	16	22	31	43	62	75	87

PROTEIN INTAKE (g), AGES 6 MO–74 YR, UNITED STATES, 1976–80—cont'd

| Income Level, Sex, and Age | No. Examined | Mean | Percentile | | | | | | |
			5th	10th	25th	50th	75th	90th	95th
INCOME ABOVE POVERTY LEVEL*									
Male									
6 mo–74 yr	8084	94	35	43	60	84	115	156	189
6-11 mo	121	41	16	19	30	38	51	65	75
1-2 yr	551	48	21	25	33	45	58	75	88
3-5 yr	892	58	26	32	42	55	70	86	98
6-8 yr	336	74	39	44	54	69	87	111	123
9-11 yr	356	82	38	47	59	75	98	127	147
12-14 yr	399	92	34	46	63	83	117	148	169
15-17 yr	418	114	36	48	72	101	139	200	248
18-24 yr	770	118	45	55	75	104	139	199	238
25-34 yr	945	109	43	52	71	99	132	174	218
35-44 yr	658	98	39	48	64	88	120	155	191
45-54 yr	603	94	37	47	63	88	116	150	179
55-64 yr	1048	85	37	43	58	80	104	133	161
65-74 yr	987	74	30	39	52	68	90	117	139
Female									
6 mo–74 yr	8036	61	23	29	41	56	75	96	115
6-11 mo	135	39	18	22	28	39	48	59	66
1-2 yr	505	46	20	25	32	43	56	67	80
3-5 yr	815	53	24	30	39	51	64	79	89
6-8 yr	308	63	31	38	48	60	77	92	100
9-11 yr	307	68	32	37	48	63	83	105	119
12-14 yr	363	66	29	38	46	63	82	104	117
15-17 yr	342	63	21	29	43	58	79	103	120
18-24 yr	771	66	20	28	44	61	81	108	132
25-34 yr	982	63	22	29	41	59	78	101	126
35-44 yr	702	63	25	31	42	58	77	103	118
45-54 yr	655	59	23	30	40	54	73	91	110
55-64 yr	1071	56	23	28	37	52	70	91	106
65-74 yr	1080	52	21	26	36	49	63	81	93

PROTEIN INTAKE (g/1000 kcal), AGES 6 MO–74 YR, UNITED STATES, 1976–80

Income Level, Sex, and Age	No. Examined	Mean	5th	10th	25th	50th	75th	90th	95th
					Percentile				
ALL INCOMES									
Male									
6 mo–74 yr	9981*	39	23	26	31	38	45	54	61
6-11 mo	179	41	21	23	34	42	46	56	62
1-2 yr	745	37	23	25	31	37	43	49	53
3-5 yr	1219	36	23	26	30	35	41	46	51
6-8 yr	428	37	24	27	31	37	42	48	51
9-11 yr	457	37	24	26	31	37	42	48	55
12-14 yr	504	37	23	26	30	36	43	49	54
15-17 yr	534†	39	22	26	31	38	46	54	61
18-24 yr	988	39	23	26	31	38	45	54	63
25-34 yr	1067	40	23	25	31	38	46	56	64
35-44 yr	745	40	23	26	31	39	46	55	62
45-54 yr	690	40	25	28	32	38	46	55	61
55-64 yr	1226†	41	24	27	33	40	47	56	66
65-74 yr	1199	41	25	28	33	40	47	55	62
Female									
6 mo–74 yr	10,337*	39	22	25	30	37	45	55	63
6-11 mo	177	39	21	23	31	40	48	55	59
1-2 yr	672	38	23	26	31	37	43	50	53
3-5 yr	1126	36	23	26	30	35	41	47	51
6-8 yr	415	36	22	25	30	35	40	46	50
9-11 yr	425	37	22	25	30	36	42	50	54
12-14 yr	487	36	22	24	30	35	42	48	53
15-17 yr	449	37	19	23	29	35	44	54	59
18-24 yr	1065†	39	21	24	30	37	45	55	62
25-34 yr	1169†	40	21	24	30	37	47	58	66
35-44 yr	844	40	23	25	30	38	46	58	63
45-54 yr	763	41	24	27	32	39	48	60	69
55-64 yr	1329	40	24	27	31	38	47	57	63
65-74 yr	1416	40	23	26	32	38	47	57	65
INCOME BELOW POVERTY LEVEL‡									
Male									
6 mo–74 yr	1538†	38	22	26	31	37	44	52	57
6-11 mo	48	—	—	—	34	39	45	—	—
1-2 yr	170	39	24	26	34	39	45	51	52
3-5 yr	298	35	24	26	29	35	41	46	51
6-8 yr	82	37	24	28	31	36	40	48	57
9-11 yr	88	38	23	26	31	37	42	49	57
12-14 yr	89	36	25	27	30	35	41	45	51
15-17 yr	89	39	18	26	31	36	45	54	62
18-24 yr	178	39	22	25	30	37	45	54	65
25-34 yr	91	37	14	21	30	36	43	51	57
35-44 yr	63	—	—	—	31	37	43	—	—
45-54 yr	46	—	—	—	32	36	43	—	—
55-64 yr	128†	38	21	23	28	38	45	54	56
65-74 yr	168	42	22	26	33	41	48	57	70

*Excludes two persons with 0 kcal.
†Excludes one person with 0 kcal.
‡Excludes persons with unknown income.

PROTEIN INTAKE (g/1000 kcal), AGES 6 MO–74 YR, UNITED STATES, 1976–80—cont'd

Income Level, Sex, and Age	No. Examined	Mean	5th	10th	25th	50th	75th	90th	95th
						Percentile			

Income Level, Sex, and Age	No. Examined	Mean	5th	10th	25th	50th	75th	90th	95th
INCOME BELOW POVERTY LEVEL‡—cont'd									
Female									
6 mo–74 yr	1909†	37	22	24	29	36	43	52	58
6-11 mo	36	—	—	—	—	32	—	—	—
1-2 yr	153	38	23	25	32	38	44	49	51
3-5 yr	272	37	24	2d	30	36	41	49	52
6-8 yr	95	35	23	26	29	35	40	46	49
9-11 yr	102	37	25	27	30	35	41	50	56
12-14 yr	104	34	18	21	27	33	42	48	51
15-17 yr	88	35	21	22	29	34	42	52	55
18-24 yr	252†	37	21	22	28	36	43	52	58
25-34 yr	162	39	22	23	29	36	48	56	63
35-44 yr	119	38	22	24	29	37	45	54	61
45-54 yr	82	37	23	25	28	35	42	57	67
55-64 yr	188	39	24	27	31	36	45	55	58
65-74 yr	256	40	23	26	32	38	46	55	63
INCOME ABOVE POVERTY LEVEL‡									
Male									
6 mo–74 yr	8083†	39	24	27	31	38	45	54	61
6-11 mo	121	41	18	23	33	43	47	59	63
1-2 yr	551	37	23	25	31	37	43	48	53
3-5 yr	892	36	23	25	30	35	41	56	51
6-8 yr	336	37	24	26	31	37	42	48	50
9-11 yr	356	37	24	26	31	37	42	47	52
12-14 yr	399	37	23	26	30	36	44	49	53
15-17 yr	417†	39	23	27	32	39	46	53	57
18-24 yr	770	39	23	27	31	38	45	55	63
25-34 yr	945	40	23	26	31	39	46	57	65
35-44 yr	658	40	23	26	31	39	46	55	62
45-54 yr	603	41	26	28	32	39	47	56	61
55-64 yr	1048	42	24	28	33	40	48	57	67
65-74 yr	987	40	25	28	33	40	47	55	61
Female									
6 mo–74 yr	8035†	39	22	25	31	37	45	55	63
6-11 mo	135	41	23	25	32	41	48	55	62
1-2 yr	505	37	23	26	31	37	43	50	54
3-5 yr	815	36	22	26	30	35	41	47	51
6-8 yr	308	36	22	25	30	35	40	46	50
9-11 yr	307	37	22	24	30	36	43	50	54
12-14 yr	363	36	23	25	30	35	42	48	53
15-17 yr	342	38	19	23	29	35	45	54	62
18-24 yr	771	39	21	24	30	37	46	56	63
25-34 yr	981†	40	21	25	30	37	47	58	67
35-44 yr	702	40	23	25	30	38	46	58	64
45-54 yr	655	42	24	27	33	39	49	61	70
55-64 yr	1071	40	24	26	31	38	46	57	63
65-74 yr	1080	40	23	26	31	38	47	57	66

CARBOHYDRATE INTAKE (g), AGES 6 MO–74 YR, UNITED STATES, 1976–80

| Income Level, Sex, and Age | No. Examined | Mean | Percentile | | | | | | |
			5th	10th	25th	50th	75th	90th	95th
ALL INCOMES									
Male									
6 mo–74 yr	9983	262	101	128	176	242	322	418	487
6-11 mo	179	130	67	76	92	121	157	198	226
1-2 yr	745	166	74	91	120	159	202	256	292
3-5 yr	1219	208	100	122	157	200	249	301	344
6-8 yr	428	244	130	154	194	239	284	341	394
9-11 yr	457	276	129	161	203	261	338	404	435
12-14 yr	504	299	133	155	205	289	367	450	522
15-17 yr	535	330	121	157	217	312	412	502	598
18-24 yr	988	321	122	154	213	294	391	514	600
25-34 yr	1067	291	120	147	200	263	357	458	540
35-44 yr	745	248	105	127	174	237	309	380	431
45-54 yr	690	244	100	123	167	228	291	374	434
55-64 yr	1227	216	82	109	150	205	272	340	387
65-74 yr	1199	204	72	97	141	193	253	316	366
Female									
6 mo–74 yr	10,339	185	70	89	125	172	230	295	343
6-11 mo	177	125	63	73	89	119	153	188	208
1-2 yr	672	158	71	87	109	142	191	240	270
3-5 yr	1126	191	94	114	141	181	229	284	322
6-8 yr	415	230	120	142	173	217	278	344	369
9-11 yr	425	233	122	136	179	221	278	336	365
12-14 yr	487	224	102	120	159	215	271	335	369
15-17 yr	449	205	78	103	133	190	265	337	383
18-24 yr	1066	197	67	90	129	185	254	326	358
25-34 yr	1170	187	67	86	126	173	228	298	354
35-44 yr	844	172	59	80	119	162	215	277	323
45-54 yr	763	159	64	77	107	150	201	251	280
55-64 yr	1329	161	63	83	110	152	198	247	300
65-74 yr	1416	158	64	81	111	151	194	244	284
INCOME BELOW POVERTY LEVEL*									
Male									
6 mo–74 yr	1539	248	80	111	163	227	312	401	472
6-11 mo	48	—	—	—	92	108	145	—	—
1-2 yr	170	155	61	83	100	156	191	237	277
3-5 yr	298	207	96	114	158	199	255	300	354
6-8 yr	82	246	102	131	180	236	298	361	449
9-11 yr	88	245	96	135	175	244	310	357	399
12-14 yr	89	268	112	138	175	253	333	428	462
15-17 yr	89	284	107	123	189	256	340	470	524
18-24 yr	178	312	134	158	208	285	378	503	586
25-34 yr	91	278	114	133	170	241	345	473	609
35-44 yr	63	—	—	—	127	225	283	—	—
45-54 yr	46	—	—	—	168	238	311	—	—
55-64 yr	129	202	58	73	126	196	268	339	399
65-74 yr	168	176	44	61	115	164	221	297	326

*Excludes persons with unknown income.

CARBOHYDRATE INTAKE (g), AGES 6 MO–74 YR, UNITED STATES, 1976–80

Income Level, Sex, and Age	No. Examined	Mean	Percentile						
			5th	10th	25th	50th	75th	90th	95th
INCOME BELOW POVERTY LEVEL*—cont'd									
Female									
6 mo–74 yr	1910	185	66	84	123	171	230	303	352
6-11 mo	36	—	—	—	—	119	—	—	—
1-2 yr	153	161	71	87	106	143	201	239	285
3-5 yr	272	191	79	100	135	174	241	316	354
6-8 yr	95	233	111	144	169	215	286	352	394
9-11 yr	102	221	100	135	175	211	279	331	345
12-14 yr	104	211	101	111	149	204	266	313	369
15-17 yr	88	207	89	111	146	189	274	314	383
18-24 yr	253	193	66	86	128	179	241	319	374
25-34 yr	162	196	74	89	132	173	239	312	434
35-44 yr	119	156	34	67	100	147	201	281	321
45-54 yr	82	148	44	74	98	137	193	235	279
55-64 yr	188	150	57	72	93	138	185	244	341
65-74 yr	256	154	49	69	103	146	193	254	283
INCOME ABOVE POVERTY LEVEL*									
Male									
6 mo–74 yr	8084	265	105	131	178	244	324	420	489
6-11 mo	121	134	67	79	93	129	164	200	247
1-2 yr	551	169	77	94	122	159	205	262	296
3-5 yr	892	210	104	125	159	201	249	302	341
6-8 yr	336	245	133	155	200	240	284	341	384
9-11 yr	356	282	136	164	207	269	341	405	448
12-14 yr	399	306	133	157	215	293	374	459	523
15-17 yr	418	340	128	164	230	324	420	516	619
18-24 yr	770	325	120	152	213	298	401	519	615
25-34 yr	945	292	123	150	202	264	357	456	529
35-44 yr	658	250	106	132	177	240	310	383	433
45-54 yr	603	246	98	123	165	230	293	380	447
55-64 yr	1048	216	84	111	150	204	271	338	382
65-74 yr	987	208	81	102	145	196	256	316	371
Female									
6 mo–74 yr	8036	185	71	90	125	172	230	294	340
6-11 mo	135	125	66	75	94	119	154	188	199
1-2 yr	505	158	71	87	110	143	191	240	260
3-5 yr	815	192	102	118	144	182	227	281	312
6-8 yr	308	229	120	142	176	217	277	337	368
9-11 yr	307	237	124	143	182	225	278	339	365
12-14 yr	363	229	102	126	169	220	276	339	373
15-17 yr	342	201	78	97	131	187	257	323	369
18-24 yr	771	199	67	91	129	188	258	326	357
25-34 yr	982	186	66	84	124	173	227	293	346
35-44 yr	702	174	62	83	120	163	218	278	325
45-54 yr	655	160	67	77	108	151	202	253	280
55-64 yr	1071	163	64	85	115	154	204	251	300
65-74 yr	1080	160	67	85	113	152	194	244	286

CARBOHYDRATE INTAKE (g/1000 kcal), AGES 6 MO–74 YR, UNITED STATES, 1976–80

Income Level, Sex, and Age	No. Examined	Mean	Percentile							
			5th	10th	25th	50th	75th	90th	95th
ALL INCOMES									
Male									
6 mo–74 yr	9981*	113	69	79	95	113	130	146	156
6-11 mo	179	131	91	99	113	129	150	167	178
1-2 yr	745	128	83	95	110	128	144	160	170
3-5 yr	1219	129	91	100	115	129	143	157	165
6-8 yr	428	125	92	99	109	125	138	152	159
9-11 yr	457	126	92	99	113	127	140	154	163
12-14 yr	504	124	82	93	109	124	140	157	165
15-17 yr	534†	119	80	89	102	118	134	150	160
18-24 yr	988	109	68	77	92	109	125	138	149
25-34 yr	1067	108	64	74	90	109	125	141	150
35-44 yr	745	104	62	74	87	104	123	137	146
45-54 yr	690	105	64	73	87	105	122	136	148
55-64 yr	1226	106	62	71	88	107	124	137	145
65-74 yr	1199	112	65	78	96	113	130	147	158
Female									
6 mo–74 yr	10,337*	118	71	84	101	119	136	152	162
6-11 mo	177	128	93	98	112	127	144	157	168
1-2 yr	672	126	83	92	108	124	143	160	170
3-5 yr	1126	128	91	99	112	127	142	158	169
6-8 yr	415	127	92	100	114	127	141	154	161
9-11 yr	425	126	93	100	112	126	139	151	161
12-14 yr	487	125	87	93	110	125	142	155	166
15-17 yr	449	120	78	86	101	121	137	153	166
18-24 yr	1065†	118	72	83	100	119	137	151	161
25-34 yr	1169†	115	67	82	98	115	132	149	161
35-44 yr	844	110	60	73	93	112	129	147	157
45-54 yr	763	112	64	75	93	112	130	148	161
55-64 yr	1329	117	70	84	99	117	135	151	159
65-74 yr	1416	123	74	86	105	124	141	158	170
INCOME BELOW POVERTY LEVEL‡									
Male									
6 mo–74 yr	1538†	115	70	80	98	115	132	150	158
6-11 mo	48	—	—	—	102	127	145	—	—
1-2 yr	170	121	80	92	103	118	134	154	168
3-5 yr	298	125	86	96	111	123	139	154	167
6-8 yr	82	123	87	99	107	121	143	152	158
9-11 yr	88	125	85	92	108	128	140	157	163
12-14 yr	89	121	82	94	102	121	136	150	158
15-17 yr	89	114	72	80	96	116	132	149	153
18-24 yr	178	110	69	72	91	110	126	147	157
25-34 yr	91	109	60	76	97	107	127	149	153
35-44 yr	63	—	—	—	89	108	131	—	—
45-54 yr	46	—	—	—	92	107	126	—	—
55-64 yr	128²	109	64	74	92	112	128	138	157
65-74 yr	168	109	51	67	88	111	133	149	171

*Excludes two persons with 0 kcal.

†Excludes one person with 0 kcal.

‡Excludes persons with unknown income.

CARBOHYDRATE INTAKE (g/1000 kcal), AGES 6 MO–74 YR, UNITED STATES, 1976–80—cont'd

Income Level, Sex, and Age	No. Examined	Mean	Percentile						
			5th	10th	25th	50th	75th	90th	95th
INCOME BELOW POVERTY LEVEL‡—cont'd									
Female									
6 mo–74 yr	1909†	120	76	85	103	120	138	153	167
6-11 mo	36	—	—	—	—	125	—	—	—
1-2 yr	153	119	84	88	104	116	132	150	165
3-5 yr	272	122	78	91	107	122	136	151	163
6-8 yr	95	125	92	98	112	126	138	149	153
9-11 yr	102	125	92	97	109	125	136	147	163
12-14 yr	104	125	83	93	107	125	141	157	168
15-17 yr	88	121	71	80	95	123	142	149	176
18-24 yr	252†	122	77	88	106	121	141	157	170
25-34 yr	162	117	77	83	98	115	133	150	167
35-44 yr	119	111	59	71	89	109	137	150	172
45-54 yr	82	113	69	77	97	115	129	140	172
55-64 yr	188	119	76	82	103	118	139	153	172
65-74 yr	256	126	74	87	105	127	146	165	175
INCOME ABOVE POVERTY LEVEL‡									
Male									
6 mo–74 yr	8083†	112	68	79	95	113	130	145	156
6-11 mo	121	134	99	104	115	129	151	167	183
1-2 yr	551	129	84	97	112	130	147	161	170
3-5 yr	892	130	94	102	117	130	144	158	165
6-8 yr	336	125	92	98	110	125	137	152	159
9-11 yr	356	127	96	101	114	128	139	154	163
12-14 yr	399	126	82	93	110	124	141	158	167
15-17 yr	417†	119	86	89	104	119	134	150	162
18-24 yr	770	108	66	77	92	109	125	137	148
25-34 yr	945	107	65	75	90	109	125	139	149
35-44 yr	658	104	62	74	87	103	123	137	145
45-54 yr	603	105	63	73	87	105	122	138	149
55-64 yr	1048	105	60	71	87	106	123	136	144
65-74 yr	987	113	67	79	97	113	130	147	158
Female									
6 mo–74 yr	8035†	118	70	84	100	119	136	152	162
6-11 mo	135	129	93	98	113	129	146	158	176
1-2 yr	505	127	83	93	109	127	145	161	170
3-5 yr	815	129	94	101	113	129	144	159	170
6-8 yr	308	128	92	100	114	128	141	155	162
9-11 yr	307	126	93	101	113	127	140	153	161
12-14 yr	363	125	87	93	110	125	142	155	165
15-17 yr	342	120	78	89	101	121	136	154	166
18-24 yr	771	117	71	81	99	118	136	149	159
25-34 yr	981†	114	65	81	97	115	132	149	160
35-44 yr	702	110	60	74	93	112	128	147	155
45-54 yr	655	112	65	75	93	112	130	149	162
55-64 yr	1071	116	69	84	99	117	134	152	159
65-74 yr	1080	123	74	86	105	123	140	157	169

FAT INTAKE (g), AGES 6 MO–74 YR, UNITED STATES, 1976–80

Income Level, Sex, and Age	No. Examined	Mean	5th	10th	25th	50th	75th	90th	95th
			\multicolumn{7}{c}{Percentile}
ALL INCOMES									
Male									
6 mo–74 yr	9983	98	32	42	60	87	123	165	199
6-11 mo	179	36	10	15	22	33	44	62	76
1-2 yr	745	52	19	25	35	48	62	84	99
3-5 yr	1219	64	26	33	45	59	78	101	117
6-8 yr	428	81	38	44	58	76	96	125	137
9-11 yr	457	86	40	48	62	80	103	131	151
12-14 yr	504	99	36	44	62	90	125	165	193
15-17 yr	535	116	38	50	72	107	143	196	236
18-24 yr	988	124	38	50	75	108	152	208	264
25-34 yr	1067	111	37	47	71	103	141	179	214
35-44 yr	745	103	39	48	64	93	129	165	192
45-54 yr	690	99	32	44	64	91	125	164	194
55-64 yr	1227	86	29	40	56	79	105	141	167
65-74 yr	1199	75	27	34	49	68	93	121	141
Female									
6 mo–74 yr	10,339	64	21	28	41	59	81	105	124
6-11 mo	177	38	11	17	26	36	46	62	70
1-2 yr	672	50	19	24	35	46	62	80	91
3-5 yr	1126	60	25	31	42	56	74	93	105
6-8 yr	415	72	34	40	53	69	88	104	115
9-11 yr	425	75	34	41	53	71	91	116	134
12-14 yr	487	74	28	35	48	69	93	120	140
15-17 yr	449	73	21	32	46	68	92	120	145
18-24 yr	1066	67	18	27	42	62	85	110	127
25-34 yr	1170	68	21	28	42	63	84	112	130
35-44 yr	844	66	22	30	42	60	82	105	131
45-54 yr	763	60	19	26	38	54	74	98	109
55-64 yr	1329	57	18	23	35	52	73	95	113
65-74 yr	1416	50	16	23	33	46	62	81	99
INCOME BELOW POVERTY LEVEL*									
Male									
6 mo–74 yr	1539	92	23	35	53	78	115	164	196
6-11 mo	48	54	—	—	23	34	47	—	—
1-2 yr	170	71	19	22	36	50	67	89	101
3-5 yr	298	80	26	35	50	65	88	110	137
6-8 yr	82	81	42	46	59	78	93	121	138
9-11 yr	88	97	21	40	59	74	95	128	145
12-14 yr	89	110	34	41	58	84	124	174	197
15-17 yr	89	124	31	38	64	98	142	182	236
18-24 yr	178	103	32	45	68	103	162	209	287
25-34 yr	91	—	20	47	64	89	142	180	220
35-44 yr	63	—	—	—	48	70	113	—	—
45-54 yr	46	77	—	—	61	93	141	—	—
55-64 yr	129	66	17	21	44	71	99	126	157
65-74 yr	168		18	23	42	61	80	105	135

*Excludes persons with unknown income.

FAT INTAKE (g), AGES 6 MO–74 YR, UNITED STATES, 1976–80—cont'd

| Income Level, Sex, and Age | No. Examined | Mean | Percentile | | | | | | |
			5th	10th	25th	50th	75th	90th	95th
INCOME BELOW POVERTY LEVEL*—cont'd									
Female									
6 mo–74 yr	1910	64	18	26	39	58	82	108	133
6-11 mo	36	—	—	—	—	38	—	—	—
1-2 yr	153	58	19	28	40	54	68	92	104
3-5 yr	272	66	23	35	45	62	80	100	119
6-8 yr	95	76	37	40	55	75	93	108	140
9-11 yr	102	74	27	35	47	69	93	114	133
12-14 yr	104	72	32	34	46	62	89	115	155
15-17 yr	88	78	26	36	48	71	96	137	142
18-24 yr	253	63	17	21	38	58	83	103	120
25-34 yr	162	71	18	26	43	63	83	126	155
35-44 yr	119	63	11	21	35	53	79	118	164
45-54 yr	82	59	14	23	36	55	79	90	107
55-64 yr	188	52	16	21	32	47	65	84	99
65-74 yr	256	46	14	18	30	43	57	75	91
INCOME ABOVE POVERTY LEVEL*									
Male									
6 mo–74 yr	8084	99	33	42	60	88	124	165	201
6-11 mo	121	35	8	12	22	32	44	62	75
1-2 yr	551	51	20	25	34	47	62	82	96
3-5 yr	892	63	26	34	44	58	75	101	111
6-8 yr	336	81	38	44	58	76	96	125	137
9-11 yr	356	87	42	49	63	81	103	131	151
12-14 yr	399	99	36	44	62	92	125	165	195
15-17 yr	418	119	41	51	74	109	143	202	236
18-24 yr	770	124	38	50	76	109	150	208	262
25-34 yr	945	112	38	47	73	103	142	178	214
35-44 yr	658	106	41	50	67	95	132	170	198
45-54 yr	603	99	32	44	64	91	125	165	196
55-64 yr	1048	87	30	40	57	81	105	144	169
65-74 yr	987	76	29	35	49	69	95	122	141
Female									
6 mo–74 yr	8036	64	21	28	41	59	81	105	123
6-11 mo	135	36	11	17	25	35	45	61	68
1-2 yr	505	49	18	23	33	44	61	77	87
3-5 yr	815	59	25	31	42	55	71	89	102
6-8 yr	308	71	34	41	52	67	87	104	114
9-11 yr	307	75	36	43	54	72	90	116	134
12-14 yr	363	75	28	36	50	71	94	120	138
15-17 yr	342	71	19	31	46	67	90	118	132
18-24 yr	771	68	20	28	43	64	86	111	127
25-34 yr	982	67	21	28	42	63	84	112	129
35-44 yr	702	67	24	31	42	62	82	105	126
45-54 yr	655	60	20	27	39	54	74	98	109
55-64 yr	1071	58	19	24	36	53	74	96	115
65-74 yr	1080	51	17	23	34	47	63	83	100

FAT INTAKE (g/1000 kcal), AGES 6 MO–74 YR, UNITED STATES, 1976–80

Income Level, Sex, and Age	No. Examined	Mean	Percentile						
			5th	10th	25th	50th	75th	90th	95th
ALL INCOMES									
Male									
6 mo–74 yr	9981*	40	25	29	34	40	47	52	56
6-11 mo	179	35	13	21	27	35	43	48	51
1-2 yr	745	39	23	27	32	39	45	51	55
3-5 yr	1219	39	26	29	34	39	44	49	53
6-8 yr	428	40	27	31	35	40	45	50	53
9-11 yr	457	39	27	30	34	39	45	49	52
12-14 yr	504	40	26	28	34	40	46	52	55
15-17 yr	534†	41	28	30	35	41	46	52	55
18-24 yr	988	40	24	27	34	40	46	52	56
25-34 yr	1067	40	24	28	34	40	47	53	56
35-44 yr	745	42	26	29	36	42	48	53	56
45-54 yr	690	41	25	29	35	41	48	54	58
55-64 yr	1226²	41	24	28	35	41	47	53	57
65-74 yr	1199	41	24	27	34	41	46	53	57
Female									
6 mo–74 yr	10,337*	40	23	28	34	40	46	52	56
6-11 mo	177	37	22	24	30	39	45	49	51
1-2 yr	672	39	23	27	33	40	45	51	55
3-5 yr	1126	39	26	28	34	39	45	50	53
6-8 yr	415	40	28	30	35	40	45	49	52
9-11 yr	425	40	27	30	35	40	45	50	53
12-14 yr	487	40	26	29	35	40	46	51	55
15-17 yr	449	41	24	29	35	42	48	54	57
18-24 yr	1065†	39	22	26	33	39	46	52	55
25-34 yr	1169†	40	22	28	34	41	46	53	57
35-44 yr	844	41	24	28	35	41	47	53	57
45-54 yr	763	40	23	28	34	41	47	53	57
55-64 yr	1329	39	22	27	32	40	46	53	57
65-74 yr	1416	38	21	26	31	38	44	51	55
INCOME BELOW POVERTY LEVEL‡									
Male									
6 mo–74 yr	1538†	40	25	28	34	41	47	53	56
6-11 mo	48	—	—	—	29	38	46	—	—
1-2 yr	170	41	24	29	35	41	48	52	55
3-5 yr	298	41	26	29	36	41	46	53	55
6-8 yr	82	41	31	31	34	41	46	50	51
9-11 yr	88	40	27	29	34	40	46	50	55
12-14 yr	89	42	27	30	35	43	50	53	56
15-17 yr	89	42	26	31	36	43	48	53	58
18-24 yr	178	40	25	28	32	40	47	52	58
25-34 yr	91	39	20	26	33	39	46	54	58
35-44 yr	63	—	—	—	29	40	48	—	—
45-54 yr	46	—	—	—	33	45	48	—	—
55-64 yr	128†	41	21	27	35	41	49	55	56
65-74 yr	168	41	14	25	34	41	47	55	62

*Excludes two persons with 0 kcal.

†Excludes one person with 0 kcal.

‡Excludes persons with unknown income.

FAT INTAKE (g/1000 kcal), AGES 6 MO–74 YR, UNITED STATES, 1976–80—cont'd

Income Level, Sex, and Age	No. Examined	Mean	Percentile						
			5th	10th	25th	50th	75th	90th	95th
INCOME BELOW POVERTY LEVEL‡—cont'd									
Female									
6 mo–74 yr	1909†	40	24	28	34	41	47	53	57
6-11 mo	36	—	—	—	—	42	—	—	—
1-2 yr	153	42	24	30	36	42	48	53	55
3-5 yr	272	41	28	31	36	42	47	53	55
6-8 yr	95	41	29	32	37	40	46	49	51
9-11 yr	102	40	26	29	36	41	45	51	53
12-14 yr	104	41	28	30	36	41	47	52	54
15-17 yr	88	42	25	29	35	41	51	56	58
18-24 yr	252†	38	20	24	31	39	45	52	55
25-34 yr	162	40	24	29	35	41	48	52	55
35-44 yr	119	42	20	27	34	44	49	54	59
45-54 yr	82	43	24	29	36	44	50	58	63
55-64 yr	188	40	23	29	33	40	47	54	59
65-74 yr	256	38	22	24	29	37	45	53	57
INCOME ABOVE POVERTY LEVEL†									
Male									
6 mo–74 yr	8083†	40	25	29	34	40	46	52	56
6-11 mo	121	34	10	20	26	34	42	47	49
1-2 yr	551	38	23	27	32	39	44	51	55
3-5 yr	892	38	26	29	33	38	43	48	51
6-8 yr	336	40	27	32	35	40	45	50	54
9-11 yr	356	39	27	30	34	39	44	49	52
12-14 yr	399	39	25	28	33	40	45	52	55
15-17 yr	417†	41	28	30	35	41	46	51	54
18-24 yr	770	40	23	27	34	40	46	52	56
25-34 yr	945	40	24	28	34	41	47	52	56
35-44 yr	658	42	26	30	36	42	48	53	56
45-54 yr	603	41	25	29	35	41	48	53	58
55-64 yr	1048	41	24	29	35	41	47	52	57
65-74 yr	987	41	25	27	34	41	46	53	57
Female									
6 mo–74 yr	8035†	40	23	28	34	40	46	52	56
6-11 mo	135	36	18	24	29	38	44	48	50
1-2 yr	505	39	22	27	32	39	45	51	55
3-5 yr	815	39	25	28	34	39	44	49	52
6-8 yr	308	39	28	30	34	40	44	49	52
9-11 yr	307	40	28	30	34	39	45	50	53
12-14 yr	363	40	26	29	35	40	45	51	56
15-17 yr	342	41	24	29	35	42	47	54	57
18-24 yr	771	39	22	27	33	39	46	51	55
25-34 yr	981†	40	22	28	34	40	46	53	57
35-44 yr	702	41	24	28	35	41	47	53	57
45-54 yr	655	40	22	28	34	40	47	53	56
55-64 yr	1071	39	22	26	32	40	46	53	57
65-74 yr	1080	38	21	26	32	38	44	51	54

CALCIUM INTAKE (mg), AGES 6 MO–74 YR, UNITED STATES, 1976–80

Income Level, Sex, and Age	No. Examined	Mean	5th	10th	25th	50th	75th	90th	95th
						Percentile			
ALL INCOMES									
Male									
6 mo–74 yr	9983	979	220	303	511	829	1283	1786	2209
6-11 mo	179	951	311	409	602	912	1170	1613	1945
1-2 yr	745	786	216	285	454	714	1016	1374	1588
3-5 yr	1219	843	245	326	527	777	1086	1449	1684
6-8 yr	428	1074	417	513	710	1019	1346	1662	1971
9-11 yr	457	1116	348	466	732	1048	1423	1843	2189
12-14 yr	504	1176	288	426	703	1025	1508	2068	2464
15-17 yr	535	1333	244	371	729	1178	1720	2519	3254
18-24 yr	988	1215	215	352	605	1001	1547	2211	2984
25-34 yr	1067	968	214	281	453	805	1266	1835	2275
35-44 yr	745	858	193	264	466	716	1143	1597	1984
45-54 yr	690	841	216	294	456	733	1126	1545	1778
55-64 yr	1227	804	193	270	426	685	1053	1437	1806
65-74 yr	1199	698	186	241	370	597	915	1310	1564
Female									
6 mo–74 yr	10,339	679	146	198	337	574	907	1281	1554
6-11 mo	177	910	264	366	561	900	1199	1466	1674
1-2 yr	672	753	220	290	454	701	966	1245	1493
3-5 yr	1126	791	229	305	488	730	1029	1355	1527
6-8 yr	415	978	276	434	646	924	1230	1574	1751
9-11 yr	425	944	276	383	574	844	1227	1619	1915
12-14 yr	487	859	201	274	495	793	1140	1552	1740
15-17 yr	449	764	115	197	392	622	1000	1450	1747
18-24 yr	1066	679	126	178	313	565	915	1301	1670
25-34 yr	1170	636	137	178	295	535	858	1219	1511
35-44 yr	844	603	135	186	289	508	768	1144	1402
45-54 yr	763	576	135	190	299	474	735	1075	1261
55-64 yr	1329	561	140	178	275	475	743	1060	1250
65-74 yr	1416	542	141	181	298	475	714	1004	1156
INCOME BELOW POVERTY LEVEL*									
Male									
6 mo–74 yr	1539	956	176	254	480	826	1243	1721	2143
6-11 mo	48	—	—	—	512	748	991	—	—
1-2 yr	170	786	180	248	458	710	970	1459	1706
3-5 yr	298	811	210	310	509	754	1047	1382	1570
6-8 yr	82	1040	257	473	785	1018	1368	1616	1776
9-11 yr	88	1008	338	469	676	959	1263	1581	1923
12-14 yr	89	1025	286	374	642	885	1260	2053	2155
15-17 yr	89	992	161	181	367	936	1433	1934	2188
18-24 yr	178	1298	162	315	586	970	1642	2715	3428
25-34 yr	91	876	169	238	303	733	1158	1694	2186
35-44 yr	63	—	—	—	344	599	849	—	—
45-54 yr	46	—	—	—	478	860	1414	—	—
55-64 yr	129	709	135	225	340	638	965	1289	1595
65-74 yr	168	673	119	186	297	595	893	1355	1560

*Excludes persons with unknown income.

CALCIUM INTAKE (mg), AGES 6 MO–74 YR, UNITED STATES, 1976–80—cont'd

Income Level, Sex, and Age	No. Examined	Mean	Percentile						
			5th	10th	25th	50th	75th	90th	95th
INCOME BELOW POVERTY LEVEL*—cont'd									
Female									
6 mo–74 yr	1910	642	120	169	303	543	867	1221	1514
6-11 mo	36	—	—	—	—	734	—	—	—
1-2 yr	153	781	208	256	389	689	1029	1285	1784
3-5 yr	272	773	232	293	432	713	1038	1361	1559
6-8 yr	95	948	297	381	642	899	1175	1521	1840
9-11 yr	102	865	302	339	543	806	1098	1492	1557
12-14 yr	104	706	173	264	392	591	978	1450	1627
15-17 yr	88	623	75	145	302	519	841	1177	1515
18-24 yr	253	612	128	169	305	494	812	1151	1511
25-34 yr	162	627	118	162	256	444	763	1413	1737
35-44 yr	119	501	74	108	185	393	703	957	1241
45-54 yr	82	495	104	147	229	428	681	995	1150
55-64 yr	188	521	115	156	266	388	708	1061	1251
65-74 yr	256	540	110	160	252	477	751	1031	1258
INCOME ABOVE POVERTY LEVEL*									
Male									
6 mo–74 yr	8084	986	229	313	514	835	1290	1801	2232
6-11 mo	221	1000	311	390	690	961	1297	1749	1991
1-2 yr	551	789	224	291	454	716	1022	1324	1567
3-5 yr	892	853	250	335	535	780	1099	1457	1697
6-8 yr	336	1086	446	531	710	1020	1339	1669	2033
9-11 yr	356	1137	350	454	743	1089	1460	1857	2219
12-14 yr	399	1208	291	435	716	1045	1615	2094	2514
15-17 yr	418	1420	299	444	776	1237	1829	2705	3284
18-24 yr	770	1192	222	352	600	1007	1528	2167	2808
25-34 yr	945	979	216	293	465	816	1286	1846	2293
35-44 yr	658	881	215	284	476	744	1168	1620	2076
45-54 yr	603	846	220	298	459	731	1130	1560	1780
55-64 yr	1048	807	205	280	426	686	1046	1445	1839
65-74 yr	987	699	197	245	375	597	914	1300	1563
Female									
6 mo–74 yr	8036	687	150	201	345	583	913	1289	1564
6-11 mo	135	954	271	497	627	929	1215	1467	1693
1-2 yr	505	745	222	304	457	700	935	1233	1438
3-5 yr	815	800	240	315	499	731	1029	1359	1527
6-8 yr	308	983	276	440	646	941	1243	1541	1689
9-11 yr	307	968	276	397	593	860	1275	1665	2022
12-14 yr	363	900	203	324	535	839	1175	1589	1749
15-17 yr	342	791	119	199	403	656	1019	1470	1804
18-24 yr	771	699	126	178	313	576	949	1379	1700
25-34 yr	982	636	137	179	301	547	858	1217	1486
35-44 yr	702	619	149	200	306	528	779	1163	1448
45-54 yr	655	585	138	195	309	474	757	1077	1297
55-64 yr	1071	571	146	181	288	490	751	1062	1255
65-74 yr	1080	541	147	188	305	473	708	984	1137

IRON INTAKE (mg), AGES 6 MO–74 YR, UNITED STATES, 1976–80

Income Level, Sex, and Age	No. Examined	Mean	Percentile						
			5th	10th	25th	50th	75th	90th	95th
ALL INCOMES									
Male									
6 mo–74 yr	9983	15.54	5.54	6.96	9.72	13.77	19.23	25.54	31.03
6-11 mo	179	12.81	2.23	2.58	4.26	8.25	17.90	30.50	43.79
1-2 yr	745	8.66	2.84	3.64	5.22	7.45	10.61	14.72	18.79
3-5 yr	1219	10.51	4.23	5.20	6.99	9.23	12.91	16.99	20.45
6-8 yr	428	12.53	5.46	6.56	8.76	11.43	15.42	19.70	21.34
9-11 yr	457	14.44	5.93	7.17	9.09	13.12	17.93	25.00	28.18
12-14 yr	504	15.88	6.19	7.47	9.89	14.37	20.08	25.28	32.88
15-17 yr	535	17.45	5.64	7.23	10.56	15.01	20.84	31.47	37.54
18-24 yr	988	17.78	6.32	7.66	10.94	15.71	21.72	29.06	34.95
25-34 yr	1067	17.32	6.71	8.02	11.25	15.60	20.87	28.67	33.53
35-44 yr	745	16.06	6.55	7.90	10.77	14.68	19.57	25.65	30.68
45-54 yr	690	16.22	6.41	8.09	11.23	14.53	19.63	25.76	31.67
55-64 yr	1227	14.77	5.98	7.29	10.06	13.40	17.99	23.49	27.81
65-74 yr	1199	14.10	5.49	6.72	9.13	12.31	17.05	22.68	27.92
Female									
6 mo–74 yr	10,339	10.61	3.91	4.95	6.92	9.55	12.83	17.14	20.62
6-11 mo	177	12.88	2.21	3.37	4.83	9.36	15.80	26.90	40.18
1-2 yr	672	8.48	2.96	3.60	5.06	7.02	9.92	14.03	18.54
3-5 yr	1126	9.51	3.56	4.59	6.39	8.58	11.59	15.21	18.65
6-8 yr	415	10.85	4.92	5.91	7.84	10.09	12.78	15.75	18.84
9-11 yr	425	11.45	5.02	5.81	7.48	10.23	14.19	18.55	22.46
12-14 yr	487	10.77	4.10	5.28	6.78	9.91	12.94	17.79	21.01
15-17 yr	499	9.86	3.67	4.37	6.26	9.41	12.12	15.59	18.84
18-24 yr	1066	10.55	3.50	4.61	6.78	9.72	13.15	17.26	20.57
25-34 yr	1170	10.90	3.96	4.88	6.99	9.74	13.21	18.04	21.08
35-44 yr	844	11.23	4.17	5.32	7.52	10.02	13.09	17.58	22.72
45-54 yr	763	10.44	4.16	5.49	7.34	9.53	12.81	16.37	18.91
55-64 yr	1329	10.69	3.96	5.18	7.07	9.37	13.22	17.41	21.02
65-74 yr	1416	10.22	4.28	5.09	6.63	9.05	12.20	16.77	19.81
INCOME BELOW POVERTY LEVEL*									
Male									
6 mo–74 yr	1539	14.04	4.12	5.72	8.25	12.16	17.84	23.35	29.07
6-11 mo	48	—	—	—	4.20	8.34	14.90	—	—
1-2 yr	170	8.45	2.35	3.39	4.92	7.27	10.64	15.60	19.72
3-5 yr	298	10.86	4.14	5.10	7.00	9.47	13.09	18.14	21.54
6-8 yr	82	12.38	4.54	5.67	8.67	11.44	15.24	19.49	20.25
9-11 yr	88	12.51	4.17	6.34	7.63	11.66	15.21	21.33	23.17
12-14 yr	89	14.35	5.77	6.31	8.13	11.66	17.52	23.93	31.53
15-17 yr	89	15.50	5.26	6.58	10.19	14.34	19.69	26.01	30.39
18-24 yr	178	17.45	5.52	6.62	10.41	15.85	21.51	25.74	34.64
25-34 yr	91	15.95	5.91	6.44	9.96	15.24	19.76	25.16	33.59
35-44 yr	63	—	—	—	—	7.90	11.94	19.19	—	—
45-54 yr	46	—	—	—	—	11.12	15.45	18.03	—	—
55-64 yr	129	12.38	3.30	5.27	8.08	11.13	14.74	21.26	24.95
65-74 yr	168	11.42	3.48	4.77	7.36	10.40	14.53	18.93	21.75

*Excludes persons with unknown income.

IRON INTAKE (mg), AGES 6 MO–74 YR, UNITED STATES, 1976–80—cont'd

Income Level, Sex, and Age	No. Examined	Mean	Percentile						
			5th	10th	25th	50th	75th	90th	95th
INCOME BELOW POVERTY LEVEL*—cont'd									
Female									
6 mo–74 yr	1910	9.99	3.35	4.33	6.26	8.83	12.28	16.17	20.33
6-11 mo	36	—	—	—	—	7.82	—	—	—
1-2 yr	153	8.64	2.79	3.40	5.02	7.12	10.25	14.65	19.79
3-5 yr	272	10.10	2.72	4.41	6.35	9.05	12.30	17.26	22.01
6-8 yr	905	11.07	4.34	5.48	7.63	9.79	13.18	15.64	17.27
9-11 yr	102	11.04	4.67	5.70	6.89	9.63	13.85	17.75	23.76
12-14 yr	104	10.09	4.10	4.70	6.46	8.49	12.27	16.27	22.27
15-17 yr	88	10.22	3.98	4.95	6.77	9.82	12.38	15.62	18.05
18-24 yr	253	9.62	2.88	3.83	6.14	8.80	11.87	15.62	20.32
25-34 yr	162	11.10	3.39	4.50	6.38	10.26	13.94	18.05	21.26
35-44 yr	119	9.34	3.19	4.15	6.03	8.61	12.10	15.09	17.21
45-54 yr	82	8.74	3.17	4.49	6.04	8.41	10.69	14.64	15.53
55-64 yr	188	9.83	3.83	3.96	5.53	7.80	12.06	16.62	21.74
65-74 yr	256	9.59	3.77	4.34	6.05	7.96	11.39	16.64	22.87
INCOME ABOVE POVERTY LEVEL*									
Male									
6 mo–74 yr	8084	15.80	5.79	7.19	9.95	14.01	19.39	26.02	31.58
6-11 mo	121	13.67	2.40	2.88	4.41	9.03	18.40	31.35	45.94
1-2 yr	551	8.78	3.05	3.89	5.27	7.51	10.62	14.69	18.25
3-5 yr	892	10.47	4.24	5.23	7.00	9.22	12.77	16.77	19.96
6-8 yr	336	12.67	5.87	6.86	8.84	11.52	15.48	19.94	21.67
9-11 yr	356	14.85	5.94	7.31	9.35	13.45	18.71	25.18	29.03
12-14 yr	399	16.23	6.03	7.65	10.43	14.88	20.12	25.33	32.92
15-17 yr	418	17.99	5.64	7.23	10.81	15.47	21.48	33.13	38.14
18-24 yr	770	17.88	6.52	7.95	11.04	15.60	21.81	29.37	35.11
25-34 yr	945	17.48	6.76	8.04	11.48	15.72	20.90	28.77	33.63
35-44 yr	658	16.27	7.05	8.12	10.87	15.01	19.78	25.86	30.68
45-54 yr	603	16.34	6.45	8.08	11.24	14.48	19.84	25.78	31.22
55-64 yr	1048	15.00	6.19	7.37	10.09	13.58	18.21	23.77	28.26
65-74 yr	987	14.46	5.88	7.01	9.38	12.53	17.30	23.28	28.31
Female									
6 mo–74 yr	8036	10.72	4.02	5.09	7.06	9.67	12.90	17.29	20.85
6-11 mo	135	13.42	2.19	3.44	5.13	9.37	17.55	28.43	40.18
1-2 yr	505	8.42	3.07	3.60	5.07	7.05	9.83	13.87	18.11
3-5 yr	815	9.39	3.67	4.66	6.45	8.48	11.36	15.15	17.85
6-8 yr	308	10.73	4.98	5.90	7.84	10.08	12.53	15.46	18.83
9-11 yr	307	11.64	5.05	6.06	7.80	10.43	14.76	18.60	22.14
12-14 yr	363	10.98	4.05	5.62	7.13	10.01	13.12	17.55	20.15
15-17 yr	342	9.64	3.37	4.27	6.10	9.21	12.00	15.41	18.83
18-24 yr	771	10.83	3.64	4.85	6.95	9.95	13.51	17.67	21.44
25-34 yr	982	10.87	4.05	4.93	7.02	9.70	13.16	17.87	21.07
35-44 yr	702	11.45	4.56	5.54	7.66	10.19	13.14	18.20	22.84
45-54 yr	655	10.63	4.23	5.61	7.48	9.67	12.88	16.68	19.17
55-64 yr	1071	10.86	4.41	5.44	7.38	9.57	13.39	17.44	21.18
65-74 yr	1080	10.37	4.41	5.32	6.81	9.25	12.25	16.81	19.62

SODIUM INTAKE (mg), AGES 6 MO–74 YR, UNITED STATES, 1976–80

Income Level, Sex, and Age	No. Examined	Mean	5th	10th	25th	50th	75th	90th	95th
					Percentile				
ALL INCOMES									
Male									
6 mo–74 yr	9983	3340	1073	1377	2003	2922	4126	5773	7077
6-11 mo	179	1069	360	448	651	920	1319	1829	2308
1-2 yr	745	1902	745	899	1252	1709	2292	3219	3822
3-5 yr	1219	2253	853	1094	1522	2023	2736	3640	4322
6-8 yr	428	2683	1236	1486	1823	2572	3301	3954	4775
9-11 yr	457	3079	1442	1587	2065	2885	3666	4620	5481
12-14 yr	504	3301	1264	1551	2131	3093	4081	5337	6368
15-17 yr	535	3803	1192	1499	2205	3241	4840	7058	8320
18-24 yr	988	4084	1250	1640	2427	3521	5193	7001	8349
25-34 yr	1067	3738	1226	1527	2254	3261	4720	6500	7989
35-44 yr	745	3401	1081	1432	2137	3035	4151	5639	7063
45-54 yr	690	3549	1129	1575	2216	3110	4509	6065	7385
55-64 yr	1227	3049	1030	1339	2006	2790	3829	5069	5732
65-74 yr	1199	2894	1047	1331	1844	2583	3596	4780	5603
Female									
6 mo–74 yr	10,339	2298	729	945	1411	2060	2902	3927	4617
6-11 mo	177	1022	299	342	545	865	1246	1696	2473
1-2 yr	672	1751	613	839	1149	1541	2184	2865	3419
3-5 yr	1126	2089	864	1013	1416	1937	2609	3364	3826
6-8 yr	415	2510	1089	1301	1770	2290	3113	3966	4342
9-11 yr	425	2577	1069	1368	1754	2318	3176	4307	4912
12-14 yr	487	2567	883	1111	1632	2318	3208	4167	5048
15-17 yr	449	2405	657	911	1460	2116	3067	4249	5096
18-24 yr	1066	2383	649	944	1445	2173	3041	4127	4873
25-34 yr	1170	2401	756	927	1429	2139	3053	4148	4848
35-44 yr	844	2380	764	972	1408	2068	3028	4020	4998
45-54 yr	763	2182	701	880	1366	1955	2682	3742	4431
55-64 yr	1329	2186	717	909	1384	1965	2715	3716	4399
65-74 yr	1416	1988	678	899	1269	1812	2425	3331	3891
INCOME BELOW POVERTY LEVEL*									
Male									
6 mo–74 yr	1539	3122	701	1098	1722	2737	3915	5554	6780
6-11 mo	48	1813	—	—	528	779	1508	—	—
1-2 yr	170	2360	586	796	1107	1670	2167	3268	3789
3-5 yr	298	2699	884	1137	1524	2016	2942	4114	5113
6-8 yr	82	2715	1042	1147	2035	2681	3348	3918	4275
9-11 yr	88	3026	1001	1249	1727	2523	3352	4294	4943
12-14 yr	89	3625	796	1295	1967	2849	3861	5211	6128
15-17 yr	89	4183	978	1194	2110	3188	4644	6198	8818
18-24 yr	178	3642	911	1582	2462	3543	5440	7263	9134
25-34 yr	91	—	1009	1437	2093	3316	4605	6105	8172
35-44 yr	63	—	—	—	1305	2545	3584	—	—
45-54 yr	46	2697	—	—	2250	3260	4753	—	—
55-64 yr	129	2396	561	1080	1543	2536	3550	4873	5488
65-74 yr	168		707	908	1412	2070	3053	4179	4790

*Excludes persons with unknown income.

SODIUM INTAKE (mg), AGES 6 MO–74 YR, UNITED STATES, 1976–80—cont'd

Income Level, Sex, and Age	No. Examined	Mean	Percentile						
			5th	10th	25th	50th	75th	90th	95th
INCOME BELOW POVERTY LEVEL*—cont'd									
Female									
6 mo–74 yr	1910	2233	627	861	1388	1984	2840	3919	4748
6-11 mo	36	—	—	—	—	783	—	—	—
1-2 yr	153	1836	592	847	1146	1586	2292	2983	3908
3-5 yr	272	2252	815	1009	1556	2122	2895	3546	3941
6-8 yr	95	2700	972	1455	1921	2568	3405	4159	5173
9-11 yr	102	2440	824	1348	1754	2192	2770	4303	4808
12-14 yr	104	2670	834	1057	1613	2126	3489	4757	5563
15-17 yr	88	2421	536	840	1387	2121	3166	4801	4960
18-24 yr	253	2224	551	820	1360	1947	2862	4194	4538
25-34 yr	162	2323	677	815	1345	1985	2813	3893	5006
35-44 yr	119	2069	514	715	1232	1846	2640	3922	4707
45-54 yr	82	2074	659	889	1328	1839	2851	3762	4367
55-64 yr	188	1905	540	740	1297	1738	2386	3158	3612
65-74 yr	256	2020	676	870	1196	1825	2451	3377	4057
INCOME ABOVE POVERTY LEVEL*									
Male									
6 mo–74 yr	8084	3376	1120	1433	2045	2952	4160	5804	7104
6-11 mo	121	1066	370	457	677	942	1291	1802	2221
1-2 yr	551	1927	790	938	1276	1714	2314	3219	3929
3-5 yr	892	2234	853	1084	1523	2026	2723	3545	4154
6-8 yr	336	2687	1261	1504	1820	2565	3269	3979	5065
9-11 yr	356	3167	1504	1671	2125	3022	3715	4704	5489
12-14 yr	399	3366	1282	1611	2195	3107	4115	5373	6382
15-17 yr	418	3887	1268	1577	2265	3279	4921	7266	8376
18-24 yr	770	4076	1320	1656	2407	3536	5202	6969	8143
25-34 yr	945	3738	1246	1537	2282	3253	4747	6488	7943
35-44 yr	658	3474	1140	1506	2180	3072	4216	5812	7186
45-54 yr	603	3563	1174	1580	2228	3140	4508	6108	7257
55-64 yr	1048	3056	1079	1407	2029	2782	3827	5072	5731
65-74 yr	987	2962	1171	1397	1902	2623	3642	4825	5720
Female									
6 mo–74 yr	8036	2310	750	956	1415	2084	2918	3926	4612
6-11 mo	135	983	302	342	547	856	1273	1679	2472
1-2 yr	505	1736	613	834	1149	1526	2181	2840	3345
3-5 yr	815	2058	880	1031	1403	1904	2473	3344	3805
6-8 yr	308	2472	1094	1277	1764	2227	3076	3901	4275
9-11 yr	307	2616	1075	1367	1757	2341	3203	4308	5131
12-14 yr	363	2565	883	1129	1693	2396	3206	4108	4862
15-17 yr	342	2369	742	895	1460	2112	3043	4132	4996
18-24 yr	771	2426	755	965	1475	2224	3116	4029	4959
25-34 yr	982	2405	772	931	1430	2143	3078	4164	4844
35-44 yr	702	2419	785	1026	1414	2145	3107	4048	5032
45-54 yr	655	2190	705	881	1377	1976	2671	3687	4383
55-64 yr	1071	2238	745	957	1404	2005	2794	3765	4446
65-74 yr	1080	1994	664	899	1281	1830	2450	3361	3883

POTASSIUM INTAKE (mg), AGES 6 MO–74 YR, UNITED STATES, 1976–80

Income Level, Sex, and Age	No. Examined	Mean	Percentile						
			5th	10th	25th	50th	75th	90th	95th
ALL INCOMES									
Male									
6 mo–74 yr	9983	2867	1008	1313	1850	2609	3523	4668	5446
6-11 mo	179	1552	711	818	1151	1458	1872	2463	2697
1-2 yr	745	1787	736	851	1213	1687	2221	2804	3216
3-5 yr	1219	1998	752	984	1383	1884	2494	3179	3644
6-8 yr	428	2386	1095	1320	1710	2304	2976	3462	3966
9-11 yr	457	2633	1026	1267	1780	2481	3267	4171	4861
12-14 yr	504	2911	940	1366	1919	2683	3620	4922	5460
15-17 yr	535	3284	931	1349	1966	2905	4211	5589	6528
18-24 yr	988	3450	1052	1409	2152	3087	4255	5630	6734
25-34 yr	1067	3184	1140	1531	2121	2932	4005	5073	5819
35-44 yr	745	2984	1215	1512	2066	2851	3596	4585	5221
45-54 yr	690	2887	1165	1509	2002	2712	3521	4459	5257
55-64 yr	1227	2664	1104	1376	1821	2474	3394	4203	4665
65-74 yr	1199	2393	863	1179	1605	2261	2985	3670	4336
Female									
6 mo–74 yr	10,339	2035	747	954	1352	1899	2547	3274	3771
6-11 mo	177	1536	651	775	1088	1508	1869	2377	2860
1-2 yr	672	1674	669	837	1140	1554	2005	2545	3077
3-5 yr	1126	1822	759	936	1270	1698	2315	2852	3290
6-8 yr	415	2201	954	1209	1649	2076	2656	3285	3821
9-11 yr	425	2230	879	1142	1534	2113	2700	3452	4030
12-14 yr	487	2116	748	959	1375	1997	2723	3409	3898
15-17 yr	449	1963	594	930	1330	1783	2532	3257	3671
18-24 yr	1066	2016	604	829	1266	1851	2588	3366	4013
25-34 yr	1170	2088	711	932	1366	1950	2604	3369	3968
35-44 yr	844	2091	808	1021	1357	1938	2602	3355	3880
45-54 yr	763	2022	764	973	1372	1918	2481	3265	3652
55-64 yr	1329	2031	754	989	1400	1923	2594	3166	3649
65-74 yr	1416	1965	807	1011	1367	1857	2450	3019	3429
INCOME BELOW POVERTY LEVEL*									
Male									
6 mo–74 yr	1539	2581	718	1006	1518	2270	3237	4463	5382
6-11 mo	48	—	—	—	1040	1299	1796	—	—
1-2 yr	170	1705	698	841	1219	1580	2079	2804	3183
3-5 yr	298	2028	793	1023	1359	1844	2594	3222	3716
6-8 yr	82	2285	862	1206	1711	2191	2803	3302	3626
9-11 yr	88	2338	777	1032	1669	2285	3117	3808	4036
12-14 yr	89	2480	715	1053	1730	2345	3168	4168	4814
15-17 yr	89	2519	529	903	1350	2461	3196	4683	5485
18-24 yr	178	3460	936	1183	1940	2933	4353	5872	7512
25-34 yr	91	2888	694	935	1685	2816	3621	5032	6583
35-44 yr	63	—	—	—	1450	2474	3476	—	—
45-54 yr	46	—	—	—	2015	2776	3594	—	—
55-64 yr	129	2337	788	965	1439	2020	2995	4366	4747
65-74 yr	168	1975	626	820	1299	1927	2484	3320	3563

*Excludes persons with unknown income.

POTASSIUM INTAKE (mg), AGES 6 MO–74 YR, UNITED STATES, 1976–80—cont'd

Income Level, Sex, and Age	No. Examined	Mean	Percentile						
			5th	10th	25th	50th	75th	90th	95th
INCOME BELOW POVERTY LEVEL*—cont'd									
Female									
6 mo–74 yr	1910	1854	578	778	1171	1714	2379	3083	3573
6-11 mo	36	—	—	—	—	1263	—	—	—
1-2 yr	153	1740	565	691	1136	1567	2066	2903	3769
3-5 yr	272	1863	727	882	1225	1686	2333	3034	3641
6-8 yr	95	2223	954	1217	1691	2119	2706	3192	3656
9-11 yr	102	2068	981	1138	1399	1890	2648	3288	3487
12-14 yr	104	1889	531	808	1189	1666	2366	3398	3899
15-17 yr	88	1898	609	838	1227	1742	2593	3092	3487
18-24 yr	253	1841	547	698	1131	1651	2463	3070	3771
25-34 yr	162	2024	617	831	1271	1848	2648	3236	3850
35-44 yr	119	1736	575	713	1045	1483	2302	3095	3547
45-54 yr	82	1637	514	579	1038	1568	2078	2736	2866
55-64 yr	188	1635	539	658	1116	1538	2053	2627	3069
65-74 yr	256	1756	550	865	1156	1647	2128	2824	3381
INCOME ABOVE POVERTY LEVEL*									
Male									
6 mo–74 yr	8084	2915	1079	1378	1907	2657	3589	4718	5514
6-11 mo	121	1604	729	824	1175	1503	1919	2526	2737
1-2 yr	551	1809	751	852	1212	1721	2285	2802	3242
3-5 yr	892	1997	764	984	1395	1891	2479	3158	3641
6-8 yr	336	2417	1106	1326	1713	2387	2993	3554	4137
9-11 yr	356	2694	1073	1354	1799	2504	3283	4345	4942
12-14 yr	399	2976	1002	1407	1950	2766	3658	4973	5625
15-17 yr	418	3475	1019	1497	2182	3116	4375	5788	6759
18-24 yr	770	3452	1061	1474	2189	3111	4276	5502	6578
25-34 yr	945	3213	1250	1576	2156	2951	4025	5102	5810
35-44 yr	658	3032	1283	1596	2109	2876	3650	4602	5323
45-54 yr	603	2926	1262	1524	2020	2718	3577	4569	5260
55-64 yr	1048	2689	1176	1402	1854	2498	3411	4175	4684
65-74 yr	987	2448	909	1210	1661	2312	3023	3708	4479
Female									
6 mo–74 yr	8036	2070	794	992	1389	1933	2578	3300	3803
6-11 mo	135	1596	765	909	1130	1599	1925	2379	2817
1-2 yr	505	1660	707	854	1142	1559	1997	2492	2957
3-5 yr	815	1819	770	954	1293	1700	2317	2818	3163
6-8 yr	308	2182	978	1209	1635	2025	2637	3275	3821
9-11 yr	307	2286	880	1145	1587	2225	2774	3486	4126
12-14 yr	363	2173	768	1042	1500	2067	2752	3442	3896
15-17 yr	342	1970	585	936	1336	1783	2506	3255	3670
18-24 yr	771	2070	648	894	1308	1899	2677	3401	4090
25-34 yr	982	2097	712	964	1376	1964	2604	3395	3999
35-44 yr	702	2140	859	1074	1400	1982	2648	3376	4013
45-54 yr	655	2064	840	1009	1416	1941	2535	3305	3669
55-64 yr	1071	2088	848	1077	1456	1971	2705	3217	3678
65-74 yr	1080	2003	830	1064	1431	1902	2497	3050	3481

VITAMIN A INTAKE (IU), AGES 6 MO–74 YR, UNITED STATES, 1976–80

Income Level, Sex, and Age	No. Examined	Mean	Percentile						
			5th	10th	25th	50th	75th	90th	95th
ALL INCOMES									
Male									
6 mo–74 yr	9983	5680	779	1201	2140	3709	6360	11,005	15,510
6-11 mo	179	5567	1011	1305	2032	3370	5681	12,547	18,874
1-2 yr	745	3616	919	1256	1935	2798	4340	6631	8367
3-5 yr	1219	4074	971	1341	2138	3324	5029	7219	9703
6-8 yr	428	4893	1175	1645	2398	3675	5689	8438	11,538
9-11 yr	457	5735	1153	1523	2470	4267	6770	11,468	14,777
12-14 yr	504	5976	1025	1496	2441	4073	6972	10,020	14,632
15-17 yr	535	5988	734	1273	2202	3966	7076	10,873	14,394
18-24 yr	988	5629	631	1105	2119	3964	6510	11,753	14,856
25-34 yr	1067	5910	546	919	1871	3558	6500	11,239	17,293
35-44 yr	745	5516	708	999	2007	3528	6218	11,134	15,731
45-54 yr	690	6198	843	1197	2256	3789	6641	11,959	16,911
55-64 yr	1227	5860	832	1258	2144	3710	6757	12,430	16,553
65-74 yr	1199	6579	976	1393	2236	3929	7077	12,155	17,161
Female									
6 mo–74 yr	10,339	4637	596	909	1674	2948	5187	9122	13,306
6-11 mo	177	4237	1250	1539	2047	3052	4816	7949	13,122
1-2 yr	672	3619	971	1266	1889	2647	4489	6872	9093
3-5 yr	1126	3940	992	1261	1991	2963	4636	7445	9915
6-8 yr	415	4593	1203	1490	2236	3629	5502	8754	12,325
9-11 yr	425	4704	935	1285	2121	3193	5512	9408	12,097
12-14 yr	487	3977	677	947	1722	2900	4648	7800	10,510
15-17 yr	449	3636	419	671	1351	2616	4295	7498	10,148
18-24 yr	1066	3951	413	785	1395	2693	4791	7991	11,997
25-34 yr	1170	4665	425	773	1486	2782	5002	8778	13,140
35-44 yr	844	4820	552	787	1448	2678	5071	9595	14,353
45-54 yr	763	5219	599	894	1721	3161	5515	10,328	14,819
55-64 yr	1329	5507	634	1084	1925	3341	6149	11,315	15,869
65-74 yr	1416	5481	832	1226	1987	3346	6225	10,808	15,500
INCOME BELOW POVERTY LEVEL*									
Male									
6 mo–74 yr	1539	5197	456	950	1853	3267	5755	10,784	14,244
6-11 mo	48	—	—	—	1955	3046	4963	—	—
1-2 yr	170	3196	920	1220	1817	2518	3719	5679	7171
3-5 yr	298	4125	827	1033	2108	3095	5031	7889	11,213
6-8 yr	82	4428	1174	1635	2235	3674	5530	7069	10,815
9-11 yr	88	5371	912	1213	2135	3349	5522	10,948	13,022
12-14 yr	89	6011	473	1023	1860	3137	6262	8888	11,710
15-17 yr	89	4811	246	663	1514	2761	5929	9783	19,514
18-24 yr	178	6435	488	969	2349	4365	8558	12,873	21,464
25-34 yr	91	4259	197	467	1495	3462	5017	10,488	13,292
35-44 yr	63	—	—	—	—	1052	2610	5185	—	—
45-54 yr	46	—	—	—	—	1758	3019	5511	—	—
55-64 yr	129	5670	319	813	1831	3433	5837	13,079	23,457
65-74 yr	168	5130	252	668	1597	2722	5826	10,576	14,890

*Excludes persons with unknown income.

VITAMIN A INTAKE (IU), AGES 6 MO–74 YR, UNITED STATES, 1976–80—cont'd

| Income Level, Sex, and Age | No. Examined | Mean | Percentile | | | | | | |
			5th	10th	25th	50th	75th	90th	95th
INCOME BELOW POVERTY LEVEL*—cont'd									
Female									
6 mo–74 yr	1910	3966	334	629	1327	2502	4464	8337	12,295
6-11 mo	36	—	—	—	—	2790	—	—	—
1-2 yr	153	3775	926	1237	1792	2886	4360	6879	10,997
3-5 yr	272	4457	812	1161	1845	3058	5176	7783	12,181
6-8 yr	95	4589	961	1275	2071	3083	4396	10,115	16,911
9-11 yr	102	4154	900	1161	1754	2801	5166	9442	11,369
12-14 yr	104	3501	409	677	1081	2254	3674	7985	9744
15-17 yr	88	2654	81	316	992	2147	3249	4062	6442
18-24 yr	253	3704	259	466	1118	2421	4696	8418	13,409
25-34 yr	162	3906	341	486	1168	2270	4520	7368	11,970
35-44 yr	119	3492	151	321	1007	1739	3091	6583	9521
45-54 yr	82	4299	230	486	927	2371	4944	9691	16,548
55-64 yr	188	4398	408	690	1404	2912	5162	9673	12,450
65-74 yr	256	5287	710	1056	1797	3137	5970	12,299	15,502
INCOME ABOVE POVERTY LEVEL*									
Male									
6 mo–74 yr	8084	5745	828	1257	2188	3771	6453	11,192	15,647
6-11 mo	121	5922	1045	1305	2077	3537	5693	15,422	23,622
1-2 yr	551	3736	912	1306	1952	2903	4484	6911	9,508
3-5 yr	892	4073	1079	1426	2161	3384	5031	7015	9,190
6-8 yr	336	4961	1160	1643	2461	3676	5692	8787	11,548
9-11 yr	356	5884	1209	1632	2598	4511	7153	12,404	15,321
12-14 yr	399	6075	1142	1528	2591	4302	7156	10,448	14,661
15-17 yr	418	6339	865	1441	2433	4318	7354	11,023	15,286
18-24 yr	770	5438	673	1127	2091	3924	6245	11,183	14,412
25-34 yr	945	6057	601	967	1912	3560	6546	11,241	17,341
35-44 yr	658	5701	758	1102	2097	3664	6246	11,355	16,164
45-54 yr	603	5858	798	1182	2296	3818	6690	11,956	15,997
55-64 yr	1048	5911	906	1352	2160	3682	6835	12,889	16,565
65-74 yr	987	6835	1088	1507	2338	4013	7205	12,411	17,593
Female									
6 mo–74 yr	8036	4765	676	968	1750	3023	5340	9297	13,547
6-11 mo	135	4389	1250	1586	2021	3051	5835	8545	13,945
1-2 yr	505	3558	975	1248	1890	2589	4465	6759	8,744
3-5 yr	815	3820	1033	1313	2061	2960	4576	7243	9,686
6-8 yr	308	4545	1230	1526	2311	3667	5534	7797	11,776
9-11 yr	307	4894	951	1299	2364	3434	5597	9410	12,120
12-14 yr	363	4138	773	1007	1825	2998	4757	7937	11,895
15-17 yr	342	3871	533	746	1448	2707	4829	8065	10,261
18-24 yr	771	4045	510	822	1435	2730	4834	7958	12,000
25-34 yr	982	4787	497	814	1546	2812	5147	9173	13,539
35-44 yr	702	4938	623	877	1590	2838	5227	10,159	14,369
45-54 yr	655	5334	737	982	1778	3195	5647	10,532	14,511
55-64 yr	1071	5669	720	1130	2031	3493	6304	11,525	16,028
65-74 yr	1080	5542	893	1267	2028	3383	6298	10,748	15,182

THIAMINE INTAKE (mg), AGES 6 MO–74 YR, UNITED STATES, 1976–80

Income Level, Sex, and Age	No. Examined	Mean	5th	10th	25th	50th	75th	90th	95th
						Percentile			
ALL INCOMES									
Male									
6 mo–74 yr	9983	1.56	0.52	0.66	0.93	1.34	1.89	2.66	3.34
6-11 mo	179	0.82	0.31	0.36	0.49	0.72	0.96	1.48	1.81
1-2 yr	745	0.94	0.36	0.42	0.59	0.83	1.13	1.49	1.85
3-5 yr	1219	1.19	0.49	0.60	0.78	1.09	1.46	1.88	2.27
6-8 yr	428	1.43	0.60	0.76	1.01	1.34	1.74	2.17	2.42
9-11 yr	457	1.63	0.60	0.72	1.06	1.45	1.97	2.67	3.34
12-14 yr	504	1.73	0.63	0.80	1.13	1.57	2.13	2.74	3.50
15-17 yr	535	1.87	0.63	0.81	1.05	1.58	2.35	3.35	4.14
18-24 yr	988	1.84	0.54	0.69	1.07	1.53	2.23	3.19	4.24
25-34 yr	1067	1.69	0.54	0.67	0.95	1.40	2.04	2.90	3.79
35-44 yr	745	1.55	0.49	0.70	0.95	1.34	1.83	2.51	3.27
45-54 yr	690	1.51	0.58	0.69	0.96	1.36	1.87	2.52	3.02
55-64 yr	1227	1.40	0.50	0.64	0.92	1.28	1.70	2.32	2.73
65-74 yr	1199	1.33	0.47	0.61	0.82	1.13	1.57	2.25	2.77
Female									
6 mo–74 yr	10,339	1.06	0.35	0.46	0.65	0.92	1.29	1.77	2.16
6-11 mo	177	0.83	0.31	0.35	0.54	0.73	1.06	1.50	1.75
1-2 yr	672	0.90	0.34	0.41	0.58	0.79	1.08	1.48	1.82
3-5 yr	1126	1.09	0.42	0.53	0.75	0.98	1.30	1.72	2.08
6-8 yr	415	1.23	0.54	0.64	0.88	1.16	1.49	1.92	2.24
9-11 yr	425	1.29	0.55	0.68	0.85	1.14	1.57	2.06	2.45
12-14 yr	487	1.16	0.41	0.51	0.72	1.04	1.42	1.96	2.38
15-17 yr	449	1.08	0.34	0.46	0.64	0.95	1.39	1.88	2.17
18-24 yr	1066	1.06	0.31	0.41	0.63	0.93	1.32	1.76	2.21
25-34 yr	1170	1.08	0.33	0.42	0.63	0.92	1.32	1.82	2.15
35-44 yr	844	1.05	0.34	0.43	0.60	0.87	1.27	1.70	2.34
45-54 yr	763	0.98	0.35	0.46	0.61	0.88	1.19	1.63	1.94
55-64 yr	1329	1.00	0.34	0.43	0.64	0.88	1.19	1.62	1.98
65-74 yr	1416	0.99	0.37	0.45	0.63	0.85	1.15	1.58	1.96
INCOME BELOW POVERTY LEVEL*									
Male									
6 mo–74 yr	1539	1.48	0.43	0.56	0.85	1.26	1.89	2.70	3.38
6-11 mo	48	—	—	—	0.57	0.74	0.92	—	—
1-2 yr	170	0.89	0.35	0.38	0.54	0.79	1.10	1.46	1.93
3-5 yr	298	1.25	0.46	0.62	0.84	1.14	1.53	2.09	2.35
6-8 yr	82	1.36	0.45	0.60	0.91	1.32	1.81	2.17	2.40
9-11 yr	88	1.52	0.60	0.67	0.98	1.31	1.69	2.86	3.57
12-14 yr	89	1.61	0.63	0.77	0.91	1.36	1.99	2.99	3.70
15-17 yr	89	1.74	0.50	0.57	0.95	1.51	2.24	3.05	3.64
18-24 yr	178	1.80	0.44	0.64	1.05	1.53	2.15	3.40	4.00
25-34 yr	91	1.68	0.42	0.57	0.93	1.23	2.29	2.80	3.84
35-44 yr	63	—	—	—	0.76	1.20	1.74	—	—
45-54 yr	46	—	—	—	1.14	1.59	2.10	—	—
55-64 yr	129	1.25	0.20	0.49	0.80	1.14	1.54	2.05	2.59
65-74 yr	168	1.08	0.41	0.48	0.68	0.97	1.35	1.86	2.23

*Excludes persons with unknown income.

THIAMINE INTAKE (mg), AGES 6 MO–74 YR, UNITED STATES, 1976–80—cont'd

Income Level, Sex, and Age	No. Examined	Mean	5th	10th	25th	50th	75th	90th	95th
						Percentile			
INCOME BELOW POVERTY LEVEL*—cont'd									
Female									
6 mo–74 yr	1910	1.05	0.32	0.40	0.61	0.90	1.26	1.76	2.24
6-11 mo	36	—	—	—	—	0.62	—	—	—
1-2 yr	153	1.01	0.37	0.42	0.61	0.84	1.16	1.72	2.43
3-5 yr	272	1.15	0.35	0.49	0.73	1.08	1.46	1.83	2.17
6-8 yr	95	1.29	0.49	0.70	0.90	1.22	1.49	1.97	2.20
9-11 yr	102	1.26	0.52	0.61	0.76	1.12	1.57	2.01	2.33
12-14 yr	104	1.04	0.34	0.41	0.65	0.92	1.25	1.96	2.34
15-17 yr	88	1.07	0.29	0.48	0.68	0.93	1.39	1.78	2.26
18-24 yr	253	1.00	0.32	0.37	0.60	0.88	1.25	1.76	2.08
25-34 yr	162	1.24	0.25	0.42	0.68	0.96	1.24	1.94	3.08
35-44 yr	119	0.87	0.20	0.37	0.52	0.73	1.05	1.49	2.22
45-54 yr	82	0.89	0.30	0.37	0.58	0.86	1.13	1.41	1.68
55-64 yr	188	0.94	0.27	0.37	0.53	0.78	1.09	1.62	2.31
65-74 yr	256	0.90	0.31	0.40	0.56	0.80	1.08	1.56	2.13
INCOME ABOVE POVERTY LEVEL*									
Male									
6 mo–74 yr	8084	1.58	0.54	0.67	0.94	1.36	1.90	2.66	3.35
6-11 mo	121	0.84	0.31	0.36	0.47	0.71	1.05	1.64	1.89
1-2 yr	551	0.96	0.37	0.45	0.61	0.83	1.14	1.50	1.85
3-5 yr	892	1.18	0.51	0.61	0.78	1.08	1.45	1.85	2.27
6-8 yr	336	1.45	0.64	0.80	1.02	1.37	1.75	2.19	2.45
9-11 yr	356	1.66	0.61	0.74	1.09	1.49	2.01	2.67	3.32
12-14 yr	399	1.76	0.62	0.80	1.14	1.62	2.15	2.71	3.50
15-17 yr	418	1.92	0.69	0.85	1.06	1.64	2.38	3.43	4.20
18-24 yr	770	1.85	0.55	0.69	1.07	1.54	2.25	3.11	4.27
25-34 yr	945	1.69	0.55	0.68	0.95	1.40	2.03	2.91	3.79
35-44 yr	658	1.57	0.52	0.72	0.97	1.35	1.83	2.53	3.27
45-54 yr	603	1.52	0.59	0.69	0.97	1.35	1.87	2.55	3.02
55-64 yr	1048	1.41	0.52	0.67	0.91	1.28	1.70	2.34	2.76
65-74 yr	987	1.35	0.47	0.63	0.83	1.16	1.60	2.28	2.97
Female									
6 mo–74 yr	8036	1.07	0.36	0.46	0.65	0.93	1.30	1.78	2.15
6-11 mo	135	0.83	0.32	0.36	0.56	0.74	1.07	1.31	1.71
1-2 yr	505	0.88	0.33	0.39	0.57	0.78	1.04	1.43	1.75
3-5 yr	815	1.08	0.42	0.55	0.76	0.96	1.26	1.64	2.05
6-8 yr	308	1.22	0.54	0.64	0.87	1.15	1.49	1.92	2.24
9-11 yr	307	1.31	0.57	0.71	0.89	1.14	1.58	2.08	2.47
12-14 yr	363	1.20	0.44	0.51	0.80	1.07	1.44	1.96	2.38
15-17 yr	342	1.08	0.34	0.46	0.62	0.94	1.35	1.88	2.17
18-24 yr	771	1.08	0.31	0.42	0.66	0.93	1.35	1.77	2.23
25-34 yr	982	1.06	0.34	0.42	0.62	0.90	1.32	1.81	2.12
35-44 yr	702	1.07	0.35	0.43	0.62	0.88	1.28	1.73	2.45
45-54 yr	655	0.99	0.37	0.47	0.61	0.89	1.19	1.65	2.00
55-64 yr	1071	1.02	0.35	0.45	0.65	0.89	1.23	1.65	1.98
65-74 yr	1080	1.01	0.39	0.48	0.65	0.86	1.17	1.60	1.95

RIBOFLAVIN INTAKE (mg), AGES 6 MO–74 YR, UNITED STATES, 1976–80

| Income Level, Sex, and Age | No. Examined | Mean | Percentile | | | | | | |
			5th	10th	25th	50th	75th	90th	95th
ALL INCOMES									
Male									
6 mo–74 yr	9983	2.27	0.71	0.93	1.35	1.94	2.77	3.80	4.72
6-11 mo	179	1.83	0.57	0.85	1.28	1.65	2.21	3.18	3.55
1-2 yr	745	1.58	0.58	0.72	1.01	1.44	1.92	2.55	2.99
3-5 yr	1219	1.81	0.65	0.85	1.22	1.70	2.24	2.94	3.37
6-8 yr	428	2.24	0.95	1.22	1.65	2.13	2.73	3.38	3.70
9-11 yr	457	2.46	0.85	1.12	1.61	2.26	3.03	4.15	4.75
12-14 yr	504	2.60	0.86	1.18	1.66	2.33	3.20	4.25	5.10
15-17 yr	535	2.91	0.69	1.01	1.62	2.53	3.66	5.23	6.16
18-24 yr	988	2.76	0.81	1.01	1.56	2.37	3.28	4.70	6.15
25-34 yr	1067	2.37	0.69	0.96	1.34	2.02	2.87	3.95	5.06
35-44 yr	745	2.08	0.68	0.87	1.27	1.83	2.53	3.45	4.13
45-54 yr	690	2.07	0.74	0.93	1.32	1.78	2.45	3.31	4.39
55-64 yr	1227	1.91	0.68	0.88	1.17	1.72	2.36	3.16	3.99
65-74 yr	1199	1.84	0.57	0.76	1.08	1.56	2.25	3.03	3.97
Female									
6 mo–74 yr	10,339	1.53	0.45	0.58	0.87	1.30	1.90	2.63	3.22
6-11 mo	177	1.73	0.57	0.79	1.17	1.61	2.20	2.89	3.22
1-2 yr	672	1.49	0.55	0.69	0.99	1.39	1.82	2.42	2.90
3-5 yr	1126	1.67	0.62	0.81	1.13	1.60	2.11	2.64	2.97
6-8 yr	415	1.99	0.80	0.99	1.39	1.94	2.46	3.00	3.43
9-11 yr	425	2.01	0.74	0.85	1.28	1.80	2.57	3.32	4.01
12-14 yr	487	1.73	0.50	0.67	1.05	1.59	2.22	2.94	3.41
15-17 yr	449	1.61	0.42	0.63	0.92	1.39	2.05	2.89	3.37
18-24 yr	1066	1.52	0.43	0.57	0.87	1.29	1.90	2.69	3.29
25-34 yr	1170	1.48	0.40	0.54	0.82	1.23	1.83	2.50	3.21
35-44 yr	844	1.45	0.40	0.56	0.79	1.17	1.72	2.36	2.94
45-54 yr	763	1.37	0.42	0.55	0.78	1.14	1.60	2.26	2.90
55-64 yr	1329	1.36	0.44	0.52	0.76	1.18	1.63	2.30	3.00
65-74 yr	1416	1.36	0.42	0.54	0.79	1.13	1.60	2.26	2.88
INCOME BELOW POVERTY LEVEL*									
Male									
6 mo–74 yr	1539	2.12	0.58	0.78	1.28	1.85	2.65	3.64	4.41
6-11 mo	48	—	—	—	0.94	1.47	1.99	—	—
1-2 yr	170	1.58	0.57	0.70	0.96	1.44	1.89	2.65	3.34
3-5 yr	298	1.81	0.64	0.88	1.19	1.65	2.26	2.90	3.40
6-8 yr	82	2.16	0.59	1.06	1.58	2.00	2.77	3.39	3.70
9-11 yr	88	2.25	0.82	1.11	1.51	2.16	2.75	3.63	4.69
12-14 yr	89	2.30	0.76	0.92	1.44	1.81	2.85	3.89	5.09
15-17 yr	89	2.30	0.52	0.63	1.28	2.08	2.87	4.09	5.09
18-24 yr	178	2.82	0.63	0.88	1.54	2.43	3.38	5.25	6.02
25-34 yr	91	2.05	0.60	0.73	1.19	1.87	2.56	3.33	4.31
35-44 yr	63	—	—	—	0.97	1.50	1.99	—	—
45-54 yr	46	—	—	—	1.43	2.08	2.51	—	—
55-64 yr	129	1.66	0.47	0.53	1.02	1.43	2.18	2.65	3.64
65-74 yr	168	1.52	0.47	0.57	0.88	1.41	1.93	2.70	2.93

*Excludes persons with unknown income.

RIBOFLAVIN INTAKE (mg), AGES 6 MO–74 YR, UNITED STATES, 1976–80—cont'd

Income Level, Sex, and Age	No. Examined	Mean	Percentile						
			5th	10th	25th	50th	75th	90th	95th
INCOME BELOW POVERTY LEVEL*—cont'd									
Female									
6 mo–74 yr	1910	1.46	0.38	0.52	0.79	1.25	1.83	2.62	3.15
6-11 mo	36	—	—	—	—	1.28	—	—	—
1-2 yr	153	1.57	0.54	0.67	1.03	1.41	1.83	2.57	3.53
3-5 yr	272	1.71	0.58	0.75	1.10	1.68	2.20	2.66	2.94
6-8 yr	95	1.90	0.79	0.92	1.34	1.80	2.32	2.74	3.47
9-11 yr	102	1.84	0.67	0.78	1.16	1.77	2.39	3.01	3.26
12-14 yr	104	1.48	0.46	0.46	0.91	1.29	1.80	2.70	3.27
15-17 yr	88	1.41	0.38	0.48	0.86	1.27	1.82	2.54	3.23
18-24 yr	253	1.39	0.42	0.58	0.80	1.16	1.75	2.56	3.07
25-34 yr	162	1.53	0.38	0.51	0.75	1.18	1.68	2.98	3.44
35-44 yr	119	1.21	0.22	0.37	0.57	1.09	1.48	1.95	2.76
45-54 yr	82	1.17	0.35	0.43	0.68	0.97	1.53	1.96	2.57
55-64 yr	188	1.30	0.41	0.47	0.68	0.96	1.53	2.13	3.16
65-74 yr	256	1.33	0.36	0.48	0.66	1.15	1.68	2.55	3.08
INCOME ABOVE POVERTY LEVEL*									
Male									
6 mo–74 yr	8084	2.29	0.75	0.95	1.36	1.96	2.80	3.84	4.77
6-11 mo	121	1.92	0.56	0.87	1.36	1.79	2.33	3.38	3.61
1-2 yr	551	1.58	0.60	0.73	1.02	1.44	1.92	2.47	2.88
3-5 yr	892	1.82	0.65	0.85	1.23	1.70	2.24	3.01	3.37
6-8 yr	336	2.27	0.97	1.25	1.69	2.16	2.73	3.38	3.74
9-11 yr	356	2.51	0.83	1.13	1.62	2.35	3.10	4.23	4.81
12-14 yr	399	2.67	0.92	1.26	1.72	2.42	3.26	4.34	5.12
15-17 yr	418	3.08	0.84	1.17	1.69	2.60	3.82	5.43	6.63
18-24 yr	770	2.75	0.84	1.03	1.55	2.37	3.27	4.65	6.15
25-34 yr	945	2.40	0.71	0.99	1.36	2.04	2.89	3.96	5.11
35-44 yr	658	2.13	0.71	0.92	1.29	1.86	2.60	3.48	4.15
45-54 yr	603	2.05	0.78	0.94	1.31	1.78	2.45	3.33	4.39
55-64 yr	1048	1.93	0.73	0.91	1.18	1.72	2.36	3.20	4.03
65-74 yr	987	1.87	0.64	0.78	1.11	1.57	2.26	3.10	4.06
Female									
6 mo–74 yr	8036	1.55	0.45	0.60	0.89	1.32	1.90	2.64	3.22
6-11 mo	135	1.79	0.68	0.93	1.31	1.65	2.21	2.80	3.22
1-2 yr	505	1.47	0.55	0.69	0.99	1.38	1.81	2.35	2.70
3-5 yr	815	1.67	0.66	0.83	1.13	1.59	2.05	2.63	2.98
6-8 yr	308	2.01	0.82	1.00	1.39	1.94	2.49	3.09	3.43
9-11 yr	307	2.06	0.76	0.86	1.30	1.82	2.61	3.51	4.10
12-14 yr	363	1.80	0.53	0.79	1.13	1.69	2.30	2.94	3.48
15-17 yr	342	1.65	0.42	0.65	0.92	1.44	2.09	2.89	3.40
18-24 yr	771	1.56	0.43	0.57	0.91	1.33	1.94	2.76	3.36
25-34 yr	982	1.47	0.40	0.54	0.83	1.23	1.83	2.44	3.10
35-44 yr	702	1.48	0.42	0.60	0.82	1.20	1.77	2.37	2.91
45-54 yr	655	1.40	0.45	0.56	0.80	1.15	1.61	2.26	2.99
55-64 yr	1071	1.37	0.45	0.54	0.78	1.19	1.64	2.32	3.00
65-74 yr	1080	1.37	0.44	0.56	0.81	1.13	1.58	2.23	2.85

PREFORMED NIACIN INTAKE (mg), AGES 6 MO–74 YR, UNITED STATES, 1976–80

| Income Level, Sex, and Age | No. Examined | Mean | Percentile | | | | | | |
			5th	10th	25th	50th	75th	90th	95th
ALL INCOMES									
Male									
6 mo–74 yr	9983	23.89	7.58	9.83	14.19	20.85	29.66	41.21	49.81
6-11 mo	179	8.92	2.84	3.64	4.73	8.39	11.61	15.26	19.16
1-2 yr	745	11.00	3.58	4.62	6.73	9.72	13.50	18.49	21.90
3-5 yr	1219	14.54	5.37	7.10	9.64	13.03	18.17	23.92	28.13
6-8 yr	428	17.78	7.27	9.19	13.00	16.66	22.09	27.50	31.43
9-11 yr	457	20.66	7.52	8.96	13.31	18.59	25.52	34.31	40.32
12-14 yr	504	22.90	8.06	10.20	14.72	20.89	27.52	37.29	44.99
15-17 yr	535	26.69	8.05	10.42	14.91	22.15	32.96	48.71	65.19
18-24 yr	988	29.76	9.71	11.42	17.13	25.98	36.96	49.09	62.08
25-34 yr	1067	28.43	10.35	13.14	17.54	25.15	35.33	47.53	58.89
35-44 yr	745	25.34	9.60	11.45	16.77	23.24	31.59	40.71	48.74
45-54 yr	690	25.12	9.33	11.89	16.27	22.41	31.51	41.40	48.21
55-64 yr	1227	21.67	8.66	10.58	13.97	19.58	26.24	37.18	41.77
65-74 yr	1199	19.95	6.56	8.88	12.48	17.68	24.14	33.72	40.24
Female									
6 mo–74 yr	10,339	15.45	5.20	6.86	9.74	13.87	19.13	25.69	30.52
6-11 mo	177	8.55	2.66	3.20	4.89	7.93	11.88	14.34	16.98
1-2 yr	672	10.62	2.96	4.07	6.65	9.47	13.38	18.02	22.13
3-5 yr	1126	13.28	4.46	6.02	9.01	11.99	16.65	21.56	25.16
6-8 yr	415	14.99	6.44	7.85	10.40	13.96	18.33	23.22	27.74
9-11 yr	425	16.43	6.95	8.23	10.78	14.73	20.02	26.96	31.72
12-14 yr	487	15.26	5.43	6.82	9.62	13.65	19.02	25.99	30.67
15-17 yr	449	14.67	4.48	6.57	9.29	13.10	18.42	24.57	28.25
18-24 yr	1066	15.89	4.62	6.30	9.57	14.53	20.15	26.82	33.44
25-34 yr	1170	16.48	5.45	7.22	10.44	14.99	20.40	27.06	33.01
35-44 yr	844	16.94	6.12	7.92	10.93	15.03	20.30	27.89	33.50
45-54 yr	763	15.61	5.79	7.47	10.05	13.97	19.37	25.24	29.77
55-64 yr	1329	15.17	5.51	6.91	9.58	13.61	19.15	25.04	28.77
65-74 yr	1416	14.42	5.19	6.56	8.96	12.90	17.35	23.69	30.09
INCOME BELOW POVERTY LEVEL*									
Male									
6 mo–74 yr	1539	20.52	5.69	7.67	11.33	17.16	25.98	37.74	44.31
6-11 mo	48	—	—	—	—	6.05	8.03	11.34	—	—
1-2 yr	170	10.76	3.05	3.97	6.39	9.17	13.55	19.27	24.53
3-5 yr	298	15.02	5.30	7.05	9.64	12.99	18.19	26.16	31.75
6-8 yr	82	16.62	6.75	8.07	11.43	15.73	21.37	25.68	30.53
9-11 yr	88	18.41	5.95	8.41	10.84	18.06	23.29	28.95	34.26
12-14 yr	89	18.98	7.59	9.14	11.80	17.36	22.61	33.10	41.30
15-17 yr	89	23.11	5.54	7.96	13.62	18.48	27.94	45.07	55.43
18-24 yr	178	27.10	6.28	9.68	16.32	25.01	33.41	42.44	56.80
25-34 yr	91	25.58	9.14	10.77	15.25	19.57	34.82	46.30	52.30
35-44 yr	63	—	—	—	11.29	19.60	29.79	—	—
45-54 yr	46	—	—	—	13.94	21.65	32.09	—	—
55-64 yr	129	18.29	5.31	8.62	10.95	15.70	21.78	34.86	41.61
65-74 yr	168	14.91	4.23	5.99	10.23	14.45	18.79	23.16	27.20

*Excludes persons with unknown income.

PREFORMED NIACIN INTAKE (mg), AGES 6 MO–74 YR, UNITED STATES, 1976–80—cont'd

Income Level, Sex, and Age	No. Examined	Mean	Percentile						
			5th	10th	25th	50th	75th	90th	95th
INCOME BELOW POVERTY LEVEL*—cont'd									
Female									
6 mo–74 yr	1910	14.37	4.56	5.92	8.63	12.64	18.00	24.41	29.63
6-11 mo	36	—	—	—	—	6.24	—	—	—
1-2 yr	153	11.48	3.24	4.96	6.68	9.88	14.60	20.32	25.23
3-5 yr	272	13.92	3.85	5.22	8.70	12.84	18.16	22.95	26.04
6-8 yr	95	15.73	5.87	7.58	10.71	14.70	18.89	22.23	29.11
9-11 yr	102	16.15	6.22	8.10	10.11	14.00	20.01	26.89	31.80
12-14 yr	104	14.07	5.29	5.88	7.69	12.06	16.86	25.57	33.14
15-17 yr	88	14.64	4.76	7.93	10.20	13.03	18.29	23.53	29.36
18-24 yr	253	14.54	3.86	5.93	8.75	12.78	18.38	24.51	33.16
25-34 yr	162	16.97	5.13	6.28	9.84	14.92	22.03	27.87	32.44
35-44 yr	119	14.02	4.56	6.12	8.86	12.68	18.11	23.20	28.21
45-54 yr	82	12.36	4.90	6.20	8.12	11.85	14.81	19.88	24.46
55-64 yr	188	13.15	5.32	5.69	7.81	10.82	16.17	22.00	29.47
65-74 yr	256	12.96	3.46	5.35	7.61	11.49	15.75	22.87	28.12
INCOME ABOVE POVERTY LEVEL*									
Male									
6 mo–74 yr	8084	24.41	7.97	10.23	14.72	21.33	30.27	41.53	50.52
6-11 mo	121	9.25	2.87	3.64	4.71	9.06	11.87	15.88	19.98
1-2 yr	551	11.13	3.86	4.69	6.90	9.86	13.57	18.52	21.52
3-5 yr	892	14.51	5.46	7.26	9.74	13.17	18.18	23.44	27.03
6-8 yr	336	18.05	8.02	9.63	12.99	17.04	22.20	27.74	31.72
9-11 yr	356	21.19	7.53	9.34	13.69	18.64	27.03	36.53	41.31
12-14 yr	399	23.70	8.20	11.05	15.57	21.77	28.72	39.11	47.00
15-17 yr	418	27.59	9.02	11.10	15.55	23.75	33.54	50.33	67.84
18-24 yr	770	30.30	10.23	11.76	17.46	26.01	37.94	50.25	65.05
25-34 yr	945	28.71	10.74	13.53	17.99	25.22	35.35	47.73	59.31
35-44 yr	658	25.83	10.11	12.05	17.17	23.62	32.21	41.57	49.34
45-54 yr	603	25.37	9.36	12.19	16.45	22.70	31.57	41.42	48.68
55-64 yr	1048	22.02	9.05	10.90	14.31	20.08	26.56	37.84	41.81
65-74 yr	987	20.51	7.40	9.03	12.93	18.33	25.05	34.17	42.65
Female									
6 mo–74 yr	8036	15.67	5.28	7.07	9.98	14.14	19.35	25.90	30.75
6-11 mo	135	8.48	2.64	3.20	4.96	7.93	11.89	14.17	16.20
1-2 yr	505	10.42	2.96	3.89	6.73	9.41	12.78	17.94	21.00
3-5 yr	815	13.13	4.63	6.32	9.07	11.84	16.13	21.37	24.71
6-8 yr	308	14.79	6.44	7.85	10.33	13.72	18.32	23.20	26.93
9-11 yr	307	16.58	7.01	8.45	11.45	14.99	20.09	27.12	30.71
12-14 yr	363	15.63	5.43	7.29	10.37	13.86	19.36	26.14	30.51
15-17 yr	342	14.68	3.95	6.20	8.85	13.26	18.44	24.57	28.22
18-24 yr	771	16.30	4.73	6.48	9.96	14.86	20.69	27.53	33.53
25-34 yr	982	16.43	5.46	7.31	10.47	15.02	20.21	26.77	33.45
35-44 yr	702	17.31	6.53	8.16	11.20	15.25	20.53	28.32	34.14
45-54 yr	655	15.98	6.12	7.64	10.34	14.38	19.66	25.68	30.50
55-64 yr	1071	15.48	5.67	7.13	10.12	14.08	19.51	25.05	29.12
65-74 yr	1080	14.75	5.37	6.84	9.31	13.34	17.74	23.93	30.38

VITAMIN C INTAKE (mg), AGES 6 MO–74 YR, UNITED STATES, 1976–80

Income Level, Sex, and Age	No. Examined	Mean	Percentile						
			5th	10th	25th	50th	75th	90th	95th
ALL INCOMES									
Male									
6 mo–74 yr	9983	108	8	15	33	73	144	237	317
6-11 mo	179	63	11	14	23	51	81	120	170
1-2 yr	745	90	8	13	28	64	121	192	252
3-5 yr	1219	104	10	16	34	76	136	226	285
6-8 yr	428	105	13	19	34	68	142	222	322
9-11 yr	457	119	13	20	41	88	158	265	336
12-14 yr	504	123	11	15	32	72	167	295	384
15-17 yr	535	112	7	16	33	69	150	244	359
18-24 yr	988	129	7	14	35	76	166	303	430
25-34 yr	1067	108	8	13	31	66	138	251	340
35-44 yr	745	96	7	15	28	66	137	211	268
45-54 yr	690	102	7	13	34	76	147	215	263
55-64 yr	1227	103	8	15	34	82	144	229	273
65-74 yr	1199	100	5	11	33	79	140	212	271
Female									
6 mo–74 yr	10,339	93	6	11	27	63	130	209	273
6-11 mo	177	72	9	13	31	51	80	142	261
1-2 yr	672	86	10	13	27	64	116	186	240
3-5 yr	1126	96	10	15	29	68	131	202	284
6-8 yr	415	109	14	19	34	80	147	241	292
9-11 yr	425	94	13	17	32	59	121	218	271
12-14 yr	487	83	6	11	25	56	108	200	276
15-17 yr	449	73	4	9	21	42	99	180	229
18-24 yr	1066	92	5	9	25	59	135	201	264
25-34 yr	1170	92	5	9	24	55	121	202	292
35-44 yr	844	83	4	10	23	53	116	202	248
45-54 yr	763	97	4	9	26	69	134	224	281
55-64 yr	1329	107	7	15	35	88	148	224	281
65-74 yr	1416	105	7	13	37	90	147	220	260
INCOME BELOW POVERTY LEVEL*									
Male									
6 mo–74 yr	1539	93	4	9	23	57	124	224	298
6-11 mo	48	—	—	—	19	41	70	—	—
1-2 yr	170	73	5	9	20	46	95	181	237
3-5 yr	298	98	7	12	33	72	141	216	259
6-8 yr	82	84	8	15	26	52	149	198	286
9-11 yr	88	114	8	15	37	76	158	269	336
12-14 yr	89	98	9	12	22	51	122	231	432
15-17 yr	89	79	1	10	23	55	93	197	241
18-24 yr	178	120	8	12	36	72	162	296	376
25-34 yr	91	77	0	5	18	48	109	181	225
35-44 yr	63	—	—	—	17	46	98	—	—
45-54 yr	46	—	—	—	24	80	137	—	—
55-64 yr	129	85	2	6	23	52	107	216	275
65-74 yr	168	70	2	3	10	45	102	179	222

*Excludes persons with unknown income.

VITAMIN C INTAKE (mg), AGES 6 MO–74 YR, UNITED STATES, 1976–80—cont'd

| Income Level, Sex, and Age | No. Examined | Mean | Percentile | | | | | | |
			5th	10th	25th	50th	75th	90th	95th
INCOME BELOW POVERTY LEVEL*—cont'd									
Female									
6 mo–74 yr	1910	77	3	7	19	44	105	183	251
6-11 mo	36	—	—	—	—	51	—	—	—
1-2 yr	153	86	8	12	23	61	124	176	266
3-5 yr	272	91	6	10	24	54	136	219	277
6-8 yr	95	97	13	18	36	80	136	185	269
9-11 yr	102	71	10	13	19	43	97	183	239
12-14 yr	104	61	3	3	16	33	73	170	209
15-17 yr	88	65	1	3	14	31	80	175	246
18-24 yr	253	83	2	6	20	46	109	182	290
25-34 yr	162	77	3	7	19	36	87	202	332
35-44 yr	119	55	0	4	13	32	68	153	182
45-54 yr	82	82	2	4	15	62	118	182	238
55-64 yr	188	76	4	7	20	47	124	164	223
65-74 yr	256	94	5	8	24	71	132	223	265
INCOME ABOVE POVERTY LEVEL*									
Male									
6 mo–74 yr	8084	110	9	16	34	75	146	239	323
6-11 mo	121	66	11	16	29	55	81	120	170
1-2 yr	551	94	10	15	29	69	122	200	260
3-5 yr	892	106	12	17	35	76	133	231	308
6-8 yr	336	108	14	21	37	73	140	228	329
9-11 yr	356	120	14	20	41	90	164	265	337
12-14 yr	399	127	12	17	36	78	184	301	384
15-17 yr	418	119	7	17	35	72	162	261	398
18-24 yr	770	132	6	15	35	77	169	309	438
25-34 yr	945	110	8	14	31	67	139	262	342
35-44 yr	658	97	8	15	31	69	139	208	260
45-54 yr	603	103	8	15	34	75	149	221	288
55-64 yr	1048	105	9	15	36	86	146	229	273
65-74 yr	987	103	6	13	38	85	142	215	274
Female									
6 mo–74 yr	8036	96	6	12	28	66	134	211	275
6-11 mo	135	72	9	12	29	50	77	152	261
1-2 yr	505	86	11	15	28	68	117	186	234
3-5 yr	815	98	12	17	31	71	129	203	284
6-8 yr	308	112	15	19	33	80	155	259	341
9-11 yr	307	101	15	21	36	66	132	224	276
12-14 yr	363	88	9	13	28	60	117	207	293
15-17 yr	342	75	5	11	22	44	105	180	229
18-24 yr	771	94	6	12	26	59	143	202	253
25-34 yr	982	93	5	10	24	56	124	200	291
35-44 yr	702	88	4	11	26	55	122	210	262
45-54 yr	655	99	5	11	27	70	138	227	284
55-64 yr	1071	111	7	18	38	93	151	224	285
65-74 yr	1080	107	8	14	40	92	150	219	261

SATURATED FATTY ACID INTAKE (mg), AGES 6 MO–74 YR, UNITED STATES, 1976–80

Income Level, Sex, and Age	No. Examined	Mean	Percentile						
			5th	10th	25th	50th	75th	90th	95th
ALL INCOMES									
Male									
6 mo–74 yr	9983	36	10	14	21	31	45	63	76
6-11 mo	179	13	0	1	8	12	18	25	30
1-2 yr	745	19	6	8	12	18	24	32	39
3-5 yr	1219	24	8	11	15	22	29	39	46
6-8 yr	428	30	13	16	21	28	37	47	55
9-11 yr	457	32	13	16	22	29	40	52	60
12-14 yr	504	37	12	15	23	33	46	61	72
15-17 yr	535	44	13	17	26	37	56	78	96
18-24 yr	988	46	13	18	27	38	58	80	102
25-34 yr	1067	40	12	15	24	37	52	66	80
35-44 yr	745	37	13	16	22	33	47	63	74
45-54 yr	690	36	11	14	21	31	46	61	75
55-64 yr	1227	31	10	13	20	29	39	53	62
65-74 yr	1199	27	8	10	17	24	33	45	53
Female									
6 mo–74 yr	10,339	23	6	9	14	21	29	39	47
6-11 mo	177	14	1	3	8	14	19	25	31
1-2 yr	672	19	6	8	12	18	23	31	37
3-5 yr	1126	22	9	11	15	21	28	35	40
6-8 yr	415	26	10	14	19	25	32	40	44
9-11 yr	425	27	11	14	19	25	34	43	51
12-14 yr	487	27	8	12	17	25	35	46	54
15-17 yr	449	26	7	10	15	24	34	43	56
18-24 yr	1066	24	6	9	14	21	31	41	50
25-34 yr	1170	24	6	9	14	22	31	40	48
35-44 yr	844	23	7	9	14	21	29	40	49
45-54 yr	763	21	5	7	12	19	26	34	44
55-64 yr	1329	20	5	7	11	17	25	34	41
65-74 yr	1416	17	4	7	11	15	21	29	36
INCOME BELOW POVERTY LEVEL*									
Male									
6 mo–74 yr	1539	34	8	11	19	29	43	62	76
6-11 mo	48	—	—	—	8	14	18	—	—
1-2 yr	170	21	7	9	14	20	25	33	40
3-5 yr	298	26	8	11	18	25	33	43	51
6-8 yr	82	31	13	18	21	30	37	45	57
9-11 yr	88	30	8	14	22	29	36	47	61
12-14 yr	89	36	12	13	23	30	45	61	73
15-17 yr	89	41	9	13	22	36	55	69	85
18-24 yr	178	47	9	13	24	39	62	84	104
25-34 yr	91	38	6	17	23	34	53	65	79
35-44 yr	63	—²	—	—	15	23	38	—	—
45-54 yr	46	—	—	—	22	32	46	—	—
55-64 yr	129	27	6	8	16	24	35	48	55
65-74 yr	168	24	5	8	15	21	30	42	52

*Excludes persons with unknown income.

SATURATED FATTY ACID INTAKE (mg), AGES 6 MO–74 YR, UNITED STATES, 1976–80—cont'd

Income Level, Sex, and Age	No. Examined	Mean	Percentile						
			5th	10th	25th	50th	75th	90th	95th
INCOME BELOW POVERTY LEVEL*—cont'd									
Female									
6 mo–74 yr	1910	23	5	8	14	20	30	40	48
6-11 mo	36	—	—	—	—	14	—	—	—
1-2 yr	15	22	7	10	15	20	26	37	42
3-5 yr	272	24	10	12	16	22	30	37	44
6-8 yr	95	29	12	15	20	29	35	43	49
9-11 yr	102	27	10	11	17	25	36	46	56
12-14 yr	104	25	7	9	15	22	33	45	56
15-17 yr	88	28	8	12	16	26	36	45	53
18-24 yr	253	22	4	6	13	19	31	39	46
25-34 yr	162	25	7	8	14	21	33	43	60
35-44 yr	119	22	3	7	14	19	26	39	58
45-54 yr	82	21	4	7	13	20	28	32	39
55-64 yr	188	18	6	7	11	16	23	31	40
65-74 yr	256	16	4	5	10	15	20	27	33
INCOME ABOVE POVERTY LEVEL*									
Male									
6 mo–74 yr	8084	36	11	14	21	31	46	63	76
6-11 mo	121	13	0	0	7	11	18	25	28
1-2 yr	551	19	6	8	12	18	24	31	39
3-5 yr	892	23	8	11	15	21	28	38	44
6-8 yr	336	30	13	15	21	28	37	48	55
9-11 yr	356	32	13	16	23	29	40	53	59
12-14 yr	399	37	12	15	23	33	46	62	74
15-17 yr	418	45	14	18	27	38	57	78	98
18-24 yr	770	46	14	18	27	39	57	79	102
25-34 yr	945	40	12	15	25	37	51	67	80
35-44 yr	658	38	13	16	24	33	48	63	75
45-54 yr	603	36	11	14	21	32	45	64	75
55-64 yr	1048	31	10	13	20	29	39	54	63
65-74 yr	987	27	8	11	17	25	33	45	53
Female									
6 mo–74 yr	8036	23	6	9	14	21	29	39	46
6-11 mo	135	14	0	1	8	14	19	25	29
1-2 yr	505	18	6	8	12	17	23	30	35
3-5 yr	815	22	9	11	15	20	27	34	39
6-8 yr	308	26	10	13	18	24	31	39	43
9-11 yr	307	27	12	15	19	26	34	41	50
12-14 yr	363	28	10	13	18	25	35	46	54
15-17 yr	342	26	7	9	14	24	33	42	56
18-24 yr	771	25	7	9	14	22	31	41	51
25-34 yr	982	23	6	9	14	22	30	40	47
35-44 yr	702	23	7	9	14	21	30	40	49
45-54 yr	655	21	5	7	12	19	26	34	44
55-64 yr	1071	20	5	7	12	18	25	35	41
65-74 yr	1080	17	5	7	11	15	22	30	37

SATURATED FATTY ACID INTAKE (g/1000 kcal), AGES 6 MO–74 YR, UNITED STATES, 1976–80

Income Level, Sex, and Age	No. Examined	Mean	Percentile						
			5th	10th	25th	50th	75th	90th	95th
ALL INCOMES									
Male									
6 mo–74 yr	9981*	15	7	9	12	15	18	20	22
6-11 mo	179	13	0	1	9	14	18	21	22
1-2 yr	745	15	6	9	12	15	18	21	23
3-5 yr	1219	14	8	9	12	14	17	19	21
6-8 yr	428	15	9	10	12	15	17	20	22
9-11 yr	457	15	8	10	12	14	17	20	21
12-14 yr	504	15	8	9	12	15	17	20	22
15-17 yr	534†	15	8	10	13	15	18	21	22
18-24 yr	988	15	8	9	12	15	18	21	23
25-34 yr	1067	14	7	9	11	14	17	20	22
35-44 yr	745	15	8	9	12	15	18	21	23
45-54 yr	690	15	8	9	12	15	18	21	23
55-64 yr	1226†	15	8	9	12	15	18	21	23
65-74 yr	1199	14	7	8	11	14	17	20	22
Female									
6 mo–74 yr	10,337*	14	6	8	11	14	17	20	22
6-11 mo	177	14	1	3	10	14	19	22	23
1-2 yr	672	15	6	9	12	15	18	21	23
3-5 yr	1126	15	8	9	12	14	17	20	21
6-8 yr	415	14	8	9	12	15	17	20	21
9-11 yr	425	15	9	10	12	15	17	20	21
12-14 yr	487	15	8	9	11	14	18	20	22
15-17 yr	449	15	7	9	12	15	18	21	22
18-24 yr	1065†	14	6	8	10	14	17	20	21
25-34 yr	1169†	14	6	8	11	14	17	20	22
35-44 yr	844	14	7	8	11	14	18	20	22
45-54 yr	763	14	6	8	11	14	17	20	22
55-64 yr	1329	14	6	8	10	13	17	19	21
65-74 yr	1416	13	6	7	10	13	16	19	21
INCOME BELOW POVERTY LEVEL‡									
Male									
6 mo–74 yr	1538†	15	7	9	12	15	18	21	23
6-11 mo	48	—	—	—	12	15	19	—	—
1-2 yr	170	16	8	10	13	16	19	22	24
3-5 yr	298	15	8	10	12	15	18	21	22
6-8 yr	82	16	10	11	13	15	18	20	21
9-11 yr	88	15	9	10	12	16	17	20	22
12-14 yr	89	16	8	9	12	16	19	21	24
15-17 yr	89	16	8	10	12	16	19	22	23
18-24 yr	178	15	7	9	12	15	19	21	23
25-34 yr	91	14	6	9	11	14	18	20	22
35-44 yr	63	—	—	—	9	14	17	—	—
45-54 yr	46	—	—	—	12	15	18	—	—
55-64 yr	128†	15	7	8	12	15	17	20	22
65-74 yr	168	15	5	7	12	15	18	22	24

*Excludes two persons with 0 kcal.
†Excludes one person with 0 kcal.
‡Excludes all persons with unknown income.

SATURATED FATTY ACID INTAKE (g/1000 kcal), AGES 6 MO–74 YR, UNITED STATES, 1976–80—cont'd

| Income Level, Sex, and Age | No. Examined | Mean | Percentile | | | | | | |
			5th	10th	25th	50th	75th	90th	95th
INCOME BELOW POVERTY LEVEL‡—cont'd									
Female									
6 mo–74 yr	1909†	14	7	8	11	14	18	20	22
6-11 mo	36	—	—	—	—	15	—	—	—
1-2 yr	153	16	9	11	12	16	19	22	23
3-5 yr	272	15	8	10	12	15	18	20	23
6-8 yr	95	15	9	11	13	15	17	20	22
9-11 yr	102	15	8	10	12	15	17	20	22
12-14 yr	104	14	5	8	11	14	18	20	21
15-17 yr	88	15	7	9	11	14	18	21	22
18-24 yr	252†	13	6	8	10	13	16	19	21
25-34 yr	162	14	6	7	12	14	18	20	22
35-44 yr	119	15	5	9	12	15	18	22	24
45-54 yr	82	15	6	9	13	15	18	21	22
55-64 yr	188	14	8	9	11	13	17	19	22
65-74 yr	256	13	5	7	10	12	16	19	22
INCOME ABOVE POVERTY LEVEL‡									
Male									
6 mo–74 yr	8083†	15	7	9	12	15	18	20	22
6-11 mo	121	12	0	1	7	13	18	21	22
1-2 yr	551	14	6	9	11	14	17	21	23
3-5 yr	892	14	8	9	11	14	16	19	21
6-8 yr	336	15	9	10	12	15	17	20	22
9-11 yr	356	14	8	10	12	14	17	20	21
12-14 yr	399	15	8	9	12	14	17	20	22
15-17 yr	417†	15	8	10	13	15	18	21	22
18-24 yr	770	15	8	9	12	15	18	21	23
25-34 yr	945	14	7	9	11	14	17	20	22
35-44 yr	658	15	8	9	12	15	18	21	23
45-54 yr	603	15	8	9	12	15	18	21	23
55-64 yr	1048	15	8	9	12	15	18	21	23
65-74 yr	987	14	7	8	11	14	17	20	22
Female									
6 mo–74 yr	8035†	14	6	8	11	14	17	20	22
6-11 mo	135	14	1	2	9	14	19	22	23
1-2 yr	505	15	6	8	12	15	18	21	23
3-5 yr	815	14	7	9	12	14	17	20	21
6-8 yr	308	14	7	9	12	14	17	19	21
9-11 yr	307	15	9	10	12	14	17	20	21
12-14 yr	363	15	8	9	12	15	18	20	22
15-17 yr	342	15	7	9	12	15	18	21	22
18-24 yr	771	14	7	8	11	14	17	20	22
25-34 yr	981†	14	6	8	11	14	17	20	22
35-44 yr	702	14	7	8	11	14	17	20	22
45-54 yr	655	14	6	8	11	14	17	20	22
55-64 yr	1071	13	6	8	10	13	17	19	21
65-74 yr	1080	13	6	7	10	13	16	19	20

OLEIC ACID INTAKE (g), AGES 6 MO–74 YR, UNITED STATES, 1976–80

Income Level, Sex, and Age	No. Examined	Mean	Percentile						
			5th	10th	25th	50th	75th	90th	95th
ALL INCOMES									
Male									
6 mo–74 yr	9983	36	10	14	21	32	46	63	76
6-11 mo	179	10	0	0	5	9	13	21	28
1-2 yr	745	18	6	8	12	17	23	30	36
3-5 yr	1219	23	8	11	16	21	29	38	44
6-8 yr	428	30	13	15	20	27	35	47	53
9-11 yr	457	31	12	16	22	29	37	49	57
12-14 yr	504	36	11	15	22	33	46	62	74
15-17 yr	535	43	14	17	26	38	55	75	90
18-24 yr	988	46	13	18	26	40	57	80	100
25-34 yr	1067	41	13	16	25	37	53	70	84
35-44 yr	745	38	13	16	24	34	48	64	73
45-54 yr	690	37	11	14	23	33	47	63	72
55-64 yr	1227	33	10	14	21	30	39	55	65
65-74 yr	1199	28	9	12	18	25	36	47	56
Female									
6 mo–74 yr	10,339	23	6	9	14	21	30	40	47
6-11 mo	177	10	1	2	5	9	14	22	25
1-2 yr	672	18	6	7	12	17	23	30	34
3-5 yr	1126	22	8	10	15	20	27	34	40
6-8 yr	415	26	11	12	19	25	32	40	45
9-11 yr	425	27	11	14	18	25	34	42	50
12-14 yr	487	27	9	11	17	25	35	42	50
15-17 yr	449	27	7	10	16	23	34	45	53
18-24 yr	1066	24	6	8	14	22	31	41	48
25-34 yr	1170	25	7	10	15	23	31	42	50
35-44 yr	844	24	7	10	14	22	30	40	49
45-54 yr	763	22	5	9	13	20	28	36	44
55-64 yr	1329	21	6	8	12	19	26	37	44
65-74 yr	1416	18	5	7	12	17	23	32	38
INCOME BELOW POVERTY LEVEL*									
Male									
6 mo–74 yr	1539	34	8	12	19	29	44	65	78
6-11 mo	48	—	—	—	5	10	17	—	—
1-2 yr	170	19	5	8	13	18	25	34	36
3-5 yr	298	26	8	12	17	24	32	43	52
6-8 yr	82	29	14	16	21	28	35	45	56
9-11 yr	88	30	8	11	20	28	37	49	60
12-14 yr	89	37	10	16	22	30	49	67	78
15-17 yr	89	42	12	18	26	37	55	74	80
18-24 yr	178	46	11	16	24	36	62	83	107
25-34 yr	91	39	9	17	23	32	53	76	85
35-44 yr	63	—	—	—	16	24	41	—	—
45-54 yr	46	—	—	—	21	38	54	—	—
55-64 yr	129	30	6	8	16	29	38	52	61
65-74 yr	168	26	7	8	15	23	32	43	53

*Excludes persons with unknown income.

OLEIC ACID INTAKE (g), AGES 6 MO–74 YR, UNITED STATES, 1976–80—cont'd

| Income Level, Sex, and Age | No. Examined | Mean | Percentile | | | | | | |
			5th	10th	25th	50th	75th	90th	95th
INCOME BELOW POVERTY LEVEL*—cont'd									
Female									
6 mo–74 yr	1910	24	6	9	14	21	31	40	51
6-11 mo	36	—	—	—	—	10	—	—	—
1-2 yr	153	21	8	10	14	19	26	36	39
3-5 yr	272	24	9	12	16	24	30	38	45
6-8 yr	95	28	11	13	21	27	33	40	51
9-11 yr	102	27	10	12	16	24	36	45	49
12-14 yr	104	26	5	9	16	24	35	42	59
15-17 yr	88	29	9	11	18	24	38	51	53
18-24 yr	253	23	5	7	14	21	31	39	47
25-34 yr	162	27	7	10	16	24	33	52	63
35-44 yr	119	24	4	7	13	19	29	45	62
45-54 yr	82	22	5	8	14	21	29	34	39
55-64 yr	188	19	6	7	12	18	24	33	43
65-74 yr	256	17	5	6	10	16	22	29	37
INCOME ABOVE POVERTY LEVEL*									
Male									
6 mo–74 yr	8084	36	11	14	22	32	46	63	77
6-11 mo	121	9	0	0	5	9	13	20	26
1-2 yr	551	18	6	8	11	16	23	30	36
3-5 yr	892	23	8	11	15	21	28	36	43
6-8 yr	336	30	13	15	20	27	35	48	53
9-11 yr	356	31	13	16	22	29	37	48	57
12-14 yr	399	36	11	15	22	33	46	62	74
15-17 yr	418	44	14	17	26	39	55	77	97
18-24 yr	770	46	13	18	27	40	56	80	100
25-34 yr	945	42	13	16	25	37	54	71	84
35-44 yr	658	39	13	17	24	35	50	65	74
45-54 yr	603	37	11	15	23	32	47	61	71
55-64 yr	1048	33	10	14	21	30	39	56	65
65-74 yr	987	29	10	12	19	25	36	47	55
Female									
6 mo–74 yr	8036	23	7	9	14	21	30	39	46
6-11 mo	135	10	1	2	4	9	14	22	24
1-2 yr	505	17	6	7	11	16	22	29	33
3-5 yr	815	21	9	10	14	20	26	33	38
6-8 yr	308	26	11	12	19	24	32	40	44
9-11 yr	307	27	12	14	19	25	33	41	50
12-14 yr	363	27	9	12	18	26	34	42	50
15-17 yr	342	26	7	10	15	23	33	44	49
18-24 yr	771	24	6	8	15	22	31	41	47
25-34 yr	982	24	7	10	15	22	31	41	48
35-44 yr	702	24	7	10	15	22	31	40	48
45-54 yr	655	22	5	9	13	20	28	36	44
55-64 yr	1071	21	6	8	13	19	26	37	45
65-74 yr	1080	19	5	8	12	17	23	32	39

OLEIC ACID INTAKE (g/1000 kcal), AGES 6 MO–74 YR, UNITED STATES, 1976–80

Income Level, Sex, and Age	No. Examined	Mean	Percentile						
			5th	10th	25th	50th	75th	90th	95th
ALL INCOMES									
Male									
6 mo–74 yr	9981*	15	8	9	12	15	18	20	22
6-11 mo	179	10	0	1	5	10	14	16	18
1-2 yr	745	14	7	8	11	14	17	19	21
3-5 yr	1219	14	8	9	11	14	16	19	21
6-8 yr	428	15	9	11	12	14	17	19	20
9-11 yr	457	14	8	9	12	14	16	18	20
12-14 yr	504	15	8	9	12	14	17	20	22
15-17 yr	534†	15	9	10	12	15	18	20	22
18-24 yr	988	15	8	9	12	15	17	20	22
25-34 yr	1067	15	8	9	12	15	18	21	23
35-44 yr	745	15	8	10	12	15	18	21	22
45-54 yr	690	15	8	10	12	15	18	21	23
55-64 yr	1226†	15	8	10	13	15	18	21	22
65-74 yr	1199	15	7	9	12	15	18	21	23
Female									
6 mo–74 yr	10,337*	14	7	9	12	14	17	20	22
6-11 mo	177	10	1	3	6	10	14	16	17
1-2 yr	672	14	7	8	11	14	17	19	21
3-5 yr	1126	14	8	9	12	14	17	19	21
6-8 yr	415	14	8	10	12	14	17	19	21
9-11 yr	425	14	8	9	12	14	16	19	20
12-14 yr	487	14	8	9	12	14	17	19	21
15-17 yr	449	15	8	9	12	15	18	21	22
18-24 yr	1065†	14	6	8	11	14	17	20	22
25-34 yr	1169†	15	7	9	12	15	18	20	22
35-44 yr	844	15	7	9	12	15	18	21	22
45-54 yr	763	15	6	9	12	15	18	21	23
55-64 yr	1329	14	7	8	11	14	18	20	22
65-74 yr	1416	14	6	8	11	14	17	20	22
INCOME BELOW POVERTY LEVEL‡									
Male									
6 mo–74 yr	1538†	15	8	10	12	15	18	21	23
6-11 mo	48	—	—	—	7	11	15	—	—
1-2 yr	170	15	7	9	12	15	18	20	22
3-5 yr	298	15	9	10	13	15	18	20	22
6-8 yr	82	15	10	11	12	15	17	19	20
9-11 yr	88	15	8	9	12	14	17	19	21
12-14 yr	89	16	10	11	13	16	19	21	23
15-17 yr	89	16	10	11	14	16	19	20	21
18-24 yr	178	15	8	9	12	15	19	20	22
25-34 yr	91	15	6	9	11	15	18	22	24
35-44 yr	63	—	—	—	11	15	17	—	—
45-54 yr	46	—	—	—	13	18	19	—	—
55-64 yr	128†	16	7	10	12	16	19	22	23
65-74 yr	168	16	6	8	12	16	19	23	25

*Excludes two persons with 0 kcal.
†Excludes one person with 0 kcal.
‡Excludes all persons with unknown income.

OLEIC ACID INTAKE (g/1000 kcal), AGES 6 MO–74 YR,
UNITED STATES, 1976–80—cont'd

Income Level, Sex, and Age	No. Examined	Mean	Percentile						
			5th	10th	25th	50th	75th	90th	95th
INCOME BELOW POVERTY LEVEL‡—cont'd									
Female									
6 mo–74 yr	1909†	15	7	9	12	15	18	21	22
6-11 mo	36	—	—	—	—	11	—	—	—
1-2 yr	153	15	8	10	13	15	17	19	21
3-5 yr	272	15	10	11	13	15	18	20	22
6-8 yr	95	15	10	10	13	15	17	19	20
9-11 yr	102	15	7	10	13	15	17	19	21
12-14 yr	104	15	6	9	12	15	18	20	23
15-17 yr	88	15	7	10	12	15	19	22	23
18-24 yr	252†	14	6	8	11	14	17	20	22
25-34 yr	162	16	8	10	12	15	19	20	22
35-44 yr	119	16	7	9	12	16	20	22	24
45-54 yr	82	16	10	10	13	16	19	23	24
55-64 yr	188	15	7	9	12	15	19	21	23
65-74 yr	256	14	6	7	10	14	18	21	23
INCOME ABOVE POVERTY LEVEL‡									
Male									
6 mo–74 yr	8083†	15	8	9	12	15	18	20	22
6-11 mo	121	9	0	1	5	9	13	15	16
1-2 yr	551	13	7	8	11	13	16	19	21
3-5 yr	892	14	8	9	11	14	16	18	20
6-8 yr	336	15	9	11	12	14	17	19	21
9-11 yr	356	14	8	9	11	14	16	18	19
12-14 yr	399	14	7	9	12	14	17	19	22
15-17 yr	417†	15	9	10	12	15	17	20	22
18-24 yr	770	15	8	9	12	15	17	20	23
25-34 yr	945	15	8	9	12	15	18	21	22
35-44 yr	658	15	8	10	12	15	18	21	22
45-54 yr	603	15	8	9	12	15	18	21	23
55-64 yr	1048	15	8	10	13	15	18	21	22
65-74 yr	987	15	8	9	12	15	18	21	23
Female									
6 mo–74 yr	8035†	14	7	9	11	14	17	20	22
6-11 mo	135	10	1	3	5	10	14	16	17
1-2 yr	505	14	7	8	11	14	16	19	21
3-5 yr	815	14	8	9	11	14	17	19	20
6-8 yr	308	14	8	9	12	14	17	19	21
9-11 yr	307	14	9	10	12	14	16	18	20
12-14 yr	363	14	8	9	12	14	17	19	21
15-17 yr	342	15	8	9	12	15	18	20	22
18-24 yr	771	14	6	8	11	14	17	20	22
25-34 yr	981†	15	7	9	12	15	17	20	22
35-44 yr	702	15	7	9	12	15	18	21	22
45-54 yr	655	15	6	9	12	15	18	21	23
55-64 yr	1071	14	6	8	11	14	18	20	22
65-74 yr	1080	14	6	8	11	14	17	20	22

LINOLEIC ACID INTAKE (g), AGES 6 MO–74 YR, UNITED STATES, 1976–80

Income Level, Sex, and Age	No. Examined	Mean	Percentile						
			5th	10th	25th	50th	75th	90th	95th
ALL INCOMES									
Male									
6 mo–74 yr	9983	13	3	4	6	11	17	25	31
6-11 mo	179	3	0	0	1	2	4	8	9
1-2 yr	745	6	1	2	3	5	8	12	15
3-5 yr	1219	8	2	3	5	7	11	15	19
6-8 yr	428	11	3	4	6	9	14	18	22
9-11 yr	457	11	3	4	6	9	14	19	25
12-14 yr	504	14	3	4	7	11	17	25	32
15-17 yr	535	15	3	4	8	12	20	28	37
18-24 yr	988	17	3	4	8	13	22	33	39
25-34 yr	1067	15	3	4	9	14	21	28	33
35-44 yr	745	14	3	4	8	12	18	26	31
45-54 yr	690	13	3	4	7	11	17	25	29
55-64 yr	1227	12	3	3	6	10	15	21	26
65-74 yr	1199	10	2	3	5	8	13	18	23
Female									
6 mo–74 yr	10,339	9	2	3	5	8	12	17	22
6-11 mo	177	3	0	0	1	2	5	8	10
1-2 yr	672	6	1	2	3	5	8	12	14
3-5 yr	1126	8	2	3	4	7	10	14	18
6-8 yr	415	9	3	3	6	8	12	16	19
9-11 yr	425	10	3	4	6	9	13	18	22
12-14 yr	487	11	2	3	6	10	14	20	27
15-17 yr	449	11	1	3	6	9	14	20	26
18-24 yr	1066	9	2	2	5	8	13	17	22
25-34 yr	1170	10	2	3	5	8	13	19	25
35-44 yr	844	10	2	3	5	8	13	18	23
45-54 yr	763	9	1	2	5	8	11	16	19
55-64 yr	1329	8	2	2	4	7	11	15	18
65-74 yr	1416	8	1	2	4	6	10	13	17
INCOME BELOW POVERTY LEVEL*									
Male									
6 mo–74 yr	1539	12	2	3	5	9	15	24	30
6-11 mo	48	—	—	—	1	3	7	—	—
1-2 yr	170	6	1	2	3	5	9	12	16
3-5 yr	298	9	2	3	5	8	12	18	25
6-8 yr	82	9	2	4	6	9	12	16	20
9-11 yr	88	10	2	4	5	9	13	18	24
12-14 yr	89	13	4	5	7	11	17	24	30
15-17 yr	89	13	2	2	6	10	19	26	36
18-24 yr	178	16	3	4	7	12	21	36	38
25-34 yr	91	12	2	3	6	10	17	24	30
35-44 yr	63	—	—	—	5	9	16	—	—
45-54 yr	46	—	—	—	7	11	18	—	—
55-64 yr	129	10	1	2	5	9	13	16	21
65-74 yr	168	8	1	2	4	7	11	14	16

*Excludes persons with unknown income.

LINOLEIC ACID INTAKE (g), AGES 6 MO–74 YR, UNITED STATES, 1976–80—cont'd

Income Level, Sex, and Age	No. Examined	Mean	Percentile						
			5th	10th	25th	50th	75th	90th	95th
INCOME BELOW POVERTY LEVEL*—cont'd									
Female									
6 mo–74 yr	1910	9	1	2	4	8	12	18	22
6-11 mo	36	—	—	—	—	4	—	—	—
1-2 yr	153	8	1	2	4	6	10	14	18
3-5 yr	272	9	2	3	5	7	11	16	20
6-8 yr	95	10	3	3	6	10	13	17	21
9-11 yr	102	10	2	4	6	8	13	20	27
12-14 yr	104	11	1	2	5	10	15	20	28
15-17 yr	88	12	2	4	5	10	15	25	27
18-24 yr	253	9	1	2	4	8	12	17	21
25-34 yr	162	11	2	3	6	9	14	19	25
35-44 yr	119	9	1	2	4	7	12	20	25
45-54 yr	82	9	1	2	4	8	11	16	19
55-64 yr	188	7	1	2	4	6	9	14	19
65-74 yr	256	6	1	2	3	5	8	12	14
INCOME ABOVE POVERTY LEVEL*									
Male									
6 mo–74 yr	8084	13	3	4	7	11	17	26	31
6-11 mo	121	3	0	0	1	2	3	6	9
1-2 yr	551	6	1	2	3	5	8	12	15
3-5 yr	892	8	2	3	5	7	11	15	18
6-8 yr	336	11	4	4	6	9	14	18	24
9-11 yr	356	11	3	4	7	10	15	20	25
12-14 yr	399	14	3	4	7	11	17	26	32
15-17 yr	418	16	4	5	8	12	20	30	38
18-24 yr	770	17	3	4	8	14	22	33	39
25-34 yr	945	16	3	5	9	14	21	28	34
35-44 yr	658	14	3	5	8	12	19	27	32
45-54 yr	603	13	3	4	7	11	17	25	30
55-64 yr	1048	12	3	4	6	10	15	22	27
65-74 yr	987	10	3	3	5	9	13	19	24
Female									
6 mo–74 yr	8036	9	2	3	5	8	12	17	21
6-11 mo	135	3	0	0	1	2	5	9	10
1-2 yr	505	6	1	2	3	5	8	12	13
3-5 yr	815	8	2	3	4	7	10	14	17
6-8 yr	308	9	3	3	6	8	12	16	18
9-11 yr	307	10	3	4	6	9	12	17	21
12-14 yr	363	11	2	3	6	10	14	20	25
15-17 yr	342	10	2	3	6	9	14	18	23
18-24 yr	771	10	2	2	5	8	13	17	22
25-34 yr	982	10	2	3	5	8	13	19	25
35-44 yr	702	10	2	3	5	8	13	18	23
45-54 yr	655	9	2	3	5	7	11	16	19
55-64 yr	1071	8	2	2	4	7	11	15	18
65-74 yr	1080	8	1	3	4	6	10	14	17

LINOLEIC ACID INTAKE (g/1000 kcal), AGES 6 MO–74 YR, UNITED STATES, 1976–80

Income Level, Sex, and Age	No. Examined	Mean	Percentile						
			5th	10th	25th	50th	75th	90th	95th
ALL INCOMES									
Male									
6 mo–74 yr	9981*	5	2	2	3	5	7	9	11
6-11 mo	179	3	0	0	1	2	4	7	8
1-2 yr	745	5	1	2	3	4	6	8	9
3-5 yr	1219	5	2	2	3	5	6	8	10
6-8 yr	428	5	2	3	4	5	6	9	10
9-11 yr	457	5	2	2	3	4	6	8	10
12-14 yr	504	5	2	2	4	5	7	9	10
15-17 yr	534†	5	2	2	3	5	7	8	10
18-24 yr	988	5	2	2	3	5	7	9	10
25-34 yr	1067	6	2	2	4	5	7	9	11
35-44 yr	745	6	2	2	3	5	8	10	11
45-54 yr	690	5	2	3	3	5	7	9	10
55-64 yr	1226	6	2	2	3	5	7	9	11
65-74 yr	1199	5	2	2	3	5	7	10	11
Female									
6 mo–74 yr	10,337*	6	2	2	4	5	7	10	12
6-11 mo	177	3	0	0	1	2	4	7	11
1-2 yr	672	5	1	2	3	4	6	8	9
3-5 yr	1126	5	2	3	3	5	6	8	10
6-8 yr	415	5	2	2	3	5	6	8	9
9-11 yr	425	5	2	3	3	5	7	9	11
12-14 yr	487	6	2	3	4	5	8	10	11
15-17 yr	449	6	2	2	4	6	8	11	12
18-24 yr	1065†	6	1	2	3	5	7	10	11
25-34 yr	1169†	6	2	2	4	6	8	10	13
35-44 yr	844	6	2	2	4	6	8	10	12
45-54 yr	763	6	2	2	4	5	8	10	12
55-64 yr	1329	6	2	2	3	5	7	10	12
65-74 yr	1416	6	2	2	3	5	7	10	12
INCOME BELOW POVERTY LEVEL‡									
Male									
6 mo–74 yr	1538†	5	2	2	3	5	6	8	10
6-11 mo	48	—	—	—	1	4	5	—	—
1-2 yr	170	5	1	2	3	4	6	8	9
3-5 yr	298	5	2	2	3	5	7	9	10
6-8 yr	82	5	2	2	3	4	6	8	9
9-11 yr	88	5	2	2	3	4	6	8	10
12-14 yr	89	6	2	3	4	5	7	10	11
15-17 yr	89	5	1	2	3	4	6	9	10
18-24 yr	178	5	2	2	3	5	6	9	11
25-34 yr	91	5	1	1	3	4	6	8	9
35-44 yr	63	—	—	—	3	5	7	—	—
45-54 yr	46	—	—	—	3	5	7	—	—
55-64 yr	128†	6	1	2	4	5	7	10	10
65-74 yr	168†	5	1	2	3	4	6	8	10

*Excludes two persons with 0 kcal.

†Excludes one person with 0 kcal.

‡Excludes all persons with unknown income.

LINOLEIC ACID INTAKE (g/1000 kcal), AGES 6 MO–74 YR, UNITED STATES, 1976–80—cont'd

Income Level, Sex, and Age	No. Examined	Mean	5th	10th	25th	50th	75th	90th	95th
INCOME BELOW POVERTY LEVEL‡—cont'd									
Female									
6 mo–74 yr	1909†	6	1	2	3	5	7	10	11
6-11 mo	36	—	—	—	—	3	—	—	—
1-2 yr	153	5	2	2	3	4	7	10	11
3-5 yr	272	5	2	2	3	5	7	9	10
6-8 yr	95	5	2	2	3	5	7	8	10
9-11 yr	102	6	2	3	4	5	7	8	10
12-14 yr	104	6	1	2	4	6	8	12	15
15-17 yr	88	6	2	3	4	6	9	11	14
18-24 yr	252†	5	1	2	3	5	7	9	11
25-34 yr	162	6	2	3	4	6	8	11	12
35-44 yr	119	6	1	2	4	6	8	10	12
45-54 yr	82	6	2	2	4	5	8	10	12
55-64 yr	188	5	1	2	3	5	7	10	11
65-74 yr	256	5	1	2	3	5	7	8	10
INCOME ABOVE POVERTY LEVEL‡									
Male									
6 mo–74 yr	8083†	5	2	2	3	5	7	9	11
6-11 mo	121	3	0	0	1	2	3	6	7
1-2 yr	551	5	1	2	3	4	6	8	9
3-5 yr	892	5	2	2	3	5	6	8	10
6-8 yr	336	5	2	3	4	5	6	8	10
9-11 yr	356	5	2	2	3	4	6	8	10
12-14 yr	399	5	2	2	3	5	7	9	10
15-17 yr	417†	5	2	2	3	5	7	8	10
18-24 yr	770	5	2	2	3	5	7	10	11
25-34 yr	945	6	2	2	4	5	7	9	11
35-44 yr	658	6	2	2	4	5	8	10	11
45-54 yr	603	5	2	2	3	5	7	9	11
55-64 yr	1048	6	2	2	3	5	7	9	11
65-74 yr	987	6	2	2	3	5	7	10	11
Female									
6 mo–74 yr	8035†	6	2	2	4	5	7	10	12
6-11 mo	135	3	0	0	1	2	4	6	10
1-2 yr	505	5	1	2	3	4	6	8	9
3-5 yr	815	5	2	3	3	5	6	8	10
6-8 yr	308	5	2	2	4	5	7	8	9
9-11 yr	307	5	2	2	3	5	7	9	11
12-14 yr	363	6	2	3	4	5	7	9	11
15-17 yr	342	6	2	2	4	5	8	10	12
18-24 yr	771	6	1	2	4	5	7	10	11
25-34 yr	981†	6	2	2	4	6	8	10	13
35-44 yr	702	6	2	2	4	6	8	10	12
45-54 yr	655	6	2	2	4	5	8	10	12
55-64 yr	1071	6	2	2	4	5	7	10	12
65-74 yr	1080	6	2	2	4	5	7	10	12

SERUM CHOLESTEROL LEVELS

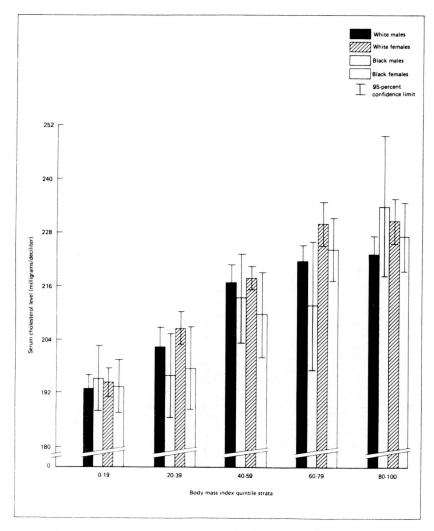

Mean serum cholesterol levels in quintile strata of body mass index for adults 18-74 years of age by race and sex: United States, 1971-74, National Center for Health Statistics, March 1983.

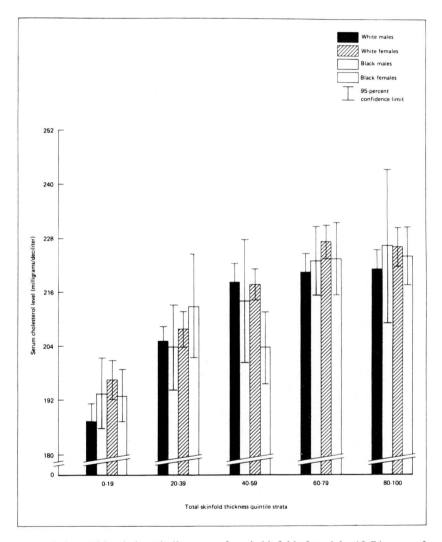

Mean serum cholesterol levels in quintile strata of total skinfolds for adults 18-74 years of age by race and sex: United States, 1971-74, National Center for Health Statistics, March 1983.

CHOLESTEROL INTAKE (mg), AGES 6 MO–74 YR, UNITED STATES, 1976–80

| Income Level, Sex, and Age | No. Examined | Mean | Percentile | | | | | | |
			5th	10th	25th	50th	75th	90th	95th
ALL INCOMES									
Male									
6 mo–74 yr	9983	405	75	107	178	307	552	826	988
6-11 mo	179	159	0	7	38	118	202	367	525
1-2 yr	745	224	40	59	89	149	340	481	613
3-5 yr	1219	250	53	71	114	180	343	538	660
6-8 yr	428	301	81	104	153	226	387	598	797
9-11 yr	457	304	91	113	158	246	397	599	725
12-14 yr	504	360	72	104	177	269	464	711	905
15-17 yr	535	419	88	125	198	319	566	847	1069
18-24 yr	988	491	89	130	214	354	663	982	1308
25-34 yr	1067	451	97	133	215	351	603	913	1073
35-44 yr	745	432	93	122	197	326	610	892	1029
45-54 yr	690	447	93	116	200	370	647	874	1046
55-64 yr	1227	426	82	113	194	361	627	822	964
65-74 yr	1199	387	65	95	167	318	567	748	905
Female									
6 mo–74 yr	10,339	266	46	68	115	194	363	580	699
6-11 mo	177	174	4	12	51	132	263	372	448
1-2 yr	672	231	33	54	93	164	336	488	644
3-5 yr	1126	240	54	72	107	169	341	533	636
6-8 yr	415	255	63	82	134	194	325	476	652
9-11 yr	425	248	72	89	132	193	329	487	581
12-14 yr	487	252	48	77	127	188	320	499	688
15-17 yr	449	247	48	72	112	185	313	505	712
18-24 yr	1066	272	32	58	117	194	375	620	723
25-34 yr	1170	278	44	68	118	201	374	619	731
35-44 yr	844	296	55	75	126	215	407	636	749
45-54 yr	763	283	52	70	116	212	389	622	710
55-64 yr	1329	266	48	66	107	195	362	577	706
65-74 yr	1416	240	37	58	97	169	344	500	606
INCOME BELOW POVERTY LEVEL*									
Male									
6 mo–74 yr	1539	423	55	93	169	305	595	896	1094
6-11 mo	48	—	—	—	30	115	190	—	—
1-2 yr	170	227	37	65	119	222	412	549	654
3-5 yr	298	282	54	74	140	217	393	585	666
6-8 yr	82	318	104	134	176	221	429	573	897
9-11 yr	88	330	55	112	144	273	452	675	761
12-14 yr	89	436	43	97	187	293	557	905	1191
15-17 yr	89	433	55	98	184	315	658	911	1167
18-24 yr	178	556	63	119	191	378	734	1130	1525
25-34 yr	91	471	58	128	191	426	657	927	985
35-44 yr	63	—	—	—	157	296	599	—	—
45-54 yr	46	—	—	—	207	449	846	—	—
55-64 yr	129	422	57	100	176	341	643	832	903
65-74 yr	168	390	58	73	162	319	567	726	1014

Excludes persons with unknown income.

CHOLESTEROL INTAKE (mg), AGES 6 MO–74 YR, UNITED STATES, 1976–80—cont'd

Income Level, Sex, and Age	No. Examined	Mean	Percentile						
			5th	10th	25th	50th	75th	90th	95th
INCOME BELOW POVERTY LEVEL*—cont'd									
Female									
6 mo–74 yr	1910	281	31	56	111	195	394	644	743
6-11 mo	36	—	—	—	—	159	—	—	—
1-2 yr	153	272	46	84	113	197	379	604	707
3-5 yr	272	297	55	81	122	223	448	618	700
6-8 yr	95	267	82	108	143	219	334	539	712
9-11 yr	102	271	57	81	131	187	402	587	708
12-14 yr	104	259	26	40	97	179	342	635	802
15-17 yr	88	265	36	45	112	184	338	712	742
18-24 yr	253	287	25	42	100	191	414	678	743
25-34 yr	162	313	34	57	115	217	470	716	852
35-44 yr	119	300	18	31	102	219	499	712	777
45-54 yr	82	286	43	64	112	223	433	635	663
55-64 yr	188	266	41	60	100	172	378	569	805
65-74 yr	256	246	24	43	94	171	362	585	671
INCOME ABOVE POVERTY LEVEL*									
Male									
6 mo–74 yr	8084	402	78	108	179	308	550	821	983
6-11 mo	121	143	0	5	38	111	202	332	462
1-2 yr	551	211	40	53	84	141	312	450	599
3-5 yr	892	241	50	69	109	170	325	518	649
6-8 yr	336	298	81	103	145	226	378	607	796
9-11 yr	356	299	93	113	158	246	386	571	725
12-14 yr	399	344	72	108	176	263	449	681	854
15-17 yr	418	419	92	125	202	319	565	845	1075
18-24 yr	770	479	92	137	215	346	652	958	1215
25-34 yr	945	450	98	133	216	348	602	905	1074
35-44 yr	658	431	101	125	202	326	611	900	1028
45-54 yr	603	442	93	113	201	369	633	865	1047
55-64 yr	1048	425	83	115	196	363	626	807	965
65-74 yr	987	387	66	100	167	307	568	748	898
Female									
6 mo–74 yr	8036	263	49	70	116	193	358	561	685
6-11 mo	135	166	1	11	40	113	257	372	430
1-2 yr	505	220	31	51	89	155	335	467	625
3-5 yr	815	226	56	72	103	160	306	481	601
6-8 yr	308	253	58	79	133	187	321	477	649
9-11 yr	307	241	73	91	132	194	321	416	512
12-14 yr	363	253	59	84	130	195	324	484	682
15-17 yr	342	239	51	74	112	187	300	486	621
18-24 yr	771	266	39	65	122	196	357	591	697
25-34 yr	982	272	44	68	117	198	368	607	706
35-44 yr	702	293	60	81	128	210	391	629	748
45-54 yr	655	285	52	70	116	216	392	623	711
55-64 yr	1071	266	48	68	107	196	366	591	702
65-74 yr	1080	239	39	60	97	170	340	488	582

CHOLESTEROL INTAKE (mg/1000 kcal), AGES 6 MO–74 YR, UNITED STATES, 1976–80

| Income Level, Sex, and Age | No. Examined | Mean | Percentile | | | | | | |
			5th	10th	25th	50th	75th	90th	95th
ALL INCOMES									
Male									
6 mo–74 yr	9981*	174	50	64	92	132	223	345	424
6-11 mo	179	158	0	10	46	114	178	426	581
1-2 yr	745	172	43	56	81	119	243	372	442
3-5 yr	1219	155	43	54	79	113	201	317	393
6-8 yr	428	149	53	62	90	121	190	291	358
9-11 yr	457	142	49	64	84	117	156	259	339
12-14 yr	504	149	50	63	83	118	168	300	386
15-17 yr	534†	149	49	64	91	123	165	269	350
18-24 yr	988	160	49	66	91	124	203	312	370
25-34 yr	1067	169	49	62	94	135	207	324	409
35-44 yr	745	182	52	69	94	141	235	355	436
45-54 yr	690	196	57	71	100	151	259	372	447
55-64 yr	1226†	214	55	74	103	173	290	406	478
65-74 yr	1199	223	49	68	103	165	302	436	560
Female									
6 mo–74 yr	10,337*	174	43	58	86	126	214	366	445
6-11 mo	177	184	7	17	54	132	278	399	488
1-2 yr	672	191	38	56	82	125	275	431	523
3-5 yr	1126	162	47	58	82	113	216	332	416
6-8 yr	415	143	43	54	81	114	155	287	377
9-11 yr	425	135	51	59	79	113	158	254	299
12-14 yr	487	138	38	53	78	112	162	258	335
15-17 yr	449	145	37	52	85	111	162	276	380
18-24 yr	1065†	167	34	52	81	124	198	352	431
25-34 yr	1169†	173	44	58	86	125	207	371	456
35-44 yr	844	192	51	64	93	140	257	395	493
45-54 yr	763	198	51	63	95	144	262	400	507
55-64 yr	1329	194	49	64	92	135	260	407	494
65-74 yr	1416	194	40	58	85	134	262	404	511
INCOME BELOW POVERTY LEVEL‡									
Male									
6 mo–74 yr	1538†	196	45	64	95	140	256	398	472
6-11 mo	48	—	—	—	45	111	217	—	—
1-2 yr	170	220	55	69	98	168	325	441	524
3-5 yr	298	172	51	61	90	123	235	318	426
6-8 yr	82	160	62	81	96	122	203	298	341
9-11 yr	88	165	49	66	90	137	199	313	383
12-14 yr	89	182	53	65	88	140	219	388	472
15-17 yr	89	167	38	62	93	131	214	278	414
18-24 yr	178	174	40	62	94	132	245	336	408
25-34 yr	91	192	48	59	94	143	266	390	433
35-44 yr	63	—	—	—	94	128	282	—	—
45-54 yr	46	—	—	—	92	207	362	—	—
55-64 yr	128†	246	50	79	120	194	336	478	551
65-74 yr	168	249	45	67	120	208	347	516	584

*Excludes two persons with 0 kcal.

†Excludes one person with 0 kcal.

‡Excludes all persons with unknown income.

CHOLESTEROL INTAKE (mg/1000 kcal), AGES 6 MO–74 YR, UNITED STATES, 1976–80—cont'd

Income Level, Sex, and Age	No. Examined	Mean	Percentile						
			5th	10th	25th	50th	75th	90th	95th
INCOME BELOW POVERTY LEVEL‡—cont'd									
Female									
6 mo–74 yr	1909†	188	36	53	86	129	238	407	493
6-11 mo	36	—	—	—	—	183	—	—	—
1-2 yr	153	202	40	72	95	145	297	421	451
3-5 yr	272	192	57	69	94	140	270	409	471
6-8 yr	95	151	52	67	86	121	163	334	379
9-11 yr	102	146	53	62	85	115	173	254	397
12-14 yr	104	149	18	41	73	115	181	305	427
15-17 yr	88	149	23	35	80	109	157	397	421
18-24 yr	252†	186	26	46	74	130	227	402	474
25-34 yr	162	183	37	61	87	132	211	373	456
35-44 yr	119	212	22	41	105	149	286	443	566
45-54 yr	82	222	47	53	93	161	278	462	536
55-64 yr	188	222	46	66	100	153	292	431	634
65-74 yr	256	227	33	53	86	129	304	475	595
INCOME ABOVE POVERTY LEVEL‡									
Male									
6 mo–74 yr	8083†	171	50	64	91	131	218	337	412
6-11 mo	121	146	0	7	45	107	176	346	515
1-2 yr	551	160	42	54	75	113	223	358	429
3-5 yr	892	149	42	53	78	108	187	314	376
6-8 yr	336	147	52	61	86	116	176	291	358
9-11 yr	356	138	49	63	83	114	151	249	326
12-14 yr	399	142	50	63	81	114	157	281	356
15-17 yr	417†	145	49	63	89	120	161	262	339
18-24 yr	770	157	49	66	90	124	194	307	369
25-34 yr	945	167	50	63	93	133	203	321	408
35-44 yr	658	176	54	69	93	142	232	334	418
45-54 yr	603	192	57	70	101	150	252	368	445
55-64 yr	1048	212	56	74	103	172	288	399	470
65-74 yr	987	220	49	68	100	159	294	435	558
Female									
6 mo–74 yr	8035†	172	44	59	85	125	210	356	443
6-11 mo	135	175	1	15	48	126	253	438	488
1-2 yr	505	187	35	54	79	119	268	444	524
3-5 yr	815	153	46	55	79	109	195	317	391
6-8 yr	308	142	35	51	80	110	155	281	377
9-11 yr	307	131	50	58	78	110	153	246	290
12-14 yr	363	136	42	58	78	111	160	252	319
15-17 yr	342	144	44	60	88	112	161	263	331
18-24 yr	771	161	37	56	81	123	183	329	417
25-34 yr	981†	171	44	57	85	125	204	371	447
35-44 yr	702	188	52	65	92	137	247	383	459
45-54 yr	655	197	51	63	97	144	263	389	497
55-64 yr	1071	189	49	64	91	135	258	401	491
65-74 yr	1080	188	41	59	85	133	252	392	480

APPENDIX VII

U.S. General Accounting Office Report to the Committee on Agriculture, Nutrition, and Forestry, United States Senate

Mean Birth Weight Quantitative Summary
Percentage Low Birth Weight Quantitative Summary
Energy Intake Reported on 24-Hour Recall
Protein Intake Reported on 24-Hour Recall
The Percentage of WIC with Low Hemoglobin at the
    Start of Participation and After 12 Months

An evaluation of the Special Supplemental Program for Women, Infants, and Children (WIC) was carried out by the U.S. General Accounting Office (GAO) to determine the program's effect on the following five outcomes:

1. Infant birth weight
2. Miscarriages, stillbirths, and neonatal deaths
3. Maternal nutrition
4. Anemia in infants and children
5. Mental retardation in infants and children

The GAO analyzed relevant scientific reports, both published and unpublished. They reviewed their design, methodology, and analysis, judging the relative worth of the contributions to the scientific literature. The GAO then attempted to respond to the five identified outcome measures of WIC effectiveness.

Does Participating in WIC Affect Infant Birth Weight?

The GAO report on birth weights found six studies that were of high or medium quality and that somewhat supported (but not conclusively) the assertion that WIC has the positive effect of increasing the birth weights of the infants whose mothers participated in WIC. Five of the six studies that examined the proportion of low birth weight infants—i.e., infants weighing less than 2500 g at birth—showed that participation in WIC is associated with some improvement. Of the women participating in WIC, 7.9% gave birth to low–birth-weight infants compared to about 9.5% of the women in the non-WIC comparison groups. Related calculations suggest a decrease of 16%-20% in the proportion of infants who were thought to have health risks at birth because of their weight. The effect of WIC on mean birth weights seems positive also. The GAO estimates is that the average benefit for WIC participants is 30 to 50 g, which is a 1%–2% increase in mean birth weight. However, both WIC and non-WIC infants averaged about 3200 g at birth, which exceeds the 2500 g boundary below which neonatal and infant health problems are expected. (See tables, p. 907.)

Does Participating in WIC Affect Fetal and Neonatal Mortality?

Both the quantity and the credibility of the results on fetal and neonatal mortality are substantially lower than those on birth weight. The favorable results reported from several evaluations are low in credibility. The GAO considers

MEAN BIRTH WEIGHT QUANTITATIVE SUMMARY

| Study | Year and Location | Reported Birth Weight (g)* | | Quantitative Indicators | | |
		WIC	Non-WIC	Raw Difference	% Differ-ence†	Statistically Significant
Kotelchuck	1978	3281	3260	21.0	0.6	Marginally
	Mass.	(4126)	(4126)			
Metcoff	1980–82	3254	3163	91.0‡	2.9	Yes
	Oklahoma City	(238)	(172)			
Stockbauer	1979–81	3254	3238	16.0	0.5	Yes
	Mo.	(6657)	(6657)			
Silverman	1971–77	3189	3095	94.0	3.0	Yes
	Allegheny County, Pa.	(1047)	(1361)			
Bailey	1980	3229	3276	−47.0	−1.4	No
	2 Fla. counties	(37)	(42)			
Kennedy	1973–78	3261.4	3138.9	122.5	3.9	Yes
	Mass.	(897)	(400)			
Summary						
Average		3244.7	3195.1	49.6	1.55§	
Weighted average‖		3257.8	3225.9	31.3	0.97§	
Range lowest		3189.0	3095.0	−47.0	−1.4	
highest		3281.0	3276.0	122.5	3.9	

*The numbers in parentheses are sample sizes.
†Raw difference divided by non-WIC birth weight.
‡Adjusted.
§Average raw difference divided by average non-WIC birth weight.
‖Each mean is weighted by the number of participants or controls in its group and an overall average is obtained by dividing by the total number of participants or controls in the six studies. The raw difference is based on the total of participants and controls.

PERCENTAGE LOW BIRTH WEIGHT QUANTITATIVE SUMMARY

| Study | Year and Location | Reported Low Birth Weight (%)* | | Quantitative Indicators | | |
		WIC	Non-WIC	Raw Difference	% Differ-ence†	Statistically Significant
Kotelchuck	1978	6.9	8.7	−1.8	−20.7	Yes
	Mass.	(4126)	(4126)			
Metcoff	1980–82	8.7	6.9	1.8	26.1	No
	Oklahoma City	(242)	(174)			
Stockbauer	1979–81	8.5	9.4	−0.9	−9.6	Yes
	Mo.	(6657)	(6657)			
Silverman	1971–77	9.7	13.0	−3.3	−25.4	Yes
	Allegheny County, Pa.	(1047)	(1361)			
Bailey	1980	5.4	9.5	−4.1	−43.1	No
	2 Fla. counties	(37)	(42)			
Kennedy	1973–78	6.0	8.8	−2.8	−31.8	Yes
	Mass.	(833)	(375)			
Summary						
Average		7.53	9.38	−1.85	−19.7‡	
Weighted average§		7.92	6.50	−1.58	−16.6	
Range lowest		5.4	6.9	1.8	26.1	
highest		9.71	13.0	−4.1	−43.1	

*Low birth weight = Less than 2500 g. (Numbers in parentheses are sample sizes.)
†Raw difference divided by non-WIC low birth weight percentage.
‡Average raw difference divided by average non-WIC low birth weight rate.
§Each birth weight rate is weighted by the number of participants or controls in its group, and an overall average is obtained by dividing by the total number of participants or controls in the six studies.

ENERGY INTAKE REPORTED ON 24-HOUR RECALL

Study	Year and Location	Measure*	Reported Data†		Quantitative Indicators		
			WIC	Non-WIC	Raw Difference	% Difference‡	Statistically Significant
Bailey	1980	Mean kcal	2390	2496	−106	−4.2	No
	Two Fla.	Mean % RDA	104	108	−4	−3.7	No
	counties		(41)	(37)			
Metcoff	1980–82	Mean kcal	1965	1883	82	4.4	No
	Oklahoma City	Mean % RDA	—	—	—	—	—
			(145)	(125)			
Endres	FY 1978	Mean kcal	—	—	—	—	—
	Ill.	Mean % RDA	77	68	9	13.2	Yes
			(115)	(651)			
NDDA	FY 1979	Mean kcal	—	—	—	—	—
	Ill.	Mean % RDA	76	70	6	8.6	Yes
			(341)	(1064)			
NDDA	FY 1980	Mean kcal	1888	1780	108	6.1	—
	Ill.	Mean % RDA	80	75	5	6.7	Yes
			(873)	(2277)			

*Percentage RDA calculated with 1974 RDA standards, except 1980 NDDA (calculated with 1980 RDA standards).

† The numbers in parentheses are sample sizes.

‡ The difference attributable to WIC or what would have been expected in the absence of WIC: $\dfrac{WIC - non\text{-}WIC}{non\text{-}WIC}$

PROTEIN INTAKE REPORTED ON 24-HOUR RECALL

Study	Year and Location	Measure*	Reported Data†		Quantitative Indicators		
			WIC	Non-WIC	Raw Difference	% Difference‡	Statistically Significant
Bailey	1980	Mean grams	90	105	−15	−14.3	No
	Two Fla.	Mean % RDA	118	138	−20	−14.5	No
	counties		(41)	(37)			
Metcoff	1980–82	Mean grams	79.3	71.8	7.5	10.4	Yes
	Oklahoma City	Mean % RDA	—	—	—	—	—
			(145)	(124)			
Endres	FY 1978	Mean grams	—	—	—	—	—
	Ill.	Mean % RDA	105	91			
			(115)	(651)			
NDDA	FY 1979	Mean grams	—	—	—	—	—
	Ill.	Mean % RDA	101	93	8	8.6	Yes
			(341)	(1064)			
NDDA	FY 1980	Mean grams	79	73	6	8.2	—
	Ill.	Mean % RDA	106	98	6	8.2	Yes
			(873)	(2277)	8		

*Percentage RDA calculated with 1974 RDA standards, except 1980 NDDA (calculated with 1980 RDA standards).

† The numbers in parentheses are sample sizes.

‡ The difference attributable to WIC or what would have been expected in the absence of WIC: $\dfrac{WIC - non\text{-}WIC}{non\text{-}WIC}$

PERCENTAGE OF WIC CHILDREN WITH LOW HEMOGLOBIN AT THE START OF PARTICIPATION AND AFTER 12 MONTHS

Study and Age Group	Visit*		
	1	2	3
Edozien†	12.9	6.6	5.3
6–23 mo‡	(8996)	(5437)	(1961)
24–47 mo§	18.8	10.3	10.0
	(9326)	(4876)	(2949)
CDC	14.2	6.1	2.7
6–23 mo‡	(450)	(450)	(450)
24–47 mo§	28.9	8.9	9.6
	(260)	(260)	(260)

*Visit 1 was the first clinical visit; visits 2 and 3 were about 6 and 11–12 months after that. The numbers in parentheses are the total number of participants.

†The composition of the groups changed; the analysis was adjusted for age, gender, race, and income.

‡Hemoglobin lower than 10 g/dl.

§Hemoglobin lower than 11 g/dl.

them to be insufficient to support the assertion that WIC reduces the incidence of fetal and neonatal deaths.

Does Participating in WIC Affect Maternal Nutrition?

The quality and the quantity of evidence from WIC evaluations on how WIC changes maternal nutrition are lower than those on birth weight. Six studies, of moderate quality, differ in many important aspects, including the rigor with which they rule out alternative explanations and the measurements they report. The GAO report found it is difficult to synthesize the results of these studies. It is not yet possible to make firm conclusions, but there is some evidence to suggest that participation in WIC is associated with some improvements in nutritional well-being, especially in diet, iron, and weight. (See tables, p. 908.)

Does Participating in WIC Affect Anemia in Infants and Children?

The GAO found limited evidence to give support to the claims that the WIC program reduces the chances that infants and children will have anemia. Evidence from two studies of only moderate quality suggests that WIC is associated with improving the levels of iron in the blood of children classified as anemic when they enter the program. The GAO reports this evidence is inconclusive. (See table, above.)

Does Participating in WIC Affect Mental Retardation in Infants and Children?

Virtually nothing is known about whether WIC has an effect on the incidence of mental retardation. No WIC evaluation has specifically addressed the question. The GAO reports only one study focused on the cognitive development of infants and children in WIC, but limitations in its study design and execution reduce confidence in its favorable conclusions.

Does Participating in WIC Benefit Some Groups More Than Others?

Regarding the different effects that WIC may be having for different groups of WIC participants, the GAO found information suggesting that they have moderate, but not high, confidence. WIC appears to have greater positive effects on infant birth weights among pregnant teenagers, black women, and women with multiple nutritional and health-related risks. The lack of sufficient and consistent information prohibits making informed judgments about the differences in WIC's effect on fetal and neonatal mortality, maternal nutrition, and anemia in infants and children. The GAO analysis concludes that there is some evidence suggesting that participating in WIC for longer than 6 months is associated with increases in average birth weight and decreases in the proportion of infants who are born at low birth weights. Evidence suggests, furthermore, that longer participation improves iron levels in a mother's blood. As for anemia in children, the limited information suggests that its incidence is reduced most during the first 6 months of participation. However, there are flaws in the evaluations, which makes this information inconclusive. Little evidence is available regarding the separate effects of the three components of the WIC program.

REFERENCES

Argeanas S, Harrille I: Nutrient intake of lactating women participating in the Colorado WIC program. Nutr Rep Int, December 1979, pp. 805–10.

Arizona WIC data: 1976–77 survey of participant nutrition and pregnancy outcomes. Transmitted to GAO from Food and Nutrition Service, Washington, DC, August 1983.

Arizona WIC data: 1977–78 evaluation of health intervention and nutrition education. Transmitted to GAO from Food and Nutrition Service, Washington, DC, August 1983.

Bailey LB, Mahan CS, Dimperio D: Folacin and iron status in low-income pregnant adolescents and mature women. Am J Clin Nutr, 33 (September 1980), pp. 1997–2001.

Bailey LB, et al: Vitamin B₆, iron and folacin status of pregnant women, Nutr Res **3** (1983), 783–93.

Baxter J (Tennessee Department of Public Health, Nashville): Reduced frequency of low weight births among women receiving WIC in Tennessee. Attachment to letter to National WIC Evaluation, Food and Nutrition Service, Alexandria, VA, June 21, 1983.

Belshaw J: WIC among the Navajos. Commun Nutritionist, **1**:3 (May-June 1982), 10–12.

Bendick M, et al: Efficiency and Effectiveness in the WIC Program Delivery System, Washington, DC: The Urban Institute, September 1976.

Berkerfield J, Schwartz JB: Nutrition intervention in the community: The WIC program, N Engl J Med, **302**:10 (March 1980), 579–81.

Brevard County Health Department: "Report of WIC Data," Rockledge, FL, July 25, 1977.

Caan B, Marger S: Evaluating evaluations. University of California, Department of Social and Administrative Health Sciences, School of Public Health, Berkeley, CA, 1983.

California WIC data: 1980 survey of nutrition education. Transmitted to GAO from Food and Nutrition Service, Washington, DC, August 1983.

Carabello D, et al: An evaluation of WIC, Masters thesis, Yale School of Medicine, Department of Epidemiology and Public Health, New Haven, CT, May 1978.

Centers for Disease Control: Analysis of Nutrition Indices for Selected WIC Participants, Atlanta: December 1977.

Centers for Disease Control: Nutrition Surveillance: Annual Summary 1980, Atlanta: November 1982.

Christie DD, Gale LB: WIC program involvement in the prevention of mental retardation, New Jersey State Department of Health, Trenton, NJ, 1979.

Collins T, Leeper D, DeMellier S: Integration of WIC program with other infant mortality programs. Final report, Appalachian Region Commission Report, University of Alabama, University, September 30, 1981.

Cook JD: Iron deficiency: Methods to measure prevalence and evaluate interventions. Nutrition Intervention Strategies in National Development, pp. 257–63, New York: Academic Press, 1983.

Deterding J, Wickiser A, Smith JL: The benefits of the WIC program in three Indian communities, University of Nebraska Medical Center, Omaha, May 1983.

Development Associates: Evaluation of the WIC Migrant Demonstration Project: A final report. N.p., May 1979.

Drayton PKD: Evaluation of the WIC Nutrition Education Intervention Program for high-risk pregnant women in Illinois. Ph.D. thesis, Southern Illinois University, Carbondale, 1982.

Dwyer J: Case study of a national supplementary feeding program: The WIC program in the United States. In BA Underwood (ed), Nutrition Intervention Strategies in National Development, Cambridge, MA: Massachusetts Institute of Technology, 1983.

Edozien JC, Switzer BR, Bryan RB: Medical Evaluation of the Special Supplemental Food Program for Women, Infants and Children (WIC), 6 vols. Chapel Hill, NC: University of North Carolina, School of Public Health, July 15, 1976.

Edozien JC, Switzer BR, Bryan RB: UNC medical evaluation of WIC, Am J Clin Nutr, **32** (March 1979), 677–92.

Endres J, Casper J: Dietary assessment of pregnant women in a supplemental food program, Am Diet Assoc J, **79**:8 (August 1981), 121–26.

Endres J, Sawicki M: Food and nutrient intake of 7,728 Illinois infants and children, 1978–1979. Supplementary report, Southern Illinois University, NDDA Laboratory, Carbondale, August 1980.

Evaluation Research Society: Standards for Program Evaluation, Washington, DC: May 1980.

Fleshood H, et al: Is WIC reducing the prevalence of LBW and infant mortality? Paper presented at the annual meeting of the American Public Health Association, Los Angeles, October 1978.

Food and Nutrition Service: Evaluating the Nutrition and Health Benefits of the Special Supplemental Food Program for Women, Infants and Children, Washington, DC: U.S. Department of Agriculture, Advisory Committee on Nutrition Evaluation, November 1977.

Food and Nutrition Service: State and local agency evaluations of the WIC program. Report on the Special Supplemental Food Program, U.S. Department of Agriculture, Washington, DC [November 1977].

Food and Nutrition Service: Evaluation of the Effectiveness of WIC. Washington, DC: U.S. Department of Agriculture, 1981.

Food and Nutrition Service: A Response to Graham's Review of the Supplemental Food Program for Women, Infants, and Children (WIC). Washington, DC: U.S. Department of Agriculture, Office of Policy, Planning, and Evaluation, December 1981.

Friends of the Earth: Would the Federal Government Make a Profit by Doubling the Budget of the WIC Program for Pregnancy? Washington, DC: February 1983.

General Accounting Office: Preliminary Report on the Special Supplemental Food Program, B-176994. Washington, DC: September 1973.

General Accounting Office: Observations on Evaluation of the Special Supplemental Food Program, Food and Nutrition Service, CED-75-310. Washington, DC: December 18, 1975.

General Accounting Office: National Nutrition Issues, CED-78-7. Washington, DC: December 1977.

General Accounting Office: The Special Supplemental Food Program for Women, Infants, and Children (WIC): How Can It Work Better? CED-79-55. Washington, DC: February 1979.

General Accounting Office: Comments on Evaluation Studies of WIC. Testimony for the Chairman, Senate Subcommittee on Agriculture. Rural Development and Related Agencies, Washington, DC, 1981.

General Accounting Office: The Evaluation Synthesis. Institute for Program Evaluation Methods Paper I. Washington, DC: April 1983.

George NN: Prepregnancy weights, weight gains and other factors related to birthweight of infants born to overweight women. Masters thesis. Bowling Green State University, Bowling Green, Ohio, June 1982.

Georgia Department of Human Resources: WIC nutrition survey. Atlanta, April 1982.

Goldberg H: An evaluation of the effectiveness of the WIC program in terms of height, birthweight, weight, and hematocrit. Paper on Harlem Hospital Medical Center (N.J.) WIC program, privately circulated, May 17, 1982.

Hawaii WIC data: 1982 survey of participant nutrition. Transmitted to GAO from Food and Nutrition Service, Washington, DC, August 1983.

Hayes CD: Making Policies for Children: A Study of the Federal Process. Washington, DC: National Academy Press, 1982.

Healthwise, Inc: WIC nutrition education evaluation. Final report. Boise, Idaho, September 30, 1980.

Heimendinger J: The effect of WIC on growth of children. Ph.D. thesis, Harvard University School of Public Health, Nutrition Department, Boston, 1981.

Heimendinger J, Lairde N: Growth changes: Measuring the effect of an intervention. Eval Rev 7:1 (February 1983), 80–95.

Hicks LE, Langham RA, Takenaka J: Cognitive and health measures following early nutritional supplementation: A sibling study. Am J Publ Health, 72 (October 1982), 1110–18.

Hicks LE, Langham RA, Takenaka J: Interpretation of behavioral findings in studies of nutritional supplementation. Am J Publ Health, 73 (June 1983), 695–97.

Horgen DM, Loris PA, Rose DM: Retrospective study of the Special Supplemental Food Program for Women, Infants, and Children (WIC). California Department of Health Services, Community Health Service Division, Sacramento, Calif., April 1982.

Hunterdon Medical Center: Innovative workshops in nutrition education. Final report, Flemington, NJ, October 1982.

Jarka E, Maass J, Elridge S: Nutritional risks identified in pregnant adolescents participating in the Illinois WIC program. Illinois Department of Public Health, Springfield, 1981.

Kautz L, Harrison GG: Comparison of body proportions of one-year-old Mexican American and Anglo children. Am J Publ Health, 71 (March 1981), 280–82.

Kennedy ET, Austin JE, Timmer CP: Cost/benefit and cost/effectiveness of WIC. Privately circulated, n.p., n.d.

Kennedy ET, Gershoff S: Effect of WIC supplemental feeding on hemoglobin and hematocrit of prenatal patients. J Am Diet Assoc, 80:3 (March 1982), 227–30.

Kennedy ET, et al: Evaluation of the effect of WIC supplemental feeding on birth weight. Am Diet Assoc J. 80:3 (March 1982), 220–27.

Kotelchuck M, et al. 1980 Massachusetts Special Supplemental Food Program for Women, Infants, and Children (WIC) evaluation project. Massachusetts Department of Public Health. Division of Family Health Services, Boston 1981.

Kotelchuck M, et al: Massachusetts Special Supplemental Food Program for Women, Infants, and Children (WIC) follow-up study. Massachusetts Department of Public Health, Division of Family Health Services, Boston 1982.

Langham RA, et al: Impact of the WIC program in Louisiana. Privately circulated, n.p., n.d.

Lawrence JES, et al: Evaluation of the WIC Program: Predesign Activities Phase I Final Report. Washington, DC: U.S. Department of Agriculture, Food and Nutrition Service, and Research Triangle Institute, August 1981.

Leddy P: Improving diet assessment methods of pregnant and breastfeeding women. University of Rhode Island, Kingston, RI, 1982.

Mahan CS: Revolution in obstetrics: Pregnancy nutrition. J Florida Med Assoc 66:4 (April 1979), 367–72.

Mahan CS, Sharbaugh C: North Central Florida WIC evaluation. Centers for Disease Control, Nutrition Surveillance, Atlanta, June 1976.

Massachusetts Department of Public Health: 1983 Massachusetts Nutrition Survey. Boston, October 1983.

Mauer AM: The WIC program tying supplemental foods to nutritional needs. J Florida Med Assoc 66:4 (April 1979), 453–56.

Metcoff J, et al: Nutrition in pregnancy (NIP). Final report, University of Oklahoma Health Science Center, Oklahoma City, December 1982.

Michigan Department of Public Health: Evaluation of health services utilization in rural areas and among migrant farmworkers. Lansing, MI, 1980.

Montana Department of Health and Environmental Services: WIC teenage pregnancy outcome project. Report on U.S. Department of Agriculture Grant 59-3198-9-82, Helena, MT. January 1982.

National Research Council: Nutrition Services in Perinatal Care. Washington, DC: National Academy Press, 1981.

NDDA Laboratory, Human Development (Food/Nutrition): Report of nutritional factors of pregnant women in the Illinois Department of Public Health Special Supplemental Food Program for WIC. Southern Illinois University, Carbondale, August 1980.

Norad D, et al: Evaluation of the Commodity Supplemental Food Program Final Report: Health and Nutrition of Three Local Projects. Washington, DC: U.S. Department of Agriculture, Food and Nutrition Service, 1982.

Northrop P: Perceptions and knowledge of breastfeeding among WIC and non-WIC pregnant women. University of Alabama, University, 1982.

Nutt PC, Wheeler M, Wheeler RA: Social program evaluation revisited: The WIC program. Ohio State University, Graduate Program in Hospital and Health Services Administration, Columbus.

Paige DM: Medical assistance cost and utilization patterns in WIC enrollees. A joint study of John Hopkins University, School of Hygiene and Public Health, and Maryland Department of Health and Mental Hygiene, Baltimore, June 1983.

Paige DM: Evaluation of the WIC program for infants on the Eastern Shore of Maryland. Johns Hopkins University, Baltimore, 1983.

Pelto JM: Results of a nutrition intervention program: The WIC program in Alaska. Alaska Med, **24**:2 (March-April 1982), 14–17.

Pestronk RM: Reasons for enrollment in the Michigan WIC program. Michigan Department of Public Health, Lansing, 1982.

Pollitt E, Lorimor R: Effects of WIC on cognitive development. Am J Publ Health, **73** (June 1983), 698–700.

Robbins GA: Surveillance of nutritional status in the United States. Public Health Currents (Ross Labs), **20**:2 (March-April 1980), 5–8.

Rosenberg MJ, McCarthy BJ, Terry JS: The effect of the WIC program on infant mortality in rural Georgia. Centers for Disease Control, Atlanta, 1981.

Rush D: Effects of changes in protein and calorie intake during pregnancy on the growth of the human fetus. In M Enkin, I Chalmers (eds), Effectiveness and Satisfaction in Antenatal Care. Philadelphia: Lippincott, 1982.

Rush D: The behavioral consequences of protein-energy deprivation and supplementation in early life: An epidemiologic perspective. In JR Galler (ed) Nutrition and Behavior. New York: Plenum Publishing, 1982.

Rush D: Is WIC worthwhile? Am J Publ Health, **72** (October 1982), 1101–03.

Rush D: In response to Hicks, et al. Am J Publ Health, **73** (June 1983), 700–01.

Rye J, White M, Majchrzak M: Does objective based health education effect positive changes in the health status of WIC program clients? Preliminary report. State Department of Health Service, Bureau of Nutrition Services, Phoenix, AZ, April 7, 1978.

Schelzel G, Britton MA: An assessment of the WIC program in Pennsylvania. Pennsylvania Health Department, Pittsburgh, January 1978.

Schramm WF: WIC prenatal participation and its relationship to newborn Medicaid costs in Missouri: A cost/benefit analysis. Draft report, Missouri Center of Health Statistics, Jefferson City, April 26, 1983.

Schuster K, Bailey L, Mahan C: Vitamin B_6 status of low-income adolescent and adult pregnant women and the condition of their infants at birth. Am J Clin Nutr, **34** (September 1981), 1731–35.

Shanklin DS: What has WIC accomplished? U.S. Department of Agriculture, Food and Nutrition Service, Washington, DC, October 1981.

Silverman PR: Allegheny County, Pa., Health Department WIC evaluation. Pittsburgh, PA, December 1981.

Slonim A, Kolasa K, Bass M: The cultural appropriateness of the WIC program in Cherokee, North Carolina. Am Diet Assoc J, **79**:8 (August 1981), 164–68.

Stockbauer J: Evaluation of the prenatal participation component of the Missouri WIC Program. Draft report, Missouri Division of Health, Jefferson City, April 26, 1983.

Thenen SW: Folacin content of supplemental foods for pregnancy. Am Diet Assoc J, **80**:3 (March 1982), 237–41.

Thomason CF (Louisiana Department of Health and Human Resources, New Orleans): Low birth weight study. Attachment to letter to National WIC Evaluation, Food and Nutrition Service, Alexandria, VA, May 16, 1983.

U.S. Senate, Committee on Agriculture, Nutrition, and Forestry: Compilation of Selected Federal Nutrition Studies, 96th Cong., 1st sess. Washington, DC: January 1979, pp. 77–80.

U.S. Senate, Committee on Agriculture, Nutrition, and Forestry. Subcommittee on Nutrition: Oversight on Federal Nutrition Programs, 97th Cong., 2nd sess. Washington, DC: February 22–23, 1982.

U.S. Senate: Oversight on Nutritional Status of Low-Income Americans in the 1980's, 98th Cong., 1st sess. Washington, DC: April 1983.

U.S. Senate, Subcommittee on Rural Development, Oversight, and Investigations: Oversight on Federal Nutrition Programs, 98th Cong., 1st sess. Washington, DC: March 1983.

U.S. Senate, Select Committee on Nutrition and Human Needs: WIC program survey 1975. Working paper, 94th Cong., 1st sess., Washington, DC, April 1975.

U.S. Senate: Medical evaluation of the Special Supplemental Food Program for Women, Infants and Children, 94th Cong., 2nd sess., Washington, DC, August 1976.

Weiler P, et al: Anemia as a criterion for evaluation of WIC. Pediatrics, **63** (April 1979), 584–90.

Wholey JS, Wholey MS: Toward improving the outcome of pregnancy: Implications for the statewide prenatal program. Report for the Tennessee Department of Public Health. Wholey Associates, Arlington, VA, June 1982.

Williams J: Wyoming WIC evaluation. State Department of Health and Social Services, Cheyenne, WY, 1982.

INDEX

Page numbers in *italics* indicate illustrations.
Page numbers followed by *t* indicate tables.